# AMA Manual of Style

## A Guide for Authors and Editors

*11th Edition*

# AMA Manual of Style

## A Guide for Authors and Editors

# 11<sup>th</sup> Edition

JAMA Network Editors

**JAMA** Network™

OXFORD
UNIVERSITY PRESS

# JAMA Network™

# OXFORD
## UNIVERSITY PRESS

Oxford University Press is a department of the University of Oxford. It furthers the University's objective of excellence in research, scholarship, and education by publishing worldwide. Oxford is a registered trade mark of Oxford University Press in the UK and certain other countries.

Published in the United States of America by Oxford University Press
198 Madison Avenue, New York, NY 10016, United States of America.

© American Medical Association 2020

Tenth Edition published in 2007

Library of Congress Cataloging-in-Publication Data
Names: American Medical Association.
Title: AMA manual of style : a guide for authors and editors / JAMA Network editors.
Other titles: Manual of style
Description: 11th edition / Stacy L. Christiansen, Cheryl Iverson, Annette Flanagin, Edward H. Livingston, Lauren Fischer, Connie Manno, Brenda Gregoline, Tracy Frey, Phil B. Fontanarosa, Roxanne K. Young. | New York : Oxford University Press, [2020] | Includes bibliographical references and index.
Identifiers: LCCN 2019028351 (print) | LCCN 2019028352 (ebook) |
ISBN 9780190246556 (hardback) | ISBN 9780190246563 (hardback) | ISBN 9780190246594 (epub)
Subjects: LCSH: Medical writing—Handbooks, manuals, etc. | Authorship—Style manuals.
Classification: LCC R119.A533 2020  (print) | LCC R119  (ebook) | DDC 808.06/661—dc23
LC record available at https://lccn.loc.gov/2019028351
LC ebook record available at https://lccn.loc.gov/2019028352

9 8 7 6 5

Printed by LSC Communications, United States of America

# Foreword

Identifying the benchmark, the "gold standard," in any discipline, is difficult. There are often numerous reference books and well-recognized and validated measures of diseases and disorders, but that single best resource can be elusive. However, the *AMA Manual of Style*, since its inaugural version in 1962, and with this 11th edition, is truly the standard, and in the words of one colleague, "the bible of medical publishing." Written by the editorial staff at *JAMA* and the JAMA Network—including physicians, manuscript editing managers, and current and former managing editors—it is the single most comprehensive text focused solely on medical publishing.

In 2018 I traveled to a meeting held at a start-up that was involved in health and wellness marketing. What did I see—5 copies of the *AMA Manual of Style*. When I asked why so many copies, the response was, "They are always in use; it has everything related to medical publishing. What more could we need?"

Dangling participles, malapropisms, misuse of hyphens and commas, and capitalization errors: I commit each of these sins daily. Is it *two* or *2, affect* or *effect, which* or *that*? Are book titles set in roman or italic type? How do you capitalize and punctuate *email*? When is causal language appropriate to be used in a research report? Do I use an SI unit or a conventional unit? What is the best way to display data? How do I handle an author dispute or determine if permission to republish part of a figure is needed? Was the correct statistical analysis used for a specific study? These puzzling questions come up every day in medical publishing and manuscript editing. The *AMA Manual of Style* answers these questions and thousands more.

Communication of medical information has changed radically over the past decade. The emergence of the internet and digital publishing changed forever how information is communicated. Reliance on a print copy of a journal is no more. The content of many journals is now "pushed" to many audiences via the internet, social media, news media, and email (or e-mail, which is it? see chapter 8.3). Transmission of information, which used to be confined to the printed word, now includes online synopses of articles, podcasts, videos, visual abstracts, and content translated into other languages. In the chapters on Manuscript Preparation; References; Editorial Assessment and Processing; Editing, Proofreading, Tagging, and Display; and the Glossary of Publishing Terms many of these new forms of communication are discussed.

The book is comprehensive. Since the publication of the last edition, old issues, including conflict of interest and scientific misconduct, have reemerged with additional and important concerns. New and evolving issues, such as open access, preprint servers, team science, open peer review, data sharing, and new rules for protecting participants' rights in research have come to the fore. These and related issues are discussed in depth in the chapter Ethical and Legal Considerations and are also addressed in the chapters on Manuscript Preparation and Editorial Assessment and Processing.

For an author, editor, or publisher working in the field of medical publishing, the 23 chapters in this volume should help answer questions that arise in daily work as well as those that occur infrequently. There is guidance on citing sources; data displays (graphical and tabular); grammar, punctuation, plurals, and capitalization; correct and preferred usage; abbreviations; nomenclature (from genetics to organisms to oncology); copyright, licensing, and permissions; units of measure; numbers, study design, and statistics; equations; and electronic editing and proofreading. The book concludes with a list of other resources that may be helpful to authors and editors.

During my tenure I have had the good fortune of working with some great writers—Don Berwick, Tony Fauci, Phil Fontanarosa, Larry Gostin, Mary McDermott, Abraham Verghese, and Jody Zylke. For them I suspect writing comes naturally; they are simply gifted communicators. But for most people, writing—particularly medical writing—is a learned skill. There are many nuances, including high-level organizational structure, reporting standards, and correct usage of medical terminology, as well as paragraph transitions, syntax, word choice, verb tense, and punctuation use. For the vast majority of authors and editors of scientific communication, this edition of the *AMA Manual of Style* will be of great assistance.

It has been my privilege to work with the authors of this book. They have taught me much about medical editing and publishing. In the field of medical journalism and communication, the *AMA Manual of Style* is indispensable. It should be on the shelf of every editor and publisher and available to authors worldwide.

Howard Bauchner, MD
Editor in Chief
*JAMA* and the JAMA Network

# Preface

Opening any new book can be cause for excitement. But for an editor, opening a new edition of a style manual has an added frisson. What is new? Have gaps been filled? Have policies that may have seemed outdated or stodgy been freshened?

These questions can only be answered by frequent use, but to provide a quick overview here is a short list of what you will find in this 11th edition of the *AMA Manual of Style*.

- The hyphen has been removed from *email*, although it is retained for other *e*-combinations (eg, e-cigarette).

- Both *internet* and *website* are lowercased (and the former *Web site* is now one word).

- The mandate for a single corresponding author has been relaxed. Two corresponding authors may be listed if justified, with one author designated as the primary point of contact responsible for all communication about the manuscript and article. This person will be listed first in the Corresponding Author section of the published article.

- Because it has become increasingly common for authors to request "co–first authorship" or "co–senior authorship," such designations will now be allowed, but one person's name will need to go first in the byline.

- The death dagger in the byline for a deceased author has been discontinued. If it is desired to note the death of an author, this may be done in the Acknowledgment section.

- Location of the publisher for books and reports is no longer required in references.

- Location of the manufacturer of drugs and equipment and devices is no longer required in text.

- A DOI (digital object identifier) should be included for journal references if available.

- Because the ability to easily and accurately copy and paste DOIs is important, a period should not be included after the DOI; the risk of the period becoming a part of the DOI itself is too great and could create problems with linking.

- When a URL is included for references, it should be preceded by the date the reference was published and/or last updated and accessed. This would make the URL the last item in the reference citation and, as with DOIs, it should not be followed by a period to avoid confusion with linking.

- Guidance on citing preprints, databases, data repositories, podcasts, apps and interactive games, and popular social media (eg, Facebook, blogs, YouTube, and Twitter) has been added to the References chapter.

- In tables and figures, sentence-style capitalization will be used in all elements except the title (eg, axis labels, column headings). This makes long phrases easier to read.

- In the chapter on Tables, Figures, and Multimedia, new examples of the following types of figures have been added: hybrid graph (2 techniques are overlaid), flowchart for a clinical trial in which participants were allocated vs randomized, funnel plot, genetic heat map, network map, gel electrophoresis images, magnetic resonance images, radiographs, ultrasonographic images. Color has been added throughout the chapter where appropriate.

- Guidance on publishing statements about data sharing has been added.

- Additional detail about public access, open access, article processing charges (APCs), open access journals, and updates on copyright, licensing, and Creative Commons (CC) licenses have been added.

- A new correction option allows retraction and replacement of an article in cases in which pervasive, but inadvertent, error(s) resulted in incorrect data throughout an article and a significant change in the findings, yet the underlying science is still reliable and important.

- Hyphens are not used in some combinations of words that are commonly read together; for example, *open access journals, health care system.*

- The singular *they* is permitted when rewriting a sentence as plural would be awkward or unclear.

- The terms *first world/third world* and *developed/developing* are not recommended as descriptors when comparing countries or regions.

- Labeling people with their socioeconomic status (eg, *the poor* or *the unemployed*) should be avoided in favor of language such as *individuals with low income* or *no income.*

- New terms related to addiction have been added: avoid *addict, alcoholic;* favor *person with opiate addiction, a person with alcohol use disorder.*

- Other new terms have been added to Correct and Preferred Usage, with clarification on use or when to avoid use, eg, *nauseous, nauseated; foreign-born; elicit, illicit, solicit; alternative, alternate; cerebrovascular accident, stroke, stroke syndrome; life expectancy, life span; substance use, substance abuse.*

- A new section on spelling and spacing variations has been added to Correct and Preferred Usage (eg, *ante mortem/antemortem, post mortem/postmortem, heart beat/heartbeat*). And yes, we still prefer *health care* over either *healthcare* or *health-care.*

- Some standards on grammar in social media have been added to the Grammar chapter to ensure clarity.

- In author bylines, all fellowship designations (eg, FRCP, FRCPC) and honorary degrees will no longer be included. Degrees below the master's level (eg, BS, BA) will only be included if they are the highest degree held.

- The Manuscript Preparation chapter adds guidance on the inclusion of figures or tables in the structured abstract, ancillary educational and promotional material (eg, audio, video, quizzes), and online-only supplements (text, tables, or figures).

- Use of aliases/nicknames for genes and proteins is strongly discouraged, although it may be necessary to dual report for aliases well-entrenched in use: *ERBB2* (previously *HER2/neu).

- Following the recommendation of the Human Genome Variation Society, the terms *mutation* and *polymorphism* should be avoided, preferring instead the terms *sequence variant, sequence variation, alteration,* or *allelic variant.* Related to this recommendation, SNV (single-nucleotide variation) is now preferred to SNP (single-nucleotide polymorphism). To aid in readers' understanding during this transition, at first mention SNV may be used, with SNP in parentheses: SNV (formerly SNP).

- The difference between *genome* and *genome assembly* is elucidated, as well as the importance of the GenBank identifier.

- In the discussion of human chromosomes, the movement from the study of structural variation from the perspective of direct visualization of bands, using staining techniques, to sophisticated fluorescent technologies to probe for structural variations is emphasized.

- Material on plant genetics (specifically corn, rice, and soybeans) has been added.

- Guidance on *Salmonella* nomenclature has been updated. Traditional binomial species designations are no longer applied to serotypes; now *Salmonella* Typhi, not *Salmonella typhi.*

- Currencies have been updated, including African denominations such as the Ethiopian birr, the Ghanaian cedi, the Malawian kwacha, the Nigerian naira, the Ugandan shilling, and the Zimbabwe dollar.

- Per SI convention, we no longer close up degree symbols in temperature with degrees Celsius and degrees Fahrenheit, but use a space after the number: a temperature of 37.5 °C (not 37.5°C).

- The SI conversion table has been updated, and it no longer includes laboratory reference values because of differences among laboratories worldwide.

- The chapter on indexing has been dropped.

- The abbreviation CI (for confidence interval) will no longer require expansion.

- Many new terms have been added to the Glossary of Publishing Terms, eg, cloud, Creative Commons, open access, hybrid open access, IP (International Protocol) address, JATS (Journal Article Tag Suite), JSON (JavaScript Object Notation), LaTeX, NISO (National Information Standards Organization), Unicode.

- A new section on Guidelines (eg, COPE, EQUATOR Network, ICMJE, WAME) has been added to the Resources chapter.

- A list of specific study types and definitions, with links to reporting guidelines, has been added to the chapter on article types.

- There is an expanded definition of *bias*, with many examples of types of bias, in the Study Design and Statistics chapter.

- The distinction between *multivariable* and *multivariate* is clarified.

- In displaying forms of statistical analysis, terms should not be shown as subscripts (eg, $P_{\text{interaction}} < .001$). Instead, use $P < .001$ for interaction.

- The Mathematical Composition chapter includes more examples of complicated forms of fences in equations.

- Use a thin space (a space usually ⅕ or ⅙ the width of an em dash: Unicode value is 2009) before and after mathematical symbols when they are used as verbs, conjunctions, or operators: ±. =, <, >, ≥, ≤, +, −, ≈.

- XML (discussion and tagging examples) rules for naming and defining parts of a document and their relationship to each other has been added, as well as a discussion of JATS tagging.

- The basic workflow of a manuscript has been updated to show single-source workflow. In this process, content remains in the original document format (eg, Word) and is stored with the XML file and related content (eg, supplemental files, multimedia). Because XML is the basis of this workflow and content, any changes required (before, during, or even after publication) must be made in the source document and new XML generated.

There may be long stretches between editions of a style manual, but an online version of the manual provides the opportunity to not only correct errors but also to provide updates and new policies. These are published on the Updates page of the online manual, which is freely available to everyone: https://www.amamanualofstyle.com/page/updates. Regular communication via Twitter (@AMAManual) and posts to our blog (http://amastyleinsider.com/) provide additional enhancements.

We have continued to work with a committee, dividing the work at the outset, doing independent research and writing, obtaining critiques from outside peer reviewers, and providing critiques on all of each other's material. Often, several cycles of writing, reviewing, and rewriting were necessary. As with the last edition, each chapter is attributed to a principal author. Others who added strength to the work are listed in the Acknowledgments section. And special thanks is due to Laura King, MA, MFA, ELS, who copyedited the entire book.

We welcome your comments on the manual, whether they are suggestions for improvements, alerts to possible corrections, or questions. Write to stylemanual@jamanetwork.org.

Cheryl Iverson, MA
Stacy L. Christiansen, MA
Co-chairs, *AMA Manual of Style* Committee

# Acknowledgments

The authors of this work did not go it alone; we are indebted to many individuals for their thoughtful critiques, comments, suggestions, and advice during the revision process. All named below reviewed and commented on one or more chapters of the manual.

Karen Adams-Taylor, MS
JAMA Network

David Antos
JAMA Network

Deanna Bellandi, MPH
JAMA Network

Robin L. Bennett, MS
CGC Division of Medical Genetics,
University of Washington, Seattle

Sara Billings, MPH
JAMA Network

Karen Boyd
formerly with JAMA Network

Neil M. Bressler, MD
*JAMA Ophthalmology* and Retina
Division, Johns Hopkins Medicine,
Baltimore, Maryland

Kevin Brown, BA
JAMA Network

Karen Bucher, MA
JAMA Network

Diane L. Cannon
formerly with JAMA Network

Cheong-Hee Chang, PhD
Department of Microbiology and
Immunology, University of Michigan,
Ann Arbor

Miriam Y. Cintron, BA
*JAMA*

Michael T. Clarke, MA
Clarke & Esposito,
Washington, DC

Helene M. Cole, MD
formerly with *JAMA*

Gregory Curfman, MD
*JAMA*

Gabriel Dietz, MA
JAMA Network

Mary L. (Nora) Disis, MD
*JAMA Oncology* and University of
Washington, Seattle

Jennifer Eberhart
*Radiology*, Oak Brook, Illinois

Amanda Ehrhardt, MA
JAMA Network

Garth D. Ehrlich, PhD
Center for Advanced Microbial
Processing, Drexel University College
of Medicine, Philadelphia,
Pennsylvania

Emmanuel A. Fadeyi, MD
Wake Forest Baptist Medical Center,
Winston-Salem, North Carolina

Ferric C. Fang, MD
University of Washington, Seattle

W. Gregory Feero, MD, PhD
*JAMA* and Maine-Dartmouth Residency,
Augusta, Maine

Nicole FioRito, BA
*JAMA*

Barbara Gastel, MD, MPH
Texas A&M University,
College Station

Paul Gee, BA
JAMA Network

Julie T. Gerke, ELS
IQVIA, Parsippany, New Jersey

Carissa A. Gilman, MA
American Cancer Society, Atlanta,
Georgia

Richard M. Glass, MD
formerly with *JAMA*

Donald C. Goff, MD
*JAMA* and Department of Psychiatry,
NYU Langone Medical Center,
New York, New York

Lawrence O. Gostin, JD
O'Neill Institute for National and
Global Health Law, Georgetown
University Law Center, Washington, DC

Timothy Gray, PhD
JAMA Network

David Green, MD, PhD
Feinberg School of Medicine of
Northwestern University, Chicago,
Illinois

Heather Green, BA
JAMA Network

Emily A. Greenhow, BA
*JAMA*

Philip Greenland, MD
*JAMA* and Northwestern University,
Chicago, Illinois

Irina Grigorova, PhD
Department of Microbiology and
Immunology, University of Michigan,
Ann Arbor

Sasha Grossman, BA
JAMA Network

Lila Haile, BA
Medical Council of Canada, Ottawa
formerly with *JAMA*

Stephan Heckers, MD, MSc
Department of Psychiatry and
Behavioral Sciences, Vanderbilt
University, Nashville, Tennessee
formerly with *JAMA Psychiatry*

James G. Hodge Jr, JD, LLM
Sandra Day O'Connor College of Law,
Arizona State University, Phoenix

Joy K. Jaeger, BA
*JAMA*

Erin Kato, BA
JAMA Network

Lou S. Knecht, MLS
formerly Deputy Chief,
Bibliographic Services Division,
National Library of Medicine,
Bethesda, Maryland

Hope J. Lafferty, AM, ELS
Hope J. Lafferty Communications,
Marfa, Texas

Thomas A. Lang, MA
Tom Lang Communications and
Training International, Kirkland,
Washington

Trevor Lane, MA, DPhil
Edanz Group, Fukuoka, Japan

Frances E. Likis, DrPH, NP, CNM
*Journal of Midwifery & Women's
Health*, Nashville, Tennessee

Iris Y. Lo, BA
JAMA Network

Rochelle Lodder, ELS
formerly with JAMA Network

Preeti Malani, MD, MSJ
*JAMA* and Department of Internal
Medicine, University of Michigan,
Ann Arbor

Ana Marušić, MD, PhD
University of Split School of
Medicine, Split, Croatia and
*Journal of Global Health*

John J. McFadden, MA
JAMA Network

Chris Meyer
JAMA Network

Joseph Clayton Mills, MA
Neuroscience Publications, Barrow
Neurological Institute, Phoenix,
Arizona

Monica Mungle, BA
JAMA Network

Christopher C. Muth, MD
*JAMA*

George T. O'Connor, MD, MS
*JAMA* and Boston University School of
Medicine, Boston, Massachusetts

Sean O'Donnell
JAMA Network

Peter J. Olson, ELS
Sheridan Journal Services, Waterbury,
Vermont

Juliet A. Orellana, MA, MLIS
JAMA Network

Debra Parrish, JD
Parrish Law Offices, Pittsburgh,
Pennsylvania

Boris C. Pasche, MD, PhD
Wake Forest Baptist Medical Center,
Winston-Salem, North Carolina

Kim S. Penelton-Campbell, BS
*JAMA*

Eric D. Peterson, MD, MPH
*JAMA* and Duke University School of
Medicine, Durham, North Carolina

Malini Raghavan, PhD
Department of Microbiology and
Immunology, University of Michigan,
Ann Arbor

Rita F. Redberg, MD, MSc
*JAMA Internal Medicine* and Women's
Cardiovascular Services, University of
California, San Francisco

Frederick P. Rivara, MD, MPH
*JAMA Network Open* and University of
Washington, Seattle

June K. Robinson, MD
Department of Dermatology,
Northwestern University
Feinberg School of Medicine,
Chicago, Illinois
formerly with *JAMA Dermatology*

Roger N. Rosenberg, MD
Department of Neurology, University
of Texas Southwestern, Dallas
formerly with *JAMA Neurology*

Paul Ruich, BA
JAMA Network

Jeffrey L. Saver, MD
*JAMA* and Geffen School of Medicine
at UCLA, Los Angeles, California

Valerie Schneider, PhD
National Center for Biotechnology
Information, Bethesda, Maryland

David Schriger, MD, MPH
*JAMA* and Department of Emergency
Medicine, University of California,
Los Angeles

Lisa M. Schwartz, MD, MS
Center for Medicine and Media and
The Dartmouth Institute for Health
Policy and Clinical Practice, Lebanon,
New Hampshire

Jamie Scott, BA
JAMA Network

Philip Sefton, MS, ELS
*JAMA*

Stephanie C. Shubat, MS
USAN Program, American Medical
Association, Chicago, Illinois

Kirby Snell, MFA
JAMA Network

Nicole Netter Snoblin
NextWord Communications,
Lake Forest, Illinois

David Song
JAMA Network

Shannon Sparenga, MS
JAMA Network

Beverly L. Stewart, MSJ
*JAMA*

Joseph P. Thornton, JD
JAMA Network and American Medical
Association

Elizabeth Wager, PhD
Sideview, Princes Risborough,
England

Sam Wilder, MFA
formerly with JAMA Network

Steven Woloshin, MD, MS Center
for Medicine and Media and The
Dartmouth Institute for Health
Policy and Clinical Practice,
Lebanon, New Hampshire

Elizabeth H. Zak, PhD
American Medical Association, Chicago,
Illinois

Sara Zimmerman
JAMA Network

Jody W. Zylke, MD
*JAMA*

We also extend sincere thanks to *JAMA* and JAMA Network Editor in Chief
Howard Bauchner, MD, for his generous support of this effort and the countless
hours of staff time it required.

## In Memoriam: Paul Frank (1960-2015)

In tribute to a member of this committee, a caring and devoted colleague.

With our thanks for 30 years of contributions to medical journal writing, editing, technology, and publishing.

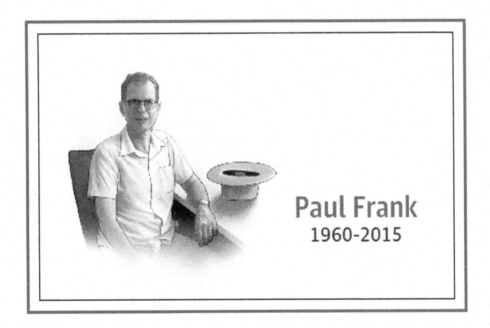

Paul Frank
1960-2015

# Contents

Contents

Contents

Contents

# 1.0 Types of Articles

**1.0** ▮▮▮▮ **Types of Articles.** Effective communication of scientific information requires consideration of the content, intended message, audience, and article format. To facilitate effective communication, editors of biomedical journals and other scientific publications use various article types, formats, and sections. However, most articles in scientific journals usually can be classified into 1 of the following general categories: Research Reports, Reviews, Other Substantive Articles (ie, nonresearch, nonreview), Opinion Articles, Correspondence, and Other Articles. For example, in the JAMA Network journals, major articles are classified into 3 main categories: research, clinical review and education, and opinion. These journals also use the following categories online to help users search by article type: research, review, opinion, case report, news, and humanities.

Editors and journals should provide clear and consistent guidance to authors about article types and requirements for each, such as in the instructions for authors. For example, JAMA Network Instructions for Authors include a section on Categories of Articles, which provides detailed information about the description and requirements for each type of article published in the journal.[1]

**1.1** ▮▮▮▮ **Research Reports.** Articles that report the results of original research investigations are perhaps the most important types of articles published by scientific journals. These articles advance scientific knowledge and, in medical journals, help inform clinical practice and advance patient care. Journals often categorize reports that present data from scientific research as Original Investigations (or Original Articles, Research Reports, or a similar designation) to emphasize the new findings these articles communicate.

Subcategories of Research articles may have specific designations based on other criteria. For instance, the JAMA Network journals may use designations based on (1) the nature of the findings, such as Preliminary Communication to indicate articles that report preliminary findings and signal the need for further investigation; (2) the topic of the research, such as Caring for the Critically Ill Patient to identify research in a specific clinical or scientific area, or Less Is More, to identify studies on how overuse of medical care may result in harm and how less intervention may lead to better health; or (3) article length, such as Brief Report to designate short reports of original studies or novel reports that involve small studies, or Research Letters to designate focused concise reports published as Correspondence.

Research reports may involve a wide range of study designs and methods, including randomized clinical trials, other intervention studies, cohort studies, case-control studies, epidemiologic investigations, surveys, meta-analyses, cost-effectiveness analyses, decision analyses, screening studies, diagnostic test evaluations, prognostic models, genetic and genomic studies, laboratory investigations, case series, case reports, and other designs. Data and information included in research reports must be original and should be as timely and current as possible. See **Box 1.1-1** for a list of common study types, descriptions, and requirements as used by the JAMA Network journals.

Research reports in biomedical journals generally follow a similar format that consists of the following sections: Title, Abstract, Introduction, Methods, Results, and Discussion, along with References, Tables and Figures, Article Information, Acknowledgments, online-only Supplemental content, and perhaps Multimedia content (see 2.5, Abstract, and 2.8, Parts of a Manuscript, Headings, Subheadings, and Side Headings, for guidance in preparing these sections). Some journals encourage use of reporting guidelines for research articles.[2] For example, guidelines for reporting clinical trials (Consolidated Standards of Reporting Trials [CONSORT]), observational studies (Strengthening the Reporting of Observational Studies in Epidemiology [STROBE]), or meta-analyses (Preferred Reporting Items for Systematic Reviews and Meta-Analyses [PRISMA]) or for other types of studies help ensure that key details related to the specific study design, methods, and results are included in the article. Box 1.1-1 also includes reporting guidelines for each of the study types listed.

**1.2**     **Reviews.** Review articles identify, synthesize, and summarize the available evidence and information about a specific topic. In biomedical journals, clinically based reviews have practical importance because practitioners may use these articles as guides for staying current with clinical information and helping inform decisions that involve clinical diagnosis and treatment. Depending on the journal, reviews can range from a rigorous, in-depth, systematic assessment of the literature to a less formal review based on a combination of selective evidence and expert opinion, similar to chapters in some textbooks. Journals generally have 2 types of reviews based on the scope of the review and level of analysis of the evidence and supporting literature.[1]

**1.2.1**     **Systematic Reviews.** Systematic reviews are critical assessments of the literature and data sources that pertain to clinical topics and often include information about the etiology, epidemiology, diagnosis, prognosis, therapy, or prevention of a disease or condition. These reviews involve a complete and up-to-date systematic search of the literature using multiple databases, covering many years, and grading the quality of the available evidence. Many journals encourage authors of systematic reviews to follow recommended reporting guidelines.[2] Systematic reviews without meta-analysis are generally published as Reviews. Systematic reviews that include meta-analysis of the available evidence and provide novel information, such as new estimates of effect size, may be published as Research articles.

Systematic reviews in biomedical journals generally follow a consistent format, although article sections may vary, depending on the specific type of review article. For example, Systematic Reviews in the JAMA Network journals usually include the following sections: Title, Abstract, Introduction, Methods, Results, and Discussion, along with References, Tables and Figures, Article Information, Acknowledgments, online-only Supplemental content, and perhaps Multimedia content (see 2.5.1.3, Structured Abstracts for Systematic Reviews [Without Meta-analysis]).

**1.2.2** **Narrative Reviews.** Narrative reviews in medical journals provide an up-to-date review that involves a specific question or issue relevant for clinical practice from the perspective of recognized experts in the topic. Although a systematic review of the literature is not necessarily required, recommendations should be supported with current evidence and based on recent research, systematic reviews, and guidelines.

Narrative reviews might include the following sections: Title, Abstract, Introduction, perhaps a Methods section, Observations, Discussion, with or without topic-specific subheadings, along with References, Tables and Figures, Article Information, Acknowledgments, online-only Supplemental content, and perhaps Multimedia content.

**1.3** **Other Substantive Article Types (Nonresearch, Nonreview).** Articles that present substantive content but do not include the methodologic approaches used in original research reports or the comprehensiveness of systematic reviews are common in biomedical journals. For instance, the Clinical Review and Education section of the JAMA Network journals includes a variety of diverse types of articles, ranging from longer, detailed reports that summarize available evidence on a topic to shorter reports that have an educational focus.

More detailed articles, which may be designated as Special Communications (or Special Articles or specific article types) to differentiate them from Research articles and Reviews, address important topics in clinical medicine, public health, health policy, or medical research in a scholarly, thorough, well-referenced, and evidence-based manner and summarize existing data and information. In biomedical journals, these articles may address major issues (eg, health care policy of ethical issues in a specific country or global comparisons) or may represent authoritative reports directly relevant to clinical practice (eg, clinical practice guidelines, consensus statements, or recommendation statements from governmental agencies). These articles usually have a structured Abstract (although the format may vary, depending on the nature and topic of the article), along with the following sections: Introduction, Methods (if applicable, eg, explaining the methods for guideline development), Results/Recommendations, and Discussion, along with References, Tables and Figures, Article Information, Acknowledgments, online-only Supplemental content, and perhaps Multimedia content.

Other substantive nonresearch, nonreview articles may present educational content or other information using various article formats according to the specific topic and usually consist of brief, focused articles. For instance, Clinical Guidelines Synopsis articles provide a succinct summary of recent guidelines from authoritative sources; Guide to Statistics and Methods articles present a concise explanation of a focused statistical concept, often based on that statistical approach as used in a related research report; and Clinical Challenge articles present a case-based clinical dilemma with diagnostic and treatment options in a question and answer format.

These and other articles provide useful information about relevant topics for journal readers and may serve as useful educational material for students and trainees. Because of the variability of the content of these brief articles, there is no standard format for these educational reports.

**1.4** **Opinion Articles.** Opinion articles are a major component of many journals and may serve many purposes, such as addressing topics of interest to readers, serving as a forum for discussion and debate of controversial issues, presenting authoritative and informative commentary on timely topics, providing insight and context about other published articles, and communicating information about the journal or about important topics from the editors. By communicating and highlighting important issues, opinion articles impart timeliness and vibrancy to a journal. In general, to be most effective, opinion articles should be focused, present a logical argument, and be brief. As the focus decreases, as the argument becomes less compelling, and as the length increases, the level of reader interest in the opinion article will most likely decline.

For example, the JAMA Network journals publish several types of Opinion articles, such as Viewpoints, Editorials, and Invited Commentaries, as well as articles that present personal vignettes and reflections.

**1.4.1** **Viewpoints (Also Called Commentaries or Perspectives).** These articles may address virtually any important topic relevant to the readers of the journal and may involve issues in medicine, clinical care, public health, research, ethics, health policy, or health law. These articles generally are not linked to another specific concurrently published article and should be well focused, scholarly, and clearly presented. Dueling Viewpoints (or Point, Counterpoint articles) involve 2 scholarly opinion articles that address a controversial current topic of interest. The articles address the same question, with one article usually presenting the yes answer and the other presenting the no answer, thereby providing balance and insights on both sides of controversial topics.

**1.4.2** **Editorials (or Invited Commentaries).** Editorials represent important opinion articles in scientific journals and generally serve 2 primary purposes.[3] Editorials written by the editor of the journal or a member of the editorial staff may communicate information about the journal or about journal policies or procedures or may present the views of the editors or editorial staff about an issue relevant to journal readers or about an article the journal has published. Editorials also may be written by authors who are not members of the editorial staff but who are invited to provide an authoritative discussion and opinion about an accompanying article or about another topic. In most cases, these invited Editorials (also referred to as Invited Commentaries in some journals) accompany research articles or other articles being published by the journal and ordinarily serve to provide balance, additional context, and caveats about the importance and implications of the accompanying article. At times, invited editorialists may be asked to comment on separate topics of interest to the journal readers or editors.

**1.4.3** **Personal Vignettes and Reflections.** Opinion articles based on personal experiences, anecdotes, or vignettes represent the importance of including narrative in scientific and biomedical journals and may be used to illustrate teaching points. For instance, most essays published as A Piece of My Mind articles in *JAMA* or as On My Mind articles in *JAMA Pediatrics* are based on personal vignettes that explore the dynamics of the patient-practitioner relationship and the wide-ranging experiences in medicine and health care or may express views and opinions about issues that affect the medical profession and other health care professionals. Articles published as Teachable Moments in *JAMA Internal Medicine* bring attention to the harms that can result from overuse of clinical care, such as with certain tests and treatments, and from underuse of needed clinical interventions.

**1.5** **Correspondence.**

**1.5.1** **Letters.** "Responsible debate, critique and disagreement are important features of science, and journal editors should encourage such discourse ideally within their own journals about the material they have published," according to the International Committee of Medical Journal Editors.[4] The correspondence section can include letters to the editor, responses from authors, and online comments and should provide readers with a mechanism for submitting comments, questions, or criticisms about published articles.[4] As part of the responsibility that authors assume in return for having their articles published, they are held accountable for responding to critical points from readers.[5] This type of interaction is an important part of postpublication peer review and helps foster responsible scientific dialogue (see 5.11.8, Ethical and Legal Considerations, Editorial Responsibilities, Roles, Procedures, and Policies, Correspondence [Letters to the Editor]).[5]

Letters that raise reasonable and important questions about the scientific, clinical, or ethical aspects of a study or appropriate interpretation, along with scholarly replies from the authors, can make for informative, useful, and lively exchanges. Another form of postpublication exchange between readers and authors of published articles involves online commenting and responses, with the exchanges posted on journal websites or other venues rather than published as letters in journals.

**1.5.2** **Research Letters.** Some journals also include brief articles that report original research data in a concise manner. For example, the JAMA Network journals classify these as Research Letters.[6] These reports contain brief Introduction, Methods, Results, and Discussion sections; are peer reviewed and subject to editorial review, like other research reports; and have limitations for length, number of references, and numbers of tables and figures. Research letters are indexed in bibliometric databases and may be an effective way for authors to publish concise, focused reports of studies.[6]

**1.6** **Other Article Types.** Journals also publish other articles and items that are relevant for their readers and may not fit into any of these categories. Examples may include news articles, educational articles, quizzes, book/media reviews, or poetry; articles intended for use by other potential readers, such as information for the public or for patients; or information in other formats, such as video, audio, and interactive material. Each of these other types of articles and material should follow consistent structure and format.

**Box 1.1-1.** Study Types, Descriptions, Requirements, and Reporting Guidelines[1]

**Randomized Clinical Trial**

A trial that prospectively assigns participants to intervention or comparison groups to study the cause-and-effect relationship between an intervention and a health outcome. Interventions include but are not limited to drugs, surgical procedures, devices, behavioral treatments, educational programs, dietary interventions, quality improvement interventions, process-of-care changes, and the like.

- 3000-3500 words
- ≤5 tables and/or figures, including CONSORT flow diagram
- 50-75 references
- Structured abstract
- Key Points
- Subtitle should be "A Randomized Clinical Trial"
- Trial registration and ID
- Trial protocol
- CONSORT checklist
- Data Sharing Statement
- Follow CONSORT Reporting Guidelines

**Parallel-Design, Double-blind Trial**

A randomized trial that prospectively assigns participants to 2 or more groups to receive different interventions. Participants and those administering the interventions are unaware of which intervention individual participants are receiving.

- 3000-3500 words
- ≤5 tables and/or figures, including CONSORT flow diagram
- 50-75 references
- Structured abstract
- Key Points
- Subtitle should be "A Randomized Clinical Trial"
- Trial registration and ID
- Trial protocol
- CONSORT checklist
- Data Sharing Statement
- Follow CONSORT Reporting Guidelines

**Crossover Trial**

A trial in which participants receive more than 1 of the treatments under investigation, usually in a randomly determined sequence, and with a prespecified amount of time (washout period) between sequential treatments.

- 3000-3500 words
- ≤5 tables and/or figures, including CONSORT flow diagram
- 50-75 references
- Structured abstract

**Box 1.1-1.** Study Types, Descriptions, Requirements, and Reporting Guidelines[1] *(continued)*

- Key Points
- Subtitle should be "A Randomized Clinical Trial"
- Trial registration and ID
- Trial protocol
- CONSORT checklist
- Data Sharing Statement
- Follow CONSORT Reporting Guidelines

**Equivalence and Noninferiority Trial**

A trial designed to assess whether the treatment or intervention under study (eg, a new intervention) is no worse than an existing alternative (eg, an active control). In these trials, authors must prespecify a margin of noninferiority that is consistent with all relevant studies and within which the new intervention can be assumed to be no worse than the active control.

- 3000-3500 words
- ≤5 tables and/or figures, including CONSORT flow diagram
- 50-75 references
- Structured abstract
- Key Points
- Subtitle should be "A Randomized Clinical Trial"
- Trial registration and ID
- Trial protocol
- CONSORT checklist
- Data Sharing Statement
- Follow CONSORT Reporting Guidelines

**Cluster Trial**

A trial that includes random assignment of groups rather than individuals to intervention and control groups.

- 3000-3500 words
- ≤5 tables and/or figures, including CONSORT flow diagram
- 50-75 references
- Structured abstract
- Key Points
- Subtitle should be "A Randomized Clinical Trial"
- Trial registration and ID
- Trial protocol
- CONSORT checklist
- Data Sharing Statement
- Follow CONSORT Reporting Guidelines

**Nonrandomized Controlled Trial**

A trial that prospectively assigns groups or populations to study the efficacy or effectiveness of an intervention but in which the assignment to the intervention occurs through self-selection or administrator selection rather than

*(continued)*

**Box 1.1-1.** Study Types, Descriptions, Requirements, and Reporting Guidelines[1] *(continued)*

through randomization. Control groups can be historic, concurrent, or both. This design is sometimes called a quasi-experimental design.

- 3000-3500 words
- ≤5 tables and/or figures, including CONSORT flow diagram
- 50-75 references
- Structured abstract
- Key Points
- Subtitle should be "A Nonrandomized Controlled Trial"
- Trial registration and ID
- Trial protocol
- CONSORT checklist
- Follow TREND Reporting Guidelines

**Trial Protocol**

A document that describes the organization and plan for a randomized clinical trial, including the trial's objective(s), design, methods, outcomes to be measured, and statistical analysis plan.

- 3000-3500 words
- ≤5 tables and/or figures
- 50-75 references
- Structured abstract
- Key Points
- Subtitle should be "A Trial Protocol"
- Trial registration and ID
- Trial protocol
- Follow SPIRIT Reporting Guidelines

**Meta-analysis**

A systematic review that includes a statistical technique for quantitatively combining the results of multiple studies that measure the same outcome into a single pooled or summary estimate.

- 3000-3500 words
- ≤5 tables and/or figures
- 50-75 references
- Structured abstract
- Key Points
- Subtitle should include "A Systematic Review and Meta-analysis"
- Follow PRISMA or MOOSE Reporting Guidelines

**Cohort Study**

An observational study that follows a group (cohort) of individuals who are initially free of the outcome of interest. Individuals in the cohort may share some underlying characteristic, such as age, sex, diagnosis, exposure to a risk factor, or treatment.

**Box 1.1-1.** Study Types, Descriptions, Requirements, and Reporting Guidelines[1] *(continued)*

- 3000-3500 words
- ≤5 tables and/or figures
- 50-75 references
- Structured abstract
- Key Points
- Follow STROBE Reporting Guidelines

**Case-Control Study**

An observational study designed to determine the association between an exposure and outcome in which study participants are selected by outcome. Those with the outcome (cases) are compared with those without the outcome (controls) with respect to an exposure or event. Cases and controls may be matched according to specific characteristics (eg, age, sex, or duration of disease).

- 3000-3500 words
- ≤5 tables and/or figures
- 50-75 references
- Structured abstract
- Key Points
- Follow STROBE Reporting Guidelines

**Cross-sectional Study**

An observational study of a defined population at a single point in time or during a specific interval in which exposure and outcome are ascertained simultaneously.

- 3000-3500 words
- ≤5 tables and/or figures
- 50-75 references
- Structured abstract
- Key Points
- Follow STROBE Reporting Guidelines

**Case Series**

An observational study that describes a selected group of participants with similar exposure or treatment and without a control group. A case series may also involve observation of larger units, such as groups of hospitals or municipalities, as well as smaller units, such as laboratory samples.

- 3000-3500 words
- ≤5 tables and/or figures
- 50-75 references
- Structured abstract
- Key Points
- Follow Reporting Guidelines

**Economic Evaluation**

A study using formal, quantitative methods to compare 2 or more treatments, programs, or strategies with respect to their resource use and expected

*(continued)*

**Box 1.1-1.** Study Types, Descriptions, Requirements, and Reporting Guidelines[1] *(continued)*

outcomes. This includes cost-effectiveness, cost-benefit, and cost-minimization analyses.

- 3000-3500 words
- ≤5 tables and/or figures
- 50-75 references
- Structured abstract
- Key Points
- Follow CHEERS Reporting Guidelines

**Decision Analytical Model**

A mathematical modeling study that compares consequences of decision options by synthesizing information from multiple sources and applying mathematical simulation techniques, usually with specific software. Reporting should address the relevant noncost aspects of the CHEERS guideline.

- 3000-3500 words
- ≤5 tables and/or figures
- 50-75 references
- Structured abstract
- Key Points
- Follow CHEERS Reporting Guidelines

**Comparative Effectiveness Research**

A study that compares different interventions or strategies to prevent, diagnose, treat, and monitor health conditions to determine which work best for which patients and under what circumstances and which are associated with the greatest benefits and harms.

- 3000-3500 words
- ≤5 tables and/or figures
- 50-75 references
- Structured abstract
- Key Points
- Follow ISPOR Reporting Guidelines

**Genetic Association Study**

A study that attempts to identify and characterize genomic variants that may be associated with susceptibility to multifactorial disease.

- 3000-3500 words
- ≤5 tables and/or figures
- 50-75 references
- Structured abstract
- Key Points
- Follow STREGA Reporting Guidelines

**Diagnostic/Prognostic Study**

A prospective study designed to develop, validate, or update the diagnostic or prognostic accuracy of a test or model.

**Box 1.1-1.** Study Types, Descriptions, Requirements, and Reporting Guidelines[1] *(continued)*

- 3000-3500 words
- ≤5 tables and/or figures
- 50-75 references
- Structured abstract
- Key Points
- Follow STARD Reporting Guidelines or TRIPOD Reporting Guidelines

**Quality Improvement Study**

A study that uses data to define, measure, and evaluate a health care practice or service to maintain or improve the appropriateness, quality, safety, or value of that practice or service.

- 3000-3500 words
- ≤5 tables and/or figures
- 50-75 references
- Structured abstract
- Key Points
- Follow SQUIRE Reporting Guidelines

**Survey Study**

A survey study includes a representative sample of individuals who are asked to describe their opinions, attitudes, or behaviors. Survey studies should have sufficient response rates (generally ≥60%) and appropriate characterization of nonresponders to ensure that nonresponse bias does not threaten the validity of the findings.

- 3000-3500 words
- ≤5 tables and/or figures
- 50-75 references
- Structured abstract
- Key Points
- Follow AAPOR Reporting Guidelines
- Optional: Survey instrument as supplemental file

**Qualitative Study**

A study based on observation and interview with individuals that uses inductive reasoning and a theoretical sampling model and that focuses on social and interpreted, rather than quantifiable, phenomena and aims to discover, interpret, and describe rather than to test and evaluate. This includes mixed-methods studies that combine quantitative and qualitative designs in a sequential or concurrent manner.

- 3000-3500 words
- ≤5 tables and/or figures
- 50-75 references
- Structured abstract
- Key Points
- Follow SRQR Reporting Guidelines or COREQ Reporting Guidelines

**Principal Author:** Phil B. Fontanarosa, MD, MBA

## ACKNOWLEDGMENT

Thanks to the following for reviewing this chapter and providing comments: Helene Cole, MD, formerly of *JAMA*; Trevor Lane, MA, DPhil, Edanz Group, Fukuoka, Japan; Peter J. Olson, ELS, Sheridan Journal Services, Waterbury, Vermont; Fred Rivara, MD, MPH, *JAMA Network Open* and University of Washington, Seattle; and Jody W. Zylke, MD, *JAMA*.

## REFERENCES

1. Instructions for Authors. *JAMA Network Open*. Accessed June 15, 2019. https://jamanetwork.com/journals/jamanetworkopen/pages/instructions-for-authors
2. Equator Network website. Accessed September 22, 2019. http://www.equator-network.org/
3. Fontanarosa PB. Editorial matters: guidelines for writing effective editorials. *JAMA*. 2014;311(21):2179-2180. doi:10.1001/jama.2014.6535
4. International Committee of Medical Journal Editors website. Accessed September 22, 2019. http://www.icmje.org/recommendations/
5. Golub RM. Correspondence course: tips for getting a letter published in *JAMA*. *JAMA*. 2008;300(1):98-99. doi:10.1001/jama.300.1.98
6. Zylke JW. Research letters in *JAMA*: small but mighty. *JAMA*. 2013;310(6):589-590. doi:10.1001/jama.2013.8102

# 2.0 Manuscript Preparation for Submission and Publication

**2.0** **Manuscript Preparation for Submission and Publication.** Preparation of a scholarly manuscript requires thoughtful consideration of the topic and anticipation of the reader's needs and questions. Certain elements are standard parts of all manuscripts or are used so often as to merit special discussion and instruction. These elements are discussed in this section in the order in which they appear in the manuscript. References are discussed separately in chapter 3 and tables, figures, and boxes in chapter 4. Some guidance is directed specifically to authors for manuscript preparation and submission, some is directed to editors for manuscript publication, and some to both authors and editors.

The preparation of any manuscript for publication should take the requirements of the intended journal into account, as well as reporting guidelines (EQUATOR Network: http://www.equator-network.org); this may enhance the chances of acceptance and expedite publication. Failure to do so may result in return without review. For the author, manuscript preparation requires familiarity with the journal to which the manuscript is submitted. Journals should publish instructions for authors, which serve as useful guides; some journals' instructions for authors contain a manuscript checklist. Some publishers also publish style manuals, which provide in-depth instruction (see 23.0, Resources), or rely on in-house guides, the *AMA Manual of Style*, or a combination of such resources. For journals that follow the International Committee of Medical Journal Editors (ICMJE) Recommendations for the Conduct, Reporting, Editing, and Publication of Scholarly Work in Medical Journals,[1] as the JAMA Network journals do, adherence to these guidelines will be acceptable, although the individual journal may require more than the ICMJE recommendations or make changes to suit its house style.

Most journals require submission of material through a web-based manuscript submission and peer review system (see 6.2, Editorial Processing).

**2.1** **Titles and Subtitles.** Titles should be concise, specific, and informative and should contain the key points of the work. Population type should be specified in the title, when possible (eg, Men With Atrial Fibrillation). For scientific manuscripts (eg, reports of research), neither overly general titles nor "cute" titles are desirable; these may be better suited to subtitles of opinion pieces (eg, Early Palliative Care in Advanced Illness: Do Right by Mama) (but see also 2.1.7, Names of Cities, States, Counties, Provinces, and Countries). Avoid the use of causal language in titles of articles reporting the results of observational research; cause-and-effect wording is best reserved for reports of randomized trials and laboratory-based controlled experiments (see 19.1.4, Results). Consult the journal's instructions for authors regarding any limitations on length of titles.

| | |
|---|---|
| *Avoid:* | Cocaine Use and Homicide |
| *Better:* | Association of Cocaine Use With Homicide Among Men in New York City |
| *Avoid:* | Obesity and Severe Obesity Among Children |
| *Better:* | Prevalence and Trends in Obesity and Severe Obesity Among Children in the United States, 1999-2012 |
| *Avoid:* | Reliability and Validity of Mobile Teledermatology |
| *Better:* | Assessment of Reliability and Validity of Mobile Teledermatology in HIV-Positive Patients in Botswana |
| *Avoid:* | Trauma Surveillance |
| *Better:* | Trauma Surveillance in Cape Town, South Africa |

Note: The shorter, more general title might be appropriate for an editorial or other opinion piece.

The key terms in a title should be given in order, from (1) exposure to (2) outcome to (3) population to (4) study type, as in the examples below:

Association of Exposure to Antibiotics During the First 6 Months of Life With Weight Gain During Childhood

Effect of Inhaled Xenon on Damage to Cerebral White Matter in Comatose Survivors of Out-of-Hospital Cardiac Arrest: A Randomized Clinical Trial

Screening Yield of HIV Antigen-Antibody Combination and Pooled HIV RNA Testing for Acute HIV Infection in a High-Prevalence Population

Effect of Behavioral Interventions on Inappropriate Antibiotic Prescribing Among Primary Care Practices: A Randomized Clinical Trial

Similarly, although the subtitle is frequently useful in expanding on the title, it should not contain key elements of the study as a supplement to an overly general title.

*Avoid:* Psychiatric Disorders: A Rural-Urban Comparison

*Better:* Rural-Urban Differences in the Prevalence of Psychiatric Disorders

*Avoid:* Multiple Sclerosis: Sexual Dysfunction and Response to Medications

*Better:* Sexual Dysfunction and Response to Medications in Patients With Multiple Sclerosis

*Avoid:* Hospitalization for Congestive Heart Failure: Explaining Racial Differences

*Better:* Assessment of Racial Differences in Hospitalization Rates for Congestive Heart Failure

*Avoid:* Breastfeeding in Children of Women Taking Antiepileptic Drugs: Cognitive Outcomes at 6 Years of Age

*Better:* Cognitive Outcomes at 6 Years of Age in Children of Breastfeeding Women Taking Antiepileptic Drugs

*Avoid:* Health Care at the US Department of Veterans Affairs: Recommendations for Change

*Better:* Recommendations for Improving Health Care at the US Department of Veterans Affairs

*Avoid:* Cardiovascular Evaluation of Competitive Athletes: Medical and Legal Issues

*Better:* Medical and Legal Issues in the Cardiovascular Evaluation of Competitive Athletes

However, too much detail also should be avoided. Subtitles should complement the title by providing supplementary information that will supply more detail about the content that will also aid in information retrieval. Several examples of informative title and subtitle combinations follow:

Effect of Naltrexone-Bupropion on Major Adverse Cardiovascular Events in Overweight and Obese Patients With Cardiovascular Risk Factors: A Randomized Clinical Trial

Prevalence of Cutaneous Adverse Effects of Hairdressing: A Systematic Review

Subtitles of scientific manuscripts may be used to amplify the title; however, the main title should be able to stand alone (ie, the subtitle should not be a continuation of the title or a substitute for a succinct title):

*Avoid:*  An Unusual Type of Pemphigus: Combining Features of Lupus Erythematosus

*Better:*  Assessment of an Unusual Type of Pemphigus With Features of Lupus Erythematosus

*Avoid:*  Von Hippel–Lindau Disease: Affecting 43 Members of a Single Kindred

*Better:*  Von Hippel–Lindau Disease in 43 Members of a Single Kindred

For observational studies in which causation cannot be demonstrated, titles should not include cause-and-effect terms. Other phrases, such as "association of," are preferred. In randomized clinical trials, in which causality can be demonstrated, the use of such phrases as "effects of" is appropriate.

Effects of Intake of Protein, Monounsaturated Fat, and Carbohydrate on Blood Pressure and Serum Lipids: Results of the OmniHeart Randomized Trial

Effects of Promoting High-Quality Staff Interactions on Fall Prevention in Nursing Homes: A Cluster Randomized Trial

Association Between Psychological Interventions and Chronic Pain Outcomes in Older Adults: A Systematic Review and Meta-analysis

Declarative sentences are used frequently as titles of news stories and opinion pieces (eg, "World Bank Pledges $200 Million to Stem Ebola Outbreak in West Africa," "Lifestyle Counseling Advised for Overweight Adults With Other Cardiovascular Risk Factors"). However, declarative sentences or phrases in scientific article titles tend to overemphasize a conclusion and should not be used.

*Avoid:*  Fibromyalgia Is Common in an Obesity Clinic

*Better:*  Prevalence of Fibromyalgia in Obese Patients

Similarly, questions should not be used for titles of scientific (research) manuscripts.

*Avoid:*  Is Television Viewing Associated With Social Isolation? Roles of Exposure Time, Viewing Context, and Violent Content

*Better:*  Association Between Television Viewing and Social Isolation: Roles of Exposure Time, Viewing Context, and Violent Content

Questions are generally more appropriate for titles of editorials, commentaries, and opinion pieces, all of which may be less scholarly, and perhaps more provocative, than research articles:

Can the Learning Health Care System Be Educated With Observational Data?

Hospital Consolidation, Competition, and Quality: Is Bigger Necessarily Better?

Why Should High-Income Countries Help Combat Ebola?

Contralateral Prophylactic Mastectomy: Is It a Reasonable Option?

Is Big Data the New Frontier for Academic-Industry Collaboration?

Toward Improved Glycemic Control in Diabetes: What's on the Horizon?

Postradiotherapy Pelvic Fractures: Cause for Concern or Opportunity for Further Research?

Randomized clinical trials should be described as such in the subtitle because this alerts readers to the level of evidence and the study design and is helpful to readers and researchers:

Effect of Behavioral Interventions on Inappropriate Antibiotic Prescribing Among Primary Care Practices: A Randomized Clinical Trial

Effect of Darapladib on Major Coronary Events After an Acute Coronary Syndrome: The SOLID-TIMI 52 Randomized Clinical Trial

Administrative Data Feedback for Effective Cardiac Treatment: The AFFECT Cluster Randomized Trial

Other aspects of study design or methods may be included in the title or subtitle:

Clinical and Safety Outcomes Associated With Treatment of Acute Venous Thromboembolism: A Systematic Review and Meta-analysis

Depression, Apolipoprotein E Genotype, and Incidence of Mild Cognitive Impairment: A Prospective Cohort Study

Physician Variation in Management of Low-Risk Prostate Cancer: A Population-Based Cohort Study

Antibiotic Exposure, Infection, and Development of Pediatric Psoriasis: A Nested Case-Control Study

Sometimes a subtitle will contain the name of the group responsible for the study, especially if the study is large and best known by its group name or acronym (this is particularly true in some specialties, such as cardiology, oncology, and ophthalmology) or if it is a part of a series of reports from the same group (see 2.1.5, Abbreviations, and 13.9, Collaborative Groups):

Association of Dietary Intake of Fat and Cholesterol With Elevated Low-Density Lipoprotein Cholesterol Levels in Children: The Dietary Intervention Study in Children (DISC)

Antibiotic Resistance Among Ocular Pathogens in the United States: Five-Year Results From the Antibiotic Resistance Monitoring in Ocular Microorganisms (ARMOR) Surveillance Study

Antihypertensive Drug Treatment to Prevent Stroke in Older Patients With Isolated Systolic Hypertension: Final Results of the Systolic Hypertension in the Elderly Program (SHEP)

Some journals, such as *JAMA*, do not include the study name in the title or subtitle for any but the original report of outcomes or secondary analyses that provide unique information.

Low-Fat Dietary Pattern and Risk of Invasive Breast Cancer: The Women's Health Initiative Randomized Controlled Dietary Modification Trial

However, the JAMA Network specialty journals include the study name in the subtitle if authors prefer to include it. For most secondary analyses, having the study name in the abstract is sufficient for information retrieval.

**2.1.1** **Quotation Marks.** If quotation marks are required in the title or subtitle, they should be double, not single (see 8.6.3, Titles).

Encouraging Patients to Ask Questions: How to Overcome "White Coat Silence"

Mandatory Extended Searches in All Genome Sequencing: "Incidental Findings" and Patient Autonomy

How Can Errors Be Avoided in Medicine? Above All "Do No Harm"

**2.1.2** **Numbers.** Follow the style for numbers included in titles as described in 18.0, Numbers and Percentages.

Educational Programs in US Medical Schools, 2012-2013

Three-Day Antimicrobial Regimen for Treatment of Acute Cystitis in Women: A Randomized Clinical Trial

Comparison of 2 Methods to Detect Publication Bias in Meta-analyses

Skin Reactions in Patients With Stage IV Melanoma Treated With T-Lymphocyte Antigen 4 Monoclonal Antibody

Primary and Secondary Prevention in 20 Years of Clinical Practice

If numbers appear at the beginning of a title or subtitle, they—and any unit of measure associated with them—should be spelled out.

Primary and Secondary Prevention Services in Clinical Practice: Twenty Years' Experience in Development, Implementation, and Evaluation

Two-Year Changes in Refractive Error and Related Biometric Factors in an Adult Chinese Population

Exceptions may be made for years (see 18.2.1, Beginning a Sentence, Title, Subtitle, or Heading).

US Adult Illicit Cannabis Use, Cannabis Use Disorder, and Medical Marijuana Laws: 1991-1992 to 2012-2013

**2.1.3** **Drugs.** If drug names appear in the title or subtitle, (1) use the approved generic or nonproprietary name, (2) omit the nonbase moiety unless it is required (see 14.4, Nomenclature, Drugs), and (3) avoid the use of proprietary names unless *(a)* several products are being compared, *(b)* the article is specific to a particular formulation of a drug (eg, the vehicle, not the active substance, caused adverse reactions), or *(c)* the number of ingredients is so large that the resulting title would be clumsy and a generic term, such as "multivitamin tablet," would not do.

> Effect of Aliskiren on Progression of Coronary Disease in Patients With Prehypertension: The AQUARIUS Randomized Clinical Trial

> Efficacy of Rofecoxib, Celecoxib, and Acetaminophen in Osteoarthritis of the Knee: A Randomized Clinical Trial

> Risk of Hospitalization for Myocardial Infarction Among Users of Rofecoxib, Celecoxib, and Other NSAIDs: A Population-Based Case-Control Study

**2.1.4** **Genus and Species.** Genus and species should be expanded and italicized in the title or subtitle and an initial capital letter should be used for the genus but not the species name, just as in the text (see 14.14.1, Biological Nomenclature).

> Reconsidering Isolation Precautions for Endemic Methicillin-Resistant *Staphylococcus aureus* and Vancomycin-Resistant *Enterococcus*

> Prevalence of *Chlamydia trachomatis* Genital Infection in Teenaged Girls

> Elimination of a Community-Acquired Methicillin-Resistant *Staphylococcus aureus* Infection in a Nurse With Atopic Dermatitis

In experimental studies in animals, the type of animal studied should be included in the title.

> Human Induced Pluripotent Stem Cell–Derived Motor Neuron Transplant for Neuromuscular Atrophy in a Mouse Model of Sciatic Nerve Injury

**2.1.5** **Abbreviations.** Avoid the use of abbreviations in the title and subtitle, unless space considerations require an exception or unless the title or subtitle includes the name of an entity or a group that is best known by its acronym. In both cases, the abbreviation should be expanded in the abstract and at the first appearance in the text (see 10.6, Acronyms, and 13.0, Abbreviations).

> Epidemiology of *DSM-5* Generalized Anxiety Disorder Across the Globe

> Discriminative Accuracy of Physician and Nurse Predictions for Survival and Functional Outcomes 6 Months After ICU Admission

> Accuracy of Airflow Obstruction Thresholds for Predicting COPD-Related Hospitalization and Mortality

Reporting of Noninferiority and Equivalence Randomized Trials: An Extension of the CONSORT Statement

Implementing the USPSTF Recommendations on Prevention of Perinatal Depression

**2.1.6** **Capitalization.** Capitalize the first letter of each major word in titles and subtitles. Do not capitalize subsequent articles (eg, *a, an, the*), prepositions of 3 or fewer letters (including *per*), coordinating conjunctions *(and, or, for, nor, but)*, or the *to* in infinitives. Do capitalize a 2-letter verb, such as *Is* or *Be*. Exceptions are made for some expressions, such as compound non-English and phrasal verbs. Note the following examples (from opinion pieces and news articles):

Risk Factors for Heart Disease in Rural Uganda Go Up With Urbanization

High Rotavirus Vaccination Rates Continue to Pay Off

Ethical Questions Concerning In Vitro Fertilization

Permanent Duplex Surveillance of In Situ Saphenous Vein Bypasses

Choice of Stents and End Points for Treatment of De Novo Coronary Artery Lesions

Weighing In on Bariatric Surgery

Researchers Size Up the Risks of Nanotechnology

Universal Screening for Tuberculosis Infection: School's Out!

See 10.0, Capitalization, for overall guidelines. For capitalization of hyphenated compounds, see 10.2, Titles and Headings.

**2.1.7** **Names of Cities, States, Counties, Provinces, and Countries.** Include cities, states, counties, provinces, or countries in titles only when essential, especially for results that may not be generalizable to other locations (eg, results unique to that site).

Prevalence and Incidence Trends for Diagnosed Diabetes Among Adults Aged 20 to 79 Years, United States, 1980-2012

Providing Conditional Economic Compensation and Uptake of Voluntary Male Circumcision in Kenya: A Randomized Clinical Trial

Mortality Related to Severe Sepsis and Septic Shock Among Critically Ill Patients in Australia and New Zealand, 2000-2012

Prevalence of War-Related Conditions of Mental Health and Association With Displacement Status in Postwar Jaffna District, Sri Lanka

Equity of Use of Home-Based or Facility-Based Skilled Obstetric Care in Rural Bangladesh

Identification of a New Serogroup Clone of *Neisseria meningitidis* From Anhui Province, China

Comparison of Stage at Diagnosis of Melanoma Among Hispanic, Black, and White Patients in Miami–Dade County, Florida

Gender Disadvantage and Reproductive Health Risk Factors for Common Mental Disorders in Women: A Community Survey in India

In other cases, include this geographic information in the abstract and the text only (see 13.5, Cities, States, Counties, Territories, Possessions, Provinces, Countries).

*Avoid:* Pertussis Infection in Adults With Persistent Cough in Nashville, Tennessee

*Better:* Pertussis Infection in Adults With Persistent Cough

*Avoid:* Hospitalization Charges, Costs, and Income for Trauma-Related Injuries at the University of California, Davis, Medical Center in Sacramento

*Better:* Hospitalization Charges, Costs, and Income for Trauma-Related Injuries at a University Trauma Center

*Avoid:* Prevalence of Erectile Dysfunction in Men Seen by Primary Care Physicians in Canada

*Better:* Prevalence of Erectile Dysfunction in Men Seen by Primary Care Physicians

**2.2** **Author Bylines and End-of-Text Signatures.** For manuscript submission, the complete names of all authors should be included in the manuscript, preferably on the title page(s), following the title, or as individual journals specify in their instructions for authors. In major articles, authors are listed in a byline, which typically appears immediately below the title or subtitle in print and online. For articles that have a large number of authors (eg, more than 50), there may not be space to list all authors below the title in the print or PDF version of the article, and the names may be listed at the end of the article. If authorship cannot appear on the first page of the print/PDF version of an article, an explicit statement about where to locate the complete list of authors should appear on page 1. For the print or PDF versions of some types of articles (eg, letters, editorials, book reviews, essays, poems, news stories), some journals may list the authors' names as signatures (or in signature blocks) at the end of the text, rather than below the title. Authors' names should not be presented with initials only, unless that is their preference. The JAMA Network journals publish complete author names and academic degrees for all authors. Some journals publish initials for first names and do not include academic degrees. Authors should consult specific journals for style and format and for instructions on how to list authors in submitted manuscripts (see 5.1, Authorship Responsibility).

**2.2.1** **Authors' Names.** The byline or signature block should contain each author's full name (unless initials are preferred to full names), including, for example, Jr, Sr, II,

III, and middle initials, and highest academic degree(s). Authors should be consistent in the presentation of their names in all published works so that they can be recognized by indexers, bibliometric databases, repositories, search engines, and readers.

If the byline includes names of Chinese, Japanese, Vietnamese, Korean, or Hungarian origin, or other names in which the family name is traditionally given first, some journals—and some authors—may "westernize" the order and give the surname last. For example, an author whose name is conventionally given as Zhou Jing, where Zhou is the surname, might list his name as Jing Zhou for publication in a Western journal, or the journal might elect to publish it that way regardless of the author's preference. For journals that choose to follow the author's preference in presentation of the order of first name (given name, familiar name) and surname and that therefore might retain the conventional (ie, non-Western) presentation of such names in the byline, the surname may be distinguished from the first name by capital letters (eg, ZHOU Jing)[2] or some other typographic distinction (eg, **Zhou** Jing or ZHOU Jing).

The JAMA Network journals favor following the authors' preferences on presentation of their names and recommend querying the author at the editing stage to ensure that the surname is properly identified. Identifying first and last names in the document tagging (eg, XML) is critical for accurate publication, indexing, and searching. For example, for the name Jing Zhou, where Jing is the given name and Zhou is the surname, if it is presented in typical Western style (ie, Jing Zhou), the name would be coded in JATS DTD XML as follows:

```
<name><surname>Zhou</surname><given-names>Jing</given-names>
</name>
```

If it is instead presented with the surname *first,* it would be coded as follows:

```
<name   name-style="eastern"><surname>Zhou</surname><given-names>Jing
</given-names></name>
```

See 2.10.19, Preferred Citation Format, and 21.1.1, Editing With XML. See also the *Chicago Manual of Style* for more details on conventional presentations of names from various cultures.[3]

Some journals have begun to request or require authors to provide unique identifiers that will link their names with a persistent record of their identities. ORCID (Open Researcher and Contributor ID)[4] and ISNI (International Standard Name Identifier)[5] are 2 such examples. As some have suggested, these records may help resolve the problem of name ambiguity in search and discovery[6] (see 5.1.1, Authorship: Definition, Criteria, Contributions, and Requirements).

**2.2.2** **Authorship.** All persons listed as authors should qualify for authorship (see 5.1, Ethical and Legal Considerations, Authorship Responsibility, and 5.1.2, Ethical and Legal Considerations, Authorship Responsibility, Guest and Ghost Authors and Other Contributors), and the authors' names should be consistently presented in all versions of the full text. The order of authors should be determined by the authors themselves (see 5.1.1, Authorship: Definition, Criteria, Contributions, and Requirements, and 5.1.5, Order of Authorship). According to the ICMJE,[1]

> Authorship should be based on the following 4 criteria: (1) substantial contributions to the conception or design of the work, or the acquisition, analysis, or interpretation of data for the work; AND (2) drafting the work or revising it critically for important intellectual content; AND (3) final approval of the version to be published; AND (4) agreement to be accountable for all aspects of the work in ensuring that questions related to the accuracy or integrity of the work are appropriately investigated and resolved.

Some journals (including all JAMA Network journals, *BMJ*, and *The Lancet*) may publish authors' specific contributions (see 2.10.8, Author Contributions).

Some authors may request that the Author Contributions note those authors who contributed equally to the work.

> **Author Contributions:** Drs Y. Zhang and J. Zhang contributed equally and are considered co–senior authors of this work. In addition, they had full access to all the data in the study and take responsibility for the integrity of data and accuracy of the data analysis.

> **Author Contributions:** Drs Li and Huang contributed equally to this work.

Persons who made other contributions but do not qualify for authorship (see 5.1.1.1, Authorship: Definition, Criteria, Contributions, and Requirements, Authorship Definition and Criteria, Box 5.1-1. Common Terms: Contributor, Author, and Collaborator) may be listed in the Acknowledgment section (see 2.10.17, Additional Contributions), with their permission (see 5.2, Acknowledgments). See 2.2.4, Multiple Authors, Group Authors.

**2.2.3** **Academic Degrees.** Journals should establish their own policies on the inclusion of authors' academic degrees. The policy of the JAMA Network journals is as follows: The highest degree or professional certification follows each author's name. If an author holds 2 doctoral degrees (eg, MD and PhD, MD and JD), either or both may be used, in the order preferred by the author. If the author has a doctorate, degrees at the master's level are not usually included, although exceptions may be made when the master's degree represents a specialized field or a field different from that represented by the doctorate (eg, MD, MPH).

Academic degrees below the master's level are usually omitted unless these are the highest degree held. Exceptions are made for specialized professional certifications, degrees, and licensure (eg, RN, RD, COT, PA) and for specialized bachelor's or master's degrees (eg, BSN, BPharm, MPA, MBA, MSJ) and combination degrees (eg, BS, M[ASCP], BNurs, MHA).

Fellowship designations (eg, FACP, FACS, FRCP, FRCS, FRCPC) and honorary degrees (eg, PhD[Hon]) are omitted (see 13.1, Academic Degrees, Certifications, and Honors, for the rationale for this policy).

**2.2.4**  **Multiple Authors, Group Authors.** When the byline contains more than 1 name, use semicolons to separate the authors' names (see 5.1.9, Group and Collaborative Authorship).

**2.2.4.1**  **Multiple Authors.** The following examples show bylines with multiple authors.

> Melvin H. Freedman, MD; E. Fred Saunders, MD; Louise Jones, MD, PhD; Kurt Grant, RN

> John E. Ware Jr, PhD; Martha S. Bayliss, MSc; William H. Rogers, PhD; Mark Kosinski, MA; Alvin R. Tarlov, MD

> Varun K. Phadke, MD; Robert A. Bednarczyk, MS, PhD; Daniel A. Salmon, MPH, PhD; Saad B. Omer, MBBS, MPH, PhD

**2.2.4.2**  **Individual Authors *for* a Group.** When a byline or signature contains 1 or more individuals' names and the name of a group (not all members of which meet the qualifications for authorship), use *for* followed by the name of the group if the specific individuals named qualify for authorship and are writing *for* the group.

> William A. Tasman, MD; for the Laser ROP Study Group

In the example above, those listed in the article as members of the group may be identified as nonauthor collaborators (see 2.10.12, Group Information [Including List of Participants in a Group] and 5.1.9, Group and Collaborative Authorship).

**2.2.4.3**  **Individual Authors *and* a Group.** When a byline or signature contains 1 or more individuals' names and the name of a group (all members of which meet the qualifications for authorship), use *and* followed by the name of the group if the individuals as well as all the members of the group qualify for authorship. In this case, every member of the group must qualify for authorship, and for journals with specific authorship criteria, like the JAMA Network journals, each member of the group must complete an authorship form indicating that he or she has met the criteria for authorship (see 2.10.12, Group Information [Including List of Participants in a Group], 5.1.9, Group and Collaborative Authorship, and 13.9, Collaborative Groups).

> Debra L. Hanson, MS; Susan Y. Chu, PhD; Karen M. Farizo, MD; John W. Ward, MD; and the Adult and Adolescent Spectrum of HIV Disease Project Group

**2.2.4.4**  **Subgroups as Author.** Occasionally a specific subgroup of a larger group will be listed as the author:

> The Writing Committee of the NORDIC Idiopathic Intracranial Hypertension Study Group

> Executive Committee for the Symptomatic Carotid Atherosclerotic Study

> The Writing Group for the DISC Collaborative Research Group

In this case, the names of the members of the subgroup should be clearly listed as authors (eg, at the end of the article) and each member of the subgroup must sign a statement indicating that he or she met the authorship criteria.

**2.2.4.5** **Group Name in Byline, With All Group Members Qualifying as Authors.** If each member of the group qualifies for authorship, the group name may be listed alone in the byline or signature block (see 2.3.3, Author Affiliations, and 2.10.12, Group Information [Including List of Participants in a Group]). The group members (authors and any nonauthor collaborators) would be listed separately at the end of the article and would be identified as authors or collaborators (see 2.10.12, Group Information [Including List of Participants in a Group], and 5.1.9, Group and Collaborative Authorship).

> Global Burden of Disease Pediatrics Collaboration

**2.3** **Author Footnotes.** The footnotes discussed below are intended for editors and production staff who manage placement of notes that may appear at the bottom of the first print or PDF page of major articles. On the journal's website or for online-only journals, these are typically displayed in an Article Information section at the end of the article. Authors preparing manuscripts for submission may follow this general guidance as well and include this information on the title page(s) or Acknowledgment at the end of the manuscript (see 2.10, Acknowledgments). For authors preparing manuscripts, footnotes should not be used within the body of the article. Such explanatory material can usually be incorporated into the text parenthetically. Note: These footnotes are different from the superscript numbers used to indicate specific author affiliations. See 2.3.3, Author Affiliations.

**2.3.1** **Order of Footnotes for Print or PDF Page.** The preferred order of types of footnotes at the bottom of the first print/PDF page of an article in the JAMA Network journals is as follows (see 21.0, Editing, Proofreading, Tagging, and Display). Note: Not all articles will include all types. In addition, many journals, including the online-only journal *JAMA Network Open*, simply combine all footnotes and list them all at the end of the article.

- Author affiliations
- Information about members of a group (see 2.10.12, Group Information [Including List of Participants in a Group])
- Corresponding author contact information

> *Byline:* John A. Doe, MD; Myrtle S. Coe, MD; Simon T. Foe, RN; for the XYZ Group
>
> *Footnotes:*
>
> **Author Affiliations:** Department of Pediatrics, Baylor College of Medicine, Houston, Texas (Doe, Foe); Department of Internal Medicine, Baylor College of Medicine, Houston, Texas (Coe).
>
> A list of the XYZ Group authors and collaborators appears at the end of this article.
>
> **Corresponding Author:** John A. Doe, MD, Department of Pediatrics, Baylor College of Medicine, 1 Baylor Plaza, Houston, TX 77030 (jdoe@baylor.edu).

**2.3.2** **Death of Author(s).** The policy of using a "death dagger" (†) after the author's name in the byline if an author has died before an article is published has been discontinued. If desired, this information can be included in the Acknowledgment section at the end of the article under the heading Additional Information. For example,

> **Additional Information:** Coauthor John Doe, MD, died January 30, 2017.

**2.3.3** **Author Affiliations.** For manuscript submission, the affiliations of all authors should be provided on the title page(s) or in the Acknowledgment section at the end of the manuscript.

For publication, the institutions with which an author is professionally affiliated, including locations, are given in a footnote in the print or PDF version of an article (see 13.5, Cities, States, Counties, Territories, Possessions, Provinces, Countries). The authors' last names are given parenthetically in the footnote following their respective institutions. On the journal's website, affiliations or links to affiliations often appear just below the byline. Note that no honorary titles precede the surname (eg, Dr or Mr). If 2 or more authors share the same last name, their initials should be used in addition to the last name to allow readers to distinguish them.

*Print or PDF Version*

*Byline:* Sherry Kit Wa Chan, MRCPsych; Stephanie Wing Yan Chan, BSc; Herbert H. Pang, PhD; Kang K. Yan, MSc; Christy Lai Ming Hui, PhD; Wing Chung Chang, MRCPsych; Eric Yu Hai Chen, MD

**Author Affiliations:** Department of Psychiatry, Li Ka Shing Faculty of Medicine, The University of Hong Kong, Hong Kong (S. K. W. Chan, S. W. Y. Chan, Hui, Chang, Chen); The State Key Laboratory of Brain and Cognitive Sciences, The University of Hong Kong, Hong Kong (S. K. W. Chan, Chang, Chen); School of Public Health, Li Ka Shing Faculty of Medicine, The University of Hong Kong, Hong Kong (Pang, Yan).

If 2 or more authors share the same initials and last name, then their full first and last names are included. Title and academic rank are not included in this footnote. If all authors in the byline are affiliated with the same department and institution, there is no need to include their names in the footnote.

List the affiliations in the order of the authors' names as given in the byline.

*Print or PDF Version*

*Byline:* Anita Kohli, MD, MS; Ashton Shaffer, BA; Amy Sherman, MD; Shyam Kottilil, MD, PhD

**Author Affiliations:** Clinical Research Directorate/Clinical Monitoring Research Program, Leidos Biomedical Research Inc, Frederick National Laboratory for Cancer Research, Frederick, Maryland (Kohli); Critical Care Medicine Department, Clinical Research Center, National Institutes of Health, Bethesda, Maryland (Kohli); Laboratory of Immunoregulation, National

Institute of Allergy and Infectious Diseases, National Institutes of Health, Bethesda, Maryland (Shaffer, Sherman, Kottilil).

*Online Version*

*Byline:* Anita Kohli, MD, MS[1,2]; Ashton Shaffer, BA[3]; Amy Sherman, MD[3]; Shyam Kottilil, MD, PhD[3]

*Links to Affiliations:*

[1]Clinical Research Directorate/Clinical Monitoring Research Program, Leidos Biomedical Research Inc, Frederick National Laboratory for Cancer Research, Frederick, Maryland

[2]Critical Care Medicine Department, Clinical Research Center, National Institutes of Health, Bethesda, Maryland

[3]Laboratory of Immunoregulation, National Institute of Allergy and Infectious Diseases, National Institutes of Health, Bethesda, Maryland

*Print or PDF Version*

*Byline:* Jerry A. Shields, MD; Renelle Pointdujour-Lim, MD; Sara E. Lally, MD; Ralph C. Eagle, MD; Carol L. Shields, MD

**Author Affiliations:** Ocular Oncology Service, Wills Eye Hospital, Thomas Jefferson University, Philadelphia, Pennsylvania.

*Online Version*

*Byline:* Jerry A. Shields, MD[1]; Renelle Pointdujour-Lim, MD[1]; Sara E. Lally, MD[1]; Ralph C. Eagle, MD[1]; Carol L. Shields, MD[1]

*Links to Affiliations:*

[1]Ocular Oncology Service, Wills Eye Hospital, Thomas Jefferson University, Philadelphia, Pennsylvania

*Print or PDF Version*

*Byline:* Jeremiah Brown Jr, MD; John H. Fingert; Chris M. Taylor; Max Lake, MD; Val C. Sheffield, MD, PhD; Edwin M. Stone, MD, PhD

**Author Affiliations:** Department of Ophthalmology, University of Iowa College of Medicine, Iowa City (Brown, Fingert, Taylor, Stone); Private practice, Salina, Kansas (Lake); Department of Pediatrics, University of Iowa College of Medicine, Iowa City (Sheffield).

*Online Version*

*Byline:* Jeremiah Brown Jr, MD[1]; John H. Fingert[1]; Chris M. Taylor[1]; Max Lake, MD[2]; Val C. Sheffield, MD, PhD[3]; Edwin M. Stone, MD, PhD[1]

*Links to Affiliations:*

[1]Department of Ophthalmology, University of Iowa College of Medicine, Iowa City

[2]Private practice, Salina, Kansas

[3]Department of Pediatrics, University of Iowa College of Medicine, Iowa City

**Single Author, Single Affiliation**

If there is a single author and a single institution with which the author is affiliated, use the singular for the Author Affiliation head:

*Byline:* James R. Keane, MD

**Author Affiliation:** Department of Neurology, University of Southern California Medical School, Los Angeles.

**Single Author, Multiple Affiliations**

If an author is affiliated with multiple institutions or different departments at the same institution, this information should be indicated parenthetically in the print or PDF version and with unique superscript numbers in the online version.

*Print or PDF Version*

*Byline*: Carlos del Rio, MD; Wendy S. Armstrong, MD

**Author Affiliations**: Hubert Department of Global Health, Rollins School of Public Health, Atlanta, Georgia (del Rio); Division of Infectious Diseases, Department of Medicine, Emory University School of Medicine, Atlanta, Georgia (del Rio, Armstrong); Emory Center for AIDS Research, Atlanta, Georgia (del Rio, Armstrong).

*Online Version*

*Byline*: Carlos del Rio, MD[1,2,3]; Wendy S. Armstrong, MD[2,3]

*Links to Affiliations*:

[1]Hubert Department of Global Health, Rollins School of Public Health, Atlanta, Georgia

[2]Division of Infectious Diseases, Department of Medicine, Emory University School of Medicine, Atlanta, Georgia

[3]Emory Center for AIDS Research, Atlanta, Georgia

The affiliation listed in the article, including departmental affiliation if appropriate, should reflect the author's institutional affiliation at the time the work was done. If the author has since moved, the current affiliation also should be provided.

*Print or PDF Version*

*Byline:* Jonathan S. Lee, MD; Daniel L. Giesler, MD, PharmD; Walid F. Gellad, MD, MPH; Michael J. Fine, MD, MSc

**Author Affiliations:** Division of General Internal Medicine, Department of Medicine, University of Pittsburgh School of Medicine, Pittsburgh, Pennsylvania (Lee, Giesler, Gellad, Fine); Now with Division of General Internal Medicine, Department of Medicine, University of California, San Francisco (Lee);

Center for Health Equity Research and Promotion, Veterans Affairs Pittsburgh Healthcare System, Pittsburgh, Pennsylvania (Gellad, Fine).

*Online Version*

*Byline:* Jonathan S. Lee, MD[1,2]; Daniel L. Giesler, MD, PharmD[1]; Walid F. Gellad, MD, MPH[1,3]; Michael J. Fine, MD, MSc[1,3]

*Links to Affiliations:*

[1]Division of General Internal Medicine, Department of Medicine, University of Pittsburgh School of Medicine, Pittsburgh, Pennsylvania

[2]Now with Division of General Internal Medicine, Department of Medicine, University of California, San Francisco

[3]Center for Health Equity Research and Promotion, Veterans Affairs Pittsburgh Healthcare System, Pittsburgh, Pennsylvania

**Group Author Affiliations**

For large groups, the name of the group may be given in the byline, and the affiliation footnote may refer the reader to the end of the article, a supplement online, or another publication for a complete listing of the participants, although preference is for these group members to be listed at the end of the article and tagged (or coded) as "authors" or "nonauthor collaborators" (see 2.2.4, Multiple Authors, Group Authors, and 2.10.12, Group Information [Including List of Participants in a Group]).

> *Preferred:* The POST (Parents From the Other Side of Treatment) Investigators are listed at the end of this article.

> *Preferred:* A complete list of the members of the Human Fetal Tissue Working Group appears at the end of this article.

**2.4** **Running Head, Running Foot in Print/PDF.** For publication, print or PDF pages customarily carry the bibliographic information for the article (journal name or abbreviation, year of publication, volume number, issue number, inclusive page numbers, and DOI, as well as the date published online, if applicable). Successive pages may also include a shortened version of the article title, called a running title or a short title (see 2.4.2, Title of the Article). When this information appears at the top of the page, it is called a running head; when it appears at the bottom of the page, it is called a running foot. In the JAMA Network journals, the following information is published on the first page of the article. Successive pages carry an abbreviated version:

> **Bibliographic Information on First Page:**

> *JAMA Neurol.* 2014;71(8):961-970. doi:10.1001/jamaneurol.2014.803

> Published online June 2, 2014.

> **Running Foot on Successive Pages:**

> *JAMA Neurology* August 2014 Volume 71, Number 8

Note: On the journal's website, this bibliographic information often appears at the top of the article.

In the JAMA Network journals, the shortened version of the article title, as well as the type of article, appears in the running head of major scientific articles (eg, reports of research) in print and PDF pages. These short titles may also be used on homepages, tables of contents, or social media posts. In the JAMA Network journals, the editorial department or article type (eg, Opinion, Original Investigation, Research, Clinical Review & Education, Letters) may also be included in the running head or foot.

| Maternal BMI, Stillbirth, Fetal and Infant Death | Original Investigation | Research |
| Blood Pressure Control in Chronic Kidney Disease | Original Investigation | Research |
| Medical Therapies for Adult Chronic Sinusitis | Review | Clinical Review & Education |
| Management of Sickle Cell Disease | Special Communication | Clinical Review & Education |

For some smaller types of articles, or if multiple shorter articles by different authors are compiled into a section or a department, the running head includes the article type or department but omits shortened titles:

Letters

Opinion        Perspective

Opinion        A Piece of My Mind

The running heads and feet are typically added during the editing and production process, and authors are not usually required to submit such information (see 21.0, Editing, Proofreading, Tagging, and Display).

**2.4.1** **Name of the Publication.** Use the accepted abbreviation of the journal name (see 13.10, Names of Journals) and the following forms, as applicable to the journal involved.

Note that journals differ in the amount of information included in running heads and running feet and that the style for abbreviations may differ slightly from that used elsewhere in the publication.

**2.4.2** **Short Title of the Article.** The shortened version of the title (ie, short title, running head) should be kept brief but should emphasize the main point of the article, not just repeat the first few words of the title. Different journals have different limits (eg, approximately 70 to 100 characters and spaces in the JAMA Network journals). No punctuation follows the running foot or head.

*Title:*        Proportion of US Adults Potentially Affected by the 2014 Hypertension Guideline

*Short Title:*  US Adults Potentially Affected by New Hypertension Guideline

*Title:*        Validation of the Atherosclerotic Cardiovascular Disease Pooled Cohort Risk Equations

|                |                                                                                                                                                            |
| -------------- | ---------------------------------------------------------------------------------------------------------------------------------------------------------- |
| *Short Title:* | Equations for Risk of Cardiovascular Disease                                                                                                               |
| *Title:*       | Everolimus Plus Endocrine Therapy for Postmenopausal Women With Estrogen Receptor–Positive, Human Epidermal Growth Factor Receptor 2–Negative Advanced Breast Cancer |
| *Short Title:* | Everolimus Plus Endocrine Therapy in Advanced Breast Cancer                                                                                                 |
| *Title:*       | Observational Modeling of Strict vs Conventional Control of Blood Pressure in Patients With Chronic Kidney Disease                                          |
| *Short Title:* | Blood Pressure Control in Chronic Kidney Disease                                                                                                            |

Careful use of abbreviations may help meet space limitations.

|                |                                                                                                           |
| -------------- | --------------------------------------------------------------------------------------------------------- |
| *Title:*       | Effect of Metformin on Left Ventricular Function After Acute Myocardial Infarction in Patients Without Diabetes |
| *Short Title:* | Metformin and LV Function After Acute MI in Patients Without Diabetes                                      |

**2.5** **Abstract.** In this age of electronic data dissemination and retrieval, in which abstracts are indexed and freely available, a well-written abstract is important in directing readers to articles of potential clinical and research interest and also for discoverability via online searching. The abstract of a research report summarizes the main points of an article: (1) the study objective or importance, (2) the study design and methods, (3) the primary results, and (4) the principal conclusions. Some journals may include funding at the end of the abstract or in the Methods section; others, like the JAMA Network journals, include this information in the Acknowledgment section (see 2.10.10, Funding/Support). For scientific studies and systematic reviews, narrative expressions, such as "X is described," "Y is discussed," "Z is also reviewed," do not add meaning and should be avoided. Results should be presented in quantitative fashion, but authors and editors should be scrupulous in verifying the accuracy of all data and numbers reported and ensuring consistency with the results published in the full article.[7]

**2.5.1** **Structured Abstracts.** For reports of original research, systematic reviews, and clinical reviews, structured abstracts (abstracts that use section heads) are recommended. Specific advice taken from *JAMA*'s Instructions for Authors,[8] adapted from Haynes et al,[9] is given here. Note that Design, Setting, and Patients or Other Participants subsections may be combined, depending on the description. If no intervention was performed, that heading may be omitted. Many journals limit the number of words in abstracts; the JAMA Network journals, for example, allow 350 words for reports of original research and for systematic reviews.

**2.5.1.1** **Structured Abstracts for Reports of Original Data (Including Systematic Reviews With Meta-analysis).** In reports of original research, include an abstract of no more than 350 words using the headings suggested below. For brevity, phrases rather than complete sentences may be used. Include the following content in each section:

Importance: Begin the abstract with a sentence or 2 explaining the clinical or research importance of the study question.

**Objective:** State the precise objective or study question addressed in the report (eg, "To determine whether . . . "). If more than 1 objective is addressed, indicate the main objective and state only key secondary objectives. If an a priori hypothesis was tested, state that hypothesis.

**Design:** Describe the basic design of the study (eg, randomized clinical trial, cohort study, cross-sectional study, case-control study, case series, meta-analysis). State the years of the study, the duration of follow-up, and the date of the current analysis if the data are older than 3 years. If applicable, include the name of the study (eg, the Framingham Heart Study). Note: The JAMA Network journals usually combine the following 3 sections as Design, Setting, and Participants during editing for publication. As relevant, indicate whether observers were aware or unaware of patient groups or allocations, particularly for subjective measurements.

**Setting:** Describe the study setting to assist readers in determining the applicability of the report to other circumstances, for example, general community, primary care or referral center, private or institutional practice, or ambulatory or hospitalized care. If the actual name of the institution is relevant, it may be given here.

**Participants:** State the clinical disorders, important eligibility criteria, and key sociodemographic features of patients. Provide the numbers of participants and how they were selected (see below), including the number of otherwise eligible individuals who were approached but declined to participate. If matching was used for comparison groups, specify the characteristics that were matched. In follow-up studies, indicate the proportion of participants who completed the study. In intervention studies, provide the number of patients who withdrew from the study because of adverse effects. For selection procedures, use the following terms, if appropriate: *random sample* (where *random* refers to a formal, randomized selection in which all eligible individuals have a fixed and usually equal chance of selection), *population-based sample, referred sample, consecutive sample, volunteer sample,* or *convenience sample.*

**Intervention(s) or Exposure(s):** Describe the essential features of any interventions or exposures, including their method and duration. Name the intervention or exposure by its most common clinical name, and use nonproprietary names of drugs or medical devices.

**Main Outcome(s) and Measure(s):** Indicate the primary study outcome measurement(s) as planned before data collection began. If the manuscript does not report the main planned outcomes of a study, state this fact and indicate the reason. State clearly whether the hypothesis being tested was formulated during or after data collection. Explain outcomes or measurements unfamiliar to a general medical readership.

**Results:** Report and quantify the main outcomes of the study, including baseline demographic characteristics and final included and analyzed sample. Include absolute numbers and measures of absolute risks (eg, increase, decrease, or absolute differences between groups), along with effect sizes and appropriate measures of uncertainty such as CIs. Use means and SDs for normally distributed data and medians and ranges or interquartile ranges (IQRs) for data that are not normally distributed. Avoid solely reporting the results of statistical hypothesis testing, such as $P$ values, which fail to convey important quantitative information. For most studies, $P$ values should follow the reporting of comparisons of absolute numbers or rates and measures of uncertainty (eg, 0.8%, 95% CI −0.2% to 1.8%; $P=.13$). $P$ values should never be presented alone without the data that are being compared. Approaches such as number needed to treat to achieve a unit of benefit may be mentioned when appropriate. Measures of relative risk (eg, relative risk, hazard ratios) may also be reported and should include CIs. Studies of screening and diagnostic tests should report sensitivity, specificity, and likelihood ratio. If predictive value or accuracy is reported, prevalence or pretest likelihood should be given as well. All randomized clinical trials should include the results of intention-to-treat analysis and adverse effects. All surveys should include response rates.

**Conclusions and Relevance:** Provide only conclusions of the study that are directly supported by the results. Give equal emphasis to positive and negative findings of equal scientific merit. In addition, provide a statement of clinical relevance, indicating implications for clinical practice or health policy and avoiding speculation and overgeneralization. The relevance statement may also indicate whether additional study is required before the information should be used in clinical settings.

**Trial Registration:** For clinical trials, provide the name of the trial registry, the registration number, and the URL of the registry.

**2.5.1.2** **Structured Abstracts for Meta-analysis** Manuscripts reporting the results of meta-analyses should include an abstract of no more than 350 words using the headings listed below. The text of the manuscript should also include a section describing the methods used for data sources, study selection, data extraction, and data synthesis. Each heading should be followed by a brief description:

**Importance:** Begin the abstract with a sentence or 2 explaining the importance of the systematic review question that is used to justify the meta-analysis.

**Objective:** State the precise primary objective of the meta-analysis. Indicate whether the systematic review for the meta-analysis emphasizes factors such as cause, diagnosis, prognosis, therapy, or prevention and include information about the specific population, intervention, exposure, and tests or outcomes that are being analyzed.

**Data Sources:** Succinctly summarize data sources, including years searched. The search should include the most current information possible, ideally with the search being conducted within several months before the date of manuscript submission. Potential sources include computerized databases and published indexes, registries, meeting abstracts, conference proceedings, references identified from bibliographies of pertinent articles and books, experts or research institutions active in the field, and companies or manufacturers of tests or agents being reviewed. If a bibliographic database is used, state the exact indexing terms used for article retrieval, including any constraints (eg. English language or human study participants). If abstract space does not permit this level of detail, summarize sources in the abstract including databases and years searched, and place the remainder of the information in the Methods section.

**Study Selection:** Describe inclusion and exclusion criteria used to select studies for detailed review from among studies identified as relevant to the topic. Details of selection should include particular populations, interventions, outcomes, or methodological designs. The method used to apply these criteria should be specified (eg. blinded review, consensus, multiple reviewers). State the proportion of initially identified studies that met selection criteria.

**Data Extraction and Synthesis:** Describe guidelines (eg, PRISMA, MOOSE) used for abstracting data and assessing data quality and validity (such as criteria for causal inference and whether data were pooled using a fixed-effect or random-effects model). The method by which the guidelines were applied should be stated (eg. independent extraction by multiple observers).

**Main Outcome(s) and Measure(s):** Indicate the primary study outcome(s) and measurement(s) as planned before data collection began. If the manuscript does not report the main planned outcomes of a study, this fact should be stated and the reason indicated. State clearly if the hypothesis being tested was formulated during or after data collection. Explain outcomes or measurement unfamiliar to a general medical readership.

**Results:** Provide the number of studies and patients/participants in the analysis and state the main quantitative results of the review. When possible, present numerical results (eg, absolute numbers and/or rates) with appropriate indicators of uncertainty, such as CIs. Use means and SDs for normally distributed data and medians and ranges or interquartile ranges (IQRs) for data that are not normally distributed. Avoid solely reporting the results of statistical hypothesis testing, such as $P$ values, which fail to convey important quantitative information. For most studies, $P$ values should follow the reporting of comparisons of absolute numbers or rates and measures of uncertainty (eg, 0.8%, 95% CI −0.2% to 1.8%; $P = .13$). $P$ values should never be presented alone without the data that are being compared. Meta-analyses should state the major outcomes that were pooled and include odds ratios or effect sizes and, if possible, sensitivity analyses. Evaluations of screening and diagnostic tests should include sensitivity, specificity, likelihood ratios, receiver operating characteristic curves, and predictive values. Assessments of prognosis should summarize survival characteristics and related variables. Major identified sources of variation between studies should be stated, including differences in treatment protocols, co-interventions, confounders, outcome measures, length of follow-up, and dropout rates.

**Conclusions and Relevance:** The conclusions and their applications (clinical or otherwise) should be clearly stated, limiting interpretation to the domain of the review.

**2.5.1.3** **Structured Abstracts for Systematic Reviews (Without Meta-analysis).** In manuscripts that are critical assessments of the literature and data sources pertaining to clinical topics, include an abstract of no more than 350 words, using the headings (which are included in the word count) suggested below. In the text of the manuscript, include a section describing the methods used for searching for data sources, study selection, data extraction, and data synthesis. Follow each heading with a brief description.

> **Importance:** Include 1 or 2 sentences describing the clinical question or issue and its importance in clinical practice or public health.

> **Objective:** State the precise primary objective of the review. Indicate whether the review emphasizes factors such as cause, diagnosis, prognosis, therapy, or prevention and include information about the specific population, intervention, exposure, and tests or outcomes that are being reviewed.

> **Evidence Review:** Describe the information sources used, including the search strategies, years searched, and other sources of material, such as subsequent reference searches of retrieved articles. Methods used for inclusion and exclusion of identified articles and for assessment of quality of included articles should be explained.

> **Findings:** Include a brief summary of the number of articles included, numbers of various types of studies (eg, clinical trials, cohort studies), and numbers of patients or participants represented by these studies. Summarize the major findings of the review of the clinical issue or topic in an evidence-based, objective, and balanced fashion, with the highest-quality evidence available receiving the greatest emphasis. Provide quantitative data.

> **Conclusions and Relevance:** The conclusions should clearly answer the questions posed if applicable, should be based on available evidence, and should emphasize how clinicians might apply current knowledge. Conclusions should be based only on results described in the abstract Findings subsection.

**2.5.1.4** **Structured Abstracts for Narrative Reviews.** Narrative Reviews on clinical topics provide an up-to-date review for clinicians on a topic of general common interest from the perspective of internationally recognized experts in these disciplines. Include an abstract of no more than 300 words using the headings listed below.

> **Importance:** An overview of the topic and discussion of the main objective or reason for this review.

> **Observations:** The principal observations and findings of the review.

> **Conclusions and Relevance:** The conclusions of the review that are supported by the information, along with clinical applications. How the findings are clinically relevant should be specifically stated.

**2.5.2** **Unstructured Abstracts.** For other major manuscripts, include an unstructured abstract (a paragraph without headings) of no more than 200 words that summarizes the objective, main points, and conclusions of the article. Abstracts are not required for opinion pieces, letters, and special features, such as news articles, although many journals include short 1-sentence précis summarizing these articles. Consult the journal's instructions for authors for special requirements in individual publications.

**2.5.3** **Tables and/or Figures in Abstracts.** Ways to make the structured abstract even more informative continue to evolve. Among these is the inclusion of a small table in the Results subsection in selected abstracts. This approach debuted in the February 6, 2013, issue of *JAMA*.[10] Other journals have also begun experimenting with inclusion of tables or figures in abstracts (graphical abstracts).[11]

**2.5.4** **Clinical Trial Registration Identifier in Abstracts.** The JAMA Network journals require that for all manuscripts that report the results of clinical trials, the trial must be registered at an appropriate online public registry that is owned by a not-for-profit entity, is publicly accessible, and requires the minimum registration data set as described by the ICMJE.[1] The numerical identifier issued by the trial registry should be listed at the end of the abstract, along with the name and URL of the trial registry. The numerical identifier and the trial registry URL should be checked for accuracy by the manuscript editor. Acceptable trial registries include the Australian New Zealand Clinical Trials Registry (http://www.anzctr.org.au), ClinicalTrials.gov (http://www.clinicaltrials.gov), ISRCTN Registry (http://isrctn. org), Nederlands Trial Register (http://www.trialregister.nl/trialreg/index.asp), University Hospital Medical Information Network Clinical Trials Registry (http:// www.umin.ac.jp/ctr), and others listed at the Clinical Trial Registry Platform of the World Health Organization (http://www.who.int/ictrp/network/primary/en).

**2.5.5** **General Guidelines.** A few specific guidelines to consider in preparing a structured or an unstructured abstract follow. Above all, keep in mind that the abstract is meant to stand alone, independent of the main manuscript.

- Consult the journal's instructions for authors.

- Use the journal's specific headings when preparing a structured abstract.

- Do not begin the abstract by repeating the title.

- Do not cite references or URLs in the body of the abstract.

- Do not cite figures or tables in the abstract (but see also 2.5.3, Tables and/or Figures in Abstracts).

- Present numerical results (eg, absolute numbers and/or rates) with appropriate indicators of uncertainty, such as CIs. Use means and SDs for normally distributed data and medians and ranges or interquartile ranges (IQRs) for data that are not normally distributed. Avoid solely reporting the results of statistical hypothesis testing, such as $P$ values, which fail to convey important quantitative information. For most studies, $P$ values should follow the reporting of comparisons of absolute numbers or rates and measures of uncertainty (eg, 0.8%, 95% CI −0.2% to 1.8%; $P=.13$). $P$ values should never be presented alone without the data that are being compared (see 19.1, The Manuscript: Presenting Study Design, Rationale, and Statistical Analysis).

- Include major terms and describe databases and study groups (related to the subject under discussion) in the abstract because the text of the abstract can be searched in many retrieval systems.

- Include the hypothesis or study question, if applicable.

- Ensure that all concepts and data mentioned in the abstract are also included in the text.

- Include the active moiety of a drug at first mention (see 14.4, Drugs).

- Avoid proprietary names or manufacturers' names unless they are essential to the study (see 14.5, Equipment, Devices, Reagents, and Software).

- Spell out abbreviations at first mention and avoid use of abbreviations unless they appear numerous times (see 13.0, Abbreviations).

- If an isotope is mentioned, spell out the name of the element when first used and provide the isotope number on the line (see 14.9, Isotopes).

- Provide the dates of the study or date ranges for studies and other data included in review articles.

- Verify the numbers provided in the abstract against those provided in the text, tables, and figures to ensure internal consistency.

**2.6**    **Keywords.** Some journals require authors to submit a short list (3-10) of keywords with their manuscript. These descriptors may be provided by the author as the terms the author believes represent the key topics presented in the article, although the keywords supplied by the author are not what PubMed or other bibliometric databases use. Some journals provide a standard taxonomy of terms that authors may select from when submitting their manuscript. These may also be used by some journals to categorize manuscripts and help guide the selection of peer reviewers. Many journals publish keywords, as submitted by authors or as edited by indexers or as tagged semantically (see 22.1, Glossary of Publishing Terms) for journal websites, including them with the articles, in online tables of contents, or both, to aid online search and discovery.

**2.7**    **Epigraphs.** Epigraphs, short quotations set at the beginning of an article, are rarely used in research papers. On occasion, an author will include an epigraph to suggest the theme of the article. In the JAMA Network journals, epigraphs are set in italics, with the signature set in boldface type underneath the quotation. If the work cited appears in the reference list, a superscript reference number should follow the epigraph to indicate the source. Otherwise, the title of the work should be provided.

> *The trouble with having an open mind, of course, is that people will insist on coming along and trying to put things in it.*
> **Terry Pratchett**[1]

> *Close both eyes*
> *to see with the other eye.*
> **Rumi**, *Essential Rumi* by Coleman Barks

**2.8** **Parts of a Manuscript, Headings, Subheadings, and Side Headings.** A consistent pattern of organization and a logical hierarchy for all headings should be used for original research articles (see 19.1, The Manuscript: Presenting Study Design, Rationale, and Statistical Analysis). Many research articles follow the IMRAD pattern (Introduction, Methods, Results, and Discussion). However, not all articles will conform to a single pattern format, and section headings vary with the type of article (see 21.0, Editing, Proofreading, Tagging, and Display).

**Introduction:** The introduction should provide the context for the article and state the objective of the study, the hypothesis or research question (purpose statement), how and why the hypothesis was developed, and why it is important. It should demonstrate to the expert that the authors know the subject and should fill in gaps for the novice. It should generally not exceed 2 or 3 paragraphs or 150 words.

**Methods:** The Methods section should include, as appropriate, a detailed description of the following features of the study:

1. study design or type of analysis

2. dates and period of study and follow-up and dates of subsequent analysis for older data (eg, older than 3 years)

3. institutional review board or ethics committee review and approval or waiver or exemption and informed consent (see 5.8, Protecting Research Participants' and Patients' Rights in Scientific Publication)

4. condition, factors, or disease studied

5. details of sample (eg, study participants and the setting from which they were drawn, inclusion and exclusion criteria)

6. intervention(s) or exposure(s), if any

7. primary outcomes and measures or observations, followed by secondary outcomes and measures

8. statistical analysis (for complicated statistical analyses, explain them for the average reader or provide a reference)

9. for all RCTs, a detailed power statement addressing the number of patients in each group needed to obtain a prespecified outcome

10. for reviews, exact search strategy, date run, and the name of the database or retrieval system used

Enough information should be provided to enable an informed reader to replicate the study. If a related methods article has already been published, that article should be cited and its important points summarized.

**Results:** The results reported in the manuscript should be specific and relevant to the research hypothesis or study question. The numbers and characteristics of the study participants should be described or summarized and followed by presentation of the results, which should list prespecified primary outcomes, followed by secondary and other outcomes. The Results section should not discuss implications or weaknesses of the study but should name any validation measures conducted as part of the study. Similarly, the Results section should not include or introduce additional description of methods; all methods should have been described thoroughly in the Methods section. The Results section should not discuss the rationale for the statistical procedures used. All primary outcomes/findings should be reported in the text and/or tables and not only represented graphically in figures. Otherwise, data shown in tables and figures usually should not be duplicated in the text unless the selected data are crucial for the reader (see 4.0, Tables, Figures, and Multimedia). It is important that absolute numbers for primary/main outcomes be presented in the text or in tables (and in the abstract) because figures generally show relative values, not absolute values.

**Discussion:** The Discussion section should be a formal consideration and critical examination of the study (ie, a discussion of the results in relation to the literature). The research question or hypothesis should be addressed in this section, and the results should be compared with the findings of other studies. Note: A lengthy reiteration of the results should be avoided. The study's limitations and the generalizability of the results should be discussed and unexpected findings with suggested explanations mentioned. If appropriate, the type of future studies needed should be mentioned.

**Conclusions and Relevance:** The article should end with a clear, concise conclusion that does not go beyond the findings of the study and a statement of relevance of the findings.

**2.8.1** **Levels of Headings.** A consistent style or typeface should be used for each level of heading throughout a manuscript so that the reader may visually distinguish between primary and secondary headings.

The styles used for the various levels of headings will vary from publisher to publisher, from publication to publication, and in print and online versions, even within the same publishing house. They may also vary within a single publication, from one category of article to another (see 21.0, Editing, Proofreading, Tagging, and Display). To prevent confusion, headings should be used, formatted, tagged, and displayed consistently.

Headings are often used as navigational links for online articles. Consideration should be given to their appropriateness for online use (eg, avoid long headings and avoid citing images and references within headings).

**2.8.2** **Number of Headings.** There is no requisite number of headings. However, because headings are meant to divide a primary part into secondary parts, and so on, there should usually be a minimum of 2. Exceptions may be made in specific cases, such as the inclusion of a single subheading, such as Limitations or Conclusions, under the main heading Discussion.

Headings reflect the progression of logic or the flow of thought in an article and thereby guide the reader. Headings also help break up the copy, making the article more approachable. Headings may be used even in articles such as editorials and reviews, which usually do not follow the organization described above for research articles. (Other typographic and design elements, such as pullout quotations, bullets [•], enumerations, tabulations, figures, and tables, may also be used to break up copy and reflect the progression of logic in the manuscript [see 21.0, Editing, Proofreading, Tagging, and Display].)

**2.8.3** **Some Cautions About Headings.**

- Use a single abbreviation as a heading judiciously. If the abbreviation has been introduced earlier, it may be used as a heading. Avoid use of an abbreviation as a heading if it might be misread as a word (eg, AHA) (see 13.11, Clinical, Technical, and Other Common Terms).

- Do not introduce abbreviations for the first time in a heading. Spell the term out in the heading if that is its first appearance and introduce the abbreviation, if appropriate, at the next appearance of the term (see also 13.11, Clinical, Technical, and Other Common Terms).

- Do not cite figures or tables in headings. Cite them in the appropriate place in the text that follows the heading.

- Do not cite references in headings.

**2.9** **Addenda.** Addenda may be material added to an article late in the publication process or material that is considered supplementary to the article. Note: An addendum is distinct from formal supplementary online material, although addenda may sometimes be presented as supplementary online material. For that, see 2.12, Online-Only (Supplementary) Material. For example, in the JAMA Network journals, if material is added late in the publication process, well after a manuscript has been accepted for publication (eg, extended follow-up, data or information on recent legislation or other relevant event, or additional studies that bear on the present article), it is best incorporated in the text as the final paragraph or paragraphs.

> Addendum: On January 24, a state district judge ordered John Peter Smith Hospital to grant Mr Muñoz's wishes and take Ms Muñoz off life support. Life support has since been removed.

The paragraph may be set off by extra space, hairline centered rule, or both, if desired. Any references cited for the first time in this addendum or final paragraph should follow the numbering of the existing reference list.

Note: If substantial material (eg, new figures, new tables, several additional cases) is added after acceptance of the manuscript or the conclusions change after acceptance, the editor must approve all such changes; additional peer review may be required.

**2.10** **Acknowledgments (Article Information).** *Acknowledgments* is the blanket term used to cover the information that follows the body of the article and precedes the references and is also known as Article Information. For authors preparing manuscripts for submission, the Acknowledgment section may include information about the authors that is not included on the title page(s) (eg, author contributions and conflict of interest disclosures), information about the manuscript (eg, funding and role of sponsor), acknowledgment of nonauthor collaborators or other contributors, and any previous presentation of the material. The Acknowledgment section is considered a continuation of the text, so that abbreviations introduced in the text may stand without expansion here.

For purposes of publication, if a footnote that would normally appear on the first page of the print or PDF version of an article (eg, the affiliation footnote) is too long to be placed on the first page, it may be placed here immediately after the acceptance date and, if applicable, the online publication information; if the journal does not publish acceptance dates, the affiliation footnote that did not fit on the first page would be placed first in the Acknowledgment section. Online, Acknowledgment sections are typically placed at the end of the article. The JAMA Network journals publish Acknowledgments as Article Information (see 2.3.1, Order of Footnotes for Print or PDF Page, where some additional types of acknowledgment footnotes are discussed [placement of such footnotes may vary among journals]). Examples of various parts of the Acknowledgment section (also called Article Information) follow, as used by the JAMA Network journals (see 5.2.3, Author Contributions, Box 5.2-1. Hypothetical Example of an Acknowledgment or Article Information Section, Including Order of All Possible Elements, for a list of the order of all possible elements that may appear in the Acknowledgments section).

**2.10.1** **Manuscript History: Submission and Acceptance Dates.** Some journals include the date of the manuscript's acceptance; others include the date of manuscript submission, the date the revision was received, and the date the manuscript was accepted. This is done in the interest of transparency and may be more important in the basic sciences. Examples are shown below:

> **Submitted for Publication:** December 2, 2018; accepted February 11, 2019.

> **Accepted for Publication:** September 15, 2018.

**2.10.2** **Publication Online First or Online Only.** If an article was published online first or online only, the date it was published online, along with the DOI, a unique character string that identifies an object on a digital network, should follow the acceptance date footnote (or, if the journal does not publish the acceptance date, it should be placed first).

> **Published Online:** March 4, 2019. doi:10.1001/jamapediatrics.2019.0025

> **Published Online:** March 7, 2019. doi:10.1001/jama.2019.1608

**2.10.3** **Information on Open Access.** If an article is published under an open access license, that information can be displayed as follows:

> **Open Access:** This is an open access article distributed under the terms of the CC-BY License. ©2018 Sestak I et al. *JAMA Oncology.*

**2.10.4** **Corrections.** If an article has been corrected since publication, this is noted formally in the Acknowledgment section and includes the date the error was fixed and a description of the error. Note: These notes do not replace the need for a published erratum (see 5.11.10, Corrections [Errata]).

> Correction: This article was corrected on May 20, 2014, to fix a typographical error in the abstract and on July 3, 2014, to fix a numerical error in the Secondary Outcomes subsection in the Results section.

> Correction: This article was corrected on February 28, 2019, to correct an omission of 2 reference citations and to add discussion of these related studies to the article introduction.

> Correction This article was corrected on January 13, 2019, to fix a numerical error in the first column of Table 2.

**2.10.5** **Author Affiliation Notes.** On the journal's website, author affiliation notes or a link to the notes may appear just below the author names. Limited space on the first page of a print or PDF version of an article may sometimes preclude setting the author affiliation footnote on the first page. If the author affiliation footnote does not fit there, it should appear at the end of the article, after the acceptance date and the online-first or online-only information, if applicable.

**2.10.6** **Group Information.** The place in the manuscript where the members of the group are listed should be provided.

> Group Information: The Eunice Kennedy Shriver National Institute of Child Health and Human Development Neonatal Research Network members are listed at the end of the article.

**2.10.7** **Corresponding Author Contact Information.** Contact information for the corresponding author (street address, if possible, with zip or postal code, and email address) is provided in a footnote. Even if there is only a single author, the full name of the person should be included. Follow the custom of individual countries regarding the placement of the zip or postal code. Note: For the JAMA Network journals, this information is provided on the first page of the print or PDF version of the article and at the beginning of Article Information of the online version.

> Corresponding Author: John H. Alexander, MD, MS, Box 3300, Duke University Medical Center, Durham, NC 27715 (john.h.alexander@duke.edu).

> Corresponding Author: Patrick J. Gullane, MB, University Health Network, University of Toronto, 200 Elizabeth St, Ste 8N-800, Toronto, ON M5G 2C4, Canada (patrick.gullane@uhn.on.ca).

> Corresponding Author: Christoph Kniestedt, MD, Department of Ophthalmology, Cantonal Hospital Winterthur, Brauerstrasse 15, 8400 Winterthur, Switzerland (research@kniestedt.ch).

> Corresponding Author: Tomoyuki Kawada, MD, PhD, Department of Hygiene and Public Health, Nippon Medical School, 1-1-5 Sendagi, Bunkyo-Ku, Tokyo 113-8602, Japan (kawada@nms.ac.jp).

Corresponding Author: N. J. Hall, MD, Department of Pediatric Surgery, Institute of Child Health, 30 Guilford St, London WC1N 1EH, England (n.hall@ich.ucl.ac.uk).

Corresponding Author: Jacqueline C. M. Witteman, PhD, Department of Epidemiology and Biostatistics, Erasmus Medical Center, PO Box 1738, 3000 DR Rotterdam, the Netherlands (j.witteman@erasmusmc.nl).

Although traditionally only a single author has been allowed to be designated as corresponding author, the JAMA Network journals now allow a maximum of 2 corresponding authors on a published article—with justification—provided that only 1 person be responsible for all communications during and after publication. This person will be listed first.[12]

*For authors from the same institution*:

Corresponding Authors: Jie Qiao, MD, PhD (jie.qiao@263.net), and Tianpei Hong, MD, PhD (tpho66@bjmu.edu.cn), Peking University Third Hospital, 49 N Garden Rd, Haidian District, Beijing 100191, China.

*For authors from the same institution but different departments*:

Corresponding Authors: Jie Qiao, MD, PhD, Center of Reproductive Medicine (jie.qiao@263.net), and Tianpei Hong, MD, PhD, Department of Endocrinology and Metabolism (tpho66@bjmu.edu.cn), Peking University Third Hospital, 49 N Garden Rd, Haidian District, Beijing 100191, China.

*For authors from different institutions*:

Corresponding Authors: Linhong Wang, PhD, National Center for Chronic Noncommunicable Diseases Control and Prevention, Chinese Center for Disease Control and Prevention, Beijing 100050, China (linhong@chinawch.org.cn); Yonghua Hu, MD, Department of Epidemiology and Biostatistics, School of Public Health, Peking University, Beijing 100191, China (yhhu@bjmu.edu.cn).

In the print or PDF version, for smaller items with signature blocks rather than bylines (eg, letters to the editor, book reviews), the signature block shows the authors' complete names and degrees only. In notes that follow the signature block, the Author Affiliation note indicates the authors' affiliations and the Corresponding Author note provides the complete name and address (including email address) of the corresponding author.

*Signature block*:

John C. Newman, MD, PhD
Michael A. Steinman, MD

Author Affiliations: Division of Geriatrics, University of California, San Francisco.

Corresponding Author: John C. Newman, MD, PhD, Division of Geriatrics, University of California, San Francisco, 4150 Clement St, Ste 181G, San Francisco, CA 94121 (newman@ucsf.edu).

*Print or PDF Version*

*Signature block:*

Sarah E. Sasor, MD
Naveed N. Nostrati, MD
Terrence Katona, DO
William A. Wooden, MD
Adam Cohen, MD
Imtiaz A. Munshi, MD
Sunil S. Tholpady, MD, PhD

**Author Affiliations:** Division of Plastic Surgery, Department of Surgery, Indiana University, Indianapolis (Sasor, Nostrati, Wooden, Tholpady); Richard L. Roudebush VA Medicine Center, Indianapolis, Indiana (Katona, Wooden, Cohen, Munshi, Tholpady).

**Corresponding Author:** Sunil S. Tholpady, MD, PhD, Division of Plastic Surgery, Department of Surgery, Indiana University, 705 Riley Hospital Dr, RI2514, Indianapolis, IN 46202 (stholpad@iupui.edu).

*Online Version*

*Signature Block (Byline):* Sarah E. Sasor, MD[1]; Naveed N. Nostrati, MD[1]; Terrence Katona, DO[2]; William A. Wooden, MD[1,2]; Adam Cohen, MD[2]; Imtiaz A. Munshi, MD[2]; Sunil S. Tholpady, MD, PhD[1,2]

*Links to Affiliations*

[1]Division of Plastic Surgery, Department of Surgery, Indiana University, Indianapolis

[2]Richard L. Roudebush VA Medical Center, Indianapolis, Indiana

There is no need to set the email address in italics or to precede it by the word *email*. Do not add a hyphen to the address to indicate a line break.

**2.10.8** **Author Contributions.** Editors may ask authors to describe what each author contributed to the work, and the list of contributions may be published at the editor's discretion. This is done in all JAMA Network journals (see 5.1.1, Authorship: Definition, Criteria, Contributions, and Requirements). The JAMA Network journals require authors of manuscripts reporting original research and reviews to provide an "access to data" statement (see 5.1.1, Authorship: Definition, Criteria, Contributions, and Requirements). If such a statement is provided, it is given under the head Author Contributions, before the other contributions.

> **Author Contributions:** Drs Hartnick and Raol had full access to all the data in the study and take responsibility for the integrity of the data and the accuracy of the data analysis.

*Concept and design:* De Guzman, Ballif, Hartnick.

*Acquisition, analysis, or interpretation of data:* All authors.

*Drafting of the manuscript:* De Guzman, Hartnick, Raol.

*Critical revision of the manuscript for important intellectual content:* De Guzman, Ballif, Hartnick, Raol.

*Statistical analysis:* Maurer, Hartnick, Raol.

*Administrative, technical, or material support:* De Guzman, Ballif, Hartnick, Raol.

*Supervision:* Hartnick.

**2.10.9** **Conflict of Interest Disclosures.** Authors are expected to provide detailed information about "financial interests, activities, relationships, and affiliations (other than those affiliations listed in the title page of the manuscript), employment, affiliation, funding and grants received or pending, consultancies, honoraria or payment, speakers' bureaus, stock ownership or options, expert testimony, royalties, donation of medical equipment, or patents planned, pending, or issued."[8] Following the guidelines of the ICMJE,[1] the definitions and terms of such disclosures include the following:

- any potential conflicts of interest "involving the work under consideration for publication" (during the time involving the work, from initial conception and planning to present)

- any "relevant financial activities outside the submitted work" (during the 3 years before submission)

- any "other relationships or activities that readers could perceive to have influenced, or that give the appearance of potentially influencing" what is written in the submitted work (based on all relationships that were present during the 3 years before submission)

See also 5.5, Conflicts of Interest.

Authors are expected to provide detailed information about any potential competing interests or conflicts, particularly those present at the time the research was conducted and up to the time of publication, as well as other financial interests, such as relevant filed or pending patents or patent applications in preparation, that represent potential future financial gain. Although many universities and other institutions and organizations have established policies and thresholds for reporting financial interests and other conflicts of interest, the JAMA Network journals require complete disclosure of all relevant financial relationships and potential financial conflicts of interest, regardless of amount or value. If authors are uncertain about what might constitute a potential conflict of interest, they should err on the side of full disclosure and contact the editorial office if they have questions or concerns. In addition, authors who have no relevant conflicts of interest are asked to provide a statement indicating that they have no conflicts of interest related to the material in the manuscript.

For some journals, conflict of interest disclosure information is for use in the editorial office and is not shared with peer reviewers. Other journals, such as the JAMA Network journals, require authors to include all such disclosures in the Acknowledgment section of the manuscript, which is shown to peer reviewers. For all accepted manuscripts, each author's disclosures of relevant conflicts of interest or declarations of no conflicts of interest should be published. Decisions about whether conflict of interest disclosure information provided by authors should be published, and thereby disclosed to readers, are usually straightforward. Although editors are willing to discuss publication of specific conflict of interest disclosures with authors, the policy of the JAMA Network journals is one of full disclosure of all relevant conflicts of interest.

Policies requiring disclosure of conflicts of interest should apply to all manuscript submissions, including letters to the editor, opinion pieces, informal essays, reviews of books and other media, and online comments.

Below are examples of conflict of interest disclosure statements.

> **Conflict of Interest Disclosures:** Dr Ware reported owning shares in and receiving regular income from an Australian company, Cyclotek Pty Ltd, which sells positron emission tomography radiopharmaceuticals, including fludeoxyglucose. No other disclosures were reported.

> **Conflict of Interest Disclosures:** Dr Morrow reported receiving research grant support administered via Brigham and Women's Hospital from Bayer Healthcare Diagnostics, Beckman Coulter, Biosite, Dade Behring, Merck, and Roche Diagnostics and having received honoraria for educational presentations from Bayer Healthcare Diagnostics, Beckman Coulter, and Dade Behring. Dr de Lemos reported receiving research grants and honoraria and consulting fees for speaking from Biosite and Roche. Dr Blazing reported receiving honoraria from Merck and Pfizer.

> **Conflict of Interest Disclosures:** Dr Chang reported having been a clinical investigator for studies sponsored by Lilly Infinity, Genentech, and Novartis. No other disclosures were reported.

> **Conflict of Interest Disclosures:** Dr Callen reported receiving an honorarium for consulting for GlaxoSmithKline and serving on a safety monitoring committee for Celgene. No other disclosures were reported.

> **Conflict of Interest Disclosure:** Dr Neuzil reported receiving research funding from MedImmune for participation in a multicenter trial of a live attenuated influenza vaccine in 2004-2005.

> **Conflict of Interest Disclosure:** Dr Smith reported serving as an expert witness for plaintiffs in US tobacco litigation.

Note: The conflict of interest disclosure may be a disclosure of no conflicts of interest.

> **Conflict of Interest Disclosures:** None reported.

**2.10.10** **Funding/Support.** Each author should provide detailed information regarding all financial and material support for the research and work, including but not limited to grant support, funding sources, and provision of equipment and supplies. This is outlined in the journals' instructions for authors (see 2.10.10, Manuscript Preparation for Submission and Publication, Acknowledgments, Funding/Support, and 5.5.3, Reporting Funding, Sponsorship, and Other Support).

All financial and material support for the research and work should be clearly and completely identified in the Acknowledgment section. Grant or contract numbers should be included whenever possible. The complete name of the funding institution or agency should be given.

If individual authors were the recipients of funds, their names should be listed parenthetically.

> **Funding/Support:** This study was supported in part by grant CA34988 from the National Cancer Institute, National Institutes of Health, and a teaching and research scholarship from the American College of Physicians (Dr Fischl).

> **Funding/Support:** This study was supported by the Gladstone Institute of Virology and Immunology Center for AIDS Research Evaluation and Allocation Committee, University of California, San Francisco; grant K23EY019071 from the National Institutes of Health, National Eye Institute; and That Man May See, the Littlefield Trust, the Peierls Foundation, and the Doris Duke Charitable Foundation through a grant supporting the Doris Duke International Clinical Research Fellows Program at the University of California, San Francisco. Mr Yen is a Doris Duke International Clinical Research Fellow.

> **Funding/Support:** This study was supported by grants 81170881 and U1201221 from the National Science Foundation of China, grant 2010CB529904 from the national 973 Program, Project 984 of Sun Yat-Sen University, and fundamental research funds of the State Key Laboratory of Ophthalmology (Dr Zhang).

> **Funding/Support:** This study was supported by a 2000 Special Projects Award of the Ambulatory Pediatric Association (Dr Hickson).

> **Funding/Support:** This work was supported by research grant R01 MH45757 from the National Institute of Mental Health (Dr Klein).

> **Funding/Support:** Funding for this study was provided by grant 5 U18 HS011885 from the Agency for Healthcare Research and Quality and through subcontracts with the Utah Department of Health (contract 026429) and the Missouri Department of Health and Senior Services (contract AOC02380132).

> **Funding/Support:** This study was supported by Merck and Co and Bayer Healthcare Diagnostics Division.

> **Funding/Support:** Alefacept was provided to the patients at no cost through a Biogen Idec patient assistance program.

**2.10.11** **Role of the Funders/Sponsors.** The specific role of the funding organization or sponsor in each of the following should be specified: design and conduct of the study; collection, management, analysis, and interpretation of the data; preparation, review, and approval of the manuscript; and decision to submit the manuscript for publication. For articles that do not include original research, "design and conduct of the study and collection, management, analysis, and interpretation of the data" is omitted (see 5.5.4, Reporting the Role of the Sponsor).

> Role of the Funder/Sponsor: The National Institutes of Health had no role in the design and conduct of the study; the collection, management, analysis, or interpretation of the data; the preparation, review, or approval of the manuscript; and the decision to submit the manuscript for publication.

> Role of the Funders/Sponsors: Staff from Merck assisted in monitoring the progress and conduct of the A to Z trial. Bayer Healthcare provided reagents for B-type natriuretic peptide testing. The sponsors were not involved in the biomarker testing, analysis, or interpretation of the data or in preparation of the manuscript for this substudy. Medical specialists employed by the sponsors reviewed the manuscript before submission.

**2.10.12** **Group Information (Including List of Participants in a Group).** If the study was performed by a group of persons, the names of the participants may be listed in the Acknowledgment section (see 2.3.3, Author Affiliations). It is important to separately identify and tag members of the group who are authors, members of the group who are nonauthor collaborators, and other members of the group (see 5.2.2, Group and Collaborative Author Lists).

**2.10.13** **Disclaimer.** A note of disclaimer is used to separate the views of the authors from those of employers, funding agencies, organizations, or others. Editors should generally retain the author's phrasing, especially if such phrasing is required by the policy of the entity mentioned.

> Disclaimer: The views expressed here are those of the authors and do not necessarily reflect the position or policy of the US Department of Veterans Affairs or the US government.

> Disclaimer: The opinions expressed herein are only those of the authors. They do not represent the official views of the government of India, St Michael's Hospital, the University of Toronto, or the study sponsors.

> Disclaimer: Use of trade names or names of commercial sources is for information only and does not imply endorsement by the US Public Health Service or the US Department of Health and Human Services.

> Disclaimer: Opinions in this article should not be interpreted as the official position of the International Committee of the Red Cross.

> Disclaimer: The opinions expressed herein are those of the authors and do not necessarily reflect the views of the Indian Health Service.

If the byline of a research manuscript includes an editor of the journal, the following type of disclaimer is useful.

> **Disclaimer:** Dr Bressler is the editor of *JAMA Ophthalmology*. He was not involved in the editorial evaluation of or decision to accept this article for publication.

**2.10.14** **Meeting Presentation.** The following formats are used for material that has been read or exhibited at a professional meeting. The original spelling and capitalization of the meeting name should be retained. Provide the exact date and location of the meeting (see 5.3, Duplicate Publication and Submission).

> **Meeting Presentation:** This study was presented at the Society of Critical Care Medicine's 48th Critical Care Congress; February 18, 2019; San Diego, California.

> **Meeting Presentation:** This work was presented at the annual meeting of the Association for Research in Vision and Ophthalmology; May 5, 2013; Seattle, Washington; at the annual meeting of the American Society of Retina Specialists; August 25, 2013; Toronto, Canada; and at the 47th Annual Meeting of the Microbiology and Immunology Group; November 15, 2013; New Orleans, Louisiana.

> **Meeting Presentation:** This study was presented at the Annual Heart Rhythm Society Scientific Sessions; May 10, 2018; Boston, Massachusetts.

**2.10.15** **Previous Posting.** For manuscripts and articles that have been previously posted to a preprint server, the following formats may be used. The original spelling and capitalization of the preprint server name should be retained. A URL or DOI link to the posting date may also be included (see 5.6.2, Public Access and Open Access in Scientific Publication).

> **Previous Posting:** This article was posted as a preprint on bioRxiv.org.

> **Previous Posting:** This manuscript was posted as a preprint on bioRxiv.org on November 9, 2018. doi:https://doi.org/10.1101/465013

> **Previous Posting:** This manuscript was posted as a preprint on PeerJPreprints. 2018;6:e26857v4. doi:https://doi.org/10.7287/peerj.preprints.26857v4

**2.10.16** **Data Sharing Statement.** For reports of randomized clinical trials, ICMJE recommends that authors of clinical trials provide a data sharing statement with submitted manuscripts and indicate if data, including individual patient data, a data dictionary that defines each field in the data set, and supporting documentation, will be made available to others; when, where, and how the data will be available; types of analyses that are permitted; and if there will be any restrictions on the use of the data.[13] This follows a previous ICMJE requirement for authors of clinical trials to also include trial protocols with submitted manuscripts and published articles. Data sharing statements may also be submitted for reports of other types of studies, but the ICMJE member journals only require this for reports of clinical trials.

The data sharing statements should address the following items:

**Data** Will the data collected for your study, including individual patient data and a data dictionary defining each field in the data set, be made available to others? Yes or no. (If no, authors may explain why data are not available.)
List all data that will be made available:

- Deidentified participant data

- Participant data with identifiers

- Data dictionary

- Other (please specify)

List where to access these data. Provide complete URL if data will be available in a repository or website, or provide complete email address if request for data must be sent to an individual.

List the beginning date and end date (if applicable) when these data will be available. If the beginning date of data availability will be when the article is published, please indicate "with publication."

- With publication

- At a date different from publication

  • Beginning date

  • End date (if applicable)

**Supporting Documents** If your manuscript is accepted for publication, the journal will publish your trial protocol, including the statistical analysis plan, and any amendments as online supplements. Please list any other supporting documents that you wish to make available (eg, statistical/analytic code, informed consent form).

- Statistical/analytic code

- Informed consent form

- None

- Other (please specify)

List where to access these documents. Provide complete URL if the documents will be available in a repository or website, or provide complete email address if request for documents must be sent to an individual.

List the beginning date and end date (if applicable) when these data will be available. If the beginning date of data availability will be when the article is published, please indicate "with publication."

- With publication

- At a date different from publication

  • Beginning date

  • End date (if applicable)

*Additional Information* Indicate the types of analyses for which the data will be made available (eg, for any purpose or for a specified purpose).

Indicate the mechanism by which the data will be made available (eg, with investigator support, without investigator support, after approval of a proposal, or with a signed data access agreement).

List any additional restrictions on the use of the data or any additional information.

If you would like to offer context for your decision not to make the data available, please enter it below (optional).

*Examples of Data Sharing Statements*

- Example when data are not available

Data

Data available: No

**Explanation for why data are not available:** Data were collected before 2018 and the institutional review board did not approve the sharing of patient data.

- Example when data are available without any restrictions

Data

Data available: Yes

**Data types:** Deidentified participant data and data dictionary

**How to access the data:** Deidentified participant data and data dictionary have been deposited in Xyz Repository (xyzrepository.org/doi:10.1234/xyz.5abc123).

**When available:** With publication.

Supporting Documents

**Document types:** Statistical code and informed consent form

**How to access documents:** Statistical code has been deposited in Xyz Repository (xyzrepository.org/doi:10.1234/xyz.5abc123). Informed consent form included in Supplement 4.

**When available:** With publication.

Additional Information

**Who can access the data:** Anyone

**Types of analyses:** Any purpose

**Mechanism of data availability:** Without investigator support

**Any additional restrictions:** None

- Example when data are available with restrictions

Data

**Data available:** Yes

**Data types:** Deidentified participant data and data dictionary

**How to access the data:** Statistical code and informed consent form available from the corresponding author (authorname@email.edu).

**When available:** At a date different from publication: beginning month, day, year.

**Supporting Documents**

**Document types:** Statistical code and informed consent form

**How to access documents:** Statistical code and informed consent form available from the corresponding author (authorname@email.edu).

**When available:** At a date different from publication: beginning month, day, year.

**Additional Information**

**Who can access the data:** Researchers whose proposed use of the data has been approved

**Types of analyses:** For a specified purpose

**Mechanism of data availability:** With investigator support following a signed data access agreement

**Any additional restrictions:** Credit to the authors of the original study reporting these data required.

**2.10.17**  **Additional Contributions.** Acknowledgment of other contributions and forms of assistance (eg, statistical review, preparation of the report, performance of special tests or research, editorial or writing assistance, or clerical assistance) also should be included. When individuals are named, their given names and highest academic degrees (see 2.2.3, Degrees) are listed, and it is recommended that their specific contributions and affiliations and whether they received compensation beyond their salaries for their assistance also be listed. Locations of the named institutions need not be included. For any individual named as providing additional contributions, the author should obtain written permission from that person indicating the person's authorization to be so named (see 5.2.1, Acknowledging Support, Assistance, and Contributions of Those Who Are Not Authors, and 5.2.9, Permission to Name Individuals).

> **Additional Contributions:** Talman Arad and Smardar Zaidman, PhD, Irving and Cherna Moskowitz Center for Nano and Bio-Nano Imaging, Weizmann Institute of Science, conducted the electron microscopy studies. Ana Tovar, MD,

Institute of Pathology, Beilinson Hospital, assisted with electron microscopy data analysis. There was no financial compensation for these contributions.

**Additional Contributions:** Ellen Maki, PhD, assisted with statistical analysis, Michelle V. Lee, RN, obtained photographic data, and Hanna Fadzeyeva assisted in data collection. Dr Maki and Ms Fadzeyeva received financial compensation for their contributions.

**Additional Contributions:** The Branch Retinal Vein Occlusion Study Group is grateful for the contributions of the many referring ophthalmologists, without whom this study could not have been performed, and to the study patients, whose faithfulness to the study led to conclusions that promise hope for others with branch vein occlusion.

**Additional Contributions:** We thank Phani Darineni, MSc, Bruce Wollison, MSc, Sam Hunter, PhD, and Ryan Abo, PhD, for bioinformatics assistance. They were not compensated for their contributions beyond their established salaries.

**Additional Contributions:** The manuscript was copyedited by Linda J. Kesselring, MS, ELS, technical editor/writer, Department of Emergency Medicine, University of Maryland School of Medicine. She received no compensation beyond her salary for this contribution.

Many journals require authors to disclose any substantial writing and editing assistance and to recognize persons responsible for such assistance. Whether compensation was received for such assistance should be a part of the disclosure. This information should be included in the Acknowledgment section, and permission to be identified should be obtained from all named individuals (see 5.2.1, Acknowledging Support, Assistance, and Contributions of Those Who Are Not Authors). In such cases, institutional affiliations may be included.

**Additional Contributions:** We thank Heather Spielvogle, PhD, and Alexis Coatney, BA, Seattle Children's Research Institute, for their assistance in editing and preparing the final manuscript as paid staff for the study.

**Additional Contributions:** We thank Petra Macaskill, PhD (School of Public Health, Sydney, Australia), for her comments on an early draft of the manuscript and her suggestions for its improvement. Dr Macaskill did not receive any compensation.

**Additional Contributions:** Lucia Taddio, BA, Erwin Darra, and Omar Parvez (all from The Hospital for Sick Children) provided assistance with data collection. Ms Taddio and Mr Darra received compensation from the study sponsor.

**Additional Contributions:** We thank Keijo Leivo, RN (Turku University Hospital; who was compensated for his contribution), and Tuukka Tikka, RN (Helsinki University Hospital; who was compensated for his contribution), for taking care of the logistics in this study. We thank Michael E. Moseley, PhD (Stanford University, Stanford, California; who received no compensation), for his invaluable advice and comments during preparation of the manuscript.

If identifiable patients are included in the article, their permission for publication should be obtained and such permission should be noted as follows (see 5.8.3, Patients' Rights to Privacy and Anonymity and Consent for Identifiable Publication).

> **Additional Contributions:** We thank the patient for granting permission to publish this information.

**2.10.18** **Additional Information (Miscellaneous Acknowledgments).** Occasionally, other types of information may be provided in the Acknowledgment section. However, permission or credit for reproduction of a figure or a table, even if modified, should be given in the figure legend or the table footnote, not in the Acknowledgment section (see 4.0, Tables, Figures, and Multimedia).

> **Additional Information:** This is report 54 in a series on chronic disease in former college students.

> **Additional Information:** This article has been reviewed by the Publications Committee of the Collaborative Study of Depression and has its endorsement.

> **Additional Information:** This article is dedicated to the memory of my mentor, friend, and father, Clifford C. Lardinois Sr, MD.

> **Additional Information:** A complete list of documents surveyed is available on request from the corresponding author.

> **Additional Information:** The original data set is available from the New York State Department of Health, Albany.

> **Additional Information:** The *P sojae* and *P ramorum* whole-genome shotgun projects have been deposited at DDBJ/EMBL/Genbank under the project accession numbers AAQY00000000 and AAQX00000000, respectively.

> **Additional Information:** These documents are also available online (https://www.library.ucsf.edu/archives/tobacco/ ).

> **Additional Information:** Additional studies are available from the UK Cochrane Centre, National Health Service Research and Development Programme, Summertown Pavillion, Middleway, Oxford OX2 7LG, England (ichalmers@cochrane.co.uk).

> **Additional Information:** This article is the first of a 3-part series. The second part will appear next month.

**2.10.19** **Preferred Citation Format.** Some journals may choose to list a preferred citation format for each article to ensure correct citation. Some may do this only for articles for which citation problems or questions are likely to arise (eg, articles with group authors) (see 2.2.1, Authors' Names, and 2.2.4, Multiple Authors, Group Authors). This information may be placed in the Article Information at the end of the print or PDF version of an article or on the article title page on the journal's website. In many cases, this information is readily available online for specific articles or through links to online reference managers.

**2.11** **Appendixes.** Some journals publish appendixes, at least occasionally, for material that might be considered ancillary to the content of the article itself (eg, derivation of a complex formula used in the article, a survey instrument used in a study, statistical modeling details). The JAMA Network journals generally do not use appendixes. If the material is worthy of inclusion because it contains important information, it could be considered for online supplemental content (see 2.12, Online-Only [Supplementary] Material).

Information contained in appendixes becomes part of the article; it is published under the imprimatur of the journal and therefore should undergo editorial evaluation and peer review and should receive the same attention to detail in the editorial and production processes as the main body of the article.

**2.12** **Online-Only (Supplementary) Material.** Publishing online-only content permits inclusion of audio, video, and interactive content. In addition, to conserve use of print pages and editorial resources and yet allow interested readers access to supplementary material (eg, additional tables, figures, or references, derivation of complex equations, appendixes, detailed description of methods, trial protocols, large amounts of relevant but detailed data), some journals may publish online-only material to supplement the content that appears in the main article. Each element included in the online supplemental content should be cited in the text of the main manuscript (eg, eTable in the Supplement) and numbered in order of citation in the text (eg, eTable 1, eTable 2, eFigure 1, eFigure 2, eMethods).[8]

The JAMA Network journals offer authors specific guidance on preparing online-only supplements (text, tables, and figures) as well as audio and video files that may be useful for other journals and all authors. See, for example, the section Online-Only Supplements and Multimedia in the *JAMA* Instructions for Authors at https://jamanetwork.com/journals/jama/pages/instructions-for-authors#SecOnline-OnlySupplementsandMultimedia.

In the JAMA Network journals, this call-out appears on the first page of the print or PDF version of the article (with a link embedded to the online-only content) and in a prominent navigational link in the online version:

⊞ Supplemental content

⊞ Video

and is called out at the appropriate place in the text:

(eFigure 1 in the Supplement)

(Video)

In addition, many journals, including the JAMA Network journals, post copies of protocols and statistical analysis plans for clinical trials as online supplemental material.

The National Information Standards Organization (NISO), together with the National Federation of Advanced Information Services, has described such online supplementary material as "items essential to the understanding of the work" (ie, "integral") or "nonessential [to the work]" (ie, "additional"). NISO counsels that "content that is a critical part of the evidence for the article's conclusions can be lost to future readers if it is indiscriminately grouped with other less crucial materials surrounding the article. Thus, it is important for authors and editors to think carefully about Supplemental Materials."[14] See NISO's *Recommended Practices for Online Supplemental Journal Article Materials* for additional guidance.[14]

NISO recommends that "supplemental materials be described (and cited and linked) at the same level as a table or figure that is contained within the article."[14]

It is the policy of the JAMA Network journals that online supplemental content is published under the imprimatur of the journal and so should undergo editorial evaluation. However, this content may not be edited or formatted and may be posted as submitted by the authors. For example, the JAMA Network journals publish the following disclaimer with supplementary online content:

> This supplementary material has been provided by the authors to give readers additional information about their work.

**2.13** **Ancillary Educational and Promotional Material.** Many journals, in addition to educational and online supplemental content, may publish ancillary promotional materials, such as audio, video, and quizzes. In the JAMA Network journals, for example, these materials are called out on the first page of the print or PDF version of the article with a related link in the online version.

⊞ Animated Summary Video

⊞ Author Video Interview

⊞ CME Quiz at jamanetworkcme.com

**Principal Author:** Cheryl Iverson, MA

ACKNOWLEDGMENT

Thanks to the following for reviewing and providing comments to improve the manuscript: Lou S. Knecht, MLS, formerly with Bibliographic Services Division, National Library of Medicine, Bethesda, Maryland; Trevor Lane, MA, DPhil, Edanz Group, Fukuoka, Japan; Frederick P. Rivara, MD, MPH, *JAMA Network Open* and University of Washington, Seattle; Michael G. Sarr, MD, Mayo Clinic, Rochester, Minnesota; Helene M. Cole, MD, Des Moines, Iowa, formerly with *JAMA*; Diane L. Cannon, formerly with JAMA Network; Miriam Y. Cintron, *JAMA*; and Peter J. Olson, ELS, Sheridan Journal Services, Waterbury, Vermont.

REFERENCES

1. International Committee of Medical Journal Editors (ICMJE). Recommendations for the Conduct, Reporting, Editing, and Publication of Scholarly Work in Medical Journals. Updated December 2018. Accessed March 9, 2019. http://www.icmje.org/recommendations/
2. Sun X-L, Zhou J. English versions of Chinese authors' names in biomedical journals: observations and recommendations. *Sci Editor*. 2002;25(1):3-4.
3. *The Chicago Manual of Style: The Essential Guide for Writers, Editors, and Publishers*. 17th ed. University of Chicago Press; 2017:461-467.
4. ORCID. Accessed March 9, 2019. http://orcid.org
5. ISNI. Accessed May 25, 2017. http://www.isni.org/
6. Butler D. Scientists: your number is up. *Nature*. 2012;485(7400):564. doi:10.1038/485564a

7. Pitkin RM, Branagan MA. Can the accuracy of abstracts be improved by providing specific instructions? a randomized controlled trial. *JAMA*. 1998;280(3):267-269. doi:10.1001/jama.280.3.267

8. *JAMA* Instructions for Authors. Updated July 15, 2019. Accessed September 23, 2019. https://jamanetwork.com/journals/jama/pages/instructions-for-authors

9. Haynes RB, Mulrow CD, Huth EJ, Altman DG, Gardner MJ. More informative abstracts revisited. *Ann Intern Med*. 1990;113(1):69-76. doi:10.7326/0003-4819-113-1-69

10. Bauchner H, Henry R, Golub RM. The restructuring of structured abstracts: adding a table in the Results section. *JAMA*. 2013;309(5):491-492. doi:10.1001/jama.2013.76

11. Graphical abstracts. Accessed May 25, 2017. http://www.elsevier.com/journal-authors/graphical-abstract

12. Fontanarosa P, Bauchner H, Flanagin A. Authorship and team science. *JAMA*. 2017;318(24):2433-2437. doi: 10.1001/jama.2017.19341

13. Taichman DB, Sahni P, Pinborg A, et al. Data sharing statement for clinical trials: a requirement of the International Committee of Medical Journal Editors. *JAMA*. 2017;317(24):2491-2492. doi:10.1001/jama.2017.6514

14. National Information Standards Organization; National Federation of Advanced Information Services. *Recommended Practices for Online Supplemental Journal Article Materials*. January 2013. Accessed June 17, 2019. https://www.niso.org/publications/niso-rp-15-2013-recommended-practices-online-supplemental-journal-article-materials

# 3.0 References

**3.0** ▮▮▮▮ **References.** References serve 3 primary purposes—documentation, acknowledgment, and directing or linking the reader to additional resources. Authors may cite a reference to support their own arguments or lay the foundation for their theses (documentation), to credit the work of other authors (acknowledgment), or to direct the reader to more detail or additional resources (directing or linking).

References are a critical element of a scientific manuscript, and, as such, the reference list demands scrutiny by authors, editors, peer reviewers, manuscript editors, and proofreaders. Authors bear primary responsibility for all reference citations. Editors and peer reviewers should examine manuscript references for completeness, accuracy, and relevance. Manuscript editors and proofreaders are responsible for assessing the completeness of references, ensuring that references are presented in proper style and format, and checking to make sure that any reference links are accurate and functional.

Much has been written about problems with bibliographic inaccuracies[1] (eg, an author's name is misspelled, the journal's name is incorrect, the year of publication or the volume, issue, or page numbers are incorrect). Such errors make it difficult to retrieve the documents cited. An even more serious problem is inappropriate citation, for example,

- a speculative commentary cited in a way that implies proved causality;

- an article's results generalized beyond what the data support;

- a retracted article cited without acknowledging the retraction in the citation;

- an article from a predatory journal cited.

Not only is accuracy critical for the integrity of the individual document, but because authors may sometimes rely on secondary rather than primary sources, an inaccurate citation in a document's reference list may be replicated in subsequent articles whose authors do not consult the primary source. Authors should always consult the primary source and should never cite a reference that they themselves have not read[2] (see 3.11.10, Abstracts Taken From Another Source).

**3.1** ▮▮▮▮ **Reference Style and Recommendations.** For greater uniformity in technical requirements for manuscripts submitted to their journals, the International Committee of Medical Journal Editors (ICMJE) developed in 1978 the Uniform Requirements for Manuscripts Submitted to Biomedical Journals (URMs).[3] (The ICMJE was originally referred to as the Vancouver group because the first meeting was in Vancouver, Canada; thereafter, the term *Vancouver style* was coined for the author-number system of reference citations.) In 2013, the Uniform Requirements was renamed to the ICMJE Recommendations for the Conduct, Reporting, Editing, and Publication of Scholarly Work in Medical Journals (or ICMJE Recommendations).[3]

Suggested formats for bibliographic style have been developed for uniformity by the US National Library of Medicine (NLM) and are available as sample references on the NLM website in the document "Samples of Formatted References for Authors of Journal Articles,"[4] as mentioned in the ICMJE Recommendations. Details for this document, including "fuller citations and explanations," are provided in *Citing Medicine: The NLM Style Guide for Authors, Editors, and Publishers*,[5] which is also published by the NLM and is frequently updated. The recommended style is based on the National Information Standards Organization (NISO) standard for Bibliographic References, ANSI/NISO Z39.29-2005 (R2010),[6] and the NLM has adapted these standards for scientific material in its databases.

These documents[3-6] (see **Box 3.1-1**) are intended to aid authors in the preparation of their manuscripts for publication and are not meant to dictate reference style to journal editors, although many journal editors have modified their reference styles to more or less follow these guidelines.[3] Many journals will accept manuscripts for consideration using these reference styles but will reformat them to their own style before publication. Authors and publishers may use reference management software to help ensure reference accuracy.

The reference style followed by the JAMA Network journals is also based on recommendations described in *Citing Medicine*.[5] The reference style of the JAMA Network journals and that of the ICMJE Recommendations represent modifications of the NLM style but follow the general principles outlined in *Citing Medicine*. Note: *Citing Medicine* follows the NISO Bibliographic References standard, but NLM practice does not always follow the NISO standard in MEDLINE/PubMed citations.[7]

Whatever reference style is followed, consistency throughout the document and throughout the publication (journal, book, website) is critical.

**Box 3.1-1.** Recommendation Documents

| Year released | Last updated | Title | Organization |
|---|---|---|---|
| 2013 | 2019 (annually) | Recommendations for the Conduct, Reporting, Editing, and Publication of Scholarly Work in Medical Journals (updates the URMs) | ICMJE |
| 2007 | 2015 | *Citing Medicine: The NLM Style Guide for Authors, Editors, and Publishers* | NLM |
| 2005 | 2010 | ANSI/NISO Z39.29-2005 (R2010) Bibliographic References | NISO |
| 2003 | 2016 | Samples of Formatted References for Authors of Journal Articles | NLM |
| 1978 | | Uniform Requirements for Manuscripts Submitted to Biomedical Journals (URMs) | ICMJE (the Vancouver group) |

**3.1.1** **Bibliographic Grouping.** Each reference is divided with periods into bibliographic groups (see 3.4, Minimum Acceptable Data for References, for an illustration of these for the principal types of references). The period serves as a field delimiter, making each bibliographic group distinct and establishing a sequence of bibliographic elements in a reference. Bibliographic elements are the items within a bibliographic group. Bibliographic elements may be separated by the following punctuation marks:

- **A comma:** if the items are subelements of a bibliographic element or a set of closely related elements (eg, the authors' names in the reference list)

- **A semicolon:** if the elements in the bibliographic group are different (eg, between the publisher's name and the copyright year) or if there are multiple occurrences of logically related elements within a group; also, before volume identification data

- **A colon:** between the title and the subtitle and after a connective and/or descriptive phrase (eg, "In," "Presented at," "Video supplement to," "Interactive feature for," "Videocast available at," "Retracted in"); also, before page numbers and article IDs or e-locators

**3.2** ████ **Reference List.** Reference to information that is retrievable is appropriately made in the reference list. This information includes but is not limited to articles published in scholarly or mass-circulation print or electronic journals, magazines, or newspapers; books; studies and abstracts presented at professional meetings; theses; films, videos, audio, and other multimedia; package inserts or a manufacturer's documentation; monographs; reports from government agencies or working groups; databases and websites; blogs; legal cases; patents; and news releases.

References should be listed in numerical order at the end of the manuscript (except as specified in 3.3, References Given in Text, and 3.5, Numbering). Two references should not be combined under a single reference number.

References to material not yet accepted for publication or to personal communications (oral, written, or email) are not acceptable as listed references and instead should be included parenthetically in the text (see 3.3, References Given in Text; 3.15, Electronic References; and 3.13.9, Special Materials, Meeting Presentations and Other Unpublished Material). According to the Council of Science Editors, "Many publishers do not permit placing any form of unpublished material in the end references"[8(p639)]; the reason for this is because these references typically are not retrievable.

**3.3** ████ **References Given in Text.** Parenthetical citation in the text of references that meet the criteria for inclusion in a reference list should be restricted to circumstances in which reference lists would not be used, such as news articles. Note that in the text (1) the author(s) may not be named, (2) the title may not be given, (3) the name of the journal is abbreviated only when enclosed in parentheses, and (4) inclusive page numbers are given. Some resources, such as URLs, may be listed in the text when it is the website itself that is referred to rather than content on the site. The examples below are from news stories, which tend to not have formal end-of-article reference lists.

> Davis et al recently reported that an apple a day does not keep the doctor away (*JAMA Intern Med.* 2015;175[5]:777-783. doi:10.1001/jamainternmed.2014.5466).

> The effect of eating an apple a day on number of physician visits was reported in a recent issue of *JAMA Internal Medicine* (2015;175[5]:777-783. doi:10.1001/jamainternmed.2014.5466).

The *JAMA Internal Medicine* article (2015;175[5]:777-783) on the effects of eating an apple a day received widespread publicity (eg, *Time*. March 30, 2015. http://time.com/3763878/apple-pharmacist-doctor-study/).

In July, a second case of *E coli* with the *mcr-1* gene was reported by Castanheira et al in a human patient in New York (*Antimicrob Agents Chemother*. Published online July 11, 2016. doi:10.1128/AAC.01267-16).

**3.4** ■ **Minimum Acceptable Data for References.** To be acceptable, a reference must include certain minimum data. The information varies among source material. Consult the specific section in this chapter devoted to that form for more complete requirements. The summary below represents only a skeleton for quick reference.

*Journal articles*

*Print:*      Author(s). Article title. *Abbreviated Journal Name.* Year;vol(issue No.):inclusive pages. DOI, if provided (see note below)

*Online:*      Authors(s). Article title. *Abbreviated Journal Name.* Publication date. DOI, if provided (see note below)

*Books*

*Print:*      Author(s). *Book Title.* Edition number (if it is the second edition or later). Publisher's name; copyright year.

*Online:*      Author(s). *Book Title.* Edition number (if it is the second edition or later). Publisher's name; copyright year. Accessed [date]. URL (or DOI, if provided; see note below)

*Website*      Author (or, if no author is available, the name of the organization responsible for the site). Title (or, if no title is available, the name of the organization responsible for the site). Name of the website. Published [date]. Updated [date]. Accessed [date]. URL

Enough information to identify and retrieve the material should be provided. More complete data (see 3.11.1, References to Journal Articles, Complete Data; 3.12.1, References to Books, Complete Data; 3.15, Electronic References; and 3.13.9, Special Materials, Meeting Presentations and Other Unpublished Material) should be used when available. Note: A DOI should be included if available and if provided (ie, by the author) or if inserted by XML editing software.

**3.5** ■ **Numbering.** References should be numbered consecutively with arabic numerals in the order in which they are cited in the text.

Unnumbered references, in the form of a resource or reading list, are rarely used in the JAMA Network journals. When they are used, these references appear alphabetically, by the first author's last name, in a list separate from the specifically cited reference list. The difference between this type of bibliography and a reference list is that the reference list is only composed of references to those items cited in the manuscript.

**3.6** **Citation.** Each reference should be cited in the text, figures, tables, or boxes in consecutive numerical order by means of superscript arabic numerals. It is acceptable for a reference to be cited only in a figure, table, or box and not in the text if it is in sequence with references cited in the text. For example, if Table 2 contains reference 13, which does not appear in the text, this is acceptable as long as the last reference cited (for the first time) before the first text citation of Table 2 is reference 12.

Use arabic superscript numerals *outside* periods and commas, *inside* colons and semicolons (see 8.0, Punctuation, and 4.0, Tables, Figures, and Multimedia). When more than 2 references are cited at a given place in the manuscript, use hyphens to join the first and last numbers of a closed series; use commas without space to separate other parts of a multiple citation.

As reported previously,[1,3-8,19]

The derived data were as follows[3,4]:

Avoid placing a superscript reference citation immediately after a number or an abbreviated unit of measure to avoid any confusion between the superscript reference citation and an exponent.

*Avoid:* The 2 largest studies to date included $26^2$ and $18^3$ patients.

*Better:* The 2 largest studies to date included 26 patients[2] and 18 patients.[3]

The 2 largest studies[2,3] to date included 26 and 18 patients, respectively.

*Avoid:* The largest lesion found in the first study was 10 cm.[2]

*Better:* The largest lesion found in the first study[2] was 10 cm.

Authors or editors may wish to reorder references to avoid long reference strings. For example, try to present references in digit spans to encompass a large number of citations.

Note: In tables, if a cell in the table involves citation of a reference number *and* a footnote symbol, give the reference number first, followed by a comma and the footnote symbol (eg, Patient characteristics[3,a]) (see 4.1.4, Table Components).

If the author wishes to cite different page numbers from a single reference source at different places in the text, the page numbers are included in the superscript citation and the source appears only once in the list of references. Note that the superscript may include more than 1 page number, citation of more than 1 reference, or both and that all spaces are closed up.

These patients showed no sign of protective sphincteric adduction.[3(p21),9]

Westman[5(pp3,5),9] reported 8 cases in which vomiting occurred.

In listed references, do not use *ibid* or *op cit*.

**3.7** **Authors.** In reference lists, use the author's surname followed by initials without periods. In listed references, the names of all authors should be given unless there are more than 6, in which case the names of the first 3 authors are used followed by "et al." Note: The guidelines in *Citing Medicine*[5] do not limit the number of authors listed in a MEDLINE/PubMed citation record, but, for space considerations, many journals truncate the list of authors' names in references and online bylines (but often with the ability to expand to view the full list).

Note spacing and punctuation. Do not use *and* between names. Roman numerals and abbreviations for Junior (Jr) and Senior (Sr) follow authors' initials. Note: Although NLM uses "2nd," "3rd," and "4th," the JAMA Network journals prefer II, III, and IV, unless the author prefers arabic numerals.

| | |
|---|---|
| 1 Author | Doe JF. |
| 2 Authors | Doe JF, Roe JP III. |
| 6 Authors | Doe JF, Roe JP III, Coe RT Jr, Loe JT Sr, Poe EA, van Voe AE. |
| >6 Authors | Doe JF, Roe JP III, Coe RT Jr, et al. |
| 1 Author *for* or *and* a group | Doe JF; Laser ROP Study Group. |
| >6 Authors *for* or *and* a group | Doe JF, Roe JP III, Coe RT Jr, et al; Laser ROP Study Group. |
| Group | Laser ROP Study Group. |

When mentioned in the text, only surnames of authors are used. For a 2-author reference, list both surnames; for references with more than 2 authors or authors and a group, include the first author's surname followed by "et al," "and coauthors," or "and colleagues."

Doe[7] reported on the survey.

Doe and Roe[8] reported on the survey.

Doe et al[9] reported on the survey.

Note: Do not use the possessive form *et al's*; rephrase the sentence.

"Doe et al's[9] data support our findings." should be changed to "The data in the study by Doe et al[9] support our findings."

In shorter nonresearch and nonclinical articles (eg, opinion pieces, book reviews, historical features, letters to the editor), the author's first name or honorific may be used at first mention:

We agree with Dr Tayeb that the prevalence of domestic violence is difficult to determine.

In *Growing Up Fast*, Joanna Lipper profiles 6 teenaged mothers living in Pittsfield, Massachusetts, at the turn of the 21st century.

**3.7.1** **Group Authors.** Although the JAMA Network journals and many other journals make a distinction between a group of individuals writing *for* a group and a group of individuals writing *as* a group or *in addition to* (ie, *and*) a group in bylines, this distinction is not retained in the NLM database and is not displayed in MEDLINE/PubMed citation records (see 5.1.9, Authorship Responsibility, Group and Collaborative Authorship). The following examples show this difference in by-line presentation.

Journal website:

## Effects of Group Psychotherapy, Individual Counseling, Methylphenidate, and Placebo in the Treatment of Adult Attention-Deficit/Hyperactivity Disorder
### A Randomized Clinical Trial

Alexandra Philipsen, MD; Thomas Jans, PhD; Erika Graf, PhD; Swantje Matthies, MD; Patricia Borel; Michael Colla, MD; Laura Gentschow; Daina Langner, PhD; Christian Jacob, MD; Silke Groß-Lesch, MD; Esther Sobanski, MD; Barbara Alm, MD; Martina Schumacher-Stien; Michael Roesler, MD; Wolfgang Retz, MD; Petra Retz-Junginger, PhD; Bernhard Kis, MD; Mona Abdel-Hamid, PhD; Viola Heinrich; Michael Huss, MD; Catherine Kornmann; Arne Bürger; Evgeniy Perlov, MD; Gabriele Ihorst, PhD; Michael Schlander, MBA; Mathias Berger, MD; Ludger Tebartz van Elst, MD; for the Comparison of Methylphenidate and Psychotherapy in Adult ADHD Study (COMPAS) Consortium

PubMed citation record:

**Effects of Group Psychotherapy, Individual Counseling, Methylphenidate, and Placebo in the Treatment of Adult Attention-Deficit/Hyperactivity Disorder: A Randomized Clinical Trial.**

Philipsen A[1], Jans T[2], Graf E[3], Matthies S[4], Borel P[4], Colla M[5], Gentschow L[5], Langner D[5], Jacob C[6], Groß-Lesch S[6], Sobanski E[7], Alm B[7], Schumacher-Stien M[7], Roesler M[8], Retz W[9], Retz-Junginger P[8], Kis B[10], Abdel-Hamid M[11], Heinrich V[11], Huss M[12], Kornmann C[12], Bürger A[12], Perlov E[4], Ihorst G[3], Schlander M[13], Berger M[4], Tebartz van Elst L[4]; Comparison of Methylphenidate and Psychotherapy in Adult ADHD Study (COMPAS) Consortium.

⊕ **Collaborators (60)**

Therefore, references should use the individuals named and the group name without *for* or *and*. Note that the group name is preceded by a semi-colon rather than a comma (to show, as noted in 3.1, References, Reference Style and Recommendations, that the information that follows is related to what precedes it but somehow distinct) and that articles (eg, *the)* in the group name are removed.

**3.7.2** **Group Author Names With or Without Individually Named Authors in the Byline.** Reference may be made to material that was authored by a committee or other group or that has no named author (see 5.1.9, Authorship Responsibility, Group and Collaborative Authorship). The following forms are used:

1. Writing Committee for the Diabetic Retinopathy Clinical Research Network. Panretinal photocoagulation vs intravitreous ranibizumab for proliferative diabetic retinopathy. *JAMA*. 2015;314(20):2137-2146. doi:10.1001/jama.2015.15217

2. World Medical Association. World Medical Association Declaration of Helsinki: ethical principles for medical research involving human subjects. *JAMA*. 2013;310(20):2191-2194. doi:10.1001/jama.2013.281053

3. Global Burden of Disease Cancer Collaboration. The global burden of cancer 2013. *JAMA Oncol.* 2015;1(4):505-527. doi:10.1001/jamaoncol.2015.0735

References may also have bylines that contain the names of individuals and the name of a group or several groups (see 5.1.9, Authorship Responsibility, Group and Collaborative Authorship).

4. Guggenheim JA, Williams C; UK Biobank Eye and Vision Consortium. Role of educational exposure in the association between myopia and birth order. *JAMA Ophthalmol.* 2015;133(12):1408-1414. doi:10.1001/jamaophthalmol.2015.3556

5. Taylor Z, Nolan CM, Blumberg HM; American Thoracic Society; Centers for Disease Control and Prevention; Infectious Diseases Society of America. Controlling tuberculosis in the United States: recommendations from the American Thoracic Society, CDC, and the Infectious Diseases Society of America. *MMWR Recomm Rep.* 2005;54(RR-12):1-81.

In examples 4 and 5 above, a semicolon, not a comma, precedes the group name in the author field and no articles (eg, *the*) are included with the group names.

In certain instances, an article may not have an author. In other instances, the author may remain anonymous (see 5.1.9, Authorship Responsibility, Group and Collaborative Authorship). However, the word "Anonymous" should not be used in a reference unless that word was published in the article's byline. Note: There is no need to repeat the word "Anonymous" to represent a first name and a surname.

6. Anonymous. Care can't get better until complaints are heard. *BMJ.* 2012;345:e4511. doi:10.1136/bmj.e4511

7. Incorrect percentages in the abstract. *JAMA Oncol.* 2017;3(12):1742. doi:10.1001/jamaoncol.2017.4368

**3.8 Prefixes and Particles.** Surnames that contain prefixes or particles (eg, von, de, La, van) are spelled and capitalized according to the preference of the persons named.

1. van Gylswyk NO, de la Valle CI.
2. Van Rosevelt RF, Bakker JC, Sinclair DM, Damen J, Van Mourik JA.
3. Al-Faquih SR.
4. Kang S, Kim KJ, Wong TY, et al.

Note: NLM does not retain the hyphen in the representation of initials for first (given) names, whereas hyphens are retained for surnames. When a given name contains a hyphen, such as Ka-Wai Tam, both initials appear, without a hyphen: Tam KW. Also, if the second part of a hyphenated name is lowercased, as in Korean hyphenated given names, the same style is applied: Hyun-seok Kim would appear in the reference as Kim HS.

**3.9 Titles.** In titles of articles, books, parts of books, and other material, retain the spelling, abbreviations, and style for numbers used in the original. Note: Numbers that begin a title are spelled out (although exceptions are made for years; see 2.1.2, Titles and Subtitles, Numbers).

### 3.9.1 English-Language Titles.

**3.9.1.1 Journal Articles and Parts of Books.** In English-language titles, capitalize only (1) the first letter of the first word, (2) proper names, (3) names of clinical trials or study groups (eg, Community health worker home visits for adults with uncontrolled asthma: the HomeBASE Trial randomized clinical trial), and (4) abbreviations that are ordinarily capitalized (eg, DNA, EEG, VDRL). Do not enclose article and book chapter titles in quotation marks. However, if a book, book chapter, or article title contains quotation marks in the original, retain them as double quotation marks (unless both double and single quotation marks are used).

**3.9.1.2 Books, Government Bulletins, Documents, and Pamphlets.** In English-language titles, italicize the titles of books, government bulletins, documents, and pamphlets and capitalize the first letter of each major word. Do not capitalize articles, prepositions of 3 or fewer letters (*as, off, out, per, up, via*), coordinating conjunctions (*and, or, for, nor, but, yet, so*), or the *to* in infinitives (see 2.1.6, Manuscript Preparation for Submission and Publication, Titles and Subtitles, Capitalization, for exceptions). Do capitalize a 2-letter verb, such as *Is* and *Be*.

### 3.9.2 Non–English-Language Titles.

**3.9.2.1 Capitalization.** In non–English-language titles, capitalization does not necessarily follow the same rules as in English-language titles. For example, in German titles (articles and books), all nouns and only nouns are capitalized; typically, in French, Spanish, and Italian book titles, capitalize only the first word, proper names, and abbreviations that are capitalized in English. As with English-language books, government bulletins, documents, and pamphlets, italicize the title.

**3.9.2.2 Translation.** Non–English-language titles may be given as they originally appeared, without translation:

1. Rubbert-Roth A. Differenzialdiagnostik der frühen Polyarthritis. *Dtsch Med Wochenschr*. 2015;140(15):1125-1130. doi:10.1055/s-0041-103627

2. Ray JC, Kusumoto F, Goldschlager N. A case of P-wave mimicry: *cherchez le P. JAMA Intern Med*. Published online August 3, 2015. doi:10.1001/jamainternmed.2015.3342

If non–English-language titles are translated into English, indication of the original language should follow the title:

3. Shimura M. Looking to the future: treatment for retinal vascular disease. Article in Japanese. *Nippon Ganka Gakkai Zasshi*. 2014;118(11):905-906.

If the non–English-language title and the translation are provided, both may be given. In the example below, the article was published in 3 languages, and all translations are provided.

4. Becerra-Posada F, Hennis A, Lutter C. Prevention of childhood obesity through trilateral cooperation. Prevención de la obesidad infantil a través de una cooperación trilateral. Prévention de l'obésité infantile grâce à la coopération trilatérale. *Rev Panam Salud Publica.* 2016;40(2):76-77.

Non–English-language titles should be verified from the original when possible. Consult a dictionary in the appropriate language for accent marks, spelling, and other particulars.

Reference to the primary source is always preferable, but if the non–English-language article is not readily available or not accessible, the translated version is acceptable. The citation should always be to the version consulted.

Such words as *tome* or *Band* (volume), *fascicolo* or *Teil* (part), *Seite* (page), *Auflage* (edition), *Abteilung* (section or part), *Heft* (number), *Beiheft* (supplement), and *Lieferung* (part or number) should be translated into English.

**3.9.3** **Names of Organisms.** In all titles, follow the style recommended for capitalization and use of italics in scientific names of organisms (see 10.3.6, Proper Nouns, Organisms, and 14.14, Organisms and Pathogens). Use roman type for genus and species names in book titles.

1. Gerding DN, Meyer T, Lee C, et al. Administration of spores of nontoxigenic *Clostridium difficile* strain M3 for prevention of recurrent *C difficile* infection: a randomized clinical trial. *JAMA.* 2015;313(17):1719-1727. doi:10.1001/jama.2015.3725

2. Khatri A, Naeger Murphy N, Wiest P, et al. Community-acquired pyelonephritis in pregnancy caused by KPC-producing *Klebsiella pneumoniae. Antimicrob Agents Chemother.* 2015;59(8):4375-4378. doi:10.1128/AAC.00553-15

3. American Academy of Pediatrics. *Clostridium difficile.* In: Kimberlin DW, Brady MT, Jackson MA, Long SS, eds. *Red Book: 2015 Report of the Committee on Infectious Diseases.* American Academy of Pediatrics; 2015:298-301.

4. Mullany P, Roberts AP, eds. Clostridium difficile: *Methods and Protocols.* Humana Press; 2010.

**3.9.4** **Non-English Words and Phrases.** In all titles, follow the guidelines recommended for use of italics or roman in non-English words and phrases (see 12.1.1, Non-English Words, Phrases, and Titles, Use of Italics). For example, even if *In Vivo* or *In Vitro* were set italic in a cited title, the JAMA Network journals would set these in roman type.

**Subtitles.** Style for subtitles follows that for titles (see 3.9, Titles) for spelling, abbreviations, numbers, capitalization, and use of italics, except that for journal articles the subtitle begins with a lowercase letter. A colon and space separate title and subtitle, even if a period was used in the original. Do not change an em dash to a colon. When the title ends with a question mark, the question mark is retained in the reference and replaces the colon as the delimiter. If the subtitle is numbered, as is common when articles in a series have the same title but different—numbered—subtitles, use a comma after the title, followed by a roman numeral immediately preceding the colon. If the title or subtitle ends with a closing quotation mark, the ending period should appear after the quotation mark because the end punctuation is not part of the original content.

1. Musch DC, Janz NK, Leinberger RL, Niziol LM, Gillespie BW. Discussing driving concerns with older patients, II: vision care providers' approaches to assessment. *JAMA Ophthalmol.* 2013;131(2):213-218. doi:10.1001/2013.jamaophthalmol.106

2. Champigneulle B, Merceron S, Lemiale V. What is the outcome of cancer patients admitted to the ICU after cardiac arrest? results from a multicenter study. *Resuscitation.* 2015;92(7):38-44. doi:10.1016/j.resuscitation.2015.04.011

3. Jackson LG. Prenatal diagnosis: Down syndrome or more? *Hum Mutat.* 2017;38(7):749. doi:10.1002/humu.23242

4. Ahn HS, Kim HJ, Welch HG. Korea's thyroid-cancer "epidemic". *N Engl J Med.* 2014;371(19):1765-1767. doi:10.1056/NEJMp1409841

Note: Capitalization is retained if the first word of the subtitle is a proper noun, as shown in example 3 above.

### 3.11 References to Journal Articles.

**3.11.1 Complete Data.** A complete reference to a journal article includes the following:

- Authors' surnames and initials (the names of all authors should be given unless there are more than 6, in which case the names of the first 3 authors are used, followed by "et al")
- Title of article and subtitle, if any
- Abbreviated name of journal (see 13.10, Abbreviations, Names of Journals)
- Year (or online publication date [month and day, year] if article is published online first and has yet to appear in a paginated issue or is published in an online-only journal)
- Volume number
- Issue number
- Part or supplement number, when pertinent
- Location (page[s] or e-locator)
- DOI (if supplied)

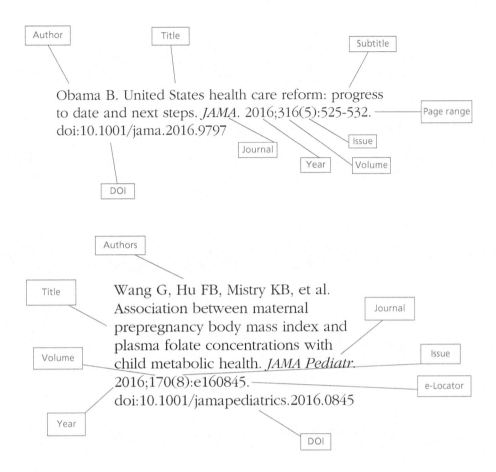

**Names of Journals.** Abbreviate and italicize names of journals. Use initial capital letters. Abbreviate according to the listing in the National Center for Biotechnology Information (NCBI) NLM Catalog database (https://www.ncbi.nlm.nih.gov/nlmcatalog/journals) (see 13.10, Names of Journals). Some publishers may have access to reference managers or other databases that provide guidance, journal title abbreviations, and tools for automated validation. For journals or publishers that do not have such resources, journal names for journals not cited in PubMed may be expanded to avoid possible confusion. Another resource is the NLM Fact Sheet "Construction of the National Library of Medicine Title Abbreviations," which can be found at https://www.nlm.nih.gov/tsd/cataloging/contructitleabbre.html.

Include parenthetical designation of a geographic location if it is included in the PubMed abbreviation, for example, *Intern Med (Tokyo, Japan)*, *Pediatr Nephrol (Berlin, Germany)*. Information enclosed in brackets should be retained without brackets (eg, *J Comp Physiol A* for *J Comp Physiol [A]*).

If the name of a journal has changed since the time the reference was published, use the name of the journal at the time of publication. For example, before January 2013, *JAMA Internal Medicine* was *Archives of Internal Medicine*. If a citation is to an article published in the older-named journal, do not change the journal name to the newer name (eg, *JAMA Intern Med)*; use the former title (eg, *Arch Intern Med)*. When the name has not changed but the abbreviation used by PubMed has changed (eg, *Br Med J* to *BMJ)*, use the abbreviation in use by PubMed at the time the reference was published (eg, *Br Med J* through 1987; *BMJ* from 1988 forward). This policy will ensure that the online links to the citation will work.

**3.11.3 Year, Volume, Issue, Location (Page Numbers), and Dates.** The year, followed by a semicolon; the volume number and the issue number (in parentheses), followed by a colon; the initial page number, a hyphen, and the final page number, followed by a period, are set without spaces. Do not omit digits from inclusive page numbers. The DOI should be included if provided. The DOI should be the final element and is not followed by a period (see 3.15, Electronic References, for more information on DOIs).

1. Quiroz YT, Schultz AP, Chen K, et al. Brain imaging and blood biomarker abnormalities in children with autosomal dominant Alzheimer disease: a cross-sectional study. *JAMA Neurol.* 2015;72(8):912-919. doi:10.1001/jamaneurol.2015.1099

2. Sunderam S, Kissin DM, Crawford SB, et al. Assisted reproductive technology surveillance—United States, 2012. *MMWR Surveill Summ.* 2015;64(suppl 6):1-29.

3. Fanin M, Angelini C. Progress and challenges in diagnosis of dysferlinopathy. *Muscle Nerve.* Published online August 8, 2016. doi:10.1002/mus.25367

**3.11.4 Online Journal Articles, Preprints, and Manuscripts.** A complete reference to a journal article online includes the following:

- Authors' surnames and initials (the names of all authors should be given unless there are more than 6, in which case the names of the first 3 authors are used, followed by "et al")

- Title of article and subtitle, if any

- Abbreviated name of journal (see 13.10, Abbreviations, Names of Journals)

- Year (or online publication date [month, day, year] if article is published online first and has yet to appear in a paginated issue or is published in an online-only journal)

- Location (pagination)

- DOI (if a DOI is not available for an online journal article, a URL and accessed date may be used; do not include a URL and accessed date for articles for which a DOI is available)

- Accessed [date]

- URL (verify that the link still works as close as possible to publication)

If including a URL in a reference citation, use the URL that will take the reader directly to the article; do not include a long search string, and also Better a short, more general URL (eg, one to the publisher's homepage). Always include "http://" or "https://" before the URL to help ensure proper linking; most sites with "http://" have changed to the more secure "https://" and note that URLs do not always require "www." The URL is not followed by a period. Verify that the link still works as close as possible to publication.

> *Avoid:*  using a URL from a search result:
>
> http://www.nature.com/search?journal=mp&q=A%20mega-analysis%20of%20genome-wide%20association%20&q_match=all&sp-a=sp1001702d&sp-m=0&sp-p-1=phrase&sp-sfvl-field=subject%7Cujournal&sp-x-1=ujournal&submit=go
>
> *Better:*  http://www.nature.com/mp/journal/v18/n4/full/mp201221a.html
>
> *Avoid:*  URLs with unnecessary characters after a delimiter (ie, hashtag, question mark, virgule):
>
> http://jama.jamanetwork.com/article.aspx?articleid=2556124#tab12
>
> *Better:*  http://jama.jamanetwork.com/article.aspx?articleid=2556124
>
> https://www.clinicaltrials.gov/ct2/show/NCT02116010?term=phago burn&rank=1
>
> https://www.clinicaltrials.gov/ct2/show/NCT02116010

NISO published The OpenURL Framework for Context-Sensitive Services standard in 2010. OpenURL uses a standardized format to encode descriptions of a website into core components (eg, character encoding, serialization, constraint language, ContextObject format, metadata format, namespace, transport, and community profile). For example, the JAMA Network journals' URLs are organized using an OpenURL format that permits any article to be easily linked to using its DOI:

> https://jamanetwork.com/journals/[journal name]/fullarticle/[DOI]
>
> https://jamanetwork.com/journals/jamaoncology/fullarticle/10.1001/jamaoncol.2016.3662

In reference citations, a DOI is preferable to a URL if one is available; a DOI should be available for most journal articles. No accessed date is required for the DOI because it is a permanent identifier; it is presented as the last item in the reference.

Note: The DOI is provided immediately after "doi:" and is set closed up to it, per convention, and is not followed by a period. For example, in reference 2 below, the DOI would not be presented as http://doi.org/10.1542/peds.2015-2488 because that is a web address and not a DOI. DOIs should not be a part of a web address in reference citations unless the DOI is being used specifically in a URL, as indicated above.

1. van der Kam S, Roll S, Swarthout T, et al. Effect of short-term supplementation with ready-to-use therapeutic food or micronutrients for children after illness for prevention of malnutrition: a randomised controlled trial in Uganda. *PLoS Med*. 2016;13(2):e1001951. doi:10.1371/journal.pmed.1001951

2. Allison MA, Hurley LP, Markowitz L, et al. Primary care physicians' perspectives about HPV vaccine. *Pediatrics*. 2016;137(2):e20152488. doi:10.1542/peds.2015-2488

3. Saeb S, Zhang M, Karr CJ, et al. Mobile phone sensor correlates of depressive symptom severity in daily-life behavior: an exploratory study. *J Med Internet Res*. 2015;17(7):e175. doi:10.2196/jmir.4273

4. Frazer K, Callinan JE, McHugh J, et al. Legislative smoking bans for reducing harms from secondhand smoke exposure, smoking prevalence and tobacco consumption. *Cochrane Database Syst Rev*. 2016;(1):CD005992. doi:10.1002/14651858.CD005992.pub3

5. Metcalfe K, Gershman S, Ghadirian P, et al. Contralateral mastectomy and survival after breast cancer in carriers of BRCA1 and BRCA2 mutations: retrospective analysis. *BMJ*. 2014;348:g226. doi:10.1136/bmj.g226

In the following example, the citation is to supplemental content (ie, not to the article itself) that appears with the online article.

6. Meeker D, Linder JA, Fox CR, et al. Effect of behavioral interventions on inappropriate antibiotic prescribing among primary care practices: a randomized clinical trial. Supplement 1. Study protocol and changes to analysis plan. *JAMA*. 2016;315(6):562-570. Accessed June 18, 2019. https://www.jamanetwork.com/journals/jama/fullarticle/2488307

An article that appears online before print publication may be edited, tagged, composed, and posted as it will appear in print or in a PDF form but before the print publication (with or without print pagination), or an article may be edited, tagged, composed, and published as part of a specific online issue of the journal. Examples are given below:

7. Tamburini S, Shen N, Chih Wu H, Clemente JC. The microbiome in early life: implications for health outcomes. *Nat Med*. Published online July 7, 2016. doi:10.1038/nm4142

In the preceding example, the article has not yet been paginated in an issue (which may be published in print, online, or both), and the DOI serves as the unique identifier for the article. If the article is subsequently published in an issue with page numbers, the following citation can be used:

8. Tamburini S, Shen N, Chih Wu H, Clemente JC. The microbiome in early life: implications for health outcomes. *Nat Med*. 2016;22(7):713-722. doi:10.1038/nm.4142

**3.11.4.1** **Preprints and Publication of Unedited Manuscripts.** Preprints are another online method for publication in which a manuscript is uploaded by authors to a public server, without editing or formatting, and typically without peer review.[9] A preprint may be a predecessor to publication in a peer-reviewed journal; it is "archived" and citable. Preprint servers include arXiv.org, bioRxiv.org, MedRxiv, and many others. Preprints were initially used more often in the physical sciences than in medicine, but they are becoming more common in the biological sciences.[10] Preprints may have DOIs and can follow this citation format:

1. Bloss CS, Wineinger NE, Peters M, et al. A prospective randomized trial examining health care utilization in individuals using multiple

smartphone-enabled biosensors. *bioRxiv*. Preprint posted online October 28, 2015. doi:10.1101/029983

If a preprint is subsequently published in a peer-reviewed journal, the reference citation should include complete data as outlined in this chapter. Note: The version cited should be the version used.

2. Bloss CS, Wineinger NE, Peters M, et al. A prospective randomized trial examining health care utilization in individuals using multiple smartphone-enabled biosensors. *PeerJ*. 2016;4:e1554. doi:10.7717/peerj.1554

Some publishers post early unedited versions of manuscripts before publication of the final version of an article.

3. Collins-McMillen D, Stevenson EV, Heon Kim J, et al. HCMV utilizes a nontraditional STAT1 activation cascade via signaling through EGFR and integrins to efficiently promote the motility, differentiation, and polarization of infected monocytes. *J Virol*. Accepted manuscript. Published online October 11, 2017. doi:10.1128/JVI.00622-17

4. Atkins M, Coutinho AD, Nunna S, Gupte-Singh K, Eaddy M. Confirming the timing of phase-based costing in oncology studies: a case example in advanced melanoma. *J Med Econ*. Accepted manuscript. Published online October 12, 2017. doi:10.1080/13696998.2017.1391818

In the examples below, the authors have published version 1 of their article a week after acceptance in a peer-reviewed journal. The full version of the same article was published in its entirety 4 weeks later. The version of the manuscript that is cited needs to be indicated.

5. Roberts-Galbraith RH, Brubacher JL, Newmark PA. A functional genomics screen in planarians reveals regulators of whole-brain regeneration. *eLife*. Accepted manuscript, version 1. Published online September 9, 2016. doi:10.7554/eLife.17002

6. Roberts-Galbraith RH, Brubacher JL, Newmark PA. A functional genomics screen in planarians reveals regulators of whole-brain regeneration. *eLife*. 2016;5:e17002. doi:10.7554/eLife.17002

**3.11.4.2** **Repositories.** Papers (manuscripts and articles) in online repositories (eg, escholarship.org [University of California]) may be cited as follows.

**3.11.4.2.1** Manuscripts and Articles in an Institutional Repository.

1. Tseng V. Effect of noise reduction methods in the ICU on sleep quality. UC Irvine. June 8, 2016. Accessed August 17, 2016. http://escholarship.org/uc/item/190551hq

2. Vodyanoy V, Pustovyy O, Globa L, Sorokulova I. Evaluation of a new vasculature by high resolution light microscopy: primo vessel and node. Cornell University Library. August 15, 2016. Accessed August 17, 2016. https://arxiv.org/abs/1608.04276v1

**3.11.4.2.2** Data Repository. When citing data from a repository, cite the original source for the data.

> 3. Cutter AD, Gray JC. Data from: Ephemeral ecological speciation and the latitudinal biodiversity gradient. *Dryad Digital Repository.* Deposited August 17, 2016. doi:10.5061/dryad.734v9

The data package or data set should be cited in the original publication to link the publication and the data. Examples of citations to a data package follow:

> 4. Francuzik W. Data from: Skin microbiome in atopic dermatitis: 16S gene sequence data. *figshare.* 2016. doi:10.6084/m9.figshare.4028943
>
> 5. Levy I, Maor Y, Mahroum N, et al. Data from: Missed opportunities for earlier diagnosis of HIV in patients that presented with advanced HIV disease: a retrospective cohort study. *Dryad Digital Repository.* 2016. doi:10.5061/dryad.73c003.11.5

**3.11.5** Discontinuous Pagination. For an article with discontinuous pagination in a single issue, follow the style shown in the examples below:

> 1. Buster KJ, Stevens EI, Elmets CA. Dermatologic health disparities. *Dermatol Clin.* 2012;30(1):53-59, viii. doi:10.1016/j.det.2011.08.002
>
> 2. Baldwin HE. Systemic therapy for rosacea. *Skin Therapy Lett.* 2007;12(2):1-5, 9.

**3.11.6** Journals Without Volume or Issue Numbers. In references to journals that have no volume or issue numbers, use the issue date, as shown in example 1 below. If there is an issue number but no volume number, use the style shown in example 2 below.

> 1. Flyvholm MA, Susitaival P, Meding B, et al. Nordic occupational skin questionnaire—NOSQ-2002: Nordic questionnaire for surveying work-related skin diseases on hands and forearms and relevant exposure. *TemaNord.* April 2002:518.
>
> 2. Johnson CL, Dohrmann SM, Kerckove VD, et al. National Health and Nutrition Examination Survey: National Youth Fitness Survey estimation procedures, 2012. *Vital Health Stat 2.* 2014;(168):1-25.

**3.11.7** Parts of an Issue. If an issue has 2 or more parts, the part cited should be indicated in accordance with the following example:

> 1. MacSweeney M, Cardin V. What is the function of auditory cortex without auditory input? *Brain.* 2015;138(pt 9):2468-2470. doi:10.1093/brain/awv197

**3.11.8** Special Issue or Theme Issue. The JAMA Network journals refer to issues published to commemorate an event or to bring together articles on the same subject as *theme issues*. References to the complete contents of a special or theme issue of a journal should be cited as follows:

1. Zylke JW, ed. Child health. *JAMA*. 2015;313(15, theme issue):1489-1584.

2. 2015 AHNS. *JAMA Otolaryngol Head Neck Surg*. 2015;141(12, theme issue):1039-1148.

Special or theme issues may also be published as supplements (see 3.11.9, References, References to Journal Articles, Supplements, for the recommended style for these).

**3.11.9** **Journal Supplements.** The following example illustrates the basic format for styling references to journal supplements:

1. Johnson EM, Wortman MJ, Lundberg PS, Daniel DC. Orderly steps in progression of jc virus to virulence in the brain. *Brain Disord Ther*. 2015;4(suppl 2):2003. doi:10.4172/2168-975X.S2-003

Often, the supplement is numbered and there is no issue number.

2. Cao Y, Steffey S, He J, et al. Medical image retrieval: a multimodal approach. *Cancer Inform*. 2015;13(suppl 3):125-136. doi:10.4137/CIN.S14053

If the supplement is numbered and there is an issue number, use the form below:

3. Viriyasiripong S. Laparoscopic radical cystoprostatectomy, surgical technique and result: a case report. *J Med Assoc Thai*. 2015;98(11)(suppl 10):S154-S157.

When numbered supplements have several parts, denoted by "pt 1" or by letters, each supplement having independent pagination, use the following form:

4. Kleinman JT, Mlynash M, Zaharchuk G, et al. Yield of CT perfusion for the evaluation of transient ischaemic attack. *Int J Stroke*. 2015;10(suppl A100):25-29. doi:10.1111/j.1747-4949.2012.00941.x

5. Kurowski BG, Pomerantz WJ, Schaiper C, Ho M, Gittelman MA. Impact of preseason concussion education on knowledge, attitudes, and behaviors of high school athletes. *J Trauma Acute Care Surg*. 2015;79(3)(suppl 1):S21-S28. doi:10.1097/TA.0000000000000675

Note: It is common for page numbers in supplements to include letters as well as numbers (eg, S21-S28 in example 5 above). Also, example 4 has no issue number.

Supplemental material published as an entire issue (eg, all the abstracts presented at a meeting) may be cited as follows:

6. Abstracts of the 51st Workshop for Pediatric Research. *Mol Cell Pediatr*. 2015;2(suppl 1):A1-A30. Accessed October 14, 2016. http://www. molcellped.com/supplements/2/S1/all

In the example below, the entire supplement has a DOI.

7. Abstracts of the 50th Congress of the European Society for Surgical Research, June 10-13, 2015, Liverpool, United Kingdom. *Eur Surg Res*. 2015;55(suppl 1):1-167. doi:10.1159/000381839

See 3.13.9.1, References, Special Materials, Meeting Presentations and Other Unpublished Material, Items Presented at a Meeting.

**3.11.10** **Abstracts From Another Source.** Several types of published abstracts may be cited: (1) an abstract of a complete article republished from another publication (perhaps accompanied by a commentary), (2) an abstract of an online-only article published in the print version of a journal to alert print-only readers, (3) a translated abstract published with full-text article in a different language, and (4) an abstract published in the society proceedings or other collection of a journal. (For examples of abstracts presented at meetings, published or unpublished, see 3.13.3, Special Materials, Serial Publications, and 3.13.9, Special Materials, Meeting Presentations and Other Unpublished Material.)

Ideally, a reference to any of these types of abstracts should be permitted only when the original article is not readily available (eg, non–English-language articles or papers presented at meetings but not yet published). If an abstract is published in the society proceedings section of a journal, the name of the meeting during which the abstract was presented need not be included, but see example 4 below if this information is included.

Abstract of a complete article republished from another publication:

1. Yang EL, Macy TM, Wang KH, et al. Economic and demographic characteristics of cerumen extraction claims to Medicare. *JAMA Otolaryngol Head Neck Surg.* 2016;142(2):157-161. Abstract republished in: *JAMA.* 2016;315(19):2128.

Abstract of an online-only article published in the print version of a journal:

2. Kelly MS, Benjamin DK, Puopolo KM, et al. Potential cytomegalovirus infection and the risk for bronchopulmonary dysplasia. *JAMA Pediatr.* 2015;169(12):e153785. Abstract republished in: *JAMA Pediatr.* 2015;169(12):1095.

Translated abstract with full-text article in a different language:

3. Siqueira MM, Araujo CA, Roza BA, Schirmer J. Indicadores de eficiência no processo de doação e transplante de órgãos: revisão sistemática da literatura. Abstract in English. *Rev Panam Salud Publica.* 2016;40(2):90-97.

Abstract of a paper published in the society proceedings of a journal:

4. Richardson J, Hendrickse C, Gao-Smith F, Thickett D. Characterisation of systemic neutrophil function in patients undergoing colorectal cancer resection. *Eur Surg Res.* 2015;55(suppl 1):4. European Society for Surgical Research abstract OP-4.

Note: In example 4, the abstract number is also provided.

**3.11.11** **Special Department, Feature, or Column of a Journal.** When reference is made to material from a special department, feature, or column of a journal, the department could be identified only in the following cases.

The cited material has no byline or signature. Note: This is preferable to citing Anonymous, unless "Anonymous" or something similar was actually used (see 2.2, Author Bylines and End-of-Text Signatures).

1. A plan to protect the world—and save WHO. Editorial. *Lancet.* 2015;386(9989):103. doi:10.1016/S0140-6736(15)61225-9

The column or department name might help the reader identify the nature of the article and this is not apparent from the title itself. Note: In these cases, the inclusion of the department or column name is optional and should be used as needed, at the editor's discretion.

2. Harris JC. Cunningham Dax Collection. Art and Images in Psychiatry. *JAMA Psychiatry.* 2014;71(12):1316-1317. doi:10.1001/jamapsychiatry.2013.2771

3. Ross JS, Krumholz HN. Open access platforms for sharing clinical trial data. Letter. *JAMA.* 2016;316(6):666. doi:10.1001/jama.2016.8794

4. O'Rourke K, VanderZanden A, Shepard D, Leach-Kemon K; Institute for Health Metrics and Evaluation. Cardiovascular disease worldwide, 1990-2013. JAMA Infographic. *JAMA.* 2015;314(18):1905. doi:10.1001/jama.2015.14994

5. Assessing and referring complications following bariatric surgery. *BMJ* Infographic. Accessed June 18, 2019. https://www.bmj.com/content/352/bmj.i945/infographic

Identification of other special departments, features, or columns may not require additional notation (eg, book or journal reviews) because their identity may be apparent from the citation itself:

6. Bevans SE, Larrabee WF Jr. Review of: *Local Flaps in Facial Reconstruction. JAMA Facial Plast Surg.* 2015;17(2):151. doi:10.1001/jamafacial.2014.1440

**3.11.12** **Discussants.** If a reference citation in the text names a discussant specifically rather than the author(s), eg, "as noted by Easter,[1]" the following form is used:

1. Easter DW. In discussion of: Farley DR, Greenlee SM, Larson DR, Harrington JR. Double-blind, prospective, randomized study of warmed humidified carbon dioxide insufflation vs standard carbon dioxide for patients undergoing laparoscopic cholecystectomy. *Arch Surg.* 2004;139(7):739-744.

Note: This convention is not used as widely now. Separately indexed opinion pieces, such as commentaries, editorials, or editor's notes, are more common.

**3.11.13** **Online Comments.** Some journals allow readers to post an online response to articles (eg, *BMJ*'s Rapid Responses, https://www.bmj.com/rapid-responses). In the first 2 examples, "Re:" precedes the title of the original article.

1. Cooke PA. Re: Primary care management of patients after weight loss surgery. Rapid Response. *BMJ.* March 15, 2016. Accessed June 18, 2019. https://www.bmj.com/content/352/bmj.i945/rr-1

2. Zinsstag J. Re: The prevention and management of rabies. Rapid Response. *BMJ.* February 10, 2016. Accessed June 18, 2019. https://www.bmj.com/content/350/bmj.g7827/rr-5

These examples provide a unique title for the comment itself:

3. Donzelli A. A reform of rewarding systems to fight against disease mongering. *PLoS Med*. March 31, 2009. Accessed February 25, 2016. http://journals.plos.org/plosmedicine/article/comment?id=info%3Adoi %2F10.1371%2Fannotation%2F2e7ecf53-c1f5-44b4-bb9c-5fb71d702320

4. Magee M. Incrementalism and voluntary standards are not enough. *JAMA*. March 8, 2019. Accessed March 10, 2019. https://jamanetwork. com/journals/jama/fullarticle/2728102

In addition, nonjournal data repositiories, blogs, and websites also allow readers to post comments on articles.

5. Curry S. Re: How to manipulate a citation histogram. Comment online. *Scholarly Kitchen* blog. August 8, 2016. Accessed August 15, 2016. https://scholarlykitchen.sspnet.org/2016/08/08/how-to-manipulate-a-citation-histogram/

**3.11.14** **Corrections.** If the reference citation is to an article with a published correction, citing the article as usual is probably sufficient, as follows:

1. Gale CR, Batty GD, Osborn DPJ, Tynelius P, Whitley E, Rasmussen F. Association of mental disorders in early adulthood and later psychiatric hospital admissions and mortality in a cohort study of more than 1 million men. *JAMA Psychiatry*. 2012;69(8):823-831. doi:10.1001/arch genpsychiatry.2011.2000

If necessary, a reference citation to the correction notice would appear as follows:

2. Errors in text and tables 2 and 3. Correction. *JAMA Psychiatry*. 2015;72(12):1259. doi:10.1001/jamapsychiatry.2015.0077

**3.11.15** **Retractions and Expressions of Concern.** If the reference citation is to an article that has since been retracted or retracted and replaced, to an article for which there is an expression of concern, or to the retraction notice itself, use the appropriate example below. The ICMJE Recommendations note, "Ideally, the authors of the retraction should be the same as those of the article, but if they are unwilling or unable the editor may under certain circumstances accept retractions by other responsible persons, or the editor may be the sole author of the retraction or expression of concern."[5(p8)] (see 5.4.4, Editorial Policy and Procedures for Detecting and Handling Allegations of Scientific Misconduct).

1. Notice of retraction: Ahimastos AA, et al. Effect of perindopril on large artery stiffness and aortic root diameter in patients with Marfan syndrome: a randomized controlled trial. *JAMA*. 2007;298(13):1539-1547. *JAMA*. 2015;314(24):2692-2693. doi:10.1001/jama.2015.16678

2. Lopes AC, Greenberg BD, Pereira CAB, Norén G, Miguel EC. Notice of retraction and replacement: Lopes et al. Gamma ventral capsulotomy for obsessive-compulsive disorder: a randomized clinical trial. *JAMA*

*Psychiatry.* 2014;71(9):1066-1076. *JAMA Psychiatry.* 2015;72(12):1258. doi:10.1001/jamapsychiatry.2015.0673

3. Expression of concern: Low concentration of interleukin-1β induces FLICE-inhibitory protein-mediated β-cell proliferation in human pancreatic islets. *Diabetes.* 2006;55:2713-2722. *Diabetes.* 2016;65(8):2462. doi:10.2337/db16-ec08a

Citing the retracted article:

4. Ahimastos AA, Aggarwal A, D'Orsa KM, et al. Effect of perindopril on large artery stiffness and aortic root diameter in patients with Marfan syndrome: a randomized controlled trial. *JAMA.* 2007;298(13):1539-1547. Retracted in: *JAMA.* 2015;314(24):2692-2693. doi:10.1001/jama.2015.16678

5. Lopes AC, Greenberg BD, Canteras MM, et al. Gamma ventral capsulotomy for obsessive-compulsive disorder: a randomized clinical trial. *JAMA Psychiatry.* 2014;71(9):1066-1076. Retracted and replaced in: *JAMA Psychiatry.* 2015;72(12):1258. doi:10.1001/jamapsychiatry.2015.0673

6. Schopfer DW, Takemoto S, Allsup K, et al. Cardiac rehabilitation use among veterans with ischemic heart disease. *JAMA Intern Med.* 2014;174(10):1687-1689. Retracted and replaced in: *JAMA Intern Med.* October 10, 2016. doi:10.1001/jamainternmed.2016.5831

In example 6, a shortened version of the reference to the retracted and replaced article is used (date and DOI only); this style may be necessary for articles that have not been published and paginated in an issue in journals with online first and print publication.

Note: DOIs do not follow the citation of the retracted article.

**3.11.16** **Duplicate Publication.** The following form is suggested for citation of a notice of duplicate publication (see 5.3, Ethical and Legal Considerations, Duplicate Publication and Submission).

1. Shariat SF, Roehrborn CG, Lamb DJ, Slawin KM. Notice of duplicate publication: Potentially harmful effect of a testosterone dietary supplement on prostate cancer growth and metastasis. *Arch Intern Med.* 2008;168(2):235-236. *Arch Intern Med.* 2008;168(18):2046-2047. doi:10.1001/archinte.168.18.2046-b

**3.12** **References to Books.**

**3.12.1** **Complete Data.** A complete reference to a book includes the following:

- Chapter authors' surnames and initials (the names of all authors should be given unless there are more than 6, in which case the names of the first 3 authors are used, followed by "et al")
- Chapter title (when cited)

- Book authors' and/or editors' (and translator, if any) surnames and initials (the names of all authors should be given unless there are more than 6, in which case the names of the first 3 authors are used, followed by "et al")
- Title of book and subtitle, if any
- Volume number and volume title, when there is more than 1 volume
- Edition number (do not indicate first edition)
- Name of publisher
- Year of copyright
- Page numbers, when specific pages are cited

With this edition of the manual, we no longer recommend including the publisher's location for several reasons: many publishers have more than 1 location and determining which location is appropriate to include can be challenging; location can be difficult to determine if looking at an online resource (eg, an e-book); and publisher location is not a necessary piece of information in retrieving the reference.

**3.12.2** **References to an Entire Book.** When referring to an entire book, rather than pages or a specific section, use the following format (see 3.7, References, Authors).

1. Etzel RA, Balk SJ, eds. *Pediatric Environmental Health.* American Academy of Pediatrics; 2011.

2. Adkinson NF Jr, Bochner BS, Burks W, et al, eds. *Middleton's Allergy: Principles and Practice.* 8th ed. Saunders; 2014.

3. Sacks O. *Hallucinations.* Alfred A Knopf; 2012.

4. Patterson JW. *Weedon's Skin Pathology.* 4th ed. Churchill Livingstone; 2016.

5. Australian Technical Advisory Group on Immunisation (ATAGI). *The Australian Immunisation Handbook.* 10th ed. Australian Government Dept of Health; 2015.

The following 2 examples are also available as e-books online:

6. World Health Organization. *Health Worker Roles in Providing Safe Abortion Care and Post-abortion Contraception.* World Health Organization; 2015. Accessed August 15, 2016. https://srhr.org/safeabortion/

7. Guyatt G, Rennie D, Meade MO, Cook DJ. *Users' Guides to the Medical Literature: A Manual for Evidence-Based Clinical Practice.* 3rd ed. McGraw-Hill Education; 2015. Accessed August 15, 2016. https://jamaevidence.mhmedical.com/book.aspx?bookID=847

**3.12.3** **References to Monographs.** References to monographs (typically a detailed, scholarly work on a single subject written by a single author who is a specialist on that subject; per *Webster's*, "a learned treatise on a small area of knowledge"[11]) should be styled the same as references to books.

1. de Pina-Cabral J. *World: An Anthropological Examination*. Malinowski Monographs. Hau Books; 2016.

**3.12.4** **References to a Chapter in a Book.** When citing a chapter of a book, capitalize as for a journal article title (see 3.9.1.1, English-Language Titles, Journal Articles and Parts of Books); do not use quotation marks. Inclusive page numbers of the chapter should be given (see 3.12.10, Page Numbers or Chapter Number).

1. Prince M, Glozier N, Sousa R, Dewey M. Measuring disability across physical, mental, and cognitive disorders. In: Regier DA, Narrow WE, Kuhl EA, Kupfer DJ, eds. *The Conceptual Evolution of* DSM-5. American Psychiatric Publishing Inc; 2011:189-227.

2. Boushey CJ. Application of research paradigms to nutrition practice. In: Coulston AM, Boushey CJ, Ferruzzi MG, eds. *Nutrition in the Prevention and Treatment of Disease*. 3rd ed. Academic Press; 2013:99-105.

Note that in example 2 above, the author of the chapter is also an editor of the book. In cases like this, names are given in both places: as authors of the chapter and as editors of the book. The same policy would apply if the authors of a particular chapter and the editors of the book were identical.

**3.12.5** **Editors and Translators.** Names of editors, translators, translator-editors, or executive, consulting, and section editors are given as follows:

1. Plato. *The Laws*. Taylor EA, trans-ed. JM Dent & Sons Ltd; 1934:104-105.

[Plato is the author; Taylor is the translator-editor.]

2. Blumenthal DK, Garrison JC. Pharmacodynamics: molecular mechanisms of drug actions. In: Bunton LL, ed. Chabner BA, Knollmann BC, associate eds. *Goodman and Gilman's The Pharmacological Basis of Therapeutics*. 12th ed. McGraw-Hill Education; 2011:41-72.

[Blumenthal and Garrison are the authors of a chapter in a book edited by Bunton, for which Chabner and Knollmann were the associate editors.]

In the following 3 examples, no book authors are named (in example 5, the chapter author is given). Each book has an editor or editors and is part of a series. Note: The name of the series, if any, is given in the final field. If the book has a number within a series, the number is also given in the final field.

3. Eagle KA, Baliga RR, Isselbacher EM, Nienaber CA, eds. *Aortic Dissection and Related Syndromes*. Springer; 2007. *Developments in Cardiovascular Medicine*; vol 260.

4. Kaufman HL, Mehnert JM, eds. *Melanoma*. Springer; 2016. Rosen ST, ed. *Cancer Treatment and Research*; vol 167.

5. Kleinman K. Darwin and Spenser on the origin of music: is music the food of love? In: Altenmüller E, Finger S, Boller F, eds. *Music, Neurology, and Neuroscience: Evolution, the Musical Brain, Medical*

*Conditions, and Therapies.* Elsevier; 2015:3-15. *Progress in Brain Research*; vol 217.

**3.12.6** **Volume Number.** Use arabic numerals for volume numbers if the work cited includes more than 1 volume, even if the publisher used roman numerals.

If the volumes have no separate titles, merely numbers, the number should be given after the general title.

1. Kasper DL, Fauci AS, Hauser S, Longo D, Jameson JL, Loscalzo J. *Harrison's Principles of Internal Medicine.* Vol 2. McGraw-Hill Professional; 2015.

If the volumes have separate titles, the title of the volume referred to should be given first, with the title of the overall series of which the volume is a part given in the final field, along with the name of the general editor and the volume number, if applicable.

2. Christiansen H, Christiansen NM, eds. *Progressive Neuroblastoma: Innovation and Novel Therapeutic Strategies.* Karger; 2015. Kiess W, ed. *Pediatric and Adolescent Medicine*; vol 20.

In example 2 above, *Pediatric and Adolescent Medicine* is the name of the entire series; *Progressive Neuroblastoma: Innovation and Novel Therapeutic Strategies* is the 20th volume.

When a book title includes a volume number or other identifying number, use the title as it was published. Note: The volume number does not need to be repeated in its customary place after the year if it is included in the book's title.

3. *Field Manual 4–02.17: Preventive Medicine Services.* US Dept of the Army; 2000.

4. Riley-Tillman TC, Burns MK, Gibbons K. *RTI Applications, Volume 2: Assessment, Analysis, and Decision Making.* Guilford Press; 2013.

**3.12.7** **Edition Number.** Use arabic numerals to indicate an edition, even if the publisher has used roman numerals, but do not indicate a first edition. If a subsequent edition is cited, the number should be given. Abbreviate "New revised edition" as "New rev ed," "Revised edition" as "Rev ed," "American edition" as "American ed," and "British edition" as "British ed."

1. Braverman LE, Cooper D, eds. *Werner and Ingbar's The Thyroid: A Fundamental and Clinical Text.* 10th ed. Lippincott Williams & Wilkins; 2012.

2. Lareau A. *Unequal Childhoods: Class, Race, and Family Life, With an Update a Decade Later.* 2nd ed. University of California Press; 2011.

3. Katz JR, Carter CJ, Lyman Kravits S, Bishop J, Block J. *Keys to Nursing Success.* 3rd rev ed. Prentice Hall; 2009.

4. *The Chicago Manual of Style: The Essential Guide for Writers, Editors, and Publishers.* 17th ed. University of Chicago Press; 2017. Accessed January 25, 2019. https://www.chicagomanualofstyle.org/

5. Smeltzer SC, Bare BG, Hinkle JL, Cheever KH. *Brunner & Suddarth's Textbook of Medical-Surgical Nursing.* American ed. Wolters Kluwer/ Lippincott Williams & Wilkins; 2009.

**3.12.8** **Publishers.** The full name of the publisher (publisher's imprint, as shown on the title page) should be given, abbreviated in accordance with the style used by the JAMA Network journals (see 13.7, Commercial Firms) but without any punctuation. Even if the name of a publishing firm has changed, use the name that was given on the published work.

The following are examples of the format for a book with a joint imprint:

1. Green L. *W. Barns-Graham: A Studio Life.* 2nd ed. Lund Humphries/ Ashgate Publishing; 2011.

2. Taylor K. *Philip Evergood: Never Separate From the Heart.* Center Gallery, Bucknell University Press/Associated University Presses; 1987.

3. Style Manual Committee, Council of Science Editors. *Scientific Style and Format: The CSE Manual for Authors, Editors, and Publishers.* 8th ed. University of Chicago Press/Council of Science Editors; 2014.

Consult Books in Print (https://www.booksinprint.com/), WorldCat (https://www. worldcat.org/), or the Library of Congress catalog (https://catalog.loc.gov/) to verify names of publishers.

If there is no publisher's name available, use "Publisher unknown" in the place of the publisher's location and name.

**3.12.9** **Year of Publication.** If the book has been published but there is no year of publication available, use "date unknown" in the place of the year. Use the full year (eg, 2016), not an abbreviated form (eg, not 16 or '16).

1. American Psychiatric Association. *Diagnostic and Statistical Manual of Mental Disorders.* 5th ed. American Psychiatric Association; 2013.

**3.12.10** **Page Numbers or Chapter Number.** Use arabic numerals, unless the pages referred to use roman pagination (eg, the preliminary pages of a book).

1. Rudolph KD, Flynn M. Depression in adolescents. In: Gottlib IH, Hammen CL, eds. *Handbook of Depression.* 3rd ed. Guilford Press; 2014:391-409.

2. Harper RD. Preface. In: *The Chicago Manual of Style.* 16th ed. University of Chicago Press; 2010:xi-xiii.

If a book uses separate pagination within each chapter, follow the style used in the book. Notice that in the example below, because the page numbers contain hyphens, an en dash is used to separate them rather than the usual hyphen.

3. Weil AA, Hyle EP, Basgoz N. Infectious diseases. In: Sabatine MS, ed. *Pocket Medicine.* 5th ed. Lippincott Williams & Wilkins; 2013:6-1–6-22.

Inclusive page numbers are preferred. The chapter number may be used instead if the author does not provide the inclusive page numbers, even after being queried, or if the page numbers are not available because of the format used (eg, audiobook).

> 4. Kwon DS, Walker BD. Immunology of human immunodeficiency virus infection. In: Paul WE, ed. *Fundamental Immunology.* 7th ed. Lippincott Williams & Wilkins; 2012:chap 42.

**3.12.11**  **Electronic Books, Books Online, Audiobooks, and Books on Tape or CD.** The basic format for references to books published via media other than print is as follows:

- Authors' surnames and initials (the names of all authors should be given unless there are more than 6, in which case the names of the first 3 authors are used, followed by "et al") or name of the group if the author is a group

- Chapter title (Note: If the reference is to the entire book, the information about chapter title is not included.)

- In: Editor(s)

- *Book Title*

- Edition number (if it is the second edition or higher; mention of first edition is not necessary; eg, 2nd ed)

- Book medium

- Publisher's name

- Copyright year or publication date

- Chapter number (or inclusive pages if available)

- Accessed [date]

- URL (verify that the link still works as close as possible to publication)

> 1. Style Manual Committee, Council of Science Editors. *Scientific Style and Format: The CSE Manual for Authors, Editors, and Publishers.* 8th ed. University of Chicago Press/Council of Science Editors; 2014. Accessed June 18, 2019. https://www.scientificstyleandformat.org

> 2. Sudarsky L. Gait and balance disorders. In: Kasper DL, Fauci AS, Longo DL, Hauser SL, Jameson JL, Loscalzo J, eds. *Harrison's Principles of Internal Medicine.* 19th ed. McGraw-Hill; 2015:chap 32. Accessed February 10, 2016. http://www.harrisonsim.com/index.php

> 3. Patrias K, Wendling DL, ed. *Citing Medicine: The NLM Style Guide for Authors, Editors, and Publishers.* 2nd ed. National Library of Medicine; 2007-. Updated October 2, 2015. Accessed August 11, 2016. http://www.nlm.nih.gov/citingmedicine

Titles of books on CD-ROM follow the capitalization style of print book titles and are italicized. Note: If the title of the book (eg, *Cecil Textbook of Medicine on CD-ROM*) indicates the medium, no mention of the medium is necessary.

> 4. Alberts B, Johnson A, Lewis J, Raff M, Roberts K, Walter P. *Molecular Biology of the Cell.* 5th ed. CD-ROM. Garland Science; 2007.

5. O'Neill LAJ. The innate immune system. In: Paul WE, ed. *Fundamental Immunology.* 7th ed. CD-ROM. Lippincott Williams & Wilkins; 2012: chap 15.

Citations for other book versions, including for e-readers and audiobooks or books on CD, can take the following formats:

6. Skloot R. *The Immortal Life of Henrietta Lacks.* Kindle e-Book. Random House; 2010:chap 31.

7. Skloot R. *The Immortal Life of Henrietta Lacks.* Audiobook. Random House Audio; 2010:chap 31.

8. Skloot R. *The Immortal Life of Henrietta Lacks.* Audio CD. Random House Audio; 2010:chap 31.

Note: The version used is the version that should be cited.

**3.13** **Special Materials.** Many of the special materials covered in this section may also be accessed (and cited) in an online format. To see examples of these citation formats, see 3.15, Electronic References. The version used (print or online) is the version that should be cited.

**3.13.1** **News Publications.** References to news publications, including newspapers (print and online) and blogs, should include the following, in the order indicated: (1) name of author (if given), (2) title of article, (3) name of newspaper, (4) date of newspaper or date of publication online, (5) section (if applicable), (6) page number (if applicable), (7) online accessed date (if applicable), and (8) website address (if applicable). Note: Newspaper names are not abbreviated. If a city name is not part of the newspaper name, it may be added to the official name for clarity, as with *Minneapolis* in example 1.

1. Tevlin J. Minneapolis street doctor dispenses care with a dose of dignity. *Minneapolis Star Tribune.* January 23, 2016. Accessed January 28, 2016. http://www.startribune.com/minneapolis-street-doctor-dispenses-care-with-a-dose-of-dignity/366313741/

2. Schencker L. Peanut allergy relief? *Chicago Tribune.* September 22, 2019:C1.

3. Ubelacker S. CAMH to "wind down" controversial gender iden-tity clinic services. *Globe and Mail.* December 15, 2015. Accessed January 28, 2016. http://www.theglobeandmail.com/news/toronto/camh-to-wind-down-controversial-gender-identity-clinic-services/article27766580/

4. Liptak A. Yale finds error in legal stylebook: contrary to claim, Harvard didn't create it. *New York Times.* December 8, 2015:A24.

5. Narula SK. WHO has only declared three public health emergencies in its history—Zika virus just became the fourth. *Quartz* blog. February 1, 2016. Accessed August 16, 2016. http://qz.com/607331

6. Guber S. When music is the best medicine. *New York Times.* September 26, 2019. Accessed September 30, 2019. https://www.nytimes.com/2019/09/26/well/live/music-therapy-cancer.html

Note: In the previous 2 examples, the web addresses provided by the blogs were shortened versions. Shortened web addresses may be used in reference citations as long as the shortened link functions properly and directs readers to the correct web page.

**3.13.2** **Government or Agency Reports.** References to reports published by departments or agencies of a government should include the following information, in the order indicated: (1) name of author (if given); (2) title of bulletin; (3) name of issuing bureau, agency, department, or other governmental division (note that in this position, Department should be abbreviated Dept; also note that if the US Government Printing Office is supplied as the publisher, it would be preferable to obtain the name of the issuing bureau, agency, or department); (4) date of publication; (5) page numbers (if specified); (6) publication number (if any); (7) series number (if given); (8) online accessed date (if applicable); and (9) web address (if applicable).

1. Johnston LD, O'Malley PM, Bachman JG, Schulenberg JE, Miech RA. *Monitoring the Future: National Survey Results on Drug Use, 1975-2014: College Students and Adults Ages 19-55*. Vol 2. National Institute on Drug Abuse, US Dept of Health and Human Services; 2014.

2. *Health, United States, 2014: With Special Feature on Adults Aged 55-64*. National Center for Health Statistics; 2015.

3. Sondik EJ. Foreword. In: *Healthy People 2010: Final Review*. National Center for Health Statistics; 2012:iii.

4. Grall T. *Census 2010 Report No. P60-255: Custodial Mothers and Fathers and Their Child Support: 2013*. US Census Bureau; 2016.

5. National Institute of Arthritis and Musculoskeletal and Skin Diseases. *Questions and Answers About Sprains and Strains*. National Institutes of Health; 2015. NIH publication 15-5328. Accessed January 28, 2016. http://www.niams.nih.gov/Health_Info/Sprains_Strains/default.asp

6. Government of Nepal. Central Bureau of Statistics. *Statistical Year Book of Nepal–2013*. Central Bureau of Statistics; 2013.

7. World Health Organization. *World Health Report 2013: Research for Universal Health Coverage*. World Health Organization; 2013.

8. United Nations High Commissioner for Refugees. *Women on the Run: First-Hand Accounts of Refugees Fleeing El Salvador, Guatemala, Honduras, and Mexico*. UNHCR: UN Refugee Agency; 2015. Accessed August 16, 2016. http://www.unhcr.org/5630f24c6.pdf

9. National Institute of Public Health. *Importance of Blood Donation: Requirements and Restrictions*. Published in Spanish. National Institute of Public Health of Mexico; 2015.

**3.13.3** **Serial Publications.** If a monograph or report is part of a series, include the name of the series and, if applicable, the number of the publication.

1. Ministry of Health. *National AIDS Control Programme*. Ministry of Health, United Republic of Tanzania; 2013. HIV/AIDS/STI Surveillance Report 23.

2. Chinnadurai S, Snyder K, Sathe NA, et al. *Diagnosis and Management of Infantile Hemangioma: Comparative Effectiveness Review No. 168*. Agency for Healthcare Research and Quality; 2016. AHRQ publication 16-EHC002-EF.

3. US Department of Commerce. *Population Division: Income, Poverty and Health Insurance in the United States, 2012*. US Bureau of the Census; 2012. Annual Social and Economic Supplement. Accessed January 28, 2016. https://www.census.gov/library/publications/2013/demo/p60-245.html

**3.13.4** **Theses and Dissertations.** Titles of theses and dissertations are given in italics. References to theses should include the name of the university (or other institution) and year of completion of the thesis. If the thesis has been published, it should be treated as any other book reference (see 3.12.1, References to Books, Complete Data).

1. Maiti N. *Association Between Bullying Behaviors, Health Characteristics, and Injuries Among Adolescents in the United States*. Dissertation. Palo Alto University; 2010.

2. Ghanbari S. *Integration of the Arts in STEM: A Collective Case Study of Two Interdisciplinary University Programs*. Dissertation. University of California; 2014. Accessed October 14, 2016. http://escholarship.org/uc/item/9wp9x8sj

3. Neel ST. *A Cost-Minimization and Policy Analysis Comparing Immediate Sequential Cataract Surgery and Delayed Sequential Cataract Surgery From Payer, Patient, Physician, and Surgical Facility Perspectives in the United States*. Master's thesis. London School of Economics and Political Science; 2013.

**3.13.5** **Special Collections.** References to material available only in special collections of a library, as in this example of a monograph written in 1757, take this form:

1. Hunter J. An account of the dissection of morbid bodies: a monograph or lecture. 1757;No. 32:30-32. Located at: Library of the Royal College of Surgeons, London, England.

**3.13.6** **Package Inserts.** Package inserts, patient information, and prescribing information (the material about the use and effects of the product) may be cited as follows:

1. Zithromax. Prescribing information. Pfizer; 2017. Accessed June 23, 2019. https://www.pfizermedicalinformation.com/en-us/zithromax

2. Azilect. Package insert. Teva Pharmaceuticals Inc; 2014.

**3.13.7** **Patents.** Patent citations take the following form. Example 1 is for a patent that has been issued, example 2 is for a patent application, and example 3 is for a European patent. See the US Patent and Trademark Office website (https://www.uspto.gov/) or the European Patent Office website (https://www.epo.org) for further details.

1. Hu D, Fong K, Pinto M, et al, inventors; Spiracur Inc, assignee. Reduced pressure therapy of the sacral region. US patent 8,361,043. January 29, 2013.

2. Gustafsson J, inventor; Cochlear Ltd, assignee. Bone conduction magnetic retention system. US patent application 20,160,037,273. February 4, 2016.

3. Menke A, Binder EB, Holsboer F, inventors; Max Planck Gesellschaft, assignee. Means and methods for diagnosing predisposition for treatment of emergent suicidal ideation. European patent EP2166112 (B1). May 6, 2013.

Note: In examples 1 and 2 above, the commas are retained; do not use thin spaces in the patent numbers (see 18.1.1, Use of Numerals, Numbers of 4 or More Digits to Either Side of the Decimal Point).

**3.13.8** **Conference Proceedings Online, Webinars, and Other Presentations.** These are treated much the same as a "presented at" reference (see 3.13.9, Special Materials, Meeting Presentations and Other Unpublished Material), with the addition of the accessed date and the URL.

1. Morales M, Zhou X. Health practices of immigrant women: indigenous knowledge in an urban environment. Paper presented at: 78th Association for Information Science and Technology Annual Meeting; November 6-10, 2015; St Louis, MO. Accessed March 15, 2016. https://dl.acm.org/doi/10.5555/2857070.2857108

2. Botkin J, Menikoff J. Opening remarks presented at: Secretary's Advisory Committee on Human Research Protections Meeting; December 4, 2015; Rockville, MD. http://www.hhs.gov/ohrp/sachrp/mtgings/2015%20Dec%20Mtg/december3-4,2015sachrpmeeting.html. Accessed March 15, 2016. Videocast available at: https://videocast.nih.gov/

The presentation in example 2 did not have a title; hence, the "title" field and the "presented at" field were combined. In addition, a webcast of the meeting is available for the presentation in example 2, and that information is also included in the reference. See example 3 below for how to cite a videocast.

3. Labor, Health and Human Services Subcommittee Hearing. National Institutes of Health: Investing in a Healthier Future. October 7, 2015. Accessed March 15, 2016. Videocast available at: http://www.appropriations.senate.gov/hearings/labor-hhs-subcommittee-hearing-national-institutes-of-health-investing-in-a-healthier-future

A transcript from a teleconference is cited as follows:

4. Volkow N, Botticelli M, Johnston LD, Miech RA. Monitoring the Future: Teleconference 2015. December 16, 2015. Accessed March 15, 2016. Transcript available at: https://www.drugabuse.gov/news-events/podcasts/2015/12/monitoring-future-teleconference-2015#content-area

A webinar is cited as follows:

5. Gunn E, Kendall-Taylor J, Vandenburg B. Taking author instructions to the next level. Council of Science Editors webinar. September 10, 2015. Accessed March 15, 2016. http://www.councilscienceeditors. org/resource-library/past-presentationswebinars/past-webinars/ 2015-webinar-3-taking-author-instructions-to-the-next-level/

**3.13.9** **Meeting Presentations and Other Unpublished Material.** References to unpublished material may include articles or abstracts that have been presented at a society meeting and published as part of the meeting proceedings or materials.

**3.13.9.1** **Items Presented at a Meeting.** These oral or poster presentations take the following form:

1. Pasternak B. Carvedilol vs metoprolol succinate and risk of mortality in patients with heart failure: national cohort study. Paper presented at: European Society of Cardiology Congress; August 31, 2014; Barcelona, Spain.

2. Minocchieri S, Berry CA, Pillow J. Nebulized surfactant for treatment of respiratory distress in the first hours of life: the CureNeb study. Abstract presented at: Annual Meeting of the Pediatric Academic Society; May 6, 2013; Washington, DC. Session 3500.

3. Nevidomskyte D, Meissner MH, Tran N, Murray S, Farrokhi E. Influence of gender on abdominal aortic aneurysm repair in the community. Poster presented at: Vascular Annual Meeting; June 5-7, 2014; Boston, MA.

Once these presentations are published, they take the form of reference to a book, journal, or other medium in which they are ultimately published, as in example 5 (see 3.12.1, References to Books, Complete Data, and 3.11.1, References to Journal Articles, Complete Data):

4. Huang G-M, Huang K-Y, Lee T-Y, Tzu-Ya Weng J. An interpretable rule-based diagnostic classification of diabetic nephropathy among type 2 diabetes patients. *BMC Bioinformatics*. 2015;16(suppl 1):S5. Selected articles from the Thirteenth Asia Pacific Bioinformatics Conference (APBC 2015). doi:10.1186/1471-2105-16-S1-S5

In example 4, the entire journal supplement is dedicated to publishing articles from a meeting.

5. Resnick ML. The effect of affect: decision making in the emotional context of health care. In: *Proceedings of the 2012 Symposium on Human Factors and Ergonomics in Health Care: Bridging the Gap.* Human Factors and Ergonomics Society; 2012:39-44.

**3.13.9.2** **Material Accepted for Publication but Not Yet Published.** Some journals may include material that has been accepted for publication but not published. However, the JAMA Network journals and other journals ordinarily will not include these materials as formal references, particularly forthcoming journal articles that have not yet been published. Reasons not to include forthcoming journal articles in a reference list include (1) citing a forthcoming article might break the journal's embargo policy, (2) publication may not occur as planned, and (3) these references are not retrievable. (The term *forthcoming* is preferred to *in press* because *in press* is an outdated term.[5,8])

The following examples are provided for books, but this is not recommended for journal articles:

6. Lewis M. *The Undoing Project: A Friendship That Changed Our Minds.* WW Norton & Co. Forthcoming 2016.

7. Christiansen SL, Iverson C, Flanagin A, et al. *AMA Manual of Style: A Guide for Authors and Editors.* 11th ed. Oxford University Press. Forthcoming 2019.

Note: Publications that permit citation of forthcoming journal articles may require authors to verify acceptance for publication (authors sometimes confuse *submitted* with *accepted*).[5,8]

**3.13.9.3** **Material Submitted for Publication but Not Yet Accepted.** In the list of references, do not include material that has been submitted for publication but has not yet been accepted. This material, with its date, should be noted in the text as "unpublished data," as follows:

These findings have recently been corroborated (H. E. Marman, MD, unpublished data, January 2015).

Similar findings have been noted by Roberts[6] and H. E. Marman, MD (unpublished data, 2015).

However, it is not best practice to cite unpublished data as a source, and these may be better noted as personal communications.

**3.13.10** **Personal Communications.** Personal communications should not be included in the list of references. Personal communications (cited in text) should be used judiciously, and documentation should be provided to support personal communication. Oral communication should be supported in writing. The following forms may be used in the text:

According to a letter from H. E. Marman, MD, in August 2015 …

Similar findings have been noted by Roberts[6] and by H. E. Marman, MD (email, August 15, 2015).

According to the manufacturer (H. R. Smith, PhD, Pharma International, written communication, May 1, 2015), the drug became available in Japan in January 2014.

The author should provide the date of the communication and indicate how it was documented (eg, letter, email, document). The person's highest academic degree(s) should also be given. If the affiliation of the person would better establish the relevance and authority of the citation, it should be included (see the example above, where H. R. Smith is identified as working for the drug's manufacturer; see also 3.15.9, Electronic References, Email and Electronic Mailing List [LISTSERV] Messages).

Some journals, including the JAMA Network journals, require that the author obtain written permission from the person whose unpublished data or personal communication is thus cited[3,8] (see 5.2.9, Acknowledgments, Permission to Name Individuals).

**3.13.11** **Classical References.** References to classical works may deviate from the usual forms in some details. In many instances, the facts of publication are irrelevant and may be omitted. Date of publication should be given when available and pertinent.

1. Shakespeare W. *A Midsummer Night's Dream*. Act 2, scene 3, line 24.
2. Donne J. *Second Anniversary*. Verse 243.

For classical references, *The Chicago Manual of Style*[12] may be used as a guide.

3. Aristotle. *Metaphysics*. 3. 2.966b 5–8.

In biblical references, do not abbreviate the names of books. The version may be included parenthetically if the information is provided (see example 4). References to the Bible are usually included in the text.

The story begins in Genesis 3:1.

Paul admonished against succumbing to temptation (I Corinthians 10:6-13).

Occasionally they may appear as listed references at the end of the article.

4. I Corinthians 10:6-13 (RSV).

**3.14** **Other Media.**

**3.14.1** **Video.** Occasionally, references may include citation of audio or video recordings or DVDs. The form for such references is as follows:

1. Smith R. *Evidence-Based Medicine: An Oral History*. The JAMA Network and the *BMJ*. 2014. Accessed October 14, 2016. https://ebm.jamanetwork.com/
2. Moyers B. *On Our Own Terms: Moyers on Dying*. DVD. Thirteen/WNET; 2000. https://billmoyers.com/series/on-our-own-terms-moyers-on-dying/
3. Bernstein Fant B, Fant L. *The American Sign Language Phrase Book With DVD*. McGraw-Hill Education; 2011.

Note that the host may be given as the author and the distributor may be given as the publisher. In addition, if the medium is given in the title of the work, it is not necessary to repeat after the title (see example 3).

For citation format for electronic books or books on CD, see 3.12.11, References to Books, Electronic Books, Books Online, Audiobooks, and Books on Tape or CD, and for audio presentations available online, see 3.13.8, Special Materials, Conference Proceedings Online, Webinars, and Other Presentations.

**3.14.2**   **Podcasts and Other Audio.** The JAMA Network frequently publishes online podcast interviews with authors. The following are suggested citation formats:

1. Interview with Charles Harding, author of "Breast Cancer Screening, Incidence, and Mortality Across US Counties," and Joann G. Elmore, author of "Effect of Screening Mammography on Cancer Incidence and Mortality". *JAMA Intern Med*. July 6, 2015. Accessed June 18, 2019. https://edhub.ama-assn.org/jn-learning/audio-player/11054180

2. Bauchner H. Editor's audio summary. *JAMA*. March 5, 2019. Accessed March 10, 2019. https://edhub.ama-assn.org/jn-learning/audio-player/17356045

3. Nate. *The Show About Science*. Butterflies with Doug Taron. October 11, 2016. Accessed January 10, 2019. https://itunes.apple.com/us/podcast/the-show-about-science/id1046413761

For citation format for audiobooks, see 3.12.11, References to Books, Electronic Books, Books Online, Audiobooks, and Books on Tape or CD.

**3.14.3**   **Apps and Interactive Games.** The suggested format for citing apps and video games follows:

1. JN Listen app. American Medical Association. Updated March 1, 2019.

2. Davis's Drug Guide With Updates & Calculators app. Version 1.18. Unbound Medicine Inc. Updated September 25, 2015.

3. *That Dragon, Cancer*. Numinous Games. 2016. Accessed August 17, 2016. http://www.thatdragoncancer.com/

**3.14.4**   **Other Multimedia.** A multimedia component can be cited as a supplement to an article or as a stand-alone item with its own DOI or URL, as shown in examples 4, 5, and 6. Citation of multimedia components to online articles, including videos, can be formatted as follows:

1. Modeled estimates of HIV incidence, prevalence, and mortality worldwide and in 188 countries, 1990-2013. Accessed August 17, 2016. https://edhub.ama-assn.org/jn-learning/interactive/13984801. Interactive feature for: Leach-Kemon K, Shepard D, O'Rourke K, VanderZanden A; Institute for Health Metrics and Evaluation. *JAMA*. 2015;314(15):1552. doi:10.1001/jama.2015.12936

2. The global burden of cancer 2013. May 28, 2015. Accessed October 13, 2016. https://jamanetwork.com/learning/video-player/10626961. Author video interview for: Global Burden of Disease Cancer Collaboration. *JAMA Oncol*. doi:10.1001/jamaoncol.2015.0735

3. Kaiser Family Foundation. A snapshot of US global health funding. Visualizing Health Policy infographic. *JAMA*. 2014;311(16):1601. Accessed October 13, 2016. doi:10.1001/jama.2014.3890

In example 3, the department name (ie, Visualizing Health Policy) is given in the reference because it helps identify the nature of what is being cited, information that is not apparent from the title (see 3.11.11, References to Journal Articles, Special Department, Feature, or Column of a Journal). However, it is sufficient to provide the title, dates, and URL for multimedia as shown in examples 4 and 5 below.

4. Middle ear aspiration. November 3, 2016. Accessed September 30, 2019. https://edhub.ama-assn.org/jn-learning/video-player/13673838

5. Association between income and life expectancy in the United States. April 10, 2016. Accessed October 13, 2016. http://jamanetwork.com/learning/video-player/12647873

6. Lee PY, Costumbrado J, Hsu CY, Kim YH. Agarose gel electrophoresis for the separation of DNA fragments. *J Vis Exp*. 2012;62:e3923. Accessed October 13, 2016. doi:10.3791/3923

**3.14.5** **Transcripts of Audio, Video, Television, or Radio Broadcasts or Television Commercials.** Citation of transcripts to television or radio broadcasts or other audio or video and television commercials takes the following form:

1. Families describe how they felt hearing about an autism diagnosis. Transcript. *Weekend Edition Saturday*. National Public Radio. January 16, 2016. Accessed October 20, 2016. http://www.npr.org/2016/01/15/463221381/families-describe-how-they-felt-hearing-about-an-autism-diagnosis

2. Heroin in the heartland. Transcript. *60 Minutes*. CBS television. January 24, 2016. Accessed October 20, 2016. http://www.cbsnews.com/news/heroin-in-the-heartland-60-minutes/

3. Device reduces risk of brain injury after heart valve replacement. Video script. JAMA Report Video. August 9, 2016. Accessed August 18, 2016. https://media.jamanetwork.com/news-item/device-reduces-risk-of-brain-injury-after-heart-valve-replacement/#

4. Celebrex commercial. Body in motion. Transcript. Pfizer. Advertisement by Kaplan Thaler Group. Last aired September 18, 2014. Accessed July 13, 2016. https://www.ispot.tv/ad/7V7z/celebrex-body-in-motion

**3.15** **Electronic References.** Electronic references are much more common since the publication of the 10th edition of this manual. Many journal articles are now published online before appearing in a printed publication with traditional pagination and volume and issue numbers. The internet has allowed publishers to use more innovative means to disseminate information, including interactive content, supplements, podcasts, and videos. Because electronic references are ubiquitous, examples have been integrated throughout this revised chapter where appropriate. *Citing Medicine*[5] also provides extensive guidelines for citing electronic content for medical research.

It is important to consider the unique requirements for electronic citation.

Websites and URLs may be evanescent, vanishing much faster than books go out of print. Addressing this phenomenon, *Citing Medicine*[5] states in chapter 22, "… many Internet items are updated or otherwise modified several times after the date of publication. The latest date of update/revision should therefore be included along with the date cited, ie, the date the person doing the citing saw the item on the Internet. This is necessary in the volatile Internet environment, where changes can be easily made and an item seen one day may not be the same in crucial ways when viewed the next day. Producing a **print** or **other copy** for future reference is strongly recommended."

In preparing a reference list, authors should check to make sure any URLs they cite are still valid; editors should check these again. Many reference managers (eg, BibTex, EndNote, ProCite, Reference Manager, RefWorks, Zotero) assist with this. Because typographical errors render URLs invalid, validation may be required several times in the publication process. Although it is desirable to have functional links, it is to be expected that, over time, some links may break as websites cease to exist or are restructured. Any updating of URLs to try to "fix" a link should be done with care, ensuring that the material that was cited originally still exists on the revised link.

**3.15.1**    **DOI.** Many publishers are using other less transient identifiers instead of, or in addition to, URLs. Among these are the DOI (digital object identifier) and the PMID (PubMed identification number). The DOI system "provides an infrastructure for persistent unique identification of objects of any type."[14] Unlike a URL, which is transient and can change, a DOI is permanent and will not change over time.

The DOI may be used to identify not only individual journal articles but also any piece of content (eg, a single figure, a multimedia component) within or associated with an article. DOIs may also be assigned to books, monographs, video, audio—any form of content.

The DOI system was announced at the Frankfurt Book Fair in 1997 and was initiated by the International DOI Foundation in 1998.[14] The first application of the DOI system, citation linking of electronic articles by the Crossref Registration Agency, was launched in 2000, the same year that the syntax of the DOI was standardized through NISO. Subsequently, other registration agencies were launched (eg, DataCite for data and other agencies for non-English languages).[14] In 2010, the DOI system was approved as a standard by the International Organization for Standardization.[14]

The International DOI Foundation has the following useful definitions[14]:

DOI is an acronym for "digital object identifier," meaning a "digital identifier of an object" rather than an "identifier of a digital object."

The unqualified term "DOI" alone (which was used in the early years of the system's development) is now deprecated, as a potential source of confusion, and the preferred usage is with a qualifier to refer to either specific components of the DOI system (eg, "DOI name": the string that specifies a unique referent within the DOI system); or the system as a whole ("DOI system": the functional deployment of DOI names as the application of identifiers in computer sensible form through assignment, resolution, referent description, administration, etc, as prescribed by the specification).

The ability to easily and accurately copy and paste DOIs is important. Because of this, a period or other punctuation should not be included after the DOI; the risk of the punctuation becoming a part of the DOI itself is too great and would create problems with linking. Online linking is one of the key reasons to have a DOI. It is also important to be aware of any programming (eg, widgets, java scripts, stylesheets) or web conversions that may inadvertently break DOIs (by reformatting, adding invisible characters, etc).

Because a DOI is assigned to a single object, a reference likewise must contain only a single DOI. In addition, DOIs should never be used in titles (eg, in retractions) because this would create the potential for a reference to have more than 1 DOI.

The DOI has 2 elements, separated by a forward slash: the prefix and the suffix:

10.1038/nature02312

The prefix is assigned by a DOI registration agency (an organization may have multiple prefixes) and the suffix identifies the particular item. Note: Some publishers use other identifiers as a part of the suffix. All DOIs begin with 10. The DOIs can be any length and, once assigned, are not changed. To find an article using the DOI, a reader can enter the DOI in the search box found at the International DOI Foundation website (https://doi.org/)[15] or most search engines. In some browsers, a standard web search using the DOI will also allow a reader to find an article. As close as possible to publication, it is advisable to check all DOIs to make sure that they resolve (ie, link to the article or object).

Publishers have options for presentation style of DOIs, and pros and cons should be considered. Publishers may present DOIs as a metadata element of a citation (eg, doi:10.1001/jama.2017.13737) or as a URL linking through a registration agency, such as Crossref (eg, https://doi.org/10.1001/jama.2017.13737).

The Crossref website provides a list of advantages (https://www.crossref.org/display-guidelines/) to displaying the DOI as a resolvable URL. Styling DOIs for a journal article as a URL per Crossref recommendations allows linking for the DOI to the article or object to be resolved through the Crossref website, one of the DOI registration agencies that manages DOIs. However, a DOI presented as metadata links users directly to the permanent article or object the DOI is identifying.

The *AMA Manual of Style* recommends presenting DOIs as metadata (eg, doi:10.1001/jama.2017.13737).

**3.15.2** **PMID.** The PMID is assigned to the journal articles cited in PubMed and is a part of the PubMed citation. To find an article, a reader can enter the PMID in the "search" box on the PubMed website (https://www.ncbi.nlm.nih.gov/PubMed/). The PII (publisher item identifier) is a unique identifier used by some journal publishers to identify documents. Although the DOI is commonly published with an article or online element, the PMID and the PII usually are not published but may exist as behind-the-scenes identifiers.

Some journals and books may be available in print and online, but these versions may not be identical: the differences may be as minor as the online correction of a typographical error in the print journal or as major as 2 different versions of the same article appearing online and in print, or additional material might only be available online (eg, multimedia, web supplements). Books are often adapted for the web to enhance interactivity for readers and add features. Because of these possible differences among various versions, it is critical that authors cite the version consulted.

**3.15.3** **Websites.** In citing data from a website, include the following elements, if available, in the order shown:

- Authors' surnames and initials, if given (the names of all authors should be given unless there are more than 6, in which case the names of the first 3 authors are used, followed by "et al"), or name of the group

- Title of the specific item cited (if none is given, use the name of the organization responsible for the site)

- Name of the website

- [Date published]

- Updated [date]

- Accessed [date]

- URL (verify that the link still works as close as possible to publication)

1. International Society for Infectious Diseases. ProMED-mail. Accessed February 10, 2016. http://www.promedmail.org

2. Charlton G. Internal linking for SEO: examples and best practices. SearchEngineWatch. Accessed February 10, 2016. https://searchenginewatch.com/sew/how-to/2428041/internal-linking-for-seo-examples-and-best-practices

3. Zika travel information. Centers for Disease Control and Prevention. January 26, 2016. Updated August 11, 2016. Accessed June 18, 2019. https://wwwnc.cdc.gov/travel/page/zika-travel-information

4. Sample size calculation. Grapentine Co Inc. Accessed December 6, 2005. http://www.grapentine.com/calculator.htm

5. Scientific Responsibility, Human Rights & Law Program. American Association for the Advancement of Science. Accessed June 18, 2019. https://www.aaas.org/program/scientific-responsibility-human-rights-law

6. Recommendations for primary care practice. US Preventive Services Task Force. Accessed March 9, 2019. https://www.uspreventiveservicestaskforce.org/Page/Name/recommendations

**3.15.4** **Social Media.** As new modalities of social media have emerged, a mechanism for citing these different outputs is useful. Social media are fluid and temporary, and in scientific reporting, a better citation is likely available.

Some suggestions for citing various popular social media follow.

▩ Facebook

1. Mayo Clinic Sports Medicine Facebook page. #RotatorCuff tears are among the most common shoulder injuries, particularly in individuals who engage in activities that require repetitive arm motions. Discover the possible treatment options for a torn rotator cuff: https://mayocl.in/2H6AR3P. Accessed March 4, 2019. https://www.facebook.com/mayoclinicsportsmedicine

▩ Blog

2. Gray T. Advice after mischief is like medicine after death. *AMA Style Insider* blog. February 11, 2019. Accessed March 10, 2019. https://amastyleinsider.com/2019/02/11/advice-after-mischief-is-like-medicine-after-death/

▩ YouTube

3. Khan Academy health and medicine YouTube page. Accessed February 10, 2016. https://www.youtube.com/user/khanacademymedicine

▩ Twitter

4. @AMAManual. Double negatives can be used to express a positive, but this yields a weaker affirmative than the simpler positive and may be confusing. "Our results are not inconsistent with the prior hypothesis." "That won't do you no good." And the classic: "I can't get no satisfaction." March 7, 2019. Accessed March 10, 2019. https://twitter.com/AMAManual/status/1103678998327017483

In some of the examples above, note that instead of a title, the entire post is given.[16]

**3.15.5** **Government/Organization Reports.** These reports are treated much like electronic journal and book references: use journal style for articles and book style for monographs. Note: Of the dates published, updated, and accessed, often only the accessed date will be available.

1. Federal Interagency Forum on Aging-Related Statistics. Older Americans 2012: key indicators of well-being. Accessed March 3, 2016. http://www.agingstats.gov

2. World Medical Association. Declaration on alcohol. Updated October 2015. Accessed March 3, 2016. https://www.wma.net/policies-post/wma-declaration-on-alcohol/

3. US Department of Health and Human Services. Protection of human subjects. 45 CFR §46. Revised July 19, 2018. Accessed June 23, 2019. https://www.hhs.gov/ohrp/regulations-and-policy/regulations/revised-common-rule-regulatory-text/index.html

4. World Health Organization. Infection prevention and control: recovery plans and implementation: Guinea, Liberia, and Sierra Leone inter-country meeting: July 20-22, 2015. Accessed March 3, 2016. http://apps.who.int/iris/bitstream/10665/204370/1/WHO_HIS_SDS_2015.23_eng.pdf

In the 2 examples below, the number of the working paper (example 5) and the publication number (example 6) provide information in addition to the URL and could prove helpful should the URLs change.

5. Carpenter CS, McClellan CB, Rees DI. Economic conditions, illicit drug use, and substance use disorders in the United States. National Bureau of Economic Research working paper 22051. February 2016. Accessed March 3, 2016. http://www.nber.org/papers/w22051

6. Johnson DL, O'Malley PM, Bachman JG, Schulenberg JE. *HIV/AIDS: Risk & Protective Behaviors Among American Young Adults, 2004-2008.* National Institute on Drug Abuse; 2010. *Monitoring the Future.* NIH publication 10-7586. June 2010. Accessed March 3, 2016. http://www.monitoringthefuture.org/pubs/monographs/hiv-aids_2010.pdf

**3.15.6** **Software.** To cite software, use the following form:

1. *Epi Info.* Version 7.1.5. Centers for Disease Control and Prevention; 2015. Accessed March 14, 2016. http://www.cdc.gov/epiinfo

2. *Stata 14.* Version 14. StataCorp; 2015. Accessed March 14, 2016. http://www.stata.com/

Software need not always be cited in the reference list; for example, it may be cited in the text if it is mentioned in the Statistical Analysis subsection of the Methods section. The following is an example of an in-text citation for software:

All analyses were conducted using SAS version 9.4 (SAS Institute Inc).

**3.15.7** **Software Manual or Guide.** In citing a software manual or guide, use the following form, which follows that for citation of a book (see 3.12.1, References to Books, Complete Data).

1. Siechert C, Bott E. *Inside Out: Microsoft Office 2013 Edition.* Microsoft Press; 2013.

**3.15.8** **Databases.** The international consortium known as DataCite released the *DC Data Citation Principles*[17] and recommends the following for data citation:

1. Importance

   Data should be considered legitimate, citable products of research. Data citations should be accorded the same importance in the scholarly record as citations of other research objects, such as publications.

2. Credit and Attribution

   Data citations should facilitate giving scholarly credit and normative and legal attribution to all contributors to the data, recognizing that a single style or mechanism of attribution may not be applicable to all data.

3. Evidence

   In scholarly literature, whenever and wherever a claim relies upon data, the corresponding data should be cited.

4. Unique Identification

   A data citation should include a persistent method for identification that is machine actionable, globally unique, and widely used by a community.

5. Access

   Data citations should facilitate access to the data themselves and to such associated metadata, documentation, code, and other materials as are necessary for both humans and machines to make informed use of the referenced data.

6. Persistence

   Unique identifiers, and metadata describing the data, and its disposition, should persist—even beyond the lifespan of the data they describe.

7. Specificity and Verifiability

   Data citations should facilitate identification of, access to, and verification of the specific data that support a claim. Citations or citation metadata should include information about provenance and fixity sufficient to facilitate verifying that the specific timeslice, version, and/or granular portion of data retrieved subsequently is the same as was originally cited.

8. Interoperability and Flexibility

   Data citation methods should be sufficiently flexible to accommodate the variant practices among communities, but should not differ so much that they compromise interoperability of data citation practices across communities.

In citing data from an online database, include the following elements, if applicable, in the order shown:

- Authors' surnames and initials, if given (the names of all authors should be given unless there are more than 6, in which case the names of the first 3 authors are used, followed by "et al"), or name of the group

- Title of the database

- Publisher, or database owner or host

- Year of publication and/or version number

- Updated [date]

- Accessed [date]

- URL (verify that the link still works as close as possible to publication)

Additional notes that might be helpful or of interest to the reader (eg, date the site was updated or modified) may also be included.

1. PDQ: NCI's Comprehensive Database. National Cancer Institute; 2015. Updated July 17, 2015. Accessed March 16, 2016. http://www.cancer.gov/publications/pd

2. HUGO Gene Nomenclature Committee (HGNC). Human Gene Nomenclature database search engine. Accessed March 14, 2016. http://www.genenames.org/

3. Symbol Report: BRAF. HUGO Gene Nomenclature Committee. Accessed August 17, 2016. http://www.genenames.org/cgi-bin/gene_symbol_report?hgnc_id=HGNC:1097

4. Online Mendelian Inheritance in Man (OMIM). Johns Hopkins University School of Medicine; 2016. Updated March 13, 2016. Accessed March 14, 2016. http://www.ncbi.nlm.nih.gov/omim

5. Evaluation of phage therapy for the treatment of *Escherichia coli* and *Pseudomonas aeruginosa* wound infections in burned patients (PHAGOBURN). ClinicalTrials.gov identifier: NCT02116010. Updated July 23, 2015. Accessed October 13, 2016. https://www.clinicaltrials.gov/ct2/show/NCT02116010

**3.15.9** **Email and Electronic Mailing List (LISTSERV) Messages.** References to email and electronic mailing list messages, like those to other forms of personal communications (see 3.13.9, Special Materials, Meeting Presentations and Other Unpublished Material), should be listed parenthetically in the text rather than in the reference list and should include the name and highest academic degree(s) of the person who sent the message, his/her affiliation, and the date the message was sent. Note: As with all personal communications, permission should be obtained from the author.

An example of an email citation, appearing in running text, is given below:

Similar findings have been noted by Roberts[6] and by H. E. Marman, MD (email communication, August 1, 2015).

An electronic mailing list (listserve or LISTSERV) message cited in running text would be given as in the example below:

The style committee for the *AMA Manual of Style* is currently preparing an update to address additional electronic reference citation formats (Annette Flanagin, CITINGMED LISTSERV, February 2, 2016).

A LISTSERV message or discussion thread with reliable linking could be cited in the reference list as in the example below:

1. Retroactive open access (under the author-pays model). CSE-L LISTSERV discussion. March 14-15, 2016. Accessed March 15, 2016. http://lists.resourcenter.net/read/messages?id=27905

**3.15.10** **News Releases.** Citations to news releases take the following format:

1. Dying in pursuit of the news. News release. Associated Press; March 30, 2015.

2. Device reduces risk of brain injury after heart valve replacement. News release. JAMA For the Media. August 4, 2016. Accessed August 18, 2016. https://media.jamanetwork.com/news-item/device-reduces-risk-of-brain-injury-after-heart-valve-replacement/

The news release in example 2 was also released as a video. See example 3:

3. Cerebral protection device effects on brain lesions after TAVI. The JAMA Report. August 9, 2016. Accessed August 18, 2016. https://www.youtube.com/watch?v=fsAHMq9eHdc

4. Use of wearable fitness technology does not improve weight loss. The JAMA Report. September 20, 2016. Accessed October 14, 2016. https://media.jamanetwork.com/news-item/use-of-wearable-device-does-not-improve-weight-loss/

5. Antidepressant may improve cognitive symptoms in people with HIV. News release. Johns Hopkins Medicine; February 25, 2016. Accessed March 18, 2016. http://www.hopkinsmedicine.org/news/media/releases/antidepressant_may_improve_cognitive_symptoms_in_people_with_hiv

6. External beam RT & brachytherapy for selected patients with intermediate-risk prostatic carcinoma. Patient brochure. Radiation Therapy Oncology Group. Accessed March 18, 2016. https://www.rtog.org/LinkClick.aspx?fileticket=n3tL9pa_Ow4%3d&tabid=213

**3.15.11** **Legal References.** Legal references cited online contain the same basic information as legal references cited in print (see 3.16, US Legal References), with the addition of the URL and the accessed date.

1. Drug Quality and Security Act, HR 3204, 113th Cong (2013). Pub L No. 113-54. Accessed September 15, 2015. https://www.congress.gov/bill/113th-congress/house-bill/3204

**3.16** **US Legal References.** A specific style variation is used for references to legal citations. Because the system of citation used is complex, with numerous variations for different types of sources and among various jurisdictions, only a brief outline can be presented here. For more details, consult *The Bluebook: A Uniform System of Citation.*[18]

**3.16.1** **Method of Citation.** A legal reference may be included in the reference list in full, with a numbered citation in the text, or it may be included in the text parenthetically and not included in the reference list. In scholarly articles, a full citation in the reference list is preferred, but in a news article or book review, for example, a parenthetical citation in the text might be adequate.

■ Full Citation

In a lawsuit regarding criminal transmission of HIV,[1] the Iowa Supreme Court stated . . . .

In the case of *Rhoades v State*[1] . . . .

This reference would then appear in the reference list as follows:

1. *Rhoades v State*, 848 NW2d 22 (Iowa 2013).

▥ Parenthetical In-Text Citation

> In a leading decision on criminal transmission of HIV (*Rhoades v State*, 848 NW2d 22 [Iowa 2013]), the Iowa Supreme Court stated . . . .

> In the case of *Rhoades v State* (848 NW2d 22 [Iowa 2013]) . . . .

**3.16.2** **Citation of Cases.** The citation of a case (ie, a court opinion) generally includes the following, in order:

▥ The name of the case (including the *v*) in italics; to shorten the case name, use only the name of the first party; omit "et al" and "the"; use only the last names of individuals

▥ The volume number, abbreviated name, and series number (if any) of the reporter (bound volume of collected cases)

▥ The page in the volume on which the case begins and, if applicable, the specific page or pages on which the point for which the case is being cited is discussed

▥ In parentheses, the name of the court that rendered the opinion (unless the court is identified by the name of the reporter) and the year of the decision; if the opinion is published in more than 1 reporter, the citations to each reporter (known as parallel citations) are separated by commas; note that *v* (for *versus*), 2d (for *second*), and 3d (for *third*) are standard usage in legal citations

> 1. *Canterbury v Spence*, 464 F2d 772, 775 (DC Cir 1972).

This case is published in volume 464 of the *Federal Reporter*, second series. The case begins on page 772, and the specific point for which it was cited is on page 775. The case was decided by the US Court of Appeals, District of Columbia Circuit, in 1972.

The proper reporter to cite depends on the court that wrote the opinion. Table T1.3 in *The Bluebook*[18] contains a complete list of all current and former state and federal jurisdictions for the United States. The 20th edition of *The Bluebook* also has many examples of non-US cases.

**13.16.2.1** **US Supreme Court.** Cite to *US Reports* (abbreviated as US). If the case is too recent to be published there, cite to *Supreme Court Reporter* (SCt), *US Reports, Lawyer's Edition* (LEd), or *US Law Week* (USLW)—in that order. Do not include parallel citation. The format for these references includes the following, in the order specified (the punctuation is noted; where none is given after a bulleted item, none is used):

▥ *First party v Second party*,

▥ Reporter volume number

▥ Official reporter abbreviation

▥ First page of case, specific pages used

▥ (Year of decision).

Some examples follow:

2. *Ledbetter v Goodyear Tire and Rubber Company*, 550 US 618 (2007).

3. *Addington v Texas*, 441 US 418, 426 (1979).

4. *King v Burwell,* 576 US ___ (2015).

**13.16.2.2** **US Court of Appeals.** Cite to *Federal Reporter*, original or second series (F or F2d). These intermediate appellate-level courts hear appeals from US district courts, federal administrative agencies, and other federal trial-level courts. Circuits are referred to by number (1st Cir, 2d Cir, etc) except for the District of Columbia Circuit (DC Cir) and the Federal Circuit (Fed Cir), which hears appeals from the US Claims Court and from various customs and patent cases. Divisions are denoted by ED (Eastern Division), WD (Western Division), ND (Northern Division), and SD (Southern Division). Citations to the *Federal Reporter* must include the circuit designation in parentheses with the year of the decision. The format for these references includes the following, in the order specified (the punctuation is noted; where none is given after a bulleted item, none is used):

- *First party v second party,*

- Reporter volume number

- Official reporter abbreviation

- First page of case, specific page used

- (Deciding circuit court and year of decision).

Some examples follow:

5. *United States vs Newman,* 773 F3d 438 (2nd Cir 2014).

6. *Scoles v Mercy Health Corp*, 887 F Supp 765 (ED Pa 1994).

7. *Bradley v University of Texas M. D. Anderson Cancer Ctr*, 3 F3d 922, 924 (5th Cir 1993).

8. *Doe v Washington University*, 780 F Supp 628 (ED Mo 1991).

**13.16.2.3** **US District Court and Claims Courts.** Cite to *Federal Supplement* (F Supp). (There is only the original series so far.) These trial-level courts are not as prolific as the appellate courts; their function is to hear the original cases rather than review them. There are more than 100 of these courts, which are referred to by geographic designations that must be included in the citation (eg, the Northern District of Illinois [ND Ill], the Central District of California [CD Cal], but District of New Jersey [D NJ] because New Jersey has only 1 federal district).

9. *Sierra Club v Froehlke*, 359 F Supp 1289 (SD Tex 1973).

**13.16.2.4** **State Courts.** Cite to the appropriate official (ie, state-sanctioned and state-financed) reporter (if any) and the appropriate regional reporter. Most states have separate official reporters for their highest and intermediate appellate courts (eg, *Illinois Reports* and *Illinois Appellate Court Reports*), but the regional reporters include cases from both levels. Official reporters are always listed first, although an increasing number of states are no longer publishing them. The regional reporters are the *Atlantic Reporter*

(A or A2d), *North Eastern Reporter* (NE or NE2d), *South Eastern Reporter* (SE or SE2d), *Southern Reporter* (So or So2d), *North Western Reporter* (NW or NW2d), *South Western Reporter* (SW or SW2d), and *Pacific Reporter* (P or P2d). If only the regional reporter citation is given, the name of the court must appear in parentheses with the year of the decision. If the opinion is from the highest court of a state (usually but not always known as the supreme court), the abbreviated state name is sufficient (except for Iowa and Ohio). The full name of the court is abbreviated (eg, Ill App, NJ Super Ct App Div, NY App Div). A third, also unofficial, reporter is published for a few states; citations solely to these reporters must include the court name (eg, *California Reporter* [Cal Rptr], *New York Supplement* [NYS or NYS2d]). The format for these references includes the following, in the order specified (the punctuation is noted; where none is given after a bulleted item, none is used).

- *First party v second party*,

- Reporter volume number

- Official state reporter abbreviation

- First page of case, specific page used

- Regional reporter and page number

- (Year of decision).

Some examples follow:

10. *Szafranski v Dunston,* 373 Ill Dec 197, 993 NE2d 502 (Ill App Ct 2013).
11. *Reber v Reiss,* 42 A3d 1131, 1135 (Pa Super Ct 2012).
12. *In re Marriage of Witten,* 672 NW2d 768, 777 (Iowa 2003).
13. *Baxter v Montana.* 2009 MT 449, 354 Mont 234, 224 P3d 1211 (Mont 2009).
14. *Planned Parenthood v Casey,* 505 US 833 (1992).

WL is Westlaw (www.westlaw.com), a legal citation database. A version of Westlaw's database also exists for countries other than the United States (eg, www.westlaw.co.uk for the United Kingdom).

When a case has been reviewed or otherwise dealt with by a higher court, the subsequent history of the case should be given in the citation. If the year is the same for both opinions, include it only at the end of the citation. The phrases indicating the subsequent history are set off by commas, italicized, and abbreviated (eg, *aff'd* [affirmed by the higher court], *rev'd* [reversed], *vacated* [made legally void, annulled], *appeal dismissed, cert denied* [application for a writ of certiorari, ie, a request that a court hear an appeal has been denied]).

15. *Kerins v Hartley*, 21 Cal Rptr 2d 621 (1993) (*vacated* and remanded for reconsideration), 28 Cal Rptr 2d 151 (1994).
16. *Glazer v Glazer,* 374 F2d 390 (5th Cir), *cert denied,* 389 US 831 (1967).

This opinion was written by the US Court of Appeals for the Fifth Circuit in 1967. In the same year, the US Supreme Court was asked to review the case in an application for a writ of certiorari but denied the request. This particular subsequent history is important because it indicates that the case has been taken to the highest court available and thus strengthens the case's value as precedent for future legal decisions.

**3.16.3** **Legislative Materials.** US Government Publishing Office Federal Digital System website (https://www.gpo.gov/fdsys/) and the website for the US Congress (https://www.congress.gov) are valuable resources for looking up US federal bills and laws.

**13.16.3.1** **Citation of Congressional Hearings.** Include the full title of the hearing, the subcommittee (if any) and committee names, the number and session of the US Congress, the date, and a short description if desired.

1.  *Hearing Before the Subcommittee on Research & Technology; Committee on Science, Space, and Technology,* 114th Cong, 1st Sess (2015) (testimony of Victor J. Dzau, MD, president, Institute of Medicine, The National Academy of Sciences). Accessed March 18, 2016. https://www.gpo.gov/fdsys/pkg/CHRG-114hhrg97564/html/CHRG-114hhrg97564.htm

2.  *Discrimination on the Basis of Pregnancy, 1977, Hearings on S 995 Before the Subcommittee on Labor of the Senate Committee on Human Resources,* 95th Cong, 1st Sess (1977) (statement of Ethel B. Walsh, vice-chairman, Equal Employment Opportunity Commission).

**13.16.3.2** **US Federal Bills and Resolutions.** Legislation not yet enacted should include the name of the bill (if available), the abbreviated name of the US House of Representatives (HR) or the US Senate (S), the number of the bill, the number of the legislative body, the session number (if available), the section (if any), and the year of publication.[18]

3.  21st Century Cures Act, HR 6, 114th Cong (2015). Accessed April 12, 2016. https://www.congress.gov/bill/114th-congress/house-bill/6

4.  Stop All Frequent Errors (SAFE) in Medicare and Medicaid Act of 2000, S 2378, 106th Cong, 2nd Sess (2000).

5.  HR Rep No. 99-253, pt 1, at 54 (1985).

6.  Koepge C. The Road to Industrial Peace: A Ten Year Study, HR Doc 82-563 (1953).

**13.16.3.3** **US Federal Statutes.** Once a bill is enacted into law by the US Congress, it is integrated into the US Code (USC). Citations of statutes include the official name of the act, the title number (similar to a chapter number), the abbreviation of the code cited, the section number (designated by §), and the date of the code edition cited. If the law is available online, the URL may also be included.

7.  Female Genital Mutilation, 18 USC §116 (2012). Accessed March 18, 2016. https://www.gpo.gov/fdsys/granule/USCODE-2011-title18/USCODE-2011-title18-partI-chap7-sec116

The above example cites section 116 of title 18 of the US Code.

A specific section of a bill or law may also be cited within the text:

The Drug Supply Chain Security Act states that dispensers "shall not accept ownership of a product, unless the previous owner prior to, or at the time of, the transaction, provides transaction history, transaction information, and a transaction statement" (§582[d][1][A]).

If a federal statute has not yet been codified, cite to Statutes at Large (abbreviated Stat, preceded by a volume number, and followed by a page number), if available, and the Public Law number of the statute.

8. Pub L No. 112-34, 125 Stat 369.

The name of the statute may be added if it provides clarification.

9. Patient Protection and Affordable Care Act, Pub L No. 111-148, 124 Stat 119 (2010).

**13.16.3.4** **US Federal Administrative Regulations.** US federal regulations are published in the *Federal Register* and then codified in the *Code of Federal Regulations*. These references to the *Federal Register* are now treated as journal references. If a URL is available, that may also be included.

10. Importation of fruits and vegetables. *Fed Regist.* 1995;60(51):14202-14209. To be codified at 7 CFR §300.

11. Payment for Drugs, Definitions. 42 CFR §447.502 (2015).

12. Authority to Bill Third Party Payers for Full Charges. 42 CFR §411.31 (1996).

Regulations promulgated by the Internal Revenue Service retain their unique format. Temporary regulations must be denoted as such.

13. Treas Reg §1.72 (1963).

14. Temp Treas Reg §1.338 (1985).

**13.16.3.5** **Bills and Resolutions for Individual States.** Legislation should include the name of the bill or resolution (if available), the abbreviated name of the US House of Representatives (HR) or the US Senate (S), the number of the bill, the number of the legislative body, the session number, and the state abbreviation and the year of enactment.[18] Some bills will also have a URL associated with them, which may also be included.

15. An Act Relative to Substance Use Treatment, Education and Prevention, HR 4056, 189th Leg (Mass 2016). April 12, 2016. Accessed October 16, 2017. https://malegislature.gov/Bills/189/House/H4056

16. End of Life. S 128. 2015-2016 Session (Ca 2015).

**13.16.3.6** **State Statutes.** Table T1.3 in *The Bluebook*[18] lists examples for each state and the District of Columbia.

17. Ill Rev Stat ch 38, §2 (1965).

This is section 2 of chapter 38 of the Illinois Revised Statutes.

18. Fla Stat §202 (2001).

This is section 202 of the Florida Statutes.

19. Mich Comp Laws §700.5506 (1998).

This is section 700.5506 of Michigan Compiled Laws.

> 20. Wash Rev Code §26.16.010 (2003).

This is section 26.16.010 of Revised Code of Washington.

> 21. Cal Corp Code §300 (West 1977).

This is section 300 of California Corporations Code and West is the name of the publisher.

Citation forms for state administrative regulations are especially diverse. Again, Table T1.3 in *The Bluebook* lists the appropriate form for each state.

**13.16.3.7** **Legal Services.** Many legal materials, including some reports of cases and some administrative materials, are published by commercial services (eg, Commerce Clearing House), often in loose-leaf format. These services attempt to provide a comprehensive overview of rapidly changing areas of expertise (eg, tax law, labor law, securities regulation) and are updated frequently, sometimes weekly. The citation should include the volume number of the service; its abbreviated title; the publisher's name (also abbreviated); the paragraph, section, or page number; and the date.

> 22. 7 Sec Reg Guide (P-H) ¶2333 (1984).

The above example cites volume 7, paragraph 2333, of the *Securities Regulation Guide*, published by Prentice-Hall in 1984.

> 23. 54 Ins L Rep (CCH) 137 (1979).

This is volume 54, page 137, of *Insurance Law Reports*, published by Commerce Clearing House in 1979.

> 24. 4 OSH Rep (BNA) 750 (1980).

This is volume 4, page 750, of the *Occupational Safety and Health Reporter*, published by Bloomberg BNA in 1980.

**13.16.3.8** **Law Journals.** Law journal references follow the same rules as medical journal references. List the authors (if any), the title of the article, the name of the journal, the volume number, issue number (or date, if there is no issue number), and page numbers.

> 25. *Doe v Westchester County Med Center, NY State Division of Human Rights*. *N Y Law J*. December 26, 1990;91:30.
> 26. Kim J. Patent infringement in personalized medicine: limitations of the existing exception mechanisms. *Wash Univ Law Rev*. 2018;96(3):623–647. Accessed September 26, 2019. https://openscholarship.wustl.edu/law_lawreview/vol96/iss3/4/

**3.17** **Non-US Legal References.** Cases tried in countries outside the United States are presented as follows:

> 1. *Ramakrishnan v State of Kerala*, AIR 1999 Kerala HC 385 (India).
> 2. *Scholem v Department of Health*, Case No. 40830/86 (Dist Ct NSW, Australia 1992).

3. *McTear v Imperial Tobacco Ltd*, CSOH 69 (Scotland).

4. *Canada v JTI-Macdonald Corp*, SCC 30 (Canada 2007).

**Principal Authors:** Lauren Fischer and Paul Frank

## ACKNOWLEDGMENT

Thank you to the following, who provided insight and careful review for this chapter: David Antos, JAMA Network; Sara Billings (who styled and ordered the references), JAMA Network; Robin Dunford, PhD, Dunford Consulting, Wantage, Oxfordshire, England; Paul Gee, JAMA Network; Emily Greenhow, *JAMA*; Lou S. Knecht, MLS, formerly Deputy Chief, Bibliographic Services Division, National Library of Medicine; Trevor Lane, MA, DPhil, Edanz Group, Fukuoka, Japan; Monica Mungle, JAMA Network; Peter J. Olson, Sheridan Journal Services, Waterbury, Vermont (who provided DOIs); Joe Thornton, JD, JAMA Network; and Sam Wilder, formerly of JAMA Network.

Additional Information: Coauthor Paul Frank died in 2015.

## REFERENCES

1. Meyer CA. Reference accuracy: best practices for making the links. *J Electron Publ.* 2008. doi:10.3998/3336451.0011.206

2. On citing well. *Nat Chem Biol.* 2010;6(2):79. doi:10.1038/nchembio.310

3. International Committee of Medical Journal Editors. Recommendations for the Conduct, Reporting, Editing, and Publication of Scholarly Work in Medical Journals. Updated December 2018. Accessed June 23, 2019. http://www.icmje.org/icmje-recommendations.pdf

4. Samples of formatted references for authors of journal articles. National Library of Medicine. Updated May 25, 2016. Accessed August 5, 2016. https://www.nlm.nih.gov/bsd/uniform_requirements.html

5. Patrias K, Wendling DL, eds. *Citing Medicine: The NLM Style Guide for Authors, Editors, and Publishers.* 2nd ed. National Library of Medicine; 2007-. Updated October 2, 2015. Accessed August 11, 2016. https://www.nlm.nih.gov/books/NBK7526

6. ANSI/NISO Z39. 29-2005 (R2010) Bibliographic References. National Information Standards Organization. Approved June 9, 2005, by the American National Standards Institute; reaffirmed May 13, 2010. Accessed August 5, 2016. https://www.niso.org/apps/group_public/download.php/12969/239_29_2005_R2010.pdf

7. Appendix F. Notes for Citing MEDLINE/PubMed. In: Patrias K, Wendling DL, ed. *Citing Medicine: The NLM Style Guide for Authors, Editors, and Publishers.* 2nd ed. National Library of Medicine; 2007-. Updated August 11, 2015. Accessed August 11, 2016. https://www.ncbi.nlm.nih.gov/books/NBK7243/

8. Style Manual Committee, Council of Science Editors. *Scientific Style and Format: The CSE Manual for Authors, Editors, and Publishers.* 8th ed. University of Chicago Press/Council of Science Editors; 2014.

9. Preprint FAQ. ASAP bio. Accessed August 15, 2016. http://asapbio.org/preprint-info/preprint-faq

10. Marcus E. Let's talk about preprint servers. *Crosstalk* blog. June 3, 2016. Accessed August 15, 2016. http://crosstalk.cell.com/blog/lets-talk-about-preprint-servers

11. Armato D. What was a university press? *Against the Grain*. December 2012–January 2013; 24(6):58-62. doi:10.7771/2380-176X.6247

12. *The Chicago Manual of Style: The Essential Guide for Writers, Editors, and Publishers*. 17th ed. University of Chicago Press; 2017.

13. Books and other individual titles on the internet. In: Patrias K, Wendling DL, ed. *Citing Medicine: The NLM Style Guide for Authors, Editors, and Publishers*. 2nd ed. National Library of Medicine; 2007- :chap 22. Updated August 11, 2015. Accessed November 23, 2016. https://www.ncbi.nlm.nih.gov/books/NBK7269

14. International DOI Foundation. DOI Handbook. Introduction. Updated October 17, 2015. Accessed October 13, 2017. https://www.doi.org/doi_handbook/1_Introduction.html

15. The Digital Object Identifier System. International DOI Foundation (IDF). Updated December 8, 2015. Accessed March 18, 2016. https://www.doi.org/

16. Christiansen SL. Citations a-twitter. *AMA Style Insider* blog. August 23, 2011. Accessed August 16, 2016. https://amastyleinsider.com/2011/08/23/citations-a-twitter/

17. Martone M, ed. Data Citation Synthesis Group. Joint Declaration of Data Citation Principles. FORCE11. 2014. Accessed December 14, 2017. https://www.force11.org/group/joint-declaration-data-citation-principles-final

18. *The Bluebook: A Uniform System of Citation*. 20th ed. Harvard Law Review Association; 2015. Accessed March 18, 2016. http://www.legalbluebook.com

# 4.0 Tables, Figures, and Multimedia

**4.0** **Tables, Figures, and Multimedia.** Tables and figures show relationships among data and other types of numerical, textual, or visual information. Text may be preferred if the information can be presented concisely (**Box 4.1-1**). For qualitative information, small amounts of data with a few simple comparisons should usually be presented in words, whereas large amounts of data with several comparisons should usually be presented in tables, graphs, or illustrations. For quantitative information, a table should be used when the display of exact values is important, whereas a figure (eg, a line or bar graph) should be used to show patterns or trends. Tables also are often preferable to graphics for small data sets and are preferred when data presentation requires many specific comparisons. However, primary outcomes should not be presented in a figure only or referred to in the text only with a general statement. For those findings, absolute numbers and measures of variance should also be included in the text.

Priorities in the creation and publication of tables and figures are to emphasize important information and to ensure that each table and figure makes a clear point. In addition to presenting study results, tables and figures can be used to explain or amplify the methods or highlight other key points in the article. Like a paragraph, each table or figure should be cohesive and focused. To be most effective, tables and figures should present ideas and information in a logical sequence. The relationship of tables and figures to the text and to each other should be considered in manuscript preparation, editorial evaluation and peer review, manuscript editing and tagging, and article layout and display for print/PDF and online.

When used properly, tables and figures add variety to article layout and are visually compelling and distinct components of scientific publications. However, authors and editors of scientific publications should avoid using tables and figures simply to break up text or to impart visual interest.

**Box 4.1-1.** Guidelines for Using Text, Tables, and Figures to Display Numerical Data

---

**Uses of text**

Present quantitative data that can be given concisely and clearly

Describe simple relationships among data

**Uses of tables**

Present more than a few precise numerical values

Present large amounts of detailed quantitative information in a smaller space than would be required in the text

Show detailed item-to-item comparisons

Display many numbers simultaneously

Display individual data values precisely

Show complex relationships among the data

**Uses of figures**

Highlight patterns or trends in data

Show changes or differences over time

Display complex relationships among quantitative variables

Aid decision-making

---

Multimedia (video, audio, interactive files), although available only online, can enhance understanding of an article's content.

**4.1** **Tables.** Because of their ability to present detailed information effectively and in ways that text alone cannot, tables are an essential component of many scientific articles. Tables can summarize, organize, and condense complex or detailed data and therefore are routinely used to present study results.

The purpose of a table is to present data or information and support statements in the text. Information in the table must be accurate and consistent with that in the text in content and style. A properly designed and constructed table should be able to stand independently, without requiring undue reference to the text.

**4.1.1** **Types of Tables.**

**4.1.1.1** **Table.** A table displays information arranged in columns and rows (see 4.1.4, Table Components and **Table 4.1-1**) and is used most commonly to present numerical data. Each table should have an object identifier (eg, Table) and a title, be numbered consecutively as referred to in the text, and be positioned as closely as possible to its first mention in the text. Formal tables usually are framed by horizontal rules, boxes, or white space. Some journals add background shading.

**4.1.1.2** **Matrix.** A matrix is a tabular structure that uses numbers, short words (eg, no, yes), symbols (eg, bullets, check marks), or shading to depict relationships among items in columns and rows and to allow comparisons among entries. A matrix may also be processed as a figure, depending on the complexity of the construction and the need for multiple colors or shading (**Table 4.1-2**).

**4.1.1.3** **Boxes, Sidebars, and Other Nontabular Material.** Information that is complementary to the text (eg, lists) can be set off in a box or sidebar within the article (see 4.3, Nontabular Material).

**4.1.2** **Organizing Information in Tables.** For a table to have maximum effectiveness, the information it contains must be arranged logically and clearly so that the reader can quickly understand the key point and find the specific data and comparisons of interest.

During the planning and creation of a table, the author should consider the primary purpose of the table: what data need to be included, compared, or emphasized.

**Table 4.1-1.** Basic Table, Including Title, Columns, Rows, and Footnotes

**Table.** Characteristics of Heat Waves During the Study Period, 1999-2010[a]

| Heat wave definition | | Counties with ≥1 heat wave event, No. (%) | Frequency of heat waves, mean No. per year (IQR) | Duration of heat waves, mean (IQR), d | Temperature, mean (IQR), °C | |
|---|---|---|---|---|---|---|
| No. of days | Temperature percentile | | | | During heat wave days | During non–heat wave days |
| ≥2 | >97 | 1943 (100) | 2.6 (2.4-2.8) | 3.3 (3.0-3.6) | 28.3 (26.9-30.1) | 23.1 (21.0-25.5) |
| ≥2 | >98 | 1943 (100) | 1.8 (1.6-1.9) | 3.1 (2.8-3.3) | 28.8 (27.4-30.5) | 23.1 (21.1-25.5) |
| ≥2 | >99 | 1943 (100) | 0.9 (0.8-1.0) | 2.8 (2.5-3.0) | 29.5 (28.1-31.1) | 23.1 (21.2-25.5) |
| ≥4 | >97 | 1942 (99.9) | 0.8 (0.7-0.9) | 5.5 (4.8-6.0) | 28.5 (27.0-30.4) | 23.2 (21.2-25.6) |
| ≥4 | >98 | 1935 (99.6) | 0.5 (0.3-0.6) | 5.1 (4.5-5.6) | 29.0 (27.5-30.8) | 23.2 (21.3-25.5) |
| ≥4 | >99 | 1723 (88.7) | 0.2 (0.1-0.2) | 4.2 (4.0-5.0) | 29.6 (28.1-31.4) | 23.2 (21.1-25.8) |

Abbreviation: IQR, interquartile range.
[a]Heat waves are defined as at least 2 or at least 4 consecutive days with temperatures exceeding the 97th, 98th, or 99th percentile of a county's daily temperatures, 1999-2010. The heat wave definition used in the main analysis was at least 2 days' duration with temperatures exceeding the 99th percentile of the county's daily temperatures. Non–heat wave days are not in the heat wave period but are matched by county and week.

**Table 4.1-2.** Matrix That Is Presented as a Figure

**Figure.** Paired Grading Class Comparison for Paravalvular Regurgitation (PVR)

| PVR at 30 d | PVR at 1 y | | | | | | Total |
|---|---|---|---|---|---|---|---|
| | None | Trace | Mild | Mild to moderate | Moderate | Severe | |
| None | 267 | 57 | 26 | 2 | 0 | 0 | 352 |
| Trace | 112 | 150 | 56 | 5 | 0 | 0 | 323 |
| Mild | 55 | 96 | 207 | 45 | 4 | 0 | 407 |
| Mild to moderate | 1 | 7 | 34 | 49 | 7 | 0 | 98 |
| Moderate | 0 | 3 | 6 | 14 | 7 | 1 | 31 |
| Moderate to severe | 0 | 0 | 0 | 1 | 1 | 0 | 2 |
| Total | 435 | 313 | 329 | 116 | 19 | 1 | 1213 |

■ Worse ■ Better ■ Same

115

**Table 4.1-3.** Two Tables With Identical Information Present the Use of a Vertical Format for the Primary Outcome vs a Horizontal Format

**Table.** Relative Risk for Death After Onset of Heart Failure Defined by the Framingham Criteria[a]

|  | Men by age, y | | | Women by age, y | | |
|---|---|---|---|---|---|---|
| Year | 60 | 70 | 80 | 60 | 70 | 80 |
| 1996-2000 | 1 [Reference] | 1 [Reference] | 1 [Reference] | 1 [Reference] | 1 [Reference] | 1 [Reference] |
| 2001-2005 | 0.84 (0.69-1.02) | 0.84 (0.73-0.97) | 0.85 (0.72-1.00) | 0.80 (0.63-1.03) | 0.91 (0.77-1.06) | 1.02 (0.90-1.15) |
| 2006-2010 | 0.63 (0.50-0.80) | 0.74 (0.63-0.88) | 0.88 (0.75-1.04) | 0.95 (0.73-1.24) | 0.99 (0.83-1.18) | 1.03 (0.90-1.17) |
| 2011-2015 | 0.48 (0.36-0.64) | 0.59 (0.49-0.71) | 0.72 (0.61-0.87) | 0.67 (0.48-0.92) | 0.79 (0.64-0.98) | 0.94 (0.82-1.09) |

[a]Data are presented as relative risk (95% CI).

**Table.** Relative Risk for Death After Onset of Heart Failure Defined by the Framingham Criteria

|  | Relative risk (95% CI) | | | |
|---|---|---|---|---|
| Age, y | 1996-2000 | 2001-2005 | 2006-2010 | 2011-2015 |
| **Men** | | | | |
| 60 | 1 [Reference] | 0.84 (0.69-1.02) | 0.63 (0.50-0.80) | 0.48 (0.36-0.64) |
| 70 | 1 [Reference] | 0.84 (0.73-0.97) | 0.74 (0.63-0.88) | 0.59 (0.49-0.71) |
| 80 | 1 [Reference] | 0.85 (0.72-1.00) | 0.88 (0.75-1.04) | 0.72 (0.61-0.87) |
| **Women** | | | | |
| 60 | 1 [Reference] | 0.80 (0.63-1.03) | 0.95 (0.73-1.24) | 0.67 (0.48-0.92) |
| 70 | 1 [Reference] | 0.91 (0.77-1.06) | 0.99 (0.83-1.18) | 0.79 (0.64-0.98) |
| 80 | 1 [Reference] | 1.02 (0.90-1.15) | 1.03 (0.90-1.17) | 0.94 (0.82-1.09) |

Because the English language is read first horizontally (from left to right) and then vertically (from top to bottom), the primary comparisons should be shown horizontally across the table. Data that depict cause-and-effect correlations, before-and-after relationships, or trends (eg, change over time) should be arranged from left to right if space allows or, alternatively, from top to bottom. Information being compared (such as numerical data) should be juxtaposed within adjacent columns to facilitate comparisons among items of interest.[1] The tables in **Table 4.1-3** present the same information. In the first table, the values for the dependent variable (years of study) are placed in the row headings, and the data for each independent variable must be compared vertically, up and down rows. Reversing the axes of the table so that the values for the dependent variable are placed in the column headings allows the data to be compared horizontally, between columns.

Although tables frequently are used to present many quantitative values, authors should remember that tabulating all collected study data is unnecessary and actually may distract and overwhelm the reader. Data presented in a table should be pertinent and meaningful. However, it is preferable for demographic data to be reported as comprehensively and transparently as possible. For example, when reporting the sex or gender of participants, do not choose to report only data for the most prevalent category; instead, report data on all participants as possible (eg, a row for women, a row for men, and a row for data not reported or unknown, or for gender variables if studied).[2] When reporting on other demographic variables, including racial and ethnic information, be as specific and comprehensive as possible (see 11.12, Inclusive Language).

The length of the table should also be considered. For ease of reading print journals and PDFs as well as for practical reasons, a table that would span more than a printed page horizontally or run vertically onto a second page should, if possible, be recast into 2 or more smaller tables. If this is not possible, the table may be set in smaller type. Another option is to publish the table as supplementary material in electronic form only, with a note in the print publication, but the same difficulty in following column headings down the table or losing one's place while scrolling wide tables occurs online as well. Yet another option is to run a table in landscape format, requiring the print reader to turn the article sideways to view (these are usually rotated online).

**4.1.3** **Tables in Online Journals.** For the JAMA Network journals online, tables appear as downloadable images, whereas other journals may use HTML tables for the online version of an article. The advantage of using tables that are images is that the table's appearance, such as the design and data alignment, can be controlled and allows for consistent presentation of the data, which is an important consideration for larger, more complex tables. The use of HTML tables has its advantages as well, the first being that a graphic file need not be downloaded to view the table, making the data more immediately accessible on any electronic device (smartphone, tablet, or computer). In addition, the table's text is searchable, and hyperlinks can be included within the table, such as reference citations that link to the reference in the list of all references at the end of the file or in a bibliography.

**4.1.4** **Table Components.** Formal tables in scientific articles conventionally contain 6 major elements: object identifier, title, column headings, stubs (row headings), body (data field) consisting of individual cells (data points), and footnotes (Table 4.1-1). Details pertaining to elements of style for table construction vary among publications; what follows is based on the general style of the JAMA Network journals.

**4.1.4.1** **Object Identifier.** Each table should be formally identified as such, and if there is more than 1 in an article, the tables should be numbered consecutively according to the order in which they are mentioned in the text (Table 1, Table 2, etc). If the article contains only 1 table, it is referred to in the text as "Table."

**4.1.4.2** **Title.** Each table should have a brief, specific, descriptive title, usually written as a phrase rather than as a sentence, that distinguishes the table from other data displays in the article. The title should convey the topic of the table succinctly but should not provide detailed background information or summarize or interpret the results.

The word "Table" and the table number are part of the title. The capitalization style used in article titles should be followed for table titles (see 10.2, Titles and Headings). The following are examples of table titles:

Table 4. Ten-Year Prevalence of Fractures, Falls, or Musculoskeletal Injuries Among Beneficiaries With Disorders of Binocular Vision

**Table 3.** Adjusted Relative Risks for Asthma and Asthma Duration Predicting 4-Year Incidence of Obstructive Sleep Apnea

Certain article types have required tables, such as a baseline characteristics table in a randomized clinical trial or a listing of studies included in a meta-analysis; the table titles should reflect this content:

**Table 1.** Baseline Characteristics of Patients in the HOME Trial

**Table.** Characteristics of Studies Included in the Meta-analysis

**4.1.4.3**   **Column Headings.** The main categories of information in the table should be contained in separate columns. In tables for studies that have independent and dependent variables, the independent variables conventionally are displayed in the left-hand column (row heading) and the dependent variables in the columns to the right. Each column should have a brief heading that identifies and applies to all items listed in that column. Terms used in the text should be consistently used in table headings as well. It is important to label groups consistently to avoid confusing readers.[1] For example, "placebo," "control," and "untreated" should not be used to describe the same group of individuals; instead, use the same term in tables as can be found in the abstract, text, and figures. When possible, use highly descriptive terms (eg, "Metronidazole group" is preferable to "Treatment group").

It is acceptable to omit the heading for the first column if the entries are different or the entries do not need further explanation (**Table 4.1-4**).[3]

Units of measure should be indicated in the column heading, unless provided in the row heading, and are preceded by a comma (Table 4.1-1).

**Table 4.1-4.** Omitted Heading for First Column

**Table.** Baseline Characteristics of Study Participants by Ferritin Level

| | Low ferritin (≤26 ng/mL) | | Higher ferritin (>26 ng/mL) | |
|---|---|---|---|---|
| | Iron (n = 51) | No iron (n = 50) | Iron (n = 60) | No iron (n = 54) |
| Women, No. (%) | 33 (64.7) | 31 (62.0) | 38 (63.3) | 34 (63.0) |
| Age ≥60 y, No. (%) | 12 (23.5) | 11 (22.0) | 17 (28.3) | 12 (22.2) |
| Age, mean (SD), y | 47.5 (15.5) | 45.9 (15.7) | 49.3 (14.6) | 48.1 (14.6) |
| Weight, mean (SD), kg | 75.9 (16.4) | 76.8 (15.8) | 81.5 (16.4) | 77.9 (16.2) |
| Hemoglobin, mean (SD), g/dL | 13.2 (1.0) | 13.7 (1.3) | 14.1 (1.0) | 14.3 (1.2) |
| Ferritin, mean (SD), ng/mL | 14.9 (5.8) | 15.2 (6.0) | 54.0 (24.3) | 58.9 (32.9) |
| sTfR, mean (SD), mg/L | 4.0 (1.33) | 3.9 (1.19) | 3.1 (0.65) | 3.1 (0.62) |
| Estimated blood volume, mean (SD), L | 4.59 (0.8) | 4.66 (0.91) | 4.79 (0.84) | 4.64 (0.84) |

Abbreviation: sTfR, soluble transferrin receptor.
SI conversion factor: To convert ferritin to pmol/L, multiply by 2.247.

Column headings are set in boldface type. If necessary, column subheadings may be used. For more complex headings, braces (or spanning rules) may be used or additional explanatory information may be provided in the footnotes (Table 4.1-1).

If all elements in a column are identical (eg, if all studies in a review used the same assay in the study methods), this information could be provided in a footnote or in the table title and the column deleted (**Table 4.1-5**).[3]

In column headings, style guidelines regarding numbers (eg, use of ordinals) and abbreviations may be relaxed somewhat to save space, with abbreviations expanded in a footnote. However, when space allows spelled-out headings, expansions are preferable to abbreviations. Column and row headings are set in sentence case (only an initial cap), similar to axis labels in figures (see 4.2.6.2, Axis Labels).

**Table 4.1-5.** Use of a Footnote to Convey Information That Would Have Been Identical for Each Row (See Footnote *a*)

**Table.** Cases of MOG-IgG–Associated Seizures Identified on Literature Review[a]

| Source | No. of patients | Age, y/sex | Ethnicity | Other antibodies | Type of seizure | Clinical syndrome |
|---|---|---|---|---|---|---|
| Hino-Fukuyo et al,[9] 2015 | 3 | 12/M; 14/M; 5/M | Japanese | None | NA | ADEM |
| Tsuburaya et al,[10] 2015 | 1 | 7/M | Japanese | None | Partial (eye deviation and L arm clonic seizures) | ADEM, ON |
| Ramberger et al,[11] 2015 | 22[b] | NA | NA | None | NA | ADEM |
| Titulaer et al,[12] 2014 | 1 | 4/F | Hispanic | NMDAR | NA | Seizures, hemiparesis; later: mutism, chorea, and orofacial dyskinesia |
| Ogawa et al,[13] 2017 | 4 | 39/M; 36/M; 23/M; 38/M | Japanese? | None | GTC; GTC; GTC + focal; GTC | Encephalopathy, ON; seizure, ON; encephalopathy; seizure, aphasia, and R hemiparesis |
| Fujimori et al,[14] 2017 | 1 | 46/M | Japanese | None | Focal progressed to secondary generalized | Encephalopathy, paraplegia |

Abbreviations: ADEM, acute disseminated encephalomyelitis; FLAIR, fluid-attenuated inversion recovery; GTC, generalized tonic-clonic; L, left; MOG, myelin oligodendrocyte glycoprotein; MRI, magnetic resonance imaging; NA, not available; NMDAR, *N*-methyl-D-aspartate receptor; R, right; ON, optic neuritis.

[a] All studies used a cell-based assay for MOG antibody testing.

[b] Represents patients who presented with 1 or a combination of cognitive impairments or seizures. It is unclear how many of these patients had seizures.

**4.1.4.4**   **Row Headings.** The left-most column of a table contains the row headings, which apply to all items in that row. If a unit of measure is not included in the column heading, it should be included here. Row headings are capitalized according to the style for sentences, not titles. Therefore, if a symbol (such as %), an arabic numeral, or a lowercase Greek letter (such as β) begins the entry, the first major word to follow should be capitalized. Row headings are left-justified, and indents are typically used to depict hierarchical relationships (**Table 4.1-6**). However, some publications use bold or shading instead.

For a table that may be readily divided into parts to enhance clarity or for 2 closely related tables that would be better combined, cut-in headings may be used. A cut-in heading may be set in boldface type to draw the reader's attention. It is placed above the table columns but below the column heads and applies to all the tabular material in the portion of the table immediately below it (**Table 4.1-7**). The cells with "NA" (under "Chronic pancreatitis") indicate "not applicable" because the training cohort had no individuals and hence contributed no data.

In some publications, cut-in headings are centered. However, centered cut-in headings may interfere with downward scanning and may not be as readable and thus should be used with care.[3,4]

Both column headings and row headings should be consistent in style and presentation between tables in the same article.

**Table 4.1-6.** Hierarchy of Stubs (Row Headings)

**Table.** Characteristics of Men With Androgen Deprivation Therapy Use

| Characteristic | Data value |
| --- | --- |
| No. of men | 35 487 |
| Age at index date, y | |
|    Mean (SD) | 75.67 (5.93) |
|    Median (IQR) | 75 (71-80) |
| Income quintile, No. (%) | |
|    1 (Lowest) | 5093 (14.4) |
|    2 | 5959 (16.8) |
|    3 | 5866 (16.5) |
|    4 | 5954 (16.8) |
|    5 (Highest) | 6455 (18.2) |
| Living in rural area, No. (%) | 6160 (17.4) |
| Prior diagnosis of osteoporosis, No. (%) | 1387 (3.9) |
| Prior fragility fracture, No. (%) | 774 (2.2) |
| Charlson Comorbidity Index score, median (IQR) | 0 (0-0) |

Abbreviation: IQR, interquartile range.

**Table 4.1-7.** Cut-in Headings Divide the Table Into Related Sections

**Table.** Demographics of Patients and Healthy Participants in the Discovery, Training, and Validation Cohorts[a]

| | No. (%) of patients and healthy participants[b] | | |
|---|---|---|---|
| | Discovery cohort (n = 230) | Training cohort (n = 379) | Validation cohort (n = 137) |
| **Pancreatic cancer** | 143 (62) | 180 (47) | 86 (63) |
| Sex | | | |
|   Men | 88 (61.5) | 102 (56.7) | 49 (57) |
|   Women | 55 (38.5) | 78 (43.3) | 37 (43) |
| Age, median (range), y | 65 (38-75) | 68 (37-89) | 67 (46-86) |
| Resection of tumors | | | |
|   Yes | 23 (16.0) | 10 (5.6) | 11 (12.8) |
|   No | 120 (84.0) | 170 (94.4) | 75 (87.2) |
| Cancer stage | | | |
|   IA | 3 (2.1) | 2 (1.1) | 1 (1.2) |
|   IB | 2 (1.4) | 2 (1.1) | 0 |
|   IIA | 11 (7.7) | 7 (3.9) | 1 (1.2) |
|   IIB | 14 (9.8) | 15 (8.3) | 12 (14.0) |
|   III | 26 (18.2) | 44 (24.4) | 22 (25.6) |
|   IV | 87 (60.8) | 107 (59.4) | 50 (58.1) |
|   Unknown | 0 | 3 (1.7) | 0 |
| Serum CA19-9, median (range), kU/L | 791 (3-608 500) | 508 (1-467 000) | 435 (2-182 300) |
| **Chronic pancreatitis** | 18 (8) | 0 | 7 (5) |
| Sex | | | |
|   Men | 13 (72.2) | NA | 3 (42.9) |
|   Women | 5 (27.8) | NA | 4 (57.1) |
| Age, median (range), y | 54 (33-67) | NA | 56 (47-85) |
| Serum CA19-9, median (range), kU/L | 27 (3-1134) | NA | 41 (3-159) |
| **Healthy participants** | 69 (30) | 199 (53) | 44 (32) |
| Sex | | | |
|   Men | 31 (44.9) | 95 (47.7) | 22 (50.0) |
|   Women | 38 (55.1) | 104 (52.3) | 22 (50.0) |
| Age, median (range), y | 53 (33-66) | 50 (18-66) | 55 (41-65) |
| Serum CA19-9, median (range), kU/L | NA | NA | 4 (3-40) |

Abbreviation: CA19-9, cancer antigen 19-9; NA, not applicable.

[a] More information is provided in the Supplement (see Patients).

[b] Unless otherwise indicated.

**4.1.4.5** **Field.** The field or body of the table presents the data. Each data entry point is contained in a cell, which is the intersection of a column and a row. Table cells may contain numerals, text, symbols, or a combination of these. However, all data must be consistent with their row and column headings. Data in the field should be arranged logically, either by sensibly ordering the rows and column headings, which helps readers find the value of interest, or by ordering the values, which can help reveal patterns in the data. For instance, time order should be used for data collected in sequence (Table 4.1-1). Similar types of data should be grouped. Numbers that are summed or averaged should be placed in the same column. Text in the field cells should be capitalized in sentence style (ie, the first word is capitalized and all words that follow in the cell are lowercased except proper nouns). Justified margins are not recommended because the spacing between words can be uneven, impairing readability.[1] For example, the JAMA Network journals set columns with text and numbers primarily flush left.

Missing data and blank space in the table field (ie, an empty cell) may create ambiguity and should be avoided, unless an entry in a cell does not apply (eg, a column head does not apply to one of the stub items).[4] Use of ellipses in cells is also ambiguous and should be avoided. The numeral 0 should be used only to indicate that the value of the data in the cell is zero. Designations such as NA (for "not available," "not analyzed," or "not applicable") may be used, provided their meaning is explained in a footnote.

Blank cells may be acceptable when an entire section of the table does not contain data, or the use of "NA" is acceptable.

**4.1.4.6** **Merged Cells.** In some tables, values may apply across multiple rows of the table, either because they belong to various subgroups or because the analysis was performed across categories. One of the ways this can be illustrated is by merging the cells (usually in the right-most column) to depict this relationship (see the last 4 columns in **Table 4.1-8**).

**4.1.4.7** **Totals.** Totals and percentages in tables should correspond to values presented in the text and abstract and should be verified for accuracy. Any discrepancies (eg, because of rounding) should be explained in a footnote.

Boldface type for true totals (ie, those that represent sums of values in the table) should be used with discretion, although the JAMA Network journals typically do not do this. Boldface should not be used to overemphasize data in the table (eg, significant odds ratios or $P$ values).

**4.1.4.8** **Alignment of Data.** Horizontal alignment (across rows) must be considered in setting tables. If the table row heading column contains lines of text that exceed the width of the column (*runover lines*) and the cell entries in that row do not, the field entries should be aligned across the first or top line of the entry (Table 4.1-9). This top-line alignment of data applies to tables that have numbers, words, or both as cell entries. If some entries within the table field contain information that cannot be contained on a single line in the cell (runover lines in the

**Table 4.1-8.** Rows Merged Vertically to Show That the Adjusted Mean Differences, Accompanying 95% CIs, and P Values Were Computed Across Subcategories

**Table.** Unadjusted and Adjusted Difference Scores of BREAST-Q Patient-Reported Outcomes (PROs)

| BREAST-Q survey | Cohort | Unadjusted scores, mean (SD) | | | Adjusted mean difference (95% CI)[a] | | | |
|---|---|---|---|---|---|---|---|---|
| | | Baseline | 1 y Postoperative | 2 y Postoperative | 1 y Postoperative | P value | 2 y Postoperative | P value |
| Satisfaction with breast | Fat grafted | 58.7 (21.5) | 60.1 (16.7) | 65.6 (17.1) | −4.74 (−8.21 to −1.28) | .008 | −0.68 (−4.42 to 3.06) | .72 |
| | No fat graft | 59.2 (22.5) | 66.1 (17.2) | 66.0 (18.3) | | | | |
| Psychosocial well-being | Fat grafted | 68.4 (18.7) | 67.2 (19.3) | 73.2 (19.2) | −3.87 (−7.33 to −0.40) | .03 | −0.59 (−3.92 to 2.74) | .73 |
| | No fat graft | 68.8 (18.5) | 73.5 (19.2) | 75.3 (19.1) | | | | |
| Physical well-being | Fat grafted | 77.2 (16.0) | 72.5 (13.5) | 74.8 (15.2) | −1.23 (−3.71 to 1.25) | .33 | −0.50 (−3.36 to 2.36) | .73 |
| | No fat graft | 78.4 (14.7) | 76.2 (14.9) | 76.8 (14.9) | | | | |
| Sexual well-being | Fat grafted | 55.7 (20.3) | 48.0 (20.5) | 52.8 (20.9) | −5.59 (−9.70 to −1.47) | .008 | −2.94 (−7.01 to 1.12) | .15 |
| | No fat graft | 54.4 (20.9) | 54.7 (21.0) | 55.4 (21.9) | | | | |

[a]Fat-grafted and non–fat-grafted differences based on mixed-effects regression models with each PRO measured at 1 or 2 years postoperatively as the dependent variable. Each model included an indicator for fat grafting between years 1 and 2 as the primary predictor, and included as covariates baseline PRO, age, body mass index, procedure type, laterality, indication for mastectomy, timing of reconstruction, radiotherapy, smoking history, race, ethnicity, fat grafting before year 1 PRO measures, concurrent revision procedure, cancer recurrence, and prior complication. Also included are random intercepts for study sites (hospitals) and an interaction variable between fat grafting and concurrent revision procedures. Analyses were performed and combined using 10 imputed data sets.

**Table 4.1-9.** Alignment of Data With the First Line in the Stub Entry

**Table.** Response of IOP at Final Follow-up at 6 Months

| Outcome | SLT (n = 50) | PGA (n = 50) | Mean difference (95% CI) | P value |
|---|---|---|---|---|
| BCVA | | | | |
|   Mean (SD), logMAR | 0.12 (0.12) | 0.09 (0.12) | −0.02 (−0.07 to 0.03) | .57 |
|   Mean Snellen equivalent | 20/32 | 20/25 | | |
| IOP, mean (SD), mm Hg | 19.5 (3.3) | 18.1 (2.4) | −1.2 (−2.5 to −0.15) | .05 |
| Mean change in IOP from baseline (95% CI), mm Hg | 4.0 (3.2 to 4.8) | 4.2 (3.5 to 4.9) | 0.2 (−0.8 to 1.3) | .78 |
| Adjusted mean change in IOP from baseline (95% CI), mm Hg[a] | 3.7 (3.7 to 4.5) | 4.4 (3.8 to 5.2) | 0.7 (−0.3 to 1.7) | .17 |
| Change in IOP from baseline, mean (SD), % | 16.9 (12.1) | 18.5 (10.6) | 1.5 (−2.9 to 6.0) | .52 |

Abbreviations: BCVA, best-corrected visual acuity; IOP, intraocular pressure; PGA, prostaglandin analogue; SLT, selective laser trabeculoplasty.

[a] Adjusted for baseline differences in IOP.

table field), the table entries in that row also should be aligned across on the first line of the row heading entry (Table 4.1-5).

Vertical alignment within each column of a table is important for the visual presentation of data. In some publications, data are aligned on common elements, such as decimal points, plus or minus signs, hyphens (used in ranges), virgules, or parentheses.

For an explanation of the use of "to" vs a hyphen in ranges with negative numbers (Table 4.1-9), see 8.3.1.3, Expressing Ranges and Dimensions.

However, in some journals, including the JAMA Network journals, all columns are set flush left whether the cell contains text or data.

**4.1.4.9** **Rules and Shading.** Some journals add rules and shading during the production process. For example, the JAMA Network journals use horizontal rules to separate rows of data. Other journals use shading for the same purpose (**Table 4.1-10**). The JAMA Network journals request that tables be submitted without rules drawn in (as opposed to table borders, which are appropriate) or shading. If these elements are included they will be manually removed during the editing process (see 4.1.10, Guidelines for Preparing and Submitting Tables).

**4.1.4.10** **Footnotes.** Footnotes may contain information about the entire table, portions of the table (eg, a column), or a discrete table entry. The order of the footnotes is determined by the placement in the table of the item to which the footnote refers. The letter for a footnote that applies to the entire table (eg, one that explains the method used to gather the data or format of data presentation) should be placed after the table title. A footnote that applies to 1 or 2 columns or rows should be placed after the heading(s) to which it refers. A footnote that applies to a single

**Table 4.1-10.** Shading Used to Separate Rows of Data

**Table.** Baseline Characteristics of Study Participants by Ferritin Level

| | Ferritin ≤26 ng/mL | | Ferritin >26 ng/mL | |
| --- | --- | --- | --- | --- |
| | Iron (n = 51) | No iron (n = 50) | Iron (n = 60) | No iron (n = 54) |
| Number (%) women | 33 (64.7) | 31 (62.0) | 38 (63.3) | 34 (63.0) |
| Number (%) ≥60 y old | 12 (23.5) | 11 (22.0) | 17 (28.3) | 12 (22.2) |
| Age, mean (SD), years | 47.5 (15.5) | 45.9 (15.7) | 49.3 (14.6) | 48.1 (14.6) |
| Weight, mean (SD), kg | 75.9 (16.4) | 76.8 (15.8) | 81.5 (16.4) | 77.9 (16.2) |
| Hemoglobin, mean (SD), g/dL | 13.2 (1.0) | 13.7 (1.3) | 14.1 (1.0) | 14.3 (1.2) |
| Ferritin, mean (SD), ng/mL | 14.9 (5.8) | 15.2 (6.0) | 54.0 (24.3) | 58.9 (32.9) |
| Soluble transferrin receptor, mean (SD), mg/L | 4.0 (1.33) | 3.9 (1.19) | 3.1 (0.65) | 3.1 (0.62) |
| Estimated blood volume, mean (SD), L | 4.59 (0.8) | 4.66 (0.91) | 4.79 (0.84) | 4.64 (0.84) |

SI conversion factor: To convert ferritin to pmol/L, multiply by 2.247.

entry in the table or to several individual entries should be placed at the end of each entry to which it applies.

For both tables and figures, footnotes are indicated with superscript lowercase letters in alphabetical order (a-z). The font size of the footnote letters should be large enough to see clearly without appearing to be part of the actual data. For tables in which superscript numbers and/or letters are used to display data, care should be taken to ensure that superscript footnote letters are distinguished clearly from superscripts used for data elements. Although some publications use symbols (*, †, etc) to indicate footnotes in tables, such symbols are ordered arbitrarily and are limited in number. Use of superscript letters ensures a logical order to the entries and a much larger supply of notations (26 characters). In addition, use of letters reduces the likelihood that the symbol could be misinterpreted as an exponent or reference citation.[4]

Footnotes are listed at the bottom of the table, each on its own line. However, to save space, tables with more than a few footnotes can use 2 columns for the footnotes (**Table 4.1-11**).

Journals often have underlying grids to permit different sizes of tables to run in a standard 2- or 3-column print format. For example, tables can be sized to fill 1.5 columns of content and footnotes run in the space beside the table (**Table 4.1-12**).

Footnotes may be phrases or complete sentences and should end with a period. Any operational signs, such as <, >, or =, imply a verb. For example, $P = .01$ is considered a complete sentence ("$P$ is equal to .01.") when used as a table footnote. Footnote letters should appear before the footnote text (preferably in superscript to distinguish them from the text) and are followed by a space for clarity. In addition, in the JAMA Network journals, the abbreviations and units of measure conversion footnotes appear first and are set off with an introductory word or phrase instead of a letter. In such footnotes, abbreviations are expanded in alphabetical order, and units of measure are listed by consecutive mention in the table (**Table 4.1-13**).

## 4.1 Tables

**Table 4.1-11.** When Tables Span the Width of the Page or Have Many Footnotes, They Can Be Presented in 2 Columns Instead of With a Single Footnote on Each Line

**Table.** Univariable and Multivariable Analyses of the Association Between at Least Moderate PVR and 1-Year Outcomes

| End point | Univariable analysis | | Multivariable analysis[a] | |
|---|---|---|---|---|
| | HR (95% CI)[b] | P value | HR (95% CI) | P value |
| All-cause mortality | 2.40 (1.30-4.43) | .005 | 2.59 (1.39-4.85) | .003 |
| Cardiovascular mortality | 2.68 (1.24-5.81) | .01 | 2.87 (1.30-6.30) | .009 |
| Rehospitalization | 2.27 (1.34-3.83) | .002 | 2.27 (1.31-3.94) | .003 |
| Composite of mortality and rehospitalization | 2.35 (1.52-3.62) | .001 | 2.36 (1.50-3.69) | <.001 |
| Aortic valve reintervention | 13.14 (3.39-50.85) | <.001 | NA | NA |

Abbreviations: HR, hazard ratio; NA, not applicable; PVR, paravalvular regurgitation; STS, Society of Thoracic Surgeons.

[a] Adjusted for age, sex, body mass index, STS score, diabetes, at least moderate baseline aortic regurgitation, and at least moderate baseline mitral regurgitation.

[b] Hazard ratio is for at least moderate PVR vs less than moderate PVR. Multivariable analysis was not performed for aortic valve reintervention because there were only 10 events.

**Table 4.1-12.** A Partial-Width Table (1.5 Columns in This Publication) With the Footnotes Beside the Table, Aligned With the Bottom of the Table

**Table.** Use of the Intervention Components Among Individuals in the Intervention Group and Smoking Cessation Rates by Component

| Component use | Individuals in the intervention group who quit smoking, No./Total (%) (n = 399) | | | |
|---|---|---|---|---|
| | Used intervention component | Did not use intervention component | P value | |
| Spoke to the tobacco treatment specialist | 58/274 (21.2) | 13/125 (10.4) | .01 | |
| Received nicotine replacement patches[a] | 50/218 (22.9) | 8/56 (14.3) | .16 | |
| Received a HelpSteps.com referral[a] | 30/128 (23.4) | 28/146 (19.2) | .39 | |
| Reported using a HelpSteps.com referral[b] | 24/55 (43.6) | 34/219 (15.3) | <.001 | |

[a] Among intervention participants who spoke to the tobacco treatment specialist.

[b] Among intervention participants who spoke to the tobacco treatment specialist and received a HelpSteps.com referral.

If several tables share a detailed or long footnote that explains several abbreviations or methods, this footnote may appear in the first table for which it is applicable, and a footnote in each succeeding table for which the footnote also is applicable may refer the reader to the first appearance of the detailed information:

Study acronyms are explained in the first footnote to Table 1.

**Table 4.1-13.** The Factor for Converting Total Serum Bilirubin Values to SI Units Is Provided in a Separate Footnote

**Table.** Risk for CP Associated With Varying Elevated TSB Levels

| | No. of infants | | Absolute CP risk, % | | Absolute risk difference (95% CI), % |
|---|---|---|---|---|---|
| | CP | Exposed | | Relative risk (95% CI) | |
| Elevation of TSB level >ETT, mg/dL | | | | | |
| <0 | 86 | 104 716 | 0.1 | 1 [Reference] | [Reference] |
| 0-4.9 | 4 | 1705 | 0.2 | 2.9 (1.0 to 7.8) | 0.2 (0 to 0.5) |
| 5.0-9.9 | 1 | 102 | 1.0 | 11.9 (1.7 to 84.9) | 0.9 (0.1 to 5.3) |
| ≥10.0 | 2 | 26 | 7.7 | 93.7 (24 to 361) | 7.6 (2.1 to 24.1) |
| Peak TSB level, mg/dL | | | | | |
| <20.0 | 87 | 103 271 | 0.1 | 1 [Reference] | [Reference] |
| 20.0-24.9 | 2 | 2772 | 0.1 | 0.9 (0.2 to 3.5) | 0 (−0.1 to 0.2) |
| 25.0-29.9 | 2 | 459 | 0.4 | 5.2 (1.3 to 20.9) | 0.4 (0 to 1.5) |
| 30.0-34.9 | 0 | 32 | 0.0 | NA | −0.1 (−0.1 to 10.6) |
| ≥35.0 | 2 | 15 | 13.3 | 158.0 (43.0 to 585.0) | 13.2 (3.7 to 37.8) |

Abbreviations: CP, cerebral palsy; ETT, exchange transfusion threshold; NA, not applicable; TSB, total serum bilirubin.

SI conversion factor: To convert TSB to μmol/L, multiply by 17.104.

The reader also may be referred to a relevant discussion in the text by a footnote:

See the Statistical Analysis section for a description of this procedure.

Several of the most common uses of footnotes include the following:
To expand abbreviations:

Abbreviations: OR, odds ratio; RR, relative risk.

To designate reporting of numerical values:

[a]Scores are based on a scale of 1 to 10, with 1 indicating least severe and 10, most severe.

To provide information on statistical analyses or experimental methods:

[b]Adjusted for age, smoking status, and body mass index.

To explain a discrepancy in numerical data:

[a]Because of rounding, percentages may not total 100.

To cite references for information used in the table:

[c]*International Classification of Health Problems in Primary Care.*[45]

To acknowledge that data in the table are taken from or based on data from another source:

[a]Data from the US Census Bureau.[5]

To acknowledge credit for reproduction of a table (if the table has been reprinted or modified with permission from another source, credit should be given in a footnote):

[a]Reproduced with permission of the *AMA Manual of Style*. American Medical Association, 2020.

[a]Adapted with permission from Vega and Avner.[41]

References for information in a table or figure should be numbered and listed as if this information were part of the text. For instance, if the source from which the material referred to in the table or figure is one of the references used in the text, that reference number should be used in the table or figure. If the reference pertains only to the table or figure (ie, the source is not cited elsewhere in the text), the reference should be listed and numbered according to the first mention of the table or figure in the text (see 3.6, Citation). All references in an article should appear in the reference list.

Note that references cited at the end of table titles are ambiguous. Instead, a footnote should be added to explain the source of the data.

Adapted from. . .

Reproduced with permission from. . .

Data were derived from. . .

When both a footnote letter and reference number follow data in a table, set the reference number first, followed by a comma and the footnote letter (see 3.6, Citation):

427 Patients[5,b]

**4.1.5** **Units of Measure.** The JAMA Network journals report laboratory values in conventional units (see 13.12, Units of Measure, and 17.0, Units of Measure). In tables, units of measure, including the variability of the measurement, if reported, should follow a comma in the column or row heading:

Age, mean (SD), y

Systolic blood pressure, mean (SD), mm Hg

Body mass index, median (IQR)

Duration of hypertension, mean (SD) [range], y

Change in rate, % (95% CI)

The JAMA Network journals use a conversion footnote to indicate how to convert values to the SI or another system (Table 4.1-13). See 17.5, Conventional Units and SI Units in JAMA Network Journals.

**4.1.6** **Punctuation.** As with numbers and abbreviations, rules for punctuation may be less restrictive in tables to save space (see 8.0, Punctuation). For example, virgules may be used to present dates (eg, 4/02/17 for April 2, 2017) and hyphens may be used to present ranges (eg, 60-90 for 60 to 90) (see 18.0, Numbers and Percentages).

However, when virgules are used to present dates, consider that some international readers place the day before the month in such constructions, causing 4/02/17 to be interpreted as February 4, 2017, instead of April 2, 2017. Also, if any range in a table includes a negative number, the word *to* should replace the hyphen in all ranges in that row or column to avoid a hyphen followed by a minus sign as well as for consistent presentation within the table (eg, −13.7 to −4.3) (Table 4.1-8 and Table 4.1-9). Phrases and sentences in tables may use end punctuation if required for readability (eg, if cells contain multisentence entries).

**4.1.7** **Abbreviations.** Within the body of the table and in column and row headings, units of measure and numbers normally spelled out may be abbreviated for space considerations (see 13.12, Abbreviations, Units of Measure; 17.0, Units of Measure; and 18.0, Numbers and Percentages). However, spelled-out words should not be combined with abbreviations for units of measure. For example, "First Week" or "1st wk" or "Week 1" may be used as a column heading, but not "First wk." Abbreviations or acronyms (but not abbreviations used to indicate units of measure) should be explained in a footnote (see 4.1.4.10, Table Components, Footnotes).

**4.1.8** **Numbers.** Additional digits (including zeros) should not be added (eg, after the decimal point) to provide all data entries with the same number of digits. Doing so may indicate more precise results than actually were calculated or measured. A percentage or decimal quotient should contain no more than the number of digits in the denominator. For example, the percentage for the proportion 9 of 28 should be reported as 32% (or decimal quotient 0.32), not 32.1% (or 0.321) (see 19.4, Significant Digits and Rounding Numbers). Values reporting laboratory data should be provided and rounded, if appropriate, according to the number of digits that reflects the precision of the reported results to eliminate reporting results beyond the sensitivity of the procedure performed (see 17.4.1, Expressing Quantities).

Values for reporting statistical data, such as *P* values and CIs, also should be presented and rounded appropriately (see 19.4, Significant Digits and Rounding Numbers). Although some publications[3(p512)] suggest use of specific designations for levels of significance (eg, a single asterisk in the table to denote values for entries with $P < .05$, 2 asterisks for $P < .01$), exact *P* values are preferred, regardless of statistical significance. In most cases, *P* values should be expressed to 2 digits to the right of the decimal point unless the first 2 digits are zeros, in which case 3 digits to the right of the decimal place should be provided (eg, instead of $P < .01$, report as $P = .002$). However, values close to .05 may be reported to 3 decimal places because the .05 is an arbitrary cut point for statistical significance (eg, $P = .053$, $P = .047$). *P* values less than .001 should be designated as "$P < .001$" rather than exact values (eg, $P = .00006$). For some studies, it is important to express *P* values to more significant digits, such as genome-wide association studies, studies that involve Bonferroni correction, and other types of studies with adjustments for multiple comparisons, and when the level of significance is defined as substantially less than $P < .05$. For very small numbers, scientific notation may be used to express the value (eg, a genome-wide significant association of $P = 1.1 \times 10^{-8}$) (see 19.5, Glossary of Statistical Terms, *P* value).

For study outcomes, individual statistically significant values should not be expressed as "*P* < .05" either in the table or in the table footnote, and nonsignificant *P* values should not be expressed as "NS" (not significant). For CIs, the number of digits should correspond to the number of digits in the point estimate. For instance, for an odds ratio reported as 2.45, the 95% CI should be reported as 1.32 to 4.78, not as 1.322 to 4.784.

**4.1.9** **Tables That Contain Online-Only Supplementary Information.** Tables that contain important supplementary information that is too extensive to be published in the journal article may be made available from other sources, including the journal's website, or other means (eg, online database, institutional website). Online-only supplementary tables posted with an article on a journal's website should undergo review because they are considered part of the article's content.[5,6]

**4.1.10** **Guidelines for Preparing and Submitting Tables.** Authors submitting tables in a scientific article should consult the publication's instructions for authors for specific requirements and preferences regarding table format. Although details about preferred table construction vary among journals, several general guidelines apply. Each table should be created using the table functionality in the word processing software or spreadsheet program and inserted in the electronic manuscript file. Reduced type should not be used. For most journals, if a table is too large to be contained on 1 manuscript page, the table should be continued on another page with a "continued" line after the title on the subsequent page. Alternatively, if the table is large or exceedingly complex, the author should consider separating the data into 2 or more simpler tables. Tables should not be submitted on oversized paper, as a graphic image, or as photographic prints.

An example of table creation instructions are provided for authors submitting manuscripts to the JAMA Network journals (**Box 4.1-2**).

**4.2** **Figures.** The term *figure* refers to any graphical display used to present information or data,[4] including statistical graphs, maps, matrixes, algorithms, illustrations, digital images, photographs, and other clinical images. Figures may be used to clarify or explain methods, to present evidence and quantitative results, to highlight trends and associations or relationships among data, to clarify complex concepts, or to illustrate items or procedures. Figures should be accurate, clear, and concise. As with tables, the figure with its title and legend should be understandable without undue reference to the text.

In scientific articles, the choice of a particular type of figure depends on the purpose and type of information being displayed. Some of the most common types of figures in biomedical publications are discussed herein.

**4.2.1** **Statistical Graphs.**

**4.2.1.1** **Line Graphs.** Line graphs have 2 or 3 axes with continuous scales on which data points connected by curves show the association or relationship between 2 or more variables, such as changes over time. In general, line graphs are not ideal for displaying values where connection between points would imply continuity that may not be in evidence.[7] Line graphs usually are designed with the dependent variable on the vertical axis (y-axis) and the independent variable on the horizontal

**Box 4.1-2.** Author Instructions for Table Creation

### Creating the table

Use the table editor of the word processing software to build a table. Regardless of which program is used, each piece of data needs to be contained in its own cell in the table.

Avoid creating tables using spaces or tabs. Such tables must be retyped during the editing process, creating delays and opportunities for error. Do not try to align cells with hard returns or extra spaces. Similarly, no cell should contain a hard return or tab. Although individual empty cells are acceptable in a table, be sure there are no empty columns.

Each row of data must be in a separate row of cells:

**Table 1.** Title

| Treatment | Group A | Group B |
| --- | --- | --- |
| Medical | 500 | 510 |
| Surgical | 500 | 490 |

Note that percentages are presented in the same cell as numbers and measures of variability are in the same cell as their corresponding statistic:

**Table 2.** Title

| Characteristic | Group A (n = 50) | Group B (n = 50) | Relative risk (95% CI) |
| --- | --- | --- | --- |
| Women, No. (%) | 25 (50) | 20 (40) | 1.25 (1.11-1.57) |
| Age, mean (SD), y | 35 (8) | 37 (7) | 0.98 (0.92-1.05) |

To indicate data that span more than 1 row, merge the cells vertically and use centered vertical alignment in the merged cell as shown in the example below.

**Table 3.** Title

| Age, y | Blood pressure, mm Hg | *P* value |
| --- | --- | --- |
| 18-34 | 120/75 | |
| 35-50 | 110/80 | .08 |
| 51-80 | 125/82 | |

axis (x-axis).[4] If justified, a secondary vertical axis[8] may be used to display an additional set of data (**Figure 4.2-1** and **Figure 4.2-2**) (see 4.2.6.1, Components of Figures, Scales for Graphs).

Axes should be continuous; broken axes disrupt any correlation between the large and small values, and the data are not easy to compare. Tick marks provide reference for points on a scale. Each tick mark represents a specified number of units on a continuous scale or the value of a category on a categorical scale. Tick marks should project to the outside of the graph, and intervals between tick marks in general should be regular and predictable to avoid confusion. Data markers should align with ticks, not fall between them. When relevant, show variability of data points in both directions and ensure that what the variability represents (eg, 95% CI) is identified (see 4.2.6.3, Components of Figures, Error Bars).

**4.2.1.2**     **Survival Plots.** Survival plots of time-to-event outcomes, such as those from Kaplan-Meier survival analyses, display the proportion or percentage of individuals, represented on the y-axis, remaining free of or experiencing a specific outcome over time, represented on the x-axis. When the outcome of interest is relatively

frequent (eg, occurs in approximately ≥70% of the study population), event-free
survival may be plotted on the y-axis from 0 to 1.0 (or 0% to 100%), with the curve
starting at 1.0 (100%). When the outcome is relatively infrequent (eg, occurs in
<30% of the study population), it may be preferable to plot upward starting at 0 so

**Figure 4.2-1.**   Graph With the Dependent Variable on the Vertical Axis (y-Axis) and the
Independent Variable on the Horizontal Axis (x-Axis)

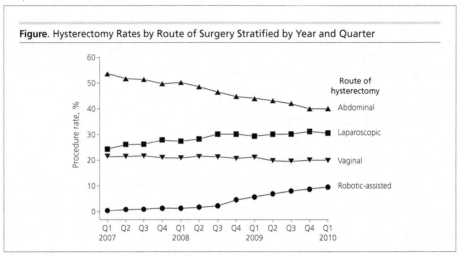

**Figure.** Hysterectomy Rates by Route of Surgery Stratified by Year and Quarter

**Figure 4.2-2.**   Graph With 3 Axes (an x-Axis, a y-Axis, and a Secondary y-Axis) to Facilitate
Comparison of Related Data

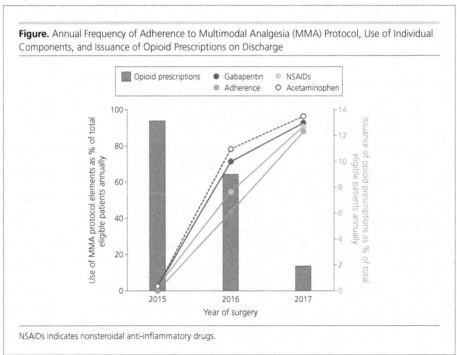

**Figure.** Annual Frequency of Adherence to Multimodal Analgesia (MMA) Protocol, Use of Individual
Components, and Issuance of Opioid Prescriptions on Discharge

NSAIDs indicates nonsteroidal anti-inflammatory drugs.

that the curves, which plot cumulative incidence,[9,10] can be seen without breaking or truncating the y-axis scale (**Figure 4.2-3**).[11] The curve should be drawn as a step function (not smoothed), and the y-axis label should specify the outcome plotted (eg, survival or disease recurrence).

The number of individuals included in the analysis at each interval (number at risk) should be shown underneath the x-axis. Time-to-event estimates become less certain as the number of individuals diminishes, so consideration should be given to not displaying data when less than 20% of the study population is still in follow-up.[11] Plots should include some indication of statistical uncertainty, such as error bars on the curves at regular time points or, when time-to-event data are being compared for 2 or more groups, an overall estimate of treatment difference, such as a relative risk (with 95% CI) or log-rank *P* value. This information can be placed within the graph (Figure 4.2-3).

**Figure 4.2-3.** Survival Curves Showing Time-to-Event Outcomes Plotted Downward (Top) or Upward (Bottom), Depending on the Frequency of the Occurrence (Variable of Interest)

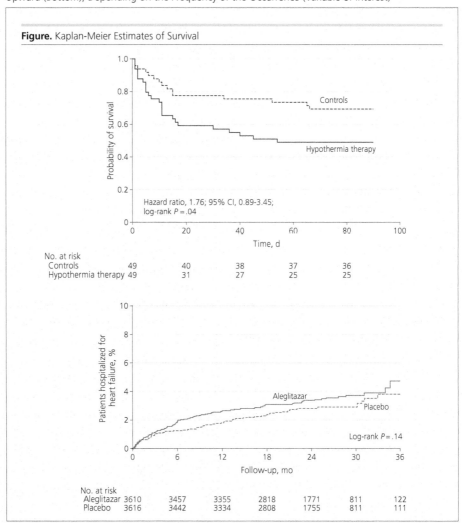

**Figure 4.2-4.**   Scatterplot With the Regression Line, Correlation Statistic, and *P* Value in the Plot

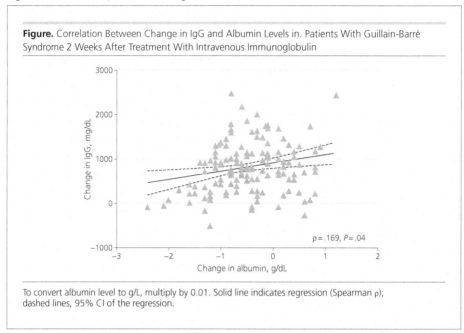

**Figure.** Correlation Between Change in IgG and Albumin Levels in. Patients With Guillain-Barré Syndrome 2 Weeks After Treatment With Intravenous Immunoglobulin

To convert albumin level to g/L, multiply by 0.01. Solid line indicates regression (Spearman ρ); dashed lines, 95% CI of the regression.

**4.2.1.3** **Scatterplots.** Scatterplots, graphs that represent bivariate data as points on a 2-dimensional Cartesian plane,[12] are useful to convey an overall impression of the relationship between 2 variables.[7] In scatterplots, individual data points are plotted according to coordinate values with continuous x- and y-axis scales. By convention, independent variables are plotted on the x-axis and dependent variables on the y-axis. Data markers are not connected by a curve, but a curve that is generated mathematically may be fitted to the data (not connecting any points but drawn through "the center") to summarize the relationship among the variables. The statistical method used to generate the curve and the statistic that summarizes the relationship or association between the dependent and independent variables, such as a correlation or regression coefficient, should be provided in the figure or legend along with the sample size, the *P* value for the slope of the line, and some indication of how the *P* value was derived[1] (**Figure 4.2-4**).

**4.2.1.4** **Histograms and Frequency Polygons.** Histograms and frequency polygons display the distribution of data in a data set by plotting the frequency (count or percentages) of observations (on the y-axis) for each interval represented on the x-axis. In both histograms and frequency polygons, the y-axis must begin at 0 and should not be broken, and the x-axis is a continuous, quantitative scale. Histograms are plotted with continuous bars of equal width determined by the x-axis intervals, in which bar height represents frequency (counts or percentages) so long as the bars are of equal width. For additional detail on these statistics, see Haighton et al.[13] No spacing is used between bars—they are either closed up or separated with a very thin white line (**Figure 4.2-5**).

Frequency polygons use data markers (representing the tops of the columns of a histogram) to represent frequency connected by a curve. Data distributions from multiple data sets that overlap can be plotted in a frequency polygon but not in a histogram (**Figure 4.2-6**). A frequency polygon (or histogram) is used to display the entire frequency distribution (counts) of a continuous variable.

**Figure 4.2-5.** Histogram Showing Frequencies for Each Period (Bar Height Represents Percentage of Cases)

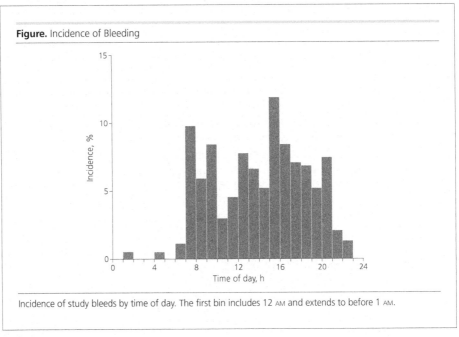

**Figure.** Incidence of Bleeding

Incidence of study bleeds by time of day. The first bin includes 12 AM and extends to before 1 AM.

**Figure 4.2-6.** Frequency Polygons Can Illustrate Distributions for Multiple Groups or, as In This Figure, Infection Types

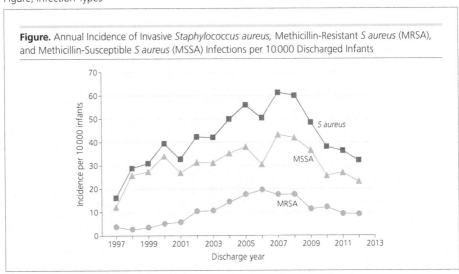

**Figure.** Annual Incidence of Invasive *Staphylococcus aureus,* Methicillin-Resistant *S aureus* (MRSA), and Methicillin-Susceptible *S aureus* (MSSA) Infections per 10 000 Discharged Infants

**4.2.1.5** **Bar Graphs.** Bar graphs are used to display frequencies (counts or percentages) according to categories shown on a baseline or x-axis. Bar graphs also allow subcategories, making it easy to compare within and between categories. Bar graphs are less ideal for showing trends over time because readers must visually connect the tops of the bars.[7] Bar graphs are not appropriate for representing summary statistics (eg, means with SDs or odds ratios with 95% CIs). A bar graph is often vertical, with frequencies shown on a vertical axis (**Figure 4.2-7**). A horizontal arrangement has advantages when the categories have long titles or when there are a large number of categories and there is insufficient space to fit all the columns required for a vertical bar chart (**Figure 4.2-8**). Data in each category are represented by a bar. Bars should have the same width, be separated by a space, and be wider than the space between them. Bar lengths are proportional to frequency, the scale on the frequency axis should begin at 0, and the axis should not be broken. All bars must have a common baseline to facilitate comparison.[14]

Categories of data should be presented in logical order and be consistent with other figures and tables in the article. The baseline of a bar graph is not a coordinate axis and therefore should not have tick marks. If the data plotted are percentages or rates, use error bars to show statistical variability (Figure 4.2-7). Because variability (error) is not always symmetrical around the values plotted, error bars should be plotted in both directions (not just above the values).[1] Note that in Figure 4.2-7 the bars are presented in the same order in each grouping and error bars show statistical variability (95% CIs).

Bar graphs may be used to compare frequencies among groups. In most cases, the number of bars in a grouped bar graph should not exceed 3. Colors or tones used to designate each group should be distinct. To ensure that bars in black-and-white figures are distinguishable, a contrast in shading of at least 30%

**Figure 4.2-7.** Vertical Bar Graph With Shading to Distinguish the 3 Groups That Are Compared

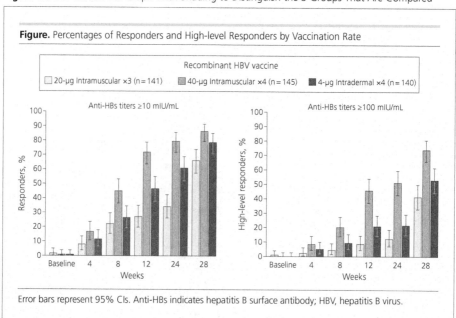

**Figure.** Percentages of Responders and High-level Responders by Vaccination Rate

Error bars represent 95% CIs. Anti-HBs indicates hepatitis B surface antibody; HBV, hepatitis B virus.

**Figure 4.2-8.** Horizontal Bar Graph With the Frequencies on the x-Axis and Categories Displayed Vertically

**Figure.** Prevalence of Albuminuria in Adults by Type of Congenital Heart Disease

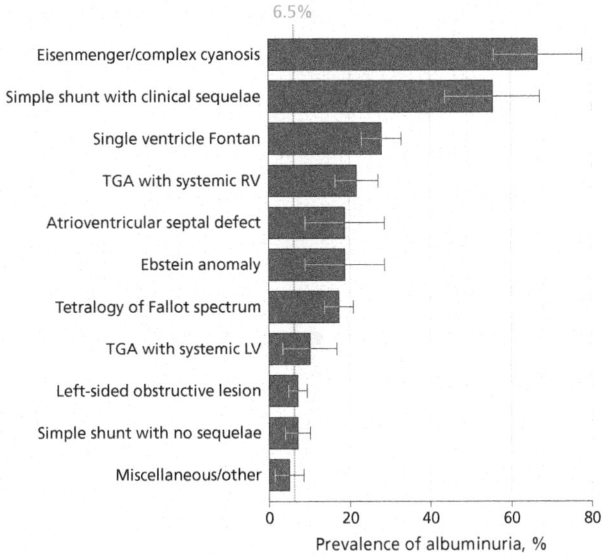

Frequency of albuminuria (defined as an albumin to creatinine ratio ≥30 mg/g) according to underlying congenital heart disease diagnosis. The solid line represents the approximate general population prevalence (6.5%). Error bars indicate 95% CIs. Subgroups included 18 patients with Eisenmenger syndrome/complex cyanosis, 18 with a simple shunt with clinical sequelae, 86 with single ventricle Fontan circulation, 60 with transposition of the great arteries (TGA) with systemic right ventricle (RV), 16 with atrioventricular septal defect, 16 with Ebstein anomaly, 126 with tetralogy of Fallot, 20 with TGA with systemic left ventricle (LV), 141 with LV obstructive lesions, 71 with a simple shunt with no sequelae, and 40 with miscellaneous other disorders.

for adjacent bars is suggested. Color or shades of gray should be used instead of patterns and cross-hatching (eg, diagonal lines) on bars (Figure 4.2-7).

**4.2.1.5.1** **Component (Stacked) Bar Graph.** Component bar graphs (or divided or stacked bar graphs) display the proportion of components constituting the total group, represented by the whole bar (**Figure 4.2-9**). Individual components are designated by distinguishing formats, such as different shading. When possible, it is preferable to use clusters of individual bars to represent each component because the only values easily interpreted in a component bar graph are the total and the end segments,[14] as is evident in Figure 4.2-9.

**4.2.1.6** **Pie Charts.** Pie charts should be avoided in scientific publications but are sometimes used in publications for lay audiences.[15] Like the component bar graph, pie charts compare relationships among component parts. Categories are represented by sections, with the area of the section being proportional to the relative frequency of each category. The angular areas of the individual components of pie

137

**Figure 4.2-9.** A Component Bar Graph

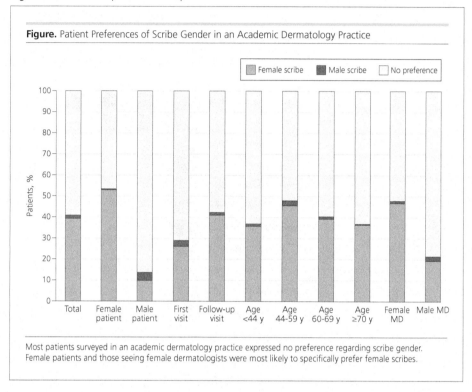

**Figure.** Patient Preferences of Scribe Gender in an Academic Dermatology Practice

Most patients surveyed in an academic dermatology practice expressed no preference regarding scribe gender. Female patients and those seeing female dermatologists were most likely to specifically prefer female scribes.

charts may be difficult to compare in series of pie charts. Usually, data depicted in pie charts can be summarized in the text or in a table.[16]

A more complex pie chart with large differences in the size of its divisions (**Figure 4.2-10**) can be reformatted as a bar graph in which the section encompassing the smaller divisions is enlarged in a second bar (**Figure 4.2-11**).

**4.2.1.7** **Dot (Point) Graphs.** Dot or point graphs display quantitative data other than counts or frequencies on a single scaled axis according to categories on a baseline (the scaled axis may be horizontal or vertical). Point estimates are represented by discrete data markers, preferably with error bars (in both directions) to designate variability (**Figure 4.2-12**).

Note the use of a baseline at y = 0 in Figure 4.2-12 when values are both positive and negative, and error bars are drawn in both directions.

**4.2.1.8** **Box and Whisker Plots.** Box and whisker plots (also known as box plots) are useful for displaying data based on their quartiles. In general, summary data presentation is best reserved for larger sample sizes; there is little point in showing data from fewer than 10 contributing sources. Box and whisker plots can provide more information about a distribution than the typical bar graph while still emphasizing the values of interest[1] and can allow readers to better compare distributions. Typically,

**Figure 4.2-10.** Example of a Complex Pie Chart

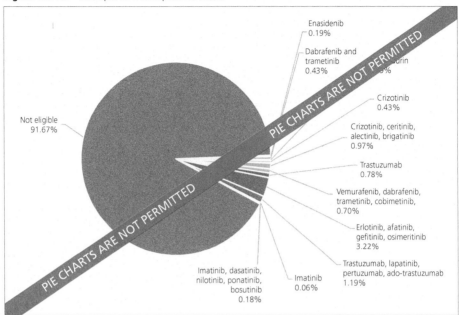

**Figure 4.2-11.** The Same Data in Figure 4.2-10 Reformatted as a Bar Graph

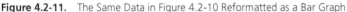
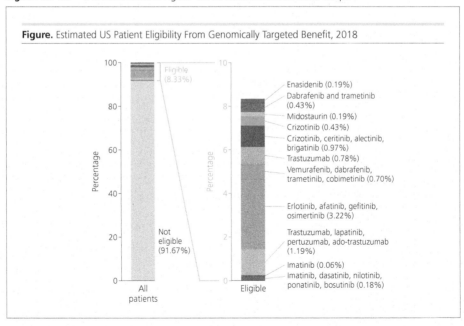

**Figure 4.2-12.** A Dot Plot (Point Estimate Graph) Depicting Categorical Data

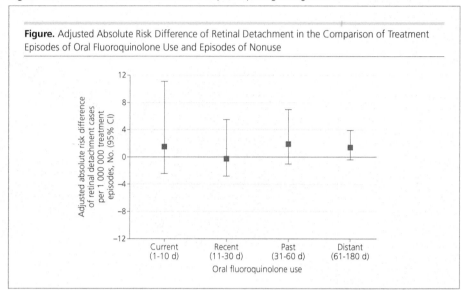

**Figure.** Adjusted Absolute Risk Difference of Retinal Detachment in the Comparison of Treatment Episodes of Oral Fluoroquinolone Use and Episodes of Nonuse

the ends of the "boxes" represent the 25th and 75th percentiles. Usually a horizontal line inside the box indicates the median or mean, and the "whiskers" represent the upper and lower adjacent values.[1] Points that fall beyond the whiskers should be shown as dots or open circles (**Figure 4.2-13**). What each element represents should be clearly indicated in the figure legend.

**4.2.1.9**  **Individual-Value Plots.** Individual values can be plotted on a graph to illustrate the full distribution of findings, for example, at different time points. The mean or median value for the group may be depicted by a horizontal line near the midpoint of the spread to illustrate the central tendency, and error bars may also be included to represent statistical variance (**Figure 4.2-14**). The horizontal lines between the upper and lower error bars in Figure 4.2-14 indicate the mean; the top and bottom error bars represent SDs.

**4.2.1.10**  **Paired Data and Spaghetti Plots.** Paired data may be plotted from each study participant and compared. Data are typically plotted at baseline and at 1 or more prespecified outcome points (**Figure 4.2-15**). If several overlapping lines with 3 or more data points each are plotted together, these graphs are called *spaghetti plots*[17,18] or *parallel coordinate line segment plots*.[19] These plots work better for a small number of study participants.[19] However, although it can be difficult to distinguish the data for the individual lines, spaghetti plots can show trends over time.[18] In Figure 4.2-15, the colored lines indicate another level of information (patients with remission are in blue).

**Figure 4.2-13.** Box and Whisker Plot With Each Element Defined in the Legend

**Figure.** Neurobehavioral Rating Scale-Agitation (NBRS-A) Subscale

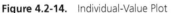

Higher NBRS-A scores indicate more severe symptoms. The horizontal bar inside the boxes indicates the median, the square in the boxes indicates the mean, and the lower and upper ends of the boxes are the first and third quartiles. The whiskers indicate values within 1.5× the interquartile range from the upper or lower quartile (or the minimum and maximum if within 1.5× the interquartile range of the quartiles) and data more extreme than the whiskers are plotted individually as outliers (shaded circles).

**Figure 4.2-14.** Individual-Value Plot

**Figure.** Association of Ticagrelor With Augmentation Index Normalized to Heart Rate

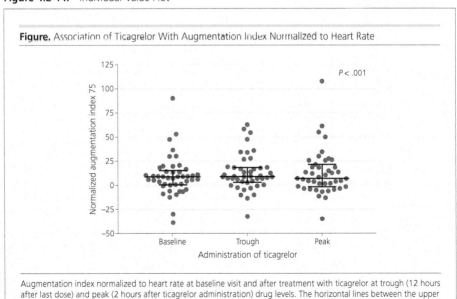

Augmentation index normalized to heart rate at baseline visit and after treatment with ticagrelor at trough (12 hours after last dose) and peak (2 hours after ticagrelor administration) drug levels. The horizontal lines between the upper and lower whisker marks indicate the mean, while the top and bottom whisker marks represent SD.

**Figure 4.2-15.** Spaghetti Plots of Scores, by Group, for Patients at Baseline and 2 Specified Measurement Times

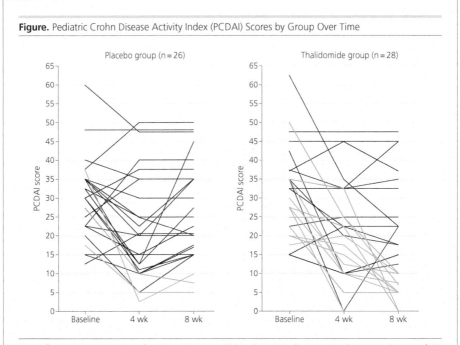

**Figure.** Pediatric Crohn Disease Activity Index (PCDAI) Scores by Group Over Time

Scores for the PCDAI can range from 0 to 95; scores higher than 10 indicate active disease, and scores of 30 or higher indicate moderate to severe disease. Blue lines represent patients with remission; black lines, patients without remission.

**4.2.1.11** **Forest Plots.** The results of meta-analyses and systematic reviews are often presented in summary figures known as forest plots.[1] Forest plots—the graphical display of individual study results and, usually, the weighted mean of studies included in a meta-analysis—are one way of summarizing the review's results for a specific outcome.[20] In these figures, the estimated effects (and 95% CIs) are presented both tabularly and graphically (**Figure 4.2-16**). The first column typically lists the sources of the data, most often previously published studies along with their publication years and citations (which should appear in the reference list of the meta-analysis with links to the originals).[20] The sources should be listed in a meaningful order, such as by date or duration of follow-up. The plot portion allows readers to see the information from the individual studies at a glance. It provides a simple visual representation of the amount of variation among the results of the studies, as well as an estimate of the overall result of all the studies together.[21] Various conventions are used in forest plots, including proportionally sized boxes to represent the weight of each study in the meta-analysis and the use of a diamond to show the overall effect at the bottom of the plot. It is important to include headers at the top of the plot to the left and right of the effect size or point estimate line (eg, 1.0 in Figure 4.2-16) to indicate which variables, interventions, exposures, or outcomes are favored. Note that the values plotted are also provided in the

**Figure 4.2-16.** Effect Sizes and Pooled (Combined) Data in a Meta-analysis, With the Size of the Data Markers Sometimes Indicating the Relative Weight of Each Study, Depending on the Software Used to Generate the Figure

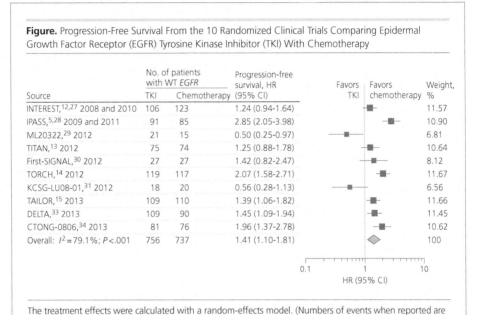

**Figure.** Progression-Free Survival From the 10 Randomized Clinical Trials Comparing Epidermal Growth Factor Receptor (EGFR) Tyrosine Kinase Inhibitor (TKI) With Chemotherapy

| Source | No. of patients with WT *EGFR* TKI | Chemotherapy | Progression-free survival, HR (95% CI) | Favors TKI | Favors chemotherapy | Weight, % |
|---|---|---|---|---|---|---|
| INTEREST,[12,27] 2008 and 2010 | 106 | 123 | 1.24 (0.94-1.64) | | | 11.57 |
| IPASS,[5,28] 2009 and 2011 | 91 | 85 | 2.85 (2.05-3.98) | | | 10.90 |
| ML20322,[29] 2012 | 21 | 15 | 0.50 (0.25-0.97) | | | 6.81 |
| TITAN,[13] 2012 | 75 | 74 | 1.25 (0.88-1.78) | | | 10.64 |
| First-SIGNAL,[30] 2012 | 27 | 27 | 1.42 (0.82-2.47) | | | 8.12 |
| TORCH,[14] 2012 | 119 | 117 | 2.07 (1.58-2.71) | | | 11.67 |
| KCSG-LU08-01,[31] 2012 | 18 | 20 | 0.56 (0.28-1.13) | | | 6.56 |
| TAILOR,[15] 2013 | 109 | 110 | 1.39 (1.06-1.82) | | | 11.66 |
| DELTA,[33] 2013 | 109 | 90 | 1.45 (1.09-1.94) | | | 11.45 |
| CTONG-0806,[34] 2013 | 81 | 76 | 1.96 (1.37-2.78) | | | 10.62 |
| Overall: $I^2 = 79.1\%$; $P < .001$ | 756 | 737 | 1.41 (1.10-1.81) | | | 100 |

0.1     1     10

HR (95% CI)

The treatment effects were calculated with a random-effects model. (Numbers of events when reported are given in eTable 1 in the Supplement.) The size of the data markers (squares) corresponds to the weight of the study in the meta-analysis. HR indicates hazard ratio; WT, wild type.

hazard ratio (HR) column. The dotted line at 1.0 represents no effect and allows for quick visualization of the effect of each study listed. The overall $I^2$ and $P$ values are provided in the figure.

In most cases, forest plots should be plotted on a log scale. Log scales are useful for presenting rates of change and are presented such that 2 equal distances represent the same percentage change.[1] For example, the distance on the x-axis between the ticks labeled 1 and 2 would be the same length as between the ticks labeled 2 and 4. Log scales begin at 1 (or a proportion thereof), not 0, and do not plot negative values (Figure 4.2-16).[1]

**4.2.1.12**    **Funnel Plots.** A funnel plot is a scatterplot of the effect size for each of the studies used in a meta-analysis vs some measure of the effect size's precision[22] and may be useful to assess the validity of the meta-analysis.[23] In the absence of bias, the plot will resemble a symmetrical inverted funnel (**Figure 4.2-17**). Conversely, if bias exists, funnel plots will often be skewed and asymmetrical.

**4.2.1.13**    **Hybrid Graphs.** Occasionally, a combination of 2 graphing techniques can provide more information than either technique alone (**Figure 4.2-18**). This figure shows the full distribution of values and also allows readers to better compare those distributions.

**Figure 4.2-17.** Funnel Plot Used to Detect Bias in a Meta-analysis

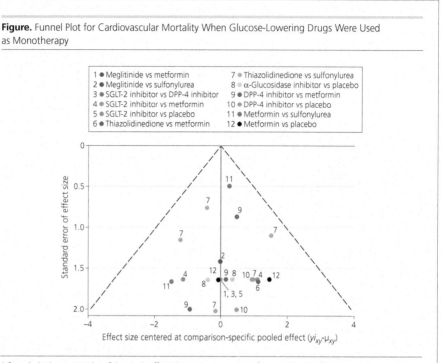

**Figure.** Funnel Plot for Cardiovascular Mortality When Glucose-Lowering Drugs Were Used as Monotherapy

A funnel plot is a scatterplot of the study effect size vs some measure of its precision, in this instance the standard error. A funnel plot that is asymmetrical with respect to the line of the summary effect (vertical red line) implies there are differences between the estimates derived from small and large studies. The studies are ordered from best to worst according to effects on cardiovascular mortality. Missing (small) studies lying on the right side of the zero line suggest that small studies tend to exaggerate the effectiveness of higher-ranked treatments compared with lower-ranked treatments. The cause of any small study effects is explored by meta-regression and is not necessarily attributable to publication bias (the absence of small, negative studies in the available literature). Red line represents the null hypothesis that the study-specific effect sizes do not differ from the respective comparison-specific pooled effect estimates. The 2 black dashed lines represent a 95% CI for the difference between study-specific effect sizes and comparison-specific summary estimates. $yi_{xy}$ is the noted effect size in study $i$ that compares $x$ with $y$. $\mu_{xy}$ is the comparison-specific summary estimate for $x$ vs $y$. Treatments are ordered by the surface under the cumulative ranking (SUCRA) curve.

### 4.2.2 Diagrams.

**4.2.2.1 Flowcharts.** Flowcharts show the sequence of activities, processes, events, operations, or organization of a complex procedure or an interrelated system of components and sometimes function as visual summaries of a study. Flowcharts are useful to depict study protocol or interventions, to demonstrate participant recruitment and follow-up such as in a randomized clinical trial (CONSORT [Consolidated Standards of Reporting Trials])[24] (**Figure 4.2-19**, and Figure 19.2-1 in 19.0, Study Design and Statistics), or to show inclusions and exclusions of samples in other types of studies, such as in systematic reviews and meta-analyses (PRISMA [Preferred Reporting Items for Systematic Reviews and Meta-analyses])[24] (**Figure 4.2-20**) and studies of diagnostic accuracy (STARD [Standards for the Reporting of Diagnostic Accuracy Studies]).[24]

**Figure 4.2-18.** Individual-Value Plots Overlaid With Box Plots

**Figure.** Box Plots and Individual Plots of Shannon Diversity Index for Skin Samples and Nose Samples of Patients With Atopic Dermatitis (AD) and Healthy Controls

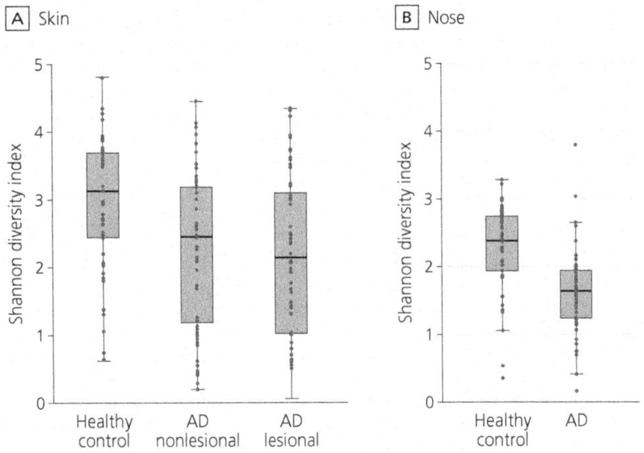

Shannon diversity index, which considers both the richness (number of different species) and evenness (how evenly the species are distributed), is shown for skin samples of patients with AD (nonlesional skin and lesional skin) (A) and healthy controls, as well as nose samples (B). Differences in microbiome diversity were found between patients with AD and healthy controls for both skin and nose. Boxes indicate the 25th percentile, median, and 75th percentile. Dots represent each sample. Whiskers show the minimum and maximum ranges.

When the assignment in an unrandomized clinical trial was not random (eg, if the treatment was allocated or assigned), a rectangle is used instead of an oval (**Figure 4.2-21**). A crossover study involves 2 or more interventions. In it, all of the study participants receive all the interventions, but those interventions are assigned in a random order[25] (**Figure 4.2-22**).

In the JAMA Network journals, the randomization point is the only oval; all other entries are rectangular. Note that the allocation point in a nonrandomized trial uses a rectangular box rather than an oval to distinguish it from a flowchart for a randomized clinical trial (Figure 4.2-21).

**4.2.2.2** **Decision Trees.** Decision trees are analytical tools used in cost-effectiveness and decision analyses.[26] The decision tree displays the logical and temporal sequence in clinical decision-making and usually progresses from left to right (**Figure 4.2-23**). A decision node is a point in the decision tree at which several alternatives can be selected and, by convention, is designated by a square. A chance node (probability node) is a point in the decision tree at which several events, determined by chance, may occur and, by convention, is designated by a circle.

**4.2.2.3** **Algorithms.** Algorithms contain branched pathways to permit the application of carefully defined criteria in the task of identification or classification,[27] such as to aid in clinical diagnosis or treatment decisions. Standard box shapes are used

**Figure 4.2-19.** Flowchart for a Randomized Clinical Trial Using CONSORT Criteria

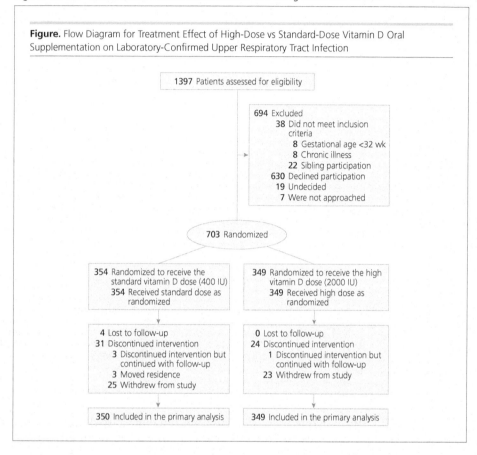

**Figure.** Flow Diagram for Treatment Effect of High-Dose vs Standard-Dose Vitamin D Oral Supplementation on Laboratory-Confirmed Upper Respiratory Tract Infection

to indicate various steps in the algorithm. For example, a diamond or hexagon indicates a decision box, which has at least 2 arrows leading to different paths in the algorithm. A rectangle or square indicates an action or decision box. Algorithms use arrows to guide readers through the process, and yes and no are marked directly on the pathways (**Figure 4.2-24**).

4.2.2.4    **Pedigrees.** Pedigrees illustrate familial relationships and are often used in the study and description of inherited disorders. Standard symbols are used to indicate each person's sex, vital status (living or dead), and whether he or she has the condition or genetic component in question, if known. Symbol shapes and lines drawn horizontally and vertically between the symbols convey information about the generations depicted and relationships among individuals,[28] with the earliest generation at the top of the figure (**Figure 4.2-25**) (see 14.6.6, Pedigrees). If the sex of each person is not relevant to the discussion and there may be a concern about identifiability or confidentiality, diamonds or other sex-neutral symbols can be substituted for the standard circles and squares (see 5.8.3, Protecting Research Participants' and Patients' Rights in Scientific

**Figure 4.2-20.** Flowchart for a Systematic Review and Meta-analysis Using PRISMA Criteria[24]

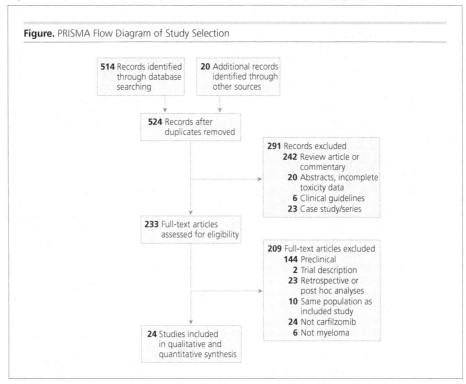

**Figure.** PRISMA Flow Diagram of Study Selection

Publication, Rights in Published Reports of Genetic Studies). A key inside the figure plot explains each symbol.

**Maps.** Maps are useful to demonstrate relationships or trends that involve location and distance or to illustrate study sampling methods (**Figure** 4.2-26). Maps may be used to demonstrate geographic relationships (eg, spread of a disease). Choropleth maps depict quantitative data (eg, relative frequencies by county, state, country, continent, province, or region), with differences in numerical data, such as rates, shown by shading or colors. Authors should verify map details to avoid misspelled or incorrect names, deleted features, distorted geographic relationships, misplaced or missing cities, and misplaced boundaries.

A heat map is a graphical representation of data that simultaneously reveals row and column hierarchical cluster structure in a data matrix.[29,30] It consists of rectangular tiling, with each tile shaded on a color scale to represent the value of the corresponding element of the data matrix. Heat maps are commonly used to display gene expression (**Figure** 4.2-27). Each row in the grid represents a gene and each column a sample. The color and intensity of the boxes are used to represent changes (not absolute values) of gene expression.[31] The heat map may also be combined with clustering methods that group genes and/or samples based on the similarity of their gene expression pattern, with similar rows and columns near

**Figure 4.2-21.** Flowchart for a Clinical Trial in Which Assignment Was Allocated

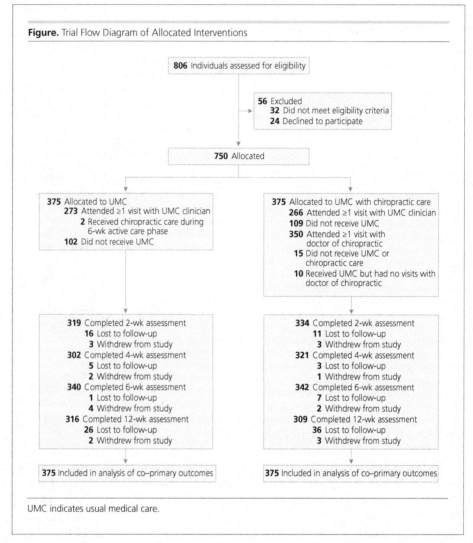

**Figure.** Trial Flow Diagram of Allocated Interventions

UMC indicates usual medical care.

each other.[29,30] Such grouping can be useful for identifying genes that are commonly regulated or biological signatures associated with a particular condition (eg, a disease or an environmental condition).[31]

Network maps, visual representations of the physical connectivity among separate points in a network,[32] can illustrate movement (**Figure 4.2-28**) or other relationships among groups or outcomes (**Figure 4.2-29**).

**4.2.4**   **Illustrations.** Illustrations may explain physiologic mechanisms, describe clinical maneuvers and surgical techniques, and provide orientation to medical imaging. Complex interactions often are easier to convey and understand in an illustration than in text or tables (**Figure 4.2-30**). It is important to apply the principles of diversity and inclusion of individuals from different racial/ethnic backgrounds, as well as age, sex/gender, and physical disabilities, to illustrations of conditions, diseases, and situations, as appropriate (see 11.12, Inclusive Language).

**Figure 4.2-22** Flowchart for a 2-Arm Crossover Study

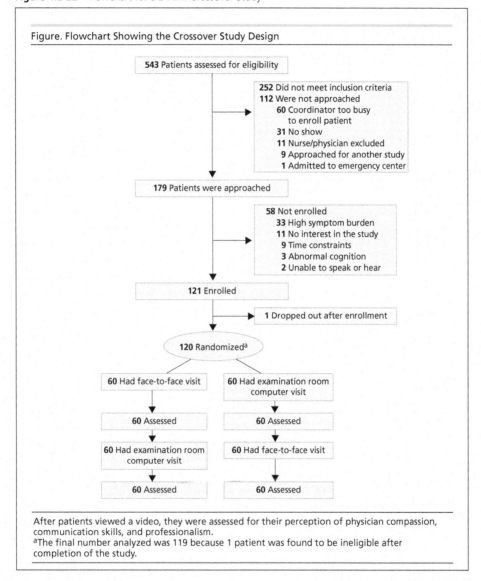

Figure. Flowchart Showing the Crossover Study Design

**543** Patients assessed for eligibility

**252** Did not meet inclusion criteria
**112** Were not approached
  **60** Coordinator too busy to enroll patient
  **31** No show
  **11** Nurse/physician excluded
  **9** Approached for another study
  **1** Admitted to emergency center

**179** Patients were approached

**58** Not enrolled
  **33** High symptom burden
  **11** No interest in the study
  **9** Time constraints
  **3** Abnormal cognition
  **2** Unable to speak or hear

**121** Enrolled

**1** Dropped out after enrollment

**120** Randomized[a]

**60** Had face-to-face visit

**60** Had examination room computer visit

**60** Assessed

**60** Assessed

**60** Had examination room computer visit

**60** Had face-to-face visit

**60** Assessed

**60** Assessed

After patients viewed a video, they were assessed for their perception of physician compassion, communication skills, and professionalism.
[a]The final number analyzed was 119 because 1 patient was found to be ineligible after completion of the study.

**4.2.5** **Photographs and Clinical Imaging.** Photographs and other images in biomedical articles are used to display clinical findings, experimental results, or clinical procedures. Such figures include radiographs (**Figure 4.2-31**) and those from other types of medical imaging (**Figure 4.2-32** and **Figure 4.2-33**), photomicrographs (**Figure 4.2-34**), and photographs of patients (**Figure 4.2-35**) and biopsy specimens (Figure 4.2-31). If an individual can be identified in a photograph, the author should obtain a signed statement granting permission to publish the photograph from the identifiable person (see 4.2.11, Consent for Identifiable Patients, and 5.8.2, Patients' Rights to Privacy and Anonymity and Consent for Identifiable Publication).

**Figure 4.2-23.** Decision Tree Showing Options and Possible Outcomes From Left to Right

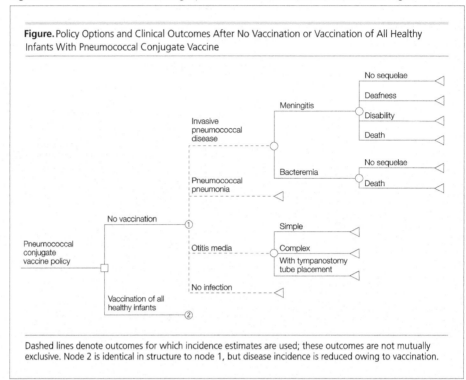

**Figure.** Policy Options and Clinical Outcomes After No Vaccination or Vaccination of All Healthy Infants With Pneumococcal Conjugate Vaccine

Dashed lines denote outcomes for which incidence estimates are used; these outcomes are not mutually exclusive. Node 2 is identical in structure to node 1, but disease incidence is reduced owing to vaccination.

The availability of digital imaging allows for enhancement of images of photographic scientific data, such as clinical images (Figure 4.2-33) or gel electrophoresis bands (**Figure 4.2-36**).[33] Such digital manipulation may produce misleading or fraudulent images (see 5.4.1, Scientific Misconduct, Misrepresentation: Fabrication, Falsification, and Omission). Some publications require that authors submit the original images; others ask authors to list image adjustments in the paper itself.[33,34]

When a figure includes labels, arrows, or other markers to identify or point out certain features, these should be explained in the figure legend (Figure 4.2-32).

**4.2.6** **Components of Figures.** Clear display of data or information is the most important aspect of any figure. For figures that display quantitative information, data values may be represented by dots, lines, curves, area, length, or shading based on the type of graph used.

**4.2.6.1** **Scales for Graphs.** The horizontal scale (x-axis) and the vertical scale (y-axis) indicate the values of the data plotted in a graph. In most graphs, values increase from left to right (on the x-axis) and from bottom to top (on the y-axis). Rarely, a third scale (secondary y-axis) may be relevant, also with values increasing from bottom

**Figure 4.2-24.**   Treatment Algorithm

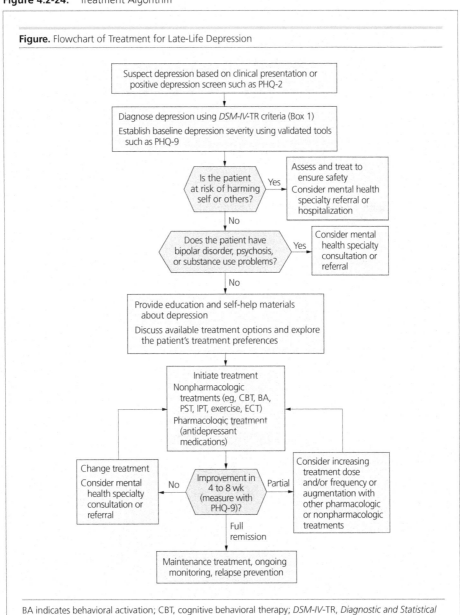

**Figure.** Flowchart of Treatment for Late-Life Depression

BA indicates behavioral activation; CBT, cognitive behavioral therapy; *DSM-IV*-TR, *Diagnostic and Statistical Manual of Mental Disorders* (Fourth Edition, Text Revision); ECT, electroconvulsive therapy; IPT, interpersonal psychotherapy; PHQ-2, Patient Health Questionnaire–2; PHQ-9, 9-item PHQ; and PST, problem-solving.

**Figure 4.2-25.** Hypothetical Pedigree of Multiple Generations in 3 Related Families, With the Probands Indicated by an Arrow

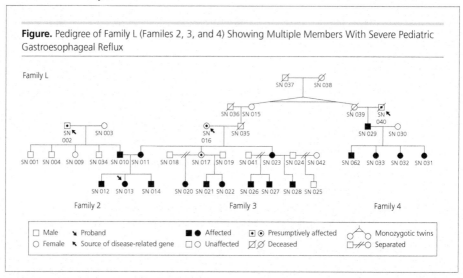

**Figure.** Pedigree of Family L (Familes 2, 3, and 4) Showing Multiple Members With Severe Pediatric Gastroesophageal Reflux

**Figure 4.2-26.** Map to Show the Distribution by Distance of Travel Time (via Ambulance) to the Treatment Site

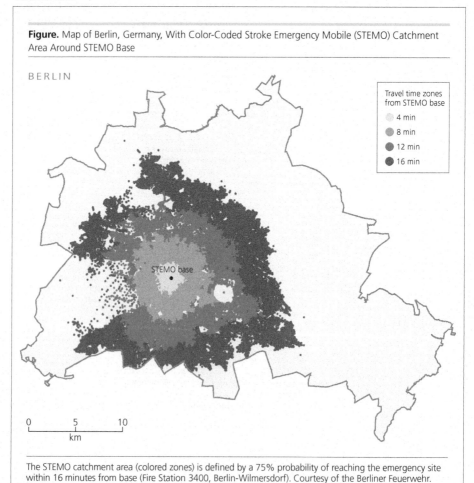

**Figure.** Map of Berlin, Germany, With Color-Coded Stroke Emergency Mobile (STEMO) Catchment Area Around STEMO Base

The STEMO catchment area (colored zones) is defined by a 75% probability of reaching the emergency site within 16 minutes from base (Fire Station 3400, Berlin-Wilmersdorf). Courtesy of the Berliner Feuerwehr.

**Figure 4.2-27.** Genetic Heat Map Showing Relative Expression Levels in 4 Clusters (Groups of Samples That Are More Closely Related to One Another[30]) Based on the Core Probe Sets

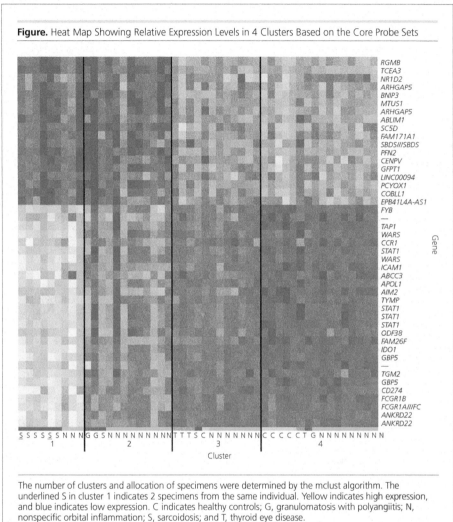

**Figure.** Heat Map Showing Relative Expression Levels in 4 Clusters Based on the Core Probe Sets

The number of clusters and allocation of specimens were determined by the mclust algorithm. The underlined S in cluster 1 indicates 2 specimens from the same individual. Yellow indicates high expression, and blue indicates low expression. C indicates healthy controls; G, granulomatosis with polyangiitis; N, nonspecific orbital inflammation; S, sarcoidosis; and T, thyroid eye disease.

to top (Figure 4.2-2). Data lines should be thicker than the scale lines to draw attention to the data.[1]

**4.2.6.1.1** **Range of Values.** The range of values on the axes should be slightly greater than the range of values being plotted, so that the entire data set can appear within the area defined by the axes and most of the possible range of values on the axes will be used. Ideally, the range should include 0 on both axes, if 0 is a possible value for the variable being plotted. In line graphs, if a large range of values is necessary but cannot be depicted with a continuous scale in a single plot, the data may be broken into separate, smaller plots or an enlarged portion of the graph may

**Figure 4.2-28.** A Network Map Shows Movement From the Point of Diagnosis to Different Areas of a Hospital by 1152 Patients With *Clostridioides difficile* (formerly *Clostridium difficile*) Infection Who Were Diagnosed in the Emergency Department During a Single Year

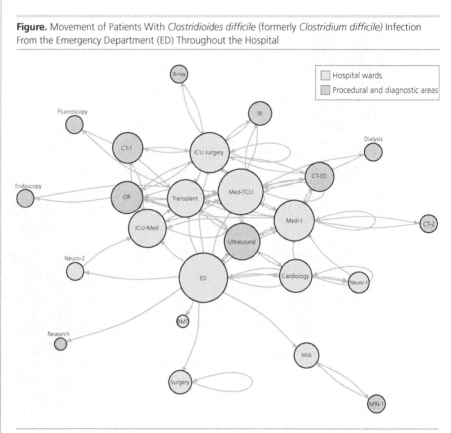

**Figure.** Movement of Patients With *Clostridioides difficile* (formerly *Clostridium difficile)* Infection From the Emergency Department (ED) Throughout the Hospital

Network graph displaying the hospital ward, procedural, and diagnostic areas in the hospital visited by a subset of patients in whom *C difficile* infection was diagnosed in the ED during a single year. The size of each circle represents the number of *C difficile*–positive patients who passed through that location. Yellow denotes bed census areas (eg, nursing units), and gray denotes procedural and diagnostic common areas. Patients with *C difficile* infection visited a mean (SD) of 4.2 (4.0) locations while hospitalized, including procedural and diagnostic common areas, representing multiple sites of potential contamination of surfaces and disease transmission. BMT indicates bone-marrow transplant unit; CT-1 and -2, computed tomographic scanner suites 1 and 2; CT-ED, CT scanner suite in the ED; ICU, intensive care unit; IR, interventional radiology; Med, medical nursing unit; MRI-1, magnetic resonance imaging suite 1; Msk, musculoskeletal unit; Neuro-1 and -2, neurology units 1 and 2; OR, operating room; and TCU, transitional care unit.

be depicted in an inset (**Figure 4.2-37**). For single-axis plots, data that exceed the limits of the axes can be indicated with an arrowhead (such as in a forest plot). Note the use of blue on the y-axes of Figure 4.2-37 to show the relationship of the range of values between the plots.

**4.2.6.1.2** **Axis Scales.** Divisions of the scales on the graph axes should be indicated by intervals chosen to be appropriate, simple multiples of the quantity plotted, such as multiples of 2, 5, or 10.[35] Numbers that represent the values on the

**Figure 4.2-29.** Network Map Illustrating Treatment Outcomes for Multiple Treatment Modalities

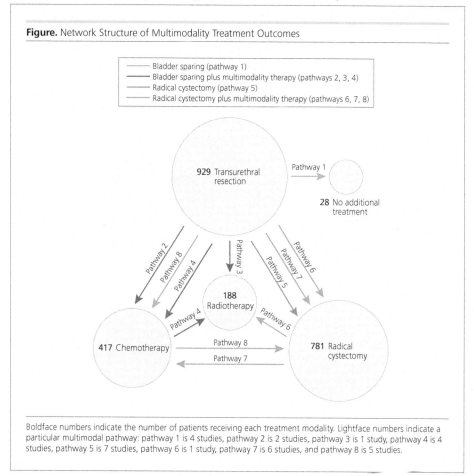

**Figure.** Network Structure of Multimodality Treatment Outcomes

Boldface numbers indicate the number of patients receiving each treatment modality. Lightface numbers indicate a particular multimodal pathway: pathway 1 is 4 studies, pathway 2 is 2 studies, pathway 3 is 1 study, pathway 4 is 4 studies, pathway 5 is 7 studies, pathway 6 is 1 study, pathway 7 is 6 studies, and pathway 8 is 5 studies.

axis scale are centered on their respective tick marks. For linear scales, the axis must appear linear, with equal intervals and equal spacing between tick marks. However, logarithmic scales may be useful to show proportional rates of change (Figure 4.2-16) and to emphasize the change rate rather than the absolute amount of change when absolute values or baseline values for data series vary greatly. Tick marks and scale numbers should be placed outside the data field, just left of the y-axis and just below the x-axis, and centered on their respective tick marks. For numbers less than 1, include the digit zero before the decimal.[4]

**4.2.6.2** **Axis Labels.** Axes should be labeled with the type of data plotted and the unit of measure used. Data may represent numerical values, percentages, or rates. For numerical data, customary units of measure and their respective abbreviations or symbols should be used (see 13.12, Units of Measure). In single-axis graphs, categories should be clearly labeled along the baseline (Figure 4.2-9).

**Figure 4.2-30.** Illustration Depicting Anatomy and Surgical Techniques

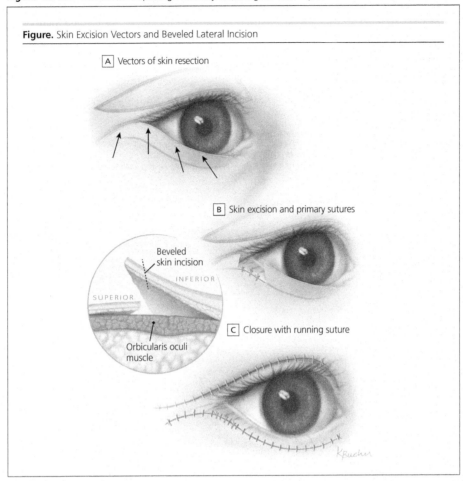

**Figure.** Skin Excision Vectors and Beveled Lateral Incision

A Vectors of skin resection

B Skin excision and primary sutures

Beveled skin incision

INFERIOR

SUPERIOR

Orbicularis oculi muscle

C Closure with running suture

**Figure 4.2-31.** Radiographs Showing 2 Views of a Patient's Left Femur Alongside an Immunohistochemically Stained Biopsy Specimen

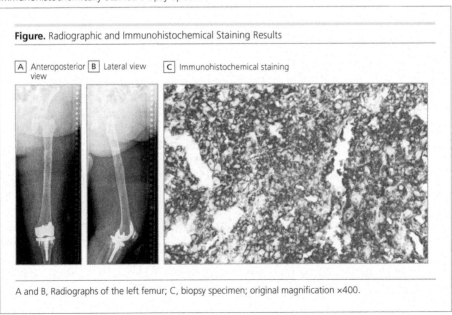

**Figure.** Radiographic and Immunohistochemical Staining Results

A Anteroposterior view  B Lateral view  C Immunohistochemical staining

A and B, Radiographs of the left femur; C, biopsy specimen; original magnification ×400.

**Figure 4.2-32.** A Series of Magnetic Resonance Images Captured at Different Times Can Show Structural Changes Resulting From Disease or Treatment

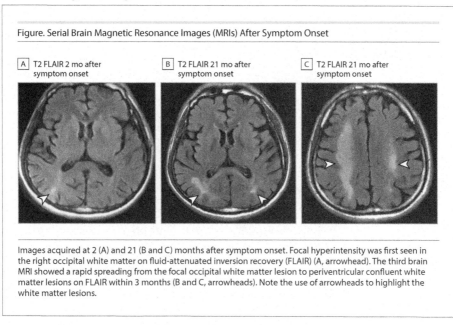

Figure. Serial Brain Magnetic Resonance Images (MRIs) After Symptom Onset

A  T2 FLAIR 2 mo after symptom onset
B  T2 FLAIR 21 mo after symptom onset
C  T2 FLAIR 21 mo after symptom onset

Images acquired at 2 (A) and 21 (B and C) months after symptom onset. Focal hyperintensity was first seen in the right occipital white matter on fluid-attenuated inversion recovery (FLAIR) (A, arrowhead). The third brain MRI showed a rapid spreading from the focal occipital white matter lesion to periventricular confluent white matter lesions on FLAIR within 3 months (B and C, arrowheads). Note the use of arrowheads to highlight the white matter lesions.

**Figure 4.2-33.** Clinical and Ultrasonographic Images of Brachial Artery Pseudoaneurysm Originating From the Profunda Brachii Artery

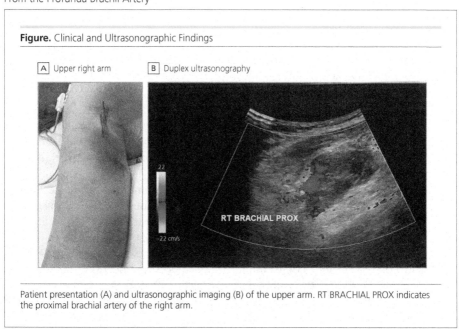

Figure. Clinical and Ultrasonographic Findings

A  Upper right arm
B  Duplex ultrasonography

Patient presentation (A) and ultrasonographic imaging (B) of the upper arm. RT BRACHIAL PROX indicates the proximal brachial artery of the right arm.

**Figure 4.2-34.** Photomicrograph of a Biopsy Specimen Illustrates the Use of Laser-Assisted Mass Spectrometry to Confirm Deposition of Gadolinium in Sclerotic Bodies of Gadolinium-Associated Plaques

**Figure.** Photomicrograph of Lesional Biopsy Specimen

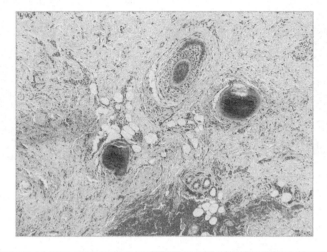

This specimen reveals round, amorphous, eosinophilic sclerotic bodies in the dermis with osteoid-like lacunae (hematoxylin-eosin, original magnification ×100).

Axis labels should follow sentence-style capitalization, in consistency with other areas of the figure (such as in the figure key or direct labeling of lines). Phrases that appear on axes are generally easier to read in sentence style than when all major words are capitalized.

**4.2.6.2.1** **Symbols, Patterns, Colors, and Shading.** Symbols, line styles, colors, and shading characteristics used in the figure must be explained, preferably by direct labeling of components in the figure or, if infeasible, in a key. Alternatively, this information may be included in the legend. For a series of figures within an article, the types of symbols, line styles, colors, and shading should be used consistently. For example, if data for the intervention group and for the control group are designated as a heavy line and as a lighter line, respectively, then these same line styles should be used for similar data for these groups in subsequent figures. When lines cross or nearly do, line styles should be applied to ensure that they are easy to discriminate.

When data points are plotted, symbols should be distinguished easily by shape and color or shade. For example, if 2 symbols are needed, the recommended symbols are ○ and ●,[35] although □ and ■ or △ and ▲ may be used. A combination of these symbols can be used when 3 or more symbols are required. The shading or color of the symbols can designate specific data. For instance, in all figures in an article, ○ may indicate data for the placebo group and ● for the intervention group. A key to the different symbols can appear in the figure. In line

**Figure 4.2-35.** Photographs Showing Nasal Size Distortion in a Short-Distance Photograph Above a Diagram Illustrating How the Extent of Distortion Is Calculated

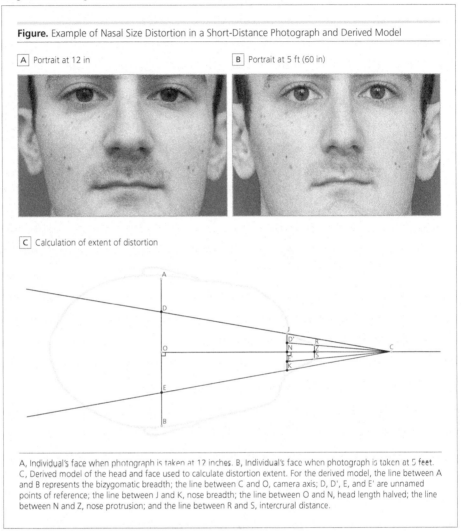

**Figure.** Example of Nasal Size Distortion in a Short-Distance Photograph and Derived Model

A, Individual's face when photograph is taken at 12 inches. B, Individual's face when photograph is taken at 5 feet. C, Derived model of the head and face used to calculate distortion extent. For the derived model, the line between A and B represents the bizygomatic breadth; the line between C and O, camera axis; D, D', E, and E' are unnamed points of reference; the line between J and K, nose breadth; the line between O and N, head length halved; the line between N and Z, nose protrusion; and the line between R and S, intercrural distance.

graphs with connected data points, the curves should be labeled directly if there is room. Colors can be used to accentuate or deemphasize data groups.

In bar charts and other figures (such as maps), shading is preferable to cross-hatching and other patterns to distinguish groups. Patterns can be difficult to read both in print and online. Shades should be of appropriate gradations to show contrast (eg, 10%, 40%, and 70% black).

**4.2.6.3** **Error Bars.** For plotted data, error bars (depicting SD, SE, range, interquartile range, or CIs) are an efficient way to display variability in the data.[36] Error bars should be drawn to encompass the entire range of variability, not in just one direction

**Figure 4.2-36.** Gel Electrophoresis Shows Protein Aggregation in Central Nervous System Tissue From a BL6 Mouse (A), a Rat (B), and a Human (C)

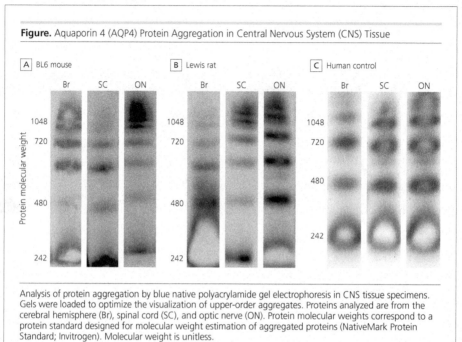

**Figure.** Aquaporin 4 (AQP4) Protein Aggregation in Central Nervous System (CNS) Tissue

Analysis of protein aggregation by blue native polyacrylamide gel electrophoresis in CNS tissue specimens. Gels were loaded to optimize the visualization of upper-order aggregates. Proteins analyzed are from the cerebral hemisphere (Br), spinal cord (SC), and optic nerve (ON). Protein molecular weights correspond to a protein standard designed for molecular weight estimation of aggregated proteins (NativeMark Protein Standard; Invitrogen). Molecular weight is unitless.

**Figure 4.2-37.** Data With Widely Ranging Values

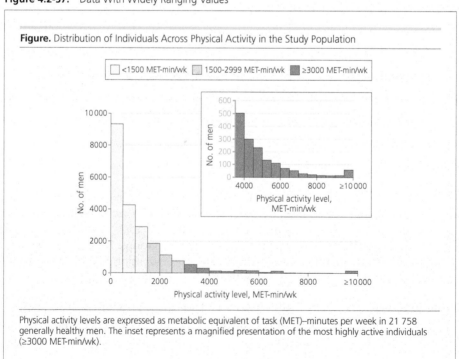

**Figure.** Distribution of Individuals Across Physical Activity in the Study Population

Physical activity levels are expressed as metabolic equivalent of task (MET)–minutes per week in 21 758 generally healthy men. The inset represents a magnified presentation of the most highly active individuals (≥3000 MET-min/wk).

(Figure 4.2-7) unless the prespecified analysis plan called for 1-sided hypothesis testing. Error bars should always be defined, either in the legend or on the plot itself.

**4.2.6.4** **Three-Dimensional Figures.** In most cases, figures should not be presented in 3-dimensional format. A 3-dimensional presentation is inappropriate for any figures that contain only 2 dimensions of data. Many software programs allow users to add enhancing elements to figures, but 3-dimensional display may confuse readers or distract from important graphical relationships. For instance, it may be difficult to read from the bar to the correct value on the axis. Most 3-dimensional presentations can be replotted into more straightforward graphics.

**4.2.7** **Titles, Legends, and Labels.** Many journals, including the JAMA Network journals, use separate titles and legends (also known as captions) to describe and clarify figures. Others combine the title and legend underneath the figure.

**4.2.7.1** **Titles.** The figure title follows the designation "Figure" numbered consecutively (ie, Figure 1, Figure 2) and does not appear in the figure itself. Articles that contain a single figure use the designator "Figure" (not "Figure 1"). The title is a succinct clause or phrase (perhaps 10-15 words) that identifies the specific topic of the figure or describes what the data show. In the JAMA Network journals, each major word in a figure title is capitalized and follows the same rules as for article titles (see 10.2, Titles and Headings). Some publications print the figure title above the figure and others place it under the figure, in sentence style.

Titles of figures, including diagrams, photographs, and line drawings, generally should not begin with a phrase identifying the type of figure:

> *Avoid:* Photograph Showing Prominent Physical Signs of Familial Hypercholesterolemia
>
> *Better:* Prominent Physical Signs of Familial Hypercholesterolemia

However, a description of the type of figure may be required in certain circumstances to provide context and avoid confusion.

> **Figure 3.** Fluorescein Angiogram Showing Widespread Retinal Capillary Nonperfusion and Marked Optic Nerve Head Leakage
>
> **Figure 4.** Autoradiograph Demonstrating Loss of Heterozygosity at the 3p25 Locus in Preneoplastic Foci and Corresponding Invasive Cancer

An exception would be a hybrid graph, in which identification of the graphing techniques may be helpful (Figure 4.2-35).

**4.2.7.2** **Legends.** The figure legend (caption) is written in sentence format and printed below or next to the figure. The legend contains information that describes the figure beyond the figure title, and it should provide sufficient detail to make the figure comprehensible without undue reference to or being overly duplicative of the text. Although the recommended maximum length for figure legends is 40 words, longer legends may be necessary for figures that require more detailed explanations or for multipart figures. Figure legends should contain expansions of abbreviations and footnotes for information too cumbersome to include in the figure itself. Legends that contain multiple paragraphs should use footnote symbols (a, b, c, etc) in accordance with table footnotes (see 4.1.4.10, Tables, Figures, and Multimedia, Tables, Table Components, Footnotes).

**4.2.7.2.1** **Composite Figures.** Composite figures consist of several parts and should have a single legend that contains necessary information about each part. Direct labeling of individual parts is recommended unless such phrasing distracts from the image. Each component of the figure is described in the legend, usually by a separate clause or sentence beginning with the designation for the part, followed by a comma (eg, A, Pretreatment infantile hemangioma). If the parts share much of the same explanation, parenthetical mention of each part is appropriate.

Capital letters (A, B, C, D, etc) should be used to label the parts of a composite figure. These letters should be placed in a small inset box that is positioned above each figure part. The figure legend should refer to each of the figure components and the letter designators in a clear and consistent format (**Figure 4.2-38**).

**Figure 4.2-38.** Multipart Figure With Each Panel Labeled Above the Image and Including a Brief Description

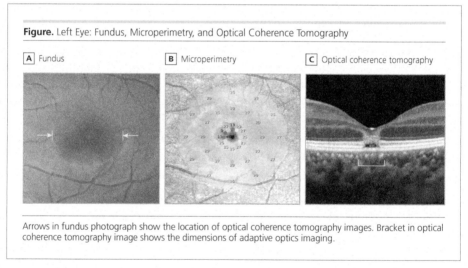

**Figure.** Left Eye: Fundus, Microperimetry, and Optical Coherence Tomography

A Fundus  B Microperimetry  C Optical coherence tomography

Arrows in fundus photograph show the location of optical coherence tomography images. Bracket in optical coherence tomography image shows the dimensions of adaptive optics imaging.

**4.2.7.2.2** **Information About Methods and Statistical Analyses.** Statements regarding methodologic details are unnecessary for each figure if this information is provided in the Methods section of the article and the text that refers to the figure clearly indicates the source of the data. Reference to the Methods section or to other figures that contain this information may be appropriate. At times, brief inclusion of methodologic details in the legend may be necessary for understanding the figure.

For data that have been analyzed statistically, pertinent analyses and significance values may be included in the figure or its legend.[37] Values for data displayed in the figure (eg, mean or median values) should be indicated in the figure or in the legend. The meaning of error bars should be explained in the legend or in the plot itself (Figure 4.2-16).

**4.2.7.2.3** **Photomicrographs.** Legends for photomicrographs should include details about the type of stain used. In figures with 2 or more parts, the stains relevant to each part should be noted after its description. To indicate scale, photomicrographs should include scale bars or rulers. If the original image has been modified (enlarged or reduced), the original magnification should be noted (Figure 4.2-34).

> Histopathologic images of the nevi, neither of which shows any histopathologic criteria for melanoma (hematoxylin-eosin; scale bars = 200 μm).

Electron micrograph legends do not require information about the stain:

> *Haemophilus influenzae* microcolonies of middle ear mucosa 24 hours after inoculation (original magnification ×5000).

**4.2.7.2.4** **Visual Indicators in Illustrations or Photographs.** Visual indicators provided in illustrations or photographs, such as a reference bar or ruler denoting a measure of dimension (eg, length) in a photomicrograph, arrows, arrowheads, or other markers, should be clearly defined in the figure or described in the figure legend (Figure 4.2-38).

**4.2.7.2.5** **Capitalization of Labels and Other Text.** Capitalization should be kept to a minimum within the body of the figure, including axis labels.[3] Capitalizing each major word can make comprehension difficult, especially when phrases or clauses are used. Sentence-style capitalization is easier to read.[4]

**4.2.7.2.6** **Abbreviations.** Abbreviations in figures should be consistent with those used in the text and defined in the title or legend or in a key as part of the figure. Abbreviations may be expanded individually in the text of the legend or may be expanded collectively at the beginning or end of the legend:

> Patients could be excluded for more than 1 reason; the primary reason for exclusion in each case is shown. CABG indicates coronary artery bypass graft; ICD, implantable cardioverter-defibrillator; LVEF, left ventricular ejection fraction; MRI, magnetic resonance imaging; PCI, percutaneous coronary intervention; and STEMI, ST-segment elevation myocardial infarction.

If several illustrations share many of the same abbreviations and symbols, full explanation may be provided in the first figure legend or in a table footnote, with subsequent reference to that legend or table footnote (see 4.1.4.10, Tables, Figures, and Multimedia, Tables, Table Components, Footnotes). This practice works relatively well in print but can make understanding figures in online articles more difficult because readers may have to open separate figure files to find the legend.

**4.2.8** ■ **Placement of Figures in the Text.** In print/PDF versions of articles, figures should be placed as close as possible to their first mention in the text. Figures should be cited in consecutive numerical order in the text, and references to figures should include their respective numbers. For example:

> Patient participation and progress through the study are shown in Figure 1.

> Figure 1 shows patient participation and progress through the study.

> Patient participation and progress through the study were monitored by the investigators (Figure 1).

Given the potential for variability in the page layout and online publication process, the text of a manuscript should not refer to figures by position on the page or by other designators, such as "the figure opposite," "the figure on this page," or "the figure above."

**4.2.9** ■ **Figures Reproduced or Adapted From Other Sources.** It is preferable to use original figures rather than those already published. When use of a previously published illustration, photograph, or other figure is necessary, written permission to reproduce it must be obtained from the copyright holder (usually the publisher). The original source should be acknowledged in the legend. If the original source in which the illustration has been published is included in the reference list, the reference may be cited in the legend, with the citation number for the reference corresponding to its first appearance in the text, tables, or figures (see 4.1.4.10, Tables, Figures, and Multimedia, Tables, Table Components, Footnotes, and 3.6, References, Citation). Permission should be obtained to reproduce the material in print, online, and in all licensed versions (eg, reprints). Content published under a Creative Commons (CC) license may not require permission, depending on the license type (see 5.6.5, Ethical and Legal Considerations, Intellectual Property: Ownership, Access, Rights, and Management, Copyright Assignment or License). It may be necessary to include additional information to comply with specific language required by the organization (usually a publisher) granting permission to republish the figure (see 5.6.8, Ethical and Legal Considerations, Intellectual Property: Ownership, Access, Rights, and Management, Permissions for Reuse).

> Reprinted with permission from the American Academy of Pediatrics.[5]

**4.2.10** ■ **Guidelines for Preparing and Submitting Figures.** The preferred format for submitting figures varies among scientific journals. Authors who submit figures with a scientific manuscript should consult the instructions for authors of the publication for specific requirements. For example, many journals require all files to be submitted through a web-based submission system. The JAMA Network journals provide detailed instructions to authors that cover, for example, image integrity, acceptable file formats, titles and legends, and labeling included within the figure (https://jamanetwork.com/journals/jama/pages/instructions-for-authors#SecFigures).[38]

**4.2.11** ■ **Consent for Identifiable Patients.** For photographs or videos in which an individual can be identified (by himself/herself or others), the author should obtain and submit a signed statement from the identifiable person that grants permission to publish the photograph. Previously used measures to attempt to conceal the identity of an individual in a photograph, such as placing black bars over the person's eyes, are not effective and should not be used (see 5.8.2, Ethical and Legal Considerations, Protecting Research Participants' and Patients' Rights in Scientific Publication, Patients' Rights to Privacy and Anonymity and Consent for Identifiable Publication). Individuals can be identified in photographs that show minimal body parts, usually from identifying features (eg, hair, scars, moles, tattoos, clothing). To avoid identifiability in such cases, photographs should be cropped if possible. Otherwise, permission must be obtained from the individual in the photograph.

For figures that depict genetic information, such as pedigrees or family trees, informed consent is required from all persons who can be identified. Authors should not modify the pedigree (eg, by changing the number of persons in the generation, varying the number of offspring in families, or providing inaccurate information about the sex of pedigree members) in an attempt to avoid potential identification. If knowledge of the sex of pedigree members is not essential for scientific purposes, individuals may be designated by diamonds or other sex-neutral symbols (see 4.2.2.4, Pedigrees, and 5.8.3, Rights in Published Reports of Genetic Studies).

**4.2.12** **Multimedia.** Some journals allow supporting multimedia to accompany an article for online-only publication, such as video, audio, or interactive files. For example, the JAMA Network journals include such content when it is important to readers' understanding of a report, to illustrate a point made or demonstrate a process described in an article, to aid in learning, or to provide a useful summary in another format. Detailed guidelines on acceptable video and audio file formats, optimal video quality, and filming and copyright considerations are provided in online instructions for authors.[39] If an individual could be identified (by himself/herself or others), authors should obtain a signed statement from the identifiable person that grants permission to publish the material (see 4.2.11, Consent for Identifiable Patients and 5.8.2, Protecting Research Participants' and Patients' Rights in Scientific Publication, Patients' Rights to Privacy and Anonymity and Consent for Identifiable Publication).

**4.3** **Nontabular Material.**
Nontabular material does not contain cells of individual data. Usually it is set off from the text by a box, rules, shading, or other elements. Sometimes the box or sidebar is cited in the text (following the citation rules for tables) and other times it is not. Any references that appear in nontabular material should also appear in the reference list and be numbered in order of their appearance (see 4.1.4.10, Tables, Figures, and Multimedia, Tables, Table Components, Footnotes).

**4.3.1** **Boxes.** A textual table or box contains words, phrases, or sentences, often in list form. Boxes are used to emphasize key points, summarize information, and/or reduce the narrative text (**Box 4.3-1**).

In this example, the box provides information in a list-type format, which allows for easier reading than the same content in prose form.

**Box 4.3-1.** Box or Textual Table of Content Set Off From the Text

> **Box 2.** Features of Irritable Bowel Syndrome
>
> **Typical features**
>
> Loose/frequent stools
>
> Constipation
>
> Bloating
>
> Abdominal cramping
>
> Abdominal discomfort
>
> Symptom brought on by food intake/specific food sensitivities
>
> Symptoms dynamic over time (change in pain location, change in stool pattern)
>
> **Concerning features for organic disease**
>
> Symptom onset after age 50 y
>
> Severe or progressively worsening symptoms
>
> Unexplained weight loss
>
> Nocturnal diarrhea
>
> Family history of organic gastroenterological diseases, including colon cancer, celiac disease, or inflammatory bowel disease
>
> Rectal bleeding or melena
>
> Unexplained iron-deficiency anemia

**4.3.2** **Sidebars.** Sidebars typically contain supplementary information, including related topics or lists of sources for further reading (**Box 4.3-2** and **Box 4.3-3**). They are

**Box 4.3-2.** Sidebar From a News Story on Antibiotic-Resistant Bacteria

> **Antibiotic-Resistant Bacteria Posing the Greatest Threats**
> At least 2 million people each year become infected with bacteria that are resistant to antibiotics, and at least 23 000 people die as a direct result. Additional patients die of conditions complicated by antibiotic-resistant infection, according to a 2013 report from the Centers for Disease Control and Prevention (CDC).
>
> The CDC report classifies *Clostridioides difficile* (formerly *Clostridium difficile*), carbapenem-resistant Enterobacteriaceae, and drug-resistant *Neisseria gonorrhoeae* as urgent threats. Methicillin-resistant *Staphylococcus aureus*, vancomycin-resistant *Enterococcus,* and 10 others are classified as serious threats. Vancomycin-resistant *S aureus*, erythromycin-resistant Group A *Streptococcus*, and clindamycin-resistant Group B *Streptococcus* are concerning threats.

**Box 4.3-3.** Sidebar of Sources for Further Reading

---

**Related guidelines and other resources**

Chaikof EL, Brewster DC, Dalman RL, et al. The care of patients with abdominal aortic aneurysm: the Society for Vascular Surgery practice guidelines. *J Vasc Surg.* 2009;50:S2-S49

Mastracci TM, Cinà CS. Screening for abdominal aortic aneurysm in Canada: review and position statement of the Canadian Society for Vascular Surgery. *J Vasc Surg.* 2007;45(6):1268-1276

Moll FL, Powell JT, Fraedrich G, et al. Management of abdominal aortic aneurysms: clinical practice guidelines of the European Society for Vascular Surgery. *Eur J Vasc Endovasc Surg.* 2011;41(suppl 1):S1-S58

---

often not called out in the text (eg, "Box 1") but instead are placed within the article in a logical place for best comprehension.

**Principal Authors:** Stacy Christiansen, MA, and Connie Manno, ELS

## ACKNOWLEDGMENT

Thanks to the following for reviewing this chapter and providing important comments: Hope Lafferty, AM, ELS, Hope Lafferty Communications, Marfa, Texas; Trevor Lane, MA, DPhil, Edanz Group, Fukuoka, Japan; Thomas A. Lang, MA, Tom Lang Communications, Kirkland, Washington; Chris Meyer, JAMA Network; Joseph Clayton Mills, MA, Neuroscience Publications, Barrow Neurological Institute, Phoenix, Arizona; David Schriger, MD, MPH, *JAMA*, and David Geffen School of Medicine at UCLA, Los Angeles, California.

## REFERENCES

1. Lang T. *How to Report Statistics in Medicine: Annotated Guidelines for Authors, Editors, and Reviewers.* 2nd ed. American College of Physicians; 2006.
2. International Committee of Medical Journal Editors. Selection and description of participants. ICMJE Recommendations for the Conduct, Reporting, Editing, and Publication of Scholarly Work in Medical Journals. Updated December 2019. Accessed April 27, 2021. http://www.icmje.org/recommendations/browse/manuscript-preparation/preparing-for-submission.html
3. *The Chicago Manual of Style.* 17th ed. University of Chicago Press; 2017.
4. Council of Science Editors. *Scientific Style and Format: The CSE Manual for Authors, Editors, and Publishers.* 8th ed. University of Chicago Press/Council of Science Editors; 2014.
5. *Recommended Practices for Online Supplemental Journal Article Materials.* National Information Standards Organization; 2013. NISO RP-15-2013. Accessed June 20, 2019. https://niso.org/publications/niso-rp-15-2013-recommended-practices-online-supplemental-journal-article-materials

6. *Best Practices for Publishing Journal Articles.* NFAIS website. Approved February 13, 2009. Accessed October 1, 2019. https://www.nfais.org/best-practices

7. Kosslyn SM. *Clear and to the Point.* Oxford University Press; 2007.

8. Customize x-axis and y-axis properties. Microsoft Power BI website. Published January 20, 2018. Accessed May 23, 2018. https://docs.microsoft.com/en-us/power-bi/power-bi-visualization-customize-x-axis-and-y-axis

9. Sullivan L. Survival analysis. Updated June 3, 2016. Accessed June 6, 2018. http://sphweb.bumc.bu.edu/otlt/MPH-Modules/BS/BS704_Survival/

10. Clark TG, Bradburn MJ, Love SB, Altman DG. Survival analysis, part I: basic concepts and first analyses. *Br J Cancer.* 2003;89(2):232-238. doi:10.1038/sj.bjc.6601118

11. Pocock SJ, Clayton TC, Altman DG. Survival plots of time-to-event outcomes in clinical trials: good practice and pitfalls. *Lancet.* 2002;359(9318):1686-1689.

12. Year 10 interactive maths—second edition: scatterplots. G S Rehill's Interactive Maths Series website. Accessed May 22, 2018. http://www.mathsteacher.com.au/year10/ch16_statistics/08_scatterplots/24scatter.htm

13. Haighton J, Haworth A, Wake G. *AS Use of Maths—Statistics: Using and Applying Statistics.* Nelson Thornes Ltd; 2003:74-76.

14. Peterson SM. *CSE GuideLines: Editing Science Graphs.* Council of Science Editors; 2000.

15. Tufte ER. *The Visual Display of Quantitative Information.* 2nd ed. Graphics Press; 2001.

16. Schriger DL, Cooper RJ. Achieving graphical excellence: suggestions and methods for creating high-quality visual displays of experimental data. *Ann Emerg Med.* 2001;37(1):75-87.

17. Hedeker D. Longitudinal data analysis, including categorical outcomes. Accessed February 12, 2018. https://hedeker-sites.uchicago.edu/

18. Wicklin R. Create spaghetti plots in SAS. Published June 2, 2016. Accessed June 1, 2018. https://blogs.sas.com/content/iml/2016/06/02/create-spaghetti-plots-in-sas.html

19. Schriger DL. Graphic portrayal of studies with paired data: a tutorial. *Ann Emerg Med.* 2018;71(2):239-246. doi:10.1016/j.annemergmed.2017.05.033

20. Schriger DL, Altman DG, Vetter JA, Heafner T, Moher D. Forest plots in reports of systematic reviews: a cross-sectional study reviewing current practice. *Int J Epidemiol.* 2010;39(2):421-429. doi:10.1093/ije/dyp370

21. Lewis S, Clarke M. Forest plots: trying to see the wood and the trees. *BMJ.* 2001;322(7300):1479-1480.

22. Sedgwick P. Meta-analyses: how to read a funnel plot. *BMJ.* 2013;346-f1342. doi:10.1136/bmj.f1342

23. Egger M, Davey Smith G, Schneider M, Minder C. Bias in meta-analysis detected by a simple, graphical test. *BMJ.* 1997;315:629. doi:10.1136/bmj.315.7109.6290

24. Equator Network. Accessed June 20, 2019. https://www.sciencemag.org/authors/science-information-authors

25. Ofori-Asenso R, Agyeman AA. Understanding cross over and parallel group studies in drug research. *Precis Med.* 2015;2:e1046. doi:10.14800/pm.1046

26. Sox HC, Higgins MC, Owens DK. *Medical Decision Making.* 2nd ed. Wiley-Blackwell; 2013.

27. Hadorn DC. Use of algorithms in clinical guideline development. In: *Clinical Practice Guideline Development: Methodology Perspectives.* US Agency for Health Care Policy and Research; 1994:93-104.

28. Bennett RL. Appendix A.1: handy reference tables of pedigree nomenclature. In: *The Practical Guide to the Genetic Family History.* 2nd ed. John Wiley & Sons Inc; 2010:287-289.

29. Wilkinson L, Friendly M. The history of the cluster heat map. *Am Stat.* 2009;63(2):179-184. doi:10.1198/tas.2009.0033

30. Kaufman L, Rousseeuw PJ. *Finding Groups in Data: An Introduction to Cluster Analysis.* John Wiley & Sons Inc; 2005.

31. Grant GR, Manduchi E, Stoeckert CJ. Analysis and management of microarray gene expression data. *Curr Protoc Mol Biol.* 2007;77:chap 19:unit 19.6. doi:10.1002/0471142727.mb1906s77

32. Keast R. How to Measure Progress & Impact: Network Mapping. Presented at: Collective Impact 2014; February 12, 2014; Melbourne, Australia. Accessed May 24, 2018. http://www.collaborationforimpact.com/wp-content/uploads/2014/03/Network-Mapping.pdf

33. Pearson H. Image manipulation: CSI: cell biology. *Nature.* 2005;434(7036):952-953. doi:10.1038/434952a

34. *Science* instructions: preparing your manuscript and figures. Accessed October 1, 2019. https://www.sciencemag.org/authors/instructions-preparing-revisedmanuscript

35. Scientific Illustration Committee of the Council of Biology Editors. *Illustrating Science: Standards for Publication.* Council of Biology Editors; 1988.

36. Cleveland WS. *The Elements of Graphing Data.* Rev ed. Hobart Press; 1994.

37. Singer PA, Feinstein AR. Graphical display of categorical data. *J Clin Epidemiol.* 1993;46(3):231-236. doi:10.1016/0895-4356(93)90070-H

38. Figures. Instructions for Authors. *JAMA* website. Accessed January 29, 2019. https://jamanetwork.com/journals/jama/pages/instructions-for-authors#SecFigures

39. Video. Instructions for Authors. *JAMA* website. Accessed February 5, 2019. https://jamanetwork.com/journals/jama/pages/instructions-for-authors#SecVideo

# 5.0 Ethical and Legal Considerations

## 5.1    Authorship Responsibility.

> *Some judge of authors' names, not works, and then*
> *Nor praise nor blame the writings, but the men.*
> Alexander Pope[1]

Nearly 70 years ago, Richard M. Hewitt, MD, then head of the Section of Publications at the Mayo Clinic, described the ethics of authorship in a *JAMA* article entitled "Exposition as Applied to Medicine: A Glance at the Ethics of It."[2] The following excerpts from Hewitt's article demonstrate an appreciation of the basic ethical responsibilities and obligations of authorship:

> Authorship cannot be conferred; it may be undertaken by one who will shoulder the responsibility that goes with it.

> The reader of a report issued by two or more authors has a right to assume that each author has some authoritative knowledge of the subject, that each contributed to the investigation, and that each labored on the report to the extent of weighing every word and quantity in it.

If we would define publication of unoriginal, repetitious medical material as a violation of medical ethics, and would officially reprove it as such, the tawdry author would be silenced and the genuine one helped.

The by-line, then, is not merely a credit-line. He who took some part in the investigation, be it ever so minor, is entitled to credit for what he did. . . . Further, the generous chap who would bestow authorship on another, perhaps without even submitting the manuscript to him, may do his colleague no favor. For the investigation is one thing, the report of it another, and, sad the day that this must be admitted: The investigation may have been excellent but the report, bad.

Since all of us necessarily adopt and absorb the ideas of others, we must be scrupulous in maintaining the spirit of acknowledgment to others. Fundamentally, your integrity is at stake. Unless you make specific acknowledgment, you claim the credit for yourself for anything that you write. In general, it is better to say too much about your sources than too little.

The author who paraphrases or refers to an article should have read it.

**5.1.1** **Authorship: Definition, Criteria, Contributions, and Requirements.** Authorship offers significant professional and personal rewards, but these rewards are accompanied by substantial responsibility. During the 1980s, biomedical editors began requiring contributors to meet specific criteria for authorship. These criteria were first developed for medical journals under the initiative of Edward J. Huth, MD,[3] then editor of the *Annals of Internal Medicine*, who cited Hewitt's work[2] during discussions at the 1984 meeting of the International Committee of Medical Journal Editors (ICMJE). The ICMJE guidelines were first published in 1985[4] and are now part of the Recommendations for the Conduct, Reporting, Editing, and Publication of Scholarly Work in Medical Journals[5] (see 2.0, Manuscript Preparation for Submission and Publication). These guidelines are reviewed, revised, and updated regularly, and numerous biomedical journals, the US National Library of Medicine,[6] and the Council of Science Editors[7,8] use them as the foundation for policies and procedures on authorship.

**5.1.1.1** **Authorship Definition and Criteria.** According to the ICMJE guidelines, all authors should have participated sufficiently in the work to take public responsibility for the content, either all the work or an important part of it. To take public responsibility, an author must be able to defend the content (all or an important part) and conclusions of the article if publicly challenged. Sufficient participation means that substantial contributions have been made in each of the following areas[5]:

1. Conception and design of the work; or acquisition, analysis, or interpretation of the data for the work; and

2. Drafting the work or revising it critically for important intellectual content; and

3. Approval of the version to be published; and

4. Agreement to be accountable for all aspects of the work in ensuring that questions related to the accuracy or integrity of any part of the work are appropriately investigated and resolved.

In 2013, the ICMJE added the fourth criterion to address concerns that all authors be accountable for the work if questions arise about its accuracy or integrity. According to the ICMJE recommendations, "an author should be able to identify which co-authors are responsible for specific other parts of the work. In addition, authors should have confidence in the integrity of the contributions of their co-authors."[5]

To justify authorship, an author must meet each of the 4 criteria. However, the term *substantial contribution* has not been adequately defined (perhaps to allow for wider application of the ICMJE criteria for authorship). As a result, the first criterion, "conception and design; or acquisition, analysis, or interpretation of the data," may be interpreted broadly. For example, an author of a nonresearch manuscript may not have analyzed data per se but may have analyzed literature, events, theories, arguments, or opinions. A *substantial contribution* may be interpreted as an important intellectual contribution, without which the work, or an important part of the work, could not have been completed or the manuscript could not have been written and submitted for publication.

The ICMJE also notes that the following contributions, alone, are not sufficient to justify authorship[5]: "acquisition of funding; general supervision of a research group or general administrative support; and writing assistance, technical editing, language editing, and proofreading" (see also 5.1.2, Ethical and Legal Considerations, Authorship Responsibility, Guest and Ghost Authors and Other Contributors). Those who do not meet the 4 authorship criteria should be acknowledged (see 5.2.1, Acknowledging Support, Assistance, and Contributions of Those Who Are Not Authors). The ICMJE notes that these criteria are "intended to reserve the status of authorship for those who deserve credit and can take responsibility for the work" and that these criteria are not intended to "disqualify colleagues from authorship who otherwise meet authorship criteria by denying them the opportunity" to participate in writing or reviewing and approving the manuscript. The ICMJE states that "all individuals who meet the first criterion should have the opportunity to participate in the review, drafting, and final approval of the manuscript."[5]

See **Box 5.1-1** for a list of common terms used for *contributor, author,* and *collaborator.*[9]

**5.1.1.2**  **Author Contributions.** Authors may not be aware of the ICMJE authorship criteria. To inform or remind authors of these responsibilities and to encourage appropriate authorship, many journals require authors to attest in writing how they qualify for authorship and to indicate their specific contributions to the work.[5,10-12] The ICMJE guidelines state, "Editors are strongly encouraged to develop and implement a contributorship policy, as well as a policy on identifying who is responsible for the integrity of the work as a whole."[5] Some journals ask authors to describe their specific contributions in an open-ended narrative format, some describe examples of various types of author contributions, and some journals provide a list of specific contributions in the form of a checklist. For example, the JAMA Network journals require all authors to complete a statement of authorship responsibility based on the ICMJE guidelines and to indicate their specific contributions from a checklist based on the ICMJE authorship criteria and empiric data from studies of authorship and author contributions. This statement is required for authors of all types of manuscripts, including editorials and letters to the editor[12] (see **Box 5.1-2**).

**Box 5.1-1.** Common Terms: Contributor, Author, and Collaborator

---

**Contributor**: Anyone—an author, a collaborator, or others—who has assisted or contributed in a meaningful way to a work.

**Author**: A contributor who has participated sufficiently in the work to take public responsibility for the content, either all the work or an important part of it, and meets defined criteria for authorship. Identification of authorship in a manuscript/article can appear in 2 ways.

**Byline author**: Author name in byline

**Nonbyline author**: Author name not in byline—listed elsewhere, typically in an Acknowledgment or Article Information section.

**Group author**: A group of individuals, usually involving multicenter study investigators, members of working groups, and official or self-appointed expert boards, panels, or committees, who wish to display a group name to indicate authorship. (Also known as corporate authorship.)

**Collaborator**: A nonauthor member of a formal group who contributes significantly to the work; often also called investigator. In these cases, a group name must be in the byline.

**Other contributors**: Anyone else who contributed in some meaningful way who is not an author and is not a nonauthor collaborator. They can be listed under Additional Contributions in an Acknowledgement or Article Information section (see 5.2, Ethical and Legal Considerations, Acknowledgments).

---

The JAMA Network journals use an authorship form for authors to indicate information about authorship responsibility, criteria, and contributions, as well as information about conflicts of interest and funding, publishing agreement and copyright license options, and an acknowledgment statement. An updated example of this authorship form is available online in the *JAMA* Instructions for Authors.[12]

Some journals publish author contributions. This practice, first suggested by Rennie et al in 1997[10,11] and endorsed by the ICMJE[5] and the Council of Science Editors,[7,8] makes the specific contributions of authors transparent to editors and readers. For example, the JAMA Network journals publish the specific contributions of each author for articles that report original data (eg, research and systematic reviews) in the Acknowledgment section at the end of the article (see 5.2, Acknowledgments).

Another initiative, following the rationale of identifying contributions that many biomedical journals used for many years, is called the Contributor Roles Taxonomy (CRediT).[13] This taxonomy "provides a high-level classification of the diverse roles performed in the work leading to a published research output in the sciences" and includes the following: conceptualization, methods, software, validation, formal analysis, investigation, resources, data curation, writing–original draft preparation, writing–review and editing, visualization, supervision, project administration, and funding acquisition.[14] The purpose of this taxonomy system is "to provide transparency in contributions to scholarly published work, to enable improved systems of attribution, credit, and accountability."[14] According to the

**Box 5.1-2.** The JAMA Network Journals Authorship Responsibility, Criteria, and Contributions Statement

Each author should meet all criteria below (A, B, C, and D) and should indicate general and specific contributions by reading criteria A, B, C, and D and checking the appropriate boxes.

☐ A. I certify that

- The manuscript represents original and valid work and that neither this manuscript nor one with substantially similar content under my authorship has been published or is being considered for publication elsewhere, except as described in an attachment, and copies of closely related manuscripts have been provided; and

- I agree to be accountable for all aspects of the work in ensuring that questions related to the accuracy or integrity of any part of the work are appropriately investigated and resolved; and

- If requested, I will provide the data or will cooperate fully in obtaining and providing the data on which the manuscript is based for examination by the editor or the editor's assignees; and

- For papers with more than 1 author, I agree to allow the corresponding author to serve as the primary correspondent with the editorial office, to review the edited manuscript and proof, and to make decisions regarding release of information in the manuscript to the media, federal agencies, or both; or, if I am the only author, I will be the corresponding author and agree to serve in the roles described above.

☐ B. I have given final approval of the submitted manuscript.

C. I have participated sufficiently in the work to take public responsibility for (check 1 of 2 below)
    ☐ part of the content.
    ☐ the whole content.

D. To qualify for authorship, you must check at least 1 box for each of the 3 categories of contributions listed below.

I have made substantial contributions to the intellectual content of the paper as described below:

1. Check at least 1 of the 2 below
    ☐ concept and design
    ☐ acquisition, analysis, or interpretation of data

2. Check at least 1 of the 2 below
    ☐ drafting of the manuscript
    ☐ critical revision of the manuscript for important intellectual content

3. Check at least 1 below
    ☐ statistical analysis
    ☐ obtained funding
    ☐ administrative, technical, or material support
    ☐ supervision
    ☐ no additional contributions
    ☐ other contributions (specify)_____

CRediT organizers, the implementation of this taxonomy is not intended to replace authorship or "define what constitutes authorship. Rather, the roles are intended to apply to all those who contribute to research that results in scholarly published works, and it is recommended that all tagged contributors be listed, whether they are formally listed as authors or named in acknowledgements"[14] (see 5.2.3, Author Contributions).

**5.1.1.3** **Additional Author Requirements.** Depending on the journal, all authors may also be required to complete a publishing agreement (transferring copyright or a publication license or opting for an open access license), identify relevant conflicts of interest or to declare no such interests, identify funding and the role of the sponsors in the work to be published, attest that they had access to the data for reports of original research, and indicate a plan for data sharing (required for reports of clinical trials; optional for reports of other study types) (see 5.6.5, Copyright Assignment or License, and 5.5.2, Requirements for Authors). Many journals send emails to all authors at various stages of the manuscript submission and evaluation processes to confirm that all are indeed authors or to have them complete authorship and disclosure forms and publishing agreements. Some journals have begun to request or require authors to provide unique researcher identifiers in an attempt to disambiguate or distinguish individual authors from other authors and improve authentication and the linking of outputs (eg, funding, published journal articles) with individual authors.[15] A common identifier is ORCID, (Open Researcher and Contributor ID), which is a universal resource identifier with a 16-digit number that is compatible with the International Organization for Standardization's Standard International Standard Name Identifier (see https://orcid.org/).

**5.1.1.4** **Access to Data and Data Sharing Statement Requirements.** The ICMJE recommends that journals ask authors to indicate whether they "had access to the study data, with an explanation of the nature and extent of access, including whether access is on-going."[5] Consistent with this recommendation, the JAMA Network journals require at least 1 named author (eg, the principal investigator), and preferably no more than 2 authors, to indicate that she or he had full access to all the data in the study and takes responsibility for the integrity of the data and the accuracy of the data analysis for all reports that contain original data (eg, research articles, systematic reviews, and meta-analyses)[12] (see 5.2.5, Access to Data Statement, and 5.5.5, Access to Data Requirement).

For reports of randomized clinical trials, the ICMJE recommends that authors of clinical trials provide a data sharing statement with submitted manuscripts and indicate if data, including individual patient data, a data dictionary that defines each field in the data set, and supporting documentation, will be made available to others; when, where, and how the data will be available; types of analyses that are permitted; and if there will be any restrictions on the use of the data.[4,16] This follows a previous ICMJE requirement for authors of clinical trials to also include trial protocols with submitted manuscripts and published articles. Data sharing statements may also be submitted for reports of other types of studies, but the ICMJE member journals only require this for reports of clinical trials.

The data sharing statements should address the following items:

**Data**

Will the data collected for your study, including individual patient data and a data dictionary defining each field in the data set, be made available to others?

Yes or No (if No, authors may explain why data are not available)

List all data that will be made available.

Deidentified participant data

Participant data with identifiers

Data dictionary

Other (please specify)

List where to access these data. Provide complete URL if data will be available in a repository or website, or provide complete email address if request for data must be sent to an individual.

List the beginning date and end date (if applicable) when these data will be available. If the beginning date of data availability will be when the article is published, please indicate "with publication."

With publication

At a date different from publication

Beginning date

End date (if applicable)

**Supporting Documents**

If your manuscript is accepted for publication, the journal will publish your trial protocol, including the statistical analysis plan, and any amendments as online supplements. Please list any other supporting documents that you wish to make available (eg, statistical/analytic code, informed consent form).

Statistical/analytic code

Informed consent form

None

Other (please specify)

List where to access these documents. Provide complete URL if the documents will be available in a repository or website, or provide complete email address if request for documents must be sent to an individual.

List the beginning date and end date (if applicable) when the documents will be available.

With publication

At a date different from publication

Beginning date

End date (if applicable)

**Additional Information**

Indicate the types of analyses for which the data will be made available (eg, for any purpose or for a specified purpose).

Indicate the mechanisms by which the data will be made available (eg, with investigator support, without investigator support, after approval of a proposal, or with a signed data access agreement).

List any additional restrictions on the use of the data or any additional information.

If you would like to offer context for your decision not to make the data available, please enter it below (optional).

**5.1.1.5** **Corresponding Author.** Every manuscript and published article should have at least 1 author who will serve as the primary contact and correspondent for all communications about the submitted work and, if it is accepted for publication, the published article. It is not efficient for editorial offices to have more than 1 formal corresponding author. However, it is helpful to provide the editorial office with contact information for coauthors in case the corresponding author becomes unavailable during the editorial and publication processes. For example, the JAMA Network journals require a corresponding author for each submitted manuscript to serve as the primary correspondent with the editorial office and, if the manuscript is accepted, to review an edited manuscript and proof, to make decisions regarding release of information in the manuscript to the news media and/or federal agencies, and to have his or her name published as corresponding author in the article.[12] Corresponding authors for the JAMA Network journals also complete a statement that they have identified all persons who have made substantial contributions to the work but who are not authors[12]:

I certify that all persons who have made substantial contributions to the work reported in this manuscript (eg, data collection, analysis, or writing or editing assistance) but who do not fulfill the authorship criteria are named with their specific contributions in an Acknowledgment in the manuscript.

I certify that all persons named in the Acknowledgment have provided me with written permission to be named.

I certify that if an Acknowledgment section is not included, no other persons have made substantial contributions to this manuscript.

(See 5.1.2, Guest and Ghost Authors and Other Contributors, and 5.2, Acknowledgments.)

**5.1.1.6** **Co–Corresponding Authors.** There have been increasing requests for multiple corresponding authors, which risks diluting the meaning of corresponding author and confusion for journal editors about which author is primarily responsible for communications before and after publication.[9] The JAMA Network journals consider requests for co–corresponding authors on a limited basis if justified but permit no more than 2 co–corresponding authors. In such cases, the journals require that a primary corresponding author be designated as the point of contact responsible for all communication about the manuscript and article, manage the tasks described above, and be listed first in the corresponding author section.[9,12]

**5.1.2  Guest and Ghost Authors and Other Contributors.** At least 1 author must be responsible for any part of an article crucial to its main conclusions, and everyone listed as an author must have made a substantial contribution to that specific article.[5] As described in 5.1.1, Authorship: Definition, Criteria, Contributions, and Requirements, many journals require authors to complete statements of authorship responsibility and to indicate specific contributions of all authors. In addition to improving the transparency of author responsibility, accountability, and credit, these policies may help eliminate guest authors and identify ghost authors.[17-24]

**5.1.2.1  Guest (Honorary) Authors.** A *guest author* or *honorary author* is a person who has not contributed substantially or at all to the published work but is listed as an author. Traditionally, supervisors, department chairs, and mentors have been given guest, or honorary, places in the byline even though they have not met all the criteria for authorship. However, this custom is not acceptable because it devalues the meaning of authorship.[17,19,22,24] The ICMJE guidelines state specifically that acquisition of funding and general supervision of the research, alone without other contributions, are not sufficient for authorship.[5] Such supervision and participation should be noted in the Acknowledgment (see 5.2, Acknowledgments). Guest authors have also included well-known persons in a particular field who have accepted money or other compensation to have their names attached to a manuscript that has already been researched and prepared by a ghost writer for an organization with a commercial interest in the subject of the paper.[17,25-27] Such practice clearly is deceitful.[17,28] Several studies[20,21,29] have documented the prevalence of guest authors in biomedical journals, ranging from 10% of research articles to 39% of review articles, in journals that were not requesting authors to disclose their specific contributions.

**5.1.2.2  Ghost Authors and Ghost Writers.** A *ghost author* is someone who has participated sufficiently in the research or analysis and writing of a manuscript to take public responsibility for the work but is not named as an author in the byline or Acknowledgment section of the published work. Studies have found prevalence rates of journal articles with ghost authors that range from 8% to 26%.[20,21,29] In biomedical publication, ghost authors have included employees of pharmaceutical companies (eg, researchers, managers, statisticians, epidemiologists), medical writers, marketing and public relations writers, and junior staff writing for elected or appointed officials.[17] As described elsewhere, ghost writers have been hired by firms with commercial interests to write reviews of specific subjects, and their authorship is not disclosed.[17,18,25-28,30]

Ghost *writers* are not necessarily ghost *authors*. For example, a writer may not have participated in the research or analysis of a study but may have been given the data and asked to draft a report for publication. If participants in the project do not meet all the criteria for authorship but have made substantial contributions to the research, writing, or editing of the manuscript, those persons should be named, with their permission, in the Acknowledgment along with their contributions and institutional affiliations, if relevant[12,17] (see 5.2, Acknowledgments). Editors and authors should not permit anyone who has participated sufficiently to meet authorship criteria or any nonauthor who has made other important contributions to not be appropriately identified in the byline or Acknowledgment, respectively (see 5.2, Acknowledgments, and 5.1.6, Changes in Authorship).

To give proper credit to medical writers and authors' editors, journal editors should require authors to identify all persons who have participated substantially in the writing or editing of the manuscript. Substantial editing or writing assistance should be disclosed to the editor at the time of manuscript submission and included in the Acknowledgment, along with the person's name, academic degrees, affiliation, type of assistance, and whether compensation for this assistance was provided[12,17] (see 5.2, Acknowledgments). The American Medical Writers Association supports this transparency in a position statement that recommends that "biomedical communicators who contribute substantially to the writing or editing of a manuscript should be acknowledged with their permission and with disclosure of any pertinent professional or financial relationships."[31]

Some journals specifically prohibit the submission of manuscripts that have been ghostwritten.[32,33] For example, the journal *Neurology* requires that "professional writers employed by pharmaceutical companies or other academic, governmental, or commercial entities who have drafted or revised the intellectual content of the paper must be included as authors."[33] Other journals require declaration and explanation of substantive writing and editing assistance. For example, corresponding authors of the JAMA Network journals attest to a statement that all persons who have made substantial contributions to the work (eg, data collection, analysis, or writing or editing assistance) but who do not fulfill the authorship criteria are named with their specific contributions in an acknowledgment in the manuscript.[12] *The Lancet* requires an additional signed statement from any medical writers or editors who provided substantial writing or editing assistance.[34]

Journal editors and manuscript editors who substantially edit a manuscript to be published in a journal generally are not specifically acknowledged if their names appear in the journal's masthead or elsewhere in the journal.

**5.1.3** **Unsigned Editorials, Anonymous Authors, Pseudonymous Authors.** The practice of publishing unsigned or anonymous editorials provides "vituperative editorialists" protection from adversaries or competitors when taking unpopular stands in the pages of their journals.[35] However, without named authors and affiliations, readers lack information to judge the objectivity and credibility of such articles. Although this practice is the norm for newspaper editorial pages, it has fallen out of use in most peer-reviewed journals. One rationale for anonymity has been that editorials, signed or not, represent the official opinion of the publication or the owner of the publication. However, such anonymity distances the real author(s) from accountability. For many years, *JAMA* published unsigned editorials. However, beginning in 1960 *JAMA* began to publish signed or initialed editorials, and since 1970 all *JAMA* editorials have been signed by their authors, including editorials written by the journal's editors. *The BMJ* began publishing signed editorials in 1981.[36] As of this writing, *The Lancet* continues to publish unsigned editorials that reflect an unstated consensus among the editors[34,37] (see 1.4, Opinion Articles).

Journals that publish unattributed editorials and unattributed scientific articles may give contradictory messages to their readers about the merits and responsibility of authorship. Authors who submit scientific papers must publicly stand by what they write, whereas unsigned editorialists can remain anonymous or hide behind a journal's masthead. Unattributed editorials may also allow the publisher or owner of the journal and influential organizations to compromise the journal's editorial independence (see 5.10, Editorial Freedom and Integrity). In addition, PubMed indicates "no authors listed" for anonymous and pseudonymous articles. Therefore, authors', names are published with all articles, including editorials in the JAMA Network journals.

Occasionally, an author may request that his or her name not be used in publication. If the reason for this request is judged to be important (such as concern for personal safety or fear of political reprisal, public humiliation, or job loss), the article could be published without that author's name. However, justification for such publication is very rare and should include careful consideration of the value of the information to be published as well as the potential risks to the author. In such rare cases, the phrase "Name withheld on request" could be used in place of the author's name, perhaps with an explanation in the Acknowledgment (see 2.2, Author Bylines and End-of-Text Signatures).

If anonymity is to be used, the author must still complete statements of authorship responsibility, conflicts of interest disclosure, and a publishing agreement (using his or her actual name), and those records must be kept confidential as part of the manuscript file (see 5.7.1, Confidentiality During Editorial Evaluation and Peer Review and After Publication). For the rare case in which withholding of an author's name is justified, the author's name should be withheld from peer reviewers and readers. However, reviewers and readers should be informed that the author has requested anonymity. Citations to such articles in PubMed will note "no authors listed" in the author field.

Pseudonyms are inappropriate in bylines of scientific reports because they are misleading and cause problems for literature citations.

**5.1.4**     **Number of Authors.** The number of authors whose names appear in the byline of scientific papers increased steadily during the second half of the 20th century.[38] Data from MEDLINE/PubMed of more than 29 million indexed articles indicate an average increase in the number of authors per article from 1.9 before 1975 to 5.81 in 2015-2019.[39] Beginning in the 1990s, articles with large numbers of authors, usually as part of a collaborative group, began to be published. According to an analysis by Aboukhalil,[40] in 1998, the first articles with more than 500 authors were published, and in 2010, articles with more than 2000 authors were published (many of these in high-energy particle physics journals). This increase occurred because of specialization, multidisciplinary and multinational collaboration, the advent of large multicenter studies, and an increase in team science. However, authorship inflation has diluted the meaning of authorship. For example, which authors in a byline that contains more than 100 names can state that they actually wrote the paper or that they participated sufficiently to take public responsibility for the work? In response to this problem, suggestions were made in the 1980s and 1990s to limit the number of authors listed in the byline and database citations.[41,42] However, such limitations may be considered as arbitrary limits and may interfere with policies to encourage transparency of author contributions. The US National Library of Medicine no longer limits the number of individual authors' names listed in an article's citation in MEDLINE/PubMed.[39,43]

For major articles (eg, research and review articles), the JAMA Network journals do not set limits on the number of authors that can be listed, as long as each author meets the journal's criteria for authorship and each author completes an authorship form that indicates specific contributions. However, the JAMA Network journals limit the number of authors for an opinion article or letter. For practical reasons, it might not be possible to list a large number of authors because of limited space available on the first page of a print/PDF article or HTML design limitations. In such cases, the names of all authors in an article with a large number of authors may be listed at the end of the article instead of in the byline at the beginning of the article (see 5.1.9, Group and Collaborative Authorship).[9] In addition, many online displays of articles present truncated lists of authors on article pages (eg, 2-3 authors and "et al") by default with the option for a reader to expand the display to the full list of authors.

Also for practical reasons, many journals limit the number of authors listed in reference list citations (see 3.7, Authors, and 5.1.9, Group and Collaborative Authorship). However, the online versions of many journal articles contain reference lists with links to original articles and to MEDLINE records in PubMed, both of which list all authors for articles.

**5.1.5**    **Order of Authorship and Shared Positions.** Before proposals for identifying authors' contributions began to be implemented, proposed guides for determining order of authorship ranged from simple alphabetical listings to mathematical formulas for assessing specific levels of individual contributions.[44-46] However, even the most systematic calculations of contribution levels will require some measure of subjective judgment, and determination of order of authors is best done by the authors' collective assessment of each author's level of contribution. Moreover, as Rennie et al[10] have argued, attempts to provide information to readers by ordering authors in particular ways are not meaningful, especially if each author's contributions are not made public. The following may help determine order of authorship[47]:

1. Only those individuals who meet the criteria for authorship may be listed as authors (see 5.1.1, Authorship: Definition, Criteria, Contributions, and Requirements).

2. The first author has contributed the most to the work, with other authors listed in descending order according to their levels of contribution. Note: Some groups of authors choose to list the most senior author(s) last, irrespective of the relative amount of their contributions.

3. Decisions about the order of authors should be made as early as possible (eg, before the manuscript is written) and reevaluated later as often as needed by consensus (see 5.1.6, Changes in Authorship).

4. Disagreement about order should be resolved by the authors, not the editor (see guidance in 5.1.8, Author Disputes).

5. Authors may provide a publishable footnote explaining the order of authorship, if there is a compelling reason.

6. Editors may request documentation of authors' specific contributions.

It has become increasingly common for authors to request "co–first author-ship," "co–senior authorship," or some other indication of equal contribution.[9] Journals will accept indication of co–first authorship, but one person's name will need to go first in the byline or author list. Requests for "co–first authorship" or "co–senior authorship" beyond 3 or 4 named authors may not be justifiable. This information can be displayed in the Acknowledgment just before the list of author contributions, such as

> Drs Brown and Jones served as co–first authors and contributed equally to the work.

**5.1.6** **Changes in Authorship.** Changes made in authorship (ie, order, addition, and deletion of authors) should be discussed and approved by all authors.[9,12] Any requests for changes in authorship after initial manuscript submission and before publication should be explained in writing to the editor in a letter signed by all authors, or if sent by email, all authors should be copied (ie, included as recipients of the email). *BMJ*'s policy for alterations in authorship of manuscripts under consideration is a useful guide for other journals: "Any change in authors and/or contributors after initial submission must be approved by all authors. This applies to additions, deletions, change of order to the authors, or contributions being attributed differently. Any alterations must be explained to the editor. The editor may contact any of the authors and/or contributors to ascertain whether they have agreed to any alteration."[48] The Committee on Publication Ethics (COPE) also has useful guidance and a flowchart for addressing changes in authorship.[49]

**5.1.7** **Deceased or Incapacitated Authors.** In the case of death or incapacitation of an author during the manuscript submission and review or publication process, a family member, an individual with power of attorney, or the corresponding author can confirm that the deceased or incapacitated person should be listed as an author. In this event, the corresponding author can forward correspondence from the individual representing the deceased author and can provide information on the deceased or incapacitated author's contributions. Designation that an author is deceased can be made in the Acknowledgment or Article Information section of the manuscript/article (see 2.3.2, Death of Author[s]).

**5.1.8** **Author Disputes.** Authorship disputes sometimes occur. For example, 10% of researchers who have received a grant from the US National Institutes of Health admitted to assigning authorship "inappropriately."[50] In surveys of plastic surgeon authors, 29% reported being involved in a dispute with a colleague over authorship issues in 2003, and 22% reported being involved in such disputes in 2011.[51] According to Karen Peterson, scientific ombudsman at the Fred Hutchinson Cancer Research Center in Seattle, Washington, 20% of the disputes adjudicated in the ombudsman office were about authorship.[52] A 2011 systematic review of 118 studies about authorship issues in various scholarly disciplines identified 4 common themes: "authorship perceptions, definitions and practices, defining order of authors on the byline, ethical and unethical authorship practices, and authorship issues related to student/non-research personnel-supervisor collaboration."[53] In meta-analysis of 14 of these studies, 29% (95% CI, 24%-35%) of researchers reported their own or others' experience with misuse of authorship.[53]

COPE lists numerous case examples of authorship disputes with relevant guidance and information on resolutions.[49] Authorship disputes are best resolved among the authors or within the institutions of the author. Useful tips for authors involved in such disputes include the following[52]:

> First try to discuss the issue amicably and try to understand the other person's point of view. For example, discuss how the idea for the work was first conceived.

> If a junior author has a dispute with a senior author, who is that person's supervisor, keep the tone inquisitive, not accusatory. Consider asking a question intended to understand how authorship was decided.

> If an individual contributor's authorship merit is in question, consider what the manuscript would have looked like without that person's contribution, and whether another author could have made or did make the same contribution.

In addition, authors can consult an intended journal's Instructions for Authors and the ICMJE criteria for authorship[5] and discuss how each author meets the criteria to help resolve any disputes.

**5.1.9**    **Group and Collaborative Authorship.** Group, collaborative, or corporate authorship usually involves multicenter study investigators, members of working groups, and official or self-appointed expert boards, panels, or committees (see Box 5.1-1). These groups can comprise hundreds of participants and often represent complex, multidisciplinary and multinational collaborations; therefore, decisions about listing group authorship pose several problems and dilemmas for authors, editors, journals, librarians, and bibliographic databases[6,9,54-57] (see 13.9, Collaborative Groups, and 2.2.4, Multiple Authors, Group Authors).

Some large clinical trials and observational studies are often best known and frequently referred to by their study name (eg, Women's Health Initiative or the Thrombolysis in Myocardial Infarction Study Group) or by their abbreviation (eg, WHI or TIMI Study Group). As a result, these groups often include the official name of the study group in an article's byline (ie, the position on an article's title page where authors are listed). However, not all members of a study group may meet authorship criteria (see 5.1.1, Authorship: Definition, Criteria, Contributions, and Requirements), and having the group name in the byline does not distinguish those members of the group who qualify for authorship from those who do not. In addition, without a single person named as author, no individual person can take responsibility and be held accountable for the work. For this reason, at least 1 individual (eg, the corresponding author or the principal investigator) should be named as primary corresponding author or guarantor (see 5.1.1.5, Corresponding Author, and 2.0, Manuscript Preparation for Submission and Publication). To address these concerns, members of a writing team or a subgroup are often identified as the authors for large groups.

For group author articles, providing appropriate credit and accountability for the many individuals involved—authors and nonauthor collaborators—and ensuring proper citation to enable online searching and retrieval of the articles are important considerations.[9,54,58] The guidelines that follow may help authors and editors determine who should be listed and where.

One or more authors may take responsibility for a group (as the authors or writing team). In this case, the names of individual authors are listed in the byline with a designation that these authors are writing on behalf of or *for* the group. Those members of the group who do not qualify for authorship would not be listed in the byline but may be listed in the Acknowledgment at the end of the article. In this case, the byline might read as follows:

> Jacques E. Rossouw, MBChB, MD; Garnet L. Anderson, PhD; for the Women's Health Initiative

*or*

> Writing Group for the Women's Health Initiative

In the latter example, the writing group members are the authors for the group, and their names should be listed in the author affiliation or Acknowledgment section (with their specific contributions identified). In these cases, the formal group author name (eg, Women's Health Initiative) should be coded in the journal's online version and in bibliographic databases so that the results of online searches for articles from this group will include articles that combine individual names or a subgroup name (eg, the Writing Group) with the formal group name in the byline.

The other nonauthor group members and their contributions may then be listed separately in the Acknowledgment section (see Box 5.1-1, Common Terms: Contributor, Author, and Collaborator and 5.2, Acknowledgments). PubMed lists these individuals in the article records as "collaborators."[6]

To ensure that authors are cited appropriately in bibliographic databases, explicit use of the term *authors* or *members of the writing group* or *writing committee for* the article is preferred. According to the National Library of Medicine, the group name must be in the byline to be reflected as an author in the MEDLINE citation.[6]

Authorship can be attributed to an entire group, although this practice may be less common than the examples given above. However, as with all articles, clear justification for all members of the group meeting all criteria and requirements for authorship must be made, and for journals that publish authors' individual contributions, all members of the group must identify their specific contributions (see 5.1.1, Authorship: Definition, Criteria, Contributions, and Requirements). In this case, the byline might read as follows:

> Clinical Outcomes Trial Investigators

In cases in which every member of a large group qualifies for authorship and the group name appears in the byline, the individual members of the study group should be listed separately in the Acknowledgment section or in a clearly identified position within the article, such as a box set off by rules (as described in 2.2.4, Multiple Authors, Group Authors).

If the group name appears in the byline, it is recommended that at least 1 person serve as the corresponding author and be named as an individual who will coordinate questions about the article. This person can be named in the affiliation footnote as corresponding author. In this case, the byline might read

> Clinical Outcomes Trial Investigators

and the affiliation footnote might read

> **Author Affiliations:** A complete list of the authors in the Clinical Outcomes Trial Investigators group appears at the end of this article.

> **Corresponding Author**: James S. Smith, MD, Department of Neurology, University of Chicago Medical School, 555 S Main St, Chicago, IL 60615 (smithjs@umc.edu).

(see 2.3.3, Author Affiliations, and 2.10.7, Corresponding Author Contact Information).

Publishing the names of all authors and their specific contributions, no matter how many, with the specific article is preferred. However, a long list of investigators and their affiliations could occupy a lot of article "space" (eg, several journal pages of print journals or PDFs or screen space online). Nevertheless, it is important to publish the name of each author with the article, for reasons of accountability and credit and to allow proper searching and retrieval of articles by individual author names in bibliographic databases. Best practice is to publish all author names in the article, even if at the end of the article in an Acknowledgment or Article Information section. Nonauthor collaborators who contribute substantially to studies (eg, investigators) should be listed in the Acknowledgment or Article Information section. A less effective option is to publish the list of nonauthor collaborators in an online-only supplement to the article, as long as this is made clear to readers. It is important to include and tag all authors and nonauthor collaborators in the article XML, otherwise, there is a risk that lists of authors or collaborators not included in the main articles may not be properly included in bibliographic databases (see 5.1.10, Standards for Electronic Editing and Tagging of Names of Authors, Collaborators, and Group Authors).

Study or other group participants should not be promised authorship status and a place in the byline merely for performing activities that alone do not qualify for authorship (eg, cooperating in a study, collecting data, attending a working conference, lending technical assistance). However, performing any of those activities in addition to writing or critically revising the manuscript and approving the version to be published would be sufficient to merit authorship (see 5.1.1, Authorship: Definition, Criteria, Contributions, and Requirements). Editors and authors should assess the need to publish lengthy lists of authors and other group participants on an individual basis, and journals should publish their policies about group authorship in their instructions for authors.[9]

**5.1.9.1** **Citation of Articles With Group Authors.** Articles with authors from a large group have been difficult to locate in bibliographic databases and have resulted in citation errors and miscalculated citation statistics.[54-56] To help resolve these problems, the following has been recommended[9,58]:

> Group author articles should identify named individual authors who accept responsibility for specific articles.

> Each group author article should clearly identify all individual authors (preferably full names, but last names and initials are acceptable) as well as the complete name of the group, whether they appear in the byline, Acknowledgement, or Article Information section.

Individual authors should be distinguished from other contributors (eg, collaborators) and participants who are not authors.

The names of individual authors and the group name should be formatted and coded for easy identifiability, searching, and retrieval of the article in print and online and in bibliographic databases (see Box 5.2-1 in 5.2, Acknowledgments).

Each group author article should clearly indicate a preferred citation (eg, in the article or in an online link from the article to a reference manager).

Search results on journal websites should clearly indicate group names as published in article bylines in addition to relevant author information.

Citation standards for group author papers should continue to be developed and followed by journals, bibliographic databases, and authors.

**5.1.10** **Standards for Electronic Editing and Tagging of Names of Authors, Collaborators, and Group Authors.** To ensure appropriate display in print and online journals as well as indexing, search, and retrieval in bibliometric databases, journals should follow standards for tagging (coding) the names of authors, non-author collaborators, and group authors. The National Information Standards Organization and the National Library of Medicine have produced the Journal Article Tag Suite (JATS) to define a set of XML elements and attributes that describe the content and metadata of journal articles.[59] JATS provides guidance on how to tag authors, nonauthor collaborators, and group authors. Consistent use of tagging within the full-text article will also enable publishers to deposit the correct metadata to databases such as PubMed and Web of Science and will improve data mining and discoverability through various search engines (see 21.0, Editing, Proofreading, Tagging, and Display).

**Principal Author:** Annette Flanagin, RN, MA

ACKNOWLEDGMENT

I thank the following for review and helpful comments: Howard Bauchner, MD, *JAMA* and JAMA Network; Carissa Gilman, American Cancer Society, Atlanta, Georgia; Timothy Gray, PhD, JAMA Network; Iris Y. Lo, JAMA Network; Lou Knecht, formerly of the National Library of Medicine, Bethesda, Maryland; Ana Marušić, MD, PhD, *Journal of Global Health* and University of Split School of Medicine, Croatia; and Fred Rivara, MD, MPH, *JAMA Network Open* and University of Washington, Seattle.

REFERENCES

1. Pope A. *An Essay on Criticism*. 1711:part II, lines 412-413.
2. Hewitt RM. Exposition as applied to medicine: a glance at the ethics of it. *JAMA*. 1954;156(5):477-479.
3. Huth EJ. Guidelines on authorship of medical papers. *Ann Intern Med*. 1986;104(2):269-274.
4. International Committee of Medical Journal Editors. Guidelines on authorship. *BMJ*. 1985;291(6947):722.
5. International Committee of Medical Journal Editors. Recommendations for the conduct, reporting, editing, and publication of scholarly work in medical journals.

Updated December 2018. Accessed July 7, 2019. http://www.icmje.org/recommendations

6. US National Library of Medicine. Fact Sheet. Authorship in MEDLINE. Updated June 22, 2018. Accessed July 7, 2019. https://www.nlm.nih.gov/bsd/policy/authorship.html

7. Council of Science Editors. *Scientific Style and Format: The CSE Manual for Authors, Editors, and Publishers.* 8th ed. University of Chicago Press/Council of Science Editors; 2014.

8. Council of Science Editors. White Paper on Publication Ethics. Updated May 2018. Accessed July 7, 2019. https://www.councilscienceeditors.org/resource-library/editorial-policies/white-paper-on-publication-ethics/

9. Fontanarosa P, Bauchner H, Flanagin A. Authorship and team science. *JAMA.* 2017;318(24):2433-2437. doi:10.1001/jama.2017.19341

10. Rennie D, Yank V, Emanuel L. When authorship fails: a proposal to make contributors accountable. *JAMA.* 1997;278(7):579-585. doi:10.1001/jama.1997.03550070071041

11. Rennie D, Flanagin A, Yank V. The contributions of authors. *JAMA.* 2000;284(1):89-91. doi:10.1001/jama.284.1.89

12. Instructions for Authors. *JAMA.* Updated January 17, 2019. Accessed January 28, 2019. https://jamanetwork.com/journals/jama/pages/instructions-for-authors

13. Brand A, Allen L, Altman M, Hlava M, Scott J. Beyond authorship: attribution, contribution, collaboration, and credit. *Learned Publishing.* 2015;28(2):151-155.

14. CASRAI. CRediT. Accessed October 11, 2019. https://casrai.org/credit/

15. ORCID. Distinguishing yourself in three easy steps. Accessed October 11, 2019. https://orcid.org

16. Taichman DB, Sahni P, Pinborg A, et al. Data sharing statements for clinical trials: a requirement of the International Committee of Medical Journal Editors. *JAMA.* 2017;317(24):2491-2492. doi:10.1001/jama.2017.6514

17. Rennie D, Flanagin A. Authorship! authorship! guests, ghosts, grafters, and the two-sided coin. *JAMA.* 1994;271(6):469-471. doi:10.1001/jama.1994.03510300075043

18. Flanagin A, Rennie D. Acknowledging ghosts. *JAMA.* 1995;273(1):73. doi:10.1001/jama.1995.03520250089041

19. Yank V, Rennie D. Disclosure of researcher contributions: a study of original research articles in *The Lancet. Ann Intern Med.* 1999;130(8):661-670.

20. Flanagin A, Carey LA, Fontanarosa PB, et al. Prevalence of articles with honorary authors and ghost authors in peer-reviewed medical journals. *JAMA.* 1998;280(3):222-224. doi:10.1001/jama.280.3.222

21. Wislar J, Flanagin A, Fontanarosa PB, DeAngelis CD. Honorary and ghost authorship in high impact biomedical journals: a cross sectional survey. *BMJ.* 2011;343:d6128. doi:10.1136/bmj.d6128

22. Davidoff F, for the Council of Science Editors Taskforce on Authorship. Who's the author? problems with biomedical authorship, and some possible solutions. February 2000. Accessed December 21, 2018. https://www.councilscienceeditors.org/wp-content/uploads/v23n4p111-119.pdf

23. Marušić A, Bates T, Anic A, Marusic M. How the structure of contribution disclosure statements affects validity of authorship: a randomized study in a general medical journal. *Curr Med Res Opin.* 2006;22(6):1035-1044.

24. Greenland P, Fontanarosa PB. Ending honorary authorship. *Science.* 2012;337(6098):1019. doi:10.1126/science.1224988

25. Smith J. Gift authorship: a poisoned chalice? *BMJ*. 1994;309(6967):1456-1457.

26. Brennan TA. Buying editorials. *N Engl J Med*. 1994;331(10):673-675.

27. Ross JS, Hill KP, Egilman DS, Krumholz HM. Guest authorship and ghostwriting in publications related to rofecoxib: a case study of industry documents from rofecoxib litigation. *JAMA*. 2008;299(15):1800-1812. doi:10.1001/jama.299.15.1800

28. DeAngelis CD, Fontanarosa PB. Impugning the integrity of medical science: the adverse effects of industry influence. *JAMA*. 2008;299(15):1833-1835. doi:10.1001/jama.299.15.1833

29. Mowatt G, Shirran L, Grimshaw JM, et al. Prevalence of honorary and ghost authorship in Cochrane reviews. *JAMA*. 2002;287(21):2769-2771. doi:10.1001/jama.287.21.2769

30. DeBakey L. Rewriting and the by-line: is the author the writer? *Surgery*. 1974;75(1):38-48.

31. Hamilton CW, Royer MG; for the AMWA 2002 Task Force on the Contributions of Medical Writers to Scientific Publications. AMWA position statement on the contributions of medical writers to scientific publications. *AMWA J*. 2003;18(1):13-16.

32. Information for Authors. *Anesthesiology*. 2018. Accessed October 21, 2018. http://anesthesiology.pubs.asahq.org/public/instructionsforauthors.aspx

33. Information for Authors. *Neurology*. Accessed October 21, 2018. http://www.neurology.org/authorship-and-disclosures

34. Information for Authors. *The Lancet*. Updated April 2018. Accessed October 21, 2018. http://www.thelancet.com/lancet-information-for-authors

35. Morgan P. *An Insider's Guide for Medical Authors and Editors*. ISI Press; 1986.

36. Lock S. Signed editorials. *BMJ*. 1981;283(6296):876.

37. *The Lancet*. Signed—*The Lancet*. *Lancet*. 1993;341(8836):24.

38. Fye WB. Medical authorship: traditions, trends, and tribulations. *Ann Intern Med*. 1990;113(4):317-325.

39. US National Library of Medicine. Number of authors per MEDLINE/PubMed citation. Updated September 7, 2018. Accessed October 11, 2019. https://www.nlm.nih.gov/bsd/authors1.html

40. Aboukhalil R. The rising trend in authorship. *Winnower*. 2014;3:e141832.26907. doi:10.15200/winn.141832.26907

41. Burman KD. "Hanging from the masthead": reflections on authorship. *Ann Intern Med*. 1982;97(4):602-605.

42. Epstein RJ. Six authors in search of a citation: villains or victims of the Vancouver convention? *BMJ*. 1993;306(6880):765-767.

43. US National Library of Medicine. MEDLINE/PubMed data element (field) descriptions. Updated July 23, 2018. Accessed October 21, 2018. https://www.nlm.nih.gov/bsd/mms/medlineelements.html

44. Schmidt RH. A worksheet for authorship of scientific articles. *Bull Ecol Soc Am*. 1987;68(1):8-10.

45. Davis PJ, Gregerman RI. Parse analysis: a new method for the evaluation of investigators' bibliographies. *N Engl J Med*. 1969;281(18):989-990.

46. Chambers R, Boath E, Chambers S. The A to Z of authorship: analysis of influence of initial letter of surname of order of authorship. *BMJ*. 2001;323(7327):1460-1461.

47. Riesenberg D, Lundberg GD. The order of authorship: who's on first? *JAMA*. 1990; 264(14):1857. doi:10.1001/jama.1990.03450140079039

48. Authorship & contributorship. *BMJ*. Accessed October 21, 2018. http://www.bmj. com/about-bmj/resources-authors/article-submission/authorship-contributorship

49. Committee on Publication Ethics. Accessed October 11, 2019. https:// publicationethics.org/

50. Martinson BC, Anderson MS, de Vries R. Scientists behaving badly. *Nature*. 2005;435:737-738. doi:10.1038/435737a

51. Reinisch JF, Li WY, Yu DC, Walker JW. Authorship conflicts: a study of aware- ness of authorship criteria among academic plastic surgeons. *Plast Reconstr Surg*. 2013;132(2):303e-310e. doi:10.1097/PRS.0b013e3182958b5a

52. Dance A. Authorship: who's on first? *Nature*. 2012;489:591-593. doi:10.1038/ nj7417-591a

53. Marušić A, Bošnjak L, Jerončić A. A systematic review of research on the meaning, ethics and practices of authorship across scholarly disciplines. *PLoS ONE*. 2011;6(9):e23477. doi:10.1371/journal.pone.0023477

54. Flanagin A, Fontanarosa PB, DeAngelis CD. Authorship for research groups. *JAMA*. 2002;288(24):3166-3168. doi:10.1001/jama.288.24.3166

55. Dickersin K, Scherer R, Suci EST, Gil-Montero M. Problems with indexing and cita- tion of articles with group authorship. *JAMA*. 2002;287(21):2772-2774. doi:10.1001/ jama.287.21.2772

56. Errors in citation statistics. *Nature*. 2002;415(6868):101.

57. Cherfas J. With missing citations reported: *Nature* genome paper jumps. *Sci Watch*. 2002;13(1):8.

58. Flanagin A, Wrobel P, Barbour V, et al. CSE recommendations for group-author ar- ticles in scientific journals and bibliometric databases. Accessed October 21, 2018. http://www.councilscienceeditors.org/resource-library/editorial-policies/ cse-policies/approved-by-the-cse-board-of-directors/cse-recommendations-for-group- author-articles-in-scientific-journals-and-bibliometric-databases/

59. National Center for Biotechnology Information. Journal Article Tag Suite. Accessed October 11, 2019. https://jats.nlm.nih.gov/faq.html

## 5.2 Acknowledgments.

> *If you wish your merit to be known, acknowledge that of other people.*
> Proverb

In scientific publication, Acknowledgments typically are used to list grant or funding support, donors of equipment or supplies, technical assistance, and impor- tant specific contributions from individuals who do not qualify for authorship (see 2.10, Acknowledgments [Article Information], and 5.1.1, Authorship: Definition, Criteria, Contributions, and Requirements). Sufficient space should be provided in publications, either in print or online, for acknowledgments so that authors can properly credit all important contributions.

### 5.2.1 Acknowledging Support, Assistance, and Contributions of Those Who Are Not Authors. In the Acknowledgment, authors identify important sources of fi- nancial and material support and assistance and give credit to all persons who have

made substantial contributions to the work but who are not authors.[1,2] Contributions commonly recognized in the Acknowledgment section include the following:

General advice, guidance, or supervision
Critical review of the manuscript
Critical review of study proposal, design, or methods
Data collection
Data analysis
Statistical assistance or advice
Technical assistance or advice
Research assistance or advice
Writing assistance
Editorial assistance
Bibliographic assistance
Clerical assistance
Manuscript preparation
Financial support
Material support
Grant support

Acknowledgments should identify anyone who has made substantial intellectual contributions to manuscripts but does not meet the criteria for authorship, including medical writers and author's editors[1-4] (see 5.1.2, Guest and Ghost Authors and Other Contributors, and 5.1.9, Group and Collaborative Authorship). For example, the JAMA Network journals require the corresponding author to identify writing and editorial assistance in the Acknowledgment section of the manuscript. These journals also publish the names, specific contributions or roles, affiliations, and funding of individuals who contribute to manuscripts but who are not authors. Such disclosure is supported by the American Medical Writers Association[3] and the European Medical Writers Association[4] because it is more helpful to editors, reviewers, and readers than are vague statements about writing or editorial assistance that give no indication about specific contributions, affiliations, or financial relationships. As an example, the Acknowledgment might read as follows:

> **Additional Contribution:** We thank Joan Smart, PhD, for research and editing assistance, and John Smith, PhD, for assistance with statistical analysis; both are employed by Medical Bibliometrics Inc and received payment from the study's sponsor.

The JAMA Network journals also require the corresponding author of all manuscripts to complete an Acknowledgment statement (on the authorship form) that reads as follows:

> I certify that all persons who have made substantial contributions to the work reported in the manuscript (eg, data collection, analysis, or writing or editing assistance) but do not fulfill authorship criteria are named with their specific contributions in an acknowledgment in the manuscript.

> I certify that all persons named in the Acknowledgment have provided me with written permission to be named.

I certify that if an Acknowledgment section is not included, no other persons have made substantial contributions to this manuscript.

Nonspecific group acknowledgments, such as "the house staff," "the nurses in the emergency department," or "patient participants" are often used to thank groups of individuals. However, if specific individuals are identifiable, permission to include them would be needed (see 5.2.9, Permission to Name Individuals). Acknowledgment of unidentifiable groups, such as "the anonymous peer reviewers," is not informative, and with current policies encouraging greater transparency, acknowledging any anonymous contributions is best avoided.

**5.2.2** **Group and Collaborative Author Lists.** A list of participants in a collaborative group may also be included in the Acknowledgment[5,6] (see 5.1.9, Group and Collaborative Authorship). However, a lengthy acknowledgment may occupy an excessive amount of article space, especially for print journals with set page budgets or limits. Some have previously proposed limits on the length of an acknowledgment (eg, 1 column of a journal page or 600 words of reduced type),[7] but such limits seem contrary to commitments to greater transparency of the contributions to scientific publication, and journals should carefully evaluate the appropriateness of any limits on the length of acknowledgments. However, the need to credit assistance from individuals, especially in reports of large multicenter clinical trials, and research networks varies considerably. Thus, the editor and corresponding author should determine the length of published acknowledgments on a case-by-case basis. Although not best practice, especially given that PubMed includes lists of nonauthor collaborators in PubMed records,[8] if it is determined that there is not sufficient space in a print or PDF article to include a long list of collaborative participants, the list can be published in an online supplement to the article with a note indicating so in the Acknowledgment or Article Information section:

> A list of study investigators and participating centers of the European Diabetes Intervention Trial is available online at http://archinte.ama-assn.org/cgi/content/full/165/22/2495.

In such cases, it is important to include and tag authors and nonauthor collaborators in the article XML. See also "Group Information" example in **Box 5.2-1** and 5.1.10, Standards for Electronic Editing and Tagging of Names of Authors, Collaborators, and Group Authors.

**5.2.3** **Author Contributions.** The International Committee of Medical Journal Editors (ICMJE) encourages authors and journals to disclose authors' individual contributions to the work reported in published articles.[9] Following this and other recommendations, a number of journals publish lists of author contributions in the article's Acknowledgment or Article Information section.[10,11] For example, the JAMA Network journals publish each author's contributions to all reports of research, as shown in the example in Box 5.2-1.

**5.2.4** **Authors' Conflict of Interest Disclosures.** Authors' conflict of interest disclosure statements should be published with articles in a consistent manner.[9] For example, some journals include authors' conflict of interest disclosures in the Acknowledgment section at the end of the article. These journals require authors to include all potential conflicts of interest, including specific financial interests and relationships and affiliations (other than those affiliations listed on the title page of the manuscript) relevant to the subject of their manuscript, in the Acknowledgment section at the time the manuscript is submitted. Authors without conflicts of interest, including specific financial interests and relationships and affiliations relevant to the subject of their manuscript, should include a statement of no such conflicts of interests in the Acknowledgment section of the manuscript[11-13] (see Box 5.2-1 and 5.5.3, Reporting Funding, Sponsorship, and Other Support).

Many journals require authors to complete the ICMJE Form for Disclosure of Potential Conflicts of Interest[9] or include the wording of the ICMJE form in their journal authorship forms.[11] An example of such a disclosure in the Acknowledgment section is shown in Box 5.2-1. Some journals include links to online PDF copies of these disclosure forms for each author or links to databases with disclosures for authors in the Acknowledgment or Article Information sections.

**5.2.5** **Access to Data Statement.** The ICMJE recommends that journals ask authors whether they "had access to the study data, with an explanation of the nature and extent of access, including whether access is on-going."[9] Consistent with this recommendation, the JAMA Network journals require at least 1 named author (eg, the principal investigator), and preferably no more than 2 authors, to indicate that she or he had full access to all the data in the study and takes responsibility for the integrity of the data and the accuracy of the data analysis for all reports that contain original data (eg, research articles, systematic reviews, and meta-analyses). This information should be published in the Acknowledgment section (see 5.1.1.4, Access to Data and Data Sharing Statement Requirements). The JAMA Network journals publish this information just before the list of author contributions.

Author Contributions: Drs Smith and Jones had full access to all the data in the study and take responsibility for the integrity of the data and the accuracy of the data analysis.

**5.2.6** **Funding and Role of Funders and Sponsors.** Information about funding, sponsorship, or other financial or material support should also be clearly and completely identified in the Acknowledgment section.[9-11] Some journals require this to be reported in the Methods section. For all manuscripts that are funded by commercial, governmental, or private entities, a description of the role of the sponsor(s) in the work reported and the preparation, submission, and review of the manuscript should be published as well. For example, for all funded manuscripts, including letters to the editor, the JAMA Network journals require the corresponding author to indicate the role of the funder or sponsor in each of the following:

Design and conduct of the study

Collection, management, analysis, and interpretation of the data

Preparation, review, or approval of the manuscript

Decision to submit the manuscript for publication

If the funder or sponsor had no role in the above activities, that information should be indicated. If authors are employees of a funder or sponsor, this information

**Box 5.2-1.** Hypothetical Example of an Acknowledgment or Article Information Section, Including Order of All Possible Elements

Note: Not all of the elements listed below are relevant for all manuscripts, and they are not published by all journals. Asterisk (*) indicates items that may normally appear on page 1 of a print or PDF article but would otherwise appear here in this order in an Acknowledgment or Article Information section.

Some of these elements would be submitted by authors (eg, author affiliations), and others would be added by manuscript or production editors (eg, acceptance and publication dates).

**For an Article With the Following Byline:**
Jack Kroll, MD; Kathryn Smith, RN, PhD; Jake Otter, MPH; Henry Jones, MD; for the Stress Intervention Trial Investigators

**Accepted for Publication:** November 17, 2017.
**Published Online:** January 5, 2018. doi:10.1001/jama.2017.57418
**Correction:** This article was corrected on February 20, 2018, to fix an error in the legend of Figure 1.
**Open Access:** This article is published under the journal's open access model and is free to read on the day of publication.
OR
This article is published under a CC BY open access license and is free to read on the day of publication.
*Corresponding Author:** Jack Kroll, MD, Division of Cardiovascular Medicine, University of Florida College of Medicine, 25 Main St, Gainesville, FL 32601 (krollj@ufcm.edu).
*Author Affiliations:** Division of Cardiovascular Medicine, University of Florida College of Medicine, Gainesville (Kroll); Department of Behavioral Science, University of Pittsburgh Medical Center, Pittsburgh, Pennsylvania (Smith); Department of Psychiatry, University of Oxford, Oxford, England (Otter).
*Group Information**: The Stress Intervention Trial Investigators are listed at the end of this article.
**Author Contributions:** As principal investigator, Dr Kroll had full access to all the data in the study and takes responsibility for the integrity of the data and the accuracy of the data analysis.
*Study concept and design:* All authors.
*Acquisition of data:* Kroll, Otter.
*Analysis and interpretation of data:* All authors.
*Drafting of the manuscript:* Kroll.
*Critical revision of the manuscript for important intellectual content:* All authors.
*Statistical analysis:* Kroll, Smith.
*Obtained funding:* Kroll.
*Administrative, technical, or material support:* Kroll.
*Study supervision:* Kroll.
**Conflict of Interest Disclosures:** Dr Kroll reported receiving research grants from and is a paid consultant to Progen International Inc, manufacturer of the neurochemical assay used in this study, and research grants from the International Society of Stress Research. No other disclosures were reported.

*(continued)*

**Box 5.2-1.** Hypothetical Example of an Acknowledgment or Article Information Section, Including Order of All Possible Elements (*continued*)

**Funding/Support:** This study was funded by Progen International Inc and the International Society of Stress Research.

**Role of the Funder/Sponsor:** Progen International Inc supplied the neurochemical assay used in this study and funded the study. Through Dr Kroll, Progen International Inc participated in the design and conduct of the study; in the collection, analysis, and interpretation of the data; and in the preparation of the manuscript. Progen International Inc reviewed the manuscript before submission and paid for editing assistance. The International Society of Stress Research had no role in the design and conduct of the study; collection, analysis, and interpretation of the data; preparation, review, or approval of the manuscript; and decision to submit the manuscript for publication.

**Group Information: The Stress Intervention Trial Investigators:** *Steering Committee:* Jeff Brown, MD, David Chillow, MD, Jane Marshall, MBBS, Lionell J. Roew, MD, Gilberto Felosa, MD, Ulrich Teich, MD, Li Wang, MD, MPH, Alexandra Zeer, PhD; *Data and Safety Monitoring Committee:* Janice Frank, MD, chair; Michelle Dickersin, MD, William Malden, MD, Adam Skowrenski, PhD, Anita Toole, MD; *Research Coordinators:* Michael Billings, MPH, Timothy Downing, PharmD, Laura Grower, RN, Kenneth Morrisey, MD, Frederic McLendon, RN, Wanda Smythe, MS, Anne Trafford, PhD.

**Disclaimer:** The views expressed in this article are those of the authors and do not necessarily reflect the opinions of the authors' institutions.

**Meeting Presentation:** Presented in part at the 12th International Stress Management Congress; February 15, 2017; Chicago, Illinois.

**Data Sharing Statement:** See Supplement 3.

Note: Some journals may publish a complete data sharing statement in the Acknowledgment or Article Information section.

**Additional Contributions:** We thank Joan Simpson, MS, of Write Services, who was paid by Progen International Inc for editing the manuscript. We thank the 3 patients with serious adverse events, who reviewed the submitted manuscript, for granting permission to include the details about their cases in this article.

**Additional Information:** Coauthor Henry Jones died April 11, 2019.

Note: Some journals may also publish a Preferred Citation in the Acknowledgment or Article Information section:

**Preferred Citation:** Kroll J, Smith H, Otter J; Stress Intervention Trial Investigators. An intervention to reduce stress. Published online January 5, 2018. *JAMA.* 2018;319(22):1553-1559. doi:10.1001/jama.2017.57418

should include any role of the funder of sponsor above and beyond the contributions of the specific sponsor-employed authors. Some journals publish this information in the Methods section. The JAMA Network journals publish it in the Acknowledgment section (see 5.5.2, Requirements for Authors, and the following examples).

**Role of the Funder/Sponsor:** The Centers for Disease Control and Prevention had no role in the design and conduct of the study or the collection, management, analysis, and interpretation of the data; it reviewed and approved the manuscript for submission.

**Role of the Funder/Sponsor:** The Deutsche Krenbhilfe had no role in the design and conduct of the study; the collection, management, analysis, and interpretation of the data; and the preparation, review, approval, or decision to submit the manuscript. Authors who are employees of Biopharm Company participated in each of these activities. The National Institutes of Health reviewed and approved the study before funding.

**Role of the Funder/Sponsor:** The Medicines Co and the REPLACE-2 Steering Committee designed the trial, developed the protocol, and determined the statistical analysis plan by consensus. Data were collected through an internet-based electronic case-report form managed by Etrials. The sponsor had no access to the database or the randomization code, which were housed at Etrials and Integrated Clinical Technologies Inc, respectively, until finalization of the database. Data management and site monitoring were performed by International HealthCare. The finalized database was electronically transferred simultaneously to the Cleveland Clinic Cardiovascular Coordinating Center and to The Medicines Co, where unblinding and statistical analyses were separately performed. All analyses for scientific publication were performed by the study statistician at the Cleveland Clinic, independently of the sponsor. Dr Lincoff wrote all drafts of the manuscript and made revisions based on the comments of the study chairman, the Steering Committee, coauthors, and the trial sponsor. The study contract specified that the sponsor had the right to review all publications before submission and could delay submission of such publications for up to 60 days if necessary to make new patent applications but could not mandate any revision of the manuscript or prevent submission for publication.

**5.2.7** **Data Sharing Statement.** For reports of randomized clinical trials, the ICMJE recommends that authors of clinical trials provide a data sharing statement with submitted manuscripts and indicate if data, including individual patient data, a data dictionary that defines each field in the data set, and supporting documentation, will be made available to others; when, where, and how the data will be available; types of analyses that are permitted; and if there will be any restrictions on the use of the data.[9] This follows a previous ICMJE requirement for authors of clinical trials to also include trial protocols with submitted manuscripts and published articles. Data sharing statements may also be submitted for reports of other types of studies, but the ICMJE member journals only require this for reports of randomized clinical trials.

The data sharing statements should address the following items:

Data

Will the data collected for your study, including individual patient data and a data dictionary defining each field in the data set, be made available to others?

Yes or No (if No, authors may explain why data are not available)

List all data that will be made available.

Deidentified participant data

Participant data with identifiers

Data dictionary

Other (please specify)

List where to access these data. Provide complete URL if data will be available in a repository or website, or provide complete email address if request for data must be sent to an individual.

List the beginning date and end date (if applicable) when these data will be available. If the beginning date of data availability will be when the article is published, please indicate "with publication."

With publication

At a date different from publication

Beginning date

End date (if applicable)

### Supporting Documents

If your manuscript is accepted for publication, the journal will publish your trial protocol, including the statistical analysis plan, and any amendments as online supplements. Please list any other supporting documents that you wish to make available (eg, statistical/analytic code, informed consent form).

Statistical/analytic code

Informed consent form

None

Other (please specify)

List where to access these documents. Provide complete URL if the documents will be available in a repository or website, or provide complete email address if request for documents must be sent to an individual.

List the beginning date and end date (if applicable) when the documents will be available.

With publication

At a date different from publication

Beginning date

End date (if applicable)

### Additional Information

Indicate the types of analyses for which the data will be made available (eg, for any purpose or for a specified purpose).

Indicate the mechanisms by which the data will be made available (eg, with investigator support, without investigator support, after approval of a proposal, or with a signed data access agreement).

List any additional restrictions on the use of the data or any additional information.

If you would like to offer context for your decision not to make the data available, please enter it below (optional).

**5.2.8** ▨ **Acknowledgment Elements and Order of Elements.** An example of the Acknowledgment section, including all possible elements, as it would appear in the JAMA Network journals is shown in Box 5.2-1. In print or PDF versions of journal articles, author affiliations and correspondence information typically are published on the title page (or first page) of an article. However, in some cases (eg, articles with lengthy abstracts and author bylines) and in some journals (due to design considerations), there may not be sufficient room for all this information, and it may be published in the Acknowledgment section at the end of the article with a note indicating such on the first page of the article. Online, the author information and Acknowledgment section usually appear at the end of the article before the reference list and may be hyperlinked from the list of authors at the beginning of the article. These sections have various names, such as Acknowledgment, Article Information, and Endnotes.

**5.2.9** ▨ **Permission to Name Individuals.** Identification of individuals in an Acknowledgment may imply their endorsement of the article's content. Thus, persons should not be listed in an acknowledgment without their knowledge and consent. For this reason, the ICMJE and the JAMA Network journals require the corresponding author to obtain written permission from any individuals named in the Acknowledgment section and to certify in writing to the editor that such permission has been obtained.[2,9,11] However, these permissions do not need to be submitted to the journal.

**5.2.10** ▨ **Personal Communication and Credit Lines.** Following the rationale that including a person's name in an acknowledgment may imply endorsement of a manuscript's content, citing an individual's name in a personal communication citation may carry the same implication. The ICMJE recommends that authors who name an individual as a source for information in a personal communication, whether through conversation, telephone call, or a letter sent by electronic communication, obtain written permission from that individual to be named.[9] The JAMA Network journals follow the ICMJE recommendation and require authors to confirm that permission has been obtained from all those named in personal communications. The same policy might apply to identifying names in credit lines in the legends of illustrations and photographs; however, obtaining such permission from the owner of the illustration or photograph would be part of obtaining permission to include such works as required under the auspices of copyright law (see 5.6.7, Copying, Reproducing, Adapting, and Other Uses of Content).

**5.2.11** ▨ **Standards for Tagging Metadata in Acknowledgments.** To ensure appropriate display in print and online journals as well as indexing, search, and retrieval in bibliometric databases, journals should follow standards for tagging (coding) to identify the Acknowledgment or Article Information section and important elements, such as author conflict of interest disclosures, funding or sponsorship information, lists of nonauthor collaborators, and group author information. The National Information Standards Organization (NISO) and the National Library of Medicine have produced the Journal Article Tag Suite (JATS)[14] to define a set of XML elements and attributes that describe the content and metadata of journal articles, including the Acknowledgment and elements in it. Consistent use of tagging within the full-text article will also enable the correct data mining by the publisher to submit specific metadata to databases such as PubMed and Web of Science and will enhance discoverability via search engines (see 21.0, Editing, Proofreading, Tagging, and Display).

**Principal Author:** Annette Flanagin, RN, MA

## ACKNOWLEDGMENT

I thank the following for review and helpful comments: Howard Bauchner, MD, *JAMA* and JAMA Network; Carissa Gilman, American Cancer Society, Atlanta, Georgia; Timothy Gray, PhD, JAMA Network; Iris Y. Lo, JAMA Network; Lou Knecht, formerly of the National Library of Medicine, Bethesda, Maryland; and Ana Marušić, MD, PhD, *Journal of Global Health* and University of Split School of Medicine, Croatia.

## REFERENCES

1. Rennie D, Flanagin A. Authorship! authorship! guests, ghosts, grafters, and the two-sided coin. *JAMA*. 1994;271(6):469-471. doi:10.1001/jama.1994.03510300075043
2. Flanagin A, Rennie D. Acknowledging ghosts. *JAMA*. 1995;273(1):73. doi:10.1001/jama.1995.03520250089041
3. Hamilton CW, Royer MG; for the AMWA 2002 Task Force on the Contributions of Medical Writers to Scientific Publications. AMWA position statement on the contributions of medical writers to scientific publications. *AMWA J*. 2003;18(1):13-16.
4. Jacobs A, Wager E. European Medical Writers Association (EMWA) guidelines on the role of medical writers in developing peer-reviewed publications. *Curr Med Res Opin*. 2005;21(2):317-321. doi:10.1185/030079905X25578
5. Flanagin A, Fontanarosa PB, DeAngelis CD. Authorship for research groups. *JAMA*. 2002;288(24):3166-3168. doi:10.1001/jama.288.24.3166
6. Fontanarosa P, Bauchner H, Flanagin A. Authorship and team science. *JAMA*. 2017;318(24):2433-2437. doi:10.1001/jama.2017.19341
7. Kassirer JP, Angell M. On authorship and acknowledgments. *N Engl J Med*. 1991;325(21):1510-1512. doi:10.1056/NEJM199111213252112
8. US National Library of Medicine. Authorship in MEDLINE. Updated June 22, 2018. Accessed December 21, 2018. https://www.nlm.nih.gov/bsd/policy/authorship.html
9. International Committee of Medical Journal Editors. Recommendations for the conduct, reporting, editing, and publication of scholarly work in medical journals. Updated December 2018. Accessed December 21, 2018. http://www.icmje.org/recommendations

10. Rennie D, Flanagin A, Yank V. The contributions of authors. *JAMA*. 2000;284(1):89-91. doi:10.1001/jama.284.1.89

11. Instructions for Authors. *JAMA*. Updated June 10, 2019. Accessed July 7, 2019. https://jamanetwork.com/journals/jama/pages/instructions-for-authors

12. Fontanarosa PB, Flanagin A, DeAngelis CD. Implementation of the ICMJE form for reporting potential conflicts of interest. *JAMA*. 2010;304(13):1496. doi:10.1001/jama.2010.1429

13. Bauchner H, Fontanarosa PB, Flanagin A. Conflicts of interests, authors, and journals: new challenges for a persistent problem. *JAMA*. 2018;320(22):2315-2318. doi:10.1001/jama.2018.1759310

14. National Center for Biotechnology Information. Journal Article Tag Suite. Accessed July 7, 2019. https://jats.nlm.nih.gov/faq.html

## 5.3 Duplicate Publication and Submission.

*Wasteful publication includes dividing the results in a single study into two or more papers ("salami science"); republishing the same material in successive papers (which need not have identical format and content); and blending data from one study with additional data to extract yet another paper that could not make its way on the second set of data alone ("meat extenders").*
Edward J. Huth, MD[1]

*Duplicate publication* is the simultaneous or subsequent reporting of essentially the same information, article, or major components of an article 2 or more times in 1 or more forms of media (either print or electronic format) by 1 or more of the same authors.[2-9] Duplicate reporting includes duplicate submission and may apply to both published and unpublished works (eg, 1 or more manuscripts not yet published but under consideration by another or multiple journals). Other terms used to describe this practice include *redundant, prior, repetitive, overlapping, related, multiple, dual, parallel, fragmented,* and *secondary* publication.[3,8,9] The term *self-plagiarism* is best avoided to describe duplication by the same author(s) given that plagiarism is a form of theft and authors cannot steal from themselves (see 5.4.2, Misappropriation: Plagiarism and Breaches of Confidentiality).

Duplicate submission or publication is not necessarily unethical, but failure to disclose the existence of duplicate articles, manuscripts, or other related material to editors and readers (covert duplication) is unethical and may represent a violation of copyright law. Moreover, reports of the same data in multiple articles waste publishing resources (ie, those of editors, reviewers, and readers as well as journal pages or space),[1] pollute the literature with redundant information of dubious additional value, may result in double counting of data or inappropriate weighting of the results of a study and thereby distort the available evidence,[2] cause problems for researchers and those who conduct systematic reviews and meta-analyses,[10,11] and may damage the reputation of authors[12] (see 5.3.1, Secondary Publication, for a discussion of legitimate secondary publication).

Duplicate publication usually involves 1 or more of the same authors, but the number of authors and order of authors may differ among the duplicate reports. Duplication occurs when there is substantial overlap in 1 or more elements of an article or manuscript. For reports of research, duplicative elements may include any or all of the following: the introduction, design, methods, samples or subsamples, data, outcomes, tables, graphics and illustrative material, discussion, or conclusions. Inclusion of the same or similar wording for Design and Methods sections in reports of follow-up studies or to describe samples or data sets in reports of secondary analyses is acceptable provided that the primary study is cited in the follow-up and secondary publications. Duplication also occurs in other types of articles (eg, reviews, case reports, opinion pieces, letters to the editor, and blog posts). Postpublication news summaries and brief summaries via social media are not typically considered duplicate publication in the context of scholarly publishing; citation of (or linking to) the primary article or reference in these summaries is recommended.

There is no widely accepted method of classifying the amount of acceptable overlap or duplication. Authors and editors often disagree on how to define and quantify duplication and whether duplicate articles are justified.[13] Researchers in 2 studies of duplicate publication classified an article as duplicative of another if 10% or more of the content was identical or highly similar.[7,14] Others have described levels and patterns of duplicate publication for research articles that emanate from 1 study, such as reporting identical samples and identical outcomes, identical samples and different outcomes, increasing or decreasing sample sizes and identical outcomes, and different subsamples from the same overall large study and different outcomes.[12,15] Studies have also found that most duplicate articles are published within 1 year of the publication of the first report.[12,16]

A number of studies of the prevalence of duplicate publication in various fields, using the various levels and definitions of duplication noted in the above paragraph, have found that 1.4% to 28% of published articles were classified as duplicative of other articles.[7,8,10,14,16-23] In addition, these studies reported that as many as 5% to 61% of duplicative articles did not include a citation or reference to the original or primary article (covert duplication).[7,10,14,18,21,22]

Following the recommendations of the International Committee of Medical Journal Editors (ICMJE),[2] a policy that prohibits or discourages duplicate submission and publication does not preclude consideration of manuscripts that report on research that has been presented at a professional society or scientific meeting as abstracts or posters, orally, or in slides or other digital media. This policy applies whether the presentation is made in person or via webcast or an online meeting presentation. However, publication of complete manuscripts in proceedings of such meetings in print or online may preclude consideration for publication in a primary-source journal. The ICMJE cautions authors to "consider how dissemination of their findings outside of scientific presentations at meetings may diminish the priority journal editors assign to their work."[2]

News reports that cover presentations of data at scheduled professional meetings would not necessarily violate this policy, but authors should avoid distributing copies of their complete manuscripts, tables, graphs, and illustrations during such meetings. Preliminary release of information directly to the news media, usually through press conferences or news releases, and dissemination of that information in news reports or social media should be considered by journal editors during the evaluation of a submitted manuscript and could jeopardize an author's chances for publication in a primary-source journal.[24] However, exceptions are made when a government health agency determines that there is an immediate public need for such information[8,24] (see 5.13.1, Release of Information to the Public).

Manuscripts that are based on the same data or report analyses of the same data sets are acceptable when these are from different authors. The ICMJE recommends that such manuscripts be handled independently because they "may differ in their analytic methods, conclusions, or both."[2] Authors of reports of secondary analyses should cite the primary analysis and publication, clearly describe the database on which the analysis and report are based, and indicate any overlap in data. This information should also be summarized in the cover letter that accompanies the submitted manuscript. Editors should make decisions on these types of papers based on their editorial priorities and the strengths of the individual analyses and reports and, if all are relatively equal, perhaps give primacy to the manuscript submitted first or consider the merits if the secondary report is an important replication study.

Authors may also publish multiple articles using the same data from very large studies but addressing different questions. In these cases, authors should clearly cite previous related articles and should inform editors of any related manuscripts under consideration elsewhere or in preparation.

See **Box 5.3-1** for examples of duplicate reports that may be acceptable and necessary.

**5.3.1** **Secondary Publication.** Secondary publication is the subsequent republication, or simultaneous publication (sometimes called dual or parallel publication), of an article in 2 or more journals (in the same or another language) by mutual consent of the journal editors. Secondary publication can be beneficial. For example, the editors of an English-language journal and a non–English-language journal may agree to secondary publication in translated form for the benefit of audiences who speak different languages.

The ICMJE approves secondary publication if all the following conditions are met[2]:

1. The authors have received approval from the editors of both journals (the editor concerned with secondary publication must have access to the primary version).

2. The priority of the primary publication is respected by a publication interval negotiated by both editors with the authors.

3. The paper for secondary publication is intended for a different group of readers; an abbreviated version could be sufficient.

4. The secondary version faithfully reflects the authors, data, and interpretations of the primary version.

5. The secondary version informs readers, peers, and documenting agencies that the paper has been published in whole or in part elsewhere–for example, with a note that might read: "This article is based

**Box 5.3-1.** Duplicate Reports That May Be Acceptable[a]

**Summaries or Abstracts of Findings Reported in Conference Proceedings**

Editors do not discourage authors from presenting their findings at conferences or scientific meetings, but they recommend that authors refrain from distributing complete copies of their papers, which might later appear in some form of publication without their knowledge. Previous presentation(s) should be noted in submitted manuscripts (see 2.10, Manuscript Preparation for Submission and Publication, Acknowledgments [Article Information], Meeting Presentation).

**News Media Reports of Authors' Findings**

Typically, editors do not discourage authors from reporting their findings at conferences covered by the news media, but they discourage authors from distributing their full papers, tables, or figures, which might later appear printed in a newspaper, a newsletter, or the news section of a magazine. Editors do not discourage authors from participating in interviews with the news media after a paper has been accepted but before it is published. However, authors should remind reporters that most journals have an embargo policy that prohibits media coverage of the manuscript under consideration and the article before it is published (see 5.13, Release of Information to the Public and Relations With the News Media).

**Fragments or Sequential Reports of Studies**

Editors make decisions about these types of duplicative research reports on a case-by-case basis. For all such papers, editors ask that authors properly reference previously reported parts of a study and send copies of these papers or articles along with their submitted manuscript.

**Detailed Reports Previously Distributed to a Narrow Audience**

The scope of this audience and the nature of distribution (eg, small print run, time-limited placement on closed website) would determine whether editors would publish a duplicative report. For all such papers, editors ask that authors properly reference all such previous publications and send copies of these along with their submitted manuscript.

**Short Reports in Print and Longer, More Detailed Reports Online**

Some journals publish shorter versions of articles in print and longer versions online. The existence of multiple versions of the same article should be made clear to readers and bibliographic databases.

**Executive Summaries and Evidence Synopses**

Concise overviews or summaries of large, detailed reports, documents, or guidelines or synopses of evidence-based analyses or systematic reviews that are regularly updated are handled on a case-by-case basis. For all such summaries, editors ask that authors properly reference the larger, more detailed report.

**Reports From Government Documents or Reports in the Public Domain**

Decisions regarding republication of government documents or other reports in the public domain are based on the importance of the message, priority for the journal's readers, and availability of the information. For example, a journal may publish reports from the Centers for Disease Control and Prevention that were initially published in the *Morbidity and Mortality Weekly Report,* or a journal may publish a report from a governmental agency after the public

*(continued)*

**Box 5.3-1.** Duplicate Reports That May Be Acceptable (*continued*)

release of a draft report (eg, from the US Preventive Services Task Force) or a required data release (eg, from the US Security and Exchange Commission). The existence of multiple versions of the same report should be made clear to readers.

**Translations of Reports in Another Language**
Translations are usually acceptable as long as they give proper attribution to the original publication (see 5.3.1, Secondary Publication). Translations should be faithful to the original, should not introduce any new content or authors, and should not omit any content or authors. Translators should be acknowledged.

**Announcements Shared Across Journals**
Simultaneous publication of editorial announcements, policies, or reporting

guidelines are acceptable provided that indication of the nature of the simultaneous publication is indicated (see 5.3.1, Secondary Publication).

**Reports Based on the Same Data or Data Sets**
Reports from different authors that are based on the same data or analyses of the same data sets are acceptable because they may differ in their methods, analysis, interpretation, or conclusions.

For each of these cases, a query to the editorial office is recommended, asking whether any previous publication or release of information jeopardizes a chance for subsequent publication in a specific journal.

<sup></sup>ªUpdated from Blancett et al.[7]

on a study first reported in the [journal title, with full reference]"–and the secondary version cites the primary reference.

6. The title of the secondary publication should indicate that it is a secondary publication (complete or abridged republication or translation) of a primary publication. Of note, the NLM does not consider translations to be "republications" and does not cite or index them when the original article was published in a journal that is indexed in MEDLINE.

MEDLINE includes a language field for identifying multiple languages in which an article, or its abstract, is published. Thus, when the same journal simultaneously publishes an article, or its abstract, in multiple languages, the MEDLINE citation will include the multiple languages if the publisher supplies this information to PubMed.[25] For example, the citation for this article in 3 languages appears in PubMed as follows:

Transcultural adaptation and validation of the Conditions of Work Effectiveness-Questionnaire-II instrument.

Bernardino E, Dyniewicz AM, Carvalho KL, Kalinowski LC, Bonat WH.

Rev Lat Am Enfermagem. 2013 Sep-Oct;21(5):1112-8. doi:10.1590/S0104-11692013000500014. English, Portuguese, Spanish.

PMID: 24142220

Simultaneous publication may appear in more than 1 journal for general announcements or new shared policies or reporting guidelines. See, for example, the following:

> Taichman DB, Sahni P, Pinborg A, et al. Data sharing statements for clinical trials: a requirement of the International Committee of Medical Journal Editors. *JAMA*. 2017;317(24):2491-2492. doi:10.1001/jama.2017.6514

In the above cited example, the following note is included at the end of the article:

> **Note:** This article is being published simultaneously in *Annals of Internal Medicine, BMJ (British Medical Journal), Bulletin of the World Health Organization, Deutsches Ärzteblatt (German Medical Journal), Ethiopian Journal of Health Sciences, JAMA, Journal of Korean Medical Science, New England Journal of Medicine, New Zealand Medical Journal, PLOS Medicine, The Lancet, Revista Médica de Chile (Medical Journal of Chile)*, and *Ugeskrift for Laeger (Danish Medical Journal)*.

**5.3.2** **Editorial Policy for Preventing and Handling Allegations of Duplicate Publication.** Covert duplicate publication violates the ethics of scientific publishing and may constitute a violation of copyright law or publication licenses and agreements. Editors have a duty to inform prospective authors of their policies on duplicate publication, which should be published in their instructions for authors. Reviewers should notify editors of the existence of duplicate articles discovered during their review. Authors should provide copies of duplicate or overlapping articles and manuscripts with their submitted manuscripts. Authors should also include citations to highly similar articles and any reports from the same study under their authorship in the reference list of the submitted manuscript. When in doubt about the possibility of duplication or redundancy of information in articles based on the same study or topic, authors should inform and consult the editor.

The editors of *JAMA* and the JAMA Network journals have adopted the following policies to prevent the practice of duplicate publication or minimize the risk of its occurrence. At the time a manuscript is submitted, the author must inform the editor in the event that any part of the material (1) has been or is about to be published elsewhere in any form or (2) is under consideration by another journal or publisher. In the case of a highly similar article or manuscript, the author should provide the editor with a copy of the other article(s) or manuscript(s) so the editor can determine whether the contents are duplicative and whether such duplication affects the editorial priority of the submitted manuscript.

Preprints are not considered duplicate publications, but authors should inform editors of previously posted preprints (see 5.6.2, Public Access and Open Access in Scientific Publication). All authors are required to complete an authorship criteria and responsibility statement, which includes the following declaration:

> Neither this manuscript nor another manuscript with substantially similar content under my authorship has been published or is being considered for publication elsewhere, except as described in an attachment, and copies of related manuscripts are provided.

In addition, many journals require authors to transfer copyright ownership or grant a publication license to the journal as a condition of publication (see 5.6.5, Copyright Assignment or License). In the case of duplicate submission, copyright or publication right is likely owned by the first journal to publish the manuscript, depending on whether copyright ownership or an exclusive publication license was transferred. Journals that require authors to grant a license to publish a manuscript, including those that rely on Creative Commons licenses, also expect authors to inform editors and prospective readers of any duplicative material (see 5.6.5, Copyright Assignment or License).

Some journals may use software to screen submitted manuscripts to help identify content that may overlap with content that has been previously published in other journals.[26] This software may also be used to help identify plagiarism. Such similarity-checking software relies on screening of public and private bibliometric databases and may result in false-positive results that require editors to review for type and extent of duplication (see 5.4.2, Misappropriation: Plagiarism and Breaches of Confidentiality).

In a case of suspected duplicate submission or publication, editors should first contact the corresponding author and request a written explanation. Additional actions that may be considered are described below.

The Committee on Publication Ethics (COPE) provides flow diagrams that editors may find helpful when assessing how best to address duplicate submission or publication.[27]

**5.3.2.1** **Duplicate Submission.** If an author submits a duplicate manuscript without notifying the editor, the editor should act promptly when evidence of duplicate submission is discovered.[2] If duplicate submission of a manuscript is suspected before publication, the editor should notify the corresponding author and ask for a copy of the potentially duplicative material, if not already in hand, as well as copies of any other similar articles and manuscripts, and request a written explanation. After reviewing all material, the editor will then decide whether to continue to consider or to reject the submitted manuscript. If the manuscript is rejected because of duplicate submission, this reason should be indicated clearly in the decision letter.

**5.3.2.2** **Duplicate Publication.** If an editor suspects that duplicate publication has occurred, the editor should contact the corresponding author and all coauthors and request a written explanation. If necessary, the editor (possibly with the benefit of additional expert opinion) may consult the editor of the other journal in which the material appeared. If both editors agree that duplication has occurred, the editor of the second journal to publish the article should inform the author of the intention to publish a notice of duplicate publication in a subsequent issue of the journal. It is preferable that this notice be signed by the author or be accompanied by a letter of explanation from the author, but a notice of duplicate publication should be published without the author's explanation or approval if none is forthcoming.[2] Depending on the situation, the editor may also choose to notify the author's institutional supervisor (eg, department chair, dean) to request an evaluation of the duplication or request assistance with acquisition of an appropriate letter from the author.

**5.3.2.3** **Notice of Duplicate Publication.** The notice of duplicate publication should be published formally in print and/or online and listed in the table of contents or online index of the journal in a citable format to ensure that the notice will be indexed appropriately in literature databases. The notice should be labeled or titled as "Notice of Duplicate Publication" and it may be published as correspondence or as a correction or erratum. The US National Library of Medicine identifies duplicate articles in its bibliographic database by adding a publication type of "Duplicate Publication" to the record of each duplicate article and links subsequently published notices of duplicate publication to the citations of the duplicate articles.[22]

It is preferable to publish an explanation from the author(s) of the duplicate article with the notice, but this is not always possible or necessary. The words *Duplicate Publication* should be included in the title of the notice, which should include complete citations to all duplicate articles (because there may be more than 1). Examples of Notices of Duplicate Publication published as Letters from the authors or editors are as follows:

> Xi B. Notice of duplicate publication: "Performance of the Simplified American Academy of Pediatrics Table to Screen Elevated Blood Pressure in Children." (*JAMA Pediatr.* doi:10.1001/jamapediatrics.2018.1923). *JAMA Pediatr.* 2018; 172(12):1198-1199. doi:10.1001/jamapediatrics.2018.4068

> Freischlag J. Notice of duplicate publication: "Pathogenesis of Barrett Esophagus: Deoxycholic Acid Up-regulates Goblet-Specific Gene *MUC2* in Concert With *CDX2* in Human Esophageal Cells" (*Arch Surg.* 2007;142 [6]:540-545). *Arch Surg.* 2008;143(8):807. doi:10.1001/archsurg. 143.8.807-a

**Box 5.3-2** provides an example of such a notice (wording would depend on the circumstances in each case), and **Box 5.3-3**, an example of a table of contents listing. Note: The examples in Boxes 5.3-2 and 5.3-3 are hypothetical and are intended to show all the elements needed for a published notice of duplicate publication and to ensure appropriate identifiability and indexing of such notices.

All journals should develop and publish policies on duplicate submission and publication. In addition, journals should develop procedures for evaluating possible violations of such policy and actions to be taken once a violation has been determined to have occurred. Such procedures include requesting an explanation from the author(s) and, if duplicate publication is determined to have occurred, notifying the other journal(s) involved, considering notifying the author's dean, director, or supervisor (this may be necessary if the author does not provide a satisfactory explanation), and publishing a notice of duplicate publication. As noted previously, COPE has useful flow diagrams that recommend steps to take if duplicate submission or publication is suspected.[27] Some journals in specific fields have decided to notify each other about cases of proved duplicate publication and sanction or ban the offending author(s) from publishing in their journals for a specified period.[28,29]

**Box 5.3-2.** Hypothetical Example of a Notice of Duplicate Publication From the Journal

---

Correction: Notice of Duplicate Publication: "Report of Multidrug-Resistant *Mycobacterium tuberculosis* Among Residents of a Long-term Care Facility" (*Arch Infect Dis*. 2014;270[12]:2008-2012.)

The article "Report of Multidrug-Resistant *Mycobacterium tuberculosis* Among Residents of a Long-term Care Facility" that I published in the December 2014 issue of the *Archives of Infection and Disease*[1] is virtually identical to an article describing the same 35 cases in similar words, that I published in the *Journal of New Results*, September 2014.[2]

I offer my sincere apologies to the readers of the *Archives of Infection and Disease*. I did not understand that my 2 manuscripts would be considered duplicative at the time I submitted them. I thought that since the 2 journals are read by different groups, some overlap in wording would be acceptable.

Anthony S. Smith, MD
Main University School of Medicine
Chicago, Illinois

**References**

1. Smith AS. Report of multidrug-resistant *Mycobacterium tuberculosis* among residents of a long-term care facility. *Arch Infect Dis*. 2014;270(12):2008-2012.

2. Smith AS. Multidrug-resistant tuberculosis among the elderly: an epidemiological assessment. *J New Results*. 2014;32(9):150-154.

---

**Box 5.3-3.** Hypothetical Example of a Duplicate Publication Notice Listing in a Journal's Table of Contents

---

**Letter**

Smith AS. Notice of duplicate publication: "Report of Multidrug-Resistant *Mycobacterium tuberculosis* Among Residents of a Long-term Care Facility" (*Arch Infect Dis*. 2014;270[12]:2008-2012.)

---

**Principal Author:** Annette Flanagin, RN, MA

## ACKNOWLEDGMENT

I thank the following for review and helpful comments: Howard Bauchner, MD, *JAMA* and JAMA Network; Carissa Gilman, American Cancer Society, Atlanta, Georgia; Timothy Gray, PhD, JAMA Network; Iris Y. Lo, JAMA Network; Ana Marušić, MD, PhD, *Journal of Global Health* and University of Split School of Medicine, Croatia; Fred Rivara, MD, MPH, *JAMA Network Open* and University of Washington, Seattle; and Elizabeth Wager, PhD, Sideview, Princess Risborough, England.

## REFERENCES

1. Huth EJ. Irresponsible authorship and wasteful publication. *Ann Intern Med.* 1986;104(2):257-259.

2. International Committee of Medical Journal Editors. Publishing and editorial issues: overlapping publications: In: Recommendations for the conduct, reporting, editing, and publication of scholarly work in medical journals. Updated December 2018. Accessed October 11, 2019. http://www.icmje.org

3. Broad WJ. The publishing game: getting more for less. *Science.* 1981;211(4487):1137-1139. doi:10.1126/science.7008199

4. Angell M, Relman AS. Redundant publication. *N Engl J Med.* 1989;320(18):1212-1214. doi:10.1056/NEJM198905043201812

5. Flanagin A, Glass RM, Lundberg GD. Electronic journals and duplicate publication: is a byte a word? *JAMA.* 1992;267(17):2374. doi:10.1001/jama.1992.03480170100039

6. Council of Science Editors. White Paper on Publication Ethics. Updated May 2018. Accessed July 7, 2019. https://www.councilscienceeditors.org/resource-library/editorial-policies/white-paper-on-publication-ethics/

7. Blancett SS, Flanagin A, Young RK. Duplicate publication in the nursing literature. *Image J Nurs Sch.* 1995;27(1):51-56. https://doi.org/10.1111/j.1547-5069.1995.tb00813.x

8. Huston P, Moher D. Redundancy, disaggregation, and the integrity of medical research. *Lancet.* 1996;347(9007):1024-1026. doi: 10.5555/uri:pii:S0140673696901531

9. Susser M, Yankauer A. Prior, duplicate, repetitive, fragmented, and redundant publication and editorial decisions. *Am J Public Health.* 1993;83(6):792-793.

10. von Elm E, Poglia G, Walder B, Tramèr MR. Different patterns of duplicate publication: an analysis of articles used in systematic reviews. *JAMA.* 2004;291(8):974-980. doi:10.1001/jama.291.8.974

11. Tramer MR, Reynolds DJ, Moore RA, McQuay HJ. Impact of covert duplicate publication on meta-analysis: a case study. *BMJ.* 1997;315(7109):635-640.

12. DeAngelis CD. Duplicate publication, multiple problems. *JAMA.* 2004;292(14):1745-1746. doi:10.1001/jama.292.14.1745

13. Yank V, Barnes D. Consensus and contention regarding redundant publications in clinical research: cross-sectional survey of editors and authors. *J Med Ethics.* 2003;29(2):109-114. doi:10.1136/jme.29.2.109

14. Bailey BJ. Duplicate publication in the field of otolaryngology–head and neck surgery. *Otolaryngol Head Neck Surg.* 2002;126(3):211-216. doi:10.1067/mhn.2002.122698

15. Melander H, Ahlqvist-Rastad J, Meijer G, Beermann B. Evidence b(i)ased medicine—selective reporting from studies sponsored by pharmaceutical industry: review of studies in new drug applications. *BMJ.* 2003;326(7400):1171-1173. doi:10.1136/bmj.326.7400.1171

16. Rosenthal EL, Masdon JL, Buckman C, Hawn M. Duplicate publications in the otolaryngology literature. *Laryngoscope.* 2003;113(5):772-774. doi:10.1177/2333794X14564442

17. Waldron T. Is duplicate publishing on the increase? *BMJ.* 1992;304(6833):1029.

18. Barnard H, Overbeke JA. Duplicate publication of original articles in and from the *Nederlands Tijdschrift voor Geneeskunde*. Article in Dutch. *Ned Tijdschr Geneeskd.* 1993;137(12):593-597.

19. Mojon-Azzi SM, Jiang X, Wagner U, Mojon DS. Redundant publications in scientific ophthalmology journals: the tip of the iceberg? *Ophthalmology.* 2004;111(5):853-866.

20. Gwilym SE, Swan MC, Giele H. One in 13 "original" articles in the *Journal of Bone and Joint Surgery* are duplicate or fragmented publications. *J Bone Joint Surg Br.* 2004;86(5):743-745.

21. Cheung VW, Lam GO, Wang YF, Chadha NK. Current incidence of duplicate publication in otolaryngology. *Laryngoscope.* 2014;124(3):655-658. doi:10.1002/lary.24294

22. Schein M, Paladugu R. Redundant surgical publications: tip of the iceberg? *Surgery.* 2001;129(6):655-661. doi:10.1067/msy.2001.114549

23. Errami M, Garner H. A tale of two citations. *Nature.* 2008;451(7177):397-399. doi:10.1038/451397a

24. Fontanarosa PB, Flanagin A, DeAngelis CD. Update on *JAMA*'s policy on release of information to the public. *JAMA.* 2008;300(13):1585-1587. doi:10.1001/jama.300.13.1585

25. US National Library of Medicine. Errata, retractions, and other linked citations in PubMed. Accessed October 11, 2019. https://www.nlm.nih.gov/bsd/policy/errata.html

26. Kleinert S. Checking for plagiarism, duplicate publication, and text recycling. *Lancet.* 2011;377(9762):281-282. doi:10.1016/S0140-6736(11)60075-5

27. Committee on Publication Ethics. What to do if you suspect redundant (duplicate) publication. In: Flowcharts, Resources. November 2015. Accessed December 21, 2018. https://publicationethics.org/resources/flowcharts

28. Bier DM, Fulginiti VA, Garfunkel JM, et al. Duplicate publication and related problems *Pediatrics.* 1990;86(6):997-998.

29. Samman N, Brennan PA, Wiltfang J, Lingen MW, Hupp JR. Journal alliance to address issues of dual submission and plagiarism. *Int J Oral Maxillofac Surg.* 2013;42(1):1. doi:10.1016/j.ijom.2012.09.007

## 5.4     **Scientific Misconduct.**

> *We should ignore whining about the supposedly awful*
> *pressures of "publish or perish" when we have little cred-*
> *ible evidence on what motivates misconduct, nor on*
> *what motivates the conduct of honest, equally stressed*
> *colleagues. Laziness, desire for fame, greed, and an*
> *inability to distinguish right from wrong are just as*
> *likely to be at the root of the problem.*
> Drummond Rennie[1]

In scientific publication, the phrase *scientific misconduct* (specifically termed *research misconduct* by US government regulations and commonly known as *fraud*) has ethical and legal connotations for researchers, authors, editors, and publishers. A few studies (with limited methods) have estimated the prevalence of scientists who have participated in scientific misconduct to range from 1% to 2%.[2-4] In a 2002 survey[5] of a random sample of 3247 scientists funded by the National Institutes of Health, participating scientists reported engaging in a number of unethical behaviors, including falsifying research data (0.3%), using another's ideas without permission or credit (1.4%), and inadequate record keeping related to research projects (27.5%). A 2009 meta-analysis[4] of 18 surveys published between 1987 and 2008 evaluated the frequency with which researchers admitted to fabricating or falsifying data. These surveys included a combined total of 11 647 researchers, primarily from the United States and the United Kingdom; 1 survey was conducted in Australia, and 2 surveys were multinational. In the meta-analysis, a pooled weighted mean of 1.97% of the researchers admitted to having "fabricated, falsified or modified data or results at least once," and 34% admitted to "other questionable research practices," such as subtle distortion, selective reporting, and selective publication of data that support one's expectations, biases, or conflicts of interest. In those surveys that asked researchers about the behavior of their colleagues, 14% responded that their colleagues had fabricated, falsified, or modified data or results.[4]

A 2018 analysis of 10 500 retracted journal articles listed in the Retraction Watch database found that the number of retractions has increased from fewer than 100 annually before the year 2000 to almost 1000 in 2014.[6] However, this analysis concluded that much of this increase appears to be associated with improved oversight at a growing number of journals. Only about 4 of every 10 000 articles have been retracted.[6]

Although inadequate record keeping and other questionable research practices are not technically forms of misconduct, they could permit misconduct to occur and make investigations of misconduct difficult to conduct. Legal determinations of scientific misconduct in biomedical publication are uncommon, although, when discovered, such misconduct results in serious questions about the validity of scientific research and the credibility of authors and journals. Proven cases of misconduct in the published literature as well as allegations and concerns that do not result in an official finding of misconduct raise important ethical questions and impose duties on authors and editors to protect and correct the literature.

Various definitions of scientific misconduct have been suggested by US and international government agencies, academic institutions, and funders, especially after highly publicized incidents of fraudulent research in the United States in the mid-1970s and early 1980s.[7-9] In 1989, the US Public Health Service released the following definition of scientific misconduct: "fabrication, falsification, plagiarism, or other practices that seriously deviate from those that are commonly accepted within the scientific community for proposing, conducting, or reporting research."[10] This definition was considered a practical tool for recognizing and dealing with allegations of scientific misconduct during the manuscript submission, review, and publication processes.[11] However, controversy grew over various interpretations of the definition (eg, How narrow or broad should the definition be? Does the definition address intent or levels of seriousness of offense? Can the definition stand up in court? Can the definition serve multiple scientific disciplines?).

In the wake of this controversy, the US Public Health Service appointed a Commission on Research Integrity in 1993. One of the charges of the commission was to develop a better definition of scientific misconduct. In 1995, the commission released a detailed report that included a recommendation that the definition be amended to include offenses that constitute research misconduct: misappropriation, interference, and misrepresentation.[12] This definition replaced the word *plagiarism* with the broader term *misappropriation*, replaced the words *fabrication* and *falsification* with the term *misrepresentation*, and added the term *interference* to address instances "in which a person's research is seriously compromised by the intentional and unauthorized taking, sequestering, or damaging of property he or she used in the conduct of research."[12] In this context, *property* included apparatus, reagents, biologic materials, writings, data, and software.

The commission's definition was not adopted by the US Public Health Service for many reasons, including protests from scientists and some science groups to which the government responded that it wanted a definition that would work for all governmental departments (eg, both the US Public Health Service and the National Science Foundation, which at the time had different definitions).[11,13] In 1996, the National Science and Technology Council, a unit within the Office of Science and Technology Policy responsible for coordinating policy among multiple government research agencies, drafted a common definition, which, after review and comment, was approved and released in 2000.[14] This definition no longer contained a category of misconduct that was in the original 1989 definition, namely, "other practices that seriously deviate from those that are commonly accepted within the scientific community for proposing, conducting, or reporting research."[14]

The revised common definition was reviewed again in 2004 and reissued without substantial change in 2005 by the US Department of Health and Human Services (DHHS) (although there were other changes to correct errors and improve clarity in the overall policy).[15]

The DHHS common definition of research misconduct remains in effect as follows[15]:

> Research misconduct is defined as fabrication, falsification, or plagiarism in proposing, performing, or reviewing research or in reporting research results.
>
> Fabrication is making up data or results and recording or reporting them.
>
> Falsification is manipulating research materials, equipment, or processes or changing or omitting data or results such that the research is not accurately represented in the research record.
>
> Plagiarism is the appropriation of another person's ideas, processes, results, or words without giving appropriate credit.

Research misconduct does not include honest error or differences of opinion.

A finding of research misconduct requires that:

there be a significant departure from accepted practices of the relevant research community; and

the misconduct be committed intentionally, or knowingly, or recklessly; and

the allegation be proven by a preponderance of evidence.

None of the definitions of scientific misconduct include honest error or differences in interpretation (see 5.4.6, Retraction and Replacement for Articles With Pervasive Errors). They also do not include or pertain to violations of human or animal experimentation requirements (see 5.8, Protecting Research Participants' and Patients' Rights in Scientific Publication), financial mismanagement or misconduct, or other acts covered by existing laws, such as sexual harassment, copyright, confidentiality, libel (see 5.6.3, Copyright: Definition, History, and Current Law; 5.7, Confidentiality; and 5.9, Defamation, Libel), or other concerns, such as authorship disputes, duplicate publication, or conflicts of interest (see 5.1, Authorship Responsibility; 5.3, Duplicate Publication and Submission; and 5.5, Conflicts of Interest).

The DHHS common definition of research misconduct[15] is intended to apply to US government–funded research. Academic and research institutions that accept US government funding must comply with the definition and associated regulations. However, this definition and the associated regulations have become de facto rules for US academic and other research institutions and are applied to any work performed by their employees or under their aegis regardless of the source of funding. These institutions often have other rules that cover "other practices that seriously deviate from those that are commonly accepted within the scientific community for proposing, conducting, or reporting research."[10]

Similar definitions have also been accepted by research and funding institutions in other countries, and some have adopted broader definitions. For example, research integrity definitions in other countries include what may be considered questionable research practices. The UK-based Wellcome Trust defines research misconduct as "behaviour or actions that fall short of the standards of ethics, research and scholarship required to ensure that the integrity of research is upheld" including "fabrication, falsification, plagiarism or deception in performing or reviewing research, and in reporting research outputs."[16] The Canadian National Research Council defines major research misconduct as fabrication, falsification, and plagiarism but also includes other wrongdoings typically covered by other regulations and policies (eg, duplicate publication, invalid authorship or contributions, peer review abuse, and mismanagement of conflicts of interest).[17] The International Committee of Medical Journal Editors (ICMJE) states that scientific misconduct "includes but is not necessarily limited to data fabrication; data falsification including deceptive manipulation of images; and plagiarism."[18] The ICMJE also notes that "failure to publish the results of clinical trials and other human studies" may also be considered as a serious form of omission-based misconduct.[18] The US Office of Research Integrity (ORI), which has jurisdiction only of US government–funded research, has a list of case summaries in which findings or research misconduct has been found against individuals with active administrative actions.[19] The ORI website also has policies and procedures for detection and investigation of allegations of research misconduct.[19]

**5.4.1** **Misrepresentation: Fabrication, Falsification, and Omission.** Fabrication, falsification, and omission are forms of misrepresentation in scientific publication. Fabrication includes stating or presenting a falsehood and making up data, results, or facts that do not exist. Falsification includes manipulation of materials or processes, changing data or results, or altering the graphic display of data or digital images in a manner that results in misrepresentation (see 5.4.3, Inappropriate Manipulation of Digital Images). Omission is the act of deliberately not reporting specific or selected information to achieve a desired outcome in the report. Data fabrication, falsification, and omission occur when an investigator or author creates, alters, manipulates, selects, or presents selected information or fails to report selected information for a desired outcome that distorts the interpretation of the original data, the research record, or the truth.[12-15]

**5.4.2** **Misappropriation: Plagiarism and Breaches of Confidentiality.** Misappropriation in scientific publication includes plagiarism and breaches of confidentiality during the privileged review of a manuscript[12-15,20] (see 5.7.1, Confidentiality During Editorial Evaluation and Peer Review and After Publication). In plagiarism, an author documents or reports ideas, words, data, or graphics, whether published or unpublished, of another as his or her own without giving appropriate credit or attribution.[12] Plagiarism of published work violates standards of honesty and collegial trust and may also violate copyright law (if the violation is shown to be legally actionable) (see 5.6.7, Copying, Reproducing, Adapting, and Other Uses of Content). The term *self-plagiarism* is erroneously included in discussions of plagiarism. The term refers to the practice of an author republishing his or her work or portions thereof without citation to the previous work. However, because this practice does not include misappropriation or theft of another's work, it is better described as a form of duplicate publication or duplicate submission, and the term *self plagiarism* should be avoided (see 5.3, Duplicate Publication and Submission).

Four common kinds of plagiarism have been identified[21]:

1. Direct plagiarism: Verbatim lifting (copying) of passages without enclosing the borrowed material in quotation marks and crediting the original author.

2. Mosaic: Borrowing the ideas and opinions from an original source and a few verbatim words or phrases without crediting the original author. In this case, the plagiarist intertwines his or her own ideas and opinions with those of the original author, creating a "confused, plagiarized mass."

3. Paraphrase: Restating a phrase or passage, providing the same meaning but in a different form without attribution to the original author.

4. Insufficient acknowledgment: Noting the original source of only part of what is borrowed or failing to cite the source material in a way that allows the reader to know what is original and what is borrowed.

The common characteristic of these kinds of plagiarism is the failure to attribute words, ideas, or findings to their true authors, whether or not the original work has been published. Such failure to acknowledge a source properly may on occasion be caused by careless note taking or ignorance of the canons of research and authorship. The best defense against allegations of plagiarism is careful note taking, record keeping, and documentation of all data observed and sources used. Those who review manuscripts that are similar to their own unpublished work may be especially at risk for charges of plagiarism. Reviewers who foresee such a potential conflict of interest should consider returning the manuscript to the editor without reviewing it. This recommendation may be stipulated in the letter that accompanies each manuscript sent for review (see 5.5.6, Requirements for Peer Reviewers, and 6.0, Editorial Assessment and Processing). Some have reported that the internet and subsequent rapid and widespread dissemination of findings and publications have resulted in an increase in plagiarism; however, text-based plagiarism software provides editors and publishers with tools to detect plagiarism and inappropriate duplication in submitted papers[22,23] (see 5.3, Duplicate Publication and Submission).

**5.4.3** **Inappropriate Manipulation of Digital Images.** Image-processing software, such as Adobe Photoshop, has made it relatively easy for authors to manipulate images to highlight a specific outcome or feature by cropping; deleting items; adjusting color, brightness, or contrast; or cloning/copying images. These same applications can be used by journal staff to screen digital images for evidence of inappropriate manipulation and fraudulent manipulation.[24,25] Some enhancements to figures, such as cropping or adjusting color of the entire image, may be appropriate if such manipulations do not alter the interpretation of the original data or omit or obscure important data. However, any manipulation that results in a change in how the original data will be interpreted or that selectively reports, omits, or obscures important data (such as adding or altering a data element or adjusting tone or compression of an image to make it appear as a uniquely different image) is considered scientific misconduct.[24,25] Authors should indicate any changes or enhancements that have been made to digital images in the legend that accompanies the image (see also 4.2.10, Guidelines for Preparing and Submitting Figures). These same principles apply to images included in video files.

Journals that regularly publish digital images should have policies and procedures in place for screening these images.[24,25] If resources are limited, screening can be reserved for those images that are included in papers that have been accepted for publication. The *Journal of Cell Biology* has a policy and guidelines for authors that are a good model for other journals.[26] During a 3-year period of screening images in all manuscripts accepted for publication, the *Journal of Cell Biology* had to revoke acceptance of 1% of papers after detecting "fraudulent image manipulation that affected interpretation of the data."[24] In addition, 25% of the accepted manuscripts had at least 1 figure that had to be remade because of inappropriate manipulation that did not affect the interpretation of the data but that violated the above guidelines.

The JAMA Network journals have the following policy on image integrity in all journal Instructions for Authors.[27]

Preparation of scientific images (clinical images, radiographic images, micrographs, gels, etc) for publication must preserve the integrity of the image data.

Digital adjustments of brightness, contrast, or color applied uniformly to an entire image are permissible as long as these adjustments do not selectively highlight, misrepresent, obscure, or eliminate specific elements in the original figure, including the background.

Selective adjustments applied to individual elements in an image are not permissible. Individual elements may not be moved within an image field, deleted, or inserted from another image.

Cropping may be used for efficient image display or to deidentify patients but must not misrepresent or alter interpretation of the image by selectively eliminating relevant visual information.

Juxtaposition of elements from different parts of a single image or from different images, as in a composite, must be clearly indicated by the addition of dividing lines, borders, and/or panel labels.

When inappropriate image adjustments are detected by the journal staff, authors will be asked for an explanation and will be requested to submit the image as originally captured prior to any adjustment, cropping, or labeling. Authors may be asked to resubmit the image prepared in accordance with the above standards.

**5.4.4** **Editorial Policy and Procedures for Detecting and Handling Allegations of Scientific Misconduct.** Detection of scientific misconduct in publishing has often been the result of the alertness of coworkers or other authors of the same manuscript and less commonly detected by editors, peer reviewers, or general readers. However, postpublication forensic statistical analysis and other replication techniques have begun to be used by peers and other experts to identify and expose scientific misconduct in published reports.

If an allegation of scientific misconduct is made in relation to a manuscript under consideration or published, the editor has a duty to ensure confidential and timely pursuit of that allegation, but the editor is not responsible for conducting the investigation.[28] This recommendation is supported by the ICMJE,[18] the World Association of Medical Editors,[29] the Council of Science Editors,[30] and the Committee on Publication Ethics (COPE).[31] COPE has a set of useful flowcharts and retraction guidelines to help editors address allegations of scientific misconduct that involve submitted or published papers.[32] In addition, the Council of Science Editors has a list of retraction resources that includes links to guidance and other information related to the handling of retractions.[33]

A 2012 study[34] of 399 high-impact journals in 27 biomedical categories found that only 35% of journals had a publicly available definition of scientific misconduct and 45% had publicly available policies that described procedures for handling allegations of misconduct. In this study, the prevalence of misconduct policies was higher in journals that endorsed any type of policy from professional editors' associations, the US ORI, or professional societies compared with those that did not refer to adherence to policies of these organizations. Editors have a duty to develop and follow a policy on handling allegations of scientific misconduct and retractions. Thus, the recommendations in this section are intended to help editors with such policies.

An editor's first step after receiving an allegation of falsified, fabricated, or plagiarized work published in her or his journal is to attempt to assess the validity or rationale for the allegation by requesting supporting documentation from the person who has made the allegation while maintaining confidentiality. If the allegation then appears to have merit, the editor should consider contacting the corresponding author, depending on the circumstances, to request an explanation while maintaining confidentiality. This initial contact can be made by telephone or email marked confidential (see 5.7.2, Confidentiality in Allegations of Scientific Misconduct). If the explanation received from the author is satisfactory and if guilt is admitted, the editor should request a letter of explanation and formal retraction from the author (preferably signed by the author and all coauthors); the editor should also notify the author's institution and inform the author of this notification.[28] If the explanation allays any concerns about misconduct, the editor may inform the person making the allegation that no misconduct has occurred. If the explanation received is not satisfactory or leads to additional concerns or if no explanation is received, the editor should contact the author's institutional authority to request a formal investigation and should notify the author of this plan.

The responsibility to conduct an investigation lies with authorities at the author's institution where the work was done (eg, dean, president, or ethical conduct/research integrity officer), with the funding agency, or with a national agency charged to investigate such allegations, such as the US ORI or the Danish Committees on Scientific Dishonesty. Many countries do not have such national agencies to investigate allegations of scientific misconduct or enforce regulations. In such cases, the journal editor must pursue an author's local institution for an appropriate response.[28,35] Editors should expect a prompt acknowledgment of their notification of an allegation of misconduct from institutional leaders.[36,37] The acknowledgment should include a plan for the inquiry or investigation into the matter and a timeline that specifies when the editor will be informed of the outcome. A checklist developed by a working group (comprising university and institutional leaders and research integrity officers, government officials, researchers, journal editors, journalists, and attorneys representing respondents, whistle-blowers) can be used by institutions to follow reasonable standards to investigate an allegation of scientific misconduct and to provide an appropriate and complete report following the investigation.[37] The editor cannot conduct the investigation because he or she does not have the appropriate institutional access or authority or an employment relationship with the author or other relationship, such as that between the author and a governmental funding agency. If the editor does not receive a satisfactory or timely reply (eg, within 2 months) from the investigational authority, the editor should consider contacting the authority again to request follow-up information. The US DHHS policy recommends that institutions complete their initial inquiry to determine whether an official investigation is warranted within 60 days of its initiation unless circumstances clearly warrant a longer period.[15]

The editor should take great care to maintain confidentiality during any communication about the allegation. However, the editor needs to identify the person or persons about whom the allegation is made when contacting the relevant institutional, funding, or governmental authority to request an investigation. This is best done by a telephone call or a brief formal letter sent by mail or attached to email and marked confidential. During such investigations, editors should avoid including details of the cases in emails that can be widely circulated and should avoid posting details, even if rendered anonymous, in email discussion forums or blogs (see 5.7.2, Confidentiality in Allegations of Scientific Misconduct). Journal editors should keep information about manuscripts, authors, and blinded reviewers confidential; however, if there is clear evidence that shows that articles in other journals may have been subject to the same misconduct, it would be acceptable for editors of these journals to discuss the matter in a confidential manner.

**5.4.5** **Retractions and Expressions of Concern.** After receiving confirmation from the author or authors and/or a report from the author's institution or other agency indicating that fabrication, falsification, or plagiarism has occurred, the journal should promptly publish a retraction. Preferably this retraction will be a signed letter from the corresponding author and all coauthors. If none of the authors will agree to publish a signed retraction, the editor may request such a retraction from the investigating institution, or the editor may issue a retraction on behalf of the journal. In each case, the editor should inform the author(s) and institutional authority of the plan to publish a retraction. See **Boxes 5.4-1** and **5.4-2** for examples of retraction notices.

A study that included a search of the internet to locate copies of 1779 retracted articles (identified in MEDLINE) that were originally published between 1973 and 2010 found that copies of retracted articles were publicly available on nonpublisher websites (ie, external to the journals that originally published the articles).[38] These nonpublisher websites provided 321 publicly accessible copies for 289 retracted articles. Of these, 304 (95%) were copies of the publishers' versions and 13 (4%) were final manuscripts. However, only 5% of these article copies included the relevant retraction notice. Moreover, studies have found that retracted articles continue to be cited in the literature, also without indication of their retracted status.[39,40] Editors are encouraged to follow the procedures outlined below to ensure that readers, researchers, authors, and librarians are aware of the status of retracted articles.

A retraction should include a complete citation to the original article and should indicate the reason for retracting the original article. The retraction, whether a formal letter or notice, should be labeled as a "Retraction," be listed in the table of contents, be published in a section of the journal (eg, the Correspondence/ Letters or Editorial section), and be published in a format that will permit a formal citation so that it can be identified easily by indexers and included in bibliographic databases (see 3.11.15, Retractions and Expressions of Concern).

**Box 5.4-1.** Examples of Hypothetical Published Retraction Notices

---

### Retraction Notices From Authors

**Notice of Retraction: Falsification of Data in "Effects of Low-Fat Diet on Risk of Breast Cancer" (*J Med Res*. 2016;242[1]:135-139)**

*To the Editor.*—We write to retract the article "Effects of Low-Fat Diet on Risk of Breast Cancer,"[1] published in the January 3, 2016, issue of the *Journal of Medical Research*. Two participants in the low-fat diet group were intentionally misclassified as not having breast cancer by one of us (J.S.). Had the reporting of these 2 cases not been falsified, our multivariate analysis would not have shown statistically significant results. We regret any problems our article and actions may have caused, and we retract the article from the literature.

John Smith
Jane Doe
Medical University
Chicago, Illinois

1. Smith J, Doe J. Effects of low-fat diet on risk of breast cancer. *J Med Res*. 2016;242(1):135-139.

**Notice of Retraction: Plagiarism in "Effects of Low-Fat Diet on Risk of Breast Cancer" (*J Med Res*. 2016;242[1]:135-139)**

*To the Editor.*—We regret that the first 3 paragraphs in the Discussion section of our article, "Effects of Low-Fat Diet on Risk of Breast Cancer,"[1] published in the January 3, 2016, issue of the *Journal of Medical Research*, were taken from another source without proper attribution. We should have cited the following article as the original source of the information contained in those paragraphs: Scott RB. Low-fat diets and cancer risk. *J Med Nutr Diet*. 2015;20(8):1450-1455. We regret any problems our article[1] may have caused, and we retract it from the literature.

John Smith
Jane Doe
Medical University
Chicago, Illinois

1. Smith J, Doe J. Effects of low-fat diet on risk of breast cancer. *J Med Res*. 2016;242(1):135-139.

### Retraction Notice From Institution

**Notice of Retraction: Falsification of Data in "Effects of Low-Fat Diet on Risk of Breast Cancer" (*J Med Res*. 2016;242[1]:135-139)**

*To the Editor.*—An official investigation conducted by the Research Integrity Review Panel of Medical University of the data reported by John Smith and Jane Doe in the article "Effects of Low-Fat Diet on Risk of Breast Cancer,"[1] published in the January 3, 2016, issue of the *Journal of Medical Research*, has confirmed falsification in the reporting. Two participants in the low-fat diet group were intentionally misclassified as not having breast cancer by one of the authors (J.S.). As a result, we retract this article from the literature. The review panel's investigation did not reveal any additional research misconduct in either author's previously published works.

---

*(continued)*

**Box 5.4-1.** Examples of Hypothetical Published Retraction Notices (*continued*)

Joan Brown
Dean
Medical University
Chicago, Illinois

1. Smith J, Doe J. Effects of low-fat diet on risk of breast cancer. *J Med Res.* 2016;242(1):135-139.

**Retraction Notice From Journal Editor**
**Notice of Retraction: Falsification of Data in "Effects of Low-Fat Diet on Risk of Breast Cancer" (*J Med Res.* 2016;242[1]:135-139)**
We have received confirmation from the Research Integrity Review Panel of Medical University that data reported by John Smith and Jane Doe in the article "Effects of Low-Fat Diet on Risk of Breast Cancer,"[1] published in the January 3, 2016, issue of the *Journal of Medical Research*, were falsified. Two participants in the low-fat diet group were intentionally misclassified as not having breast cancer by one of the authors (J.S.). As a result, we retract this article from the literature. The review panel's investigation did not reveal any additional research misconduct in either author's previously published works.

Mary Frank
Editor, *Journal of Medical Research*

1. Smith J, Doe J. Effects of low-fat diet on risk of breast cancer. *J Med Res.* 2016;242(1):135-139.

**Expression of Concern From Journal Editor**
**Expression of Concern: Falsification of Data in "Effects of Low-Fat Diet on Risk of Breast Cancer" (*J Med Res.* 2016;242[1]:135-139)**
In the January 3, 2016, issue of the *Journal of Medical Research*, we published "Effects of Low-Fat Diet on Risk of Breast Cancer,"[1] by John Smith and Jane Doe. On March 15, 2016, we received information that cast serious doubt on the validity of several cases that were reported in Tables 1 and 2 and that prompted us to alert the author and the author's institution and to request a formal investigation. An interim report from the Medical University's Research Integrity Review Panel, received on April 10, 2016, indicates that "data were falsified for two participants in this study" and that a formal investigation is under way. We have requested formal retractions from the authors and a final report from the university's review panel, including information about the validity of the authors' previous publication in the *Journal of Medical Research*. In the interim, we publish this expression of concern to alert our readers to the serious concerns raised about the validity of the data, interpretations, and conclusions of the article published in January 2016.[1]

Mary Frank
Editor, *Journal of Medical Research*

1. Smith J, Doe J. Effects of low-fat diet on risk of breast cancer. *J Med Res.* 2016;242(1):135-139.

**Listing of a Retraction Notice in the Table of Contents**
Letters
Notice of Retraction: Plagiarism in "Effects of Low-Fat Diet on Risk of Breast Cancer" (*J Med Res.* 2016;242[1]:135-139)—J Smith, J Doe

**Box 5.4-2.** Citations of Published Retraction Notices and Expressions of Concern

---

**Retraction Notices From Authors**

Ahimastos AA, Askew C, Leicht A, et al. Notice of retraction: Ahimastos AA, et al. Effect of ramipril on walking times and quality of life among patients with peripheral artery disease and intermittent claudication: a randomized controlled trial. *JAMA*. 2013;309(5):453-460. *JAMA*. 2015;314(14):1520-1521. doi:10.1001/jama.2015.10811

Acharya CR, Hsu DS, Anders CK, et al. Retraction: Acharya CR, et al. Gene expression signatures, clinicopathological features, and individualized therapy in breast cancer. *JAMA*. 2008;299(13):1574-1587. *JAMA*. 2012;307(5):453. doi:10.1001/jama.2012.2

Poehlman ET. Notice of retraction: final resolution. *Ann Intern Med*. 2005;142(9):798.

Poehlman ET. Retraction of Poehlman et al. *Journal of Applied Physiology*. 1994;76:2281-2287. *J Appl Physiol*. 2005;99(2):779.

[Note: In the following 2 retractions, the coauthors signed the retraction, but the author responsible for the misconduct did not.]

Cooper PK, Nouspikel T, Clarkson SG. Retraction of Cooper et al. *Science*. 275(5302):990-993. *Science*. 2005;308(5729):1740.

Warloe T, Aamdal S, Reith A, Bryne M. Retraction of: Diagnostics and treatment of early stages of oral cancer. *Tidsskr Nor Laegeforen*. 2006;126(17):2287.

**Retraction Notices From Editors**

Bauchner H. Notice of Retraction: Wansink B, Cheney MM. Super bowls: serving bowl size and food consumption. *JAMA*. 2005;293(14):1727-1728. *JAMA*. 2018;320(16):1648. doi:10.1001/jama.2018.14249

DeAngelis CD, Fontanarosa PB. Retraction: Cheng B-Q, et al. Chemoembolization combined with radiofrequency ablation for patients with hepatocellular carcinoma larger than 3 cm: a randomized controlled trial. *JAMA*. 2008;299(14):1669-1677. *JAMA*. 2009;301(18):1931. doi:10.1001/jama.2009.640

Horton R. Retraction—Non-steroidal anti-inflammatory drugs and the risk of oral cancer: a nested case-control study. *Lancet*. 2006;367(9508):382.

**Expressions of Concern From Editors**

McNutt M. Editorial expression of concern. Expression of Concern on Brantley et al. *Science* 2011;333(6049):1606-1609. *Science*. 2014;344(6191):1460. doi:10.1126/science.344.6191.1460-a

Bauchner H, Fontanarosa PB. Expression of Concern: Kiel et al. Efficacy of a hip protector to prevent hip fracture in nursing home residents: the HIP PRO randomized controlled trial. *JAMA*. 2007;298(4):413-422. *JAMA*. 2012;308(23):2519. doi:10.1001/jama.2012.14079

---

If there is a lengthy delay until the schedule for publication of a retraction in a formal issue, consideration should be given to publishing the retraction notice online first or before subsequent publication in a specific issue. The US National Library of Medicine (NLM) will index the retraction as long as it clearly states that an article in question is being retracted or withdrawn, whether in whole or in part, and is signed by an author, the author's legal counsel or institutional representative, or the journal editor.[41] Online versions of journals and bibliographic databases should provide reciprocal links to and from the notice of retraction and the retracted article. Retractions should be made freely available and accessible on a journal's website (ie, readers should not have to pay an access fee to see the retraction notice).[18,35] A retracted article should be properly labeled or watermarked as retracted in online and PDF versions of journals and should not be removed from the online journal or archive. Such labeling may include the words "Retracted Article" or "This Article Has Been Retracted" placed prominently at the top of the online article and on each page of a PDF file of the article. These labels can be hyperlinked to the published retraction. Copies of retracted articles deposited in public repositories and other databases should also be labeled prominently as retracted and should link to the published retraction notice.

If an author of a fraudulent article, or any institutional authority, refuses to submit an explanation for publication as a retraction, the editor may be able to leverage the authority and influence of his or her position and that of the journal to compel an appropriate response, keeping in mind the journal's obligation to publish a retraction.[28,35] If, however, the editor is unable to receive a satisfactory or timely response from an author or the investigating authority on the merit of the allegation, the editor may publish a notice of Expression of Concern to alert readers, librarians, and the scientific community that there are concerns that an article may include fabricated, falsified, or plagiarized work and follow this later with a formal retraction. An Expression of Concern from journal editors may also allow for timely notification while awaiting a formal investigation. This notice of concern should follow the same publication format as recommended for notices of retraction. If evidence of misconduct is sufficient and the editor cannot obtain a retraction letter from the author and is awaiting the results of an official investigation, the editor may choose to publish an expression of concern and follow this with a formal retraction once the institution has completed its investigation.

The validity of other work published in the journal by the authors responsible for the misconduct should also be questioned. The ICMJE recommends that editors ask institutions to provide assurance of the validity of earlier work published in their journals or to retract those as well. If this is not done, editors may choose to publish a notice or expression of concern stating that the validity of such previously published work is uncertain.[18]

Box 5.4-1 shows examples of retraction notices from authors, an institution, and an editor and a listing in the table of contents. Examples of recent retractions in the literature are given in Box 5.4-2. Some authors may not want to explain the reason for the retraction in a forthright manner. Editors should work with authors or their institutional authority to make these notices as accurate as possible. In some cases, publishing an author's evasive or incomplete statement might be better than publishing nothing from the author; in such a case, the journal can also publish an explanatory note from the author's institutional authority or the editor.

When an article is retracted, the original article should not be removed from a journal's website or other online archival publication. However, it should be made clear to all users of online archival material that the article has been retracted and should not be used or cited. This requirement includes clear labeling of retracted articles and 2-way linking between retraction notices and the original articles. The NLM does not remove the citation of a retracted article; the citation is updated to indicate that the article has been retracted, and links between the original citation and the citation to the retraction notice are added.[41]

**5.4.6**    **Retraction and Replacement for Articles With Pervasive Errors.** Retractions may also be used for articles that are seriously and pervasively flawed because of honest, inadvertent error that is not a result of fabrication, falsification, or plagiarism.[28,42-45] However, retraction of an article because of serious and pervasive errors should be used cautiously. Indeed, Sox and Rennie[35] have called for retractions to be reserved solely for cases of scientific misconduct. Retractions should never be used for typical errors; in these cases, a correction is appropriate[46] (see 5.11.10, Ethical and Legal Considerations, Editorial Responsibilities, Roles, Procedures, and Policies, Corrections [Errata]).

A study[47] of 395 articles retracted during the years 1982 through 2002 found that 107 (27%) reflected scientific misconduct and 244 (62%) represented unintentional errors (another 44 [11%] represented other issues or provided no information about the reasons for the retractions). Another study[48] of 1112 retracted articles, based on notifications of retraction in PubMed between 1997 and 2009, found that 55% were retracted for misconduct. Twenty percent of these retractions were attributable to some type of error, such as problems with the data (10%); error in the methods, analysis, or interpretation (7%); and problems with the sample (3%). A review[39] of 2047 retracted articles with retraction notifications in PubMed from 1977 through 2012 found similar results: 21% of the retractions were attributable to error, whereas 67% were attributable to fraud or suspected fraud and 10% were attributable to plagiarism; duplicate publication (14%) and miscellaneous or unknown reasons accounted for the remaining retractions.

The NLM does not differentiate between articles that are retracted because of serious but unintended error and those that are retracted because of scientific misconduct.[41] A *pervasive error* in a published article could result from a human or programmatic coding problem or a miscalculation, and this could cause extensive inaccuracies throughout an article (eg, abstract, methods, results, discussion, conclusions, tables, figures, and supplemental information).[42] Inadvertent publication of pervasive incorrect data that does not affect the results, interpretations, or conclusions of an article can be managed with a formal Correction notice, perhaps with a Letter of explanation from the authors published with the Correction notice and correcting the article online[45] (see 5.11.10, Corrections [Errata]). However, inadvertent pervasive errors that result in a major change in the direction or significance of the results, interpretations, and conclusions is a serious matter.[42] In such a case, the editor should request the authors to thoroughly review the published article, all underlying data, and all analyses to check for any additional errors and provide the following:

- Complete explanation for how the errors were discovered

- An itemized listing of all errors and corrections

- A marked-up copy of the original article identifying all errors and corrections (Note: A tracked-changes version of the original text of tables and figures is helpful.)

- Confirmation that there are no additional errors.

- Indication of whether the errors change the statistical direction of the results, interpretations, and conclusions

- Letter of explanation summarizing all the above from all authors to be considered for publication

The editor should then re-review the published work, authors' explanation, and marked-up copy of the original article identifying all errors and corrections. This review may include additional external peer review or statistical review. If the editor then determines that the science of the article is still reliable and important, a formal Notice of Retraction and Replacement as a Letter from the authors may be published. The JAMA Network journals and *The Lancet* journals have published such notices and have replaced or republished the original article along with on-line supplements that include a version of the original retracted article showing the original errors and a version of the replacement article showing what was corrected.[42-45] This option provides authors who have made inadvertent pervasive errors that have resulted in changes to results of published articles with a mechanism to retract the erroneous article without the "do not use" stigma associated with retractions that are reserved for acts of fabrication, falsification, and plagiarism. The ICMJE supports this option.[18]

In these cases, online versions of journals and bibliographic databases should provide reciprocal links to and from the Notice of Retraction and Replacement (or Republication) and the retracted and replaced (or republished) article. In addition, a prominent notice should appear on the online and PDF versions of the article. See the following examples:

> Lopes AC, Greenberg BD, Pereira CB, Norén G, Miguel EC. Notice of retraction and replacement. Lopes et al. Gamma ventral capsulotomy for obsessive-compulsive disorder: a randomized clinical trial. *JAMA Psychiatry.* 2014;71(9):1066-1076. *JAMA Psychiatry.* 2015;72(12):1258. doi:10.1001/jamapsychiatry.2015.0673

> Kessler RC, Duncan GJ, Gennetian LA, et al. Notice of retraction and replacement: Kessler et al. Associations of housing mobility interventions for children in high-poverty neighborhoods with subsequent mental disorders during adolescence. *JAMA.* 2014;311(9):937-947. *JAMA.* 2016;316(2):227-228. doi:10.1001/jama.2016.6187

**5.4.7**     **Allegations Involving Unresolved Questions of Scientific Misconduct.** Cases may arise in which an allegation requires the journal editor to have access to the data on which the manuscript or article in question was based. Following the recommendations of the ICMJE, *JAMA's* authorship statement includes the following language for all authors:

> I agree to be accountable for all aspects of the work in ensuring that questions related to the accuracy or integrity of any part of the work are appropriately investigated and resolved; and

> If requested, I shall produce the data or will cooperate fully in obtaining and providing the data on which the manuscript is based for examination by the editors or their assignees.

For discussion of reasonable time limits for which authors should keep their data, see 5.6.1, Ownership and Control of Data.

If an author refuses a request for access to the original data or if the author or the author's institution refuses to comply with the journal's request for information about the allegation, the journal and its editor may be left in a precarious position. The ICMJE and COPE recommend that journals publish an Expression of Concern detailing the unresolved questions regarding an allegation of scientific misconduct in their publications (see 5.4.5, Retractions and Expressions of Concern).[18,31]

**5.4.8** **Allegations Involving Manuscripts Under Editorial Consideration.** In the case of a manuscript under consideration that is not yet published in which fabrication, falsification, or plagiarism is suspected, the editor should ask the corresponding author for a written explanation. If an explanation is not provided or is unsatisfactory, the editor should contact the author's institutional authority (ie, dean, director, ethical conduct/research integrity officer) or governmental agency with jurisdiction to investigate allegations of scientific misconduct to request an investigation. In all such communications with authors and institutional authorities, the editor should take care to maintain confidentiality and should follow the same procedures described in 5.4.4, Editorial Policy and Procedures for Detecting and Handling Allegations of Scientific Misconduct. If the author's explanation or institutional investigation demonstrates that the misconduct did not occur, the editor should continue to consider the manuscript on its own merits. If the author's explanation or a formal investigation demonstrates misconduct, the editor should then reject the paper. However, rejecting and returning to an author a manuscript associated with suspected or confirmed misconduct without addressing the possible misconduct issues is inappropriate because it may result in the work being published elsewhere.[31]

**Principal Author:** Annette Flanagin, RN, MA

ACKNOWLEDGMENT

I thank the following for review and helpful comments: Howard Bauchner, MD, *JAMA* and JAMA Network; Carissa Gilman, American Cancer Society, Atlanta, Georgia; Timothy Gray, PhD, JAMA Network; Iris Y. Lo, JAMA Network; Ana Marušić, MD, PhD, *Journal of Global Health* and University of Split School of Medicine,

Croatia; Chris Meyer, JAMA Network; and Fred Rivara, MD, MPH, *JAMA Network Open* and University of Washington, Seattle.

## REFERENCES

1. Rennie D. Dealing with research misconduct in the United Kingdom: an American perspective on research integrity. *BMJ*. 1998;316(7146):1726-1728.
2. Ranstam J, Buyse M, George SL; for the ISCB Subcommittee on Fraud. Fraud in medical research: an international survey of biostatisticians. *Control Clin Trials*. 2000;21(5):415-427.
3. Steneck NH. Fostering integrity in research: definitions, current knowledge, and future directions. *Sci Eng Ethics*. 2006;12(1):53-74.
4. Fanelli D. How many scientists fabricate and falsify research? a systematic review and meta-analysis of survey data. *PLoS One*. 2009;4(5):e5738. doi:10.1371/journal.pone.0005738
5. Martinson BC, Anderson MS, de Vries R. Scientists behaving badly. *Nature*. 2005;435(7043):737-738. doi:10.1038/435737a
6. Brainard J. Rethinking retractions. *Science*. 2018;362(6413):390-393. doi:10.1126/science.362.6413.390
7. Relman AS. Lessons from the Darsee affair. *N Engl J Med*. 1983;308(23):1415-1417. doi:10.1056/NEJM198306093082311
8. Knox R. The Harvard fraud case: where does the problem lie? *JAMA*. 1983;249(14):1797-1799, 1802-1807. doi:10.1001/jama.1983.03330380003001
9. Rennie D, Gunsalus CK. Scientific misconduct: new definition, procedures, and office—perhaps a new leaf. *JAMA*. 1993;269(7):915-917. doi:10.1001/jama.1993.03500070095037
10. US Department of Health and Human Services, Public Health Service. Responsibilities of awardee and applicant institutions for dealing with and reporting possible misconduct in science: final rule. *Fed Regist*. 1989;54(151):32446.
11. National Academy of Sciences. *Responsible Science: Ensuring the Integrity of the Research Process*. National Academy Press; 1992.
12. Commission on Research Integrity *Integrity and Misconduct in Research*. Office of Research Integrity; 1995. Accessed December 21, 2018. https://ori.hhs.gov/report-commission-research-integrity-1995
13. Committee on Assessing Integrity in Research Elements, Institute of Medicine. *Integrity in Scientific Research: Creating an Environment That Promotes Responsible Conduct*. National Academy Press; 2002. Accessed December 21, 2018. https://www.nap.edu/catalog/10430/integrity-in-scientific-research-creating-an-environment-that-promotes-responsible
14. Office of Science and Technology Policy. Federal policy on research misconduct. *Fed Regist*. 2000;65(6):76260-76264. Accessed November 3, 2018. https://www.gpo.gov/fdsys/granule/FR-2000-12-06/00-30852
15. US Department of Health and Human Services. 42 CFR Parts 50 and 93. Public Health Service policies on research misconduct; final rule. *Fed Regist*. 2005;70(94):28386. Accessed December 21, 2018. https://www.gpo.gov/fdsys/pkg/FR-2005-05-17/pdf/05-9643.pdf
16. Wellcome Trust. Research misconduct. Updated October 2017. Accessed December 21, 2018. https://wellcome.ac.uk/funding/guidance/research-misconduct

17. National Research Council of Canada. Research and scientific integrity policy. Effective December 12, 2018. Accessed July 7, 2019. https://nrc.canada.ca/sites/default/files/2019-04/nrc_online_policy_e2.pdf

18. International Committee of Medical Journal Editors. Recommendations, scientific misconduct, expressions of concern, and retraction. Updated December 2018. Accessed December 21, 2018. http://www.icmje.org/recommendations/browse/publishing-and-editorial-issues/scientific-misconduct-expressions-of-concern-and-retraction.html

19. US Office of Research Integrity website. Accessed July 7, 2019. https://ori.hhs.gov

20. Marshall E. Suit alleges misuse of peer review. *Science*. 1995;270(5244):1912. doi:10.1126/science.270.5244.1912

21. Northwestern University. *Academic Integrity: A Basic Guide*. June 2018. Accessed November 3, 2018. https://www.northwestern.edu/provost/policies/academic-integrity/academic-integrity-guide-june-2018_signed-jsh-rrb_rev10-2-18v2.pdf

22. Li Y. Text-based plagiarism in scientific publishing: issues, developments and education. *Sci Eng Ethics*. 2013;19(3):1241-1254. doi:10.1007/s11948-012-9367-6

23. Eysenbach G. Report of a case of cyberplagiarism—and reflections on detecting and preventing academic misconduct using the internet. *J Med Internet Res*. 2001;2(1):e4. doi:10.2196/jmir.2.1.e4

24. Rossner M. How to guard against image fraud. *Scientist*. 2006;20(3):24. Accessed November 25, 2018. http://www.the-scientist.com/?articles.view/articleNo/23749/title/How-to-Guard-Against-Image-Fraud/

25. Rossner M, Yamada K. What's in a picture? the temptation of image manipulation. *J Cell Biol*. 2004;166(1):11-15. doi:10.1083/jcb.200406019

26. *Journal of Cell Biology*. Instructions for Authors. Editorial policies: data integrity and plagiarism. Accessed November 3, 2018. http://jcb.rupress.org/editorial-policies#data-integrity

27. Figures, image integrity. *JAMA* Instructions for Authors. Updated December 7, 2018. Accessed December 21, 2018. https://jamanetwork.com/journals/jama/pages/instructions-for-authors#SecFigures

28. Bauchner H, Fontanarosa PB, Flanagin A, Thornton J. Scientific misconduct and medical journals. *JAMA*. 2018;320(19):1985-1987. doi:10.1001/jama.2018.14350

29. World Association of Medical Editors. Recommendations on publication ethics policies for medical journals. Accessed November 3, 2018. http://wame.org/recommendations-on-publication-ethics-policies-for-medical-journals

30. Council of Science Editors. CSE's white paper on promoting integrity in scientific journal publications. March 30, 2012. Updated May 2018. Accessed November 4, 2018. https://www.councilscienceeditors.org/resource-library/editorial-policies/white-paper-on-publication-ethics

31. Committee on Publication Ethics. A code of conduct and best practice guidelines for journal editors. March 7, 2011. Accessed November 4, 2018. https://publicationethics.org/files/Code%20of%20Conduct.pdf

32. Committee on Publication Ethics. Flowcharts. Accessed November 4, 2018. https://publicationethics.org/resources/flowcharts

33. Council of Science Editors. Retraction resources. November 2013. Accessed July 7, 2019. https://www.councilscienceeditors.org/resource-library/editorial-policies/retraction-resources

34. Bosch X1, Hernández C, Pericas JM, Doti P, Marušić A. Misconduct policies in high-impact biomedical journals. *PLoS One*. 2012;7(12):e51928. doi:10.1371/journal. pone.0051928

35. Sox HC, Rennie D. Research misconduct, retraction, and cleansing the medical literature: lessons from the Poehlman case. *Ann Intern Med*. 2006;144(8):609-613. doi:10.7326/0003-4819-144-8-200604180-00123

36. National Academies of Sciences, Engineering, and Medicine. Addressing research misconduct and detrimental research practices: current knowledge and issues. In: *Fostering Integrity of Research*. National Academies Press; 2017. Accessed November 4, 2018. https://www.nap.edu/read/21896/chapter/11#107

37. Gunsalus CK, Marcus AR, Oransky I. Institutional research misconduct reports need more credibility. *JAMA*. 2018;319(13):1315-1316. doi:10.1001/jama.2018.0358

38. Davis PM. The persistence of error: a study of retracted articles on the internet and in personal libraries. *J Med Libr Assoc*. 2012;100(3):184-189. doi:10.3163/1536-5050.100.3.008

39. Fang FC, Steen RG, Casadevall A. Misconduct accounts for the majority of retracted scientific publications. *Proc Natl Acad Sci USA*. 2012;109(42):17028-17033. doi:10.1073/pnas.1212247109

40. Pfeifer MP, Snodgrass GL. The continued use of retracted, invalid scientific literature. *JAMA*. 1990;263(10):1420-1423. doi:10.1001/jama.1990.03440100140020

41. National Library of Medicine. Errata, retractions, and other linked citations in PubMed. Updated August 8, 2018. Accessed November 25, 2018. https://www.nlm. nih.gov/bsd/policy/errata.html

42. Heckers S, Bauchner H, Flanagin A. Retracting, replacing, and correcting the literature for pervasive error in which the results change but the underlying science is still reliable. *JAMA Psychiatry*. 2015;72(12):1170-1171. doi:10.1001/ jamapsychiatry.2015.2278

43. Correcting the scientific literature: retraction and republication. *Lancet*. 2015;385(9966):394. doi:10.1016/S0140-6736(15)60137-4

44. Lopes AC, Greenberg BD, Pereira CB, Norén G, Miguel EC. Notice of Retraction and Replacement: Lopes et al. Gamma ventral capsulotomy for obsessive-compulsive disorder: a randomized clinical trial. *JAMA Psychiatry*. 2014;71(9):1066-1076. *JAMA Psychiatry*. 2015;72(12):1258. doi:10.1001/ jamapsychiatry.2015.0673

45. Kessler RC, Duncan GJ, Gennetian LA, et al. Notice of retraction and replacement: Kessler RC, et al. Associations of housing mobility interventions for children in high-poverty neighborhoods with subsequent mental disorders during adolescence. *JAMA*. 2014;311(9):937-947. *JAMA*. 2016;316(2):227-228. doi:10.1001/ jama.2016.6187

46. Christiansen S, Flanagin A. Correcting the medical literature: "to err is human, to correct divine". *JAMA*. 2017;318(9):804-805. doi:10.1001/jama.2017.11833

47. Nath SB, Marcus SC, Druss BG. Retractions in the research literature: misconduct or mistakes? *Med J Aust*. 2006;7;185(3):152-154.

48. Budd JM, Coble ZC, Anderson KM. Retracted publications in biomedicine: cause for concern. 2011. Association of College and Research Libraries Conference. Accessed November 25, 2018. http://www.ala.org/acrl/sites/ala.org.acrl/files/content/conferences/confsandpreconfs/national/2011/papers/retracted_publicatio.pdf

## 5.5 ■■■■ Conflicts of Interest.

> *Of all the causes which conspire to blind*
> *Man's erring judgment, and misguide the mind,*
> *What the weak head with strongest bias rules,*
> *Is pride, the never-failing vice of fools.*
> Alexander Pope[1]

### 5.5.1 ■■■■ Definition, History, and Rationale for Journal Policies.
A conflict of interest occurs when an individual's objectivity is potentially, but not necessarily, compromised by a desire for prominence, professional advancement, financial gain, or a successful outcome. Conflicts of interest that arise from personal or financial relationships, academic competition, and intellectual passion are not uncommon in science. In biomedical publication, a conflict of interest may exist when an author (or the author's institution, employer, or funder) has financial or other relationships that could influence (or bias) the author's decisions, work, or manuscript.[2-8] However, much concern has been directed toward the financial interests of researchers and authors, perhaps because such interests often are the easiest to measure or identify, and because of the complex relationships between them and the funders of their work.[9-18] In addition, concerns have increased about author biases associated with financial ties to industry and pressures from commercial funders that result in incomplete, delayed, or suppressed publication.[8,9,12,18-21]

Journal editors strive to ensure that information published in their journals is as balanced, objective, and evidence based as possible. Because of the difficulty in distinguishing the difference between an actual conflict of interest and a perceived conflict,[22] many biomedical journals require authors to disclose all relevant potential conflicts of interest.[2,6,7] Financial interests may include but are not limited to employment, consultancies, stock ownership, honoraria, paid expert testimony, royalties, patents (filed, pending, or registered), grants, and material or financial support from industry, government, or private agencies. Nonfinancial interests include personal or professional relationships, affiliations, knowledge, or beliefs that might affect objectivity.

Many potential biases may be detected during the editorial assessment and peer review of a manuscript (eg, problems with a study's methods and analysis, inappropriate interpretation of results, unbalanced selection or citation of the literature, unjustified emphasis or overly enthusiastic language, and conclusions that go beyond a study's results) or are apparent from the author's affiliation or area of expertise. However, financially motivated biases are less easily detected. Therefore, in the 1980s biomedical journals began to require authors to disclose any financial interests in the subject of their manuscript.[23,24] During the next 20 years, authors typically included information about financial support from grant and funding agencies in their submitted manuscripts, primarily because the funding agencies require them to do so, but it was less common for authors to disclose other financial interests, unless such information had been specifically requested.

Despite many high-profile scandals and studies that demonstrated bias associated with unreported conflicts of interest,[8-12,19-21] many journals continued to have no conflict of interest policies. One of the first studies to assess the prevalence of journal policies was conducted in 1997. This study[25] of 1396 top-ranked biomedical and science journals in terms of impact factor identified only 181 journals (13%) with conflict of interest policies; those journals with policies were overrepresented by medical journals. A subsequent study[26] conducted in 2005 of the 7 highest-impact peer-reviewed journals in 12 different scientific disciplines found a higher prevalence of journals that reported having conflict of interest policies (80%), although only 33% made these policies publicly available (eg, in their instructions for authors). All the top-ranked general medical and multidisciplinary science journals had such policies, but journals in other scientific disciplines were less likely to have such policies and/or to publish them in their instructions for authors.[26] In more recent years, studies[27-31] have found continued increases in journals adopting conflict of interest disclosure policies. However, individual policies and compliance with them continue to vary among journals and disciplines.[27,28,32] Recognizing this problem, in 2009 the International Committee of Medical Journal Editors (ICMJE) created a universal author disclosure form that can be used for all authors and any journal.[2,33] With the goal of improving usability and reporting, the ICMJE form has been modified a few times and a version is available for downloading at http://www.icmje.org/.[2] Some journals have begun to consider encouraging authors to disclose interests in centralized repositories.

Most biomedical journals, including the JAMA Network journals, require disclosure of conflicts of interest from everyone involved in the editorial process, including authors, reviewers, editorial board members, and editors, and for all types of articles.[7] The JAMA Network journals also have policies for recusal of peer reviewers and editors with conflicts of interest (see 5.5.6, Ethical and Legal Considerations, Conflicts of Interest, Requirements for Peer Reviewers, and 5.5.7, Ethical and Legal Considerations, Conflicts of Interest, Requirements for Editors and Editorial Board Members). The ICMJE,[2] the Council of Science Editors (CSE),[34] the Committee on Publication Ethics (COPE),[35] and the World Association of Medical Editors (WAME)[36] support similar policies of disclosure and transparency or recusal, depending on the circumstances. Many journals also require individuals (such as editorial and publishing employees and full-time and part-time editors) who have access to material during the review and publication processes to comply with policies on conflicts of interest.

Undisclosed conflicts of interest, whether intentionally concealed or unintentionally unreported because of denial or confusing policies, are harmful to researchers and authors, journals, and the public trust in science. In a regulatory attempt to improve transparency of industry-physician relationships and to manage the bias associated with undisclosed financial interests on medical knowledge, the US Centers for Medicare & Medicaid Services released a public website in September 2014 under the Sunshine Act.[37] This website, called Open Payments, provides information on a wide range of types of payments, including research funding and general payments for consulting, honoraria, gifts, travel, education, royalties or licenses, investment, compensation for serving as faculty or speaker, and research funding and grants, made to US physicians and teaching hospitals by industry and manufacturers of drugs, devices, biologicals, or medical supplies. For the year 2017, Open Payments reported more than $8.4 billion in payments from 1525 companies to 628 000 physicians and 1158 institutions, including $2.82 billion in general payments and $4.66 billion in research payments.[38] Such regulatory efforts may result in an increase in conflict of interest disclosures on the part of US physician authors to biomedical journals.

The following discussion addresses conflict of interest policies in general as recommended by the ICMJE,[2] CSE,[34] COPE,[35] and WAME[36] and provides specific examples of policies, procedures, and terms as used by the JAMA Network journals.[7,39]

**5.5.2**    **Requirements for Authors.** Authors should disclose all conflicts of interest related to the subject in the manuscript at the time of manuscript submission (if so required by the journal), in a cover letter to the editor, or on the journal's disclosure form (if the journal uses one). Journals should define conflicts of interest and the types of disclosures required (eg, all types of conflicts of interest or only financial interests) in their instructions for authors and in any disclosure forms. For example, the JAMA Network journals require authors to include all relevant financial interests, activities, relationships, and affiliations (other than those affiliations listed on the title page of the manuscript) in the Acknowledgment section of the manuscript so that all involved in reviewing manuscripts (editors and peer reviewers) can see the disclosure.[4,7,39] The journals describe these policies in their instructions for authors and in the online manuscript submission forms.

In an attempt to remove stigma associated with the word "conflict," some journals use the term *declaration of interests*. Journals commonly require authors to provide disclosure (or declaration) statements in a cover letter or disclosure form and do not share these disclosures with peer reviewers, unless the journal routinely shares author correspondence and submission forms with peer reviewers. Whether a journal requires complete disclosure of all potential conflicts of interest or only those related to the specific manuscript and whether the disclosures are to be nonconfidential and included in the manuscript or confidential and listed only in documents and communications not shared with peer reviewers, these policies should be made clear to all prospective authors and be publicly available in easily accessible instructions for authors. However, if a manuscript is accepted, whether the journal's disclosure policy is nonconfidential or confidential during the review process, the author's disclosures should be published.

For example, at the time a revision is requested, and before acceptance, the JAMA Network journals require authors to complete an Authorship Form with a section for disclosure of potential conflict of interest that is based on the questions included in the ICMJE universal disclosure form. To help authors avoid incomplete, inaccurate, or inconsistent disclosures, each time an author answers "no" to the questions about potential conflicts of interest, a pop-up message appears asking if the author is certain that "no" is the correct answer and if the author's answer is consistent with disclosures in recently published articles.[7] The JAMA Network journals do not publish these Authorship Forms. Instead, for accepted manuscripts, each author's disclosure statement is extracted from the Authorship Form and added to the manuscript during the editing process and then published in a conflict of interest disclosure statement in the Article Information section at the end of the article. If there is inconsistency between the disclosures included in the submitted manuscript and what each individual author has declared in the Authorship Forms, a manuscript editor will query the corresponding author to confirm that the disclosures in the edited manuscript are accurate (see 5.5.2.3, Publishing Authors' Disclosure Statements).

Some journals that require the ICMJE disclosure form publish these as online supplements to articles and may or may not include the disclosures in the actual articles. Such practice makes it challenging for readers to efficiently read or access the disclosure statements when reading a specific article.

The JAMA Network journals also require all authors to report detailed information regarding all financial and material support for the research and work, including but not limited to grant support, funding sources, and provision of equipment and supplies (see 5.5.3, Reporting Funding, Sponsorship, and Other Support).

**5.5.2.1** **Definitions and Terms of Conflict of Interest Disclosures.** The JAMA Network journals require authors to provide detailed information about all relevant financial interests, activities, relationships, and affiliations (other than those affiliations listed on the title page of the manuscript), including but not limited to employment, affiliation, funding and grants received or pending, consultancies, honoraria or payment, speakers' bureaus, stock ownership or options, paid expert testimony, royalties, donation of medical equipment, or patents planned, pending, or issued.

Following the 2018 guidelines of the ICMJE,[2] the definitions and terms of such disclosures include the following:

1. Any potential conflicts of interest "involving the work under consideration for publication" (during the time involving the work, from initial conception and planning to present),

2. Any "relevant financial activities outside the submitted work" (during the 3 years before submission), and

3. Any "other relationships or activities that readers could perceive to have influenced, or that give the appearance of potentially influencing" what is written in the submitted work (based on all relationships that were present during the 3 years before submission).

Authors without conflicts of interest, including relevant financial interests, activities, relationships, and affiliations, should include a statement of no such interests in the Acknowledgment section of the manuscript and in the disclosure forms. The Instructions for Authors for the JAMA Network journals note that "failure to include this information in the manuscript may delay evaluation and review of the manuscript" and that "authors should err on the side of full disclosure and should contact the editorial office if they have questions or concerns."[7,39]

Although many universities and other institutions and organizations have established thresholds for reporting financial interests (eg, $5000, $10 000), the JAMA Network journals require complete disclosure of all relevant financial relationships and potential financial conflicts of interest, regardless of amount or value.

Decisions about whether conflict of interest information provided by authors should be published, and thereby disclosed to readers, are usually straightforward. For example, authors of a manuscript about hypertension should report all financial relationships they have with all manufacturers and owners of products, devices, tests, and services used in the management of hypertension, not only those relationships with companies whose specific products, devices, tests, and services are mentioned in the manuscript. Authors should also consider reporting affiliations with organizations, societies, or other entities that may be related to the subject of their manuscripts, such as nonpaying volunteer leadership positions in professional societies or advocacy organizations. If authors are uncertain about what constitutes a relevant conflict of interest or relationship and whether the journal would deem a specific conflict of interest relevant, they should contact the editorial office.

**5.5.2.2** **Application of Policies to Different Types of Articles.** A journal's conflict of interest policies should apply to all manuscript submissions and types of articles, including reports of research, reviews, opinion pieces (eg, editorials), educational articles, reviews of books and other media, letters to the editor, and online-only comments.[4,5]

Some journals might not accept manuscripts from authors with financial interest in the subject of the manuscript. For example, editors of some journals prefer that authors of some types of articles, such as editorials and other opinion pieces and reviews, not have relevant financial interests in the subject matter.[40,41] Unlike scientific reports, editorials and nonsystematic reviews contain no primary data and offer an evaluation of a topic from a selection and interpretation of the literature; hence, they are more susceptible to bias,[8] which accompanying financial disclosures do not obviate. Authors of opinion pieces and review articles are expected to provide an expert and authoritative perspective that is not unduly biased, which they may not be able to do if they have financial ties to products or services mentioned in the manuscript or are otherwise related (eg, within the same area, category, or topic).

However, such policies may be overly restrictive and may limit the journal's ability to publish articles from some qualified authors. Journals with concerns about the financial interests of authors of opinion pieces and review articles must balance the risk of publishing potentially biased discussion and comment against excluding potentially valuable contributions to the literature, which in some fields may be the only expert contribution available. The key is for the editor to ensure that the editorial or review is as balanced, objective, and evidence based as possible. If, after review and careful consideration, the editor believes the work is biased and that the author is unable or unwilling to revise the manuscript to eliminate such bias and prospective readers would be misled, the editor should not accept the manuscript for publication. The policy of the JAMA Network journals recognizes that conflicts of interest are common and in some cases perhaps even helpful (eg, from a knowledgeable and critical reviewer with an opposing viewpoint). This policy favors complete disclosure from all authors over a ban of authors with conflicts of interest. However, when inviting an author to write an editorial to comment on a paper to be published, the editors will ask the prospective author to disclose any relevant conflicts of interest before writing and submitting the manuscript and consider this information carefully, in light of the potential for risk from bias vs benefit from expertise, before confirming that the author is the best available person to write the editorial.

**5.5.2.3** **Publishing Authors' Disclosure Statements.** Information about relevant conflicts of interest can be published in the Acknowledgment or Article ninformation about grants and financial or material support) or on the title page of the article near the author's affiliation (see 2.10.9, Conflict of Interest Disclosures, and 5.2, Acknowledgments). The following example shows placement in the Acknowledgment (or Article Information) section:

**Author Contributions:** Dr Jones had full access to all of the data in the study and takes responsibility for the integrity of the data and the accuracy of the data analysis.

*Concept and design:* Jones, Jacques, Smith, Brown.

*Acquisition of data:* Jones, Smith, Brown.

*Analysis and interpretation of data:* Jones, Jacques, Smith, Brown.

*Drafting of the manuscript:* Jones.

*Critical revision of the manuscript for important intellectual content:* Jacques, Smith, Brown.

*Statistical analysis:* Jacques.

*Obtained funding:* Jones.

*Supervision:* Brown.

**Conflict of Interest Disclosures:** Dr Jones reported serving as a paid consultant to Wyler Laboratories. Dr Jacques owns stock in Wyler Laboratories. No other disclosures were reported.

[*Or:* **Conflict of Interest Disclosures:** None reported.]

**Funding/Support:** This study was funded in part by Wyler Laboratories.

The following example shows placement in the author affiliation footnote on the title page/screen:

**Author Affiliations:** Department of Cardiology, Ambrose University Hospital, Boston, Massachusetts (Jones, Smith), and Wyler Laboratories, Geneva, Switzerland (Jacques, Brown).

**Conflict of Interest Disclosures:** Dr Jones reported serving as a paid consultant to Wyler Laboratories. Dr Jacques owns stock in Wyler Laboratories. No other disclosures were reported.

**Corresponding Author:** John J. Jones, MD, Department of Cardiology, Ambrose University Hospital, 444 N State St, Boston, MA 01022 (jonesj@ ambroseuniv.edu).

**5.5.3** ▨ **Reporting Funding, Sponsorship, and Other Support.** In addition to individual financial conflicts of interest, authors should report all financial and material support for the work reported in the manuscript. This support includes, but is not limited to, grant support and funding, provision of equipment and supplies, and other paid contributions.[2,4] All financial and material support for the work should be indicated in the Acknowledgment section of the manuscript, along with detailed information on the roles of each funding source or sponsor (see 5.2.6, Funding and Role of Funders and Sponsors). Some journals also request that this information be included in a funding field in electronic manuscript submission systems, either in free text or with a defined taxonomy. For example, FundRef uses a standard taxonomy of funder names.[42] Journals using FundRef may also deposit the standardized names of funders for published articles in a publicly searchable registry managed by CrossRef along with grant numbers and DOIs and other metadata about the published article.

In addition, all individuals who provided other important paid contributions should be identified, with their names and affiliations listed in the Acknowledgment section of the manuscript or as authors if they meet the full criteria for authorship. These contributions include the work of employed or compensated writers, editors, statisticians, epidemiologists, and others involved with manuscript preparation, data collection or management, and analyses. Acknowledgment of such contributions should be specific and may include information on funding. For example, the JAMA Network journals require authors to include information about each nonauthor contributor's role/contribution, academic degree(s), affiliation, and indication if compensation was received for each person named in the Acknowledgment section (see 5.2.1, Acknowledging Support, Assistance, and Contributions of Those Who Are Not Authors).

**5.5.4** **Reporting the Role of the Funder/Sponsor.** In the interest of full disclosure, the ICMJE recommends that authors report how funders and sponsors have participated in the work reported in a specific manuscript.[2,43] Journals should require authors to indicate the role of the sponsor/funding organization in each of the following: "design and conduct of the study; collection, management, analysis, and interpretation of the data; preparation, review, or approval of the manuscript; and decision to submit the manuscript for publication."[39] If the sponsor or funder had no such roles, this should be stated. This information may be included in the Acknowledgment or Methods section of the manuscript[2] (see 5.2.6, Funding and Role of Funders and Sponsors). Authors should not agree to allow sponsors with a proprietary or financial interest in the outcome of a study or review article to control the author's rights to publication, although review of manuscripts by sponsors or funders is typically permitted as long as such review does not impose an unacceptable delay or suppression.[2,8,12,43] According to the ICMJE, "authors should avoid entering into agreements with study sponsors, both for-profit and non-profit, that interfere with the authors' access to all of a study's data or that interfere with their ability to analyze and interpret the data and to prepare and publish manuscripts independently when and where they choose."[2]

**5.5.5** **Access to Data Requirement.** For all reports, regardless of funding source, that contain original data (research and systematic reviews), at least 1 named author should indicate that she or he "had full access to all the data in the study and takes responsibility for the integrity of the data and the accuracy of the data analysis"[2,3,39] (see 5.1.1, Authorship: Definition, Criteria, Contributions, and Requirements). This responsibility can vest with the principal investigator, the corresponding author, or both. Although in some research groups, particularly small ones, all authors may have access to all the data, it is usually not meaningful to state generically that all authors had such access. In such cases, the JAMA Network journals prefer that no more than 2 authors are indicated as being so responsible and prefer that at least 1 author is not employed by or affiliated with the study sponsor.[39]

**5.5.6** **Requirements for Peer Reviewers.** Following the recommendations of the ICMJE, CSE, and WAME, reviewers should disclose conflicts of interest in reviewing specific manuscripts and disqualify themselves from a specific review if necessary.[2,34,36] Reviewers should never use information obtained from an unpublished manuscript to further their own interests. Following the same rationale applied to authors, reviewers should state explicitly if they have no relevant conflicts of interest to disclose.[2]

The JAMA Network journals include the following instructions regarding conflicts of interest in the letter sent requesting an individual to review a manuscript:

> While most conflicts of interest are not disqualifying, if you perceive that you have a disqualifying interest, either financial or otherwise, please contact the reviewing editor immediately (if possible, with the names of alternative reviewers). This will not affect your reviewer status.

Not all conflicts of interest are necessarily disqualifying, and in some cases the reviewer with the most expertise may also have conflicts of interest. For example, if a potential conflict of interest exists (financial or otherwise) but the editor and reviewer agree that the reviewer can provide an objective assessment, the JAMA Network journals may request that the reviewer disclose the specific conflict and provide the review. Other journals may choose to exclude any reviewer with a conflict of interest from participating in the review process. A journal's policy on conflicts of interest for peer reviewers should be communicated to the reviewer when the review is requested.

The online review system used by the JAMA Network journals also contains a field in the reviewer recommendation form that requires reviewers to disclose conflicts of interest or state that they have no relevant conflicts of interest before submitting their reviews. This information is kept confidential and is not revealed to authors or other reviewers.

Many journals will accept reviewer recommendations from authors, but editors should carefully vet any such recommendations and should avoid automatically routing papers to author-recommended reviewers. There have been cases of authors gaming electronic submission systems by recommending fictitious reviewers and then reviewing their own papers under the guise of these sham reviewers.[44]

Journals may also consider authors' requests not to send papers to specific reviewers. Authors who wish to exclude specific reviewers should explain the reasons for such requests at the time of manuscript submission. As with author-recommended reviewers, editors should carefully consider author requests to exclude specific reviewers (see 6.1.2.1, Selection of Reviewers, and 5.11, Editorial Responsibilities, Roles, Procedures, and Policies).

**5.5.7** **Requirements for Editors and Editorial Board Members.** Editors may also have their objectivity influenced or biased by conflicts of interest.[45-50] As a result, the ICMJE, CSE, and WAME recommend that editors follow policies on conflicts of interest that require disclosure of all relevant conflicts of interest (financial and nonfinancial) and that they not participate in the review of or decisions on any manuscripts in which they may have a conflict of interest.[2,34,36] Editors and journal editorial board members are prohibited from using information obtained during the review process for personal or professional gain and should refrain from making any decisions or recommendations about manuscripts in which they have a personal, professional, or financial interest. According to the ICMJE, "Editors who make final decisions about manuscripts should recuse themselves from editorial decisions if they have conflicts of interest or relationships that pose potential conflicts related to articles under consideration."[2] This recommendation applies to all editors, other editorial staff, and any editorial board members who make decisions to consider, accept, revise, or reject manuscripts. All decision-making editors and editorial board members should provide the editor in chief with conflict of interest disclosure statements at least annually, with updates for any major changes.

Editors should also consider how to handle manuscripts from an author who is from the same institution as the editor or in a field in which the editor has research funding and how to handle their own research and review articles.[6] In the event that an editor works alone and has a conflict of interest with a particular manuscript, he or she should assign that manuscript to a guest editor or a member of the editorial board and should not take part in the review and editorial decision of such manuscripts. The JAMA Network journals publish disclaimers with any research or reviews articles that have an author who is also a decision-making editor for the journal to inform readers that the author-editor was not involved in the review or editorial decision.

> **Disclaimer:** Dr Brown, the journal's deputy editor, was not involved in the editorial review of or decision to publish this article.

Editorials written by journal editors are exempt from such procedures, but it may be prudent for editors to ask other editors or editorial board members to review and comment on these types of manuscripts before publication (see 5.11, Editorial Responsibilities, Roles, Procedures, and Policies).

The JAMA Network journal editors complete an ICMJE conflict of interest disclosure form annually in which any financial interests and relationships (type, entity, and whether money is paid to the individual or their institution) are listed and which is kept confidential in the editorial office. The editors also agree to recuse themselves from reviewing, editing, or participating in editorial decisions about any manuscripts that deal with a matter in which they have a potential conflict of interest.

**5.5.8　Handling Failure to Disclose Conflicts of Interest.**

**5.5.8.1　For Authors of Manuscripts Not Yet Published.** In the event that an undisclosed conflict of interest on the part of an author is brought to the editor's attention (usually during the review process), the editor should remind the author of the journal's policy and ask the author if he or she has anything to disclose. The author's reply may affect the editorial decision on whether to publish the manuscript.

**5.5.8.2　For Authors of Published Articles.** If an editor receives information (usually from a reader) alleging that an author has not disclosed a conflict of interest in the subject of an article that has been published, the editor should contact the author and ask for an explanation. If the author admits that he or she failed to disclose the existence of a conflict of interest in the subject of the article and if that author had previously submitted a signed conflict disclosure statement that did not disclose that conflict of interest, the editor should request a written explanation from the author and an updated conflict of interest disclosure and publish this information as a Letter of explanation or notice of failure to disclose conflict of interest along with a Correction notice and correct the article online.[7] Depending on the circumstances and extent of the inaccurate disclosure, some editors may notify the offending author's institution or funder.[7] (See this example[51] and **Box 5.5-1**.) COPE has a useful flowchart, "What to do if a reader suspects undisclosed conflict of interest (CoI) in a published article."[52]

As in the case of other types of allegations of wrongdoing (eg, scientific misconduct), editors are not responsible for investigating unresolved allegations of conflict of interest in an article or manuscript. That responsibility lies with the author's institution, the funding agency, or other appropriate authority. If the editor deems the author's reply to the allegation inappropriate or incomplete, the editor may need to break confidentiality and inform the author's supervisor (eg, dean, research integrity officer, department chair, director) or representative of the funding agency.

**Box 5.5-1.** Hypothetical Example of a Notice of Failure to Disclose Conflict of Interest and Listing in the Journal's Table of Contents

---

**Failure to Disclose Financial Interest**

*To the Editor.*—I regret that at the time I submitted my manuscript "Effective Vaccine Strategies for Pertussis,"[1] published in the March 17, 2017, issue of the *Journal of Medicine*, I failed to disclose that I have served as a paid expert witness in several diphtheria-pertussis-tetanus vaccine injury–related lawsuits. I had completed the journal's conflict of interest disclosure statement, but I did not realize that expert testimony was considered a potential conflict of interest. I do not believe that my involvement in those legal proceedings biased me in any way, and I regret any confusion this may have caused. I have requested that the article be corrected to add this disclosure.[2]

V. W. Brazen, MD
Virginia State University
Arlington

**References**

1. Brazen VW. Effective vaccine strategies for pertussis. *J Med.* 2017;27(5):440-441.
2. Missing conflict of interest disclosure. *J Med.* 2018;28(1):68.

**Listing in Table of Contents**
**Correction**
Failure to Disclose Conflict of Interest.
V. W. Brazen

---

**5.5.8.3** **For Reviewers, Editors, and Editorial Board Members.** The discovery of an undisclosed conflict of interest on the part of peer reviewers may result in the journal not asking that reviewer to consult again. Failure to disclose relevant conflicts of interest on the part of editors or editorial board members is grounds for dismissal.

**Principal Author:** Annette Flanagin, RN, MA

## ACKNOWLEDGMENT

I thank the following for review and helpful comments: Howard Bauchner, MD, *JAMA* and JAMA Network; Carissa Gilman, American Cancer Society, Atlanta, Georgia; Timothy Gray, PhD, JAMA Network; Iris Y. Lo, JAMA Network; Ana Marušić, MD, PhD, *Journal of Global Health* and University of Split School of Medicine, Croatia; and Joseph P. Thornton, JD, JAMA Network and American Medical Association.

## REFERENCES

1. Pope A. *An Essay on Criticism.* 1711:part II, lines 1-4.
2. International Committee of Medical Journal Editors. Recommendations for the conduct, reporting, editing, and publication of scholarly work in medical journals. Updated December 2018. Accessed December 21, 2018. http://www.icmje.org
3. DeAngelis CD, Fontanarosa PB, Flanagin A. Reporting financial conflicts of interest and relationships between investigators and research sponsors. *JAMA.* 2001;286(1):89-91. doi:10.1001/jama.286.1.89
4. Flanagin A, Fontanarosa PB, DeAngelis CD. Update on *JAMA*'s conflict of interest policy. *JAMA.* 2006;296(2):220-221. doi:10.1001/jama.296.2.220
5. Fontanarosa P, Bauchner H. Conflict of interest and medical journals. *JAMA.* 2017;317(17):1768-1771. doi:10.1001/jama.2017.4563
6. Gottlieb JD, Bressler NM. How should journals handle the conflict of interest of their editors? who watches the "watchers"? *JAMA.* 2017;317(17):1757-1758. doi:10.1001/jama.2017.2207
7. Bauchner H, Fontanarosa PB, Flanagin A. Conflicts of interests, authors, and journals: new challenges for a persistent problem. *JAMA.* 2018;320(22):2315-2318. doi:10.1001/jama.2018.17593
8. Blumenthal D, Causino N, Campbell E, Louis KS. Relationships between academic institutions and industry in the life sciences: an industry survey. *N Engl J Med.* 1996;334(6):368-373. doi:10.1056/NEJM199602083340606
9. Stelfox HT, Chua G, O'Rourke K, Detsky AS. Conflict of interest in the debate over calcium-channel antagonists. *N Engl J Med.* 1998;338(2):101-106. doi:10.1056/NEJM199801083380206
10. Boyd EA, Bero LA. Assessing faculty financial relationships with industry: a case study. *JAMA.* 2000;284(17):2209-2214. doi:10.1001/jama.284.17.2209
11. Bekelman JE, Li Y, Gross CP. Scope and impact of financial conflicts of interest in biomedical research: a systematic review. *JAMA.* 2003;289(4):454-465. doi:10.1001/jama.289.4.454
12. Rennie D. Thyroid storm. *JAMA.* 1997;277(15):1238-1243. doi:10.1001/jama.1997.03540390068038
13. DeAngelis CD. The influence of money on medical science. *JAMA.* 2006;296(8):996-998. doi:10.1001/jama.296.8.jed60051
14. Wayant C, Turner E, Meyer C, Sinnett P, Vassar M. Financial conflicts of interest among oncologist authors of reports of clinical drug trials. *JAMA Oncol.* 2018;4(10):1426-1428. doi:10.1001/jamaoncol.2018.3738

15. Checketts JX, Sims MT, Vassar M. Evaluating industry payments among dermatology clinical practice guidelines authors. *JAMA Dermatol.* 2017;153(12):1229-1235. doi:10.1001/jamadermatol.2017.3109

16. Horn J, Checketts JX, Jawhar O, Vassar M. Evaluation of industry relationships among authors of otolaryngology clinical practice guidelines. *JAMA Otolaryngol Head Neck Surg.* 2018;144(3):194-201. doi:10.1001/jamaoto.2017.2741

17. Ziai K, Pigazzi A, Smith BR, et al. Association of compensation from the surgical and medical device industry to physicians and self-declared conflict of interest. *JAMA Surg.* 2018;153(11):997-1002. doi:10.1001/jamasurg.2018.2576

18. Lo B, Field MJ; Committee on Conflict of Interest in Medical Research, Education, and Practice; Institute of Medicine Institute of Medicine. *Conflict of Interest in Medical Research, Education, and Practice.* April 21, 2009. Accessed December 21, 2018. https://www.ncbi.nlm.nih.gov/books/NBK22942

19. Sismondo S. Ghost management: how much of the medical literature is shaped behind the scenes by the pharmaceutical industry? *PLoS Med.* 2007;4(9):e286. doi:10.1371/journal.pmed.0040286

20. Psaty BM, Kronmal RA. Reporting mortality findings in trials of rofecoxib for Alzheimer disease or cognitive impairment: a case study based on documents from rofecoxib litigation. *JAMA.* 2008;299(15):1813-1817. doi:10.1001/jama.299.15.1813

21. Ross JS, Hill KP, Egilman DS, Krumholz HM. Guest authorship and ghostwriting in publications related to rofecoxib: a case study of industry documents from rofecoxib litigation. *JAMA.* 2008;299(15):1800-1812. doi:10.1001/jama.299.15.1800

22. Friedman PJ. The troublesome semantics of conflict of interest. *Ethics Behav.* 1992;2(4):245-251. doi:10.1207/s15327019eb0204_2

23. Relman AS. Dealing with conflicts of interest. *N Engl J Med.* 1984;310(18):1182-1183. doi:10.1056/NEJM198405033101809

24. Knoll E, Lundberg GD. New instructions for authors. *JAMA.* 1985;254(1):97-98. doi:10.1001/jama.1985.03360010103037

25. Krimsky S, Rothenberg LS. Conflict of interest policies in science and medical journals: editorial practices and author disclosures. *Sci Eng Ethics.* 2001;7(2):205-218. doi:10.1007/s11948-001-0041-7

26. Ancker J, Flanagin A. A comparison of conflict of interest policies at peer-reviewed journals in multiple scientific disciplines. *Sci Eng Ethics.* 2007;13(2):147-157. doi:10.1007/s11948-007-9011-z

27. Blum JA, Freeman K, Dart RC, Cooper RJ. Requirements and definitions in conflict of interest policies of medical journals. *JAMA.* 2009;302(20):2230-2234. doi:10.1001/jama.2009.1669

28. Cooper RJ, Gupta M, Wilkes MS, Hoffman JR. Conflict of interest disclosure policies and practices in peer-reviewed biomedical journals. *J Gen Intern Med.* 2006;21(12):1248-1252. doi:10.1111/j.1525-1497.2006.00598.x

29. Meerpohl JJ, Wolff RF, Niemeyer CM, Antes G, von Elm E. Editorial policies of pediatric journals: survey of instructions for authors. *Arch Pediatr Adolesc Med.* 2010;164(3):268-272. doi:10.1001/archpediatrics.2009.287

30. Kesselheim AS, Lee JL, Avorn A, Servi A, Shrank WH, Choudhry NK. Conflict of interest in oncology publications: a survey of disclosure policies and statements. *Cancer.* 2012;118(1):188-195. doi:10.1002/cncr.26237

31. Anraku A, Jin YP, Trope GE, Buys YM. Survey of conflict-of-interest disclosure policies of ophthalmology journals. *Ophthalmology.* 2009;116(6):1093-1096. doi:10.1016/j.ophtha.2008.12.053

32. Check E. Journals scolded for slack disclosure rules. *Nature*. January 18, 2006. doi:10.1038/news060116-6

33. Drazen JM, Van Der Weyden MB, Sahni P, et al. Uniform format for disclosure of competing interests in ICMJE journals. *JAMA*. 2010;303(1):75-76. doi:10.1001/jama.2009.1542

34. Council of Science Editors. CSE's white paper on publication ethics. Updated May 2018. Accessed July 7, 2019. https://www.councilscienceeditors.org/resource-library/editorial-policies/white-paper-on-publication-ethics

35. Committee on Publication Ethics. Principles of transparency and best practice in scholarly publishing. January 15, 2018. Accessed July 7, 2019. https://publicationethics.org/files/Principles_of_Transparency_and_Best_Practice_in_Scholarly_Publishingv3.pdf

36. World Association of Medical Editors. Conflict of interest in peer-reviewed medical journals. Posted March 27, 2009. Updated July 25, 2009. Accessed December 21, 2018. http://www.wame.org/conflict-of-interest-in-peer-reviewed-medical-journals

37. Centers for Medicare & Medicaid Services. Open Payments. Accessed July 12, 2019. https://cms.gov/openpayments

38. Centers for Medicare & Medicaid Services. The facts about Open Payments Data. Accessed December 21, 2018. https://openpaymentsdata.cms.gov/summary

39. *JAMA* Instructions for Authors. Updated June 10, 2019. Accessed July 7, 2019. https://jamanetwork.com/journals/jama/pages/instructions-for-authors

40. Publishing commentary by authors with potential conflicts of interest: when, why, and how. *Ann Intern Med*. 2004;141(1):73-74. doi:10.7326/0003-4819-141-1-200407060-00020

41. James A, Horton R. *The Lancet*'s policy on conflicts of interest—2004. *Lancet*. 2004;363(9402):2-3.

42. Crossref. Funder Registry. Updated January 19, 2017. Accessed December 21, 2018. https://www.crossref.org/services/funder-registry/

43. Davidoff F, DeAngelis CD, Drazen JM, et al. Sponsorship, authorship, and accountability. *JAMA*. 2001;286(10):1232-1234. doi:10.1001/jama.286.10.1232

44. Ferguson C, Marcus A, Oranksy I. Publishing: the peer-review scam. *Nature*. 2014;515(7528):480-482. doi:10.1038/515480a

45. A medical editor's resignation. *JAMA*. 1893;21(16):582. doi:10.1001/jama.1893.02420680032009

46. Hoey J. When editors publish in their own journals. *CMAJ*. 1999;161(11):1412-1413.

47. Watson G, Watson M, Chapman S, Byrne F. Environmental tobacco smoke research published in the journal *Indoor and Built Environment* and associations with the tobacco industry. *Lancet*. 2005;365(9461):804-809. doi:10.1016/S0140-6736(05)17990-2

48. Wright IC. Conflict of interest and the *British Journal of Psychiatry*. *Br J Psychiatry*. 2002;180:82-83. doi:10.1192/bjp.180.1.82

49. Pincock S. Journal editor quits in conflict scandal. *Scientist*. August 28, 2006. Accessed December 21, 2018. https://www.the-scientist.com/daily-news/journal-editor-quits-in-conflict-scandal-47277

50. Wu AW, Kavanaugh KT, Pronovost PJ, Bates, DW. Conflict of interest, Dr Charles Denham and the *Journal of Patient Safety*. *J Patient Saf*. 2014;10(4):181-185. doi:10.1097/PTS.0000000000000144

51. Baselga J. Failure to accurately disclose conflicts of interest in articles published in *JAMA Oncology*. *JAMA Oncol*. 2019;5(1):118-119. doi:10.1001/jamaoncol.2018.5674

52. Committee on Publication Ethics. What to do if a reader suspects undisclosed conflict of interest in a published article. Updated 2013. Accessed July 7, 2019. https://publicationethics.org/guidance/flowcharts

## 5.6 Intellectual Property: Ownership, Access, Rights, and Management.

> *[Will copyright survive the new technologies?] That question is about as bootless as asking whether politics will survive democracy. The real question is what steps it will take to ensure that the promised new era of information and entertainment survives copyright. History offers a clue.*
> Paul Goldstein[1]

*Intellectual property* is a legal term for that which results from the creative efforts of the mind (intellectual) and that which can be owned, possessed, and subject to competing claims (property).[2] Three legal doctrines governing intellectual property are relevant for authors, editors, and publishers in biomedical publishing: copyright (the law protecting authorship and publication), patent (the law protecting invention and technology), and trademark (the law protecting words and symbols used to identify goods and services in the marketplace).[1] This section focuses primarily on intellectual property and copyright law as they relate to ownership, access, rights, and management of content and publication.

### 5.6.1 Ownership and Control of Data.
Conceptual application of the term *property* to scientific knowledge is not new, but advances in science and technology, economic factors, regulations, and policies have fueled disputes, concerns, and changes in attitude about data ownership, control, transparency, and access.[1-11] Data used in biomedical research are increasingly complex and include large data sets, models, algorithms, and metadata (data that provide information or characteristics about other data). With the exception of commercially owned information, scientific data are generally viewed as a public good, allowing others to benefit from knowledge of and access to the information without decreasing the benefit received by the individual who originally developed the data. However, personal, professional, financial, and proprietary interests can interfere with the altruistic goals of data sharing.[7-9,12-15]

#### 5.6.1.1 Data: Definition and Types of Ownership.
For purposes herein, *data* include but are not limited to written and digital laboratory notes, documents, research and project records, experimental materials (eg, reagents, cultures), descriptions of collections of biological specimens (eg, cells, tissue, genetic material), descriptions of methods and processes, patient or research participant records and measurements, results of bibliometric and other database searches, illustrative material and graphics, audio and video recordings, analyses, surveys, questionnaires, responses, data sets (eg, protein or DNA sequences, microassay or molecular structure data), databases, metadata (data that describe or characterize other data), and algorithms. The US National Institutes of Health (NIH) defines *digital scientific data* as "the digital recorded factual material commonly accepted in the scientific community as necessary to validate research findings including data sets used to support scholarly

publications, but does not include laboratory notebooks, preliminary analyses, drafts of scientific papers, plans for future research, peer reviews, communications with colleagues, or physical objects, such as laboratory specimens . . . The definition of digital scientific data includes data that are used to support a scientific publication as well as data from completed studies that might never be published. It may include data that support or refute a hypothesis, but does not include draft or preliminary data sets."[6] The NIH definition does not include software.

In scientific research, 3 common arenas exist for ownership of data: the government, the commercial sector, and academic or private institutions or foundations. Although perhaps a less frequent occurrence, when data are produced by a researcher or other individual without a relationship to a government agency, a commercial entity, or a private institution, the data are owned by that individual.

Any information produced by an office or employee of the US federal government during his or her employment is owned by the government.[16] The US Freedom of Information Act (FOIA), enacted in 1966, is intended to ensure public access to government-owned information (except trade secrets, financial data, national defense information, and personnel or medical records protected under the Privacy Act).[2,17] Access to documents with such data that are otherwise unavailable may be obtained through a FOIA request in the United States. Many countries have implemented similar freedom of information legislation.

Data produced by employees in the commercial sector (eg, a pharmaceutical, device, or biotechnology company, health insurance company, or for-profit hospital or managed care organization) are typically governed by the legal relationship between the employee and the commercial employer, granting all rights of data ownership and control to the employer. However, if the data have been used to secure or are funded by a government grant or contract, such data may be obtained by an outside party through a FOIA request or by a court-ordered subpoena.[3,17]

The US Bayh-Dole Act of 1980 permits universities or nonprofit institutions to have control of the intellectual property generated from federally funded research. For example, according to guidelines established by Harvard University and subsequently adopted by other US academic institutions (as well as those in other countries), data developed by employees of academic institutions are owned by the institutions.[18,19] These policies allow access to data by university scientists and allow departing scientists to take copies of data with them, but the original data remain at the institution. However, researchers do not always understand university intellectual property policies or data management plans, or who owns data, how to interpret and comply with funder mandates for data access, how long data should be retained, data depositing requirements, costs associated with data management and depositing, and a host of ethical issues related to data management, access, and sharing.[18,20]

**5.6.1.2**    **Data Transparency, Sharing, and Length of Storage.** The notion that data should be transparent and shared with others for review, criticism, and replication is a fundamental but perhaps idealistic tenet of the scientific enterprise. Sharing research data encourages scientific inquiry, permits reanalysis, promotes new research, facilitates education and training of new researchers, permits creation of new data sets when data from multiples sources are combined, and helps maintain the integrity of the scientific record.[2,4-6,10] However, the practice of data sharing has varied widely, and it was not until the early 2000s that guidelines for data sharing were developed[4,5] and only recently that more assertive calls for data transparency have been promulgated for medical research.[6,8,10,21-23]

Although data sharing is essential for research, costs and risks may result in restrictions on access to certain data imposed by the owner, initial investigator, or sponsor or funder. Potential costs and risks to the owner or initial investigator include technical and financial obstacles for data storage, reproduction, and transmission; loss of academic or financial reward or commercial profit; unwarranted or unwanted criticism; risk of future discovery or exploitation by a competitor; the discovery of error or fraud; and breaches of confidentiality and violations of rights to privacy of personal data. The discovery of error or fraud and breaches of confidentiality have important relevance in scientific publishing. Discovery of error or fraud, if corrected or retracted in the literature, is clearly beneficial. For research involving humans, epidemiologic and statistical procedures are available to maintain confidentiality for individual study participants, but challenges to protect identifying data of individual research participants remain[6,10,22] (see 5.4, Scientific Misconduct; 5.8, Protecting Research Participants' and Patients' Rights in Scientific Publication; and 5.11.10, Corrections [Errata]).

A number of research sponsors and governmental agencies have developed policies to encourage data transparency and sharing.[5,6,22-25] For example, in 2003, the NIH began requiring investigators to include a plan for data sharing in all grant applications that request $500 000 or more in direct costs.[5] That same year, the Wellcome Trust began encouraging its funded investigators to release data to the public from large-scale biological research projects, such as the International Human Genome Sequencing Consortium. The Wellcome Trust has required funded researchers to maximize the value of research with data management plans for research that "is likely to create significant research outputs that are of value to other researchers and users," such as clinical trials, longitudinal studies of patient and population cohorts, genetic studies, large-scale neuroimaging studies, computational models and simulations of neurologic, physiologic, or other biological systems, and the creation and development of databases.[24]

The 2003 NIH policy on data sharing, which is still in force, states that "data should be made as widely and freely available as possible while safeguarding the privacy of participants and protecting confidential and proprietary data."[5] In 2013, the US Office of Science and Technology Policy released a policy titled "Increasing Access to the Results of Federally Funded Scientific Research," which directs "peer-reviewed publications and digital scientific data resulting from federally-funded scientific research to be publically accessible."[26]

Focusing on clinical trials, the US Institute of Medicine (IOM), now called the National Academy of Medicine (NAM), issued a report in 2015 on data sharing that concludes with the following: "Responsible sharing of clinical trial data will allow other investigators to carry out additional analyses and reproduce published findings, strengthen the evidence base for regulatory and clinical decisions, and increase the scientific knowledge gained from investments by the funders of clinical trials. Data sharing can accelerate new discoveries by avoiding duplicative trials, stimulating new ideas for research, and enabling the maximal scientific knowledge and benefits to be gained from the efforts of clinical trial participants and investigators."[10] The IOM/NAM report also acknowledged risks, burdens, and challenges to the sharing of clinical trial data, including "the need to (1) protect the privacy and honor the consent of clinical trial participants; (2) safeguard the legitimate economic interests of sponsors (eg, intellectual property and commercially confidential information); (3) guard against invalid secondary analyses, which could undermine trust in clinical trials or otherwise harm public health; (4) give researchers who put effort and time into planning, organizing, and running clinical trials adequate time to analyze the data they have collected and appropriate recognition for their intellectual contributions; and (5) assuage the fear of research institutions that requirements for sharing clinical trial data will be unfunded mandates."[10] In addition, any policies promoting data sharing should acknowledge the financial costs associated with a priori planning of research to address the above needs and the costs associated with data deposit and maintenance. The IOM/NAM report has specific recommendations for various stakeholders, including funders and sponsors, disease advocacy organizations, regulatory and research oversight bodies, institutional review boards and research ethics committees, investigators, research institutions and universities, membership and professional societies, and journals.

Several proposals prescribe the minimum optimal time to keep data (eg, 2-7 years). However, there is no universally accepted standard for data retention by academic and research institutions. For example, the NIH requires its funded scientists to keep data for a minimum of 3 years after the closeout of a grant or contract agreement and recognizes that an investigator's academic institution may have additional policies regarding the required retention period for data.[5] The NIH also gives the right of data management, including the decision to publish, to the principal investigator.[5] The European Medicines Agency recommends that essential documents for clinical trials be retained for at least 15 years after completion or discontinuation of the trial.[25] With new policies for data transparency and recommendations for deposit in accessible repositories, data may be available for longer periods in both public and private repositories. However, length of data storage and retention in such repositories is one of the many challenges to an effective data management policy and culture (see 5.6.1.5, Record Retention Policies for Journals).

**5.6.1.3**    **Data Sharing, Deposit, and Access Requirements of Journals.** In 1985, the US Committee on National Statistics, which is part of the National Research Council (NRC),[27] released a report on data sharing that continues to serve as a useful guide for researchers, authors, editors, and journals. Among the committee's recommendations, the following have specific relevance for scientific journal publication[27]:

> Data sharing should be a regular practice.

> Initial investigators should share their data by the time of the publication of initial major results of analyses of the data except in compelling circumstances, and they should share data relevant to public policy quickly and as widely as possible.

> Investigators should keep data available for a reasonable period after publication of results from analyses of the data.

> Subsequent analysts who request data from others should bear the associated incremental costs and they should endeavor to keep the burdens of data sharing to a minimum. They should explicitly acknowledge the contribution of the initial investigators in all subsequent publications.

Journal editors should require authors to provide access to data during the peer review process.

Journals should give more emphasis to reports of secondary analyses and to replications.

Journals should require full credit and appropriate citations to original data collections in reports based on secondary analyses.

Journals should strongly encourage authors to make detailed data accessible to other researchers (although some may view this as outside the purview of a journal's responsibilities).

Similar to policies on data sharing and storage for academic and research institutions, policies for scientific journals are highly variable and not always available. In 2002, an NRC review of 56 of the most frequently cited life science and medical journals reported that 39% had policies on data sharing and 45% had no stated policy.[4] Of the 18 medical journals in this review, only 22% had policies on data sharing. In a 2009-2010 survey of 1329 scientists in a variety of disciplines, 75% reported that they share their data with others, but only 36% reported that others can easily access those data.[8] At that time, only 55% of scientists reported that their funders required that they provide a data management plan. That survey revealed multiple perceived and actual barriers to data sharing by scientists, including lack of established standards for meta-data associated with the data as well as data formatting, archiving, and depositing in repositories. In 2013-2014, a follow-up survey was conducted among 1015 of the scientists who had participated in the previous survey and after many funders had begun to implement policies that required data sharing and data management plans.[9] The follow-up survey found that scientists were more willing to share data, but perceived risks and barriers continue to challenge actual data sharing practices.

To address the lack of standard policies for data sharing among scientific journals, in 2003 the NRC recommended the following[4]:

Scientific journals should clearly and prominently state (in their instructions for authors and on their websites) their policies for distribution of publication-related materials, data, and other information.

Policies for sharing materials should include requirements for depositing materials in an appropriate repository.

Policies for data sharing should include requirements for deposition of complex data sets in appropriate databases and for the sharing of software and algorithms integral to the finding being reported.

The policies should also clearly state the consequences for authors who do not adhere to the policies and the procedure for registering complaints about noncompliance.

The NRC also proposed a set of principles that may be useful to journals developing policies on data sharing[4]:

Authors should include in their publications data, algorithms, or other information that is central or integral to the publication—that is, whatever is necessary to support the major claims of the paper and would enable one skilled in the art to verify or replicate the claims.

If central or integral information cannot be included in the publication for practical reasons (for example, because a data set is too large), it should be made freely (without restriction of its use for research purposes and at no cost) and readily accessible through other means (for example, online). Moreover, when necessary to enable further research, integral information should be made available in a form that enables it to be manipulated, analyzed, and combined with other scientific data.

If publicly accessible repositories for data have been agreed on by a community of researchers and are in general use, the relevant data should be deposited in one of these repositories by the time of publication.

Authors of scientific publications should anticipate which materials integral to their publications are likely to be requested and should state in the "Materials and Methods" section or elsewhere how to obtain them.

If material integral to a publication is patented, the provider of the material should make the material available under a license for research use.

Focusing specifically on clinical trials, the 2015 IOM/NAM report, *Sharing Clinical Trial Data: Maximizing Benefits, Minimizing Risk*,[10] recommends that journals do the following:

Require authors of both primary and secondary analyses of clinical trial data to document that they have submitted a data sharing plan at a site that shares data with and meets the data requirements of the World Health Organization's International Clinical Trials Registry Platform before enrolling participants, and

Commit to releasing the analytic data set underlying published analyses, tables, figures, and results no later than the times specified in this report (eg, the full analyzable data set with metadata no later than 18 months after study completion—with specified exceptions for trials intended to support a regulatory application—and the analytic data set supporting publication results no later than 6 months after publication); and

Require that submitted manuscripts using existing data sets from clinical trials, in whole or in part, cite these data appropriately; and

Require that any published secondary analyses provide the data and metadata at the same level as in the original publication.

While funders and governmental agencies continue to sort out practical and effective policies of data sharing, storage, and access, many journals currently encourage data sharing by the authors of articles they publish, and some journals require data sharing as a condition of publication. In 2017, the International Committee of Medical Journal Editors (ICMJE) issued a statement on sharing clinical trial data that supports the recommendations of the IOM/NAM and that indicates new requirements for sharing of deidentified individual patient data underlying the results presented in published articles.[22] For reports of randomized clinical trials, ICMJE requires authors to provide a data sharing statement that indicates if data, including individual patient data, a data dictionary that defines each field in the data set, and supporting documentation, will be made available to others; when, where, and how the data will be available; types of analyses that are permitted; and if there will be any restrictions on the use of the data. Data sharing statements may also be submitted for reports of other types of studies, but the ICMJE member journals only require this for reports of clinical trials.

Data sharing statements should address the following items:

### Data

Will the data collected for your study, including individual patient data and a data dictionary defining each field in the data set, be made available to others?

Yes or no. (If no, authors may explain why data are not available.)

List all data that will be made available:

Deidentified participant data

Participant data with identifiers

Data dictionary

Other (please specify)

List where to access these data. Provide complete URL if data will be available in a repository or website, or provide complete email address if request for data must be sent to an individual.

List the beginning date and end date (if applicable) when these data will be available. If the beginning date of data availability will be when the article is published, please indicate "with publication."

With publication

At a date different from publication

Beginning date

End date (if applicable)

### Supporting Documents

If your manuscript is accepted for publication, the journal will publish your trial protocol, including the statistical analysis plan, and any amendments as online supplements. Please list any other supporting documents that you wish to make available (eg, statistical/analytic code, informed consent form).

Statistical/analytic code

Informed consent form

None

Other (please specify)

List where to access these documents. Provide complete URL if the documents will be available in a repository or website, or provide complete email address if request for documents must be sent to an individual.

List the beginning date and end date (if applicable) when these data will be available. If the beginning date of data availability will be when the article is published, please indicate "with publication."

With publication

At a date different from publication

Beginning date

End date (if applicable)

### Additional Information

Indicate the types of analyses for which the data will be made available (eg, for any purpose or for a specified purpose).

Indicate the mechanism by which the data will be made available (eg, with investigator support, without investigator support, after approval of a proposal, or with a signed data access agreement).

List any additional restrictions on the use of the data or any additional information.

If you would like to offer context for your decision not to make the data available, please enter it below (optional).

Examples of data sharing statements are shown in 2.10.15, Data Sharing Statement.

A number of journals have had data sharing or availability polices that range from encouragement to strict requirements for different types of data for more than a decade, including *Nature, Science*, the Public Library of Science (PLOS) journals, and a number of medical journals, but policies have not been fully standardized. For example, in 2007 the *Annals of Internal Medicine* began encouraging data transparency by publishing a statement with research articles that indicates authors' willingness to share the study protocol (original and amendments), statistical code used to generate results, and the data set from which the results were derived.[28] Since that time, the journal has encouraged sharing but has not required it and notes that "access to these items may range from completely unrestricted (eg, free availability of all the items via posting on an open-access website) to restricted (eg, availability of certain portions of the items to approved individuals through written agreements with the author or research sponsor)."[29] *The BMJ* has a similar policy, and authors of original research articles are required to include a data sharing statement when submitting their article. The statement should explain what additional unpublished data from the study—if any—are available, who can access the data, and how the data can be obtained.[30] *BMJ Open* also lists examples of repositories that accept data deposits and provide permanent links to the deposits and has a useful list of resources for data management and sharing.[31] As members of the ICMJE, both journals require authors of clinical trials to include data sharing statements.

For many years, a number of scientific journals (eg, *Science,*[32] *Nature*[33]) have required authors to submit large data sets (eg, protein or DNA sequences, microarray or molecular structure data) to approved, accessible databases and to provide accession numbers as a condition of publication. It is appropriate for authors and journals to include links to public repositories for such data in the Methods or Acknowledgment sections of articles (see 2.10.18, Manuscript Preparation for Submission and Publication, Acknowledgments [Article Information], Additional Information [Miscellaneous Acknowledgments]).

However, both *Science* and *Nature* now indicate in their instructions for authors that they require authors to make materials, study protocols, and data codes necessary for study replication available to others without qualification or restriction—unless formally explained to the editors at the time a manuscript is submitted.[32,33] *Science* states the following in its information for authors[32]:

Data and Materials Availability After Publication

After publication, all data and materials necessary to understand, assess, and extend the conclusions of the manuscript must be available to any reader of a Science Journal. After publication, all reasonable requests for data, code, or materials must be fulfilled. Any restrictions on the availability of data, code, or materials, including fees and restrictions on original data obtained from other sources must be disclosed to the editors as must any Material Transfer Agreements (MTAs) pertaining to data or materials used or produced in this research, that place constraints on providing these data, code, or materials. Patents (whether applications or awards to the authors or home institutions) related to the work should also be declared.

Unreasonable restrictions on data, code, or material availability may preclude publication. Problems in obtaining access to published data are taken seriously by the Science Journals and can be reported at science_data@aaas.org.

*Nature* has a similar policy and adds, "After publication, readers who encounter refusal by the authors to comply with these policies should contact the chief editor of the journal. In cases where editors are unable to resolve a complaint, the journal may refer the matter to the authors' funding institution and/or publish a formal statement of correction, attached online to the publication, stating that readers have been unable to obtain necessary materials to replicate the findings."[33]

Some journals have other conditions of publication that require authors to deposit specific information about their research (eg, metadata, results, or both) in a public repository or archive, although this is not data sharing per se. For example, following the recommendations of the ICMJE,[34] biomedical journals that publish clinical trials require authors to have registered their trials in approved, publicly accessible trial registries and to provide registration identifiers as a condition of publication (see 2.5.1, Structured Abstracts, and 19.3.6, Meta-analyses). In addition, many funders require authors to post articles that describe the results of their funded research in publicly available repositories, such as PubMed Central or Europe PubMed Central, and many journals make these deposits on behalf of authors (see 5.6.2, Public Access and Open Access in Scientific Publication).

Some journals require authors to provide data available on request for examination by the editors or peer reviewers (see 5.4, Ethical and Legal Considerations, Scientific Misconduct). For example, the JAMA Network journals require all authors to complete an authorship form that includes the following as part of their authorship responsibility statement:

If requested, I shall produce the data on which the manuscript is based for examination by the editors or their assignees.

In addition, for reports that contain original data (eg, research articles, systematic reviews, and meta-analyses), the JAMA Network journals require at least 1 author (eg, the principal investigator) to indicate that she or he "had full access to all the data in the study and takes responsibility for the integrity of the data and the accuracy of the data analysis" (see 5.5.5, Access to Data Requirement). The ICMJE supports this requirement.[34]

With the aim to provide standards for journals, the Center for Open Science has produced a set of guidelines to promote transparency and openness in journal policies and practices.[21] The guidelines provide 8 modular transparency standards that participating journals can adopt in part or in full and by which journals are ranked according to 3 levels of transparency. The standards include journals' policies and requirements for the following[21]:

Citation of data and materials

Data transparency (eg, posting in an accessible repository)

Transparency of analytic methods and code

Transparency of research materials

Transparency of design and analysis for review and publication

Preregistration of studies

Preregistration of analysis plans

Encouragement of replication studies

**5.6.1.4** **Manuscripts Based on the Same Data.** On occasion, an editor may receive 2 or more manuscripts based on the same data (with concordant or contradictory interpretations and conclusions). If the authors of these manuscripts are not collaborators and the data are publicly available, the editor should consider each manuscript on its own merit (perhaps asking reviewers to examine the manuscripts simultaneously). Authors should attempt to resolve disputes over contradictory interpretations of the same data before submitting manuscripts to journals. When more than 1 manuscript is submitted by current or former coworkers or collaborators who disagree on the analysis and interpretation of the same unpublished data, the recipient editors are faced with a difficult dilemma. In such cases, the ICMJE recommends the following[34]:

If editors receive manuscripts from separate research groups or from the same group analyzing the same data set (for example, from a public database, or systematic reviews or meta-analyses of the same evidence), the manuscripts should be considered independently because they may differ in their analytic methods, conclusions, or both. If the data interpretation and conclusions are similar, it may be reasonable although not mandatory for editors to give preference to the manuscript submitted first. Editors might consider publishing more than one manuscript that overlap in this way because different analytical approaches may be complementary and equally valid, but manuscripts based upon the same dataset should add substantially to each other to warrant consideration for publication as separate papers, with appropriate citation of previous publications from the same dataset to allow for transparency.

Secondary analyses of clinical trial data should cite any primary publication, clearly state that it contains secondary analyses/results, and use the same identifying trial registration number as the primary trial and unique, persistent dataset identifier.

Secondary analyses of any studies should always fully describe and cite the original research and publication and explain any overlapping or previously reported data (see 5.3, Duplicate Publication and Submission).

**5.6.1.5** **Record Retention Policies for Journals.** Journals should develop and implement consistent policies for retention of records and data related to the content that they publish. Legal documents (eg, copyright transfers, publication licenses, and permissions) should be kept indefinitely. All other records should be kept for a consistent, defined period. For example, the JAMA Network journals retain electronic copies of rejected manuscripts, correspondence, and reviewer comments up to 1 year to permit consideration of appeals of decisions. Electronic copies of accepted manuscripts and related correspondence and reviews are kept for 3 years. Journals also should develop consistent policies for the retention of online metadata associated with manuscript submissions, authors, and peer reviewers. For example, the JAMA Network journals retain metadata on manuscript submissions, decisions, and processing and milestone dates indefinitely to permit monitoring and reporting of key performance indicators and trends for individual journals (see 5.7.3, Confidentiality in Legal Petitions and Claims for Privileged Information). The ICMJE recommends the following[34]:

> When a manuscript is rejected, it is best practice for journals to delete copies of it from their editorial systems unless retention is required by local regulations. Journals that retain copies of rejected manuscripts should disclose this practice in their Information for Authors.

> When a manuscript is published, journals should keep copies of the original submission, reviews, revisions, and correspondence for at least three years and possibly in perpetuity, depending on local regulations, to help answer future questions about the work should they arise.

**5.6.2** **Public Access and Open Access in Scientific Publication.** The open access movement began in the late 1990s in conjunction with technologic advances and calls for greater transparency in and availability of scientific information and following the proliferation of online journals available (both versions of print journals and journals published only online), the concurrent inability of declining library budgets to keep pace with increases in the numbers of journals and rising subscription prices, and demands to reduce information gaps and access to the results of funded research.[35-39] Broadly defined, *open access* is the free and unrestricted online availability of content.[37] In its most liberal application, open access publishing means that users have unrestricted access without typical copyright restrictions and can freely read, download, copy, distribute, print, search, or link to full text of articles, as well as reuse and modify such content in part or whole for any lawful purpose provided that authors are properly acknowledged and cited.[40,41] *Public access* is the free access to content and typically permits users to read, download, print, search, and link to content, but with some copyright restrictions or limitations on sharing and reuse.[41] Many funders require authors of funded research to publish articles as public access (eg, US National Institutes of Health)[42] or open access (eg, Wellcome Trust).[43]

There are 2 types of open access and within them several models: self-archiving (sometime called green open or public access) and open access publishing (eg, gold open access and hybrid open access). *Self-archiving* is the deposition of content in an open archive (ie, repository), sometimes before formal publication or after publication. PubMed Central is a public repository that archives full text of articles published in the biomedical and life sciences. In addition, many academic and commercial institutions and funders have their own archives or repositories. However, posts of articles in these repositories may not necessarily be open access; they may be posted for public access with limitations on reuse.

Preprint servers permit the posting and archiving of manuscripts before and after formal peer review and publication in a journal. A *preprint* is a complete manuscript that authors post to an open preprint server before publication in a journal. The preprint manuscript may be amended or updated, commented on by others, and remains on the preprint server even if subsequently published in a peer-reviewed journal. The first preprint server, arXiv, began in 1991 for the physics community. Since then, many preprint servers for other disciplines have been launched, including bioRxiv for biology and life sciences in 2013 and medRxiv for health sciences in 2019. Concerns have been expressed that self-archiving before peer review and publication may pose problems for version and quality control (eg, users may not understand the difference between an article that has not undergone peer review, revision, and editing and one that has undergone such measures to improve quality). Moreover, concerns have been raised that the posting of preprints in medicine "could lead to wide dissemination of inaccurate and potentially harmful clinical and public health information and to researchers pursuing hypotheses that are subsequently found to lack proper grounding, thereby erasing any gains made from the rapid dissemination of results."[44] However, medical and health preprints are increasing with a growing number of funders and journals accepting preprints, and some journals offering simultaneous submission with posting of manuscripts to preprint servers.

In *open access publishing*, all or part of a journal is freely open to unrestricted use and perhaps unfettered reuse. This may or may not include the data that support specific types of articles (eg, research reports). The funding model for open access publishing requires author, institution, or funding agency payments, a subsidy from the owner or publisher, and/or external grants. Open access payments for publication are called *article processing charges* (APCs) (also known as *article publication charges*). The open access financial model differs from the traditional journal publishing model, in which publication and sustainability of the publishing enterprise are based on revenue from paid subscriptions, advertising, licensing, royalties, reprints, and other forms of revenue. There are different models of open access[40,41] and a variety of practices within each model.

*Gold open access*: journals make all content freely available from the time of publication, which is typically (but not always) funded by APCs and no individual or institutional subscription, permission, or access/reuse fees (however, other sources of revenue may be available, such as via institutional agreements, grants, and advertising).

*Diamond open access*: a form of gold open access that does not include a requirement for authors to pay APCs.

*Hybrid open access*: journals with a traditional paid subscription-based economic model that offer authors of articles the option to pay a fee (APC) for immediate open access.

*Delayed public access:* journals with a traditional paid subscription-based economic model make research articles free public access without any author fees (often a delayed period, such as 6-12 months before the article is made free public access). Note: This model is not open access.

Although a few journals were published in an open access model before the 1990s, most open access journals began publication after the year 2000, when BioMed Central (BMC) launched a series of open access journals that were peer reviewed but did not undergo editorial revision and editing. In exchange for an APC payment, research articles were made immediately free open access at the time of publication. In addition, individual organizations, such as universities, could purchase a membership at a significantly greater collective fee (through prepaid or bulk-paid APCs), allowing their author-employees or affiliated authors to publish in BMC journals without having to pay the author publication fees for individual articles. In 2019, BMC, owned by Springer Nature, published more than 300 open access journals, with most journals charging APCs (varying in price from US$860 to $3680) in exchange for immediate open access to the full text of published articles.[45] BMC now indicates that the APCs cover peer review and a range of publishing services, including "provision of online tools for editors and authors, article production and hosting, liaison with abstracting and indexing services, and customer services."[46]

In 2003, PLOS launched its first in a series of open access journals with an initial $9 million grant from the Moore Foundation.[47] In addition to grants, journal operations were funded by APCs: in 2003 the author fee was $1500 to publish an article; in 2006 the fee was increased to $2500. By 2010, PLOS reported that it was financially self-sufficient based on the APC model, and in 2017 APCs ranged from $1595 to $3000.[48] During this time, PLOS launched one of the first mega journals. A *mega journal* "publishes freely accessible articles, which have been reviewed for scientific trustworthiness, but leaves it to the readers to decide which articles are of interest and importance to them."[49] These journals rely on large numbers of submissions and high acceptance rates. *PLOS ONE* launched in 2010 and published 6913 articles that year; in 2014 the journal published 30 054 articles, and the acceptance rate was 69%.[49] Since then, the number of articles, although still very high, published by *PLOS ONE* has declined annually as other mega journals (eg, *Scientific Reports)* have entered the market and more journals have offered open access options.[50]

An unanticipated exploitative outcome of open access publishing has been the swift rise of *predatory journals* that charge authors APCs to publish in journals of dubious reputation or experience and without peer review, editorial, or publishing services.[51] In some cases, authors are unaware of the deceptive nature of these journals and are duped by journal titles that resemble prominent quality journals. In other cases, authors deliberately use these dubious journals to publish articles quickly without peer review or quality checks or to build a citation ladder and later cite these articles in genuine journals to make their research appear more credible than it is. These deceptive journals have proliferated, causing concerns about the integrity of scientific scholarship as they have permeated authentic electronic databases.[52] By 2014 an estimated 8000 predatory journals were reported to have published an estimated 420 000 articles.[53]

A number of traditional journals (published by academic societies and/or commercial publishers) offer hybrid open access options to permit authors to comply with funder mandates for open access. Between 2015 and 2017, the numbers of fully open access journals increased by 11%, hybrid journals increased by 17%, and subscription-only journals decreased by 37%.[54] Open access advocates and some funders require authors to publish in fully open access journals.

The Directory of Open Access Journals was launched in 2003 with 300 open access (gold) journals.[55] In July 2019, the Directory of Open Access Journals listed 13 500 journals that have published more than 4.1 million articles.[55] Advocates of open access publishing cite the benefits of widespread dissemination of research: universal access, enhanced global collaboration, improved transparency of research, and the belief that open access articles will be read, used, and cited more frequently than articles published in traditional journals with access controls.[35,37,38,43,45] Others express concern about the quality of literature published in a system that may favor those who pay or that uses limited peer review and editorial curation and raise other concerns, such as unfairness of the author-pays model for researchers with limited funds, confusion about evolving policies among authors and journals, risk for exploitation of researchers and authors, risk of unfettered commercial reuse, and risks to the financial stability of journals with business models based on more diversified, traditional sources of revenue and to their owners.[39,40,50-53]

Coupled with the open access movement, in 2005 funding agencies (eg, NIH and the Wellcome Trust) began requesting or requiring funded investigators to permit articles that describe results of their funded research to be posted in publicly accessible repositories (such as PubMed Central).[42,43] Negotiations between these agencies and publishers resulted in another form of access: delayed public access.[26] In this model, which has been in wide use by scientific and biomedical publishers (especially those owned by not-for-profit professional societies) for many years, research articles are made freely available after a defined interval, such as 6 months, 1 year, or 2 years. The interval, which may be influenced by the frequency of journal publication, is intended to protect subscription, licensing, advertising, and other traditional forms of journal revenue.

Many journals offer authors a range of public access and open access options, with and without fees, including public access for research articles after a specified time without author fees, immediate open access for research articles or all articles based on APCs and perhaps other processing or publication fees, permitting deposits in public repositories with a specified delay or without such delay, and permitting self-archiving in authors' individual or institutional repositories. Open access publishing models are proliferating with some funder mandates threatening traditional publishing models, and debate continues over which models might be sustainable in the long term.[40,41,56] Each model has advantages and disadvantages. A combination of models may be appropriate for publishers and journals that seek to balance the advantages of open access with the financial requirements of sustainable, quality publication.

In addition, journals and funders are developing and experimenting with different publication licenses in lieu of standard copyright transfers to permit various access and use rights for articles published under public access and open access models. According to the Association of Learned and Professional Scholarly Publishers (ALPSP), although many publishers still require some form of copyright transfer, the proportion of small and large publishers that use publication licenses increased from 15% and 17%, respectively, in 2005 to 18% and 40%, respectively, in 2012[57] (see 5.6.5, Ethical and Legal Considerations, Intellectual Property: Ownership, Access, Rights, and Management, Copyright Assignment or License). A subsequent survey of 240 publisher members of ALPSP in 2015 reported that 80% of publishers continued to rely on a subscription or content licensing business model, with 83% also offering some form of APC option that included use of a publication license (69% had hybrid open access journals and 17% had fully open access journals).[58] These models continue to evolve.

In parallel with the open access movement, Creative Commons (CC), a nonprofit organization, was created in 2001 and developed copyright licenses known as CC licenses that are intended to permit a wide range of permissions, sharing, and reuse without fees and often without individual point-of-use permissions.[59] Six copyright license types are available, ranging from Attribution (CC BY) to Attribution-NonCommercial-NoDerivs (CC BY-NC-ND). The CC BY license permits others to copy, distribute, transform, and build on work for any purpose, even commercially, as long as they credit the original creator. This is the most liberal of the 6 licenses and is recommended for maximum dissemination and use of licensed materials. The CC BY-NC-ND license, which is the most restrictive of the CC licenses, permits others to download works and share them as long as they credit the original creator but does not permit alteration or commercial reuse of the work without additional permission. Additional information is available on the Creative Commons website[59] (see 5.6.5, Copyright Assignment or License).

**5.6.3** **Copyright: Definition, History, and Current Law.** *Copyright* is a term used to describe the legal right of authors to control the communication and reproduction of their original works of authorship, and in the United States, it has its basis in the US Constitution.[1,16] Copyright law provides for the protection of rights of parties involved in the creation and dissemination of intellectual property. While a variety of people and entities derive benefits from copyright laws (authors, publishers, editors, composers, artists, and the producers of video and audio broadcasts and programs, films, websites, computer programs, applications, and software), few thoroughly understand the law and its basic applications. This section discusses current copyright laws and applications in scientific publishing. Copyright laws, scope, and protections vary by country (see 5.6.11, International Copyright Protection). The discussion in this section addresses US copyright law except where specifically indicated. This section is intended to explain copyright law as it applies to scientific publication; it is not intended to serve as legal advice. A media lawyer should be consulted for any specific concerns about rights, protections, infringements, or remedies.

Copyright is a form of legal protection provided to the author of published and unpublished original works.[16(§102,§104),60,61] The author, or anyone to whom the author transfers copyright, is the owner of copyright in the work. Current law gives the owner of copyright the following exclusive rights[16(§102,§103)]:

257

- To reproduce the work in copies

- To prepare derivative works based on the copyrighted work

- To distribute, perform, or display the work publicly

A copyrightable work must be fixed in a tangible medium of expression and includes the following[16(§102),62]:

- Literary works (which include computer software and works produced in digital formats)

- Musical works, including any accompanying words

- Dramatic works, including any accompanying music

- Pantomimes and choreographic works

- Pictorial, graphic, and sculptural works

- Motion pictures and other audiovisual works

- Sound recordings

- Architectural works

The following are not protected by copyright, although they may be covered by patent and trademark laws[16(§102),60,63] (see 5.6.14, Patents, and 5.6.15, Trademark):

- Ideas, methods, and systems. Examples include

  Inventions (inventions meeting certain requirements may be patentable)

  Recipes

- Names, titles, and short phrases. Examples of names, titles, or short phrases that do not contain a sufficient amount of creativity to support a claim in copyright include

  The name of an individual (including pseudonyms, pen names, or stage names)

  The title or subtitle of a work, such as a book, a song, or a pictorial, graphic, or sculptural work

  The name of a business or organization

  The name of a band or performing group

  The name of a product or service

  A domain name or URL

  The name of a character

  Catchwords or catchphrases

  Mottos, slogans, or other short expressions

▪ Typeface, fonts, and lettering

▪ Blank forms. Examples of blank forms include

Time cards

Graph paper

Account books

Diaries

Bank checks

Scorecards

Address books

Report forms

Order forms

Date books and schedulers

▪ Familiar symbols and designs. Examples of familiar symbols and designs include but are not limited to

Letters, punctuation, or symbols on a keyboard

Abbreviations

Musical notation

Numbers and mathematical and currency symbols

Arrows and other directional or navigational symbols

Common symbols and shapes, such as a spade, club, heart, diamond, star, yin and yang, or fleur-de-lis

Common patterns, such as standard chevron, polka dot, checkerboard, or houndstooth

Well-known and commonly used symbols that contain a minimal amount of expression or are in the public domain, such as the peace symbol, gender symbols, or simple emoticons

Industry designs, such as the caduceus, barber pole, food labeling symbols, or hazard

Warning symbols

Familiar religious symbols

Common architecture moldings

Some of the more common provisions of US copyright law as well as problems encountered by scientific authors, editors, and publishers are discussed in sections 5.6.4 through 5.6.10.

**5.6.3.1** **History of Copyright Law.** Copyright law evolved after Gutenberg's movable type reduced the cost and labor required to make copies of written and printed works.[1,62,64] During the early 18th century, copyright became the mediator between the author or publisher and the marketplace. In 1710, England created the Statute of Anne, the first copyright act, which addressed exact copies only. Article I, section 8, of the US Constitution, enacted in 1798, serves as the foundation for US copyright law, which grants the US Congress the power to "promote the progress of science and useful arts, by securing for limited times to authors and inventors the exclusive right to their respective writings and discoveries."[65,66] Since then, the US law has undergone a number of updates and general revisions in response to innovations and changes in technology, to broaden the definition and scope of copyright law, and to address mechanisms for protection among different countries.[16,66] In 1790, the United States created the first copyright law to cover magazines and books, but again, this was only for exact copies. During the 19th century, copyright law was extended to translations, works made for hire, music, dramatic compositions, photography, and works of art. During the 20th century, copyright law was extended to cover motion pictures, performance and recording of nondramatic literary works, sound recordings, computer programs, and architectural works. The US Copyright Act of 1909 added formal requirements to ensure protection, such as use of copyright notice, official registration, and renewal of copyright terms.[66]

**5.6.3.2** **US Copyright Act of 1976.** Before 1978, 2 systems of copyright coexisted in the United States. Common law copyright, regulated by individual states, protected works from creation until publication, and a separate federal law protected works from publication until 28 years thereafter (with an option for a 1-time renewal of the 28-year term).[16,60] The Copyright Act of 1976, which became effective January 1, 1978, contained the first major revisions of US copyright law in almost 70 years. This act, reversing many of the formalities required by the 1909 act, remains in force today. Thus, for all works created after 1978, current law automatically provides protection to the creator of the work at the time it is created, whether written, typewritten, or entered into a computer, whether the work is published or not, and whether the work bears a copyright notice. In addition, the 1976 act changed the terms of copyright duration, with most terms equaling the life of the author plus 50 years. In 1998, the term of copyright protection for most works was extended to the life of the author plus 70 years[16,66] (see 5.6.4, Types of Works and Copyright Duration in the United States).

**5.6.3.3** **International Conventions and Treaties.** In 1886, the Berne Convention was created by 10 European nations to protect copyright across national boundaries. The United States did not sign on to the Berne Convention until 1989.[16,67] The Universal Copyright Convention (UCC) was adopted in 1952 as an alternative for countries that disagreed with some aspects of the Berne Convention. A number of conventions and treaties adopted in the 1990s address copyright as it has been affected by new economic, social, cultural, and technological developments and by new international rules, including the Agreement on Trade-Related Aspects of Intellectual Property Rights (TRIPS), World Intellectual Property Organization

(WIPO) Copyright and Performances and Phonograms Treaty, and the WIPO Copyright Treaty.[66,67] For more details, see 5.6.11, International Copyright Protection.

**5.6.3.4**   **Copyright and New Technology.** Throughout the 20th and 21st centuries, technological advances have challenged copyright law, including photographs, motion pictures, radio, television, photocopying, cable television, computers, databases, multimedia, and the internet.[1,61,64] The most recent challenge began in the 1990s with the increase of electronic publishing and new media. Although copyright law was designed to be technology neutral, it applied only to tangible copies and to the physical distribution of these copies. Although early users of the internet sent email messages and posted information on electronic mailing lists and bulletin boards without much concern for ownership and copyright of their communications, editors and publishers became concerned about maintaining the integrity, quality, and ownership of their intellectual property once content was easily and widely digitized, published, and transmitted electronically.

In 1998, the US Digital Millennium Copyright Act (DMCA) was enacted to extend copyright protection to works created in a digital medium.[16] Interpreting the DMCA, Hart notes that "works created in digital media are considered 'fixed' if they can be perceived, reproduced, or otherwise communicated for more than a transitory period, including the fixation on a computer disc or in a computer's random access memory."[61(p190)] Among its major provisions, the DMCA implements the WIPO treaties; limits certain liability of online service providers that adhere to specific requirements through safe-harbor provisions; limits liability of libraries and archives; prohibits the circumvention of technological barriers designed to control access to content (anticircumvention); establishes penalties for such circumvention; addresses works now available through new technologies, such as distance education audio, video, and webcasts; and preserves existing rights of copyright owners.[16,61]

Since its enactment, the DMCA has addressed concerns about copyright protection and infringement in electronic publishing. However, continuing rapid advances in technology foretell future changes in copyright law, requiring the publishing community to be alert to such changes for the foreseeable future.

**5.6.4**   **Types of Works and Copyright Duration in the United States.** The length of copyright protection in the United States depends on several factors: when the work was created (key dates are before or after January 1, 1978), the number of authors (ie, single-author vs joint-author works), and the type of work (eg, work made for hire or owned by the federal government).[68,69] See **Table 5.6-1** for examples of types of works, conditions, and terms of copyright protection.[68]

**5.6.4.1**   **Works Created After 1978.** To be protected by copyright law, a work must be original. For works created by a single author, copyright belongs to that author from the instant of its creation and for 70 years after the author's death.[16(§302),68,69] See Table 5.6-1 for details on other conditions and terms and 5.6.4.3, Ethical and Legal Considerations, Intellectual Property: Ownership, Access, Rights, and Management, Types of Works and Copyright Duration in the United States, Joint Works by 2 or More Authors, and 5.6.4.4, Types of Works and Copyright Duration in the United States, Works Made for Hire.

**Table 5.6-1.** Copyright Term and the Public Domain in the United States, as of 2019[a]

| Never published, never registered works[b] | | |
|---|---|---|
| **Type of work** | **Copyright term** | **What was in public domain as of January 1, 2019[c]** |
| Unpublished works | Life of the author plus 70 years | Works from authors who died before 1949 |
| Unpublished anonymous and pseudonymous works and works made for hire | 120 Years from date of creation | Works created before 1899 |
| Unpublished works when the death date of the author is not known[d] | 120 Years from date of creation[e] | Works created before 1899[e] |
| **Works registered or first published in the United States** | | |
| **Date of publication[f]** | **Conditions[g]** | **Copyright term[c]** |
| Before 1924 | None | None. In the public domain due to copyright expiration |
| 1924 through 1977 | Published without a copyright notice | None. In the public domain due to failure to comply with required formalities |
| 1978 to March 1, 1989 | Published without notice and without subsequent registration within 5 years | None. In the public domain due to failure to comply with required formalities |
| 1978 to March 1, 1989 | Published without notice but with subsequent registration within 5 years | 70 Years after the death of author. If work of corporate authorship, 95 years from publication or 120 years from creation, whichever expires first |
| 1924 through 1963 | Published with notice but copyright was not renewed[h] | None. In the public domain due to copyright expiration |
| 1924 through 1963 | Published with notice and copyright was renewed[h] | 95 Years after publication date |
| 1964 through 1977 | Published with notice | 95 Years after publication date |
| 1978 to March 1, 1989 | Created after 1977 and published with notice | 70 Years after death of author. If work of corporate authorship, 95 years from publication or 120 years from creation, whichever expires first |
| 1978 to March 1, 1989 | Created before 1978 and first published with notice in the specified period | The greater of the term specified in the previous entry or December 31, 2047 |
| From March 1, 1989, through 2002 | Created after 1977 | 70 Years after the death of author. If a work of corporate authorship, 95 years from publication or 120 years from creation, whichever expires first |
| From March 1, 1989, through 2002 | Created before 1979 and first published in this period | The greater of the term specified in the previous entry or December 31, 2047 |
| After 2002 | None | 70 Years after the death of author. If a work of corporate authorship, 95 years from publication or 120 years from creation, whichever expires first |
| Anytime | Works prepared by an officer or employee of the US government as part of that person's official duties[i] | None. In the public domain in the United States (17 USC §105) |

**Table 5.6-1.** Copyright Term and the Public Domain in the United States, as of 2019 (*continued*)

[a]This table was adapted and reproduced from Copyright Term and the Public Domain in the United States. ©2004-2019 Peter B. Hirtle, under Creative Commons Attribution 3.0 License.[68] It was first published in Peter B. Hirtle, "Recent Changes To The Copyright Law: Copyright Term Extension," Archival Outlook, January/February 1999. This version is current as of January 1, 2019. The most recent version is found at https://copyright.cornell.edu/publicdomain. Additional information for works published outside of the United States and for sound recordings can also be found at this site. For some explanation on how to use the table and complications hidden in it, see Peter B. Hirtle, "When Is 1923 Going to Arrive and Other Complications of the US Public Domain," Searcher (September 2012). The table is based in part on Laura N. Gasaway's chart, "When Works Pass Into the Public Domain," at http://www.unc.edu/~unclng/public-d.htm, and similar charts found in Marie C. Malaro, A Legal Primer on Managing Museum Collections Smithsonian Institution Press; 1998:155-156). A useful copyright duration chart by Mary Minow, organized by year, is found at http://www.librarylaw.com/DigitizationTable.htm. A flowchart for copyright duration is found at http://sunsteinlaw.com/practices/copyright-portfolio-development/copyright-pointers/copyright-flowchart/, and a tree-view chart on copyright is at http://chart.copyrightdata.com. Several US copyright duration calculators are available online, including the Public Domain Sherpa (http://www.publicdomainsherpa.com/calculator.htm) and the Durationator (in beta at http://www.durationator.com/). Europeana's public domain calculators for 30 different countries outside of the United States (at http://www.outofcopyright.eu/). The Open Knowledge Foundation has been encouraging the development of public domain calculators for many countries: see http://publicdomain.okfn.org/calculators/. See also Library of Congress Copyright Office. Circular 15a, Duration of Copyright: Provisions of the Law Dealing with the Length of Copyright Protection (Library of Congress; 2004) at http://www.copyright.gov/circs/circ15a.pdf. Further information on copyright duration is found in chapter 3, "Duration and Ownership of Copyright," in Copyright and Cultural Institutions: Guidelines for Digitization for US Libraries, Archives, and Museums, by Peter B. Hirtle, Emily Hudson, and Andrew T. Kenyon (Cornell University Library; 2009), available for purchase at http://bookstore.library.cornell.edu/ and as a free download at http://ecommons.cornell.edu/handle/1813/14142.

[b]Treat unpublished works registered for copyright prior to 1978 as if they had been published in the United States (though note that the only formality that applied was the requirement to renew copyright after 28 years). Unpublished works registered for copyright since 1978 can be considered as if they were an "unpublished, unregistered work."

[c]All terms of copyright run through the end of the calendar year in which they would otherwise expire, so a work enters the public domain on the first of the year following the expiration of its copyright term. For example, a book published on March 15, 1923, entered the public domain on January 1, 2019, not March 16, 2018 (1923 + 95 = 2018).

[d]Unpublished works when the death date of the author is not known may still be copyrighted after 120 years, but certification from the Copyright Office that it has no record to indicate whether the person is living or died less than 70 years before is a complete defense to any action for infringement (see 17 USC §302[e]).

[e]Presumption as to the author's death requires a certified report from the Copyright Office that its records disclose nothing to indicate that the author of the work is living or died less than 70 years before.

[f]"Publication" was not explicitly defined in the Copyright Law before 1976, but the 1909 act indirectly indicated that publication was when copies of the first authorized edition were placed on sale, sold, or publicly distributed by the proprietor of the copyright or under his authority.

[g]Not all published works are copyrighted. Works prepared by an officer or employee of the US government as part of that person's official duties receive no copyright protection in the United States. For much of the 20th century, certain formalities had to be followed to secure copyright protection. For example, some books had to be printed in the United States to receive copyright protection, and failure to deposit copies of works with the Register of Copyright could result in the loss of copyright. The requirements that copies include a formal notice of copyright and that the copyright be renewed after 28 years were the most common conditions and are specified in the Table.

[h]A 1961 Copyright Office study found that fewer than 15% of all registered copyrights were renewed. For books, the figure was even lower: 7%. See Ringer B. Study No. 31: renewal of copyright. In: *Copyright Law Revision: Studies Prepared for the Subcommittee on Patents, Trademarks, and Copyrights of the Committee on the Judiciary, United States Senate, Eighty-sixth Congress, First [-Second] Session*. US Government Printing Office; 1961:220. A good guide to investigating the copyright and renewal status of published work is Demas S, Brogdon JL. "Determining Copyright Status for Preservation and Access: Defining Reasonable Effort. *Library Resources and Technical Services* 1997;41(4):323-334. See also Library of Congress, Copyright Office. *Circular 22: How to Investigate the Copyright Status of a Work*. Library of Congress, Copyright Office; 2004 (http://www.copyright.gov/circs/circ22.pdf). The Online Books Page FAQ (http://onlinebooks.library.upenn.edu/okbooks.html), especially "How Can I Tell Whether a Book Can Go Online?" and "How Can I Tell Whether a Copyright Was Renewed?" is also helpful.

[i]Contractors and grantees are not considered government employees. Generally, they create works with copyright (although the government may own that copyright). See CENDI Frequently Asked Questions About Copyright: Issues Affecting the US Government (http://www.cendi.gov/publications/04-8copyright.html). The public domain status of US government works applies only in the United States.

**5.6.4.2**  **Works Created Before 1978.** Several different rules apply to works created before 1978 and depend on whether the work was published, previous copyright duration terms, and whether the copyright has been renewed (Table 5.6-1).[68,69] For example, as of 2019, unpublished works created before 1978 are protected for the life of the author plus 70 years. Works published between 1924 and 1977 are protected for 95 years after date of publication provided that a copyright notice was published and appropriate renewals were made[68,69] (see 5.6.6, Copyright Notice and Registration). Works that were published before 1924 are now in the public domain.

**5.6.4.3**  **Joint Works by 2 or More Authors.** A joint work is a work prepared by 2 or more authors with the intention that their contributions be merged into inseparable or interdependent parts of a unitary whole. For such works, the 70-year term begins after the death of the last surviving author.[16(§302)]

**5.6.4.4**  **Works Made for Hire.** Works created by an individual who is paid by another specifically for such work are covered by a particular provision of the copyright statute. In these cases, the law recognizes the employer or the party contracting for the work as the owner of the copyright in the work. Works made for hire generally fall into 2 categories.[16(§101),70] The first category is a work prepared by an employee within the scope of her or his employment duties, such as a journal editorial written by an editor who is employed by or otherwise contracted to work as an editor by the journal's owner. The second category comprises certain specially ordered or commissioned works. Examples include a news story written by a freelance journalist or an index prepared by an individual under contract. In these cases, although a formal copyright assignment is not necessary, the parties must sign an agreement before the work is produced specifying that the work is to be a work made for hire. Copyright duration for works made for hire is 95 years from the year of first publication or 120 years from the date of the work's creation, whichever is shorter.[16(§302)]

**5.6.4.5**  **Works Created by Anonymous and Pseudonymous Authors.** The same terms of copyright duration that apply to works made for hire apply to works published by anonymous or pseudonymous authors—95 years from the year of first publication or 120 years from the date the work was created, whichever is shorter. If 1 or more authors' names are disclosed and registered with the US Copyright Office before the 95-year or 120-year term expires, the term changes to 70 years after the last surviving author's death[16(§302),69] (see 5.1.3, Unsigned Editorials, Anonymous Authors, Pseudonymous Authors).

**5.6.4.6**  **Works in the Public Domain or Created by the US Government.** A work is in the public domain if it has failed to meet the requirements of copyright protection or its copyright protection has expired. Works in the public domain may be used freely by anyone without permission. US works published before 1924 are now in the public domain.[68] In 2015, the Project Gutenberg website included more than 58 000 books that were considered free to use, mostly because copyright had expired.[71] Works created by US federal government employees in the course of their employment are also in the public domain[16(§105)] (see 5.6.1, Ownership and Control of Data, and 5.6.5.3, Exception—Works Created by Employees of the US Federal Government or That of Other Nations). However, works produced by state and local governments are subject to copyright protection.

Works created by other national governments are subject to the copyright laws of their respective countries and perhaps the Berne Convention, WIPO Copyright Treaties, or other international treaties (see 5.6.11, International Copyright Protection).

**5.6.4.7** **Collective Works.** A *collective work* comprises a number of independent contributions (usually from many authors), which constitute separate and independent works in themselves, and are assembled into a collective whole. Examples of collective works include periodicals, such as journals, magazines, multiauthored textbooks, and encyclopedias.[16(§101)] Copyright in the independent contributions is separate from copyright in the collective work as a whole and initially belongs to the individual authors until they transfer copyright to the owner of the collective work, usually a publisher. Publishers that require authors of collective works (such as authors of a journal article) to transfer copyright or a publication license should require such transfer from each author, not just the corresponding author. Editors of collective works may also be required to transfer copyright assignment or a publication license if their contributions are not already covered under work for hire or other employment agreements. Thus, both the individual articles (independent works) and the journal (collective work) can be protected by copyright.

**5.6.4.8** **Compilations and Derivative Works.** According to US copyright law, *compilations* are works "formed by the collection and assembling of preexisting materials or data that are selected, coordinated, and arranged in such a way that the resulting work as a whole constitutes original work of authorship."[16(§101)] The term *compilation* includes collective works (see 5.6.4.7, Types of Works and Copyright Duration in the United States, Collective Works). Examples of compilations include a compendium of previously published articles on a specific theme or topic or a collection of abstracts. The basis for protection of a compilation is the judgment required to select and arrange the material.[62] In this context, the 1991 US Supreme Court ruling in *Feist Publications Inc v Rural Telephone Service Co Inc* is worth noting.[72] In that case, a regional telephone company used a local telephone company's directory without its permission. The local company sued for copyright infringement and lost. The court held that the "data" in the directory (collections of public telephone numbers) had no substantial originality or creativity and that comprehensive collections of data arranged in conventional formats do not merit copyright protection.[72]

*Derivative works* are those based on 1 or more preexisting works, such as a translation, abridgment, condensation, or republication in a different format, language, or media.[16(§101)] Examples of derivative works include revised editions of books or articles that are republished, translated, or annotated individually or collected and republished in print and/or online.

Scientific journal publishers typically request that authors transfer broad rights to their work in the form of a copyright transfer or exclusive license or a nonexclusive license that includes rights to produce compilations and derivative works. Such publishers often receive royalties from the distribution and sale of compilations and derivative works. In addition, publishers who own copyright or have exclusive licenses in individual articles are legally able to address misuse or piracy of such works (see 5.6.2, Public Access and Open Access in Scientific Publication).

**5.6.4.9**    **Revised Editions.** A revised edition of a previously copyrighted work may be regarded as a separately copyrighted work if there is substantial original new work in the new edition. The *Chicago Manual of Style* defines *substantial* as change that occurs in 1 or more of the essential elements of the work, such as text, notes, appendixes, or tables and illustrations (if they are integral to the work), and notes that generally at least 20% of a new edition should consist of new or revised material.[73(§1.26)] Thus, a new foreword or preface, the addition of a few references, or corrections to the original text do not constitute a revised edition, but they may be included in subsequent printings with an explanation on the copyright notice page. For example, this edition of the *AMA Manual of Style* constitutes a major revision that results in a new copyrighted work. For revised editions, any unaltered material retained in a subsequent edition remains protected under the original copyright, and copyright applicable to the new material does not extend the duration of copyright in the old material.

The *Chicago Manual of Style* recommends that publishers use standard language to designate specific editions: 2nd edition, 3rd edition, 4th edition, and so on.[73(§1.26)] If the new edition is simply printed in a different format, eg, in paperback or in a different language through a licensing agreement, the status can be designated as "Paperback edition 2005" or "French-language edition" (see 3.12.7, References to Books, Edition Number).

Some publishers list the various dates of revisions on the copyright page as a record of publishing history. The publishing history follows the copyright notice. For example, this manual has had 11 editions:

2020, *AMA Manual of Style: A Guide for Authors and Editors*, 11th ed (Christiansen et al)

2007, *AMA Manual of Style: A Guide for Authors and Editors*, 10th ed (Iverson et al)

1998, *American Medical Association Manual of Style: A Guide for Authors and Editors*, 9th ed (Iverson et al)

1989, *American Medical Association Manual of Style*, 8th ed (Iverson et al)

1981, *Manual for Authors & Editors*, 7th ed (Barclay et al)

1976, *Stylebook/Editorial Manual of the AMA*, 6th ed (Barclay)

1971, *Stylebook/Editorial Manual of the AMA*, 5th ed (Hussey)

1966, *Stylebook and Editorial Manual*, 4th ed (Talbott)

1965, *Stylebook and Editorial Manual*, 3rd ed (Talbott)

1963, *Stylebook and Editorial Manual*, 2nd ed (Talbott)

1962, *Style Book* (Talbott)

**5.6.5** **Copyright Assignment or License.** Typically, copyright of a work vests initially with the author of the work. As copyright owner, an author may transfer rights to a publisher by copyright assignment, exclusive license, or nonexclusive license.[16,64,73] A broadly worded exclusive license may provide much of the same rights to publishers as would a copyright transfer agreement. Thus, an owner of an exclusive assignment (through either copyright transfer or broadly worded exclusive license) may produce derivative works and sublicense specific rights to others. Some publishers permit authors to retain certain rights to their works, even when assigning copyright or granting an exclusive license (such as making copies for educational purposes, posting a copy on a personal or institutional website, or depositing a copy in an institutional or other repository to comply with research funding requirements). A nonexclusive license for publication permits a publisher certain rights to publish and disseminate work, but the copyright remains with the author, who retains control over access, use, and distribution.

Journals that offer open access publication may rely on nonexclusive copyright licenses that permit a range of access and reuse options, such as those created by Creative Commons (https://creativecommons.org).[59] The Creative Commons (CC) copyright licenses permit a wide range of permissions, sharing, and reuse without fees and often without individual point-of-use permissions.[59] Creative Commons has 6 types of copyright license, ranging from Attribution (CC BY) to Attribution-NonCommercial-NoDerivs (CC BY-NC-ND) (see 5.6.2, Public Access and Open Access in Scientific Publication).

Publishers that have copyright or exclusive publication licenses also may grant others nonexclusive secondary-use licenses to use, reproduce, or disseminate content, and many grant authors the rights to post copies of research articles in approved public repositories or share copies with colleagues for noncommercial educational purposes (see 5.6.2, Public Access and Open Access in Scientific Publication). In addition, publishers may grant a 1-time nonexclusive licensee to reproduce a work in a specified manner (eg, permission to reprint or translate and distribute a specific article) (see 5.6.7, Copying, Reproducing, Adapting, and Other Uses of Content, and 5.6.9, Standards for Commercial Reprints and e-Prints).

Publishers that make substantial investments in their products may seek exclusive publication rights from authors. However, few visual artists or professional photographers will agree to such terms and more commonly grant nonexclusive rights to publishers who want to include their works. In addition, many institutions and scientific research funders encourage or require authors to transfer nonexclusive, open access, or other conditional rights of their work to publishers (see 5.6.5.4, Exception—Institutional Owners of Copyright, and 5.6.2, Public Access and Open Access in Scientific Publication). Journals that accept such limited conditional licenses need to be sure that they obtain licenses that cover all subsidiary rights that the publisher may want to exercise or sublicense (eg, online and licensed versions, reprints, e-prints, collections, and archival copies as well as versions in multiple languages and multiple types of media). Increasing demands by authors and their institutions and funders and the increasing complexity of publishing models portend much future debate among authors, institutions, and publishers with regard to copyright assignments, licenses, and publication (see 5.6.2, Public Access and Open Access in Scientific Publication).[39-44,57,58]

Common arguments in favor of copyright transfer or publication license from authors to publishers include the following:

- The publisher must have the opportunity to publish or license the publication of the work in other forms to recoup or justify the expenses associated with the editorial and peer review, editing and quality assurance, publication, distribution, online hosting, indexing, and maintenance of the original work.

- The publisher, with business and legal expertise and resources, is better able to distribute and maintain the work in print and online, protect it from misuse and piracy, and take advantage of new technologies and media.

- The publisher is better equipped to invest in the work and take the risk that the work may not be successful.

- The publisher serves the author's interest in promotion of the work and professional advancement.

Common arguments in favor of the author's retention of copyright include the following:

- Authors who retain ownership of their works can distribute their works themselves, through their institutions, repositories, or other means, or via author-pay open access publication options.

- Authors who retain ownership of their works can help to limit the increasing subscription costs of scientific journals.

- Authors deserve to receive financial reward from both the original publication and any subsequent republication or dissemination.

- Authors' retention of copyright meets the traditional need for identification of intellectual ownership.

- New technology enables misuse and theft of intellectual property and obviates the ability of publishers to protect copyright, perhaps rendering copyright obsolete.

**5.6.5.1** **Assignment of Copyright or License as a Condition of Publication.** As a condition of considering a work for publication, publishers of biomedical and scientific journals require authors to transfer copyright or an exclusive publication license or assert a CC publication license (often used with author-pay for open access publications) in the event that the work is published. This requires authors to complete a publishing agreement indicating the transfer of copyright or a publication license to the publisher. Since the transfer of copyright or publication license may not actually occur until the work is published, editors may choose to consider manuscripts submitted without a statement of copyright transfer or publication license from the author and then ask for it if a revision is requested or the manuscript is to be accepted. In the event that the work is published, the author agrees to transfer copyright or a publication license to the journal, publisher, or owner. If the work is not published, the copyright then remains with the author.

For example, the JAMA Network journals require all authors (including each coauthor) to complete a copyright transfer or publication license statement:

> **Copyright Transfer.** In consideration of the action of the American Medical Association (AMA) in reviewing and editing this submission (manuscript, tables, figures, audio, video, and other supplemental files submitted for publication), I hereby transfer, assign, or otherwise convey all copyright ownership, including any and all rights incidental thereto, exclusively to the AMA, in the event that such work is published by the AMA.

Authors of articles published in JAMA Network journals who elect to pay for an open access CC BY license complete the following publication license transfer statement:

> **Publication License.** In consideration of the action of the American Medical Association (AMA) in reviewing and editing this submission (manuscript, tables, figures, audio, video, and other supplemental files submitted for publication), I hereby transfer, assign, or otherwise convey first publication rights exclusively to the AMA, in the event that such work is published by the AMA, in addition to the attributes of a CC BY License.

Note: For both of these assignments, there are exceptions and different statements for authors who are employed by the US federal or other national government or who authored a work under a work for hire agreement (see 5.6.5.3, Ethical and Legal Considerations, Intellectual Property: Ownership, Access, Rights, and Management, Copyright Assignment or License, Exception—Works Created by Employees of US Federal Government or That of Other Nations, and 5.6.5.4, Ethical and Legal Considerations, Intellectual Property: Ownership, Access, Rights, and Management, Copyright Assignment or License, Exception—Institutional Owners of Copyright).

**5.6.5.2** **Assignment by Coauthors.** The authors of a joint work are co-owners of copyright in the work. To transfer copyright or grant a publication license in a joint work, the copyright assignment or license must be signed by each of the authors.

**5.6.5.3** **Exception—Works Created by Employees of the US Federal Government or That of Other Nations.** Because copyright does not vest in works created by the US federal government, no assignment from the author is necessary.[16(§105)] However, journals should obtain a signed statement from each author who contributed to a work as a federal government employee. What constitutes a work of a government employee as part of the person's official duties is not always clear, but generally, the application of the federal employee exception is determined by the nature of the author rather than the nature of the work or its funding. Works created by authors of other national governments may be subject to the copyright laws of their respective countries.

For example, the JAMA Network journals require all authors who contribute to a work as part of their duties as an employee of the US federal government or that of another nation to complete the following statement:

> **Federal Employment**: I was an employee of the US federal government or that of another nation when this work was conducted and prepared for publication; therefore, it is not protected by the Copyright Act, and copyright ownership cannot be transferred.

or

> **Federal Employment**: I was an employee of the US federal government or that of another nation when this work was conducted and prepared for publication; therefore, it is not protected by the Copyright Act, and a publication license cannot be transferred.

When some authors of a joint work contributed as employees of the US federal government or that of another nation and other authors did not, each government-employed author must complete the federal employment statement and all other authors must use the standard copyright transfer agreement.

**5.6.5.4** **Exception—Institutional Owners of Copyright.** On occasion, a manuscript from an author or authors from a single institution may be submitted with a copyright transfer or publication license and completed on behalf of the institution rather than by the individual authors. The institution presumably has an agreement with the authors, following the work for hire provision of the copyright law, that all work performed while the authors are employees of the institution is owned by the institution. Accordingly a representative of the institution may transfer copyright or grant a publication license (see 5.6.4, Types of Works and Copyright Duration in the United States, and 5.6.4.4, Types of Works and Copyright Duration in the United States, Works Made for Hire).

For example, the JAMA Network journals provide the following work for hire statement:

> **Work for Hire**. I am employed by an institution that considers this submission a "work made for hire" and that requires an authorized representative of the institution to assign copyright [or publication license] on my behalf.

The JAMA Network journals then require an institutional representative to complete copyright, or publication license, transfer on behalf of the author(s).

Scientific journals should be cautious about accepting limits on copyright transfers or publication licenses from institutions or commercial entities that could remove the journal's ability and authority to approve subsequent uses of a journal article, and the journal's imprimatur of that article, for commercial or promotional purposes. Journals also need to avoid the possibility of commercial or exploitative use of a work in a manner deemed unsuitable by the journal.

**5.6.6** **Copyright Notice and Registration.** Although use of a copyright notice is not required under copyright law, the US Copyright Office strongly recommends use of such a notice.[60] A copyright notice for all visual copies of a work should contain the following 3 elements[16(§401)]:

The word "Copyright," the abbreviation "Copr," or the symbol ©,

The year of first publication of the work, and

The name of the copyright owner.

*Examples:*
Copyright 2019 American Medical Association
© 2019 American Medical Association

Note: For the JAMA Network journals, the wording above includes the name of the owner of the journals (American Medical Association) not the name of the journal. It is recommended that all copyright notices be placed in such a "manner and location as to give reasonable notice of the claim of copyright."[16(§401),60] The wording and placement of copyright notices applies equally to print and online works.

The JAMA Network journals include the copyright notice with every article (in print and online) or in the Article Information section for open access licenses.

*Example:*

**Open Access:** This is an open access article distributed under the terms of the CC BY License. © 2019 Smith CT et al. *JAMA Network Open.*

See also 2.10.3, Acknowledgments [Article Information], Information on Open Access.

The year in the copyright notice should be the year of publication. Journal home pages and other main pages of journal websites should change the year of copyright notice at the beginning of each year, but back-issue content should retain the copyright year for the original year of publication.

According to the US Copyright Office, registration creates a public record of key facts that relate to the authorship and ownership of the claimed work, including the title of the work, the author of the work, the name and address of the claimant or copyright owner, the year of creation, and information about whether the work is published, has been previously registered, or includes preexisting material.[60] Registration is not required for copyright protection, and failure to register a work does not affect the copyright owner's rights in that property. However, registration does offer several benefits: it establishes a public record of the copyright claim and is a prerequisite to bringing suit for copyright infringement in US courts.[60] Registration requires a completed application form, filing fee, and the deposition of copies of the work (usually 2 copies of printed materials or the submission of identifying material for electronic publications).[16(§408)] Registration is best made within 3 months of publication.[60,73] Registration filing fees vary for single original works, serials (including journals, periodicals, newspapers, annuals, and proceedings), visual and performing arts, sound recordings, and copyright renewals and are available online from the US Copyright Office at http://www.copyright.gov.

**5.6.7** **Copying, Reproducing, Adapting, and Other Uses of Content.** To copy or reproduce an entire work without authorization from the copyright owner constitutes copyright infringement. However, a reasonable type and amount of copying of a copyrighted work is permitted under the fair use provisions of US copyright law.[16(§107)]

**5.6.7.1** **Fair Use.** What constitutes fair use of copyrighted material in a given case depends on the following 4 factors[16(§107)]:

1. Purpose and character of the use, including whether such use is of a commercial nature or is for nonprofit educational purposes
2. Nature of the copyrighted work
3. Amount and substantiality of the portion used in relation to the copyrighted work as a whole
4. Effect of the use on the potential market for or value of the copyrighted work

Although each of these factors may provide a safe haven for use of copyrighted works without permission from the owner, the fourth factor, the market value of the original work, has been considered important by the courts in copyright infringement cases.

Fair use purposes include "criticism, comment, news reporting, teaching, scholarship, or research."[16(§107)] This allows authors to quote, copy, or reproduce small amounts of text or graphic material. Appropriate credit should always be given to the original source. In the case of a direct quote, quotation marks or setting off the quoted material, with an appropriate reference or footnote to the original source, is required (see 5.4.2, Misappropriation: Plagiarism and Breaches of Confidentiality).

**5.6.7.2** **Text.** The amount of text subject to fair use is determined by its proportion of the whole, but this proportion is not measurable by word count. Contrary to popular belief, there are no specific numbers of words or lines or amount of content that may be taken without permission. The so-called 300-word rule has been cited erroneously to justify quoting passages of text without permission. This erroneous assertion probably originated with the custom of sending out review copies of books and allowing reviewers to quote passages of 300 words or less in a published review. In 1985, *The Nation* magazine lost a landmark suit for copyright infringement after publishing a 300-word excerpt from former US President Gerald Ford's 200 000-word unpublished memoir, which was to be published as a book by Harper & Row (*Harper & Row Publishers, Inc v Nation Enterprises*).[74] In this case, the trial court ruled that the excerpt "was essentially the heart of the book."[74] *The Chicago Manual of Style* recommends that a quote never extend more than a "few contiguous paragraphs" and that quotes, even if interrupted by original text, should not "overshadow the quoter's own material."[73(§4.86)] The length quoted should never be such that it would diminish the potential market for or value of the original work (see 5.3, Duplicate Publication and Submission, and 5.4.2, Misappropriation: Plagiarism and Breaches of Confidentiality).

**5.6.7.3** **Tables, Graphs, and Illustrations.** Fair use of tabular and graphic material and illustrations is more difficult to assess. Although 1 or 2 lines of information from a table might be used without permission, reprinting the entire table without permission is inappropriate and could result in a claim of copyright infringement. The same applies to graphs and illustrations. For example, the JAMA Network journals require all authors to obtain permission to adapt a major part of or republish an entire table, graph, or illustration that has been previously published (unless published under an unrestricted Creative Commons license). Unrestricted permission is needed to reproduce this material in all "print, online, and licensed versions" of the journal. Many publishers permit online users to download copies of tables, graphs, and illustrations as slides or other formats that include citation to the original work for use in teaching.

**5.6.7.4** **Photographs and Works of Art.** Photographs and works of art protected by copyright may not be reproduced, enhanced, or altered without permission of the copyright owner, who may be the photographer or artist, a museum or gallery, an academic institution, a commercial entity, or a previous publisher. For example, the JAMA Network journals obtain permission from owners of copyrights of works of art, typically museums and galleries, to reproduce these in humanities and other articles. In this case, the journal receives a nonexclusive 1-time right to reproduce the art in an article in print and online, which does not permit reuse of the artwork in other works without obtaining permission for such secondary use from the copyright owner of the work of art.

**5.6.7.5** **Unpublished Works.** Authors should not rely on the fair use provision to justify quoting from unpublished manuscripts and letters.[69,73] In several cases, the US courts have taken a conservative view toward use of extensive quotations and paraphrasing from unpublished works without permission, making it difficult to justify such use. For example, in *J. D. Salinger v Random House, Inc*,[75] the Second Court of Appeals ruled that inclusion of extensive quotes from Salinger's unpublished letters in Hamilton's unauthorized biography of Salinger was improper. In a subsequent case, *New Era Publications International, ApS v Henry Holt and Company, Inc*,[76] the trial court ruled that quotation from unpublished work was not fair use "even if necessary to document serious character defects of an important public figure." For terms and conditions of copyright protection for unpublished works, see Table 5.6-1.

**5.6.7.6** **Correspondence and Reviews Regarding Manuscripts and the Editorial Process.** All correspondence regarding a manuscript and the editorial process is considered unpublished and confidential and thus should not be used without knowledge of the owner of the correspondence. In the case of a letter, the letter writer is the owner. In the case of a manuscript review, the peer reviewer is the owner, unless the reviewer was contracted under a work-for-hire provision. Thus, authors and journals have no legal right to publish extensive quotes or paraphrases of reviews without the reviewer's consent (see 5.7.1, Confidentiality During Editorial Evaluation and Peer Review and After Publication) or of letters, not submitted for publication, without the letter writer's permission (see 5.6.7.7, Copying, Reproducing, Adapting, and Other Uses of Content, Quotes and Paraphrases

From Oral and Written Communications). In addition, to date, the courts have not allowed attempts to gain access to confidential peer review records or confidential information about manuscripts that are not published or not included in published articles (see 5.7.1, Confidentiality During Editorial Evaluation and Peer Review and After Publication).

**5.6.7.7** **Quotes and Paraphrases From Oral and Written Communications.** Many journals accept citations to personal communications (ie, oral and written communications). Court decisions regarding use of unpublished works[75,76] indicate that written communication, such as a letter or a memorandum (whether handwritten, typed, printed, or in digital format), if unpublished, may require permission from the letter or memo writer to be cited in a published work. Unless recorded, an oral communication, such as a personal or telephone conversation, cannot be copyrighted. However, authors should obtain written permission from the sources of quotations that are cited as oral and written communications in their manuscripts and should provide a copy of all such permissions to the journal[34] (see 3.13.10, Personal Communications).

**5.6.7.8** **Works in the Public Domain.** Works in the public domain (which are not protected by copyright) may be quoted freely, with proper credit given to the original source. Examples of works in the public domain include those funded completely by the US government and those works on which the copyright term has expired (see 5.6.4.6, Works in the Public Domain or Created by the US Government). Other examples are available from Project Gutenberg.[71]

**5.6.7.9** **Abstracts.** One widely debated application of fair use is the reproduction of abstracts of journal articles in other publications or databases. It can be argued that abstracts, especially structured abstracts, represent the whole work. As a result, any secondary publication or commercial use of abstracts of journal articles as derivative works in print or online without permission of the copyright owner may be considered copyright infringement.

**5.6.7.10** **Digital Images, Multimedia, and Other Works.** Fair use considerations apply equally to reproductions of copyrighted material published in digital format. That is, what is considered fair use in the print domain is likewise fair use in the electronic world. Copyright infringement is a violation of the law—whether the infringed work is photocopied, printed, or copied electronically (see also discussion of the US Digital Millennium Copyright Act in 5.6.3, Copyright: Definition, History, and Current Law). Thus, digital works (eg, digitally produced or reproduced photographs, slides, radiographs, scans, chromatographs, audio, and video) are protected under copyright law and require permission from the copyright owner to be reproduced in a publication.

With high-performance computer technology, digital images can be manipulated to enhance communication. However, digital adjustments could also be used to bias findings or to deceive. Journals should have guidelines for submission (including recommended file formats and sizes for editorial review and publication), enhancement, and publication of digital images, audio, and video that require authors to identify the software used as well as a record of how the original work was obtained and whether it was altered or manipulated.[77,78] Some journals have defined acceptable alterations (such as cropping) and proposed the use of standards for color, brightness, and scale. Others have developed mechanisms to identify inappropriate manipulation[77,78] (see 5.4.3, Inappropriate Manipulation of Digital Images, and 4.2.5, Photographs and Clinical Imaging).

**5.6.7.11** **Social Media.** Publishers, editors, and authors use social media to promote readership and encourage dialogue about articles and related content. Social media users should be aware of risks associated with unauthorized use, reuse, and sharing of content protected by copyright or trademark. Even if safe-harbor provisions protect online content providers, copyright infringement can occur, and users (publishers, editors, and authors) may be held liable for such infringement. Standard practices for obtaining rights or permissions to copyright-protected content apply in social media. Social media users should also be aware of user agreements of some commercial social media companies that claim ownership of all content posted and shared via these social media networks and sites.

**5.6.7.12** **Linking and Framing.** Linking is a fundamental feature of any electronic publication. Many online versions of articles contain hypertext links within the article (eg, to and from citations to references, tables, figures, supplemental content, and multimedia) and links external to the article (eg, to other articles or resources). Such linking is generally considered appropriate use. However, deep linking into a particular internal page of a website, especially if it permits circumvention of access restrictions or barriers, may be considered an unlawful use of the linked-to material.[61(p215)] *Framing* is the enclosure and display of another's content within a frame that has the branding and navigation of the framing site but without actually delivering the user to that site. Such framing may be argued to be the creation of a derivative work, which, if done without permission, will likely be regarded as an infringement.[61(p218)]

**5.6.7.13** **Fair Use Exclusions and Reproduction Permission/Credit Language.** If a portion of a copyrighted work is to be used in a subsequent work and such use is not fair use, written permission must be obtained from the copyright owner (see 5.6.8, Ethical and Legal Considerations, Intellectual Property: Ownership, Access, Rights, and Management, Permissions for Reuse). Examples of such portions include text, tables, graphs, illustrations, or photographs. It is never permissible to use an entire article unless permission to do so is obtained in writing or the article is not protected by copyright. If there is doubt about the copyright status of a particular work, an inquiry should be directed to the author, publisher, or national copyright office. In all cases, the material should carry a proper credit line and, if applicable, copyright notice:

Data Adapted From Table and Used in Subsequent Article

Table 1 is adapted with permission from Singer M, Deutschman CS, Seymour CW, et al. The Third International Consensus Definitions for Sepsis and Septic

Shock (Sepsis-3). *JAMA*. 2016;315(8):801-810. doi:10.1001/jama.2016.0287. Copyright 2016 American Medical Association.

Republishing Entire Article

Republished with permission from *JAMA*. 2016;315(8):801-810. doi:10.1001/jama.2016.0287. Copyright 2016 American Medical Association.

Republishing Part of on an Entire Figure

Source: The left panel of Figure 2 was reproduced with permission from the American Society of Hematology.

Republished under the Creative Commons Attribution (CC-BY 4.0).

Note: Since most publications have an online presence or may do so in the future, it is not appropriate to use the wording "reprinted with permission." All permission and credit lines should use words such as "reproduced" or "republished."

**5.6.8** **Permissions for Reuse.** The copyright owner has the right to attach conditions to giving permission for reuse whether in print or electronic format, such as requiring proper credit and copyright notice. Permission is usually granted by most publishers without charge or with a small processing fee to use portions (text, figures, or tables) of articles or other works when such use will not result in commercial gain. To expedite review of permission requests, requestors should include the following information in each request:

- Title and complete citation of the original work

- Indication of the portion of the work to be reused, if not the entire work

- Information about the secondary use or publication in which the work will appear (including commercial or noncommercial use, method of dissemination, and intended audience)

- Scope of reuse rights (eg, nonexclusive, worldwide, all languages, print, online, and licensed versions)

Many journals/publishers may use an online service for processing or requests and permissions to reproduce content. Some journals may provide authors with instructions and a form for obtaining rights for reproducing or adapting material that is owned by others. See the sample form used by the JAMA Network journals in Box 5.6-1.

**5.6.9** **Standards for Commercial Reprints and e-Prints.** Pharmaceutical and device companies, institutions, and other organizations may purchase nonexclusive rights to reproduce scientific articles as reprints or provide access to these as e-prints, single articles, or collections of articles to help market their products. A *reprint* is the republication of an article or collection of articles in which the content is unchanged from the original publication (except perhaps for the inclusion of postpublication corrections). An *e-print* is a digital reproduction of or an online link to an article or collection of articles, usually PDF file(s) (see 5.12.7, Reprints and e-Prints). These sponsored materials often are produced and

**Box 5.6-1.** Requirements for Reproducing or Adapting Copyright-Protected Material for Publication in *JAMA*: Guidelines for Authors

Permission to reproduce or adapt copyright-protected material (tables, figures, videos, or substantial portions of text) in *JAMA* must be obtained from the copyright owner.

In general, publishers hold the copyright to material previously published in journals, books, and digital media, but in some instances, especially for illustrations, photographs, and videos, the original creator of the work may retain copyright. Copyright to unpublished material is usually held by the creator of the work.

**If you wish to include copyright-protected material in your article, please provide BOTH of the following items:**

❏ 1. Written permission from the copyright owner of the material (see instructions that follow);

AND

❏ 2. For previously published material, a copy of the original publication (journal article, book chapter, etc) in which the content appeared.

**How to Request Permission**

For previously published material, direct your request for grant of permission to the permissions department of the journal or publisher. For unpublished material, contact the creator of the work to find out who owns the copyright. Request permission as soon as possible. In the event that your request cannot be granted, you will need time to substitute other material.

**Include all of the following information in your request (see attached form):**

**1. Your Contact Information**
Name, mailing address, telephone number, and email address.

**2. Information About the Material to Be Used**
**Complete Source Citation**
*For Journals*: Author(s), article title, journal title, year of publication, volume number, issue number, and inclusive page numbers.
*For Books*: Author(s) or editor(s), book title, publisher, year of copyright, and inclusive page numbers.

**Material You Wish to Use**
Specify by figure, table, or video number(s) or identify the portion of text.

**3. How the Material Is to Be Used**
Title of your article to be published in *JAMA*
Names of author(s)

**4. Terms of Use**
Use of the material in print, online, and licensed versions of *JAMA*
Nonexclusive rights
Unrestricted time
All languages
**Note: We cannot accept permissions that restrict use to one-time only or to English-language only.**

Include the permission(s) and copy(ies) of the original material with your manuscript.

*(continued)*

## Request for Permission to Reproduce or Adapt Copyright-Protected Material for Publication in *JAMA*

To:_____ Date:_____

    Copyright Owner, Publisher, or Other

I (we) request permission to reproduce or adapt the material specified below in *JAMA*. Citation to the original publication or appropriate credit will be published. A grant of permission form is included for your use.

Requestor's Contact Information

Name_____ Title_____

Organization_____

Mailing Address_____

City_____ State/Province _____Zip/Postal Code_____ Country_____

Telephone_____ Email_____

### Source Citation of Material to Be Used (Please Print)

*For Journals*: Author(s), article title, journal, year of publication, volume number, issue number, and inclusive pages.

*For Books*: Author(s) or editor(s), book title, publisher, year of copyright and inclusive pages.

_____

_____

**Description of Material**: Specify figure, table, or video number(s) or description of text and page number(s).

_____

### How the Content Is to Be Used (Please Print)

*JAMA* Manuscript Number (if known)_____

Corresponding Author:_____

Title of Article_____

Terms of use: Use in print, online, and licensed versions of *JAMA*

    Nonexclusive rights

    Unrestricted time

    All languages

Note: We cannot accept permissions that restrict use to one-time only or to English-language only.

_____

**Grant of Permission: Please complete and return this to the requestor listed above.**

I/we hold copyright to the material specified above and grant permission for its use in association with the designated *JAMA* article in print, online, and licensed versions of *JAMA* according to the terms listed above.

For previously published content, citation to the original publication will accompany the content.

For unpublished content, copyright credit should read as follows (please print):

_____

_____ Date _____

Signature of Copyright Owner or Designate

_____

Print Name of Copyright Owner or Designate

distributed by custom publishing companies and marketing agencies. To ensure the quality of these reprints and e-prints and to protect the integrity of the scientific journals that originally published the articles, the publishers and editors of the JAMA Network journals have developed standards for sponsored reprints and e-prints (**Box 5.6-2**).[79]

**Box 5.6-2.** The JAMA Network Journals Standards for Reprints and e-Prints Purchased by Organizations

**Fundamental Principles**

The JAMA Network strives to produce medical research and information that adheres to the highest professional standards. The JAMA Network editorial process is designed to ensure that all published information is timely, rigorously peer-reviewed, and clinically relevant.

Reprints may not imply endorsement of a product or influence by an organization. Each reprint request is subject to approval by the JAMA Network, which reserves the right to reject orders deemed not in keeping with our standards.

**Ownership of Copyright**

Materials published in JAMA Network journals, including subsequent translations, are owned and copyrighted by the American Medical Association (AMA), unless there is indication of copyright owned by others or that the material is under a publication license. Materials under AMA copyright remain the property of the AMA and may not be reproduced in any form without written permission from the publisher. The AMA encourages reporting of any suspected unauthorized use to the AMA. The AMA is responsible for securing all necessary permissions.

**Content**

All JAMA Network editorial content must be reproduced verbatim for a reprint or e-print. Any reprints or e-prints of content that has been corrected should incorporate that correction either at the end of the article or as a notation. No content is available for reprints or e-prints prior to publication in a JAMA Network journal. Articles published online ahead of print may be purchased as e-prints or reprints on the date they are published online, provided they meet all the criteria listed above.

In the event that a correction is necessary for an article, reprints or e-prints of the article will be unavailable until the correction is published.

**Single-Article Reprints in Paper Format**

The policies outlined below apply to paper reprints of a single JAMA Network article or multiple related articles from a single issue as indicated by an editorial notation (eg, an Original Investigation that refers to a Commentary, Editorial, etc).

**Policy and Procedures**

1. Single-article reprints are subject to JAMA Network Fundamental Principles and approval.

(*continued*)

**Box 5.6-2.** The JAMA Network Journals Standards for Reprints and e-Prints Purchased by Organizations (*continued*)

2. With rare exceptions, reprints must include a front cover that includes the following:

   • Name/logo of journal

   • JAMA Network logo

   • Title of article, complete list of authors, and issue date

   • The phrase "Reprint Article" or its translation must appear at the top of the cover. No other content is permitted on the front cover.

3. Reprints must also include the original running footer plus the following information:

   "(Reprinted) Journal Name" and copyright information.

4. Prescribing information or disclaimers required or approved by a government regulatory body (eg, US Food and Drug Administration [FDA]) or the purchasing company's inventory numbers may be included subject to JAMA Network Fundamental Principles and approval. When prescribing information is required, the printed product will consist of the article followed by a buffer page and then the prescribing information. The buffer page will include a statement similar to the following:

   "This reprint is provided courtesy of [company name], which has a financial interest in the product/topic discussed in this article. The following FDA-approved labeling has been provided by [company name]. [Journal Name] and the AMA do not assume responsibility for the content of the following information."

   Note: The above statement is permitted only on the buffer page for approved prescribing information.

5. Reprint holders and all materials contained therein (cover letters and other materials printed as part of, attached to, or surrounding a reprint) are subject to JAMA Network Fundamental Principles and approval.

6. No promotional material may be included with or attached to the reprint.

7. The following disclosure, or its translation, may be included in 8-pt type on the bottom of the noncontent back cover page.

   "This reprint is provided courtesy of [company name], which has a financial interest in the product/topic discussed in this article."

**Web and Other Electronic Formats (Green Prints)**
The policies outlined below apply to JAMA Network journals e-prints, which are currently available in 2 formats:

**Box 5.6-2.** The JAMA Network Journals Standards for Reprints and e-Prints Purchased by Organizations (*continued*)

Access via a link to the PDF that resides on our dedicated provider e-print server for a specific number of accesses or length of time
A downloadable rights-protected PDF-based e-print

**Policy and Procedures**

Organizations may purchase JAMA Network journals e-prints under the conditions outlined in the Fundamental Principles section and under the following product-specific conditions:

1. e-Print requests, including the web page or email message that links to the article, are subject to JAMA Network Fundamental Principles and approval.

2. The requested e-print must adhere to the following criteria:

   - The content of the article PDF will not be altered.

   - The web page or email message must not describe or interpret the article.

   - The link to the article(s) must be separate from any marketing or other nonjournal content (ie, separate header stating "Journal Resources" or similar).

   - The link must include the full citation to the article (ie, author, title, and journal name, year, volume, issue, pages, or DOI if the article has been published online ahead of print).

   - The name of the company sponsoring the website or email message must be clearly displayed.

   - After JAMA Network approval, the link and the information surrounding the link must not be changed without prior approval.

3. Following approval, access will be granted to the electronic article.

**Access to a PDF-Based e-Print Residing on the AMA e-Prints Dedicated Server**

Purchasing organizations wishing to link to an AMA journal article PDF may purchase access to that PDF for a specific number of accesses or length of time, provided that the above stipulations are met. A URL link will be provided to enable the purchasing organization to establish password-free access from the supporting company's linking page to the e-print PDF. The purchasing organization will maintain this link for the duration of the agreement.

**Access to a Rights-Protected, Freestanding PDF-based e-Print**

This e-print is a downloadable rights-protected PDF of the article(s) that is similar in appearance to a paper reprint.

Rights-protected PDF-based e-prints will include the cover page and running footer requirements described in the paper-format reprint section Single Article Reprint of these standards.

*(continued)*

**Box 5.6-2.** The JAMA Network Journals Standards for Reprints and e-Prints Purchased by Organizations (*continued*)

Prescribing information or disclaimers required or approved by a government regulatory body (eg, FDA) may be included with a PDF e-print subject to the JAMA Network Fundamental Principles and approval process. When prescribing information is included, a buffer page with disclaimer information (described in Single-Article Reprints, Paper Format, Item 4) will be required. Such information will be attached to the original article PDF and then locked (rights protected) prior to delivery.

The company website and specific page and/or email from which the rights-protected PDF e-print will link are subject to the JAMA Network Fundamental Principles and AMA eprint criteria.

An organization may purchase multiple e-prints on a related subject. These e-prints may be packaged together via links or bundled into a single rights-protected PDF. When these electronic packages consist of articles not related by editorial notation in the original publication, they will be subject to the JAMA Network Fundamental Principles and product-specific conditions approval process.

**The JAMA Network Journals Reprint Collections**

The policies outlined below apply to collections of articles drawn from a single issue or multiple issues of JAMA Network journals. These products may be in print or electronic format.

**Policy and Procedures**

1. JAMA Network Reprint Collections are subject to JAMA Network Fundamental Principles and approval. They must also meet the following product-specific conditions:

   - The customer selects a topic, core article, or selection of articles for a reprint collection and submits a request to the JAMA Network.

   - The JAMA Network proposal will include the selected articles, the proposed purchaser(s) and distribution mechanism(s), along with a PDF mock-up of the design for approval.

   - No promotional material for a product or activity involving the purchasing organization may be included with or attached to the Reprint Collection.

2. Prescribing information or disclaimers required or approved by a government regulatory body (eg, US Food and Drug Administration [FDA]) or the purchasing company's inventory numbers may be included subject to the JAMA Network Fundamental Principles and approval. When prescribing information is required, the printed product will consist of the article followed by a buffer page and then the prescribing information. The buffer page will include a statement similar to the following:

**Box 5.6-2.** The JAMA Network Journals Standards for Reprints and e-Prints Purchased by Organizations (*continued*)

> "This reprint is provided courtesy of [company name], which has a financial interest in the product/topic discussed in this article. The following FDA-approved labeling has been provided by [company name]. [Journal Name] and the AMA do not assume responsibility for the content of the following information."
>
> Note: The above statement is permitted only on the buffer page for approved prescribing information.
>
> 3. Reprint holders and all materials contained therein (cover letters and other materials printed as part of, attached to, or surrounding a reprint) are subject to JAMA Network Fundamental Principles and approval.

**5.6.10**     **Standards for Licensed International Editions.** A publisher may license others to publish international or translated editions of its scientific journals. To ensure the quality of these editions, the following standards are recommended:

- Copyright in the international edition and all translated articles is owned by the original publisher, unless articles or parts of articles are governed by a specific publication license (in which case such should be indicated on or within each specific article).

- Each issue must contain a minimum number of pages or amount of content.

- Articles republished from the original journal must account for a minimum of 50% of each issue's total pages or content. The remaining 50% of total pages or content may include local editorial material and local commercial content (eg, advertisements).

- The licensed publisher will appoint an editorial director (whose appointment will be approved by the editor of the original journal) to select articles from the original edition to be republished in the international edition and review the quality of translations.

- Each republished article must include a complete citation to the original article (ie, journal, year, volume and issue numbers, inclusive page numbers or e-locator, and DOI) and complete original titles, author bylines, and author affiliations.

- Abridgments or changes to original content, other than translation, are not permitted.

- Content should be republished within a minimum amount of time (eg, 6 months from date of original publication).

- International editions may include local editorial material that cannot constitute more than 50% of total pages or content. Local editorial includes the cover (if the original journal cover is not used), masthead, table of contents, editorial indexes, brief news reports, summaries of conferences, meeting calendars, announcements, commentaries, editorials, letters, and explanations of original articles.

- Local editorial does not include (1) any original clinical or scientific articles (ie, quantitative or qualitative research reports or analyses, case descriptions, clinical or product reviews, product or therapeutic comparisons, scientific abstracts) or (2) any articles previously published by other journals.

- All authors of all local editorial should have their complete names, academic degrees or credentials, and affiliations published with each article.

- For online publications, translated articles should link to the original article.

- Journals with advertising should have multiple advertisements and should not be sponsored by one commercial entity or interest.

- Advertisements in print editions should not appear adjacent to editorial content on the same topic; advertisements in online editions should follow the same policies for online advertising as the parent edition.

- Commercial content shall not be presented to appear as editorial content. Appearance, artwork, and format shall be of such a nature as to avoid confusion with the editorial content of the publication.

See 5.12, Advertisements, Advertorials, Sponsorship, Supplements, Reprints, and e-Prints.

**5.6.11** **International Copyright Protection.** There is no international copyright law.[67] Copyright law, scope, protections, and remedies are governed by individual nations and treaties among them. Thus, copyright laws do not automatically protect an author's work throughout the world. However, most countries offer protection to works from other nations.[67,80] For a detailed discussion of the copyright laws of individual countries, consult the World Intellectual Property Organization (WIPO), which is under the auspices of the United Nations in Geneva, Switzerland.[80] See 5.6.13, Copyright Resources, for contact information for WIPO.

The Berne Convention for the Protection of Literary and Artistic Works (commonly known as the Berne Convention)[81] was originally signed by 10 European countries in 1886 in Berne, Switzerland, to protect copyright across their national borders.[67,81] Today, the Berne Convention is administered by WIPO. For many years, the United States declined to sign on to the Berne Convention because of its lack of formality and its minimalist approach. For example, the Berne Convention does not require the use of a copyright notice, which was in conflict with prior US copyright law. To accommodate the US need for a minimum set of standards, the Universal Copyright Convention (UCC) was created by the United Nations Educational, Scientific, and Cultural Organization (UNESCO) in 1952. Under the UCC, works created in the United States could have multilateral protection without forfeiting the prior US requirement for copyright notice.[66]

After amending its copyright law by eliminating the requirement for copyright notice, the United States signed the Berne Convention in 1989. Most resource-rich nations and many transitional countries subscribe to this convention, and there are special provisions for resource-limited countries that wish to make use of them.[81] As of 2019, 176 nations had signed on to the Berne Convention.[81] The Berne Convention has no formal requirements. However, each signatory country agrees to protect the copyright in works created in other member countries. Although the United States no longer mandates the use of copyright notice, the US Copyright Office still encourages voluntary use (see 5.6.6, Copyright Notice and Registration). The significance of the UCC is now largely historical after the adoption of the Trade-Related Aspects of Intellectual Property Rights (TRIPS) agreement and other international agreements in the 1990s, including WIPO's Copyright and Performances and Phonograms Treaty and the WIPO Copyright Treaty. The WIPO Copyright Treaties, adopted in 1996, provide additional protections for works created in other member countries and address issues and questions raised by new economic, social, cultural, and technological developments as well as new international rules.

**5.6.12** **Moral Rights.** Moral rights, first introduced by the French as *droit moral*, is a doctrine of copyright law intended to protect individual creators' noneconomic investments in their work and the personality of the creator as it relates to the work regardless of copyright ownership or transfer.[62(§25.03),81] Two moral rights that are most often recognized are the right to attribution and the right to integrity (ie, right to prevent destruction or mutilation of work).[62(§25.03)] This doctrine is endorsed by most member countries of the Berne Convention. Although the United States is a member of the Berne Convention, US law does not provide for moral rights, except for certain visual works of art to protect them from mutilation or misattribution through the Visual Artists Rights Act of 1990.[16(§106A)] Creators of other works in the United States are provided limited moral rights protection under other federal laws (such as the Lanham Act), state laws, or contracts that include specific provisions for moral rights.[62(§25.03)] Under interpretations of relevant US laws as well as any applicable contract provisions, US editors and publishers may not give authorship credit to someone who has not written the work and may not credit an author of a written work without the author's permission (see 5.1.2, Guest and Ghost Authors and Other Contributors). In the United States, courts have also held that mutilation of a work (distortion or substantial alteration of the work without consent of the author) may result in copyright infringement.[62(§25)] However, authors are not similarly protected against unauthorized changes made during editing and publication of their work.[62(§25)] Because of the ease of manipulation and distortion of electronic works, concerns about moral rights in the context of electronic publishing are increasing in the United States and may portend changes in this area of law in the future.[62(§25)]

**5.6.13** **Copyright Resources.** Additional information about copyright law may be obtained from several sources. For a detailed legal account, consult *Perle and Williams on Publishing Law*[62] or *Nimmer on Copyright*[64] (although these resources are expensive and may be best consulted via a library that has these in its holdings). Other useful texts include the *Chicago Manual of Style* chapter "Rights, Permissions, and Copyright Administration"[73] and *Internet Law: A Field Guide*.[61] Specific information, useful guides, and forms may be obtained free of charge from the US Copyright Office.[16,60,63,66,67,69]

US Copyright Office
Library of Congress
101 Independence Ave SE
Washington, DC 20559-6000
Telephone: 202-707-3000 or 877-476-0778
www.copyright.gov

Additional useful information can also be obtained from the following:

Association of American Publishers (AAP)
455 Massachusetts Ave NW, Ste 700
Washington, DC 20001
Telephone: 202-347-3375
www.publishers.org

Association of Learned and Professional Society Publishers (ALPSP)
Egale 1, 80 St Albans Rd
Watford, Hertfordshire
WD17 1DL UK
Telephone: +44-1245-260571
Email: admin@alpsp.org
www.alpsp.org/default.htm

STM: International Association of Scientific, Technical and Medical Publishers
Prama House
267 Banbury Rd
Oxford
OX2 7HT UK
Telephone: +44-1865-339-321
https://www.stm-assoc.org/

World Intellectual Property Organization (WIPO)
34, chemin des Colombettes
CH-1211 Geneva 20, Switzerland
Telephone: 41 22 338 9111
http://www.wipo.int/portal/en/

**5.6.14** **Patents.** Patents protect different types of intellectual property than do copyright and trademark. Patent law protects invention and technology, copyright protects an original artistic or literary work (see 5.6.1, Ownership and Control of Data), and trademark protects brand names and logos used on goods and services (see 5.6.15, Trademark).

A patent is a grant of property right by the government to protect a newly created idea on the basis of its technical and legal merit.[82] In biomedicine, patents are commonly applied for and approved for new products, such as pharmaceuticals, reagents, assays, devices, equipment, procedures, and methods. Patent law is intended to encourage discovery and investment in research of new technology by rewarding an inventor with a monopoly on the right to market the new product for a specified period. This law restricts other parties from manufacturing, selling, or using the new product without the patent holder's permission, generally for a period of 20 years.[82]

The US Patent and Trademark Office (USPTO) defines 3 types of patents for invention and discoveries[82]:

*Utility patents*: for a new and useful process, machine, article of manufacture, or composition of matter, or any new and useful improvement thereof.

*Design patents*: for a new, original, and ornamental design for an article of manufacture.

*Plant patents*: for the asexual reproduction of any distinct and new variety of plant.

In the United States, patents are awarded by the USPTO. For more details, instructions, and copies of patent forms, contact the USPTO:

US Patent and Trademark Office
Department of Commerce
Washington, DC 20231
Telephone: (571) 272-1000 or (800) 786-9199
Email: usptoinfo@uspto.gov
https://www.uspto.gov/

As with copyright, there is no international patent law or protection; patents are protected by individual countries. In some regions, a regional patent office (eg, the European Patent Office or the African Regional Intellectual Property Organization) accepts and grants patent applications in the member states of that region. Several international treaties (eg, the Paris Convention for the Protection of Industrial Property and the Patent Cooperation Treaty) support cross-country rights in patent and trademark matters.[82] Detailed information about international treaties on patents is available from WIPO (for contact information, see 5.6.13, Copyright Resources).

Controversies continue over claims for patents of naturally occurring substances, medical and surgical methods, and even genetically altered cells, gene fragments, and genetically based diagnostic tests.[83-87] Desires for profit and primacy of discovery have caused delay or suppression of the publication of important medical information.[12,13,88] In 2014, the US Supreme Court ruled in favor of the Association for Molecular Pathology (*v Myriad Genetics, Inc*) and declared that isolated human genes cannot be patented.[89] However, related ethical issues and concerns about experimental reproducibility for such patent claims persist.[82,87-89] For these reasons, editors should request that authors disclose information about patents, including ownership and upcoming and pending applications for patent grants, that are related to the work included in their submitted manuscripts in their financial disclosures to journals (see 5.5, Conflicts of Interest).

**5.6.15** **Trademark.** Trademark and unfair-competition laws are designed to prevent a competitor from selling goods or services under the auspices of another. Trademark law, not copyright law, protects trademarks, service marks, and trade names.[90] *Trademarks* are legally registered words, names, symbols, designs, or any combination of these items that are used to identify and distinguish goods from those goods manufactured and sold by others and to indicate the source or origin of the goods (eg, brand names).[90] Examples of commonly recognized trademarks include the *Wall Street Journal*, NBC, and Coca-Cola. A *service mark* is the same as a trademark except that it is used to distinguish services, not goods, of a specific provider.[90] Examples of service marks include McDonald's (restaurant services), AT&T (telecommunications services), and Amazon.com (online retail services). The terms *trademark* and *mark* are often used to refer to both trademarks and service marks,[90] and some companies use both (eg, Google). *Trade names* are the names given by manufacturers or businesses to specific products or services. For example, Synthroid is the trade name (or proprietary name) for the drug levothyroxine (see 14.4.3, Proprietary Names). Trade names are not legally protected in the same manner as are trademarks. Trademark law provides legal protection for titles, logos, fictional characters, pseudonyms, and unique groupings of words, symbols, or graphics.[62,90] Whereas copyright law protects an authored work, trademark law protects the words and symbols used in the marketing of that work.

Trademarks are classified into 4 categories in order of their increasing distinctiveness: generic, descriptive, suggestive, and fanciful or arbitrary.[62] Suggestive and fanciful or arbitrary marks are more likely to receive trademark protection than are generic or descriptive marks.[62] An example of an arbitrary mark (a common word that has no specific connection to its product) is Apple (the technology company); an example of a fanciful mark (created solely for use as a trademark) is Xerox. An example of a suggestive mark is Microsoft (suggestive of *soft*ware for *micro*computers). To receive trademark status, a mark must be distinctive (ie, not similar to other marks) and not generic or merely descriptive of a category of products. For example, trademark status was not awarded to *World Book* or *Farmers' Almanac* because both were considered "merely descriptive of the contents of each publication,"[91] and *Software News* magazine was not considered protectable because it referred to a class of products of which the magazine is a member (ie, it was generic).[91] For additional information, contact the USPTO (contact information available in 5.6.14, Patents).

**5.6.15.1** **Titles.** Book titles are rarely protected under trademark law because of judicial reluctance to protect titles that are used only once.[62(§24.03)] A few exceptions to this norm have occurred with book titles that have engendered common secondary meanings, that is, become widely recognized and associated with the name of the author or publisher (eg, *Gone With the Wind*).[91] The title of a series of creative works (eg, book series, journals, magazines, newspapers, television series, or software) may more easily receive trademark protection than can the title of a single creative work.[62(§24.03),91] Thus, *JAMA* is a trademarked title. In the biomedical sciences, it may be difficult to trademark journal titles that are generic and may not be distinguishable from the science or field the journal serves, such as the journals *AIDS*, *Brain*, or *Stroke*. However, some seemingly generic titles have been trademarked, such as *Neurology* and *Pediatrics*.

**5.6.15.2** **Logos.** Logos, designs, or symbols may also receive trademark protection if they distinguish particular goods or services and identify the source of those goods and services.[62(§24.05)] Examples of such logos include the Bantam publishing house rooster and Apple computer's apple. A background design, apart from the words imposed on it, can be protected by trademark if it is of a distinctive quality and functions to identify the source of a good.[62(§24.05)]

**5.6.15.3** **Fictional Characters and Pseudonyms.** Fictional characters may be protected by trademark if they achieve secondary meaning and are widely recognized (eg, Mickey Mouse). Similarly, a pseudonym can be given trademark status.[62(§24.06)]

**5.6.15.4** **Trade Dress.** *Trade dress* is the visual or physical appearance of a product or its packaging, which, if distinct from that of other similar products, may be protected under trademark law. Trade dress is intended to prevent marketplace confusions and to protect consumers from packaging or appearance of products that are designed to imitate other products and prevent consumers from purchasing one product under the belief that it is another. For example, the Coca Cola bottle, the label on Campbell's soup, and the colors and shapes of certain pill capsules have qualified as protectable trade dress. Trade dress includes graphic elements and design, typography, shape, and color. For example, the designs, including the borders, of the print covers of the *National Geographic* and *Time* magazine have been awarded trademark status.[62(§24.03),91] Historically, trade dress protection has generally applied to goods; however, trade dress protection has been extended to cover the overall "look and feel" of a website.[92] The look and feel of a website may include elements such as borders, frames, colors, highlights, orientation, fonts, layout, images and graphics, animation, and sounds, as well as the arrangement and display of these elements. Thus, although the content of a website is likely protected under copyright law, the user interface might be protectable under trade dress application of trademark law. Some predatory or deceptive publishers have misused the likeness of well-known journals to hijack the journals and confuse prospective authors and entice them to submit to predatory or phony journals.[93] A test to determine whether the look and feel of a website has been infringed should include the following factors[92]:

1. Overall similarity
   - Fonts and formatting
   - Color scheme
   - Sounds, animations, and visual effects
   - Symbols, logos, and marks
   - Layout and arrangement
   - User experience design
2. Proximity of products or services in the relevant market(s)
3. Intentional copying
4. Likelihood of consumer confusion

**5.6.15.5** **Application and Registration for Trademark Protection.** In the United States, application for a trademark registration can be made under both federal and state laws.

A legal expert should be consulted for information about registering trademarks in other countries. However, registering a trademark is not sufficient; actual use of the trademark in a given market ensures protection (ie, the longer the actual use of the trademark, the stronger the legal protection).[62,91] Typically, the rights to a trademark belong to the first user in a specific geographic market.

Trademark protection is also governed by the national laws of individual countries and international treaties, such as the TRIPS agreement. In the United States, an application to register a trademark must be filed with the USPTO.[90] Applying for trademark protection is more complicated than applying for copyright protection. The USPTO requires a formal application to be submitted (preferably electronically), along with a drawing of the mark, samples of the mark as it has been used, and a filing fee.[90] The USPTO conducts a formal review of the application, which may take several months. The office may deny the request for registration if the mark is judged to be generic, merely descriptive, or similar to another registered mark (or a mark for which another application is under review). Registration may also be denied if the mark is not used or intended for use in interstate or international commerce. If the application is approved internally by the USPTO, a notice is published in the *Official Gazette* to make the application publicly known. During the 30 days after the *Official Gazette* notice, any third party can file a formal opposition to the application.[90]

If the application is approved, the USPTO will issue a certificate of registration if the mark is in use. If the mark is not yet in use, the applicant is required to file a statement that describes the mark's intended use and has 6 months to use the mark in commerce and submit a statement of such use or request a 6-month extension to file a statement of use.[90]

**5.6.15.6** **Trademark Symbols.** Once registered, the mark is entitled to carry the trademark symbol ®. Only those marks that are officially registered by the USPTO can use the official symbol ®. Marks that are under review may use the symbol TM or SM, but these do not have legal significance.[90]

**5.6.15.7** **Duration of Trademark Protection.** A US trademark registration extends for 10 years and may be extended indefinitely provided the owner continues to use the mark on or in connection with the applicable goods and/or services and files all required documentation with the USPTO at the appropriate times. For example, between the fifth and sixth years of the initial term and in the ninth year of every 10-year period thereafter, additional forms must be filed with the USPTO to ensure legal protection.[90]

**5.6.15.8** **Loss of Trademark Rights and Antidilution Law** A mark can lose its legal protection if the owner discontinues using it (termed *trademark abandonment*), if the owner does not file a statement that the trademark is still in use between the fifth and sixth years of the initial term, or if the owner does not renew the registration by the end of each 10-year registration period.[90] Trademark protection may also be forfeited if a mark becomes too generic or no longer identifies goods or services with a particular source (ie, the mark becomes "diluted"). In legal terms, *trademark dilution* is the reduction of the capacity of a famous mark to identify and distinguish goods and services and occurs when a mark similar or identical to a famous mark reduces the value or distinctiveness of the famous mark to identify and distinguish its goods and services.[90,94] For example, *Webster's* is no longer a registered trademark because the name lost its ability to identify a specific publisher of dictionaries, and Zipper is no longer a registered trademark for "slide fastener."

A mark used in multiple contexts by different product owners or service providers may diminish the ability of a given mark to serve as unique identifier of that product or service.[62(§24),90] Such dilution of unique trademark status is known as *blurring*. A trademark may also be diluted by *tarnishment*, when a well-known trademark is improperly associated with an inferior or offensive product or service.[62(§24)] The following factors may be considered in judging such dilution of unique trademark status of one mark by another [62(§24.03)]:

- Similarity of marks

- Similarity of the products covered by the marks

- Sophistication of consumers

- Predatory intent

- Renown of the senior mark

- Renown of the junior mark

For this reason, owners of trademarks will often send letters to editors and publishers objecting to misuse of their trademarks in publication. Such demands are intended to keep trademarks from being diluted by common use. For example, authors and editors should not use trademark names as generic verbs, nouns, or modifiers (eg, use "photocopied" rather than "xeroxed").

**5.6.15.9**   **Use of Trademarked Names in Publication.** Under the US Federal Trademark Dilution Act,[94] restricted use of trademark names applies mainly to commercial use of trademarks, not to editorial use in publication. For example, a photography magazine may not use the word "Kodak®" as part of its cover design, and a computer manufacturer may not place the word "Kodak®" on the front of a computer. However, an author or editor may include the word "Kodak"—without the trademark symbol—in an article about cameras and film development without risking trademark infringement.

The symbol ®, or the letters TM or SM, should not be used in scientific journal articles or references, but the initial letter of a trademarked word should be capitalized (see 10.3.5, Proprietary Names).

On occasion, a trademark owner will request that its trademark or trade name appear in all capital letters or a combination of capital and lowercase letters, often with the trademark symbol. Authors and editors are not required by law to follow such requests. It is preferable to use an initial capital letter followed by all lowercase letters (eg, Xerox, Kodak, Scopus, Embase) unless the trademark name is an abbreviation (eg, IBM, *JAMA, DSM-5*) or uses an intercapped construction (eg, PubMed, iTunes) (see 10.9, "Intercapped" Compounds; 13.0, Abbreviations; and 14.4.3, Proprietary Names). Online databases, if trademarked, can be listed in all capital letters (eg, MEDLINE, CINAHL, SCIE).

**5.6.15.10** **International Trademark Protection.** Like copyright law, there is no international trademark law, and trademark protections are offered by different jurisdictions in different countries. However, WIPO (www.wipo.org)[80] administers the Madrid System for the International Registration of Marks, which offers a route to trademark protection in multiple countries by filing a single application. Information is also available from the International Trademark Association (www.inta.org).

**5.6.15.11** **Trademark Protection for Domain Names.** *Domain names* are internet addresses that point to a specific website, usually a home page. They are usually easily remembered names that are linked to numeric internet protocol (IP) addresses via a domain name system (DNS). Examples include uspto.gov or harvard.edu.[62(§25.09)] Domain names include top-level domain (TLD) names (eg, ".com," ".org," ".edu") and second-level names (eg, "jama" in jama.com or "nih" in nih.gov). A domain name is not automatically entitled to protection once registered; like other trademarks, it must be used in connection with the website located at that address.[61]

Since 1998, the Internet Corporation for Assigned Names and Numbers (ICANN) has been responsible for managing the domain name system.[95] Domain names can be registered by many different companies (known as registrars) that are authorized by ICANN. Domain name registrars have different terms for renewal of domain name registration, ranging from 1- to 10-year increments.[95] ICANN registrars manage many generic TLD (gTLD) names. Anyone can register for the following gTLDs: .com, .info, .net, .org. Some gTLDs are restricted to individuals or entities that belong to a defined community, such as .aero, .asia, .cat, .coop, .edu, .gov, .mil, .mobi, .museum, .tel, and .travel. ICANN does not accredit registrars for TLDs that are restricted to specific entities and purposes, such as ".edu" for educational institutions, ".gov" for US government agencies, and ".mil" for US military sites. In addition, there are hundreds of 2-letter country code TLDs that may be obtained from host country agencies in accordance with rules determined by the Internet Assigned Numbers Authority.[96]

Disputes over ownership and rights to use domain names are considered under the principles of trademark infringement and dilution, with some specific additions to address cybersquatting and typosquatting.[61,62] *Cybersquatting* (or domain squatting) is the act of obtaining a trademark-associated domain name with the aim of benefitting from the association or selling it to the trademark owner [61,95] *Typosquatting* is "the registration of a domain name that is similar to another's for the purpose of capitalizing on typos that may lead the user to the squatter's website rather than the site the user intends to locate."[61,95] In 1999, the Anticybersquatting Consumer Protection Act was enacted to address these problems of misuse of domain names.[61,95]

To make a successful claim against use of a specific domain name, the following must be demonstrated[95]:

- the domain name is identical or confusingly similar to a trademark or service mark in which the complainant has rights,

- the registrant has no rights or legitimate interests in respect to the domain name, and

- the domain name has been registered and is being used in bad faith.

For more information on applying for and managing domain names and remedies for misuse of domain names, consult ICANN or WIPO (contact information for WIPO is available in 5.6.13, Ethical and Legal Considerations, Intellectual Property: Ownership, Access, Rights, and Management, Copyright Resources).

> Internet Corporation for Assigned Names and Numbers (ICANN)
> 12025 Waterfront Dr, Ste 300
> Los Angeles, CA 90094-2536
> Telephone: (310) 301-5800
> https://www.icann.org/

Contact information for international regional offices is also available in the Contact Us page of the ICANN website.

**Principal Author:** Annette Flanagin, RN, MA

### ACKNOWLEDGMENT

I thank the following for review and helpful comments: Howard Bauchner, MD, *JAMA* and JAMA Network; Michael Clarke, Clarke & Esposito, Washington, DC; Timothy Gray, PhD, JAMA Network; Iris Y. Lo, JAMA Network; Joseph P. Thornton, JD, JAMA Network and American Medical Association; Elizabeth Wager, PhD, Sideview, Princes Risborough, UK; and Sara Zimmerman, JAMA Network.

### REFERENCES

1. Goldstein P. *Copyright's Highway: From Gutenberg to the Celestial Jukebox.* Rev ed. Stanford University Press; 2003.
2. Nelkin D. *Science as Intellectual Property: Who Controls Scientific Research?* Macmillan Publishing Co; 1984.
3. Mishkin B. Urgently needed: policies on access to data by erstwhile collaborators. *Science.* 1995;270(5238):927-928. doi:10.1126/science.270.5238.927
4. Committee on Responsibilities of Authorship on the Biological Sciences, National Research Council. *Sharing Publication-Related Data and Materials: Responsibilities of Authorship in the Life Sciences.* National Academy of Sciences; 2003.
5. National Institutes of Health Office of Extramural Research. NIH data sharing policy and implementation guidance. Updated March 5, 2003. Accessed January 1, 2018. https://grants.nih.gov/grants/policy/data_sharing/data_sharing_guidance.htm
6. National Institutes of Health. National Institutes of Health plan for increasing access to scientific publications and digital scientific data from NIH funded scientific research. February 2015. Accessed January 6, 2019. https://grants.nih.gov/grants/NIH-Public-Access-Plan.pdf
7. Share alike. *Nature.* 2014;507(7491):140. doi:10.1038/507140a
8. Tenopir C, Allard S, Douglass K, et al. Data sharing by scientists: practices and perceptions. *PLoS One.* 2011;6(6):e21101. doi:10.1371/journal.pone.0021101
9. Tenopir C, Dalton ED, Allard S, et al. Changes in data sharing and data reuse practices and perceptions among scientists worldwide. *PLoS One.* 2015;10(8):e0134826. doi:10.1371/journal.pone.0134826
10. Institute of Medicine. *Sharing Clinical Trial Data: Maximizing Benefits, Minimizing Risk: Recommendations.* National Academies Press; 2015. Accessed January 6, 2019. http://www.nap.edu/catalog.php?record_id=18998. doi:10.17226/18998

11. US Food and Drugs Administration. Food and Drug Administration Amendments Act (FDAAA) of 2007. Updated March 29, 2018. Accessed January 1, 2019. https://www.fda.gov/regulatoryinformation/lawsenforcedbyfda/significantamendmentstothefdcact/foodanddrugadministrationamendmentsactof2007/default.htm

12. Blumenthal D, Campbell EG, Anderson MS, Causino N, Louis KS. Withholding research results in academic life science. *JAMA*. 1997;277(15):1224-1228. doi:10.1001/jama.1997.03540390054035

13. Campbell EG, Clarridge BR, Gokhall M, et al. Data withholding in academic genetics: evidence from a national survey. *JAMA*. 2002;287(4):473-480. doi:10.1001/jama.287.4.473

14. Whittington CJ, Kendall T, Fonagy P, Cottrell D, Cotgrove A, Boddington E. Selective serotonin reuptake inhibitors in childhood depression: systematic review of published versus unpublished data. *Lancet*. 2004;363(9418):1341-1345.

15. Dickersin K, Rennie D. The evolution of trial registries and their use to assess the clinical trial enterprise. *JAMA*. 2012;307(17):1861-1864. doi:10.1001/jama.2012.4230

16. US Copyright Office, Library of Congress. Copyright Law of the United States. Accessed January 6, 2019. https://www.copyright.gov/title17

17. US Department of Justice. Department of Justice Freedom of Information Act reference guide. Updated December 13, 2018. Accessed January 6, 2019. https://www.justice.gov/oip/department-justice-freedom-information-act-reference-guide

18. National Academy of Sciences. *Responsible Science: Ensuring the Integrity of the Research Process*. Vol 2. National Academy Press; 1993:127-128.

19. Harvard Office of Technology Development. Statement of policy in regard to intellectual property (IP Policy). Amended December 12, 2013. Accessed January 6, 2019. http://otd.harvard.edu/faculty-inventors/resources/policies-and-procedures/statement-of-policy-in-regard-to-intellectual-property

20. Erway R. Starting the conversation: university-wide research data management policy. *OCLC Research*. 2013. Accessed January 6, 2019. http://www.oclc.org/content/dam/research/publications/library/2013/2013-08.pdf

21. Center for Open Science. Transparency and Openness Promotion (TOP) Guidelines. Accessed January 1, 2018. https://osf.io/ud578

22. Taichman DB, Sahni P, Pinborg A, et al. Data sharing statements for clinical trials: a requirement of the International Committee of Medical Journal Editors. *JAMA*. 2017;317(24):2491-2492. doi:10.1001/jama.2017.6514

23. Wellcome. Sharing research data to improve public health: full joint statement by funders of health research. Accessed January 6, 2019. https://wellcome.ac.uk/what-we-do/our-work/sharing-research-data-improve-public-health-full-joint-statement-funders-health

24. Wellcome. Developing an outputs management plan. Accessed January 6, 2019. https://wellcome.ac.uk/funding/guidance/developing-outputs-management-plan

25. European Medicines Agency. Guideline on GCP compliance in relation to trial master file (paper and/or electronic) for content, management, archiving, audit and inspection of clinical trials. March 31, 2017. Accessed January 6, 2019. http://www.ema.europa.eu/docs/en_GB/document_library/Scientific_guideline/2017/04/WC500225871.pdf

26. Holden JP. Executive Office of the President. Office of Science and Technology Policy. Memorandum for the heads of executive departments and agencies. Increasing access to the results of federally funded scientific research. February 22,

2013. Accessed January 6, 2019. https://obamawhitehouse.archives.gov/sites/default/files/microsites/ostp/ostp_public_access_memo_2013.pdf

27. Fienberg SE, Martin ME, Straf ML. *Sharing Research Data*. National Academy Press; 1985.

28. Laine C, Goodman SN, Griswold ME, Sox HC. Reproducible research: moving toward research the public can really trust. *Ann Intern Med*. 2007;146:450-453.

29. *Annals of Internal Medicine*. Information for Authors. Accessed January 6, 2019. http://annals.org/aim/pages/authors#data-sharing-and-reproducible-research

30. *BMJ* Author Hub. Data sharing. Accessed January 6, 2019. http://authors.bmj.com/submitting-your-paper/data-sharing

31. Resources for Data Management and Sharing. *BMJ Open*. Accessed January 6, 2019. http://bmjopen.bmj.com/pages/datamanagement

32 *Science* journals: editorial policies. *Science*. Accessed January 6, 2019. http://www.sciencemag.org/authors/science-editorial-policies

33. Policies. Availability of data, material and methods. *Nature*. Accessed January 6, 2019. http://www.nature.com/authors/policies/availability.html

34. International Committee of Medical Journal Editors. Recommendations for the conduct, reporting, editing, and publication of scholarly work in medical journals. Updated December 2018. Accessed January 6, 2019. http://www.icmje.org/recommendations

35. Suber P. *Open Access*. MIT Press. 2012. Accessed January 6, 2019. https://mitpress.mit.edu/books/open-access

36. Tenopir C, King D. Trends in scientific scholarly publishing in the United States. *J Sch Publishing*. 1997;28(3):135-170. doi:10.3138/JSP-028-03-135

37. Budapest Open Access Initiative. Accessed January 6, 2019. http://www.budapestopenaccessinitiative.org/

38. Bethesda Statement on Open Access Publishing. Released June 20, 2003. Accessed January 6, 2019. http://legacy.earlham.edu/~peters/fos/bethesda.htm#definition

39. Frank M. Access to the scientific literature—a difficult balance. *N Engl J Med*. 2006;354(15):1552-1555.

40. Clark MT. Open sesame? increasing access to medical literature. *Pediatrics*. 2004; 114(1):265-268. doi:10.1542/peds.114.1.265

41. Anderson RA. Open access: meaning(s) and goal(s). *Scholarly Kitchen*. November 24, 2014. Accessed January 6, 2019. https://scholarlykitchen.sspnet.org/2014/11/24/open-access-meanings-and-goals

42. US Department of Health and Human Services. National Institutes of Health. NIH Public Access Policy. March 18, 2014. Accessed January 6, 2019. https://publicaccess.nih.gov/index.htm

43. Wellcome. Open access policy. Accessed January 6, 2019. https://wellcome.ac.uk/funding/managing-grant/open-access-policy

44. Maslove DM. Medical preprints—a debate worth having. *JAMA*. 2018;319(5):443-444. doi:10.1001/jama.2017.17566

45. BMC Research in Progress Annual Report 2018. Accessed January 6, 2019. https://figshare.com/articles/BMC_Research_in_Progress_Annual_Report_2018/7234922

46. BioMed Central. Article-processing charges. How much is BMC charging? 2019 article-processing charges. Accessed January 6, 2019. https://www.biomedcentral.com/getpublished/article-processing-charges/biomedcentral-prices

47. Gordon and Betty Moore Foundation. PLOS. Accessed January 6, 2019. https://www.moore.org/grants/list/GBMF165

48. PLOS. Publication fees. Accessed January 6, 2019. https://www.plos.org/publications/publication-fees/
49. Björk BC. Have the "mega-journals" reached the limits to growth? *PeerJ*. 2015;3:e981. doi:10.7717/peerj.981
50. Davis P. *Scientific Reports* overtakes *PLOS ONE* as largest mega journal. April 6, 2017. Accessed January 6, 2019. https://scholarlykitchen.sspnet.org/2017/04/06/scientific-reports-overtakes-plos-one-as-largest-megajournal/
51. Anderson K. "Predatory" open access publishers—the natural extreme of an author-pays model. March 6, 2012. Accessed January 6, 2019. https://scholarlykitchen.sspnet.org/2012/03/06/predatory-open-access-publishers-the-natural-extreme-of-an-author-pays-model/
52. Moher D, Shamseer L, Cobey KD, et al. Stop this waste of people, animals and money. *Nature*. 2017;549(7670):23-25. doi:10.1038/549023a
53. Shen C, Björk BC. "Predatory" open access: a longitudinal study of article volumes and market characteristics. *BMC Med*. 2015;13:230. doi.org/10.1186/s12916-015-0469-2
54. Universities UK. Monitoring the transition to open access. December 2017. Accessed July 1, 2019. https://universitiesuk.ac.uk/policy-and-analysis/reports/Documents/2017/monitoring-transition-open-access-2017.pdf
55. Directory of Open Access Journals. Accessed July 7, 2019. https://doaj.org/
56. Clarke M. Plan S: impact on society publishers. *Scholarly Kitchen*. December 5, 2018. Accessed January 6, 2019. https://scholarlykitchen.sspnet.org/2018/12/05/plan-s-impact-on-society-publishers/
57. Inger S, Gardner T. *Scholarly Journals Publishing Practice: Academic Journal Publishers' Policies and Practices in Online Publishing: Fourth Survey, 2013*. Association of Learned and Professional Scholarly Publishers; 2013.
58. University of California Libraries. Pay it forward. June 30, 2016. Revised July 18, 2016. Accessed January 6, 2019. https://www.library.ucdavis.edu/wp-content/uploads/2018/11/ICIS-UC-Pay-It-Forward-Final-Report.rev_.7.18.16.pdf
59. Creative Commons. Accessed January 6, 2019. http://creativecommons.org/
60. US Copyright Office, Library of Congress. Circular 1: copyright basics. Revised September 2017. Accessed January 6, 2019. https://www.copyright.gov/circs/circ01.pdf
61. Hart JD. *Internet Law: A Field Guide*. 6th ed. BNA Books; 2008.
62. Fischer MA, Perle EG, Williams JT. *Perle and Williams on Publishing Law*. 4th ed. Wolters Kluwer; 2015.
63. US Copyright Office, Library of Congress. Circular 33: works not protected by copyright. Revised September 2017. Accessed January 12, 2019. https://www.copyright.gov/circs/circ33.pdf
64. Nimmer D. *Nimmer on Copyright*. Vol 1–11. Matthew Bender & Co Inc; 2013.
65. US Constitution. Article I. Section 8. National Archives website. Accessed January 12, 2019. https://www.archives.gov/founding-docs/constitution-transcript
66. US Copyright Office, Library of Congress. Circular 1a: United States Copyright Office: a brief introduction and history. Accessed January 12, 2019. https://www.copyright.gov/circs/circ1a.html
67. US Copyright Office, Library of Congress. Circular 38a: international copyright relations of the United States. Revised January 2019. Accessed January 12, 2019. https://www.copyright.gov/circs/circ38a.pdf

68. Hirtle PB. Copyright term and the public domain in the United States. Updated January 3, 2019. Accessed July 7, 2019. https://copyright.cornell.edu/publicdomain

69. US Copyright Office, Library of Congress. Circular 15a: duration of copyright. Accessed January 14, 2019. https://www.copyright.gov/circs/circ15a.pdf

70. US Copyright Office, Library of Congress. Circular 30: works made for hire. Revised September 2017. Accessed January 12, 2018. https://www.copyright.gov/circs/circ30.pdf

71. Project Gutenberg. Last modified January 3, 2019. Accessed January 12, 2019. http://www.gutenberg.org

72. *Feist Publications Inc v Rural Tel Ser Co Inc*, 499 US 340 (1991).

73. *The Chicago Manual of Style*. 17th ed. University of Chicago Press; 2017. Accessed January 1, 2018. http://www.chicagomanualofstyle.org/

74. *Harper & Row Publishers, Inc v Nation Enterprises*, 471 US 539 (1985).

75. *J. D. Salinger v Random House, Inc*, 811 F2d 90 (2d Cir 1987).

76. *New Era Publications International, ApS v Henry Holt and Company, Inc*, 695F Supp 1493, 1524–1525 (SD NY 1988).

77. Rossner M. How to guard against image fraud. *Scientist*. 2006;20(3):24. Accessed January 15, 2019. https://www.the-scientist.com/?articles.view/articleNo/23749/title/How-to-Guard-Against-Image-Fraud/

78. Rossner M, Yamada K. What's in a picture? the temptation of image manipulation. *J Cell Biol*. 2004;166(1):11-15. doi:10.1083/jcb.200406019

79. JAMA Network. Standards for AMA publishing group reprints and e-prints purchased by organizations. Accessed January 12, 2019. https://jamanetwork.com/pages/reprint-orders

80. World Intellectual Property Organization. Accessed January 12, 2019. http://www.wipo.int/portal/en/

81. World Intellectual Property Organization. Berne Convention for the protection of literary and artistic works. Accessed January 12, 2019. http://www.wipo.int/treaties/en/ip/berne

82. US Patent and Trademark Office. General information concerning patents. October 2015. Accessed January 12, 2019. https://www.uspto.gov/patents-getting-started/general-information-concerning-patents

83. Gostin LO. Who owns human genes? is DNA patentable? *JAMA*. 2013;310(8):791-792. doi:10.1001/jama.2013.177833

84. Deftos LJ. *Harvard v Canada*: the myc mouse that still squeaks in the maze of biopatent law. *Acad Med*. 2001;76(7):684-692.

85. Gitter DM. International conflicts over patenting human DNA sequences in the United States and the European Union: an argument for compulsory licensing and a fair-use exemption. *N Y Univ Law Rev*. 2001;76(6):1623-1691.

86. Lawson C. Patenting genetic diagnostic methods: NGS, GWAS, SNPs and patents. *J Law Med*. 2015;22(4):846-863.

87. Sherkow JS, Greely HT. The history of patenting genetic material. *Annu Rev Genet*. 2015;49:161-82. doi:10.1146/annurev-genet-112414-054731

88. Marshall E. Dispute slows paper on "remarkable" vaccine. *Science*. 1995;268(5218):1712-1715.

89. Chandrasekharan S, McGuire AL, Van den Veyver IB. Do recent US Supreme Court rulings on patenting of genes and genetic diagnostics affect the practice of genetic screening and diagnosis in prenatal and reproductive care? *Prenat Diagn*. 2014;34(10):921-926. doi:10.1002/pd.4445

90. US Patent and Trademark Office. Trademark. Updated September 28, 2017. Accessed January 13, 2019. https://www.uspto.gov/trademark

91. Kirsch J. *Kirsch's Handbook of Publishing Law.* Acrobat Books; 1995.

92. Brown L. Bridging the gap: improving intellectual property protection for the look and feel of websites. *JIPEL.* May 1, 2014;3(2). Accessed January 12, 2019. http://jipel.law.nyu.edu/vol-3-no-2-3-brown/

93. Anderson R. Deceptive publishing: why we need a blacklist, and some suggestions on how to do it right. *Scholarly Kitchen.* August 17, 2015. Accessed January 1, 2019. http://scholarlykitchen.sspnet.org/2015/08/17/deceptive-publishing-why-we-need-a-blacklist-and-some-suggest ions-on-how-to-do-it-right/

94. Federal Trademark Dilution Act of 1996. Pub L No. 104-98, 109 Stat 985 (January 16, 1996). Codified at 15 USC 1125.

95. Internet Corporation for Assigned Names and Numbers. Accessed January 12, 2019. https://www.icann.org

96. Internet Assigned Numbers Authority. Accessed January 12, 2019. https://www.iana.org

## 5.7 Confidentiality.

> *Confidentiality promises are widely recognized as an ethical obligation, regardless of the legal duty accompanying them . . . maintenance of confidentiality promises falls within editorial discretion.*
> Jeffrey A. Richards[1]

The author-editor relationship is an alliance founded on the ethical rule of confidentiality. Confidentiality occurs when a person discloses information to another with the understanding that the information will not be divulged to others without permission.[2] In the context of scientific publication, this rule provides primarily for authors' rights to have the information they submit to a journal, whether in manuscript form or in communications to the editorial office, kept confidential and a concomitant duty of editors and reviewers to maintain their obligations to ensure that any information concerning a submitted manuscript is kept confidential. This agreement between author and editor preserves the integrity of the scientific review and publication process. Under this agreement, confidentiality may be breached only in rare circumstances, and all such breaches must be handled with care. Note: The level of confidentiality related to a submitted manuscript may be high, as occurs in journals with double-blind or single-blind peer review, or may permit wider sharing of information at different stages of the evaluation and publication processes, as occurs in journals with various forms of open peer review (see additional discussion in 5.7.1, Confidentiality During Editorial Evaluation and Peer Review and After Publication).

## 5.7.1 Confidentiality During Editorial Evaluation and Peer Review and After Publication.
Strict confidentiality regarding the review and evaluation of submitted manuscripts, related content, and all relevant correspondence and other forms of communication is essential to the integrity of the editorial process (see

6.1, Editorial Assessment). Authors must feel free to submit manuscripts that contain their unique ideas and information that may affect their reputations or careers or that may be proprietary. Thus, editors and reviewers have an ethical duty to keep information about a manuscript confidential, and authors have a right to expect that confidentiality will be maintained.[3-7] Policies that support the confidential nature of the peer review and editorial processes are well described by the International Committee of Medical Journal Editors (ICMJE),[3] the Council of Science Editors (CSE),[4] the World Association of Medical Editors (WAME),[5] and the Committee on Publication Ethics (COPE).[6] The existence of a submission of a manuscript to a journal should not be revealed (by confirmation or denial) to anyone other than the editors, editorial staff, peer reviewers, and necessary publishing staff (ie, those essential to producing the journal but not others, such as sales and marketing staff), unless and until the manuscript is released for publication (see 5.13, Release of Information to the Public and Relations With the News Media). In addition, editors should refrain from discussing any aspect of the peer review process of a particular manuscript or any unpublished manuscripts with anyone except authors, reviewers, and editorial staff.

Some journals that have formal relationships with other journals have implemented *cascading peer review* processes to redirect rejected manuscripts from one journal to another, often from a generalist or more competitive journal to a more specialized journal or one with a higher acceptance rate within the same publishing group or a consortium of journals in the same field[8] (see 5.11.5, Editorial Responsibilities, Roles, Procedures, and Policies, Editorial Responsibility for Rejection). For example, the JAMA Network journals offer authors the option to select another journal in the network and the manuscript, correspondence, and any reviews are automatically and immediately transferred to the second journal in the event that it is rejected by the first journal. A number of publishers have implemented similar cascading processes to improve efficiency and reduce time to eventual publication. Authors should be informed in advance if such options are available and if manuscripts, related content, reviews, correspondence, and decisions will be shared with other specific journals.

Even after publication, information and communications about a manuscript, its review (including reviewers' comments), or the editorial process should not be made public without consent of the author, editor, or reviewer (see 5.6.1.5, Ownership and Control of Data, Record Retention Policies for Journals, and 5.6.7, Copying, Reproducing, Adapting, and Other Uses of Content).

To maintain confidentiality, editors should deny requests or demands for confidential information during editorial evaluation, during peer review, and after publication from any third party, including readers, authors of other manuscripts, owners of the journal, publishing staff other than those essential to producing the journal in print or online, news media, advertisers, governmental agencies, academic institutions, commercial entities, and representatives of those seeking information for use in actual or threatened legal proceedings (see 5.7.3, Confidentiality in Legal Petitions and Claims for Privileged Information). Exceptions to this policy may be made in specific circumstances provided that disclosures are limited and that anyone else given access to confidential information agrees to keep the information confidential. Examples of exceptions include the following:

- A prospective author who is invited by an editor to write an opinion piece commenting on a manuscript that has not yet been published. (Note: Such authors should be reminded about the confidential nature of the unpublished work and not to consult anyone about the manuscript without prior approval of the editor, including the author of the unpublished manuscript.)

- A governmental agency representative consulted by the editor or author on a matter considered a public health emergency or a matter that by regulation requires notification (eg, serious adverse drug event).

- An attorney who is asked to advise an editor if legal concerns are raised or who represents the journal in legal proceedings.

- An institutional or funding authority requested by the editor to investigate an allegation of scientific misconduct related to a manuscript under consideration or a published article (for additional information, see 5.7.2, Confidentiality in Allegations of Scientific Misconduct, and 5.4.4, Editorial Policy and Procedures for Detecting and Handling Allegations of Scientific Misconduct).

- An author's violation of public journal policy, such as covert duplicate publication or failure to disclose conflicts of interest (see 5.3.2, Editorial Policy for Preventing and Handling Allegations of Duplicate Publication, and 5.5.8, Handling Failure to Disclose Conflicts of Interest).

- An author's refusal to address an editor's questions about serious ethical concerns, such as whether research participants provided appropriate informed consent or whether a study was appropriately reviewed and approved, or waived for approval, by an independent ethics committee (see 5.8.1.3, Ethical Review of Studies and Informed Consent, Reports of Unethical Studies).

Journals do not own or have licenses to unpublished works (because copyright and publication licenses are not typically transferred until the event of publication). Thus, editors should not keep print or electronic copies of rejected manuscripts. Copies should be destroyed and/or purged from electronic manuscript systems and databases. However, a journal may choose to keep a copy of a rejected manuscript for a predetermined, limited period (eg, 1 year) if it has a policy that allows for author appeals of editorial decisions (see 5.6.1.5, Record Retention Policies for Journals). Similarly, reviewers should not keep copies of the manuscripts they are asked to assess and should not use or appropriate information accessed during the confidential peer review process. Reviewers should destroy any copies of manuscripts and related content that they have reviewed. Reviewers should not use others' manuscripts as teaching tools or reveal any information about unpublished manuscripts in any public discourse or presentation, other communications, or social media posts because doing so would violate confidentiality.

Journals should publish details about the confidential nature of the editorial, peer review, and publication processes in their instructions for authors, and editors should inform all reviewers of the confidential nature of peer review in correspondence to and instructions for reviewers[3] (see 5.11, Editorial Responsibilities, Roles, Procedures, and Policies). If a journal uses a form of open peer review, authors and reviewers should be informed of the level of confidentiality and openness and of the stages in which more or less openness may occur (eg, before or after the editorial decision and publication).

Journals should inform reviewers in explicit terms what they mean by "confidentiality," "confidential information," and "privileged information" (ie, that not subject to disclosure). Journals should also inform reviewers and authors if the review process is single-blinded (ie, only the reviewers' identities are not disclosed), double-blinded (ie, both the reviewers' and the authors' identities are not disclosed), or open (ie, all author and reviewer identities are disclosed to all during review, and for accepted manuscripts reviewer comments may be published with or without attribution). For additional discussion of the various mechanisms of peer review (eg, single-blind, double-blind, open), see 6.1, Editorial Assessment.

**5.7.1.1** **Confidentiality Requirements During Blind (Anonymous) Peer Review.** Many medical and scientific journals, including the JAMA Network journals, use a single-blind review process, in which the authors' names and affiliations are revealed to peer reviewers but reviewers' identities are not revealed to authors. This is also referred to as anonymous review.

Peer reviewers should receive instructions reminding them to maintain confidentiality when they are invited to review and also after they agree to review (see, for example, the instructions in **Box 5.7-1** and 6.1, Editorial Assessment). Reviewers should be instructed not to keep copies of manuscripts they have reviewed and to refrain from discussing the information in the manuscript with others, without permission of the journal. Reviewers should never contact authors directly to discuss their review without explicit permission from the editor.

In some circumstances, a reviewer may wish to enlist the aid of a colleague to assist with the review. Some journals prohibit such consultation, and other journals require that editorial permission be sought in advance of the consultation. Reviewers who are uncertain about a journal's policy should contact the editorial office. For example, *JAMA* informs reviewers that they may enlist the aid of colleagues to assist with the review so long as confidentiality is maintained and all other review policies (such as those pertaining to conflicts of interest) are followed. *JAMA* reviewers are required to inform editors if such consultation has occurred.

A journal does not have an obligation to send every submitted manuscript for external peer review,[3] but editors should share copies of reviewer comments with the authors of those manuscripts that have been sent for review. For example, after an initial editorial decision (eg, rejection or revision) has been made about a reviewed manuscript, *JAMA* and the JAMA Network journals provide the corresponding author with copies of the reviewers' comments for those manuscripts that have been sent for external peer review. In addition, reviewers for *JAMA* and the JAMA Network journals are also asked to provide confidential comments to the editor, which include recommendations of acceptance, revision, or rejection; these reviewer-specific recommendations

**Box 5.7-1.** Examples of *JAMA* Instructions to Peer Reviewers

---

**Instructions for Reviewers About Maintaining Confidentiality Included in Initial Email Requesting Peer Review**

We consider this request and the information in this email to be strictly confidential. Please do not forward this email to others and please delete or destroy any copies of this email.

Note: In addition, every email correspondence includes the following: "Confidentiality Note: This communication, including any attachments, is solely for the use of the addressee, may contain privileged, confidential, or proprietary information, and may not be redistributed in any way without the sender's consent. Thank you."

**Instructions Given to Peer Reviewer Concerning Confidentiality After Reviewer Has Agreed to Conduct Review**

We consider this manuscript and your review of it to be strictly confidential. Any use or distribution of the confidential information in this manuscript for any reason beyond performing this review is prohibited. If you download any electronic files or print out copies, please delete and/or destroy these documents once you have completed your review. If you need to consult a colleague to help with the review, please do not share the hyperlink above because it will give them access to your personal account. You may, however, share a printed copy of the manuscript with a colleague so long as you inform them that the information is confidential and that you indicate such consultation has occurred and include that reviewer's name in your review.

Reviewers' identities are not revealed to authors or other reviewers. Reviewers should not contact the authors. If you have any questions about this manuscript or the review process, please contact the editor.

---

generally are not shared with the authors. However, comments directed to the editor may be summarized or excerpted and included in a decision letter to the author if necessary.

To provide reviewers with constructive feedback, journal editors should send to reviewers copies of other unnamed reviewers' comments. The ICMJE encourages editors "to share reviewers' comments with co-reviewers of the same paper, so reviewers can learn from each other in the review process."[3] Editors should inform reviewers how their reviews will be used and who will have access to the reviews and to the identities of the reviewers (see 6.1, Editorial Assessment). In blind peer review, reviewers have a right to expect that their identities will be protected and not shared with authors without their permission. Some journals that use single-blind review offer reviewers the option to reveal their identities.

An editor may occasionally choose not to send a reviewer's comments to the author, for example, when comments are considered libelous or hypercritical. Similarly, an editor may choose to remove or mask any unhelpful or derogatory comments from an otherwise valuable review.

**5.7.1.2** **Confidentiality Requirements During Double-blind Peer Review.** Double-blind peer review, although used less frequently in biomedical publication, is more commonly used in some disciplines (eg, humanities, psychology, nursing). In double-blind review, authors' and reviewers' identities are hidden from each other in an attempt to minimize implicit bias toward certain groups (eg, women, junior researchers, those from less prestigious institutions or specific geographic locations).[9] In this type of process, authors need to prepare their manuscripts in a way that does not reveal their identity and journals need to provide instructions to facilitate this process and to ensure that overtly identifying information is not included in manuscripts sent for peer review. Some journals offer authors the option to select double-blind review or single-blind review.[10]

**5.7.1.3** **Signed Reviews.** Some journals that use blind review offer reviewers the option to reveal their identities to authors. Reviewers may occasionally intentionally identify themselves in their reviews or sign their reviews, even though they know the journal's peer review process is blind and the option to sign is not formally offered. Although such identification might imply that the reviewer has waived the right to anonymity, it does not relieve the editor or the reviewer of the duty to maintain confidentiality. If the editor of a journal with a blind review process wishes to disclose the identity of a reviewer who has signed a review, the editor should first contact the reviewer to verify that the reviewer actually intended for her or his identity to be revealed. The editor should remind the reviewer and the author that any communication about the manuscript should occur through the editorial office. If the editor does not want to disclose any reviewer identities, the editor may inform the reviewer that her or his identity or signature will be removed from the review.

**5.7.1.4** **Open Peer Review.** A number of journals have experimented with and implemented forms of open review that encourage or require reviewers to identify themselves to the authors and other reviewers.[11-15] The *Medical Journal of Australia* and *Nature* conducted early trials that offered authors and reviewers the option of open peer review and found relatively low uptake or benefits over their more traditional single-blind review process.[13,14] Other journals, such as *the BMJ*,[11,12] publish signed comments from the reviewers with accepted papers. A further open-review innovation was launched by *eLife*, which uses online consultation for reviewers to collaborate with each other and the editors during review.[15] Here again, authors and reviewers should be informed of policies regarding open review and publication of reviewer comments and identities and be reminded that all communications about the peer review and editorial process should be directed to the editor and editorial staff. Journals should clearly describe such policies in instructions for authors and reviewers and in relevant correspondence to authors and reviewers.

**5.7.1.5** **Acknowledging and Crediting Reviewers.** An author may want to credit the help of peer reviewers in an acknowledgment. Public acknowledgment of anonymous reviewers is not necessary or informative. However, some journals will honor authors' requests to thank anonymous reviewers.

Many journals also publish the names of individuals who reviewed for the journal during the previous year, or other specific period, to thank them publicly. Journals can notify reviewers of this plan in their instructions for reviewers or in relevant correspondence. Journals also offer peer reviewers other rewards or forms of recognition for their effort and time: some journals pay reviewers a small stipend; others offer free online access to the journal, provide continuing education credit, or send formal letters that can be shared with employers, supervisors, or others. New services and platforms are available to permit reviewers to claim public credit for reviews with the use of DOIs and researcher identifiers assigned to their specific reviews in a public manner or in a blinded manner associated with reviews performed for specific journals.

An editor may rarely receive a request from an author to include a peer reviewer who has made substantial suggestions for a complete revision as a co-author. If the author's request appears justified, the editor should contact the reviewer to discuss the author's request, and, if appropriate, the author and the reviewer should communicate directly. If such an arrangement occurs, the request must be made early in the process (ie, before the major revision or complete rewrite), and the reviewer would then need to participate fully in the revision and to meet authorship criteria (see 5.1.1, Authorship: Definition, Criteria, Contributions, and Requirements). Such a scenario is unlikely to occur with reports of original research.

**5.7.2** **Confidentiality in Allegations of Scientific Misconduct.** Allegations of scientific misconduct (eg, fabrication, falsification, and plagiarism) must be considered carefully with regard to rules of confidentiality. In cases of credible allegations of such misconduct, an editor may need to disclose specific confidential information in a very controlled and limited manner.[3] For example, after a credible allegation of scientific misconduct, an editor may need to contact an author's or a reviewer's relevant institutional, funding, or governmental authority (eg, an academic president, dean, or ethics/integrity officer) to request a formal investigation. In this situation, the editor will need to identify the person about whom the allegation was made. All communications regarding such allegations should be indicated as confidential. During such investigations, editors should avoid posting details, even if rendered anonymous, in email lists or blogs when seeking advice from colleagues. For more details on how an editor should handle such an allegation, see 5.4.4, Editorial Policy and Procedures for Detecting and Handling Allegations of Scientific Misconduct.

**5.7.3** **Confidentiality in Legal Petitions and Claims for Privileged Information.** A number of cases in US law have served as the foundation for or have directly supported the confidential nature of the editorial and peer review process.

In 1972, the US Supreme Court ruled in *Branzburg v Hayes* that a reporter could be forced to testify if, during a news gathering, the reporter became a witness to a crime.[16] However, the court also noted that individual states could create their own standards with regard to a journalistic privilege (ie, a right) to keep sources of information confidential, allowing lower courts in subsequent rulings to support such privilege. With this understanding, many states have enacted legislation that protects the press from mandatory disclosure of sources, work product, and information.[17,18] These state "shield laws" vary in scope but may offer qualified privilege to reporters to protect confidential information in legal settings unless it can be established that (1) the information sought is relevant and/or material, (2) it is unavailable by other means or through other sources, and (3) a compelling need exists for the information.[17] However, there have been challenges to journalists' privilege to keep sources of information confidential.

After the 1993 US Supreme Court ruling in *Daubert v Merrell Dow Pharmaceuticals, Inc,*[19] concerns arose that attempts to breach the confidential nature of the editorial process would increase through subpoenas for journal records.[20] In this case, the court identified standards required for admissibility of scientific expert testimony. These standards include, among others, whether the evidence on which the expert opinion is based has been peer reviewed and published, and they have been applied to limit admissibility of unreliable junk science as evidence in specific cases.

In 1994, a legal precedent was set regarding confidentiality and protection from attempts to invade the confidential and privileged nature of the editorial process for peer-reviewed journals.[21] In *Cukier v American Medical Association,* an author whose manuscript had been rejected by *JAMA* sued to compel the journal to disclose the identity of those persons responsible for allegedly defamatory statements made to the editors concerning the author's financial interest.[21] Citing the confidential nature of the peer review process, the editors refused to disclose the source of this information. The Circuit Court of Cook County, Illinois, ruled that the editors were not required to disclose this information on the basis of the Illinois Reporter's Privilege Act,[22] which provides that members of the news media (in this case, journal editors) cannot be compelled to disclose sources unless the information cannot be obtained elsewhere and such disclosure is essential to the protection of the public interest. This decision was affirmed by the Illinois Appellate Court, and subsequently, the Illinois Supreme Court declined to hear the case.

Other cases that have supported the confidential nature of the peer review process include *Henke v US Department of Commerce and the National Science Foundation,*[23] *Cistrom Biotechnology Inc v Immunex Corp,*[24] and cases concerning subpoenas to many journals in 2007 and 2008, including *JAMA* and the *New England Journal of Medicine,* regarding a pharmaceutical company's marketing and sales practices for 2 nonsteroidal anti-inflammatory drugs and product liability litigation in the states of Illinois[25,26] and Massachusetts.[27,28] In these cases, attorneys for the pharmaceutical company (which was defending against thousands of lawsuits that alleged false representations in advertising and marketing of these drugs) issued subpoenas to the journals seeking broad categories of documents and information related to manuscripts submitted about these drugs, including "all documents regarding the decision to accept or reject manuscripts, copies of rejected manuscripts, the identities of peer reviewers and the manuscripts they reviewed, and the comments by and among peer reviewers and editors regarding manuscripts, revisions, and publication decisions."[25(p1956)] Product liability attorneys have pursued such confidential information to bolster or undermine the testimony of expert witnesses and as legal leverage. In both of these cases, the courts ruled that confidential information was irrelevant to the pending legal claims and that, given the confidentiality of the peer review process, the burden and expense of discovery required by the journals to comply with the company's broad subpoenas outweighed any benefit of such forced compliance.[25-28]

With multiple examples of case law supporting journals in successfully resisting external attempts to obtain confidential information via litigation and quashing subpoenas, journals, editors, and publishers can rely on legal precedents and principles to help them maintain confidentiality of the peer review and editorial process. Parrish and Bruns[29] have summarized the reasons journals should resist complying with subpoenas that intrude on such confidentiality as follows:

- Violation of confidentiality obligations for one case may make it more difficult to defend future intrusions, may result in perceived breach of trust that could damage a journal's reputation among authors and peer reviewers involved in a specific case as well as other current and prospective authors and reviewers, and may result in an author or reviewer suing the journal for breach of confidentiality.

- Compliance with a subpoena disrupts the journal's activities and processes and consumes the journal's time and resources.

- Substantial costs can be incurred in responding to a subpoena, collecting documents, and providing depositions.

- A subpoena may be used as a means of harassment to prevent an author or a journal from publishing.

If a journal editor receives a subpoena or request from an attorney for confidential information, the editor should consult the publisher, the journal's attorney, or both. If the subpoena or request comes to the publisher or journal owner, the editors should be informed. The disclosure of confidential information to an attorney in this context would be protected under attorney-client privilege. However, it is important to limit disclosure of such information to the publisher (eg, protecting the names of authors or reviewers). According to Parrish and Bruns,[29] in general, subpoenas are broad; therefore, editors may object to the scope and burden of having to respond to such a request as has been successfully argued and ruled in several courts.[21-28] If negotiation with a party who served the subpoena must occur, editors and their legal representatives should request a narrowing of scope of the subpoena, a redaction of all irrelevant confidential information, the destruction or return of all surrendered documents that contain any confidential information, and a limit on who can view any confidential information. In addition, the journal may seek indemnification from the authors or reviewers if they sue the journal for violation of confidentiality. If such negotiations fail or do not protect the journal properly, the journal can file a legal motion to quash the subpoena.[25-29]

The Council of Science Editors offers similar advice and notes that, unlike formal subpoenas, inquiries from law firms requesting confidential information "are probably best to politely decline, citing confidentiality."[4] The Council of Science Editors also recommends that "generally, editors should resist revealing confidential information when served a subpoena unless advised to do so by legal counsel. Not only is the requested information usually confidential, but often uncovering ALL information (for which lawyers are trained to ask) can be time-consuming, interrupt normal business, and be expensive. Citing, for example, the Avoidance of Undue

Burden or Expense Under Rule 45(c)(1) of the Federal Rules of Civil Procedure may be useful."[4] The ICMJE concurs and recommends the following: "Editors therefore must not share information about manuscripts, including whether they have been received and are under review, their content and status in the review process, criticism by reviewers, and their ultimate fate, to anyone other than the authors and reviewers. Requests from third parties to use manuscripts and reviews for legal proceedings should be politely refused, and editors should do their best not to provide such confidential material should it be subpoenaed."[3]

**5.7.4** **Confidentiality in Selecting Editors and Editorial Board Members and in Editorial Meetings.** When editors or editorial board members are interviewed and evaluated for a prospective position with a journal, all participants in the selection process should be reminded that all discussions should remain confidential. In some cases, a signed statement of confidentiality may be requested of members of search/interview committees. Without assurance of such confidentiality, professional reputations and the journal's relationship with influential academic, research, and professional society leaders may be jeopardized. In addition, editorial board members should be reminded of the confidential nature of board meetings and other editorial meetings (see 5.11.11, Role of the Editorial Board).

**Principal Author:** Annette Flanagin, RN, MA

### ACKNOWLEDGMENT

I thank the following for reviewing and providing helpful comments: Howard Bauchner, MD, *JAMA* and JAMA Network; Timothy Gray, PhD, JAMA Network; Iris Y. Lo, JAMA Network; Debra Parrish, JD, Parrish Law Offices, Pittsburgh, Pennsylvania; June Robinson, MD, Northwestern University Feinberg School of Medicine, Chicago, Illinois; and Joseph P. Thornton, JD, JAMA Network and American Medical Association.

### REFERENCES

1. Richards JA. Note: confidentially speaking: protecting the press from liability for broken confidential promises. *Washington Law Rev.* 1992;67:501.
2. Beauchamp TL, Childress JF. *Principles of Biomedical Ethics.* 6th ed. Oxford University Press; 2008.
3. International Committee of Medical Journal Editors. Recommendations for the conduct, reporting, editing, and publication of scholarly work in medical journals. Updated December 2018. Accessed January 14, 2019. http://www.icmje.org/
4. Council of Science Editors. White paper on publication ethics. Updated May 2018. Accessed July 7, 2019. https://www.councilscienceeditors.org/resource-library/editorial-policies/white-paper-on-publication-ethics
5. World Association of Medical Editors. Recommendations on publication ethics policies for medical journals. Accessed January 14, 2019. http://wame.org/recommendations-on-publication-ethics-policies-for-medical-journals
6. Committee on Publication Ethics. Core practices. Accessed December 27, 2018. https://publicationethics.org/core-practices
7. Cummings P, Rivara FP. Reviewing manuscripts for *Archives of Pediatrics & Adolescent Medicine. Arch Pediatr Adolesc Med.* 2002;156(1):11-13. doi:10.1001/archpedi.156.1.11

8. Davis P. Cascading peer-review—the future of open access? *Scholarly Kitchen*. October 12, 2010. Accessed December 27, 2018. http://scholarlykitchen.sspnet.org/2010/10/12/cascading-peer-review-future-of-open-access/

9. Cressey D. Journals weigh up double-blind peer review. *Nature News*. July 15, 2014. doi:10.1038/nature.2014.15564

10. *Nature* journals offer double-blind review. *Nature*. 2015;518(7539):274. doi:10.1038/518274b

11. Godlee F. Making reviewers visible: openness, accountability, and credit. *JAMA*. 2002;287(21):2762-2765. doi:10.1001/jama.287.21.2762

12. Resources for reviewers. *BMJ*. Accessed December 27, 2018. http://www.bmj.com/about-bmj/resources-reviewers

13. Bingham CM, Higgins G, Coleman R, Van Der Weyden M. The *Medical Journal of Australia* internet peer review study. *Lancet*. 1998;358(9126):441-445. doi:10.1016/S0140-6736(97)11510-0

14. Overview: *Nature's* peer review trial. *Nature*. 2006. doi:10.1038/nature05535

15. Sheckman R, Watt F, Weigel D. Scientific publishing: the *eLife* approach to peer review. *eLife*. 2013;2:e00799. doi:10.7554/eLife.00799

16. *Branzburg v Hayes*, 408 US 665 (1972).

17. Lening C, Cohen H. Journalists' privilege to withhold information in judicial and other proceedings: state shield statutes. *CRS Report for Congress*. Order Code RL32806. Updated June 27, 2007. Accessed December 27, 2018. https://fas.org/sgp/crs/secrecy/RL32806.pdf

18. Reporters Committee for Freedom of the Press. Introduction—legislative protection of news sources—the constitutional privilege and its limits. Accessed December 27, 2018. https://www.rcfp.org/first-amendment-handbook/introduction-legislative-protection-news-sources-constitutional-privilege-a

19. *Daubert v Merrell Dow Pharmaceuticals, Inc*, 113 S Ct 27866 (1993).

20. Gold JA, Zaremski MJ, Lev ER, Shefrin DH. *Daubert v Merrell Dow*: the Supreme Court tackles scientific evidence in the courtroom. *JAMA*. 1993;270(24):2964-2967. doi:10.1001/jama.1993.03510240076036

21. *Cukier v American Medical Association*, 630 NE 2d 1198 (Ill App 1 Dist 1994).

22. Reporter's Privilege. Chapter 7835, Illinois Compiled Statutes, Act 5, Article VIII, Part 9, Sections 901-909. 735 ILCS 5/8-901 to 909.

23. *Henke v US Department of Commerce and the National Science Foundation*, 83 F3d 1445 (US App 1996).

24. Peer review and the courts. *Nature*. 1996;384(6604):1.

25. DeAngelis CD, Thornton JP. Preserving confidentiality in the peer review process. *JAMA*. 2008;299(16):1956. doi:10.1001/jama.299.16.jed80000

26. Keys A. In *Re: Bextra and Celebrex* marketing sales practices and product liability litigation. Case No. 08 C 402. US District Court, Northern District of Illinois, Eastern Division (March 14, 2008).

27. Curfman GD, Morrissey SM, Annas GJ, Drazen JM. Peer review in the balance. *N Engl J Med*. 2008;358:2276-2277. doi:10.1056/NEJMe0803516

28. Sorokin LT. In *Re: Bextra and Celebrex* marketing sales practices and product liability litigation. No. CIV.A. 08-mc-10008-MLW. US District Court, District of Massachusetts (March 31, 2008).

29. Parrish DM, Bruns DE. US legal principles and confidentiality of the peer review process. *JAMA*. 2002;287(21):2839-2841. doi:10.1001/jama.287.21.2839

## 5.8 Protecting Research Participants' and Patients' Rights in Scientific Publication.

*An experiment is ethical or not at its inception; it does not become ethical post hoc—ends do not justify means. There is no ethical distinction between ends and means.*
Henry K. Beecher[1]

Contemporary rules for protecting the rights of individuals (namely, research participants and patients) in scientific publication have their foundations in doctrines developed during the mid-20th century: the Nuremberg Code,[2] the World Medical Association's Declaration of Geneva,[3] and the World Medical Association's Declaration of Helsinki,[4] as well as the 1979 US Belmont Report.[5] Modern research protection of such rights is governed by national and international guidelines and requirements.[4-14] In the United States, the primary policy governing biomedical research is the Regulations for the Protection of Human Subjects (45 CFR §46), also known as the Common Rule.[6]

Since its release in 1991, the Common Rule has been amended over the years and was revised substantially in 2017 (82 FR §7149),[7] with these revisions taking effect in early 2019.[15] The revisions to the Common Rule address substantial research developments, including the following[7,16]:

- An increase in the number and types of clinical trials and observational studies

- More diverse social and behavioral research that involves human participants

- Use of sophisticated analytic techniques to study human biospecimens

- Expanded use of electronic health data, other digital records, and large data sets in research

- The increased volume and availability of public and private data and biospecimens

Common Rule reforms aim to provide enhanced protections for study participants and improve efficiency for researchers, funders, research host institutions, institutional review boards (IRBs), and research participants.[16,17]

Researchers and authors have an ethical duty to follow the core foundational principles outlined in these doctrines (namely, autonomy, beneficence, and justice).[4] They must also honor individuals' rights to privacy when conducting and reporting research that involves human participants and patients with identifiable information. Journal editors have similar ethical duties when reviewing and making decisions about publishing studies that involve human or animal participants and when evaluating manuscripts that contain identifiable information about patients or study participants.[18-23] Additional privacy doctrines and laws in the United States and many other countries protect an individual's right to privacy.[9-11] Legal claims for invasion of privacy (eg, nonconsensual publication of identifying details in text, photographs, video, or audio of individuals) could be brought against an author, editor, or a journal. Privacy law differs from defamation law in that truth may not be used as a defense for invasion of privacy (see 5.9, Defamation, Libel).

**5.8.1**     **Ethical Review of Studies and Informed Consent.** To protect the safety and dignity of individuals who participate in research, academic institutions and funding agencies require any study that involves human participants be reviewed and approved by an IRB or independent ethics review committee. (Note: When referring to individuals who participate in studies, the word *participant* is preferred to *subject* [see 11.1, Correct and Preferred Usage of Common Words and Phrases]. However, a number of guidelines and regulations cited herein refer to human "subjects.")

Final revisions to the Common Rule provide the following useful definitions regarding protection of human participants in research[7]:

> *Research*: "any systematic investigation, including research development, testing and evaluation, designed to develop or contribute to generalizable knowledge. Activities which meet this definition constitute research for purposes of this policy, whether or not they are conducted or supported under a program which is considered research for other purposes. For example, some demonstration and service programs may include research activities."

> *Human subject*: "a living individual about whom an investigator (whether professional or student) conducting research: (i) Obtains information or biospecimens through intervention or interaction with the individual, and uses, studies, or analyzes the information or biospecimens; or (ii) Obtains, uses, studies, analyzes, or generates identifiable private information or identifiable biospecimens."

> *Intervention*: "includes both physical procedures by which information or biospecimens are gathered (for example, venipuncture) and manipulations of the subject or the subject's environment that are performed for research purposes."

> *Interaction*: "includes communication or interpersonal contact between investigator and subject."

> *Private information*: "includes information about behavior that occurs in a context in which an individual can reasonably expect that no observation or recording is taking place, and information which has been provided for specific purposes by an individual and which the individual can reasonably expect will not be made public (for example, a medical record)."

> *Identifiable private information*: "private information for which the identity of the subject is or may readily be ascertained by the investigator or associated with the information."

> *Identifiable biospecimen*: "a biospecimen for which the identity of the subject is or may readily be ascertained by the investigator or associated with the biospecimen."

**5.8.1.1**     **Institutional Review Board and Ethical Approval.** All reports of research involving human participants should include indication of ethical review and approval or exemption or exclusion based on institutional policies or regulations. For research conducted in the United States, according to the revised Common Rule, categories of research that involve human participants that may be exempt or excluded from IRB review are based on the level of risk posed to the study participants.[7] A list of these categories and additional specific protections for studies including pregnant women, human fetuses, neonates, children, and prisoners are available in the Final Revisions to the Common Rule.[7] In addition, the revised Common Rule indicates that the following activities, which may be reported in manuscripts submitted to medical or health journals, may be excluded or deemed outside the scope of the regulation requiring IRB review[7,17]: "scholarly and journalistic activities (eg, oral history, journalism, biography, literary criticism, legal research, and historical scholarship)" and "public health surveillance activities, including the collection and testing of information or biospecimens, conducted, supported, requested, ordered, required, or authorized by a public health authority" (eg, public health authority investigations of a major disaster, disease outbreak, or injuries from a consumer product). However, investigators should not make independent determinations of exemption or exclusion of IRB review because of the potential for conflicts of interest and should follow the formal policies of their respective institutions.[7]

An example of low-risk research that may be considered exempt from formal IRB review and informed consent requirements includes secondary research of nonidentifiable information or biospecimens from existing data sets.[7] Here again, investigators should indicate if such research has been determined to be exempt from formal IRB review by their institutions and if the data are deidentified or protected by prior consent or privacy safeguards. Research that involves the use of cadaver specimens is exempt because the Common Rule defines human study participants as "living individuals." However, other regulations may apply to research that involves cadaver specimens.[6] See also 5.8.2.1, Reporting Waivers, Exclusions, and Exemptions.

One of the efficiencies included in the revision of the Common Rule is the requirement for a single IRB to review and approve studies conducted at multiple sites or centers in the United States, unless the study is governed by other US laws or conducted in other or multiple countries.[7,16,17]

**5.8.1.2**   **Informed Consent.** The nature and purpose of all procedures and their possible risks must be fully explained to potential research participants in advance, including consent for secondary research on identifiable private information and biospecimens at the time of initial collection.[8] Participants must fully comprehend the nature of the participation and voluntarily agree to such participation. However, informed consent documents must be posted online for advance review and be simplified to include "essential information that a reasonable person should know" with additional details in an appendix to the informed consent document.[7,17] Research protocols for studies that involve human participants typically address the following minimum set of protections: risks to all participants, experimental procedures, anticipated benefits to participants (if any), consent for secondary research of private identifiable information or biospecimens, proposed consent document and process to be used, and appropriate additional safeguards if the study is to include vulnerable participants (eg, children, incapacitated adults).[6,7]

**5.8.2** **Journal Policies and Procedures.** All journals should require authors of manuscripts that report studies that involve human participants to state explicitly in the Methods section of the manuscript that an appropriate independent ethics committee or IRB approved the study protocol or project or determined that the investigation was excluded or exempt from such approval and the reasons why. The name of the ethics committee(s) or IRB(s) should be specified in the Methods section. If the study protocol was approved by several ethics committees or IRBs, as might be expected in a study conducted in more than 1 country, it is appropriate to note that review and approval were conducted by the ethics committees or IRBs of all participating centers or institutions.

Journals should also require authors to indicate in the Methods section that informed consent was obtained in a manner consistent with the Common Rule requirements (or regulations of other countries or the Declaration of Helsinki[4]) from all adult participants and from parents or legal guardians for minors or incapacitated adults and how such consent was obtained (ie, written or oral). Authors should also indicate whether research participants received compensation or were offered any incentive for participating in the study.

**5.8.2.1** **Reporting Waivers, Exclusions, and Exemptions.** Authors and investigators should not make a personal determination about whether a study is excluded or exempt from formal ethical review and approval. They should cite the exclusion or exemption policies of their institutions per the relevant provisions of the revised Common Rule[7] (or additional supporting guidance) for studies conducted in the United States or similar regulations of other countries. If an IRB or ethics committee waived or exempted the requirement for informed consent, or if a study uses publicly available deidentified data, authors should explain the reason for such waiver or exemption.

**5.8.2.2** **Policies for Studies That Involve Animals.** Ethical approval for research that involves animals and relevant animal-handling protocols should be reviewed and approved by independent animal care and use committees as required by national regulations, such as the US National Institutes of Health Office of Laboratory Animal Welfare requirements,[21] the guidelines of the International Association of Veterinary Editors,[22] or the ARRIVE (Animals in Research: Reporting In Vivo Experiments) guidelines.[23] Such review and approval or waiver should be adequately described in the Methods section of all manuscripts that report research that involves animals.

**5.8.2.3** **Policies to Guide Authors to Report Ethical Protections.** Although numerous regulations and international documents require compliance with these procedures with support from groups such as the International Committee of Medical Journal Editors (ICMJE),[18] World Association of Medical Editors,[19] and Committee on Publication Ethics (COPE),[20] authors and journals have failed to properly report information on ethical review and approval of research and participants' informed consent.[24-27] Several studies have evaluated the rate of publication of articles with and without reporting review by IRB or ethics oversight committees and participants' informed consent. Although the quality of reporting has improved over time, the proper reporting of ethical protections in research studies remains concerning. An assessment of 1133 articles that reported studies of human participants, human tissue, or identifiable personal data that were published in 5 leading general medical journals (*BMJ, The Lancet, Annals of Internal Medicine, JAMA,* and the *New England Journal of Medicine*) in 2005 and 2006 found that 36 articles (3.2%) lacked a statement of ethical approval, 62 (5.5%) lacked disclosure of informed consent, and 15 (1.3%) lacked both.[28] Other more recent evaluations of specialty medical journals found higher rates of failure to report on ethical approval and participant informed consent.[29,30] Studies that evaluated the reporting of ethics protections in clinical trials found rates of failure to report ethical protections ranging from 4% to 26% of trials.[31,32] A 2013 content analysis of 491 journals' instructions for authors found that only 203 (40%) stated that participant consent to publish identifiable information was necessary, 154 (30%) required submission of participant consent forms, and 50 (10%) had specific consent forms for publication of identifiable information.[33]

Specific guidelines regarding documentation of formal ethical review and informed consent should be included in a journal's instructions for authors, and editors should require authors to properly report on ethical protections for participants in all studies considered for publication.

A number of studies have identified discrepancies in the reporting of research methods in published articles in contrast with what is reported in study protocols. Protocols should include description of the ethical protections and informed consent provided to study participants. Clinical trial authors must submit study protocols to journals, along with their manuscripts; this practice is recommended for other types of studies. For example, the JAMA Network journals require submission of clinical trial protocols, including statistical analysis plans, with manuscripts, and if these manuscripts are accepted for publication, the trial protocol is published as an online supplement[34] (see 2.12, Online-Only [Supplementary] Material). The revised Common Rule also indicates that investigators should post copies of the generic informed consent documents and any related appendixes used in studies on funder or institutional websites.[7]

**5.8.2.4**    **Additional Regulations and Principles.** US biomedical investigators who are subject to jurisdiction of an IRB or formal ethics review committee should follow the principles described in the revised Common Rule.[6,7] Investigators outside the United States should rely on their relevant national regulations[11,12] or applicable regional guidelines, such as the Council of Europe's Convention on Human Rights and Biomedicine.[13] Investigators who are not subject to jurisdiction of an institutional ethical review committee or national or regional guidelines should rely on the international guidelines, such as the Council for International Organizations of Medical Science (CIOMS) International Ethical Guidelines for Biomedical Research Involving Human Subjects[11] or the Declaration of Helsinki.[4] The Declaration of Helsinki requires that (1) research protocols specify that the study was reviewed by a qualified research ethics committee independent of the investigator and sponsor, (2) research participants have "freely given informed consent, preferably in writing," and (3) reports of experimentation not in accordance with the basic principles described in the Declaration "should not be published."[4]

For studies conducted in a host country by investigators from another country, regulations from the host country and the investigator's home (sponsoring) country should be followed, and the IRB or ethics committees that reviewed and approved the study should be cited in the Methods section of the manuscript.[11,14,35,36] For studies conducted in multiple countries, relevant regulations of all host countries and any home or sponsoring countries and/or the Declaration of Helsinki[4] or the Universal Declaration on Bioethics and Human Rights[14] should be followed. All IRB or ethics committees that reviewed and approved the study should be cited in the Methods section. In all multinational and multicultural studies, ethical requirements for protecting the interests of the research participants should be addressed. These requirements include acquiring informed consent, avoiding harm, attending to the study participants' needs, and adhering to obligations when the study is completed.[36] Each of these considerations should be addressed in the Methods section of the manuscript. See also 5.8.2.1, Reporting Waivers, Exclusions, and Exemptions.

**5.8.2.4** **Reports of Unethical Studies.** Despite prior publications of unethical research, such practices cannot be tolerated. In a 1966 pioneering article on ethics and clinical research, Beecher[1] identified 50 unethical studies involving human participants that were published in medical journals. Beecher concluded that "an experiment should be ethical at its inception and is not made ethical by publication"[1] and that "failure to obtain publication would discourage unethical experimentation."[1] Editors should seek more information from authors of a report of an experimental investigation that involves humans or animals that lacks information about formal ethical review or appropriately obtained informed consent from human participants. Authors may have neglected to report this information because of inadvertent omission or a misunderstanding. For example, an author may not report this information because ethical review was deemed excluded or exempt by a regulatory authority or considered unnecessary (such as in a retrospective audit of publicly available data) or an informed consent requirement was formally waived by an IRB (eg, in public health surveillance). See examples of exclusions and exemptions indicated in the revised Common Rule in 5.8.1, Ethical Review of Studies and Informed Consent. In such cases, this rationale for an exclusion, exemption, or waiver should be reported in the Methods section of research reports. If a manuscript contains a secondary analysis and the information about IRB or ethical approval and/or informed consent was reported in the primary publication, this information should be included in all subsequent reports and secondary analyses.

All manuscripts, including those that report studies in which IRB or ethical approval, informed consent requirements, or both were deemed unnecessary, exempt, or previously reported, must include details about how the ethical requirements were met or why these requirements were considered unnecessary or exempt. Investigators and authors should not make personal determinations on the appropriateness of ethical review and informed consent. See 5.8.1, Ethical Review of Studies and Informed Consent.

Even when a study has been approved by an ethical oversight committee or IRB, the ethics of the reported research may be questioned by reviewers and editors. In such cases, editors are obliged to ask the authors to clarify the situation and respond to any concerns. Unless the authors can provide satisfactory responses and reassurance, editors may reject the manuscript in question for publication.

If an author refuses to address concerns about such ethical requirements, the editor may consider notifying the author's institutional or funding authority (see

5.7.2, Confidentiality in Allegations of Scientific Misconduct, and 5.4, Scientific Misconduct).

Publication of an investigation that raises ethical dilemmas may be warranted if such publication would encourage professional and public debate and reform. Such publication should be accompanied by an editorial or an editor's note that describes the ethical issues and concerns. Research that violates established ethical principles should not be published.

**5.8.3** **Patients' Rights to Privacy and Anonymity and Consent for Identifiable Publication.** *Privacy* is a state or condition of limited access to matters of a personal nature, including but not limited to personal information about individuals, their bodies, their decisions, and their familial and intimate relations, as well as their right to control such access.[37] When individuals grant others some form of access to themselves (eg, during a patient-clinician or participant-investigator encounter), they (patients and study participants) may allow limited intrusions in private matters but are not waiving all such rights. Thus, a loss of privacy depends on the kinds or amount of access, who has access, through what means, and pertaining to which aspect of a person's identity.[37] Some privacy is surrendered when individuals grant others access to their personal information, bodies, or biospecimens (eg, during encounters between patient and clinician or research participant and investigator).[37] During these encounters, confidentiality, a subset of privacy, should be maintained, and identifiable information should not be shared with others or made public without consent.

Authors and editors should ensure protection of patients' and research participants' rights to privacy, anonymity, and confidentiality in publication, including (1) withholding or deleting patients' and study participants' identifiable information from case reports and detailed descriptions in reports of studies unless they have provided permission for publication and (2) not including or removing identifiable information from text descriptions, demographic data listed in tables or displayed in figures, laboratory reports, genetic pedigrees, other data displays, photographs and other digital images, video, and audio unless the patients or research participants have provided permission for publication.[18,38-40] Photographs with black bars or other objects placed over the eyes of patients or partially obscuring part of a face should not be used in publication in print, online, video, or other multimedia. Patients can identify themselves (or be identified by others) from identifying features, dermatologic presentations, scars, and even clothing worn at the time a photograph was taken or video was recorded.[41-43] Authors must use care when submitting manuscripts that have any detailed descriptions of patients or study participants in text, tables, figures and clinical images, audio, or videos.

Case descriptions and case reports serve as important contributions to the medical literature and make up a substantial portion of some journal content, especially in some specialties. Traditionally, such reports have included specific details about patients. However, as Pitkin and Scott[44] have noted, "The degree of detail and specificity is sometimes sufficient to permit identification, and at the same time, it is often much greater than necessary for any message the author means to convey." Only those details essential for understanding and interpreting a specific case report or case series should be provided. In most instances, the description can be more general than specific to ensure anonymity, without substantive loss of meaning. Although the degree of specificity needed will depend on the context of what is being reported, specific ages, race/ethnicity, and other sociodemographic details should be presented only if clinically or scientifically relevant and important.

Patients have occasionally recognized descriptions of themselves in medical articles without accompanying photographs and even after "superfluous social details" have been removed.[39] To protect a patient's right to privacy, nonessential identifying data (eg, sex, age, race/ethnicity, occupation, and location of treatment) generally should be removed from a manuscript, unless clinically or epidemiologically relevant or important. However, omitting certain details may be problematic.[39,40] For example, omitting a patient's occupation from a case report might seem reasonable at first, but such information may be needed later during an occupational exposure assessment or an epidemiologic investigation. More important, authors and editors should not alter or falsify details in case descriptions to secure anonymity because doing so may introduce false or inaccurate data into the medical literature.[27] For example, changing the city in which the patient lived may seem innocuous, until another investigator subsequently cites the case report and the erroneous city in an epidemiologic analysis of locations of disease outbreaks. Changing specific demographic data, such as sex, could be considered falsification.

Several cases have occurred in which patients who had not consented to publication of their personal details in medical journals were recognized by themselves or others in specific articles or subsequent news coverage.[39,45] In several recent cases, retractions have been published with parts or entire articles removed from public availability.[46-48] The ICMJE and a number of medical journals have important rules for protecting patients' rights to privacy by adding a specific requirement for consent for publication from any potentially identifiable patient.[18,40-43]

Therefore, when detailed case descriptions or identifiable data, identifiable photographs, videos of faces or identifiable body parts, or patient audio that might permit any patient to be identified are included in a manuscript or online supplement to the manuscript, authors should obtain written permission from the identifiable patients (or legally authorized representatives) to publish the information and share a copy of the permission with the journal. Such consent should include an opportunity for the patient to read the manuscript before publication or waive the right to do so. Nonspecific institutional consent forms that do not include a provision for a patient to review the information to be published or waive that right are not acceptable. Although institutions often obtain consent from patients to use such information obtained in a medical encounter or research for "educational purposes or publication," such consent does not always cover publication in journals or via the internet. Some institutional consent forms permit a revocation of the consent at a later date without qualification. Accordingly, generic institutional consent forms may not be acceptable for publication of identifiable information in a journal. An example of the patient permission for publication form used by the JAMA Network journals appears in **Box 5.8-1**. The JAMA Network journals have versions of this form translated into multiple languages, which are available on request.

The ICMJE recommends that patient permission forms "be archived with the journal, the authors, or both, as dictated by local regulations or laws."[18] The JAMA Network journals store patient permission forms in a secure location that is accessible to only a few staff members. According to the ICMJE, some journals may

**Box 5.8-1.** The JAMA Network Journals' Permission for Publication of Identifying Material in the JAMA Network Journals

I give my permission for the following material to appear in the print, online, and licensed versions of the JAMA Network journals and for the JAMA Network journals to grant permission to third parties to reproduce this material.

Title or subject of article or photograph, video, or audio:_____

_____

I understand that my name will not be published but that complete anonymity cannot be guaranteed.

*Please check the appropriate box below after reading each statement.*

☐ I have read the manuscript or a general description of what the manuscript contains and reviewed all photographs, illustrations, video, or audio files in which I am included that will be published.

*or*

☐ I have been offered the opportunity to read the manuscript and to see all photographs, illustrations, video, or audio files in which I am included, but I waive my right to do so.

Signed_____         Date_____

Print name_____

If you are granting permission for another person, what is your relationship to that person?_____

choose to require authors to archive the consent form and then provide the journal with "a written statement that attests that they have received and archived written patient consent."[18]

For manuscripts accepted for publication, journals should indicate that such consent for publication from identifiable patients or study participants has been obtained, either in the Methods section, if appropriate, or in the Acknowledgment section at the end of the article as follows:

> **Methods:** This investigation was approved by the medical center's institutional review board. The 12 patients in this case series provided written informed consent for the investigation. In addition, each patient was given an opportunity to review the manuscript and consented to its publication.

> **Methods:** This study did not require institutional review board approval based on guidelines from the National Human Research Protections Advisory Committee because it was based on government-issued, deidentified, public use data.

> **Acknowledgment:** We are grateful to the 2 patients who provided permission after reviewing the manuscript to publish this.

> **Acknowledgment:** We thank the father of the child in Figure 2 for granting permission for publication of this photograph.

Some editors and authors have commented that obtaining consent from identifiable patients is too burdensome.[49-52] Asking those who so argue to consider that the identifiable person could be themselves or a close relative might help convey the rationale for this requirement. Others have argued that the process of obtaining such consent may be offending to the patient or the patient's family members.[49] However, subsequent discovery of unauthorized publication of a patient's information that results in identification or unwanted publicity could be even more disturbing[40,46-48,53] and may also violate national privacy laws, such as the US Health Insurance Portability and Accountability Act (HIPAA)[9,10] or the privacy laws of other countries.[11-13] Moreover, publication of unauthorized identifiable patient information could result in legal claims related to invasion of privacy, allegations of professional misconduct, or criminal penalties.[9,10,48,53]

Whether a manuscript contains identifiable patient information can be determined on a case-by-case basis. In some cases, potentially identifiable data can be removed from the manuscript. However, if such details are required, authors and editors should assess the risk of identifiability after considering the type and amount of detail that is needed, circumstances surrounding the clinical situation or investigation, and, if applicable, relevant identifiable information contained in previously published reports that involve the same patient(s) or news reports that have resulted in publicity.[43] (Note: Previous publication or news coverage does not eliminate a patient's right to privacy in a subsequent publication in a scientific journal and does not negate the need for patient permission.) After a manuscript has been submitted, if the editors determine that the information could result in recognition—even if only by the patient—they should ask the author to delete identifiable details and material. This can be done with most manuscripts. However, if deidentification is not possible, editors should ask the author to obtain consent from the patient, including offering the patient the opportunity to read the manuscript or review the video or audio. If the patient cannot be located or refuses to consent to publication and deidentification is not possible, the manuscript should not be published.

Authors should not create composite patients from their clinical experience and present these as actual cases, even in narrative essays. If a fictionalized or hypothetical case is presented as an example or for educational purposes, this should be indicated to readers with words such as "case scenario" or "hypothetical case" or by providing a prominent disclaimer in the article (see 5.8.5, Patients' Rights in Narrative Essays and News Reports in Biomedical Journals).

**5.8.4** **Rights in Published Reports of Genetic Studies.** The rules for ethical approval of studies and for obtaining informed consent also apply to genetic studies of family pedigrees and population-based samples. However, obtaining written consent for publication of identifiable information from all members of a large pedigree (many of whom may be deceased or unaware of the collection of family data) may be difficult or impossible. Proposals for obtaining some form of group consent and for avoiding the publication of information about identifiable family members who will not give their permission have been considered.[54] All such studies must be reviewed by an independent ethics review committee or IRB, and if the individual members of the family or population-based sample are considered to be human subjects and identifiable, consent for publication may be required; otherwise, a waiver may be granted[55,56] (see 5.8.1, Ethical Review of Studies and

Informed Consent). The Methods section of all reports of genetic studies should include statements about ethics committee or IRB review and approval or waiver and information about informed consent procedures or waivers and should include consent for publication of identifiable information if not covered by other acceptable informed consent documentation.

As with reports of other types of studies, nonessential identifying information should be removed from reports of genetic studies. However, data should not be altered or scrambled in an attempt to protect the identities of individuals or family members, although relevant information may be masked.[54] For example, in pedigree charts, diamonds or another sex-neutral symbol can be used instead of squares and circles if the sex of family members is not essential to the report (eg, if the disease is known not to be sex linked), or sections of pedigrees may be excluded from pedigree charts or not described in detail if appropriate consent could not be obtained as long as such omissions are noted (see 4.2.2, Diagrams, and 14.6.6, Pedigrees).

**5.8.5** **Patients' Rights in Narrative Essays and News Reports in Biomedical Journals.** Descriptions and photographs of individuals are often included in narrative essays and news stories in medical and health journals. However, if these descriptions or photographs identify patients or anyone in an actual patient-clinician encounter, the authors should be asked to deidentify those patients. Such deidentification should not include altering data or facts or presenting composites of multiple patients as a single case. Identifying details may be omitted but may not be altered or falsified. If patients cannot be deidentified, their written consent for publication must be obtained (Box 5.8-1). Fictionalized cases and reports generally should not be presented except in rare cases and unless this is made clear to readers (eg, a hypothetical case to explain a clinical scenario or a fictional essay in which it is made clear to the readers that it is fictional). In news stories, third-party photographs should not be used if they include identifiable patients, unless consent for publication has been obtained. Appropriately credited stock or staged photographs that depict patients or simulate a patient-clinician encounter are acceptable if made transparent to the reader.

**5.8.6** **Patients' Rights in Social Media.** Content published in journal-related social networking sites, blogs, and online discussion groups is subject to the same norms, standards, and regulations as is all other published and posted content. Thus, the principles described in 5.8.2 (Patients' Rights to Privacy and Anonymity and Consent for Identifiable Publication) apply, and permission for publication is required from all identifiable patients and research participants in all posts about them in social networking sites, blogs, and online discussion groups.

Principal Author: Annette Flanagin, RN, MA

### ACKNOWLEDGMENT

I thank the following for review and helpful comments: Howard Bauchner, MD, *JAMA* and JAMA Network; Lawrence O. Gostin, JD, O'Neill Institute for National and Global Health Law, Georgetown University Law Center, Washington, DC; Timothy Gray, PhD, JAMA Network; James G. Hodge Jr, JD, LLM, Sandra Day O'Connor College of Law, Arizona State University, Phoenix; and Iris Y. Lo, JAMA Network.

## REFERENCES

1. Beecher HK. Ethics and clinical research. *N Engl J Med*. 1966;274(24):1354-1360. doi:10.1056/NEJM196606162742405

2. The Nuremberg Code. *JAMA*. 1996;276(20):1691. doi:10.1001/jama.1996.03540200077043

3. World Medical Association. Declaration of Geneva. Updated October 14, 2017. Accessed January 14, 2019. https://www.wma.net/policies-post/wma-declaration-of-geneva/

4. World Medical Association. WMA Declaration of Helsinki: ethical principles for medical research involving human subjects. 64th WMA General Assembly, Fortaleza, Brazil. October 2013. Accessed January 14, 2019. https://www.wma.net/policies-post/wma-declaration-of-helsinki-ethical-principles-for-medical-research-involving-human-subjects/

5. National Commission for the Protection of Human Subjects of Biomedical and Behavioral Research. The Belmont Report: ethical principles and guidelines for the protection of human subjects of research. April 18, 1979. Accessed January 14, 2019. http://www.hhs.gov/ohrp/humansubjects/guidance/belmont.html

6. US Department of Health and Human Services. Regulations for the Protection of Human Subjects (45 CFR §46). January 19, 2017. Accessed December 27, 2018. https://www.gpo.gov/fdsys/pkg/FR-2017-01-19/html/2017-01058.htm

7. US Department of Health and Human Services. Final Revisions to the Common Rule. Accessed January 14, 2019. https://www.hhs.gov/ohrp/regulations-and-policy/regulations/finalized-revisions-common-rule/index.html

8. US Department of Health and Human Services, Office for Human Research Protections. Regulatory changes in ANPRM: comparison of existing rules with some of the changes being considered. Accessed December 27, 2018. https://www.hhs.gov/ohrp/regulations-and-policy/regulations/regulatory-changes-in-anprm/index.html

9. US Department of Health and Human Services. Health information privacy: summary of the HIPAA privacy rule. Accessed December 27, 2018. http://www.hhs.gov/ocr/privacy/hipaa/understanding/summary/index.html

10. Office for Civil Rights. Standards for privacy of individually identifiable health information. 45 CFR §160 and 164. Revised April 3, 2003. Accessed December 27, 2018. http://www.hhs.gov/ocr/privacy/hipaa/understanding/coveredentities/introdution.html

11. Council for International Organizations of Medical Science. *International Ethical Guidelines for Biomedical Research Involving Human Subjects*. 4th ed. 2016. Accessed December 27, 2018. https://cioms.ch/wp-content/uploads/2017/01/WEB-CIOMS-EthicalGuidelines.pdf

12. Office for Human Research Protections, US Department of Health and Human Services. International compilation of human subject research standards. Content last reviewed on March 3, 2016. Accessed December 27, 2018. https://www.hhs.gov/ohrp/international/compilation-human-research-standards/index.html

13. Council of Europe. Additional protocol to the Convention on Human Rights and Biomedicine, Concerning Biomedical Research, Strasbourg, France. Adopted January 25, 2005; entered into force September 1, 2007. Accessed December 27, 2018. https://www.coe.int/en/web/conventions/full-list/-/conventions/treaty/195

14. United Nations Educational, Scientific and Cultural Organization (UNESCO). Universal Declaration on Bioethics and Human Rights. Paris, France: UNESCO;

October 19, 2005. Accessed December 27, 2018. http://portal.unesco.org/en/ev.php-URL_ID=31058&URL_DO=DO_TOPIC&URL_SECTION=201.html

15. Baumann J. HHS research oversight rule set for one-year-delay. *Bloomberg News.* October 10, 2017. Accessed December 27, 2018. https://www.bna.com/hhs-research-oversight-n73014470727/

16. Hodge JG, Gostin LO. Revamping the US Federal Common Rule: modernizing human participant research regulations. *JAMA.* 2017;317(15):1521-1522. doi:10.1001/jama.2017.1633

17. Emanuel EJ. Reform of clinical research regulations, finally. *N Engl J Med.* 2015;373(24):2296-2299. doi:10.1056/NEJMp1512463

18. International Committee of Medical Journal Editors. Recommendations for the conduct, reporting, editing, and publication of scholarly work in medical journals. Updated December 2018. Accessed January 14, 2019. http://www.icmje.org/recommendations

19. World Association of Medical Editors. WAME recommendations on publication of ethics policies for medical journals. Accessed January 14, 2019. http://wame.org/recommendations-on-publication-ethics-policies-for-medical-journals

20. Committee on Publication Ethics. Core practices. Accessed December 27, 2018. https://publicationethics.org/core-practices

21. National Institutes of Health, Office of Laboratory Animal Welfare. PHS Policy on Humane Care and Use of Laboratory Animals. Revised 2015. Updated December 24, 2018. Accessed December 27, 2018. https://olaw.nih.gov/policies-laws/phs-policy.htm

22. International Association of Veterinary Editors. Consensus author guidelines for animal use. July 23, 2010. Accessed December 27, 2018. http://www.veteditors.org/consensus-author-guidelines-on-animal-ethics-and-welfare-for-editors/

23. Kilkenny C, Browne WJ, Cuthill IC, Emerson M, Altman DG. Improving bioscience research reporting: the ARRIVE guidelines for reporting animal research. *PLoS Biol.* 2010;8(6):e1000412. doi:10.1371/journal.pbio.1000412

24. Yank V, Rennie D. Reporting of informed consent and ethics committee approval in clinical trials. *JAMA.* 2002;287(21):2835-2838. doi:10.1001/jama.287.21.2835

25. Weil E, Nelson RM, Ross LF. Are research ethics standards satisfied in pediatric journal publications? *Pediatrics.* 2002;110(2 pt 1):364-370.

26. Myles PS, Tan N. Reporting of ethical approval and informed consent in clinical research published in leading anesthesia journals. *Anesthesiology.* 2003;99(5):1209-1213.

27. Botkin JR, McMahon WM, Smith KR, Nash JE. Privacy and confidentiality in the publication of pedigrees: a survey of investigators and biomedical journals. *JAMA.* 1998;279(22):1808-1812. doi:10.1001/jama.279.22.1808

28. Finlay KA, Fernandez CV. Failure to report and provide commentary on research ethics board approval and informed consent in medical journals. *J Med Ethics.* 2008;34(10):761-764. doi:10.1136/jme.2007.023325

29. Dingemann J, Dingemann C, Ure B. Failure to report ethical approval and informed consent in paediatric surgical publications. *Eur J Pediatr Surg.* 2011;21(4):215-219. doi:10.1055/s-0031-1277145

30. Murphy S, Nolan C, O'Rouke C, Fentron JE. The reporting of research ethics committee approval and informed consent in otolaryngology journals. *Clin Otolaryngol.* 2015;40(1):36-40. doi:10.1111/coa.12320

31. Taljaard M, McRae AD, Weijer C, et al. Inadequate reporting of research ethics review and informed consent in cluster randomised trials: review of random sample of published trials. *BMJ*. 2011;342:d2496. doi:10.1136/bmj.d2496

32. Bridoux V, Schwarz L, Moutel G, Michot F, Herve C, Tuech JJ. Reporting of ethical requirements in phase III surgical trials. *J Med Ethics*. 2014;40(10):687-690. doi:10.1136/medethics-2012-101070

33. Yoshida A, Dowa Y, Murakami H, Kosugi S. Obtaining subjects' consent to publish identifying personal information: current practices and identifying potential issues. *BMC Med Ethics*. 2013;14:47. doi:10.1186/1472-6939-14-47

34. *JAMA* Instructions for Authors. Updated December 7, 2018. Accessed January 14, 2019. https://jamanetwork.com/journals/jama/pages/instructions-for-authors

35. Kent DM, Mwamburi DM, Bennish ML, Kupelnick B, Ioannidis JP. Clinical trials in sub-Saharan Africa and established standards of care: a systematic review of HIV, tuberculosis, and malaria trials. *JAMA*. 2004;292(2):237-242. doi:10.1001/jama.292.2.237

36. Aagaard-Hansen J, Johansen MV, Riis P. Research ethical challenges in cross-disciplinary and cross-cultural health research: the diversity of codes. *Dan Med Bull*. 2004;51(1):117-120.

37. Beauchamp TL, Childress JF. *Principles of Biomedical Ethics*. 7th ed. Oxford University Press; 2012.

38. Slue WE Jr. Unmasking the Lone Ranger. *N Engl J Med*. 1989;321(8):550-551. doi:10.1056/NEJM198908243210823

39. Riis P, Nylenna M. Patients have a right to privacy and anonymity in medical publication. *JAMA*. 1991;265(20):2720. doi:10.1001/jama.1991.03460200100043

40. Smith J. Keeping confidences in published papers: do more to protect patients' rights to anonymity. *BMJ*. 1991;302(6786):1168.

41. Robinson JK, Bhatia AC, Callen JP. Protection of patients' right to privacy in clinical photographs, video, and detailed case descriptions. *JAMA Dermatol*. 2014;150(1):14-16. doi:10.1001/jamadermatol.2013.8605

42. Koch CA, Larrabee WF. Patient privacy, photographs, and publication. *JAMA Facial Plast Surg*. 2013;15(5):335-336. doi:10.1001/jamafacial.2013.1411

43. Fontanarosa PB, Glass RM. Informed consent for publication. *JAMA*. 1997;278(8):682-683. doi:10.1001/jama.1997.03550080092048

44. Pitkin RM, Scott JR. Privacy and publication. *Obstet Gynecol*. 2001;98(2):198.

45. Borg GJ. More about parkinsonism after taking ecstasy. *N Engl J Med*. 1999;341(18):1400-1401. doi:10.1056/NEJM199910283411815

46. Palus S. Patients did not okay publishing brain surgery details. *Retraction Watch*. June 30, 2016. Accessed December 27, 2018. http://retractionwatch.com/2016/06/30/patients-did-not-okay-publishing-brain-surgery-details/

47. Stern V. Authors couldn't find a patient to give consent for case report: then the patient found the report. *Retraction Watch*. February 27, 2017. Accessed December 27, 2018. http://retractionwatch.com/2017/02/27/authors-couldnt-find-patient-give-consent-case-report-patient-found-report/

48. Stern V. Authors say patient threatened legal action after being subject of scholarly paper. *Retraction Watch*. July 13, 2107. Accessed December 27, 2018. http://retractionwatch.com/2017/07/13/authors-say-patient-threatened-legal-action-subject-scholarly-paper/

49. Snider DE. Patient consent for publication and the health of the public. *JAMA*. 1997;278(8):624-626. doi:10.1001/jama.1997.03550080034018

50. Clever LH. Obtain informed consent before publishing information about patients. *JAMA*. 1997;278(8):628-629. doi:10.1001/jama.1997.03550080038019

51. Tierney E. Consent for publication of a case report. *Anaesthesia*. 2004;59(8):822-823. doi:10.1111/j.1365-2044.2004.03878.x

52. Ghai B, Saxena AK. Patient's consent for publication. *Anaesthesia*. 2005;60(3):289. doi:10.1111/j.1365-2044.2005.04126.x

53. Court C. GMC finds doctors not guilty in consent case. *BMJ*. 1995;311(7015):1245-1246. doi:10.1136/bmj.311.7015.1245

54. Emanuel EJ, Grady CC, Crouch RA, Reidar KL, Miller FG, Wendler DD. *The Oxford Textbook of Clinical Research Ethics*. Oxford University Press; 2011.

55. Botkin JR. Protecting the privacy of family members in survey and pedigree research. *JAMA*. 2001;285(2):207-211. doi:10.1001/jama.285.2.207

56. Beskow LM, Burke W, Merz JF, et al. Informed consent for population-based research involving genetics. *JAMA*. 2001;286(18):2315-2321. doi:10.1001/jama.286.18.2315

## 5.9 Defamation, Libel.

*Truth is generally the best vindication against slander.*
Abraham Lincoln[1]

*Defamation* is the act of harming another's reputation by libel or slander and thereby exposing that person to public hatred, contempt, ridicule, or financial loss.[2-7] *Libel* is false and negligent or malicious publication that involves words, pictures, or signs.[2,4] Technically and historically, libel has differed from slander in that slander was defined as defamation by oral expressions or gestures and libel was defined as defamation in writing or fixed format. For libel and slander, resulting liability depends on a third party reading or hearing the defamatory words. With the advent of modern forms of communication, the distinction between these terms has become blurred because of the mix of print and electronic text, audio, and video content in multiple forms of media.[3(§5.01),4]

Truth is considered a defense against libel in most cases.[3(§5.09)] However, the context of the alleged libelous communication; effect of the communication on an average reader; intentions and actions of the author/writer, editor, and publisher; and location of the publication have influenced liability.[3-5] For example, a statement may be truthful in isolation, but coupled with other statements or placed in a different context, the same statement could result in an overall false impression, which could result in a determination of defamation.[3(§5.09)] In contrast, a statement with minor inaccuracies or omission of inconsequential details could still be considered substantially true and thus not be determined to be defamatory.[3(§5.09)] Libel law is complex, and it is difficult for an author, editor, or publisher to know with certainty whether the text of a specific manuscript could be defended successfully in a libel lawsuit. Editors and publishers should consult lawyers with expertise in media law when concerned about risks of libel and should carry liability insurance that covers claims for libel (see 5.9.8, Defense Against Libel Suits and Claims, and 5.9.9, Minimizing the Risk of Libel).

In the United States, libel law generally requires courts to balance 2 competing values: freedom of expression vs protection of personal reputation.[3,5,8] Freedom of expression has its foundation in the First Amendment of the US Constitution, and this freedom has been generally assured in instances that involve public officials governed by US law since a landmark US Supreme Court decision in 1964.[9] In *New York Times Co v Sullivan*,[9] an elected official in Alabama sued the *New York Times* for publishing an advertisement that included statements, some of which were inaccurate, about police actions against students who participated in a civil rights demonstration; the elected official had supervisory responsibility over the police force about which the statements were made. After a series of decisions on this case in which it was demonstrated that some of the published statements were false, the US Supreme Court determined that a public official could not recover damages for publication of a false statement that relates to his or her official conduct unless it is proven that the defendant published the statement knowing it was false or with reckless disregard for whether it was false (ie, actual malice). This decision established important protections for the press against libel claims based on First Amendment protections to ensure that debate on public issues remains "uninhibited, robust, and wide open,"[4(p319),9] but decisions in US courts have not always resulted in such favorable protections for the press.[3,5]

Libel threats and suits have been used to silence those with opposing viewpoints and censor the free flow of information. For example, SLAPP suits (the acronym for *strategic lawsuit against public participation*) have been used in attempts to intimidate those who wish to publish criticism or information that could expose wrongdoing on the part of a particular industry or corporation.[3(§5.15),5] Even if the suit is groundless and the plaintiff eventually loses the case, a protracted and expensive legal battle may be damaging to an author, editor, publisher, or journal. For example, in 1984, Immuno AG, a multinational pharmaceutical company based in Austria, brought a $4 million libel suit against an unpaid editor of the *Journal of Medical Primatology*, Jan Moor-Jankowski, and the journal's publisher.[10] The lawsuit followed publication of a letter from an author who raised questions about Immuno AG's plans to conduct hepatitis research in Sierra Leone, West Africa, using chimpanzees caught in the wild. Before publication of the letter, Moor-Jankowski had sent the letter to Immuno AG for review and requested comments and a reply to be published along with the letter. The company rejected the opportunity to reply and threatened litigation. Moor-Jankowski suggested that Immuno AG contact the author for further information, but after no response was received from the company, the *Journal of Medical Primatology* published the letter. After extensive and costly legal proceedings (the publisher was uninsured), the Appellate Division of the Supreme Court of New York ruled that the statements contained in the letter were either opinion or factual statements that Immuno AG had failed to prove false. Immuno AG petitioned for hearing by the US Supreme Court, but that petition was denied in 1991.[11]

In US courts, most libel cases have been difficult for plaintiffs to win. This is not necessarily the case in other countries, and in recent years, *libel tourism*, in which lawsuits are filed in countries other than where the alleged defamation occurred or that may be more amenable to plaintiff's allegations, has become a concern.[6,12] For example, before the UK Defamation Act of 2013,[13] libel laws were known to be more favorable to plaintiffs in the United Kingdom.[8,14] The UK Defamation Act has 2 sections that help protect scholarly journals. Section 6 stipulates a protection for scientific and academic journals provided that an alleged defamatory statement "relates to a scientific or academic matter" and that it has undergone an independent review by the editor of the journal and 1 or more persons with expertise in the matter concerned.[13] Section 9 of the UK Defamation Act specifically addresses libel tourism and limits courts' geographic jurisdiction over claims.[13] In recent years, several cross-national libel cases have been dismissed or decided in favor of journal defendants.[15-18] For example, in 2012, Andrew Wakefield, whose research that claimed a relationship between MMR vaccination and autism had been discredited, sued the *BMJ* and its editor for a series of articles that reported on the discredited research that were published in 2011.[16] Wakefield filed suit for defamation against the UK-based *BMJ* in 2012 in Texas court, after he had moved from London to Texas. Texas courts denied Wakefield's suit and appeal on the grounds that he did not have standing to sue the UK-based *BMJ* in Texas. Subsequently, the Third Court of Appeals ruled in 2014 that Texas courts had no jurisdiction over this case and that "simply making an alleged article accessible on a website is insufficient to support specific jurisdictions in a defamation suit."[16,17]

Publication is an essential element for a legal action of libel.[3(§5.02)] In this context, *publication* means that the alleged libelous communication was transmitted to a third party who read, saw, or heard the alleged libelous communication.[3(§5.02)] According to Hart, "as a general matter, courts view publication of material on the Internet as equivalent to publication through traditional print media."[4(p321)]

Courts have distinguished between those who publish third-party information (ie, publishers) and those who provide facilities to third parties to transmit information (ie, online service providers). Editors and publishers of scientific journals, whether publishing information in print, online, or in both media, generally review, edit, and control the information that is transmitted and delivered, whereas online service providers may not provide such oversight and control of third-party postings.[4(p324)] In *Stratton Oakmont, Inc v Prodigy Services Co*,[19] the court held that even an online service provider could be held liable for a subscriber's defamatory statement because the online service provider exercised "sufficient control over its computer bulletin boards to render it a publisher with the same responsibilities as a newspaper." Thus, scientific journals are more vulnerable to libel suits than are online service providers because of the editorial control their editors typically exercise.

A publication is considered defamatory when it includes each of the following[3-5]:

■ A substantially false statement concerning another

■ Publication to a third party (ie, someone other than the person who made the statement or the person who is the subject of the statement) (Note: there is no legal privilege to make or repeat the false statement; however, there may be exceptions, such as in publication of testimony made during judicial or legislative proceedings; see 5.9.7, Republication and News Reporting)

■ Fault amounting to at least negligence if involving a private individual (ie, failing to meet the minimum standards that a reasonable person would have been expected to meet in researching, fact checking, writing, reviewing, and publishing the statement) or actual malice if involving a public figure (ie, publishing with knowledge that the statement is false or with reckless disregard for the truth of the statement)

▨ Injury to reputation results from the statement

**5.9.1** **Living Persons and Existing Entities.** A statement generally cannot be libelous unless it is "of and concerning" a living person or existing entity (eg, corporation, institution, or organization).[3,5] According to a 1992 case, *Gugliuzza v KCMC, Inc*, "once a person is dead, there is not extant reputation to injure or for the law to protect."[20] Even when the living person or entity is not named in the statement, if the person's or corporation's identity can be determined from other published facts, a case for libel can be made.

**5.9.2** **Public and Private Figures.** A public figure is a person who assumes a role of prominence in society, such as an elected official, a celebrity, or an infamous criminal. In cases of alleged libel, public figures are afforded less legal protection than private individuals.[3,5] In a 1964 case, *New York Times Co v Sullivan*,[9] the US Supreme Court determined that for a public official to prove defamation, the official must demonstrate that the alleged defamatory statement was made with actual malice (ie, with knowledge that the statement was false or with disregard for the truth of the statement) (see 5.9, Defamation, Libel). A private figure is defined in the negative: someone who is not a public figure.[5] In contrast, a private individual need not prove malice, only negligence, to be successful in a libel suit.[3-5]

In legal settings, biomedical authors and commentators who publish might be considered limited-purpose public figures, for example, if they publish articles or online-only comments in an attempt to influence a matter of substantial public interest, a governmental agency decision, or legislation.[3,5] In some cases, an author who publishes might be considered a limited-purpose public figure among the community represented by the readers of a specific publication, including journals, websites, blogs, social media, and email lists or forums.[4,21,22]

Answers to the following questions may aid in determining public figure status of an individual and vulnerability to a claim of defamation when a personal statement about an individual is published[3,5,7]:

▨ Is the person described someone who has assumed a role of prominence or notoriety?

▨ Does the content of the statement pertain to a matter of public controversy or public concern?

▨ If the statement refers to a public figure, does it contain references to the individual's public figure status (eg, the individual's job performance or public behavior)?

▨ If the statement refers to a public figure, will the connection between such references and the individual's public status be evident to a reasonable reader?

▨ If the reference is peripheral to the person's public figure status or responsibilities, does it involve nonrelevant, highly intimate, or embarrassing facts?

**5.9.3**     **Groups of Individuals.** Defamatory statements about groups of individuals are usually not legally actionable if the group is so large that no individual can be identified in the statements.[3,5,7] For example, broad statements about specific groups (eg, physicians) or entities (eg, the pharmaceutical industry) are not at risk for libel actions because no single individual or company is identifiable.

**5.9.4**     **Statements of Opinion.** Statements that contain pure opinion (ie, purely subjective judgment without assertion of fact) are not legally actionable because opinions cannot be proven true or false.[3(§5.08),5,6,8,23] However, an opinion that includes, asserts, or implies facts that are false and defamatory could result in liability.[5,6,24] As noted previously, publication of an expression of opinion about a public figure may be protected under the fair comment doctrine (see 5.9.2, Public and Private Figures).[5,7] Fischer et al[3(§5.08)] offer the following questions to help readers (as well as viewers and listeners) distinguish statements of fact from statements of opinion:

- Can the statement be verified or proved to be true or false?

- Are the facts on which the opinion is based fully disclosed to the reader?

- If not, are the facts on which the opinion is based obvious to a reasonable reader or readily available to the reader from other sources?

- Are both the disclosed and undisclosed facts on which the opinion is based substantially true?

- Does the context of the opinion suggest to a reasonable reader that it represents opinion and not fact?

- Have the statements that contain opinions been published in a manner that informs readers that they deal with opinion, commentary, or criticism (eg, a clearly identified editorial or opinion page)?

**5.9.4.1**     **Editorials, Letters, and Reviews.** In some publications, such as newspapers and popular magazines (whether print or online), editorials, correspondence, and reviews tend to alert the reader that the content is opinion. This is not always the case for scientific journals. No matter where the material is published, malicious criticism of an individual or entity could be considered defamatory, especially if it is demonstrated that such criticism was not based on facts.[5,24] However, criticism of a public figure or public institution or commercial entity may not be actionable if such criticism is scholarly and supported by evidence and documentation. Similarly, scholarly criticism of an individual's research, theory, opinion, or previous publication that is supported by evidence and documentation may not be actionable for libel.[6,12,17,21,22] In any case, editors and publishers should be cautious about statements critical of individuals or commercial entities made in editorials, letters, and reviews. Use of such phrases as "in my opinion" or "I believe" will not necessarily protect an author against an action for libel. Whenever possible, authors of letters, editorials, and reviews in biomedical publications should support opinions, assertions, and interpretations with documentation and/or formal references, and editors should review all such material and require authors to provide appropriate documentation and references. Editors and publishers should consider obtaining legal review of material being considered for publication that contains potentially libelous statements. In addition, publishers should have liability insurance that covers the costs of defending against suits for libel[6] (see 5.9.8, Defense Against Libel Suits and Claims, and 5.9.9, Minimizing the Risk of Libel).

**5.9.4.2** **Reviews of Books and Other Media.** For reviews of books and other media (eg, video, film, audio, journals, websites, exhibits, performance, software, applications), well-documented critical comments about the book, media, or the work of an author, editor, publisher, producer, or developer are generally acceptable, but critical comments about the specific author, editor, publisher, producer, or developer should be avoided. For example, in the 1994 seminal case of *Moldea v New York Times Co*,[25] the author of a book that received a disparaging review in the *New York Times* sued for libel after trying and failing to get the *New York Times* to publish his rebuttal letter. The book review included a number of critical comments, including a statement that the book contained "too much sloppy journalism to trust the bulk of this book's 512 pages."[8] This comment was supported with specific examples of misspellings and allegations of mischaracterization of events.[8] After an initial decision in favor of the *New York Times*, an appeal that favored the author's claim, and an unusual reversal by the appeals court, the libel suit was dismissed. The final decision in this case reaffirmed impunity from libel suits for opinion pieces and provided a "workable test for analyzing allegedly defamatory statements of opinion."[8]

**5.9.5** **Social Media.** Content published in social networking sites, blogs, and online discussion groups is subject to the same norms, standards, and regulations as is all other published and posted content. The Associated Press recommends caution in sharing content via social media and notes the following: "Because of the difficulty in verifying the authenticity of material posted on social media sites, it is important not simply to lift quotes, photos or video from social networking sites and attribute them to the domain or feed where the information was found"[5] (see 5.6.7.11, Social Media, and 5.8.3, Patients' Rights to Privacy and Anonymity and Consent for Identifiable Publication).

**5.9.6** **Works of Fiction.** Fictional accounts are not actionable for defamation unless a reasonable reader believes that the story is depicting factual events and can identify the person bringing suit in the story.[3] Humor, satire, and parody may be exempt from defamation suits as long as they are clearly works of fiction.[3]

**5.9.7** **Republication and News Reporting.** A publication, author, or journalist can be held liable for republishing a defamatory statement. For example, if an author or journalist republished a defamatory statement about a public figure knowing that the statement was false, the publisher and author could be held liable. Similarly, if the republished false statement was about a private figure, the publisher and author could be held liable for defamation even if the statement was published without knowledge of its falsity (ie, through negligence). However, under the privileges of fair reporting an author or journalist may repeat a previously published defamatory statement if it is part of official proceedings (eg, formal governmental proceedings or press conference) as long as the account is fair and accurate.[5] Under the privilege of neutral reporting, an author or journalist may republish an account of a previously published defamatory statement as long as the second account is a neutral or balanced report of a public controversy or matter of legitimate public concern[5] (see 5.9.4, Statements of Opinion). However, this privilege is not supported in all jurisdictions; thus, reporters, authors, and editors should follow the principles of careful reporting, editorial evaluation, and judgment. Scientific journal authors, reporters, and editors who rely on confidential sources for potentially defamatory statements are at risk for libel action and should carefully consider the risks and benefits of the value of publishing information from undisclosed sources. For example, in the United States, shield laws, intended to protect news reporters from being legally forced to reveal identities of sources, vary by state, and their application has been challenged in a number of cases.[3(§5.09),4(pp45-46)]

**5.9.8**    **Defense Against Libel Suits and Claims.** Truth is a defense against claims of libel in most cases (see 5.9, Defamation, Libel). Aside from consideration of the truth of damaging statements, some jurisdictions also consider whether damaging statements were made with intent to harm.[3(§5.09)] As a result, editors should query authors about any statements that criticize or imply criticism of individuals or corporate entities and ask the authors to provide evidence or documentation to support such statements. If an editor is concerned about the risk vs benefit of publishing such statements, obtaining a legal review as part of the process of peer review is recommended. The legal review should be performed by an attorney with experience in media law. Even though legal review may result in delay and several requests for revision, it may help protect the editor and publisher from a libel claim. In addition, offering those criticized an opportunity to review the material before publication, if deemed appropriate by the editor, or to respond to the criticism after publication may reduce the risk of a successful claim.

Threats of litigation and fear of libel suits have had chilling effects on some editors and journals and kept them from meeting their ethical duties to authors, readers, and the public. In a legal context, the term *chilling effect* refers to the stifling or discouragement of legitimate speech or publication by the threat of legal sanction via vague or very broad laws. For example, during the 1980s, a number of medical journals declined to publish retractions of articles by 2 researchers, Slutsky and Breuning (even though the articles had been proven to be fraudulent and even after Breuning's federal indictment), because of fear that the journals would be liable for publishing statements impugning the work of Robert Slutsky and Stephen Breuning.[26] Such defensive editorial practices should be avoided because they may impair the integrity of the journal and allow fraudulent research to continue to be read and cited.[27]

Another case that involved a claim against the *Journal of Alcohol Studies* demonstrates the need for an editor's awareness of the risks of libel and the need for legal review of potentially defamatory material before acceptance for publication.[28] In this case, an author sued the *Journal of Alcohol Studies* in 1989 claiming breach of contract after the journal did not publish an accepted manuscript. The editor had determined the manuscript to be libelous after acceptance but before publication. The journal decided to publish the manuscript following an agreement with the plaintiff/author that he would drop his lawsuit. The editor said he had no choice in light of the mounting legal fees. Ironically, a libel suit was never filed after publication of the article because the person about whom the potentially libelous statements were made believed that readers could determine that the statements made about him were not truthful.[28]

Until recently, libel laws in the United Kingdom had been reported to have significant chilling effects on journals, especially because of the resources required to defend against claims. A 2010 informal survey of 22 leading scientific and medical journals conducted by the journal *Science* found that these concerns were not uncommon, especially among medical journals in the United Kingdom.[12] Several recent but lengthy libel cases against journals, in which the cases were dismissed or awarded to journal defendants,[12,15-18] and UK legislative reform[13] have provided journals with additional legal precedents and protections from resource-draining libel threats and claims.

The *Science* survey also included reports from journals and publishers dealing with stifling libel suit threats. For example, a publisher with the American Psychological Association reported dealing with "about 20-30 threats of lawsuits related to manuscripts in prepublication status" during a 25-year period.[12]

**5.9.9** **Minimizing the Risk of Libel.** The suggestions in this section are offered to help authors, editors, and publishers reduce the risk of libel in biomedical publication. All statements of fact about individuals or commercial entities should be supported or documented and verified to be accurate in the context in which they were and are made. Similarly, statements of opinion should be supported or based on documented facts and should not be malicious. In addition, authors should disclose any conflicts of interest or concerns about the potential reactions of those criticized to the editor so that the editor and author work together to ensure responsible publication (see 5.5, Conflicts of Interest). Editors should consider offering those who are criticized in a submitted manuscript an opportunity to review the material of concern before publication, to respond to the criticism after publication, or both. Journals that publish postpublication online comments, open peer review comments, audio and video, and blogs should consider risks of libel and apply the same policies and procedures that are used for traditional manuscripts and published articles. In addition, editors should consult experienced media attorneys when necessary, and publishers should have insurance that covers claims for libel. None of these suggestions will ensure that a lawsuit—even if frivolous or groundless—will not be made, but they should help editors, authors, and publishers avoid situations in which such claims have merit.

**5.9.10** **Demands to Correct, Retract, or Remove Libelous Information.** Demands to correct or retract allegedly libelous material should be handled carefully. Removal of libelous information in print is not possible, and the standard course of action has been to publish corrections or retractions in an expeditious and prominent manner.[4,5] Online versions that are close in content and form to the printed version and online-only content should follow the same policies and procedures. Online archives, which are considered part of the original publication, may be corrected, edited, or removed, and continued posting of defamatory material in an online version of archive—without an appropriate correction or retraction—may increase the risk of liability for the author, editor, and publisher.[4] However, demands to remove libelous material must be carefully balanced against the need to preserve the integrity of the scientific record, and correction and retraction are always preferred over removal of content.[29,30] Editors should consider consulting a lawyer with expertise in media law to determine the best course of action.

Editors and publishers should follow the recommendations on publishing corrections and retractions from the International Committee of Medical Journal Editors[31] and the US National Library of Medicine[32] (see 5.4.4, Editorial Policy and Procedures for Detecting and Handling Allegations of Scientific Misconduct). If an allegation of defamation or threat to take legal action because of alleged defamation is determined to be frivolous or groundless, the editor should inform the person making the allegation that there is no merit to the allegation or threat, and no further action should be taken. If the allegation is considered to have merit, the editor may wish to consider publishing a letter from the person or representative of the entity criticized and ask the author to provide a letter of explanation or apology for publication, or the editor may choose to publish a correction or a retraction. In each case, reciprocal linking should be established between any published letters, correction, or retraction and the original article. In rare and truly extraordinary circumstances, the editor may choose to remove or obscure the libelous material from an article or other online posting provided that a brief explanation of why the material has been removed or obscured is included and is made easily accessible. If the libelous material is so inextricably embedded in the context of an article that it cannot be partially removed or obscured, an entire article may need to be removed from the online archive provided that the bibliographic citation to the article remains intact and a brief explanation of why the article has been removed is included with or linked from the citation. In each of these cases, correction or retraction is highly preferred to changing or removal of content.[31,32] In addition, republication in derivative products (eg, reprints, e-prints, collections) of articles that contain defamatory material must be avoided because these are not part of the original publication and republication of known libelous material may result in additional liability and damage claims.

**5.9.11** **Resources for Other Liability Concerns.** There are other sources of information on legal and liability matters for publishers and editors that are beyond the scope of this manual. *Perle, Williams & Fischer on Publishing Law,*[3] *Internet Law: A Field Guide,*[4] and *The Associated Press Stylebook and Briefing on Media Law*[5] are good resources for information that address many of these issues, including those related to copyright, patent, trademark, and domains (see 5.6, Ethical and Legal Considerations, Intellectual Property: Ownership, Access, Rights, and Management), privacy and consent (see 5.8, Protecting Research Participants' and Patients' Rights in Scientific Publication), advertising (see 5.12, Advertisements, Advertorials, Sponsorship, Supplements, Reprints, and e-Prints), online promotion, spam laws, data collection and privacy, circulation audits, taxation and accounting issues, electronic contracts, and employment issues.

**Principal Author:** Annette Flanagin, RN, MA

### ACKNOWLEDGMENT

I thank the following for review and helpful comments: Howard Bauchner, MD, *JAMA* and JAMA Network; Timothy Gray, PhD, JAMA Network; Iris Y. Lo, JAMA

Network; Debra Parrish, JD, Parrish Law Offices, Pittsburgh, Pennsylvania; and Joseph P. Thornton, JD, JAMA Network and American Medical Association.

## REFERENCES

1. Lincoln A. Letter to Secretary Stanton, refusing to dismiss Postmaster General Montgomery Blair, July 18, 1864. In: Bartlett J. *Familiar Quotations*. 15th ed. Little Brown & Co Inc; 1980:523.
2. *The Law Dictionary*. Accessed December 27, 2018. http://thelawdictionary.org
3. Fischer MA, Perle EG, Williams JT. *Perle, Williams & Fischer on Publishing Law*. 4th ed. Wolters Kluwer Law & Business; 2015.
4. Hart JD. *Internet Law: A Field Guide*. 6th ed. BNA Books; 2008.
5. Associated Press. *The Associated Press Stylebook and Briefing on Media Law*. Basic Books; 2017.
6. Mawer WT, Hicks GJ. Academic journals and the management of defamation and plagiarism. *Southern Law J*. 2008;18:87-98. Accessed December 27, 2018. http://www.southernlawjournal.com/2008/05_.pdf
7. Stubbs SE, Boyce WJ. The risks of libel in medical publishing. *Ann Allergy*. 1994;72(2):101-103.
8. Hershey J. Casenote: if you can't say something nice, can you say anything at all? *Moldea v New York Times Co* and the importance of context in First Amendment law. 67 U Colo L Rev 705 (Summer 1996).
9. *New York Times Co v Sullivan*, 376 US 254, 280 (1964).
10. *Immuno AG v Moor-Jankowski*, 74 NY 2d 548, 556 (1989).
11. *Immuno AG v Moor-Jankowski*, 77 NY 2d 235 (1991).
12. Wogan T. Scientific publishing: a chilling effect? *Science*. 2010;328(5984):1348-1351. doi:10.1126/science.328.5984.1348
13. Parliament of the United Kingdom. Defamation Act of 2013. Accessed December 27, 2018. http://www.legislation.gov.uk/ukpga/2013/26/contents
14. Beauchamp RW. England's chilling forecast: the case for granting declaratory relief to prevent English defamation actions from chilling American speech. *Fordham Law Rev*. 2006;74(6):3073-3145. Accessed December 27, 2018. http://ir.lawnet.fordham.edu/flr/vol74/iss6/5
15. Wilson I. The Defamation Act 2013. *Law Society Gazette*. February 24, 2014. Accessed December 27, 2018. https://www.lawgazette.co.uk/legal-updates/the-defamation-act-2013/5039959.article
16. Dyer C. Texas judge throws out Wakefield's libel action against *BMJ*. *BMJ*. 2012;345:e5328. doi:10.1136/bmj.e5328
17. *Dr. Andrew J. Wakefield, MB, BS v. The British Medical Journal Publishing Group, Ltd*.; Brian Deer; and Dr. Fiona Godlee Appeal from 250th District Court of Travis County (opinion). Texas Court of Appeals. Third District at Austin. Judgment rendered September 19, 2014. No. 03-12-00576-CV. US Law. JUSTIA. Accessed December 27, 2018. https://law.justia.com/cases/texas/third-court-of-appeals/2014/03-12-00576-cv.html
18. Cressey D. Nature Publishing Group wins long-running libel trial. *Nature News*. July 6, 2012. doi:10.1038/nature.2012.10965
19. *Stratton Oakmont, Inc v Prodigy Services Co*, No. 31063/94, NY Sup Ct (1995).
20. *Gugliuzza v KCMC, Inc*, 606 So2d 790, 20 Media La Rptr 1866 (La 1992).
21. Swartz BE. Defamation law: implications for medical authors. *Plast Reconstr Surg*. 2003;111(1):498-499.

22. *Ezrailson v Rohrich*, 09-01-038-CV, 17 TLCS 1075 (2001).

23. *Gertz v Robert Welch Inc*, 418 US 323, 347 (1974).

24. *Milkovich v Lorain Journal Co*, 497 US 1 (1990).

25. *Moldea v New York Times Co*, 793 F Supp 335, 337 (DDC 1992); Moldea I, supra note 12; Moldea II, supra note 12.

26. LaFollette MC. *Stealing Into Print: Fraud, Plagiarism, and Misconduct in Scientific Publishing*. University of California Press; 1992.

27. Whitely WP, Rennie D, Hafner AW. The scientific community's response to evidence of fraudulent publication; the Robert Slutsky case. *JAMA*. 1994;272(2):170-173. doi:10.1001/jama.1994.03520020096029

28. MacDonald KA. Rutgers journal forced to publish paper despite threats of libel suit. *Chronicle Higher Educ*. September 13, 1989:A5.

29. International Association of Scientific, Technical, and Medical Publishers. Preservation of the objective record of science: an STM guideline. March 2006. Accessed January 14, 2019. https://www.stm-assoc.org/2006_04_19_Preservation_of_the_Objective_Record_of_Science.pdf

30. International Federation of Library Associations and Institutions. IFLA/IPA joint statement on retraction or removal of journal articles from the web. Updated March 14, 2018. Accessed December 27, 2018. http://www.ifla.org/publications/iflaipa-joint-statement-on-retraction-or-removal-of-journal-articles-from-the-web

31. International Committee of Medical Journal Editors. Recommendations for the conduct, reporting, editing, and publication of scholarly work in medical journals. Updated December 2018. Accessed January 14, 2019. https://www.icmje.org/recommendations

32. US National Library of Medicine. Errata, retraction, and other linked citations in PubMed. Updated August 8, 2018. Accessed January 14, 2019. https://www.nlm.nih.gov/bsd/policy/errata.html

## 5.10    Editorial Freedom and Integrity.

> *Editorial independence is crucial for the viability of a journal and editors have many masters–the public, the readers, the authors and the owners. Negotiating the resultant minefield requires a purposeful and independent stance. This is particularly so in instances of a relatively modern phenomenon: concerted attempts by clinical groups to influence, or even abort, publication of articles, which may threaten their practice. Moreover, modern social media facilitates this manipulation. . . . To be an editor is to live dangerously!*
> **Martin B. Van Der Weyden**[1]

*Editorial freedom* is the independence an editor has to make editorial decisions without control or interference from others; it implies a range of independence, from complete absence of external restraint and coercion to merely a sense of not being unduly hampered or frustrated. *Integrity* is the state of honesty, credibility, incorruptibility, and accountability. A biomedical journal has editorial integrity if it adheres to these values, but different journals have different levels of editorial freedom. The First Amendment of the US Constitution affirms several freedoms, including the freedom of the press.[2] Thus, communication through the US press or other media is a right that should not be interfered with by the government, other institutions, or individuals. Many countries guarantee similar freedoms of the press.[3] Freedom of the press is a foundation for editorial independence, "which is the distinct right of the editor to publish any material that passes defined criteria for quality and that fits within the mission of the publication, without suffering undue interference from others."[4(p2344)]

A journal's editorial independence must be balanced against the need for appropriate authority, responsibility, and accountability as well as trust between the editor and the journal's many stakeholders: readers, authors, reviewers, deputy/associate and other journal editors, editorial staff, editorial board members, publishers, owners, subscribers, advertisers, and others[4] (see 5.11, Editorial Responsibilities, Roles, Procedures, and Policies). The level of editorial freedom differs among different biomedical journals, from maximum independence for those peer-reviewed journals in which the editor has complete authority and responsibility for the journal, its content (including all editorial and advertising content), reuse of its content, and use of the journal name and logo to no independence for those journals that are not peer reviewed or in which all authority and responsibility rests completely with others (eg, publishers or owners). Journals that are published primarily to serve business, political, or other concerns of their owners may be viewed as house organs. For some biomedical journals and editors, the level of editorial freedom may be best described as somewhere between complete editorial independence and no independence. Furthermore, editorial freedom may be assumed to exist by an editor and the journal's readers until or unless a major conflict occurs. A 1999 survey of the editors of 33 peer-reviewed medical journals owned by professional societies (10 journals represented in the International Committee of Medical Journal Editors and a random sample of 23 specialty journals with high impact factors) found that 23 of the 33 editors (70%) reported that they had complete editorial freedom, and the remainder reported that they had a high level of freedom.[5] However, many of these editors reported having received at least some pressure in recent years over editorial content from the professional society's leadership (42%), senior staff (30%), or rank-and-file members (39%).[5]

Editors and journals have experienced incursions from interpersonal, social, political, and economic forces. Editors have been dismissed from their posts and journals have ceased publication after a mere "stroke of the editorial pen."[6] In one case, the *Irish Medical Journal* was voted out of existence in 1987 after the editor published an editorial against physician strikes that angered some influential members of the Irish Medical Organisation.[6,7]

Editors of several leading general medical journals have been unwillingly removed from their positions after publishing articles that were considered inappropriate by various entities (eg, owners, publishers) and for having disagreements with owners or publishers about the editor's level of autonomy and authority over the journal's content and the journal's name and brand (eg, logo).[8-24] In these cases, long-term struggles between the editors and the owners of the journals resulted in loss of trust between the parties. Because of a lack of effective protective oversight and governance and apparent lack of an effective system for conflict resolution, precipitate decisions to remove the editors resulted in widespread criticism of the owners and threats to the integrity and continued existence of the journals (see 5.10.1, Maintaining Editorial Freedom: Cases of Editorial Interference and the Rationale for Mission, Trust, and Effective Oversight and Governance).

An earlier example of a medical editor credited for his struggles to maintain editorial freedom is Hugh Clegg, editor of the *BMJ* from 1944 to 1965. In 1956, Clegg wrote an unsigned editorial entitled "The Gold-headed Cane" in which he castigated the president of the Royal College of Physicians for taking office for the seventh successive year.[25] He also admonished the college for its failure to recognize the modern welfare state and its lack of attention to postgraduate medical education. With much difficulty, Clegg kept his editorial position and freedom and purposely published a reply from the president that rebutted all of Clegg's criticisms. Clegg believed that medical editors are the protectors of the conscience of the profession, and he is well known for his assertion that editors who maintain this ideal will often find themselves in trouble. This trouble may come in the form of incursions into editorial freedom, which editors must be able to defend. For more detailed examples, see 5.10.1, Maintaining Editorial Freedom: Cases of Editorial Interference and the Rationale for Mission, Trust, and Effective Oversight and Governance.

Editors of biomedical journals that have editorial freedom must have complete authority for determining all editorial content of their publications.[4,26-33] (Unless otherwise dictated by a journal's specific mission, this may not be the case for journals that are house organs or that have minimal editorial freedom.) Although many stakeholders may offer useful input and advice, editorial decisions must be free from restraint or interference from the publication's owner, publisher, advertisers, sponsors, subscribers, authors, editorial board or publication committee members, reviewers, and readers. Owners, publishers, boards, and publication committees may have the right to select, hire, evaluate, and dismiss the editor, but they should not interfere with day-to-day editorial decisions and policies.[4,13,27,28,33]

Without a clear delineation of editorial freedom and the authority to maintain it, an editor might not be able to ensure the integrity of the publication. Thus, owners, publishers, and editors must have a clear and mutually understood definition of the editor's level of editorial freedom, authority, responsibility, and accountability.[4,27,28] Editors of journals with complete editorial freedom should not comply with external pressure from any party—including owners, publishers, advertisers, sponsors, authors, reviewers, and readers—that may compromise their autonomy or their journal's integrity.[27,28] Examples of such inappropriate pressures include, but are not limited to, the following:

- Pressure from an owner or a politically powerful or motivated individual or group on the editor to avoid publishing certain types of articles or to publish a specific article

- Pressure or requirement of an editor by a publisher or owner to modify or suppress specific content before publication

- Demand from an owner or publisher or external group or entity to censor or remove published content deemed controversial or contrary to a specific position or that includes negative outcomes about a specific product or service

- Harassment of an editor by a reader who is motivated politically or competitively to force the journal to publish an allegation about an article or author or to retract or remove a published article before a formal investigation or for which the allegation is without merit

- Demand from an owner or publisher or external person or organization to have access to confidential editorial or peer review records (see 5.7.1, Confidentiality During Editorial Evaluation and Peer Review and After Publication)

- Demand from an author or group of authors to bypass the journal's standard editorial and peer review processes and publish their manuscript without review or revision (eg, a society demanding acceptance and publication without review or revision of its meeting abstracts, proceedings, or papers)

- Demand from an author for exceptions to a journal's editorial policies or requirements for specific manuscripts

- Attempt by an author or peer reviewer to have an editorial decision reversed by threatening the journal's editor or owner

- The use or repurposing of the journal's content or name by the publisher, owner, or external entity without the editor's knowledge and consent or in a manner that could harm the journal's editorial integrity

- Demand by an advertiser to insert an advertisement adjacent to an article about or related to the advertised product or a threat to withdraw advertising support because of publication of a specific article (see 5.12, Advertisements, Advertorials, Sponsorship, Supplements, Reprints, and e-Prints)

- An advertiser or publisher's attempt to publish an advertisement or sponsored content disguised as editorial content (advertorial) (see 5.12, Advertisements, Advertorials, Sponsorship, Supplements, Reprints, and e-Prints)

- A publisher demanding information about accepted articles in advance of publication to sell that information to advertisers or sponsors or for other commercial purposes

- A sponsor attempting to exert influence over editorial decisions or selecting specific content for publication (eg, sponsored supplements) (see 5.12, Advertisements, Advertorials, Sponsorship, Supplements, Reprints, and e-Prints)

- A publisher demanding publication of an advertisement that the editor deems inappropriate (see 5.12, Advertisements, Advertorials, Sponsorship, Supplements, Reprints, and e-Prints)

- Request from a company to an editor to purchase reprints or e-prints of an article under consideration but not yet accepted for publication

- Demands by a commercial entity or governmental agency to publish or censor specific content

▪ Compliance with governmental or other external policy to not consider manuscripts from authors based on their nationality, ethnicity, race, political beliefs, or religion (see 5.11, Editorial Responsibilities, Roles, Procedures, and Policies)

▪ Pressure from a news organization or journalist or sponsor to publish information about a journal article before the news embargo is lifted (see 5.13.3, Embargo)

▪ Social media pressure from advocates or those motivated by political or commercial interests regarding a specific published article

▪ Pressure or demands from advocates to change policies or access rules after publication

Editors may need to educate and remind the journal's various stakeholders about the fundamentals of editorial freedom and its direct relation to the publication's integrity.

**5.10.1** **Maintaining Editorial Freedom: Cases of Editorial Interference and the Rationale for Mission, Trust, and Effective Oversight and Governance.** Interference with editorial freedom has affected several prominent medical journals and has been well documented in the biomedical literature and the press. However, many other cases of such interference have not been made public or are discussed only anecdotally, privately, or via restricted electronic exchanges or posts. The experiences of *JAMA*, the *New England Journal of Medicine*, and the *Canadian Medical Association Journal (CMAJ)* are presented here for the following reasons: there is sufficient literature documenting the relevant events, effective protective oversight mechanisms and governance plans were lacking or insufficient at the time, and the mechanisms for protection of editorial freedom that were developed as a result of these events are informative and may be helpful for other journals, editors, publishers, and owners.

**5.10.1.1** **The Case of *JAMA*.** Beginning in 1982, George D. Lundberg, MD, served as editor in chief of *JAMA*, a weekly, peer-reviewed, general medical journal, and a group of specialty journals, then known as the *Archives* journals, which are owned and published by the American Medical Association (AMA). *JAMA* had operated under a set of goals and objectives that were developed by Lundberg and the journal's editorial staff and that were approved by the journal's editorial board and AMA management.[32] These goals and objectives had protected the editor on several occasions from external pressures to restrict the journal's editorial freedom, and in 1993 the AMA House of Delegates (the policy-setting and governing body of the association) passed a resolution that reaffirmed editorial independence for all its scientific journals.[33] Although *JAMA* had a defined mission that included editorial freedom that had been publicly supported by its owner, it did not have sufficient oversight and a governance plan in place to help promote a trust relationship between the editor and AMA leadership, facilitate resolution of conflicts, and help prevent interference and threats against editorial freedom and authority.

During Lundberg's editorship, there had been tension between him and representatives of the AMA leadership and executive staff related to editorials and articles that were published in *JAMA* that were controversial or contrary to AMA positions. In 1999, Lundberg was abruptly fired by the AMA after he accelerated the publication of an article in *JAMA* (after peer review and acceptance) that reported the results of college students' attitudes toward sex to coincide with the impeachment hearings of President Clinton. According to the AMA's executive vice president, the publication of that article was an act of "inappropriately and inexcusably interjecting [*JAMA*] into a major political debate that has nothing to do with science or medicine."[8-11] At the time, *JAMA* had as 2 of its objectives "to foster responsible and balanced debate on controversial issues that affect medicine and health care" and "to inform readers about nonclinical aspects of medicine and public health, including the political, philosophic, ethical, legal, environmental, economic, historical, and cultural."[32] In addition, the journal had a long history of publishing articles that were pertinent to ongoing national and international political discussions, that were directly or indirectly related to medicine or public health, and that were released at a specific time to influence those discussions.

The AMA was widely criticized for the firing, which was considered interference with the journal's editorial independence and which damaged the reputation of the journal and the AMA and harmed *JAMA*'s previously demonstrated integrity.[8-13,34] Immediately after Lundberg's firing, the journal's remaining editors, led by interim coeditors, and the editorial board published an editorial in protest.[14] The senior editorial staff considered resignation but decided to stay on to support the journal. However, 2 members of the journal's editorial board and some members of the AMA resigned, and some readers cancelled subscriptions to the journal. Many authors threatened to withhold manuscript submissions to *JAMA*, and others threatened not to serve as reviewers.

The AMA appointed an independent 9-member search committee, chaired by a member of the *JAMA* editorial board who was also an editor of one of the AMA-owned *Archives* specialty journals. Other members of the committee included leaders in academia and research who were independent of the AMA, other journal editors, and a *JAMA* deputy editor; it did not include AMA executive staff or officers. The search committee's objectives were to identify a new editor, review the journal editor's job description and reporting relationships, determine how to evaluate the editor's performance, and review existing practices and develop safeguards to ensure the journal's editorial independence, integrity, and responsibility.[35,36]

Before the search committee had completed its work, the *JAMA* editorial board (which included 9 editors of the AMA-owned *Archives* specialty journals) met with the remaining *JAMA* editors, other editorial staff, publisher and publishing staff, and AMA senior management during its regularly scheduled annual editorial board meeting. During that meeting, an executive session was called that included the editorial board members and senior editorial staff but excluded representatives of AMA senior management and the journals' publishing staff. The editorial board voted unanimously to resign en masse if the journal's complete editorial freedom and a new governance plan to repair the journal's integrity were not accepted by the AMA leadership.

After multiple discussions and negotiations between the search committee and AMA leadership, a new governance structure for *JAMA* and the *Archives* specialty journals was developed by the search committee, AMA senior management, and the AMA Board of Trustees to "insure editorial freedom and independence for

*JAMA*, the *Archives* Journals, and their Editor in Chief."[35,36] This governance structure was set in place before Catherine D. DeAngelis, MD, MPH, became editor in chief of *JAMA* and the *Archives* journals in January 2000, and it was a condition of her acceptance of the position. The governance plan was subsequently reaffirmed by AMA leadership and served the journal through DeAngelis' editorship.[37-39] The Journal Oversight Committee served DeAngelis and the journal during her position as editor in chief.

In 2011, Howard Bauchner, MD, was appointed editor in chief,[40] with similar terms and reporting to the Journal Oversight Committee for editorial administrative matters but with one modification: for business and financial matters he would report to the publisher (both positions, editor in chief and publisher, are senior vice presidents within the AMA). Illustrations of the current and previous governance models are presented in **Figure 5.10-1** for other peer-reviewed journals, editors, publishers, and owners to consider. The journal's current governance structure supports the editor in chief's editorial independence, facilitates access of the editor in chief to the decision-making body and senior management of the AMA, and provides mechanisms for review of the editor in chief's performance and conflict resolution (**Box 5.10-1**). For editorial administrative responsibilities, the editor in chief reports to the Journal Oversight Committee, which is an independent committee of the AMA. The AMA Board of Trustees approves the membership of the Journal Oversight Committee as recommended by the Journal Oversight Committee. The JAMA Editorial Board is appointed by the editor in chief and serves in an advisory capacity. The editors of the JAMA Network journals are appointed by and report to the *JAMA* editor in chief; their editorial independence flows through editorial independence of the *JAMA* editor in chief. As noted in the Editorial Governance Plan (Box 5.10-1), the editor in chief has total responsibility for editorial content and does not report to management for any aspect of the editorial content of *JAMA*, the JAMA Network journals, or other publications under his or her jurisdiction.

**5.10.1.2** **The Case of the *New England Journal of Medicine*.** Beginning in 1991, Jerome P. Kassirer, MD, served as editor in chief of the *New England Journal of Medicine*, a weekly, peer-reviewed, general medical journal that is owned and published by the Massachusetts Medical Society. In 1999, Kassirer was dismissed as editor in chief of the *New England Journal of Medicine* after a struggle over authority with leaders of the Massachusetts Medical Society could not be resolved.[15-18] Kassirer objected to the society's plans for reuse of the journal's content and cobranding of the journal name with other information providers over which he had no control or authority.[17] He also objected to plans to move the journal's editorial staff from its academically affiliated location at Harvard University to the publisher's commercial offices because he believed that these plans threatened the journal's credibility and autonomy.[17] According to Kassirer, the decision to dismiss him was made by the Massachusetts Medical Society's Committee on Administration and Management, which did so without input from the society's trustees or the Committee on Publications.[17] According to the society's bylaws, the Committee on Publications was responsible for the publication of the journal and was the authority to which the editor in chief had reported for decades.

In response to the firing of Kassirer, there was much criticism from the international medical community as well as resignations of members of the Committee

**Figure 5.10-1.** Governance Models for *JAMA*

## 2012, Reporting structure for *JAMA's* Editor in Chief

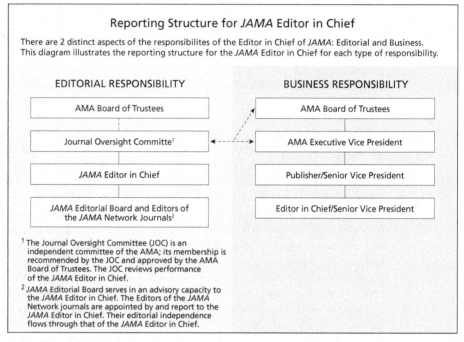

Reporting Structure for *JAMA* Editor in Chief

There are 2 distinct aspects of the responsibilites of the Editor in Chief of *JAMA*: Editorial and Business. This diagram illustrates the reporting structure for the *JAMA* Editor in Chief for each type of responsibility.

| EDITORIAL RESPONSIBILITY | BUSINESS RESPONSIBILITY |
| --- | --- |
| AMA Board of Trustees | AMA Board of Trustees |
| Journal Oversight Committe[1] | AMA Executive Vice President |
| *JAMA* Editor in Chief | Publisher/Senior Vice President |
| *JAMA* Editorial Board and Editors of the *JAMA* Network Journals[2] | Editor in Chief/Senior Vice President |

[1] The Journal Oversight Committee (JOC) is an independent committee of the AMA; its membership is recommended by the JOC and approved by the AMA Board of Trustees. The JOC reviews performance of the *JAMA* Editor in Chief.

[2] *JAMA* Editorial Board serves in an advisory capacity to the *JAMA* Editor in Chief. The Editors of the *JAMA* Network journals are appointed by and report to the *JAMA* Editor in Chief. Their editorial independence flows through that of the *JAMA* Editor in Chief.

## 2004, Reporting structure for *JAMA's* Editor in Chief[a]

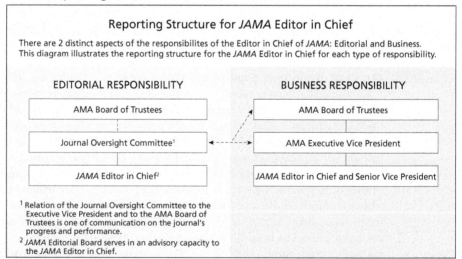

Reporting Structure for *JAMA* Editor in Chief

There are 2 distinct aspects of the responsibilites of the Editor in Chief of *JAMA*: Editorial and Business. This diagram illustrates the reporting structure for the *JAMA* Editor in Chief for each type of responsibility.

| EDITORIAL RESPONSIBILITY | BUSINESS RESPONSIBILITY |
| --- | --- |
| AMA Board of Trustees | AMA Board of Trustees |
| Journal Oversight Committee[1] | AMA Executive Vice President |
| *JAMA* Editor in Chief[2] | *JAMA* Editor in Chief and Senior Vice President |

[1] Relation of the Journal Oversight Committee to the Executive Vice President and to the AMA Board of Trustees is one of communication on the journal's progress and performance.

[2] *JAMA* Editorial Board serves in an advisory capacity to the *JAMA* Editor in Chief.

[a] Reproduced from *JAMA*. 2004;291(1):109.[37]

on Publications, the journal's editorial board, and members of the Massachusetts Medical Society.[15-19] In addition, the journal's remaining editors discussed a plan for mass resignation in response.[18] Deciding that such an action could irreversibly damage the journal, the remaining editors discussed and negotiated with the

**Box 5.10-1.** Editorial Governance Plan for *JAMA* and the JAMA Network

1. There will be a seven (7) member Journal Oversight Committee (JOC). This committee will function and be recognized not only as a system to evaluate the Editor in Chief but also as a buffer between the Editor in Chief and American Medical Association (AMA) management and as a system to foster objective consideration of the inevitable issues that arise between a journal and its parent body.

2. The JOC will prepare an annual evaluation of the Editor in Chief, which will be reported to the Executive Vice President (EVP) and to the Board of Trustees of the AMA. The Committee will have the charge to evaluate the performance of the Editor in Chief on the basis of objective criteria, and deliver that evaluation on an annual basis to the EVP and Board of Trustees of the AMA. The JOC will be responsible for determining the criteria for evaluation of the Editor in Chief. These criteria will be established in writing and made available to each member of the JOC, the *JAMA* Editorial Board, the Editor in Chief and the EVP and approved by the Board of Trustees of the AMA. The *JAMA* Editorial Board will be solicited for input to the evaluation process by the Committee. Correspondence about the performance of the Editor of *JAMA* received from constituent groups will be shared with the Committee. The Editor in Chief will be offered a five-year contract. If the Editor in Chief is dismissed during the term of the employment contract, other than for cause, the contract will be paid in full. Should such dismissal occur in year 5 of the contract, the minimum payment to the Editor in Chief shall be 12 months' salary.

3. The JOC will be charged, in addition, with reviewing and, if necessary, making additional recommendations to the AMA EVP/CEO and Board concerning governance and structural reforms necessary to ensure the AMA Journals' editorial independence. For this purpose, the Editor in Chief and SVP for Publishing will serve as advisors to the committee. This function will be ongoing.

4. The seven members of the JOC will include one member of AMA senior management, one member from outside the AMA with publishing business experience, and five members representing the scientific, editorial, peer reviewer, contributor and medical communities. The Committee members shall serve four-year staggered terms, although a new member may complete the remainder of another individual's term when a vacancy occurs. A Committee member may serve no more than two (2) full terms for a maximum tenure of eight (8) years, with the exception of the AMA senior management member, whose term shall be a continuing one, without term limits, as determined by the EVP/CEO. If a member of the JOC is completing the partial term of another individual who created a vacancy, he or she will then be eligible for one additional four-year term so that the staggering of terms remains intact.

5. No member of the JOC may be an AMA employee except for the member from AMA Senior Management. No AMA employee may be Chair of the committee, who shall be elected by the JOC.

*(continued)*

**Box 5.10-1.** Editorial Governance Plan for *JAMA* and the JAMA Network (*continued*)

6. JOC members are to be selected by the AMA Board only from a list of recommended persons submitted by the JOC. The list will include at least one alternate candidate except, if the JOC recommends an incumbent for reappointment, the JOC may recommend the incumbent alone. In the event that the Board does not select one of the submitted names, additional names will be recommended by the JOC, as necessary. Members of the JOC can be appointed or removed only by a 2/3 supermajority vote of the AMA Board of Trustees in the exercise of its oversight function.

7. Any proposal to dismiss the Editor in Chief for any reason shall be brought before the JOC for evaluation and a formal vote. The recommendations and views of the JOC shall be presented to the AMA Board along with the recommendation and views of the EVP/CEO. A supermajority (2/3) vote of the AMA Board would be required for dismissal of the Editor in Chief.

8. The Editor in Chief will report to the Senior Vice President for Publishing only for business and financial operations. The Editor in Chief will not report to management for any aspect of the editorial content of *JAMA*, the JAMA Network journals, or other AMA publications under his or her jurisdiction. Editorial independence of the Editor in Chief will be absolutely protected and respected by AMA management. In order to exercise its evaluative functions, the JOC will have full access to financial information including revenue and expense statements, budgets, and actual results. In order to have access to this proprietary information each member of the JOC who receives it will execute the AMA's standard Confidentiality and Conflict of Interest Agreements.

9. The Editor in Chief will have total responsibility for the editorial content of *JAMA* and responsibility for the performance of the JAMA Network Editors and other AMA publications under his or her jurisdiction. AMA management recognizes and fully accepts the necessity of editorial independence for the Editor in Chief at all times.

May 26, 1999
Revised: December 2001
Revised: November 2005
Revised: September 2008
Revised: April 2014

Massachusetts Medical Society a set of principles to maintain the journal's editorial independence and the editor's authority and responsibility for all content, editorial policies, use of the journal's content, name, and logo, and location of the editorial office.[18] With these assurances, Marcia Angell, MD, then the journal's executive editor, agreed to serve as editor in chief until a search committee with representation of the editorial staff and the wider academic community could identify a new editor in chief for the journal.[18] In May 2000, Jeffrey M. Drazen,

MD, was appointed editor in chief, and it was reported that the editorial freedoms negotiated previously by Angell would remain.[41] The journal's editor in chief reports to the Committee on Publications of the Massachusetts Medical Society, which is appointed by the Board of Trustees; the editor in chief also has a dotted-line relationship with the society's executive vice president, who reports to the society's Board of Trustees. Drazen served as editor in chief until 2019, when Eric J. Rubin, MD, PhD, was appointed.

**5.10.1.3** **The Case of the *Canadian Medical Association Journal* (CMAJ).** Beginning in 1996, John Hoey, MD, served as editor in chief of the *CMAJ*, a weekly, peer-reviewed general medical journal owned by the Canadian Medical Association (CMA). In 2006, the CMA abruptly fired Hoey and the journal's senior deputy editor, Anne Marie Todkill.[20,21] Initial public reasons from the publisher and CMA leadership for the dismissals were to "freshen" the *CMAJ* and because of "irreconcilable differences" between the editor in chief and the CMA, but no specific differences were cited.[20,21] Although the CMA denied that the decisions had anything to do with editorial independence, Hoey, other editors, editorial board members, and members of the journal's oversight committee have all described several examples of censorship and interference with the *CMAJ* by CMA leaders and executives dating back to 2001 or earlier.[20,21,42-44]

In 2001, *CMAJ* published an editorial supporting medical use of marijuana, which contradicted the CMA's position and for which the CMA's general counsel complained to Hoey.[23] In 2002, the *CMAJ* published an editorial criticizing Quebec physicians for not properly staffing an emergency department after a patient with a myocardial infarction died while being transported from an emergency department that had closed at midnight to a second open emergency department.[23] Members of the CMA board called the editorial irresponsible, and the CMA president called for the editorial to be retracted. The *CMAJ* editorial board responded that the CMA was threatening the *CMAJ*'s editorial independence.[23,44] Following these incidents, a journal oversight committee was established in 2002. However, the oversight committee's roles and functions were unclear and interpreted differently by the CMA leadership, the editor in chief, and even the chair of the committee.[23]

In late 2004, the CMA had reorganized its publishing services and placed the ownership and direction of the *CMAJ* under a subsidiary, CMA Holdings Inc.[45] This change reduced the editor in chief's contact with the CMA and increased his interactions with the holding company and publisher, whose primary objective was profit.[45] However, this change did not decrease the CMA's attempts to influence the editorial direction and decisions of the journal. In late 2005 and early 2006, 2 other incidents of interference and censorship by CMA leadership and executives occurred.[21-23] In one case, a *CMAJ* news story reported on the difficulty Canadian women had in obtaining nonprescription emergency contraception (Plan B) from Canadian pharmacists. Apparently, the Canadian Pharmacists Association complained to the CMA's chief executive officer and objected to *CMAJ*'s plan to run this news story after one of the *CMAJ* reporters interviewed an executive with the association. The CMA's chief executive officer took the objections to the *CMAJ* publisher, who told Hoey not to run the news story. Faced with what was thought to be an unreasonable demand and to avoid a crisis, the editors and reporters then modified the news story to address some of the objections and a revised article was published.[21-23,42] An unsigned editorial was subsequently published in the

*CMAJ* to alert readers to the incident of editorial interference and to "set in motion a process to ensure the future editorial independence of the journal."[46]

The second case of such interference involved a *CMAJ* news story that was critical of a Canadian public health official. The news story was published in the online version of *CMAJ* on February 7, 2006, and was subsequently removed from the website.[42] On February 20, Hoey and Todkill were fired, and 2 days later, a revised version of the original story was posted online that was less critical of the health official and more supportive of and beneficial to the CMA.[42]

During this time, Hoey had lost confidence in the journal's oversight committee and asked an ad hoc committee to review these events.[21,22] The ad hoc committee faulted the editors for modifying the news story on Plan B before it was published and for failing to follow the appropriate channel for conflicts (ie, the journal's oversight committee).[42] However, the ad hoc committee found more serious fault with the CMA for "blatant interference with the publication of a legitimate report" and concluded that the "*CMAJ*'s editorial autonomy is to an important degree illusory."[42]

Following the dismissals of Hoey and Todkill, the remaining editors, led by acting editor Stephen Choi, MD, published an editorial in protest of the firings.[47] Choi and colleagues drafted a proposal that included editorial independence for the *CMAJ* and aimed to ensure that the CMA and the publisher would not make decisions about editorial content.[21] The CMA did not agree to the proposal, and Choi and another editor resigned.[21] Other editors and most of the editorial board also resigned, and there were calls from academic leaders not to send papers or serve as peer reviewers for the journal.[21,48,49] The journal's former editor in chief, Bruce P. Squires, MD, was asked to serve as acting editor, but under pressure from editors of other journals, he too was unable to serve unless the CMA would agree to the journal's editorial independence.[23]

Like the events at *JAMA* and the *New England Journal of Medicine*, the abrupt firing of *CMAJ*'s editors and the refusal of the CMA to recognize the journal's editorial independence resulted in widespread news coverage of the conflicts, and a number of other leading journals published articles in support of the *CMAJ* editors.[20-22,44,48-50] In the wake of such criticism, in March 2006 the CMA announced the establishment of a panel to assess the journal's governance and management and agreed to an interim plan granting the editor in chief total responsibility for editorial content.[51] With this plan in place, Noni MacDonald, MD, agreed to serve as interim editor and Squires agreed to serve as editor emeritus.[52] The *CMAJ* governance review panel released its final report on July 14, 2006.[45] The report contained 25 recommendations, all of which were accepted by the CMA.[51-53] The recommendations included the following[45]:

- Assurance that the editor in chief would have editorial independence

- Amendment of the *CMAJ*'s mission statement to enshrine the "principle of editorial integrity, independent of any special interests"

- Confirmation that the CMA has no right to alter any editorial content but should be given the same advance notice of potentially controversial content that is given to the news media (see 5.13.3, Embargo)

- Proposal that the CMA take back direct ownership of the *CMAJ* from its for-profit holding company

▪ Proposal that the *CMAJ* editor in chief have separate and discrete reporting structures for editorial and business matters (ie, the editor in chief has access to the CMA Board of Directors if needed to defend or explain editorial positions or other concerns that cannot be resolved through administrative mechanisms, such as the journal's oversight committee; the editor in chief reports directly to an officer of the CMA rather than to the publisher about the journal's business matters; and the publisher reports to the same officer)

▪ A recommendation for a reconstituted journal oversight committee that permits it to more effectively help resolve potential disputes between the journal's owner, publisher, and editor in chief

For more details on the makeup and responsibilities of the *CMAJ's* oversight committee and the panel's other recommendations, see the *CMAJ* Governance Review Panel's final report.[45] In January 2007, Paul C. Hébert, MD, was appointed editor in chief of the *CMAJ* with assurance of the journal's independence as outlined in the *CMAJ* Governance Review Panel's report.[54] He led the journal for 5 years, and in 2012, John Fletcher, MB BChir, MPH, was appointed editor in chief,[55,56] and the journal was served by a 7-member Journal Oversight Committee and the governance plan developed in 2006.[45] In 2016, the CMA abruptly announced a "re-structuring and modernization plan," fired the editor in chief, and disbanded the journal's oversight committee.[57] Once again, public criticism ensued.[58,59] In January 2017, the *CMAJ* announced the formation of yet another new governing council, based on the previous 2006 governance plan, to protect editorial independence and facilitate "healthy communication between editors of the journal's owners."[60]

**5.10.1.4** **Other Major Medical Journals.** Editors in chief of other major medical journals owned by medical societies in Australia and Norway have been dismissed or forced to resign because of seriously different or conflicting views with the publishers or owners about the management of the journal and how and when management decisions were made.[61-64] Editors and publishers of smaller journals (in terms of size, resources, and bibliometric ranking) also need to consider the journal's organizational structure and protection for editorial independence. For example, the editors in chief of the *Croatian Medical Journal*, which is owned by 4 medical schools with a governance agreement for the journal,[65] were threatened to be removed and there was a threat to remove the journal's editorial independence from the governance agreement after complaints were lodged about how the editors handled ethical breaches by an author with an academic appointment at one of the universities.[66,67] This did not occur because the editors had previously published an article about the agreement in the journal to make it public,[65] and the editors received public support from within Croatia and internationally. In these cases, as in those described for *JAMA*, the *New England Journal of Medicine,* and *CMAJ*, concerns were raised about the integrity and perceived quality of the journals following the actual or threatened dismissals or forced resignations of the editors.

Editors have also been removed or dismissed for failing to follow best practices as recommended by the International Committee of Medical Journal Editors, Council of Science Editors, Committee on Publication Ethics, and World Association of Medical Editors. For example, in 2006 the editor in chief of *Neuropsychopharmacology* was asked to resign after he published articles in the journal for which he was an author that had commercial funding without complete publication of the commercial ties of the authors[68] (see 5.11, Editorial Responsibilities, Roles, Procedures, and Policies, and 5.5, Conflicts of Interest).

**5.10.2** **Ensuring a Trust Relationship Among Journal Editors, Publishers, and Owners.** As described by Davies and Rennie,[4] the relationship between editors and publishers/owners is interdependent and must be based on mutual trust. However, there are bound to be uncertainties, concerns, and occasional conflicts that could threaten the trust relationship.[4] To maintain trust, a formal agreement between the editor and owner should specify each party's expectations and the mission of the journal (for example, see *JAMA*'s governance plan in Box 5.10-1 and *JAMA*'s Key and Critical Objectives[69] reproduced in **Box 5.10-2**). If these expectations are not formalized in a governance plan or other document, are not mutually understood, or are intentionally disregarded (as happened in the cases described above), either party (but usually the owner) "may seek new (and possibly costly) mechanisms of accountability, reassurance, and control,"[4] which would result in loss of trust and potentially serious damage to the integrity, credibility, and reputation of both the journal and the owner.

Uncertainty, concerns, and disputes are best resolved informally through reciprocally open communication between the editor and publisher/owner and by maintaining a trust relationship. However, formal procedures for conflict resolution must be in place in the event that a dispute cannot be resolved informally.[4] These procedures should rely on the journal's mission and objectives to direct the assessment of the dispute, should require measured consideration of the facts involved (with appropriate evidence), and should not result in hasty decisions that do not consider the outcomes of such decisions for the editor, owner, and journal. In the cases described in the previous section, the continued existence and reputation of each journal was suddenly and unexpectedly put at risk because there was no effective independent mechanism to help achieve resolution of conflict or, if resolution proved impossible, allow time for an orderly change of editors. Such an orderly system and buffer and, if all else fails, such an orderly transition best serves the interests of journals, owners, publishers, and editors.[4] In a case of serious conflict, if a contract with term limit exists between editor and publisher/owner, then the publisher can opt to not renew the contract rather than abruptly dismiss the editor.

The following recommendations, many of which are supported by the International Committee of Medical Journal Editors,[27] World Association of Medical Editors,[28] Council of Science Editors,[29] and Committee on Publication Ethics,[30] may help editors, publishers, and owners develop policies for maintaining editorial freedom for their publications. Such policies should be regularly reviewed and made publicly available to the extent possible. For example, an individual editor's contract would not be made public, but a general description of the editor's level of authority, responsibility, and accountability can be published along with the journal's mission in an editorial, on the journal's masthead, or elsewhere. These recommendations are offered to help journals protect against threats to editorial freedom and integrity, but even if all these recommendations are followed, they will not provide absolute immunity from such threats.

**Box 5.10-2.** *JAMA's* Key and Critical Objectives[69]

---

**Key Objective**

To promote the science and art of medicine and the betterment of the public health.

**Critical Objectives**

1. To maintain the highest standards of editorial integrity independent of any special interests

2. To publish original, important, well-documented, peer-reviewed articles on a diverse range of medical topics

3. To foster responsible and balanced debate on issues that affect medicine, health, health care, and health policy

4. To provide physicians with continuing education in basic and clinical science to support informed clinical decisions and ongoing career development

5. To enable physicians to remain informed in multiple areas of medicine, including developments in fields other than their own

6. To improve health and health care internationally by elevating the quality of medical care, disease prevention, and research

7. To inform readers about various aspects of medicine and public health, including the political, philosophic, ethical, legal, environmental, economic, historical, and cultural

8. To recognize that, in addition to these specific objectives, the journal has a social responsibility to improve the total human condition and to promote the integrity of science

9. To achieve the highest level of ethical medical journalism and to produce a publication that is timely, credible, and enjoyable to read

10. To use technologies to drive innovation and improve the communication of journal content

---

Complete editorial freedom is recommended for all peer-reviewed biomedical journals because it ensures the highest level of editorial quality, credibility, and integrity. However, it is recognized that not all journals operate under complete editorial freedom, and achieving all the elements necessary for complete independence may not be possible or desirable for some journals. Thus, these recommendations are provided for peer-reviewed journals with complete editorial freedom (highly preferred) and those journals with limited editorial freedom.

▪ The editor should have a written contract or job description that clearly defines the editor's duties, rights, level of authority, responsibility, accountability, term of appointment, relationship to the publication's owner, reporting relationship, oversight and governance plan, objective criteria for evaluating the performance of the editor and journal, rights if removed from the position before term expiration, and procedures for conflict resolution. An explicit and mutually accepted definition of the editor's authority, responsibility, and accountability before the editor accepts the position will enable the editor to make an informed decision about accepting the position. Editors should carefully consider the ramifications of signing any nondisclosure agreements that would prevent them from speaking publicly if unwillingly removed from their positions.

- A governance plan should be in place that defines oversight and evaluation policies and procedures for the editor, conflict resolution mechanisms for the editor and owner of the journal, and the level of editorial freedom provided the editor and the journal. This plan should be published or otherwise made publicly available.

- Ideally, as in journals with complete editorial freedom, the editor should have direct access to the highest level of management in the organization or company that owns the publication. If this is not possible, as in journals with limited editorial freedom, the editor's line of authority and reporting relationship should be specified in a formal agreement.

- All journals should have a published and easily accessible mission statement that clearly defines the journal's goals and objectives; for journals with editorial freedom, the mission statement should include explicit reference to editorial freedom. The mission statement should serve as a guide for the editorial direction of the journal and should be relied on by the editor, editorial board, and members of the oversight or governance body when conflicts or disputes arise; it should be reviewed regularly by the editor and editorial board.

- An independent editorial oversight committee may help the editor establish and maintain the specified level of editorial freedom and resolve conflicts. To be independent, this committee's chair should not be a representative of the owner's employed, appointed, or elected leadership, and representation of the owner's employed, appointed, or elected leadership on the oversight committee should be limited (ideally to a single individual) or at most should have fewer voting positions on the committee than would constitute a majority. Although this may require a different appointment procedure for some societies, the importance of an independent oversight committee for helping to maintain the journal's integrity and manage contentious conflicts cannot be overstated. Note: An oversight committee differs from an editorial board, which serves to advise the editor on editorial content and policies (see 5.11.11, Role of the Editorial Board).

- In journals with complete editorial freedom, editors should have complete authority to hire, evaluate, and dismiss all editorial staff as well as the authority to appoint, evaluate, and dismiss editorial board members and peer reviewers (see 5.11, Editorial Responsibilities, Roles, Procedures, and Policies). If this arrangement is not possible for all editorial staff (eg, manuscript editors or other editorial staff employed, provided, or outsourced by the publisher), editors should at a minimum be able to review and evaluate their performance. For journals with limited editorial freedom in which the owner may make recommendations about editorial board members or peer reviewers, the editor should have final authority to approve their appointment, evaluate their performance, and terminate their appointment.

- The editor should have the opportunity to interview and comment on candidates for a new publisher being considered during the editor's term. The publisher should have the opportunity to interview and comment on candidates for a new editor being considered by the journal owner and/or search committee. For society-owned journals using outside publishers, editors should be involved in the selection and performance review of the publisher and other external commercial companies or vendors (eg, advertising, marketing, and research agencies; printers; suppliers of editorial systems; and online vendors or hosts) as well as decisions to renew or terminate publishing agreements.

- In journals with complete editorial freedom, editors should have complete authority over use and reuse of the name, logo, and content of the journal in print, online, and other media. Content includes editorial content, covers, mastheads, design, formatting, online features and linking, and approval of advertising and sponsorship. Although the editor must not be involved in the business (ie, selling) of advertisements and sponsorship, the editor should have authority over policies on appropriate types of advertisements and their placement and over policies on sponsorship activities (see 5.12, Advertisements, Advertorials, Sponsorship, Supplements, Reprints, and e-Prints). At a minimum, for journals with limited editorial freedom, the editor's level of authority and responsibility for content should be specified in a governance plan, contract, or other formal document.

- Owners and publishers should not interfere in the evaluation, review, selection, or editing of editorial content that is under the authority of the editor. For journals with complete editorial freedom, this pertains to all content. All changes and corrections made to content during production and publishing and after publication should be reviewed and approved by the editor or the editorial team reporting to the editor and production staff involved in producing the content but not the journal's owner, publisher, or sales and marketing staff.

- Editors and owners should establish mutually understood policies and procedures that guard against the influence of external commercial and political interests as well as personal self-interest on editorial decisions (see 5.5, Conflicts of Interest).

- Editors should be accountable for their editorial decisions, which should be based on the validity and credibility of the content and its relevance and importance to readers, not the commercial success of the journal or political interests of owners or other groups. Editors' decisions and communications with stakeholders should be based on competence, fairness, confidentiality, expeditiousness, and courtesy and should be governed by a policy on management of conflicts of interest (see 5.11, Editorial Responsibilities, Roles, Procedures, and Policies, and 5.5.7, Requirements for Editors and Editorial Board Members). However, editors need to understand the requirements for financial management and sustainability of their journals and they should publish content that attracts readers, authors, peer reviewers, subscribers, advertisers, and other stakeholders. Note: This does not mean that stakeholders should determine specific editorial content to publish or not to publish. For journals to maintain editorial freedom and integrity, editors should be free to express critical but responsible views without fear of retribution, even if these views are controversial or conflict with the commercial goals of the publisher or the policies, positions, or objectives of the owner or external forces.

- Editors should understand the business models that support their journals and should review financial operations with the publisher or journal owner. Any proposed changes to business models should be discussed with the editor.

- For journals with complete editorial freedom, the journal should publish a statement about its editorial independence and a prominently placed disclaimer that identifies and separates a publication's owner and sponsor from the editorial staff and content. For example, *JAMA* regularly publishes its objectives[69] (which include "to maintain the highest standards of editorial integrity independent of any special interests") and a statement that it is editorially independent of its owner and publisher. The following appears in the masthead of the journal:

  > All articles published, including opinion articles, represent the opinions of the authors and do not reflect the official policy of *JAMA*, the American Medical Association, or the institutions with which the author is affiliated, unless otherwise indicated.

  For journals that have limited or no editorial authority over specific types or sections of content (eg, pages reserved for the owning society or association or other content stipulated to be out of the editor's control), authority and responsibility for such content should be made clear to readers.

- Owners have the right to hire and fire editors. However, except for provisions contractually stipulated (eg, term limits or contract expiration), owners should dismiss editors only for substantial reasons that are incompatible with a position of trust, such as editorial mismanagement, scientific misconduct, fiscal malfeasance, undisclosed conflicts of interest that result in biased editorial decisions, unsupported changes to the long-term editorial direction or stated mission of the journal, criminal behavior, or specific activities that violate terms of a formal agreement.

- Editors should inform editorial board members, advisory committee members, owners, publishers, and editorial and publishing staff of the journal's policies on editorial freedom.

- Editors should publish articles on editorial integrity freedom when appropriate and should alert readers and the wider international community to major transgressions against editorial freedom.

**Principal Author:** Annette Flanagin, RN, MA

## ACKNOWLEDGMENT

I thank the following for review and helpful comments: Howard Bauchner, MD, *JAMA* and JAMA Network; Timothy Gray, PhD, JAMA Network; Iris Y. Lo, JAMA Network; Ana Marušić, MD, PhD, *Journal of Global Health* and University of Split School of Medicine, Croatia; Fred Rivara, MD, MPH, *JAMA Network Open* and

University of Washington, Seattle; and Joseph P. Thornton, JD, JAMA Network and American Medical Association.

## REFERENCES

1. Van Der Weyden MB. On being editor of the *Medical Journal of Australia*: living dangerously. *Mens Sana Monogr.* 2012;10(1):150-157. doi:10.4103/0973-1229.91295

2. The United States Constitution Online. Accessed December 27, 2018. https://www.usconstitution.net/const.html#Am1

3. Reporters Without Borders. 2018 Worldwide Press Freedom Index. Accessed December 27, 2018. https://rsf.org/en/ranking/2018

4. Davies HTO, Rennie D. Independence, governance, and trust: redefining the relationship between *JAMA* and the AMA. *JAMA.* 1999;281(24):2344-2346. doi:10.1001/pubs.JAMA-ISSN-0098-7484-281-24-jed90044

5. Davis RM, Mullner M. Editorial independence at medical journals owned by professional associations: a survey of editors. *Sci Eng Ethics.* 2002;8(4):513-528.

6. Death of a journal. *Lancet.* 1987;2(8573):1442. doi:10.1016/S0140-6736(87)91138-X

7. O'Brien E. Closure of the *Irish Medical Journal. Ir Med J.* 1987;80(5):247-248.

8. Goldsmith MF. George D. Lundberg ousted as *JAMA* editor. *JAMA.* 1999;281(5):403. doi:10.1001/jama.281.5.403

9. Tanne JH. *JAMA*'s editor fired over sex article. *BMJ.* 1999;318(7178):213. doi:10.1136/bmj.318.7178.213

10. Smith R. The firing of brother George. *BMJ.* 1999;318(7178):210. doi:10.1136/bmj.318.7178.210

11. Horton R. The sacking of *JAMA. Lancet.* 1999;353(9149):252-253. doi:10.1016/S0140-6736(99)00019-7

12. Davidoff F. The making and unmaking of a journal. *Ann Intern Med.* 1999;130(9):774-775. doi:10.7326/0003-4819-130-9-199905040-00019

13. Kassirer JP. Editorial independence. *N Engl J Med.* 1999;340(21):1671-1672. doi:10.1056/NEJM199905273402109

14. *JAMA* Editors, AMA *Archives* Journals Editors, *JAMA* Editorial Board Members. *JAMA* and editorial independence. *JAMA.* 1999;281(5):460. doi:10.1001/jama.281.5.460

15. Horton R. An unwilling exit from the *NEJM. Lancet.* 1999;354(9176):358. doi:10.1016/S0140-6736(99)90251-9

16. Kassirer JP. Goodbye, for now. *N Engl J Med.* 1999;341(9):686. doi:10.1056/NEJM199908263410909

17. The departure of Jerome P. Kassirer. Letters and response. *N Engl J Med.* 1999;341(17):1310-1313. doi:10.1056/NEJM199910213411712

18. Angell M. The Journal and its owner—resolving the crisis. *N Engl J Med.* 1999;341(10):752. doi:10.1056/NEJM199909023411008

19. Bloom FE. Scruples or squabbles? *Science.* 1999;285(5431):1207. doi:10.1126/science.285.5431.1207

20. Sacking of *CMAJ* editors is deeply troubling. *Lancet.* 2006;367(9512):704. doi:10.1016/S0140-6736(06)68277-9

21. Spurgeon D. Owner fails to guarantee editorial independence. *BMJ.* 2006;332(7541):565.

22. Spurgeon D. CMA draws criticism for sacking editors. *BMJ.* 2006;332(7540):503. doi:10.1136/bmj.332.7540.503

23. Shuchman M, Redelmeier DA. Politics and independence—the collapse of the *Canadian Medical Association Journal*. *N Engl J Med*. 2006;354(13):1337-1339. doi:10.1056/NEJMp068056

24. Hoey J. Editorial independence and the *Canadian Medical Association Journal*. *N Engl J Med*. 2006;354(19):1982-1983. doi:10.1056/NEJMp068104

25. The gold-headed cane. *BMJ*. 1956;1(4970):791-793.

26. Booth CC. The *British Medical Journal* and the twentieth-century consultant. In: Bynum WF, Lock S, Porter R, eds. *Medical Journals and Medical Knowledge*. Routledge Chapman Hall Inc; 1992:259-260.

27. International Committee of Medical Journal Editors. Recommendations for the conduct, reporting, editing, and publication of scholarly work in medical journals. Updated December 2018. Accessed January 14, 2019. https://www.icmje.org/recommendations

28. World Association of Medical Editors. The relationship between journal editors-in-chief and owners (formerly titled Editorial independence). Modified version posted July 2009. Accessed January 14, 2019. http://wame.org/editorial-independence

29. Council of Science Editors. Relations between editors and publishers, sponsoring societies, or journal owners. White Paper on Publication Ethics. Updated May 2018. Accessed January 14, 2019. https://www.councilscienceeditors.org/resource-library/editorial-policies/white-paper-on-publication-ethics/

30. Committee on Publication Ethics website. Accessed December 27, 2018. https://publicationethics.org/

31. Smith R. Editorial independence and the *BMJ*. *BMJ*. 2004;329(7205):272.

32. Lundberg GD. Goals for The Journal. *JAMA*. 1982;248(5):553. doi:10.1001/jama.1982.03330050035025

33. Lundberg GD. House of Delegates reaffirms editorial independence for AMA's scientific journals. *JAMA*. 1993;270(10):1248-1249. doi:10.1001/jama.1982.03330050035025

34. Kassirer J. Should medical journals try to influence political debates? *N Engl J Med*. 1999;340(6):466-467. doi:10.1056/NEJM199902113400609

35. Rosenberg RN, Anderson ER Jr. Editorial governance of the *Journal of the American Medical Association*: a report. *JAMA*. 1999;281(23):2239-2240. doi:10.1001/jama.281.23.2239

36. Signatories of the Editorial Governance Plan. Editorial governance for *JAMA*. *JAMA*. 1999;281(23):2240-2242. doi:10.1001/jama.281.23.224

37. DeAngelis CD, Maves MD. Update of the Editorial Governance Plan for *JAMA*. *JAMA*. 2004;291(1):109. doi:10.1001/jama.291.1.109

38. DeAngelis CD. *JAMA* and its editor—thinking forward. *JAMA*. 2000;283(1):105. doi:10.1001/jama.283.1.105

39. DeAngelis CD. Onward. *JAMA*. 2011;305(24):2575-2576. doi:10.1001/jama.2011.876

40. Bauchner H. My vision for *JAMA*. *JAMA*. 2011;306(1):98-99. doi:10.1001/jama.2011.936

41. Johannes L. *New England Journal of Medicine* appoints Drazen as editor in chief. *Wall Street Journal*. May 12, 2000:1.

42. Kassirer JP, Davidoff F, O'Hara K, Redelmeier DA. Editorial autonomy of *CMAJ*. *CMAJ*. 2006;174(7):945-950. doi:10.1503/cmaj.060290

43. Armstrong PW, Cashman NR, Cook DJ, et al. A letter from *CMAJ*'s editorial board to the CMA. *CMAJ*. 2002;167(11):1230.

44. Kuehn BM. *CMAJ* governance overhauled: firings, resignations, compromised independence cited. *JAMA*. 2006;296(11):1337-1338. doi:10.1001/jama.296.11.1337

45. *CMAJ* Governance Review Panel: final report. July 14, 2006. Accessed December 27, 2018. http://www.cmaj.ca/sites/default/files/additional-assets/site/pdfs/GovernanceReviewPanel.pdf

46. The editorial autonomy of *CMAJ*. *CMAJ*. 2006;174(1):9. doi:10.1503/cmaj.051608

47. Choi S, Flegel K, Kendall C. A catalyst for change. *CMAJ*. 2006;174(7):901, 903. doi:10.1503/cmaj.060276

48. Spurgeon D. Most of *CMAJ* editorial board resigns. *BMJ*. 2006;332:687.

49. Webster P. Canadian researchers respond to *CMAJ* crisis. *Lancet*. 2006;367(9517):1133-1134. doi:10.1016/S0140-6736(06)68492-4

50. Ncayiyana DJ. Journal ownership versus editorial independence tug-o'-war. *S Afr Med J*. 2006;96(6):470-471.

51. CMAJ. *CMAJ* and editorial autonomy. *CMAJ*. 2006;175(4):339. doi:10.1503/cmaj.060917

52. MacDonald N, Squires B, Hawkins D. Editorial independence for *CMAJ*: signposts along the road. *CMAJ*. 2006;175(5):453. doi:10.1503/cmaj.060985

53. Payne D. Panel gives *CMAJ* editorial independence. *The Scientist*. July 17, 2006. Accessed January 14, 2019. https://www.the-scientist.com/?articles.view/articleNo/24159/title/Panel-gives-CMAJ-editorial-independence/

54. Hébert PC. A new year and new opportunities. *CMAJ*. 2007;176(1):9.

55. Weeks C. John Fletcher to helm CMA Journal. *Globe and Mail*. January 18, 2012. Accessed December 27, 2018. https://www.theglobeandmail.com/life/health-and-fitness/john-fletcher-to-helm-cma-journal/article1358910/

56. Fletcher J. What's next for *CMAJ*? *CMAJ*. 2012;184(5):507. doi:10.1503/cmaj.120275

57. Canadian Medical Association. CMA Board of Directors announces restructuring and modernization plan for *CMAJ*. February 29, 2016. Accessed January 3, 2018. https://www.cma.ca/En/Pages/cma-board-of-directors-announces-restructuring-and-modernization-plan-for-the-cma-journal.aspx

58. Weeks C. Critics decry Canadian medical journal's "Orwellian" revamp. *Globe and Mail*. February 29, 2016. Accessed December 27, 2018. https://www.theglobeandmail.com/news/national/critics-decry-canadian-medical-journals-orwellian-revamp/article28960721/

59. Kassirer JP. A Canadian purge. *BMJ Opinion* blog. March 4, 2016. Accessed December 27, 2018. http://blogs.bmj.com/bmj/2016/03/04/jerome-p-kassirer-a-canadian-purge/

60. Kelsall D, Flegel K, Patrick K, Russell E, Sibbald B, Stanbrook MB. Renewal for *CMAJ*. *CMAJ*. 2017;189:E1. doi:10.1503/cmaj.161478

61. Kmietowicz Z. Editor in chief of *Journal of the Norwegian Medical Association* resigns. *BMJ*. 2015;350:h766. doi:http://dx.doi.org/10.1136/bmj.h766

62. Smith P. Former MJA editor files claim against AMA. *Australian Doctor*. September 10, 2012. Accessed December 27, 2018. https://www.australiandoctor.com.au/news/former-mja-editor-files-claim-against-ama

63. Scott S. Backlash over decision by Australia's top medical journal to outsource to company with history of "unethical" behavior. ABC News. May 1, 2015. Accessed December 27, 2018. http://www.abc.net.au/news/2015-05-01/academic-outrage-as-leading-health-journal-editor-sacked/6435850

64. McCook A. Editor of *Medical Journal of Australia* fired after criticizing decision to outsource to Elsevier. *Retraction Watch*. May 1, 2015. Accessed December 27, 2018.

http://retractionwatch.com/2015/05/01/editor-of-medical-journal-of-australia-fired-after-criticizing-decision-to-outsource-to-elsevier/#more-27943

65. Marušić M, Bosnjak D, Rulic-Hren S, Marušić A. Legal regulation of the *Croatian Medical Journal*: model for small academic journals. *Croat Med J.* 2003;44(6):663-673.

66. Callaham M, Sahne P, Winker M, Overbeke J, Habibzadeh F, Ferris L. World Association of Medical Editors: support of the *Croatian Medical Journal*'s editorial independence. *Croat Med J.* 2008;49(1):100. doi:10.3325/cmj.2008.1.100

67. Marušić M, Marušić A. Threats to the integrity of the *Croatian Medical Journal*: an update. *Croat Med J.* 2008;49(1):8-11. doi:10.3325/cmj.2008.1.8

68. Pincock S. Journal editor quits in conflict scandal. *Scientist.* April 28, 2006. Accessed January 14, 2019. http://www.the-scientist.com/?articles.view/articleNo/24267/title/Journal-editor-quits-in-conflict-scandal

69. For Authors. About *JAMA. JAMA*'s key and critical objectives. Updated September 2018. Accessed January 14, 2019. https://jamanetwork.com/journals/jama/pages/for-authors#fa-about

## 5.11 Editorial Responsibilities, Roles, Procedures, and Policies.

*I believe the editor is the primary source for ethical responsibility among professional publications.*
George D. Lundberg, MD[1]

Along with the autonomy and authority that come with editorial freedom are responsibility and accountability (see 5.10, Editorial Freedom and Integrity).[2-5] Editors are responsible for determining journal content, ensuring the quality of the journal, directing editorial staff and board members, developing and improving procedures, encouraging new ideas and innovation, following standards and best practices, and creating and enforcing policies that allow the publication to meet its mission and goals effectively, efficiently, and ethically and in a fiscally responsible manner.[2-7] This section focuses primarily on decision-making editors (ie, editors in chief and other editors, such as deputy, associate, assistant, contributing, section, and guest editors) who make decisions to review, reject, request revision of, and accept content for publication.

### 5.11.1 The Editor's Responsibilities. An editor's primary responsibilities are to inform and educate readers and to maintain the quality and integrity of the journal.[2,3] Thus, editors are obligated to make rational and consistent editorial decisions, select manuscripts for publication that are appropriate for their readers, ensure that the content of their journal is of high quality, and maintain standards to ensure the journal's integrity[2,3,8-10] (see 5.10, Editorial Freedom and Integrity). The editor's duty to readers often outweighs obligations to others with vested interest in the publication and may require actions that may not appear fair or suitable to authors, reviewers, owners, publishers, advertisers, or other stakeholders.

Some editors' roles may be major public positions with broad, ethically based, professional and social responsibility (eg, editors in chief of major medical or scientific journals),[2-4,7,8] whereas other editors' responsibilities are more limited (eg, other decision-making editors), more focused (eg, assistant editors or section editors), or procedural or technical (eg, manuscript editors, managing editors, production editors). These responsibilities, regardless of scope, should be clearly delineated in the editor's position description and supported by the publication's editorial mission statement (see 5.10, Editorial Freedom and Integrity).

The Council of Science Editors,[2] the Committee on Publication Ethics,[5] and the World Association of Medical Editors[3,4] have useful guides that outline best practices and responsibilities for journal editors regarding authors, reviewers, readers, and other stakeholders. Bishop,[10] Morgan,[11] and Riis[12] identified additional requisites of an editor: competence, fairness, confidentiality, expeditiousness, and courtesy.

**5.11.1.1** **Competence.** Editors must possess a general scientific knowledge of the fields covered in their publications and be skilled in the arts of writing, editing, critical assessment, negotiation, and diplomacy. In addition, editors should consider joining professional societies in their respective scientific fields as well as professional organizations for editors (eg, Council of Science Editors, European Association of Science Editors, World Association of Medical Editors, International Society of Managing & Technical Editors, American Medical Writers Association, European Medical Writers Association, Society for Scholarly Publishing, and Association of Learned and Professional Society Publishers [see 23.11, Professional Scientific Writing, Editing, and Communications Organizations and Groups]). These societies have websites, publications, policy statements, and other resources, conferences, and courses and workshops for new editors. Editors who publish original research, or reviews or interpretations of research, should be familiar with the scientific methods used, including the general principles of statistics.[12] They should encourage complete, accurate, and full reporting and advise authors to follow established reporting guidelines, such as those available from the EQUATOR (Enhancing the Quality and Transparency of Health Research) Network.[13] Editors should also rely on the expertise of others (eg, other editors associated with the journal, editorial board members, peer reviewers, statistical consultants, legal advisers) for advice and guidance, with the recognition that the editor has the ultimate authority for all editorial decisions. A competent editor will make rational editorial decisions, within a reasonable period of time, and communicate these decisions to authors in a clear and consistent manner.[2,4,8,10-12] A competent editor (whether editor in chief or manuscript editor) will also be skilled in the art of rhetoric[14] to recognize the tools of linguistic persuasion and identify and remove bias, hyperbole, inconsistent arguments, and unsupported assertions and conclusions from manuscripts. In addition, a competent editor will encourage and adapt to creativity and innovation to help improve the process and outcome of scholarly publication as well as the dissemination of and access to published content. Finally, as Bishop[10] suggests, a sense of humor should not be regarded as a trivial characteristic for an editor because a bit of humor can often avoid, or at least soften, potential conflicts between editors and authors, reviewers, owners, publishers, other stakeholders, and other editors.

**5.11.1.2** **Fairness.** Editors must act impartially and honestly,[4,5,9,12] even though they cannot always avoid the influence of all biases. Using peer review and consulting other editors during the editorial process may help control some personal biases.[8] Editors of peer-reviewed journals are responsible for maintaining the integrity of the editorial and peer review processes, developing editorial policies, and ensuring that editorial staff are properly trained in the policies and procedures involved.[2,4] Editors should document factors relevant to editorial decisions and maintain records of decisions and reviewers' recommendations and comments for a defined period so they will be prepared to deal with appeals or complaints (see 5.6.1.5, Record Retention Policies for Journals).

**5.11.1.2.1** **Appeals.** Journals should develop and maintain policies for handling appeals of decisions.[2,3,5] The Council of Science Editors has noted the following in this regard: "Despite editors' best efforts to solicit fair and unbiased reviews to evaluate manuscripts fairly, and to make decisions that are in the best interest of the journal and its readers, authors may still want to challenge editorial decisions. Often such appeals follow the rejection of a manuscript and may be based on authors' views that they can address reviewers' comments or that a reviewer did not understand or provided an inaccurate review. Editors should have a policy in place to address such appeals and complaints about editorial decisions and help resolve these issues."[15(p14)] As part of this process, editors may need to remind authors that reviewers do not make editorial decisions; they are advisers. Editorial decisions are made by the editors (see 5.11.3, Editorial Responsibility for Manuscript Assessment).

The Lancet has published a useful review of its appeals policy and procedures.[16] The Lancet has also established an independent editorial ombudsman who is assigned to review unresolved allegations of editorial mismanagement, such as delays, discourtesy, failure to follow established procedures as outlined in instructions for authors, and accusations of editorial dishonesty, conflicts of interest, or failure to handle complaints about author misconduct.[17,18] This ombudsman does not consider complaints about the substance of editorial decisions (vs the process of decisions) or editorial content or complaints about other journals. The ombudsman publishes reports that summarize these disputes and their resolutions.[18] Journals should include a description of the appeals process in their instructions for authors.

The Committee on Publication Ethics (COPE) offers services to editors of member journals and a forum to discuss specific cases, including author appeals and concerns about editorial conduct.[19] Other journals and publishing groups have independent oversight committees for which serious unresolved complaints about a journal's editor in chief can be brought. For example, the JAMA Network journals are governed by a Journal Oversight Committee, and the *New England Journal of Medicine* has a Committee on Publications Ethics. The editors in chief of *JAMA* and the *New England Journal of Medicine* report to these bodies for editorial matters (see 5.10, Ethical and Legal Considerations, Editorial Freedom and Integrity).

In resolving disputes, editors should consider all sides of an issue and avoid favoritism toward friends and colleagues or allowing editorial decisions to be influenced by powerful or threatening external forces (see 5.10, Editorial Freedom and Integrity).

**5.11.1.2.2** **Conflicts of Interest.** Editors should not have financial interests in any entity that might influence editorial evaluations and decisions and should have a formal recusal process in place if they have financial or other conflicts of interest with specific manuscripts[2,3,8,9] (see 5.5, Conflicts of Interest). Editors with other types of conflicts of interest with a specific manuscript or author that could impair objective decision-making should recuse themselves from involvement with such manuscripts and should delegate responsibility for the review and decision of such manuscripts to another editor or editorial board member.[2,3] For example, the JAMA Network journals do not permit an editor who collaborates with an author or who is employed by the same institution as an author to make decisions about that author's manuscript; the review and decision-making authority are delegated to another editor or an editorial board member without such a relationship.[9] Some journals will not consider manuscripts from authors who also serve as editors for the journal (this does not apply to editorials). Other journals will consider such submissions, but reviews of and decisions about manuscripts for which an editor is an author or coauthor are managed independently by another editor who has complete decision-making authority (including the ability to reject a manuscript in which the editor in chief is an author). In such cases, if a manuscript by an author who is also an editor for the journal is accepted for publication, a disclaimer indicating that the editor-author was not involved in the review and editorial decision should be published with the article.

**Example of Editor Recusal Statement Published With an Article**

> Dr Jagger, editor in chief of the journal, had no role in the editorial review of or decision to publish this article.

**5.11.1.3** **Confidentiality.** Most journals maintain some form of confidentiality with manuscripts under consideration (exceptions would include journals that use public open review). Editors should ensure that the journal's policies on confidentiality are made public (eg, via instructions for authors and in communications with authors and peer reviewers). For journals that use traditional forms of peer review (ie, not open to the public during review), editors must ensure that information about a submitted manuscript is not disclosed to anyone outside the editorial office, other than the peer reviewers and authors invited to write an editorial commenting on an accepted but not yet published manuscript (see 5.7, Confidentiality).[2,4] Editors should create and maintain policies about confidentiality and ensure that all current and new staff (editorial and production), authors, reviewers, and editorial board members are sufficiently educated about the journal's principles of confidentiality. The following statement may be useful when handling inquiries about manuscripts under consideration or previously rejected:

> We can neither confirm nor deny the existence of any manuscript unless and until such manuscript is published.

Editors should also establish policies and procedures to handle breaches of confidentiality by authors, peer reviewers, and editorial staff (see 5.7, Confidentiality).

**5.11.1.4** **Expeditiousness.** Although the time required to evaluate a manuscript depends on many factors (eg, complexity of a specific manuscript, overall number of submitted manuscripts, resources of the editorial office, time allocated for peer review, and availability of efficient submission and review systems), an author has a right to expect to receive a decision within a reasonable time.[11,12] Journals should publish an audit or otherwise make available to prospective authors turnaround times for manuscript decisions, peer review, and publication.[2] See, for example, the annual audit published by *JAMA*[20] and 5.11.13, Editorial Audits and Research. If the review and evaluation of a manuscript are delayed significantly beyond the journal's standard turnaround times for any reason, notifying the author of the reason for the delay is appropriate. Authors have a right to contact the editorial office to inquire about the status of their manuscripts. Many journals also offer authors the opportunity to check the progress of their submission online.

Editors should plan to accept manuscripts with knowledge of the number of accepted manuscripts awaiting publication, the number of pages allocated to the journal per year (for journals with print issues) or the number and types of articles that can be published during a year (in print, online, or both), the business model of the journal, and the resources available to evaluate, edit, and publish these articles and related content. Editors or their managers should monitor inventories of submitted and accepted manuscripts, manuscripts scheduled but not yet published, typical turnaround times for all stages of editorial processing and publication, and allocated resources (financial and human) to manage and publish the journal.

On occasion, an editor will receive a request from an author or a suggestion from a reviewer to expedite publication of a specific manuscript. The quickened pace of scientific discovery and heightened competition among scientists and journals have fostered an increase in requests for rapid review and publication, and technologic advances have facilitated the ability to do so.[21-24] Many journals have procedures for accelerated consideration and publication. For example, *JAMA* and the JAMA Network journals have procedures for expedited peer review and editorial consideration of manuscripts reporting high-quality evidence (usually randomized clinical trials) that have immediate clinical or public health importance or perhaps research that is scheduled to be presented at a major meeting.[22] Many journals routinely publish accepted manuscripts online ahead of print publication or publish articles online only. For the JAMA Network journals, such online-first and online-only publication includes appropriate procedures for editorial review and revision, editing, and proofing before online publication, as well as identification of the online publication date. This is especially important for journals that publish information that can affect clinical decisions and patient care. Other journals routinely release unedited copies of manuscripts while editing occurs and post the edited versions later. Readers should be informed whether a published manuscript has not yet been edited, and all versions should be properly identified and date stamped. For journals that do not routinely publish all content online ahead of print, a policy should be developed to allow for rapid consideration and early online publication of appropriate accepted manuscripts (eg, those with important and urgent implications for public health) that does not compromise the peer review and editorial decision processes or the integrity of the journal and does not result in the premature publication of an incomplete or inaccurate article (see 5.13, Release of Information to the Public and Relations With the News Media).

**5.11.1.5** **Courtesy.** More than a mere extension of etiquette and convention, editorial politeness requires editors and all editorial staff to deal with authors and reviewers in a respectful, fair, professional, and courteous manner.[10-12] Diplomacy, tact, empathy, and negotiation skills will help editors maintain positive relationships with authors, whether their work is accepted for publication or rejected. Note: Sections 5.11.2 through 5.11.7 focus on the editor's responsibility for manuscript processing, assessment, and decisions (see 6.0, Editorial Assessment and Processing).

**5.11.2** **Acknowledging Manuscript Receipt.** Journals should send a notice to authors to acknowledge receipt of their manuscripts and provide names and contact information of relevant editorial staff. Acknowledgment letters may be sent automatically from manuscript submission systems, usually after an author has viewed the submission and confirmed that it is complete.

**5.11.3** **Editorial Responsibility for Manuscript Assessment.** The editor should establish and maintain procedures and policies for appropriate editorial assessment and decisions to accept, request revision of, and reject manuscripts (see 6.0, Editorial Assessment and Processing).[4] The editor also establishes whether such decisions will be made unilaterally or by other editors (eg, deputy, associate, assistant, contributing, section, or guest editor) or in collaboration. However, the editor in chief has the ultimate responsibility for all editorial decisions, unless she or he is recused from the editorial process because of a conflict of interest (see 5.11.1.2.2, Conflicts of Interest, and 5.5.7, Requirements for Editors and Editorial Board Members).

Factors used to determine decisions should be made available to authors and reviewers. For example, JAMA Network journal editors use the following general criteria to evaluate manuscripts: material is original, writing is clear, study methods are appropriate, data are valid, conclusions are reasonable and supported by the data, information is important, and topic has general medical interest.[25] Through instructions for authors and online peer reviewer forms, JAMA Network journal authors and reviewers are informed that these basic criteria are used to assess a manuscript's eligibility for publication.

Depending on a journal's business model and editorial resources and the number of manuscripts received, the editor may rely on a triage process to evaluate all manuscripts before peer review. Not all manuscripts will be appropriate for the journal, and after an initial assessment the editor may decide to reject some manuscripts without sending them for external peer review. For example, *JAMA* editors reject more than 70% of the approximately 7000 major manuscripts received annually without obtaining external peer review.[20] In such cases, the editor's duty to provide a detailed review to the author of each manuscript is outweighed by the duty to reviewers (by not requesting their time to review a manuscript that has no chance of publication), owners (by not consuming resources needlessly), and other authors who have submitted manuscripts to the journal (by maintaining efficient processes) (see 6.0, Editorial Assessment and Processing). In addition, the author may be best served by a prompt notification of a rejection decision if the manuscript is unlikely to make it through the journal's review process and be considered for acceptance, thereby allowing the author to submit the manuscript to another journal without additional delay. Many journals also offer authors options to request that rejected manuscripts, with or without review, to be transferred quickly to other journals in a group (see 5.11.5.1, Journals With Cascading/Referral Systems for Rejected Manuscripts).

For manuscripts determined to be eligible for external review and additional consideration, all components of the submission should receive proper review and editorial assessment, including the manuscript text, tables, figures, and references, as well as relevant supplementary materials, documents, and multimedia files.

**5.11.4** **Editorial Responsibility for Peer Review.** Decisions about manuscripts are made by editors, not peer reviewers. Reviewers offer valuable advice, serve as consultants to the editor, and may make recommendations about the suitability of a manuscript for publication, but all editorial decisions should be made by the editors. Editors are obliged to be courteous to peer reviewers, provide them with guidance and explicit instructions (especially on the type of peer review or options used by the journal), assign only those manuscripts that are appropriate to specific reviewers (in terms of reviewer expertise and interest), maintain confidentiality if using blind or anonymous review, provide reviewers with sufficient time to conduct their review, and avoid overworking them.[2,4] Editors should ask reviewers in advance whether they are available for and interested in reviewing a specific manuscript, unless they have a prior agreement to assign manuscripts to reviewers without advanced consent (see 5.5.6, Requirements for Peer Reviewers, and 5.7.1, Confidentiality During Editorial Evaluation and Peer Review and After Publication).

Many journals publish lists of reviewers' names to acknowledge, credit, and thank them publicly for their work. Some journals offer qualifying reviewers continuing education credit, a letter of commendation that can be shared with supervisors or promotion committees, or complimentary subscriptions to the journal. Few journals offer financial compensation to peer reviewers, except perhaps those who may review a substantial number of manuscripts or perform specialized reviews (eg, statistical review). Editors should provide feedback to reviewers, such as notifying reviewers of the manuscript's final disposition, sharing copies of other reviewer comments of the same manuscript, and providing regular assessments of the quality of the reviewer's work.[2,4] As a means to promote academic credit for peer reviews, some journals and postpublication services post or permit reviewers to post their reviews online, citations to reviews, or redacted indications that reviews were completed for specific journals during specific years, often with the inclusion of reviewer's personal identifiers.

Editors should not share a specific review of a manuscript with anyone outside the editorial office, other than the authors and other reviewers, unless the journal operates a prepublication collaborative peer review system or an open peer review system that includes publication of reviewer recommendations and comments and reviewers are informed of this in advance. Editors should develop a specific policy regarding who has access to copies of a review, and this policy should be clearly communicated to all persons involved in the review process (see 6.0, Editorial Assessment and Processing, and 5.7.1, Confidentiality During Editorial Evaluation and Peer Review and After Publication).

Many journals develop databases of reviewers, including their addresses and affiliations, areas of expertise, turnaround times, and quality ratings for each manuscript review. Editors and publishers are obligated not to make secondary use of the information in the database without the prior consent of the reviewers and should never exploit the information for personal use, benefit, or profit (eg, selling a list of peer reviewers' names and contact information for promotional purposes). For example, the JAMA Network journals offer peer reviewers the option to receive email alerts with new articles published by the journal for which they are reviewing, and the reviewers can indicate before they submit their review if they do not wish to receive these alerts.

**5.11.5** | **Editorial Responsibility for Rejection.** Rejecting manuscripts may be one of the most important responsibilities of an editor. By rejecting manuscripts appropriately, an editor sets standards and defines the editorial content for the journal.[11] Decisions to reject a manuscript may be based on a wide range of factors, such as lack of originality, lack of importance or relevance to the journal's readers, poor writing, flawed methods, scientific weakness, invalid data, biased interpretations and/or conclusions, timeliness, or the specific publishing priorities of the journal.[4] A rejection letter must be carefully worded to avoid offending the author and could express regret for the outcome but also must not raise false hopes about the merits of an unsuitable manuscript. Many editors avoid use of the word *rejection* in any letters, opting instead for phrases such as "we are unable to accept" or "your paper is not acceptable for publication." However, editors should be certain that the intent of a letter of rejection is clear. If the letter sounds too much like a request for revision, the author may subsequently resubmit an irrevocably flawed manuscript, or worse, the author may resubmit a rejected manuscript, essentially unchanged, with the hope that the editor will not notice.[11]

An editor should determine on a case-by-case basis whether a standard rejection letter (form letter) or an individualized letter that explains the specific deficiencies of the manuscript should be sent to the author. Some editors recommend that for a manuscript rejected for "reasons of editorial choice (usually without outside editorial peer review), the editor has no obligation to provide the author any explanation beyond the statement that the manuscript was not considered appropriate."[8] Other editors suggest that all authors be provided a specific reason for rejection of their manuscript.[4] However, a standardized (form) rejection letter that includes an explanation for rejection based on editorial priority (especially for large journals that receive large numbers of submissions or that have very low acceptance rates) or that is accompanied by copies of detailed reviewer comments is sufficient for many manuscripts that are rejected.

Editors should develop specific policies for the rejection process, including how to handle previously rejected manuscripts resubmitted with an appeal for reconsideration (see 5.11.1.2.1, Appeals).[5,15,16] If the author's appeal provides reasonable justification, the editor should carefully consider the appeal (see 6.1.5, Appealing an Editorial Decision).

Because journals do not own unpublished works (ie, copyright or a publication license is typically transmitted in the event of publication), journal offices should not keep print or electronic copies of rejected manuscripts for any period longer than that required to deal with appeals of decisions; they should be destroyed or deleted. JAMA Network journals retain copies of rejected manuscripts for 1 year (see 5.6.1.5, Record Retention Policies for Journals, and 5.6.5, Copyright Assignment or License).

Journals with low rejection rates may be new and building an inventory of publishable articles, may be associated with a discipline/specialty that encourages barrier-free publication, or may have an author-pay business model that requires publication of a large number of articles based solely on technical soundness. However, editors of these journals also have a responsibility to review and make careful decisions about publication of manuscripts that are incomprehensible, seriously flawed, covertly duplicate, associated with research misconduct, or otherwise do not meet the standards of the journal.[26,27]

**5.11.5.1** **Journals With Cascading/Referral Systems for Rejected Manuscripts.** Some journals and publishers have developed systems to refer rejected manuscripts to other journals within the same publishing group or consortium in a specific field to improve efficiency and reduce time to eventual publication. Authors should be informed in advance if such options are available and if manuscripts, related content, reviews, correspondence, and decisions will be shared with other specific journals. Authors should be permitted to accept or decline such options (see 5.7.1, Confidentiality During Editorial Evaluation and Peer Review and After Publication).

**5.11.6** **Editorial Responsibility for Revision.** The editor's impartial focus on improving a manuscript facilitates the process of revision. According to Morgan,[11] "in letters requesting revision the editor should use an impersonal tone in criticizing." All such communication is best if the tone is objective and constructive. Editors should clearly communicate to authors what is expected in a revision; it may be helpful for editors to request that authors submit revised manuscripts with changes, additions, and deletions indicated and a cover letter that itemizes the changes made in response to each of the editor's and reviewers' comments and suggestions.

Editors are obligated to use sound editorial reasoning in requesting a revision. Editors must be skilled in arbitrating reviewer disagreements and reconciling contradictory recommendations, which may result from reviewers having diverse backgrounds, different expectations of the journal, and variable levels of expertise, diligence, or interest in the subject of the manuscript.[11] Authors object to receiving inconsistent or contradictory comments from reviewers and editors and may object to new and different criticisms of the revised manuscript submitted in response to the initial review. Although editors can never be certain that new issues will not surface at the time of resubmission, they are obligated to evaluate all reviewer comments, address any inconsistencies or unreasonable criticisms, censor any inappropriate criticisms, and guide authors in preparing their revisions.[4,8] Editors should also ensure that reviewers' recommendations do not contradict the guidance in the journal's instructions for authors, and if they do, this should be addressed in any request for revision; such direction can help prevent author confusion and frustration. Editors who make decisions about publication should not simply pass on reviewer comments without direction for the revision or by permitting reviewers' recommendations to serve as the editor's decision.

Some editors may be uncomfortable asking an author to revise a manuscript if there is a possibility that the revision will not be published. However, a revision may be needed to permit an author to provide missing data or information or to more clearly describe the study or work being reported so that the editor can properly evaluate the manuscript. The revision may also expose important weaknesses, limitations, or flaws that were not apparent in the original submission and that necessitate a decision to reject. Alternatively, a revision may introduce new issues or concerns or simply may not be satisfactory. In each of these cases, the editor's responsibility to readers outweighs any obligation to publish the author's revised manuscript. Editors should develop specific policies regarding requests for revisions, and the revision letter should state explicitly whether the author should or should not expect publication of a satisfactorily revised manuscript.[4] For example, JAMA Network journal editors include language similar to the following in their revision letters:

> If you decide to revise your manuscript along these lines, there is no guarantee that it will be accepted for publication. That decision will be based on our editorial priorities at the time, the quality of your revision, and perhaps additional peer review.

The rejection of a revised manuscript is probably best handled with a letter that tactfully explains why the revision was not acceptable. Although editors may need to ask for multiple revisions of a manuscript, such requests should include a detailed explanation to the authors. In most cases, these efforts serve to give the authors the best chance for their manuscript to reach a level of quality that is appropriate for acceptance and publication.

**5.11.7** **Editorial Responsibility for Acceptance.** Editors should follow consistent procedures to evaluate papers and make decisions regarding acceptance (see 5.11.3, Editorial Responsibility for Manuscript Assessment). Editors should inform authors of acceptance of their manuscripts in a letter that describes the subsequent process of publication, including substantive editing and any remaining queries; editing of the manuscript, tables, and figures and other content for accuracy, consistency, clarity, style, grammar, and formatting; and what material the author will be expected to review and approve before publication. Editors may also provide an approximate timetable for the publication process. If authors are given an expected date of publication, they should be informed of the likelihood of the date changing and, for journals with print versions, if the article will be published online first or online only. The acceptance letter should also remind authors of any policies regarding duplicate publication, disclosure of conflicts of interest, and restrictions on prepublication release of information to the public or the news media (see 5.3, Duplicate Publication and Submission; 5.5, Conflicts of Interest; and 5.13, Release of Information to the Public and Relations With the News Media).

Authors should avoid making substantial changes to the manuscript after acceptance, unless correcting an error, answering an editor's request for missing information, responding to an editor's or a proofreader's query, or providing an essential update. Likewise, editors should review manuscripts before acceptance and avoid asking authors for substantial changes after final acceptance.

If circumstances (eg, change in editorial strategy or clustering of certain papers for simultaneous publication or a special issue) cause a delay in publishing an accepted manuscript beyond the typical time between acceptance and publication, editors should inform the corresponding author of the reason for the delay.

Editors should not reverse decisions to accept manuscripts after the authors have been notified unless serious problems are subsequently identified with the content of the manuscript (eg, flawed methods, inconsistent or invalid data, allegations of misconduct) or the author has failed to meet the journal's publication requirements (eg, disclosure of duplicate submissions or publications, disclosure of conflicts of interest, transfer of copyright or a publication license).[5] An example of editorial discourtesy in handling accepted manuscripts occurred when an editor "unaccepted" a manuscript that his journal had accepted unconditionally 20 months earlier. The reason provided to the authors for this change of decision was that the journal's inventory of accepted manuscripts had become too large.[28] However, if a new editor inherits from the journal's previous editor a large inventory of accepted manuscripts deemed outdated or inappropriate, the new editor may have to find ways to deal with these manuscripts appropriately.[5] In such a case, the editor may request a one-time or temporary increase in journal pages or resources from the publisher. If this is not a viable option, for financial or other reasons, the editor may choose to contact the authors of accepted manuscripts that have not yet been scheduled for publication and explain that too many manuscripts had been accepted to allow publication within a reasonable period. The editor may offer the authors options to withdraw their manuscript and send it to another journal, reduce the length of their manuscript to allow it to be published in the limited number of pages allocated to the print journal, or publish their manuscript online only. However, any decisions not to publish previously accepted manuscripts should be made carefully and perhaps with the consultation of the journal's editorial board or legal adviser.

**5.11.7.1** **Provisional Acceptance.** Some editors will grant authors a provisional acceptance, offering to publish their manuscripts if certain revisions, conditions, or minor requirements are met. Some journals use provisional or conditional acceptance for revision requests when they are fairly certain that the revision will be accepted for publication. However, use of a provisional acceptance as a request for revision can cause problems if the revised manuscript is not suitable for publication. To avoid such problems, provisional acceptance decision letters should clearly communicate that acceptance is contingent on specific conditions that are clearly described for the author. If a new editorial policy requires a new condition for publication to be met by authors who submitted manuscripts before the policy took effect, a provisional acceptance can be used to permit these manuscripts to move forward without unnecessary delay.

**5.11.8** **Correspondence (Letters to the Editor).** A scholarly journal should provide a forum for readers and authors to participate in postpublication peer review and scientific dialogue and to exchange important information, responsible debate, and critical assessment, especially with regard to articles published in the journal.[2,3,24,29] A common forum for such exchange is the correspondence, or letters to the editor, section (see 1.5, Correspondence). Such letters become part of the published record and, like articles, are indexed by bibliographic databases. In the correspondence section, journal readers have the opportunity to offer relevant comments, query authors, and provide objective and scholarly criticism of published articles. Authors of articles to which the letters pertain should always be given the opportunity to respond, and editors should encourage authors to submit letters in reply and to address all criticisms. A study of 8 leading general medical journals found that the proportion of author replies to letters increased from 47% in 2002 to 63% in 2007.[30] Another study of electronic letters published in the *BMJ* between 2005 and 2007 found that authors did not respond to 45% of criticisms in these letters.[31] For journals that publish formal letters in a dedicated journal department, the letter author's comments and criticisms and the author's reply should be published in the same issue or online release to enable readers to evaluate the arguments presented. If an author chooses not to submit a reply for publication, the journal may publish a statement indicating that the author was shown the letter but declined to comment. Follow-up or later work that clarifies or amplifies a previous publication (other than a correction of an error or omission or retraction of fraud) may also be considered for publication as a letter[4] (see 5.11.10, Corrections [Errata], and 5.4, Scientific Misconduct).

Editors should establish policies and procedures for processing and evaluating letters just as they have done for handling manuscripts, and these should be published in the journal's instructions for authors or as part of the regular correspondence section. Like authors of manuscripts, authors of letters are expected to follow the same policies and procedures for authorship responsibility, disclosure of duplicate publication and submissions, disclosure of conflicts of interest, copyright or publication license transfer, research ethics, and protection of patients' rights to privacy in publication.

Journals prefer to publish letters that objectively comment on or critically assess previously published articles, offer scholarly opinion or commentary on journal content or the journal itself, or include important announcements or other information relevant to the journal's readers (although journals may have separate sections for announcements, meetings, and events). Letters that merely praise authors, the editor, or the journal rarely provide any meaningful or useful information. Likewise, ad hominem attacks should not be published. The International Committee of Medical Journal Editors (ICMJE) offers this guidance[29]: "responsible debate, critique and disagreement are important features of science, and journal editors should encourage such discourse ideally within their own journals about the material they have published. Editors, however, have the prerogative to reject correspondence that is irrelevant, uninteresting, or lacking cogency, but they also have a responsibility to allow a range of opinions to be expressed and to promote debate."

Some journals also publish short reports (eg, <500-600 words) of original research, technical comments, or novel case reports in the correspondence column. For example, the JAMA Network journals publish these as Research Letters,[32] and some of the JAMA Network journals publish short case reports as Observations in the Correspondence section. These reports should be handled as regular manuscripts, with peer review and revision, as necessary, and should follow all other editorial policies.

Many journals set limits on the length of letters that will be considered for publication (eg, ≤500 words and ≤5 references). Some journals will publish small tables or figures in letters, space permitting. To maintain timeliness, some journals also set a limit on the amount of time in which a letter sent in response to a published article must be received. For example, *JAMA* generally allows readers 4 weeks to submit a letter in response to a published article. Journals with time limits may allow exceptions for important letters that are submitted after the recommended deadline, especially for letters that identify important errors. Journals with space and time limits have been criticized for limiting postpublication scientific exchange and debate,[33,34] but such criticism does not recognize the resource limitations of journals and their editorial and production staff or the practical concerns associated with gathering all relevant submitted letters on a specific article and sending them to the author for a reply and publishing these in a timely manner.

Many journals have addressed this criticism by permitting online-only correspondence or comments to be posted without such restrictions on length and timeliness. For instance, in 1998, the *BMJ* began an experiment with an unrestricted policy for online-only response letters that included no limitations on length, timeliness, or number of online postings.[35] By 2002, the 20 000 online letters represented one-third of the journal's total online content.[36] After posting the 50 000th online-only letter in 2005, the *BMJ* recognized that the quality of some of these responses was low and commented that "the bores are threatening to take over. Some respondents feel the urge to opine on any given topic, and pile in early and often, despite having little of interest to say."[37] As a result, the *BMJ* added a maximum length requirement and raised the bar for acceptance of online letters to those that contribute "substantially to the topic under discussion."[37] Today, the *BMJ* requires all letters to the editor to first be submitted as online rapid responses, a selection of which will also be published as formal letters in the journal.[38]

Typically, a submitted letter undergoes an initial assessment, at which point it may be rejected, revised, or accepted. Some letters may be sent for peer review or accepted without external peer review. Letters on the same topic or in response to the same article should be grouped, sent to the author of the original article for reply (if necessary), and published in the same issue under one general title. Journals should cross-reference, and reciprocally link online, the original article and related letters to allow readers to identify and read the original articles and all related letters. Authors of letters should complete authorship forms, disclose conflicts of interest, and complete publishing agreements. Journals may edit accepted letters for content, length, clarity, grammar, style, and format. Authors should review and approve changes that alter the substance or tone of a letter or response.

For journals that publish online-only letters or comments, these postings may be reviewed to verify that they meet the journal's guidelines and requirements for such postings, determine that they contribute substantially to the previous publication and/or the discussion under way, and check for libel, error, and gratuitousness. If accepted, these postings may require minimal or no editing. Journals that publish online-only letters or comments should require authors of these comments to report conflicts of interest. Note: Online-only letters and comments may not be indexed by bibliographic databases.

**5.11.9** **Social Media.** Journals and editors that use social media to promote journal content or to encourage public dialogue about published articles should follow the same ethical norms, standards, and responsibilities outlined in this section and others in chapter 5. Blog posts should be managed as are traditional journal opinion pieces and letters and should follow the guidelines on authorship, duplicate publication, conflicts of interest, intellectual property, confidentiality, protecting patients' rights to privacy, and libel. Journals should review social media posts to ensure that text, images, and multimedia in posts adhere to the policies of the social media provider.

**5.11.10**    **Corrections (Errata).** Journals should publish corrections (or errata) following errors or important omissions made by authors or introduced by editors, manuscript editors, production staff, printers, or online journal platform hosts.[2,4,29,39] According to the ICMJE, journal editors have a duty to publish corrections in a timely manner[29]; however, the age of the original article in which the error was made should not be used as a reason not to publish a correction. Corrections to print publications should be published on a numbered editorial page and listed in the journal's table of contents. It is preferable to publish Correction notices in a consistent place in the journal, such as at the end of the correspondence section. If this is not possible or if corrections are routinely published in available white space in print versions of journals, these should still be listed in the journal's table of contents. Correction notices should have titles and DOIs. If easily identified, Correction notices will then be included in literature databases, such as MEDLINE, and appended to online citations to the original article that contains the error.[40] Substantive corrections made to online-only content and publications should be summarized in a Correction notice, which should also be properly labeled and identified (eg, listed in the online table of contents) and reciprocally linked to the original content. On occasion, an error may be so serious (eg, error in drug dosage) or important to the author (eg, misspelling of author's name) to warrant immediate correction online. In this case, it should be made clear in the online article that a correction has been made, and a formal Correction notice should follow. An error may be deemed appropriate to correct online (eg, a typographical error or an error in XML tagging that affects display of an article or a formatting or linking error) that does not warrant a formal Correction notice.

For all corrected articles, it should also be made clear in the online article that a correction has been made, including a brief description of what was corrected (this note can be placed in the Article Information section). The ICMJE recommends that journals post a new corrected version of the article, indicating that this is a corrected article, with details of the changes from the original version and the date(s) on which the changes were made.[29]

Example of Correction notes in Article Information of corrected articles:

> **Correction:** This article was corrected on July 24, 2018, to correct title errors in Figure 3 and Figure 4.

> **Correction:** This article was corrected on February 1, 2019, to correct typographical errors.

In online publications and online versions of print journals, corrections should reciprocally link to and from the original article. Corrections should also be appended to all derivative publications (eg, reprints). If major errors are corrected in derivative publications, a note should be included that indicates that a correction has been made and/or links to a correction.

Corrections (or errata) should not be used for Retraction notices of fraudulent articles that result from fabrication, falsification, or plagiarism (see 5.4.5, Retractions and Expressions of Concern). However, articles with pervasive errors could require a retraction and replacement of the published article.[41] For example, a pervasive error could result from miscoding of data or a miscalculation that caused extensive inaccuracies throughout an article (eg, Abstract, Methods, Results, Discussion, Conclusions, Tables, Figures, and Supplementary content). Correction of pervasive errors that result in major changes in the direction or significance of the originally published results, interpretations, and conclusions is a serious matter.[41] However, if the errors were inadvertent and the underlying science is still considered valid after subsequent review, the original article can be retracted and replaced. This can be done with a letter of explanation from the authors that is published with the retracted and replaced article and a supplement that contains a copy of the original article with the errors highlighted and a copy of the replaced article with the corrections highlighted[41] (see 5.4.6, Retraction and Replacement for Articles With Pervasive Errors).

See **Table 5.11-1** for a list of types, definitions, and publication responses for errors, corrections, and retractions.

**5.11.11**   **Role of the Editorial Board.** Editorial boards comprise leaders and experts in the subject area(s) represented by a journal. Editorial board members provide various functions, including representing the journal and providing outreach to the community of readers and authors served by the journal; advising the editor on policies, editorial content, and editorial direction of the journal; serving as peer reviewers; writing and recruiting manuscripts; and assisting the editor on editorial decisions (ie, handling manuscripts with which the editor has a conflict, serving as guest editor, or serving as section editor or editor for specific types of manuscripts). For some journals, editorial board members serve as decision-making editors who conduct initial triage of the quality and suitability of manuscripts or assign manuscripts to peer reviewers. Journals without independent oversight committees may wish to position the editorial board with the ability to help maintain the editorial freedom and integrity of the editor and journal (see 5.10, Editorial Freedom and Integrity). For some journals, the editorial board may serve as the official governing body that appoints the editor in chief; however, in such cases, lines of authority for editorial management and decisions may become challenging. Editorial boards should be working functional boards with specific roles, responsibilities, direction, a clear reporting relationship, and term limits.[10,42] Although nonworking figurehead boards may help the image or marketing of a journal, they will not provide reliable and consistent advice and assistance to the editor.

An editorial board should be independent of the publisher, owner, or other external forces, and the journal's editor in chief should serve as the chair of the editorial board. Editorial board members should be selected and appointed by the journal's editor, not the publisher or the owner.[10] However, if the editor has an agreement with the publisher or owner that permits an external group (eg, a professional society or university that owns or has a formal relationship with the journal) to nominate board members, the editor should have the final authority to appoint these individuals and to review their performance, and the number of editorial board members identified by the owner or an external group should be limited to a minority of the total board membership. Editors should maintain confidentiality and fairness when making decisions to renew or not renew a specific board member's appointment.

**Table 5.11-1.** JAMA Network Journal Policy on Corrections, Pervasive Errors, and Retractions[a]

| Type | Definition | Publication response |
|---|---|---|
| Minor errors | Inconsequential errors (eg, typographical error that could result in misunderstanding) | **Article corrected online:** An indication of correction and date of correction are added to the article information (HTML and PDF versions). |
| Substantive errors | Errors that require a Correction notice (eg, author name misspelled, incorrect numbers, important missing information) | **Correction notice published:** The article is corrected online with indication of correction and date of correction added to the article information (HTML and PDF versions). The Correction notice and corrected article are reciprocally linked. |
| Pervasive errors | Inadvertent errors that result in the need to correct important or numerous data in the abstract, text, tables, and figures (eg, a coding error) | **A. Letter and Correction:** If none of the conclusions or interpretations are affected and there are no statistically significant changes in the primary results, a Letter of explanation from the authors and a Correction notice are published; the article is corrected online with indication of correction and date added to article information (HTML and PDF versions). The Letter, Correction notice, and corrected article are linked to each other.<br><br>**B. Retraction and Replacement:** If the direction or significance of the results, interpretations, and conclusions change—and the science is still valid—a Letter of explanation from the authors is published as a Notice of Retraction and Replacement; the corrected article is replaced online with indication of correction and date added to article (HTML and PDF versions); a PDF copy of the original article with the errors highlighted and a PDF copy of the replacement article with the corrections highlighted are published in an online supplement to the corrected, replaced article; the replacement article includes a prominent note: "This article has been retracted and replaced with a corrected version." The Letter and replacement article are reciprocally linked.<br><br>**C. Retraction:** If the results, interpretations, and conclusions change—and the science is no longer valid—a Notice of Retraction is published (see below). |
| Scientific or research misconduct<br><br>or<br><br>Pervasive errors that should not be corrected or replaced | Fabrication, falsification, or plagiarism<br><br>or<br><br>Pervasive errors that invalidate the results, interpretations, conclusions, and the underlying science | **A. Retraction:** If confirmed, a Notice of Retraction as a Letter from the authors or an Editorial from the editors is published. A prominent note and watermark are added to the retracted article (HTML and PDF versions): "This article has been retracted." The Notice of Retraction and the retracted article are reciprocally linked.<br><br>**B. Expression of Concern:** If not officially confirmed by the authors or authors' institution or funders, but evidence of scientific or research misconduct is substantial, a Notice of Expression of Concern may be published as an Editorial from the editors. A prominent note is added to the HTML and the PDF versions of the article: "An Expression of Concern has been published about this article." The Notice of Expression of Concern and the article of concern are reciprocally linked. |

[a]Reproduced from *JAMA*. 2017;318(9):804-805.[39]

Editors should inform new editorial board members of their duties, responsibilities, and terms of service.[5] Editors should develop, review, and update as necessary an editorial board member position description that clearly lists roles, responsibilities, requirements, and term limits. For example, see the position description for an editorial board member for *JAMA* (**Box 5.11-1**).

A conflict of interest policy should also be established for editorial board members (see 5.5.7, Requirements for Editors and Editorial Board Members). Editorial board members should disclose all relevant conflicts of interest (financial and nonfinancial) to the editor; they should not participate in the review of or decisions on any manuscripts in which they may have a conflict of interest; and they should never use information obtained during the review process, editorial consultation, or an editorial board meeting for personal or professional gain. Editorial board members may be asked to serve multiple journals, which may pose a conflict of interest, especially for journals that represent a small community or the same field or specialty. The following questions may help editorial board members and editors decide whether holding positions with 2 journals poses a conflict of interest: Are both journals competing for the same readership, subject matter, and authors? Are the editorial positions and responsibilities similar? Can the editorial board member meet this journal's requirements as listed in the position description?

Journal editors should hold regular meetings of the editorial board, with an in-person meeting at least annually[10] and conduct regular meetings via conference call or the internet as needed. In any case, the editor should communicate

**Box 5.11-1.** Editorial Board Member Position Description

1. Attend annual meetings of their respective editorial board.
2. Permit their name to be placed on the masthead of the journal and their photo and profile to be used in marketing the journal.
3. Serve as an advisor for the editor.
4. Serve as reviewers/consultants for the journal, reviewing manuscripts as mutually agreed.
5. Serve as ambassadors to their scientific, clinical, and academic disciplines.
6. Assist in recruitment of authors, manuscripts, and reviews for the journal and help to promote the journal.
7. Write editorials, viewpoints, and other articles as mutually agreed.
8. Perform other duties as mutually agreed.
9. Not serve as a decision-making editor or editorial board member of a competing journal without the approval of the EIC.
10. Annually discloses to the editor in chief all financial interests and affiliations that could pose a conflict of interest, and promptly notifies the editor about any new potential conflicts of interest.
11. Comply with the recusal policy of the journal and promptly notify the editor in chief if a potential conflict arises.
12. Remain in good standing at their institutions and promptly notify the editor in chief if their status changes or comes under administrative review.

Board members are appointed for 2-year terms with a maximum tenure of ten (10) years, assuming consistent service and compliance with these responsibilities and expectations.

frequently with the editorial board members, ensure that board members understand their responsibilities and terms, and review the performance of each board member on a regular basis and before renewing a term.

**5.11.12** **Disclosure of Editorial Practices, Procedures, and Policies.** Underlying the ethics of editorial responsibility is the need for disclosure of editorial procedures and policies to authors, reviewers, and readers.[5] Typically, these are listed, and explained as necessary, in the publication's instructions for authors, which should be published and readily available on the journal's website (if published online). Items that should be considered for inclusion in a journal's instructions for authors or related resources for authors are listed in **Box 5.11-2**.

When an important editorial policy is first created or undergoes a major revision, it should be announced to prospective authors, reviewers, and readers. The easiest way to accomplish this is to publish an editorial note or an editorial. Editors should also draw attention to major changes in policy and procedures in the journal's instructions for authors and correspondence with authors.

Editors should also ensure that all individuals responsible for contributing to the publication are properly identified, typically in the masthead (eg, editorial and publishing staff, editorial board members, advisers, oversight bodies or publication committees, and owners). Other items that should be disclosed include any sources of financial support or other sponsorship that supports the publication.

**5.11.13** **Editorial Audits and Research.** Many journals conduct internal assessments, audits, and research into various aspects of the editorial process. For example, a journal may produce monthly or annual reports from its database of manuscripts, authors, peer reviewers, and decision-making editors to track inventory, workflow, and efficiency.[2] Editors may also rely on regular reports of article and journal key performance metrics, such as article views/downloads, citations, and news and social media coverage. Trends from these reports can help editors determine the number and types of manuscripts to accept for publication, assess the performance of specific types of articles and topics, assess staffing needs, track reviewer performance, and determine when to institute corrective action or a change in editorial strategy. For example, *JAMA* publishes an annual editorial audit that includes many performance metrics as well as the number of manuscripts received the previous year, acceptance rates, and the turnaround time for manuscripts that are reviewed, accepted or rejected, and published.[20] Many journals also publish dates of acceptance and key usage metrics with each article.

In addition, some journals systematically analyze information from submitted manuscripts as part of research to improve the quality of the editorial or peer review processes. All identifying information should remain confidential during such assessments, and any research conducted should not interfere with the review process or the ultimate editorial decision. For example, *JAMA*'s Instructions for Authors inform prospective authors that information related to their submissions may be subject to such analysis and that confidentiality will be maintained.[25] If a research project involves change in the journal's usual review process (eg, random assignment to a different review procedure), authors should be informed and given the opportunity to choose whether they want their manuscripts to be included in the study. Their decision to participate or not should not adversely affect the editorial consideration of their manuscript in any way.

**Box 5.11-2.** Items That Should Be Considered for Inclusion in a Journal's Instructions for Authors

---

**Information About the Journal**
- Name, address, telephone number, email address, and URLs of the journal's website and online submission system
- List of editors and other staff and editorial board or link to this information
- Journal's mission, goals, and objectives or link to this information
- Policies and procedures on editorial assessment, review, and processing (eg, turnaround times for reviews and decisions, type of peer review process, acknowledging receipt of submissions, editing and review of accepted manuscripts, postacceptance editing and production, appeals)
- Journal editorial and publication policies or links to these policies
- Types of manuscripts and topics or disciplines suitable for submission
- General information about the journal (ownership, affiliations)

**Requirements for Manuscript Submission**
- Name, address, telephone number, and email address of corresponding author and complete names of all coauthors, their email addresses, and institutional affiliations
- Methods and requirements for submitting manuscripts, tables, figures, multimedia, supplemental files, and cover letters
- Style and format of manuscript text, tables, figures, references, abstracts, multimedia, and supplementary material
- Specific requirements for categories of manuscripts (eg, reports of original research, reviews, letters, editorials, or journal-specific features) and any reporting guidelines
- Technical submission information (eg, figure file types and sizes, video format and sizes)

**Requirements for Manuscript Consideration and Publication**
- Policies on authorship, contributions of authors, access to data, and acknowledging assistance
- Policy on expectation of originality of submitted manuscript and notification of duplicate or closely related manuscripts or preprints
- Policy on disclosure of conflicts of interest
- Policy on disclosure of funding and the role of the sponsor
- Policies for registration of studies and data sharing
- For experimental investigations that involve human or animal participants, policy on approval by ethics committee or institutional review board and informed consent or appropriate animal care and use
- Policy on including identifiable descriptions, photographs, audio, or video of patients and relevant permissions
- Policies on obtaining permission for republishing or adapting previously published material
- Policies on embargos and prepublication release of information
- Policies on publishing agreement, transfer of copyright, or publication license
- Policies on public access and/or open access and any fees

---

**5.11.14** **Editorial Quality Review.** Quality review should be included in every journal's operations. Before and after publication, editorial and production staff and advisers should review each issue, online release, or a selection of articles and other content for errors (which, if detected, should be considered for publication as corrections), problems in presentation and format, and general appearance. All editorial and publishing staff should have the opportunity to participate in the quality review process, and all errors, problems, and suggestions for improvement should be communicated to the editor as well as those directly involved in editing and producing the publication.

**Principal Author:** Annette Flanagin, RN, MA

## ACKNOWLEDGMENT

I thank the following for review and helpful comments: Helene Cole, MD, formerly associate editor at *JAMA,* Clive, Iowa; Carissa Gilman, American Cancer Society, Atlanta, Georgia; Timothy Gray, PhD, JAMA Network; Iris Y. Lo, JAMA Network; Fred Rivara, MD, MPH, *JAMA Network Open* and University of Washington, Seattle; and Jody Zylke, MD, *JAMA.*

## REFERENCES

1. Lundberg GD. Perspective from the editor of *JAMA, The Journal of the American Medical Association. Bull Med Libr Assoc.* 1992;80(2):110-114.
2. Council of Science Editors. White Paper on Publication Ethics. Updated May 2018. Accessed January 1, 2019. https://www.councilscienceeditors.org/resource-library/editorial-policies/white-paper-on-publication-ethics/
3. World Association of Medical Editors. Recommendations on publication ethics policies for medical journals. Accessed January 1, 2019. http://wame.org/recommendations-on-publication-ethics-policies-for-medical-journals
4. World Association of Medical Editors Education Committee. A syllabus for prospective and newly appointed editors. October 26, 2001. Accessed January 1, 2019. http://www.wame.org/syllabus-for-prospective-and-newly-appointed-editors
5. Committee on Publication Ethics. Core practices. Accessed January 1, 2019. https://publicationethics.org/core-practices
6. Greenberg D, Strous RD. Ethics and the psychiatry journal editor: responsibilities and dilemmas. *Isr J Psychiatry Relat Sci.* 2014;51(3):204-210.
7. Lundberg GD. The social responsibility of medical journal editing. *J Gen Intern Med.* 1987;2(6):415-419.
8. Relman AS. Publishing biomedical research: role and responsibilities. *Hastings Cent Rep.* May/June 1990:23-27.
9. Gottlieb JD, Bressler NM. How should journals handle the conflict of interest of their editors? who watches the "watchers"? *JAMA.* 2017;317(17):1757-1758. doi:10.1001/jama.2017.2207
10. Bishop CT. *How to Edit a Scientific Journal.* ISI Press; 1984.
11. Morgan P. *An Insider's Guide for Medical Authors and Editors.* ISI Press; 1986.
12. Riis P. The ethics of scientific publication. In: European Association of Science Editors. *Science Editors' Handbook.* EASE; January 1994. Reissued June 2003.
13. The EQUATOR Network. Accessed January 1, 2019. http://www.equator-network.org/
14. Horton R. The rhetoric of research. *BMJ.* 1995;310(6985):985-987.

15. Council of Science Editors. 2.1.10, Considering appeals for reconsideration of rejected manuscripts. In: White Paper on Publication Ethics. Updated May 2018. Accessed January 1, 2019. https://www.councilscienceeditors.org/resource-library/editorial-policies/white-paper-on-publication-ethics/

16. Sperschneider T, Kleinert S, Horton R. Appealing to editors? *Lancet.* 2003;361(9373):1926.

17. Ombudsman. *The Lancet* website. Accessed January 1, 2019. http://www.thelancet.com/ombudsman

18. Molyneux M. Ombudsman's annual report for 2016. *Lancet.* 2017;389(10071):783. doi:10.1016/S0140-6736(17)30400-2

19. Committee on Publication Ethics. Accessed January 1, 2019. http://publicationethics.org/

20. Bauchner H, Fontanarosa PB, Golub RM. To *JAMA* authors, reviewers, and readers—thank you. *JAMA.* 2018;319(13):1329-1330. doi:10.1001/jama.2018.3775

21. Fontanarosa PB, DeAngelis CD. Update on JAMA-EXPRESS: rapid review and publication. *JAMA.* 2008;300(24):2920-2921. doi:10.1001/jama.2008.866

22. Rosenberg RN. Expedited publication initiative. *Arch Neurol.* 2011;68(5):563. doi:10.1001/archneurol.2010.353

23. Ghali WA, Cornuz J, McAlister FA, Wasserfallen JB, Devereaux PJ, Naylor CD. Accelerated publication versus usual publication in 2 leading medical journals. *CMAJ.* 2002;166(9):1137-1143.

24. Kalcioglu MT, Ileri Y, Karaca S, Egilmez OK, Kokten N. Research on the submission, acceptance and publication times of articles submitted to international otorhinolaryngology journals. *Acta Inform Med.* 2015;23(6):379-384. doi:10.5455/aim.2015.23.379-384

25. Instructions for Authors. *JAMA.* Updated June 10, 2019. Accessed July 7, 2019. https://jamanetwork.com/journals/jama/pages/instructions-for-authors

26. Bohannon J. Who's afraid of peer review? *Science.* 2013;342( 6154):60-65. doi:10.1126/science.342.6154.60

27. Hawkes N. Spoof research paper is accepted by 157 journals. *BMJ.* 2013;347:f5975. doi:10.1136/bmj.f5975

28. Chusid MJ, Casper JT, Camitta BM. Editors have ethical responsibilities, too. *N Engl J Med.* 1984;311(15):990-991.

29. International Committee of Medical Journal Editors. Recommendations for the conduct, reporting, editing, and publication of scholarly work in medical journals. Updated December 2018. Accessed January 1, 2019. https://www.icmje.org/recommendations

30. Von Elm E, Wandel S, Jüni P. The role of correspondence sections in post-publication peer review: a bibliometric study of general and internal medicine journals. *Scientometrics.* 2009;81(3):747-755. doi:10.1007/s11192-009-2236-0

31. Gøtzsche, PC, Delamothe T, Godlee F, Lundh A. Adequacy of authors' replies to criticism raised in electronic letters to the editor: cohort study. *BMJ.* 2010;341:c3926. doi:10.1136/bmj.c3926

32. Zylke JW. Research letters in *JAMA*: small but mighty. *JAMA.* 2013;310(6):589-590. doi:10.1001/jama.2013.8102

33. Altman DG. Poor-quality medical research: what can journals do? *JAMA.* 2002;287(21):2765-2767. doi:10.1001/jama.287.21.2765

34. Altman DG. Unjustified restrictions on letters to the editor. *PLoS Med.* 2005;2(5):e126. doi:10.1371/journal.pmed.0020126

35. Crossan L. Letters to the editor: the new order. *BMJ.* 1998;316(7142):1406-1410. doi:10.1136/bmj.316.7142.1406

36. Delamothe T, Smith R. Twenty thousand conversations. *BMJ.* 2002;324(7347):1171-1172.

37. Davies S. Revitalising rapid responses: we're raising the bar for publication. *BMJ.* 2005;330(7503):1284.

38. *The BMJ.* Resources for readers. How to respond to an article on *The BMJ*—rapid responses. Accessed January 1, 2019. https://www.bmj.com/about-bmj/resources-readers

39. Christiansen S, Flanagin A. Correcting the medical literature: "to err is human, to correct divine". *JAMA.* 2017;318(9):804-805. doi:10.1001/jama.2017.11833

40. National Library of Medicine. Errata, retractions, and other linked citations in PubMed. Updated August 8, 2018. Accessed January 1, 2019. https://www.nlm.nih.gov/bsd/policy/errata.html

41. Heckers S, Bauchner H, Flanagin A. Retracting, replacing, and correcting the literature for pervasive error in which the results change but the underlying science is still reliable. *JAMA Psychiatry.* 2015;72(12):1170-1171. doi:10.1001/jamapsychiatry.2015.2278

42. Marcovitch H, Williamson A. 1.1.3: Editorial boards. In: European Association of Editors. *Science Editors' Handbook.* EASE; June 2003.

## 5.12 Advertisements, Advertorials, Sponsorship, Supplements, Reprints, and e-Prints.

*Regardless of platform or format, the difference between editorial content and marketing messages should be clear to the average reader.*
**American Society of Magazine Editors**[1]

Commercial activities, such as advertising, sponsorship, reprints, and e prints, provide a major source of revenue for many scientific publications. With this revenue, publications can offset some of the costs of journal operations, production, and distribution; may be able to set lower subscription rates than would otherwise be possible; and can serve as a source of income for the journal's owner. Thus, some editors and publishers consider advertising a financial necessity. From a financial perspective, generating revenue is an important goal of advertisers, publishers, and editors—advertisers want to sell more products, publishers want to increase journal revenue, and editors want their journals to remain financially viable and sustainable. However, editors have a larger ethical responsibility to their readers, who must be able to rely on the editor to ensure that the journal's integrity remains intact and that the information contained in the publication is valid and objective. This responsibility includes ensuring that advertising does not influence editorial decisions or content and having policies and procedures in place that prevent such influence.

Thus, editors should have ultimate responsibility for all content published in their journals, including advertisements and sponsored content (see 5.10, Editorial

Freedom and Integrity, and 5.11, Editorial Responsibilities, Roles, Procedures, and Policies). The International Committee of Medical Journal Editors (ICMJE) recommends that editors "have full and final authority for approving print and online advertisements and enforcing advertising policy."[2] New or revised advertisements should be shown to the editor far enough in advance to ensure compliance with advertising guidelines. If an advertisement is deemed to be noncompliant, the advertiser may be offered the opportunity to revise the advertisement. However, some editors may not be able to review and approve specific ads because of limited resources (personnel and time). In these cases, someone representing the journal who understands the advertising policies and who is not in the sales or marketing department should review the ads. Nevertheless, all editors should be involved in the development, enforcement, and evaluation of formal advertising policies for print and online versions of their journals. For example, principles for advertising in print and online are developed jointly by editorial and publishing staff for the JAMA Network journals.[3] These principles are used by publishing and editorial staff to determine the suitability of advertising. Although editorial and publishing staff regularly review and discuss these policies and their applicability in specific situations, the JAMA Network journals editor in chief has final authority over all content, including advertisements, and can decide to accept or reject for publication any ads based on the advertising principles.

Advertising must not be allowed to influence editorial decisions.[1,2] All editorial decisions must be based on the quality and suitability of the editorial content and should not be influenced by potential revenue or loss of revenue from advertising, sponsorship, sales of reprints/e-prints, or related commercial activities or the influence of ad sales and marketing representatives. This policy is supported by the ICMJE,[2] World Association of Medical Editors (WAME),[4] and the Committee on Publication Ethics (COPE).[5] Complete separation of the roles and functions that determine editorial decisions and advertising sales is critical. Thus, editorial staff must not be involved in the promotion or sale of any advertisements, and the publishing staff who sell advertisements and sponsorship should not be permitted access to editorial content until it is published. Editors should have policies and procedures in place to address reader and online user concerns and complaints, assessment of such concerns, and appropriate remedy or action. The ICMJE recommends that editors consider publishing letters that raise important concerns about advertising content in the same way that they publish letters that raise concerns about articles,[2] including asking the advertiser to submit a reply.

**5.12.1**    **Advertisements.** Advertisements appear in print and online journals, email alerts, other online products and services, apps, and other types of media (such as podcasts and blogs). For biomedical publications, advertisements typically include the following:

- Advertisements that promote professional or trade-related products (primarily pharmaceuticals and medical equipment in biomedical publications), services, educational opportunities or products, or announcements (see 5.12.3, Advertorials). For print publications, these are typically called *display advertisements*. For digital publications online, online advertisements generally take the form of banner placements, including *position placements* (static, animated, or expanding) that display in fixed locations on a page/screen, *interstitial placements* (including pop-up windows and floating ads) that launch and cover page/screen content at or following page load and may require user action to close or dismiss, or *text-based ads*, such as email alerts or other online communications of information (see 5.12.6, Advertising and Sponsorship in Online Publications).

▪ Advertisements that promote products and services not specifically related to a profession or trade (such as an ad for an automobile or an airline in a medical journal).

▪ Classified or recruitment advertisements (listings of employment opportunities, educational courses, workshops, announcements, or other services).

In most cases, advertisers pay to place advertisements for their products and services in publications. Those advertisements for which a publisher does not typically charge a fee include public service announcements, ads for nonprofit organizations or charities, and house ads, which promote a product or service provided by the owner of the publication.

Important considerations for editors and publishers are whether paid advertisements and sponsorship invite potential infringements on editorial independence and whether they represent important revenue opportunities for journals in increasingly competitive markets.[6,7] The keys to maintaining editorial integrity are to achieve a balance between these seemingly opposing forces, maintain a recognizable separation between the functions and decisions of editorial and advertising departments, and have consistent and publicly available policies on advertising and sponsorship.[1-6,8-10]

Although the primary function of most journals is to educate and inform in a neutral manner and that of advertisements is to educate and inform in a promotional manner, advertisers and editors share a common goal—to influence the behavior of readers. Obvious differences between editorial text and advertising copy exist. In biomedical publication, editorial material typically comprises text composed in a consistent scholarly format with data-filled tables and figures, whereas advertisements typically contain colorful formatting, bold statements, and eye-catching graphics. Scholarly editorial material is generally intended to be objective, whereas advertisements are generally intended to be preferential, selective, and persuasive. Problems arise when the means to achieve the common goal—of influencing behavior—are outside expected norms or violate specific regulations and standards. The guidelines of the American Society of Magazine Editors (ASME) state that editors should not permit advertisers to influence or compromise editorial integrity and should not allow advertisements to deceive readers.[1]

The *Principles Governing Advertising in Publications of the American Medical Association* is a useful guide for other journals and publications and includes the following[3]:

> These principles, developed jointly by editorial and publishing staff, are applied by the American Medical Association (AMA) to ensure adherence to the highest ethical standards of advertising and to determine the eligibility of products and services for advertising in the AMA's print and digital publications.

The appearance of advertising in AMA publications is neither a guarantee nor an endorsement by the AMA or the AMA publication of the product or the claims made for the product in such advertising.

The fact that an advertisement for a product, service, or company has appeared in an AMA publication shall not be referred to in collateral advertising. As a matter of policy, the AMA will sell advertising space in its publications.

To maintain the integrity of the AMA publications, advertising (ie, promotional material, advertising representatives, companies, or manufacturers) cannot influence editorial decisions or editorial content. Decisions to sell advertising space are made independently of and without information pertinent to specific editorial content. AMA publications' advertising sales representatives have no prior knowledge of specific embargoed editorial content before it is published.

In many countries, advertisers must meet specific criteria established by national regulatory agencies. For example, drug ads are required to follow the regulations of the Food and Drug Administration in the United States,[11] the Association of the British Pharmaceutical Industry in the United Kingdom,[12] and the Pharmaceutical Advertising Advisory Board in Canada.[13] The International Federation of Pharmaceutical Manufacturers Associations[14,15] and the World Health Organization[16] have guidelines for pharmaceutical marketing practices that may be helpful for countries without well-defined regulations. However, these regulatory agencies have been criticized for not enforcing their regulations, and a number of studies[17-20] have found evidence of misleading advertisements published in biomedical journals.

**5.12.2** **Guidelines for Advertisements Directed to Physicians and Other Health Care Professionals.** The editorial and publishing staff of the JAMA Network journals have developed general eligibility requirements and guidelines for advertising copy to ensure that advertisements published in these journals are appropriate (see **Boxes 5.12-1** and **5.12-2**).[3] The ASME also has developed a set of principles for advertisements.[1]

The following criteria for print pharmaceutical ads are adapted from the guidelines prepared by the World Health Organization[16] and the International Federation of Pharmaceutical Manufacturers Associations[14]:

Advertising text should be presented legibly.

Pharmaceutical ads in print journals must include the following (in online ads, this information may be included on a website to which the ad links):

Name of the product, typically the trade (brand) name

The active ingredients, using either the international nonproprietary names or the approved generic name of the drug

The drug's main indication, precautions, most frequent or severe adverse events, contraindications, and clinically relevant interactions and warnings

Name and address of the manufacturer or distributor and how to contact them

Date of production of the advertisement

**Box 5.12-1.** Eligibility Requirements to Advertise in Journals Published by the American Medical Association (AMA)[a]

1. The AMA, in its sole discretion, reserves the right to decline any submitted advertisement or to discontinue publication of any advertisement previously accepted. By submitting ads for consideration, all advertisers agree to the *Principles Governing Advertising in Publications of the American Medical Association* and all Rate Card provisions, as amended from time to time.

2. Products or services eligible for advertising shall be germane to, effective in, and useful in (a) the practice of medicine, (b) medical education, and/or (c) health care delivery and shall be commercially available.

3. In addition to the above, products and services that are offered by responsible advertisers that are of interest to physicians, other health professionals, and consumers are also eligible for advertising.

4. Pharmaceutical products for which approval of a New Drug Application by the Food and Drug Administration (FDA) is a prerequisite for marketing must comply with FDA regulations regarding advertising and promotion.

5. Institutional advertising germane to the practice of medicine and public service messages of interest to physicians may be considered eligible for appearance in AMA publications.

6. Alcoholic beverages and tobacco products may not be advertised.

7. Equipment, Instruments, and Devices: The AMA determines the eligibility of advertising for products intended for preventive, diagnostic, or therapeutic purposes. Complete scientific and technical data concerning the product's safety, operation, and usefulness may be required. These data may be either published or unpublished. Samples of equipment, devices, or instruments should not be submitted. The AMA reserves the right to decline advertising for any product that is involved in litigation with a governmental agency with respect to claims made in the marketing of the product.

8. Food Products: (a) general-purpose foods, such as bread, meats, fruits, and vegetables, are eligible; (b) special-purpose foods (eg, foods for carbohydrate-restricted diets and other therapeutic diets) are eligible when their uses are supported by acceptable data; and (c) dietary programs: only diet programs prescribed and controlled by physicians may be eligible.

9. Dietary Supplements: Advertisements for dietary supplements and vitamin preparations are not eligible unless the safety and efficacy of the product have been reviewed and approved by the FDA for a disease claim.

10. Books: A book may be requested for review to determine its eligibility to be advertised.

11. Insurance Coverage: Claims made in advertisements for insurance coverage must conform with the following specific criteria: (a) claims relating to policy benefits, losses covered, or premiums must be complete and truthful; (b) claims made shall include full disclosure of exclusions and limitations affecting the basic provisions of policy; (c) claims incorporating quoted testimonials must meet the same standards as other claims; and (d) each advertisement for insurance products and services must include a

*(continued)*

**Box 5.12-1.** Eligibility Requirements to Advertise in Journals Published by the American Medical Association (AMA) (*continued*)

---

statement indicating either the states in which the products or services are available or the states in which the products or services are not available.

12. CME Programs: Advertisements for continuing medical education (CME) programs are not eligible unless the CME sponsor is accredited by the Accreditation Council for Continuing Medical Education and is an accredited medical school (or hospital affiliated with such a school), a state or county medical society, a national medical specialty society, or other organization affiliated with the American Board of Medical Specialties member boards.

13. Miscellaneous Products and Services: Products or services not in the above classifications may be eligible for advertising if they satisfy the general principles governing eligibility for advertising in AMA publications.

[a]Reproduced from *Principles Governing Advertising in Publications of the American Medical Association.*[3]
These guidelines are intended for advertisements for US-based companies, products, and services. See references 12 through 16 for examples of relevant guidelines for other countries

---

**Box 5.12-2.** Guidelines for Advertising Copy in Journals Published by the American Medical Association (AMA)[a]

---

1. The advertisement should clearly identify the advertiser of the product or service offered. In the case of pharmaceutical advertisements, the full generic name of each active ingredient shall appear.

2. Layout, artwork, and format shall be such as to be readily distinguishable from editorial content and to avoid any confusion with the editorial content of the publication. The word "advertisement" may be required.

3. Unfair comparisons or unwarranted disparagement of a competitor's products or services will not be allowed.

4. Advertisements will not be acceptable if they conflict with either the *Principles of Medical Ethics of the American Medical Association* or the advertising guidelines in Current Opinions of the Council on Ethical and Judicial Affairs of the American Medical Association.

5. It is the responsibility of the manufacturer to comply with the laws and regulations applicable to the marketing and sale of its products. Acceptance of advertising in AMA publications should not be construed as a guarantee that the manufacturer has complied with such laws and regulations.

6. Advertisements may not be deceptive or misleading.

7. Advertisements will not be accepted if they are offensive in either text or artwork, or contain attacks or derogations of a personal, racial, sexual, or religious nature, or are demeaning or discriminatory toward an individual or group on the basis of age, sex, race, ethnicity, religion, physical appearance, or disability.

[a]Reproduced from *Principles Governing Advertising in Publications of the American Medical Association.*[3]

---

Abbreviated prescribing information, which should include an approved indication or indications for use together with the dosage and method of use and a succinct statement of the contraindications, precautions, and adverse effects

For a "reminder" advertisement (a "short advertisement containing no more than the name of the product and a simple statement of indications to designate the therapeutic category of the product"[14]), the abbreviated prescribing information may be omitted (see 5.12.3, Advertorials).

When published studies are cited in promotional material, standard retrievable references with complete bibliographic information should be included (see 3.0, References). Information in advertisements and other promotional material, such as excerpts from the medical literature or quotations from personal communications, must not change or distort the intended meaning of the author(s) or the significance of the relevant work or study. Prepublication peer review and editorial evaluation of articles help to reduce problems associated with misleading or inappropriate information from published articles, but ads do not typically undergo the same level of evaluation before publication. Several studies[18-23] have documented problems with advertisements in medical journals, including promotional statements not being accurately supported by references, references cited to support promotional statements that are not retrievable (eg, "data on file"), and numerical distortion of data presented in tables and graphs.

According to the International Federation of Pharmaceutical Manufacturers Associations,[14] the same requirements that apply to printed materials should also apply to electronic promotional materials, including audiovisuals. Specifically, in the case of pharmaceutical product–related websites, the identity of the pharmaceutical company and of the intended audience should be readily apparent, the content and presentation should be appropriate for the intended audience, and country-specific information should comply with local laws and regulations[15] (see 5.12.6, Advertising and Sponsorship in Online Publications). Typically, an online advertisement links to a company's website, where the details about the prescribing information as listed above are provided.

The following issues should be addressed in any journal's policy on advertising:

1. Advertising to editorial content ratio
2. Advertising placement and positioning: including interspersion of ads within editorial content, advertising-editorial juxtaposition (adjacency), and placement of ads on journal covers
3. Separation of advertising sales and influence from editorial decisions
4. Appropriate advertising content

**5.12.2.1** **Advertising to Editorial Content Ratio.** For print publications that have an abundance of advertising, setting an advertising to editorial page ratio (ie, limiting the advertising content to no more than a certain proportion of total annual pages) may help protect the perceived integrity of the publication.[24] The ICMJE recommends that journals not be dominated by advertising.[2] If possible, journals should avoid publishing advertisements from only 1 advertiser; otherwise readers may perceive that the journal is sponsored by this single advertiser or that this advertiser has influenced the editor and the editorial content. For print journals, compliance with relevant postal regulations in some countries may also need to be considered if the number of ad pages exceeds the number of editorial pages. The ratio of editorial to advertising in digital versions of journals should also follow these general principles.

### 5.12.2.2 Advertising Placement and Positioning.

##### 5.12.2.2.1 Advertising Interspersion.
Placing advertisements between articles and interleaving them within articles may attract advertisers, but such practices may also diminish the perceived credibility of the publication—especially if the ads create difficulty for the reader in reading or finding editorial content. For scholarly biomedical journals, ads should not be interleaved within a scientific or clinical article in print or online. Many print publications group or stack their ads in the front and back of their journals, leaving a separate section of editorial content (an *editorial well*) in the middle of the publication for articles that are not interspersed with ads. Some advertisers may avoid journals that stack ads because they want their ads to be placed next to editorial material. For that reason, some journals place popular editorial features (such as news articles) in the front and back of the journal to allow for ad interspersion of those sections and maintain an ad-free editorial well for the original research and other major articles. Ordinarily, ads should not appear on a print journal's front cover. For discussion of online advertising interspersion, see 5.12.6, Advertising and Sponsorship in Online Publications.

##### 5.12.2.2.2 Advertising-Editorial Juxtaposition (Adjacency).
Advertisers may request placement of their ads next to related editorial content to help promote their products. Although common in consumer publishing, this practice is discouraged by the ICMJE and WAME.[2,4] The ASME offers this broad principle that applies to both print and online advertising: "advertisements should not be integrated into editorial content" to avoid the implication of editorial endorsement of the product or service promoted in the ad.[1] Ad adjacency, like interspersion, may be an impediment to readers and may diminish the perceived integrity of a scholarly publication. The *Principles Governing Advertising in Publications of the American Medical Association* state that "placement of advertising adjacent to (ie, next to or within) editorial content on the same topic is prohibited."[3] To avoid the occurrence of adjacent ads and editorial content on the same topic, even by chance, the editorial and production staff of the JAMA Network journals reviews the entire makeup (imposition or rundown) of the print issue of the journal after the ad deadlines have closed and before the journal is printed. If an ad is scheduled to appear adjacent to an article on the same or a closely related topic, the editors ask the production staff to move the ad or may decide to move the article. For those journals that permit online ads on pages with editorial content, ad adjacency policies should be developed that maintain the journal's editorial integrity. (See 5.12.6, Advertising and Sponsorship in Online Publications, for additional discussion of advertising-editorial adjacency in online publications.)

##### 5.12.2.2.3 Advertising on or Around Journal Covers.
Although advertisements ordinarily should not be placed on print journal covers, some journals permit ads to be attached to covers (with removable cover tips), around covers (with belly bands), or as

unattached ads (outserts) that are placed in a transparent polybag with the journal provided that these ads do not conceal the journal's title/logo or the postal address of the recipient if being sent through the mail.

**5.12.2.3** **Separation of Advertising Sales and Influence From Editorial Decisions.** Specific advertising and commercial content should not influence editorial decisions and content. The ICMJE states that "advertising must not be allowed to influence editorial decision."[2] COPE concurs, adding that "advertising departments should operate independently from editorial departments."[5] Providing advertising sales representatives with editorial calendars that include specific content scheduled for upcoming issues invites pressure for advertising-editorial adjacency and other attempts from industry to interfere with editorial decisions. The ASME advises that editorial content of any kind should not be submitted to advertisers for approval.[1] Recognizing the need for inherent separation between the planning and scheduling of editorial content and advertising, the ICMJE states that advertising should not be sold on the condition that it will be juxtaposed with specific editorial content.[2] Journal editors and publishers can respond to industry pressure by reminding advertisers of the importance of the journal's integrity. Advertisers understand this issue because without integrity a publication will have few readers, and without readers, the advertiser cannot reach potential users and purchasers of their products. For this reason, advertising sales staff should not have access to the specific embargoed editorial content until after publication. However, sales staff may know about general editorial plans, such as plans for theme issues, proceedings, symposia, or sponsored supplements (see 5.12.4, Sponsored Supplements).

**5.12.2.4** **Appropriate Advertising Content.** Appropriate ads must meet the following requirements[3,14,16]:

- No false claims

- No implied false claims

- Ability to substantiate claims

- No omissions of important facts

- No distortion of data

- Good taste (although this is difficult to define objectively)

- Clear identification of the advertiser of the product or services being offered

- Layout, artwork, and format that differ from those of the editorial content so that readers can clearly distinguish the advertising and editorial content

**5.12.3** **Advertorials.** An *advertorial* is an advertisement that imitates editorial content or presents content in an editorial-like format, such as using text, tables, or figures in a manner similar to the journal's editorial content. During the early 1990s, following a decline in the biomedical advertising market, advertorials became more common. The ASME principles state: "Regardless of platform or format, the difference between editorial content and marketing messages should be clear to the average reader" and that "advertisements that mimic the 'look and feel' of the print or digital publication in which they appear may deceive readers and should be avoided."[1] The ASME previously published guidelines for special advertising sections[25]; these guidelines have been replaced by general guidelines that emphasize transparency.[1] See **Box 5.12-3** for ASME guidelines relevant to special advertising sections and for differentiating editorial content and advertising.

Companies may submit advertisements that provide information on a topic that pertains to a product the company markets (or plans to market) but that do not name any commercial product. It is essential that such ads are clearly labeled

**Box 5.12-3.** ASME Guidelines to Differentiate Editorial Content and Advertising[a]

- Regardless of platform or format, the difference between editorial content and marketing messages should be clear to the average reader. On websites populated by multiple sources of content, including user-generated content, aggregated content and marketer-provided content, editors and publishers must take special care to distinguish between editorial content and advertising. Advertisements that mimic the "look and feel" of the print or digital publication in which they appear may deceive readers and should be avoided.

- Print and digital advertisements that resemble editorial content should be identified as advertising in compliance with Federal Trade Commission regulations. 73 FTC 1307 (1968) states that when a marketing message "uses the format and has the general appearance of a news feature and/or article for public information which purports [to give an] independent, impartial and unbiased view . . . the Commission is of the opinion that it will be necessary to clearly and conspicuously disclose it is an advertisement."

- The United States Postal Service also requires the labeling of editorial-like print advertisements: The USPS Domestic Mail Manual states that "under 18 USC 1734, if a valuable consideration is paid, accepted, or promised for the publication of any editorial or other reading matter in a Periodicals publication, that matter must be plainly marked 'advertisement.'"

- To ensure that such labeling is clear and conspicuous, ASME recommends the use of terms such as "Advertisement," "Advertising," and "Special Advertising Section" for print advertising units and further recommends that these terms should be printed horizontally and centered at the top of each advertising unit in readable type.

- ASME also recommends that native advertising on websites and in social media should be clearly labeled as advertising by the use of terms such as "Sponsor Content" or "Paid Post" and visually distinguished from editorial content and that collections of sponsored links should be clearly labeled as advertising and visually separated from editorial content.

[a]Reproduced with permission from the American Society of Magazine Editors.[1]

"Advertisement," have a different format from the journal's editorial content, and include a prominent display of the company name, logo, or both so that readers can quickly ascertain that the information is an advertisement from the company and not part of the journal's editorial content.

**5.12.4** **Sponsored Supplements.** Sponsored supplements are collections of articles, usually on a single topic, and are published as an extra edition or a separate section of a journal, often after a meeting or symposium. Studies have found that articles published in sponsored supplements are less likely to undergo formal peer review and are more likely to have promotional attributes, such as misleading titles, focus on a single-drug topic, and use of brand names only.[26-29] Because of the promotional and biased quality of such industry-sponsored supplements, the JAMA Network journals do not publish them. In addition, the US National Library of Medicine will not index articles in sponsored supplements unless sponsorship is clearly indicated and certain disclosure conditions regarding authors and editors are met.[30] The *BMJ* published a debate on the pros and cons of publishing sponsored content, including the following arguments[29] in favor: (1) they provide added value if safeguards are followed and (2) excluding industry is unrealistic; and opposed: (1) reader confusion, (2) risk to the journal's brand and reputation, and (3) editors cannot avoid being influenced.

Supplements can serve useful educational purposes, provided the content is objective, balanced, independent, and scientifically rigorous and sponsorship is transparent.[1,2,29,30] Sponsored supplements also may provide additional revenue to publishers. Recognizing this, the ICMJE developed a set of recommendations to guide editors when considering the publication of sponsored supplements.[2] The ICMJE recommendations, listed below, should help avoid bias in the selection of content for inclusion in industry-sponsored publications[2]:

> The journal editor must be given and must take full responsibility for the policies, practices, and content of supplements, including complete control of the decision to select authors, peer reviewers, and content for the supplement. Editing by the funding organization should not be permitted.

> The journal editor has the right to appoint one or more external editors of the supplement and must take responsibility for the work of those editors.

> The journal editor must retain the authority to send supplement manuscripts for external peer review and to reject manuscripts submitted for the supplement with or without external review. These conditions should be made known to authors and any external editors of the supplement before beginning editorial work on it.

> The source of the idea for the supplement, sources of funding for the supplement's research and publication, and products of the funding source related to content considered in the supplement should be clearly stated in the introductory material.

> Advertising in supplements should follow the same policies as those of the primary journal.

Journal editors must enable readers to distinguish readily between ordinary editorial pages and supplement pages.

Journal and supplement editors must not accept personal favors or direct remuneration from sponsors of supplements.

Secondary publication in supplements (republication of papers published elsewhere) should be clearly identified by the citation of the original paper and by the title.

The same principles of authorship and disclosure of potential conflicts of interest discussed elsewhere in this document should be applied to supplements.

**5.12.5** **Other Forms of Sponsorship.** Other forms of sponsorship include sales of bulk subscriptions or content licenses to commercial entities for distribution or access to individuals or groups, noncommercial sponsorship or grants to support specific editorial sections, and grants to support publication of journals in resource-poor communities. With each type of sponsorship, the funding source should be clearly indicated to recipients and readers/users, and all editorial content should be under the complete authority of the editor, should undergo the journal's usual editorial evaluation and peer review, and should not be influenced by the sponsor(s).

**5.12.6** **Advertising and Sponsorship in Online Publications.** Online ads are not restricted by the physical limits of a printed page. For example, an advertiser or content user can increase the type size of the prescribing information that appears in small type in an online pharmaceutical ad. Ads can rotate, expand, be animated, or pop up on or float into a screen with or without the user's initiated action. An ad for a particular drug, product, or service can be hyperlinked to the manufacturer or provider's website. In addition, ads can be targeted for specific users or a specific user experience. Online publication and technologic innovation have challenged the traditional print-based standards that separate advertising and editorial content. However, the general principles for protecting editorial integrity of print publications apply to advertising in online publications and other electronic products, such as websites, email, audio and video recordings, apps, social media and blogs, and online databases, especially for publications in clinical and health-related fields.[1,2,4,5] For example, just as a print reader can choose to read an ad or skip over it, an online user should have the same choice. Online ads should display in a distinct position that does not overlap editorial content or, when overlapping is unavoidable (eg, with interstitial ads or expanding banners), they should be easily dismissible through an automatic or user-initiated close function to not interfere with the reading and use of editorial content and should not dominate the online content. Online ads and sponsored content should be readily distinguishable from editorial content. As stated by the ASME, "on websites populated by multiple sources of content, including user-generated content, aggregated content and marketer-provided content, editors and publishers must take special care to distinguish between editorial content and advertising."[1]

**5.12.6.1** **Privacy Concerns Related to Advertising.** Privacy rights of online journal users and visitors must be maintained. If any specific or personal information about users is to be collected and specifically distributed or sold to third parties (such as advertisers), users should be informed in advance and given the opportunity to not have their information shared with others. Aggregate demographic information about numbers and types of users may be provided to advertisers to guide decisions about placing advertisements in specific journals in the same manner that circulation numbers are provided to advertisers and used for decisions to place print ads. This information may also be used by publishers to set advertisement rates and fees. Data on digital advertising metrics that do not capture or convey personally identifiable user information, such as overall numbers of users, impressions (ie, number of times an advertisement has been observed), and banner ad click-through numbers and rates (percentage of user-initiated banner clicks to impressions), generally are acceptable to share with advertisers. As digital advertising technologies evolve, new categories of activity tracking measures may allow advertisers and publishers to leverage functionality and measure user behavior (eg, views, impression downloads, interaction or hover data) as well as mitigate concerns about illegitimate data (eg, invalid increases from robotic nonhuman traffic or humans committing fraud). Wherein the function and intent of established and evolving advertising technologies do not capture or convey personally identifiable user information and provided they do not violate other journal advertising policies, user data generally can be shared with advertisers. The Interactive Advertising Bureau provides useful standards and best practices about digital advertising for advertisers, publishers, and other media, including guidelines for digital advertising display, compliance with legislation and regulation, and sharing of user data.[31]

**5.12.6.2** **Guidelines for Online Advertising and Sponsorship.** As the technology advances, online advertising will provide additional opportunities and ethical dilemmas for publishers and editors. Accordingly, guidelines for online advertising and sponsorship will also continue to evolve. The guidelines developed for use in online versions of the JAMA Network journals[3] provide guidance for advertising in online publications and appear in **Box 5.12-4**.

**15.12.6.3** **Online Sponsorship.** The ICMJE acknowledges that "various entities may seek interactions with journals or editors in the form of sponsorships, partnerships, meetings, or other types of activities" and that standards should be followed to preserve editorial independence.[2] The following recommendations are offered for journals that publish sponsored content online:

- Editorial content of any sponsored product (eg, online publications, websites, email, audio and video recordings, apps, social media and blog posts, and online databases) should be determined by the standard editorial process.

- The sponsor should have no influence over the editorial content of any sponsored product.

- Sponsorship policies should be clearly noted, either in text accompanying the product or on a disclosure page, and should clarify that the sponsor had no input into or influence over the content.

**Box 5.12-4.** Advertising in Digital Publications[a]

The current standards for ensuring the editorial integrity of print publications apply to advertising in electronic publications and derivative products, such as online journals, websites, and online databases, especially for publications in clinical and health-related fields.

In-text linking within an article to an advertisement is not permitted.

Advertisements that appear on journal website pages may coincidentally be related to the subject of an article, but such juxtaposition must be random.

Viewers will not be sent to a commercial site unless they choose to do so by clicking on an advertisement.

Expanding advertisements will expand only if a viewer scrolls over or clicks on them.

Interstitial and riser advertisements may appear for nonauthenticated audiences and may require user-initiated actions to close or dismiss the advertisements.

Advertisements with audio will play audio only if a viewer clicks on the advertisement.

A. Advertising
  1. Digital advertising may be placed on the JAMA Network journal websites.
  2. Digital advertisements must be readily distinguishable from editorial content and the word "Advertisement" must be displayed. Advertisements may link off-site to a commercial website.
  3. Digital advertisements may appear as static or animated advertisements.
  4. Digital advertisements may not be sold to be intentionally juxtaposed with, appear in line with, or appear adjacent to an article on the same topic. However, because ads rotate in various positions, adjacency may occur coincidentally or at random.
  5. JAMA Network journals' logos may not appear on commercial websites as a logo or in any other form without prior written approval by the individuals responsible for the respective areas within the AMA.
  6. Websites shall not frame the JAMA Network journal website content without express permission, shall not prevent the viewer from returning to the JAMA Network journal website or other previously viewed screens, and shall not redirect the viewer to a website the viewer did not intend to visit. The JAMA Network journals reserve the right to not link to or to remove links to other websites.
  7. All online advertising (including email advertisements) must be reviewed and approved by the JAMA Network journals' editorial and publishing staff. Such review will include the website landing page to which the advertisement links. Specific requirements are provided below.

B. Website Advertisement Requirements
  1. Articles will not include internal links to advertisements.
  2. Advertisements must follow the Guidelines for Advertising Copy and must not include unsubstantiated claims.
  3. The word "*Advertisement*" will appear adjacent to the advertisement and will be hyperlinked to a landing page that states the following: This is a paid advertising placement and the JAMA Network journals do not endorse the advertised product. Advertisements must adhere to the JAMA Network journals' Online Advertising Principles.

**Box 5.12-4.** Advertising in Digital Publications (*continued*)

4. The website URL to which the advertisement links must be provided to editorial and publishing staff for review and prior approval and must contain the following elements: (a) company sponsoring the website is clearly displayed and (b) no registration of personal information is required before reaching the website

C. Requirements for Advertisements in Email Alerts
   1. Email alerts may have HTML advertisements embedded in the email (top and/or bottom).
   2. The word "*Advertisement*" must appear adjacent to the advertisement.
   3. Advertisements must follow the Guidelines for Advertising Copy and must not include unsubstantiated claims.
   4. The website URL to which the ad links must be provided for review and must contain the following elements: (a) the company sponsoring the website is clearly displayed and (b) no registration of personal information is required before reaching the website.

ªReproduced from *Principles Governing Advertising in Publications of the American Medical Association*.[3]

■ All financial or material support for sponsored content should be acknowledged and clearly indicated (eg, on the home or landing page as well as on any packaging and collateral material included).

■ These acknowledgments should not make any claim for any supporting company product(s). The final wording and positioning of the acknowledgment should be determined by the journal, with review and approval by the editor. The wording could be similar to "Produced by [*Journal Name*] with support from [Company Name]."

■ The acknowledgment of the sponsor's support may be linked to the sponsor's website.

■ Journal names and logos should not appear on the sponsoring company website without prior written approval by the journal.

■ Journal search engines should not include content from sponsors unless the results of such searches clearly indicate the difference between sponsored and nonsponsored content. Sponsors should not receive preferential treatment in search programs and search results.

■ Journals should carefully consider the pros and cons of use of *digital native advertisements* (online ads presented in the same format as editorial content and interspersed within editorial content), and, if permitted, transparent indication of sponsored content and the name of the sponsor should be provided.

See 5.12.4, Sponsored Supplements.

**5.12.7** **Reprints and e-Prints.** Publishers of journals may sell reprints and eprints of journal articles as a source of revenue. Reprints and e-prints may be purchased by authors for personal use, by others for educational purposes, or by commercial entities for promotional purposes. In biomedical journal publishing, a *reprint* is the republication of an article or collection of articles in which the content is unchanged from the original publication (except perhaps for the inclusion of postpublication corrections). An *e-print* is a digital reproduction of or an online link to an article or collection of articles, usually PDF files(s). For example, publishers of the JAMA Network journals sell reprints to authors (at relatively low cost) as a service for authors and to the pharmaceutical industry as a source of revenue. Many journals permit authors to post e-prints of their articles (usually PDF files) on personal or other archival/institutional websites and to deposit copies in public repositories to meet requirements of funders (see 5.6.2, Public Access and Open Access in Scientific Publication), and some journals permit commercial entities to purchase and post copies of eprints on their websites. Note: Reprints and e-prints differ from *preprints*, which are print and online versions of articles/manuscripts made formally available to others before publication in a peer-reviewed journal.

Journals should establish and follow consistent policies and procedures on the production, sale, review or approval, and distribution or dissemination of reprints and e-prints. For an example of such standards, see those developed for *JAMA* in 5.6.9, Standards for Commercial Reprints and e-Prints. Editorial decisions must be free of any influence from the potential for sale of reprints and e-prints, and all such sales must not be permitted to occur until after publication of the original article. Reprinted articles should not be abridged or altered by the purchaser and should not include an advertisement or the advertiser's logo or other commercial content. A publisher may incorporate or append a correction to a previously published article in a reprint/e-print as long this is noted in the reprint/e-print.

**Principal Author:** Annette Flanagin, RN, MA

## ACKNOWLEDGMENT

I thank the following for review and helpful comments: Karen Adams-Taylor, JAMA Network; Howard Bauchner, MD, *JAMA* and JAMA Network; Carissa Gilman, American Cancer Society, Atlanta, Georgia; Timothy Gray, PhD, JAMA Network; Iris Y. Lo, JAMA Network; and Sean O'Donnell, JAMA Network.

## REFERENCES

1. American Society of Magazine Editors. ASME guidelines for editors and publishers. April 15, 2015. Accessed January 1, 2019. http://www.magazine.org/asme/editorial-guidelines

2. International Committee of Medical Journal Editors. Recommendations for the conduct, reporting, editing, and publication of scholarly work in medical journals. Updated December 2018. Accessed January 1, 2019. https://www.icmje.org/recommendations

3. American Medical Association. *Principles Governing Advertising in Publications of the American Medical Association*. Revised February 2016. Accessed January 1, 2019. https://jamanetwork.com/DocumentLibrary/Advertising/AMA_Advertising_Principles_Feb2016.pdf

4. World Association of Medical Editors. Recommendations on publication ethics policies for medical journals. Accessed January 1, 2019. http://wame.org/recommendations-on-publication-ethics-policies-for-medical-journals

5. Committee on Publication Ethics. Principles of transparency and best practice in scholarly publishing. Updated January 15, 2018. Accessed January 1, 2019. https://

publicationethics.org/resources/guidelines-new/principles-transparency-and-best-practice-scholarly-publishing

6. Fletcher RH. Adverts in medical journals: caveat lector. *Lancet.* 2003;361(9351):10-11. doi:10.1016/S0140-6736(03)12185-X

7. Tsai AC. Conflicts between commercial and scientific interests in pharmaceutical advertising for medical journals. *Int J Health Serv.* 2003;33(4):751-768. doi:10.2190/K0JG-EXG1-FB12-0ANF

8. Smith R. Medical journals and pharmaceutical companies: uneasy bedfellows. *BMJ.* 2003;326(7400):1202-1205. doi:10.1136/bmj.326.7400.1202

9. Callaham M. Journal policy on ethics in scientific publication. *Ann Emerg Med.* 2003;41(1):82-89. doi:10.1067/mem.2003.42

10. Lexchin J, Light DW. Commercial influence and the content of medical journals. *BMJ.* 2006; 332(7555):1444-1447. doi:10.1136/bmj.332.7555.1444

11. US Food and Drug Administration. Title 21: Food and Drugs. Chapter 1: Food and Drug Administration, Department of Health and Human Services. Subchapter C: drugs: general. 21CFR 202.1. Current as of April 1, 2018. Accessed January 1, 2019. https://www.accessdata.fda.gov/scripts/cdrh/cfdocs/cfcfr/cfrsearch.cfm?fr=202.1

12. Prescription Medicines Code of Practice Authority. Code of Practice for the Pharmaceutical Industry 2016. Accessed January 1, 2019. http://www.pmcpa.org.uk/thecode/Pages/default.aspx

13. Pharmaceutical Advertising Advisory Board. The PAAB code of advertising acceptance. Updated January 1, 2018. Accessed January 1, 2019. http://code.paab.ca/pdfs/paab_code_PDF_official.pdf

14. International Federation of Pharmaceutical Manufacturers Associations. IFPMA Code of Pharmaceutical Marketing Practices. 2012. Accessed January 1, 2019. https://www.ifpma.org/resource-centre/ifpma-code-of-practice/

15. Francer J, Izquierdo JZ, Music T, et al. Ethical pharmaceutical promotion and communications worldwide: codes and regulations. *Philos Ethics Humanit Med.* 2014;9:7. doi:10.1186/1747-5341-9-7

16. World Health Organization. *Ethical Criteria for the Promotion, Advertisement, and Publicity of Medicines.* World Health Organization; 2013. Accessed January 1, 2019. http://apps.who.int/medicinedocs/en/m/abstract/Js22161en/

17. Brushwood DB, Knox CA, Liu W, Jenkins KA. Evaluating promotional claims as false or misleading. *Am J Health Syst Pharm.* 2013;70(21):1941-1944. doi:10.2146/ajhp130076

18. Othman N, Vitry A, Roughead EE. Quality of pharmaceutical advertisements in medical journals: a systematic review. *PLoS One.* 2009;4(7):e6350. doi:10.1371/journal.pone.0006350

19. Korenstein D, Keyhani S, Mendelson A, Ross JS. Adherence of pharmaceutical advertisements in medical journals to FDA guidelines and content for safe prescribing. *PLoS One.* 2011;6(8):e23336. doi:10.1371/journal.pone.0023336

20. Villanueva P, Peiro A, Liberos J, Immaculada P. Accuracy of pharmaceutical advertisements in medical journals. *Lancet.* 2003;361(9351):27-32. doi:10.1016/S0140-6736(03)12118-6

21. van Winkelen P, van Denderen JS, Vossen CY, Huizinga TW, Dekker FW. How evidence-based are advertisements in journals regarding the subspecialty of rheumatology? *Rheumatology (Oxford).* 2006;45(9):1154-1157. doi:10.1093/rheumatology/kel073

22. Cooper RJ, Schriger DL. The availability of references and the sponsorship of original research cited in pharmaceutical advertisements. *CMAJ*. 2005;172(4):487-491. doi:10.1503/cmaj.1031940

23. Cooper RJ, Schriger DL, Wallace RC, Mikulich VJ, Wilkes MS. The quantity and quality of scientific graphs in pharmaceutical advertisements. *J Gen Intern Med*. 2003;18(4):294-297. doi:10.1046/j.1525-1497.2003.20703.x

24. Rennie D, Bero LA. Throw it away, Sam: the controlled circulation journals. *CBE Views*. 1990;13(13):31-35. doi:10.2214/ajr.155.4.2119127

25. American Society of Magazine Editors. *Guidelines for Special Advertising Sections*. 8th ed. American Society of Magazine Editors; July 1996.

26. Bero LA, Galbraith A, Rennie D. The publication of sponsored symposiums in medical journals. *N Engl J Med*. 1992;327(16):1135-1140. doi:10.1056/NEJM199210153271606

27. Steinbrook R, Lo B. Medical journals and conflicts of interest. *J Law Med Ethics*. 2012;40(3):488-499. doi:10.1111/j.1748-720X.2012.00681.x

28. Citrome L. Citability of original research and reviews in journals and their sponsored supplements. *PLoS One*. 2010;5(3):e9876. doi:10.1371/journal.pone.0009876

29. Wedzicha JA, Steinbrook R, Kassirer JP. Should medical journals publish sponsored content? *BMJ*. 2014;348:g352. doi:10.1136/bmj.g352

30. US National Library of Medicine. Conflict of interest disclosure and journal supplements in MEDLINE: best practices. Updated December 11, 2017. Accessed January 1, 2019. https://www.nlm.nih.gov/pubs/factsheets/supplements.html

31. Interactive Advertising Bureau. Standards, guidelines, and best practices. Accessed January 1, 2019. https://www.iab.com/guidelines/

## 5.13 Release of Information to the Public and Relations With the News Media.

> *Most people understand science and technology less through direct experience than through the filter of journalism. . . . Journalists are, in effect, brokers, framing social reality and shaping the public consciousness about science.*
> Dorothy Nelkin[1]

Public interest in health, health care, and medical science is substantial, and there are many challenges to the effective and fair communication of scientific information to professionals, news media, and the public. The quality of this communication has traditionally begun with a journal article. Flawed, incomplete, or biased research publications in journals without editorial balance or explanation set the stage for poor communication to professionals and the news media. Inaccurate, incomplete, or exaggerated news reporting can mislead the public about the importance or even the meaning of scientific information. Major changes in the media landscape undermine the quality of news. Economic pressures from declining circulation have led many newspapers to eliminate health and science news sections, resulting in a loss of news editors and journalists with expertise in the critical evaluation of medical research and a very limited number of journalists trained as scientists or health care professionals. Increasingly, science news is provided by reporters or bloggers who may have limited understanding of science, medicine, and health. The competitive nature of the business of news delivery and scientific publication has led to the expansion of online news systems, on-demand news, blogs, social media, tabloid journalism, and sponsored and deceptive journals, news sites, blogs, and websites masquerading as credible and objective providers of science and health information. Moreover, the public is often poorly prepared to think critically about science, which makes them susceptible to inaccurate or misleading news reports.

The responsible dissemination of the results of new scientific research and information to the public is critical. However, amid the burgeoning means of conveying such information, accuracy and reliability of science news coverage in the news media are not increasing proportionately. To gain a competitive edge in the information chain, news organizations may exchange complexity, analysis, background, and perspective for immediacy, brevity, and sensationalism. Thus, the need for journal editors to develop and maintain viable, appropriate, and ethical relationships with news journalists for all types of media has become even more important.

The incomplete, inconsistent, and inaccurate coverage of health, medicine, and science in the news media is well documented.[2-15] For example, HealthNewsReview.org evaluated reporting by major US news organizations on new medical treatments, tests, products, and procedures. Reviewers assessed and graded 1976 news stories from 2006 to 2015 (including newspaper articles, wire or news services stories, online stories, and network television stories) and rated most stories as unsatisfactory on 5 of 10 review criteria: costs, benefits, harms, quality of the evidence, and comparison of the new approach with alternatives.[16] As summarized by Schwitzer, "drugs, medical devices, and other interventions were usually portrayed positively; potential harms were minimized, and costs were ignored."[12(p1183)] HealthNewsReview.org continues to regularly evaluate the quality of news stories about health according to the following 10 criteria[17]:

- Does the story adequately discuss the costs of the intervention?

- Does the story adequately quantify the benefits of the treatment/test/product/ procedure?

- Does the story adequately explain/quantify the harms of the intervention?

- Does the story seem to grasp the quality of the evidence?

- Does the story commit disease-mongering?

- Does the story use independent sources and identify conflicts of interest?

- Does the story compare the new approach with existing alternatives?

- Does the story establish the availability of the treatment/test/product/procedure?

- Does the story establish the true novelty of the approach?

- Does the story appear to rely solely or largely on a news release?

HealthNewsReview.org also provides a toolkit for journalists with tips for understanding and interpreting studies, including commonly misunderstood and misreported issues, such as statistical significance, association vs causation, odds ratios, absolute vs relative risk, intention-to-treat analysis, number needed to treat, subgroup analysis, and surrogate markers.[17] The tips also include Schwitzer's 7 words that should never be used in medical news: *cure, miracle, breakthrough, promising, dramatic, hope*, and *victim*[17] (see 11.1, Correct and Preferred Usage of Common Words and Phrases). Other organizations with useful guidance include the Association of Health Care Journalists[18] and the Open Notebook.[19]

Scientific journal editors also have responsibilities regarding communicating scientific information to the public and their relationship with the news media[3,20-23]:

- Publish appropriate, accurate, reliable, timely, and accountable scientific information.

- Help authors of research articles follow quality of reporting guidelines, avoid use of causal language when reporting observational studies,[24] report findings in an objective and circumspect manner, and minimize bias in the analysis and presentation of their findings.

- Require authors to report limitations of their studies, all sources of funding, and disclosures of conflicts of interest.

- Provide editorial balance for complex, controversial, or practice-changing reports of new research by publishing explanatory editorials or invited commentary with research articles as needed.

- Inform authors and journalists about journal policies regarding release of information in manuscripts under consideration or accepted before publication and journal embargoes prohibiting news media coverage of articles before publication (see 5.13.1, Release of Information to the Public).

- Assist the news media in preparing accurate reports of the information about to be published by providing news releases that meet explicit quality standards set by journals (see 5.13.5, News Releases), answering questions, facilitating equal advanced access to the journal articles in a controlled and consistent manner, and providing access to authors or other experts as needed (see 5.13.1, Release of Information to the Public).

- Evaluate the quality of news coverage of information published in the journal. For example, if a news organization has published an inaccurate report of a particular journal article, the journal editor should consider notifying the journalist or news editor to identify the errors in the report.

Journal editors and news journalists share a common obligation—to ensure that the public receives accurate information and is not misled.[3,20] This obligation becomes particularly important when information about risk is communicated to the public. For example, failure to describe health risks accurately and in proper perspective may be misleading, can create unnecessary concern, and may result in loss of public trust in reporters, editors, and scientists. Tensions between journalists, editors, and scientists—often driven by self-interests—can do much to confuse the public. These tensions should be recognized and mitigated, and journals should seek an appropriate balance among their duties to the community of readers they serve, the integrity of the scientific literature, and public entitlement to access to important scientific information without unreasonable delay.[20]

**5.13.1** **Release of Information to the Public.** In many ways, biomedical journals and their editors act as gatekeepers for the release of scientific information to their readers and the public. However, conflicts often arise between journal editors (who have an ethical duty to ensure that the information they publish has been appropriately peer reviewed and assessed for quality) and authors and scientists (who want to disseminate their findings as widely and quickly as possible) and between editors and news reporters (who want to deliver information about new scientific developments as widely and quickly as possible). The announcement of "scientific breakthroughs" at press conferences or through press releases before the data that support the supposed advance have been evaluated and published in a peer-reviewed journal may cause confusion for the public (who may be given misleading or inaccurate information), news media (who may give undue attention to an inaccurate or incomplete claim), journal editors (who may have a policy that discourages publication of data that have already been reported in the press), and investigators (who may forfeit their chance for publication in a reputable peer-reviewed journal by choosing to publish by press conference or through news releases).[20-22]

Journal editors have developed 2 policies to discourage premature release of information to the public. The first policy, based on the Ingelfinger rule (developed in 1969 by Franz Ingelfinger, MD, then editor of the *New England Journal of Medicine*), is an understanding between authors and editors that a manuscript will be considered for publication on the condition that it has not been submitted or reported elsewhere[23] (see 5.3, Duplicate Publication and Submission). The second policy is a news embargo, which is an agreement between journalists and editors that prohibits news coverage of a journal article until it is published (see 5.13.3, Embargo). Although some authors and journalists misunderstand or disagree with the intent of the Ingelfinger rule and the news embargo,[24] many journals have found that both, if applied consistently and fairly, effectively serve all communities interested in disseminating quality scientific information to the public. The International Committee of Medical Journal Editors (ICMJE),[25] the Council of Science Editors,[26] and the World Association of Medical Editors[27] recommend that journals develop and follow policies for orderly, controlled, and consistent release of information to the public, including the use of embargoes.

There are 4 general exceptions to a journal policy that precludes prepublication release of information to the public[20]:

- Presentation of information during scientific or clinical meetings

- Release of information that is determined to be of urgent public need

- Testimony before government agencies

- Release of information that is in the public domain

A new evolving exception involves posting of manuscripts on preprint servers. Although not new to the physics and other scientific communities, preprint servers are relatively new in medical and health sciences. Preprint servers enable authors to post preprints (manuscripts) of studies for public dissemination before formal peer review and publication in a journal. Concerns about public release of research findings that could potentially cause harm to public health or patients have resulted in some journals urging caution about such posting. However, the number of preprints in medical and health sciences is increasing, and journal policies about preprints are evolving with an increasing number of funders and journals encouraging preprints (see 5.6.2, Public Access and Open Access in Scientific Publication).

**5.13.1.1** **Presentation of Information During Scientific or Clinical Meetings.** Presentation of findings during formal scientific or clinical meetings (via oral presentation or poster presentation) ordinarily does not preclude consideration of a manuscript reporting the complete findings for publication.[20,22,25] Authors may include abstracts of their findings in print or online proceedings published for these meetings and summaries of their research in meeting presentation slides or posters. However, authors should refrain from disseminating or publishing details in proceedings that are not included in the meeting abstract or presentation. Authors should not include a complete report of their findings (ie, a manuscript that they plan to submit to a journal) or distribute copies of their detailed findings or tables and figures that go beyond what is included in the meeting presentation to meeting attendees or journalists. Authors are encouraged to participate in discussion and the usual exchange with meeting attendees during their presentation. Video, audio, and social media summaries of meeting presentations also do not preclude consideration of the full manuscript for publication provided these are intended for meeting participants.

Authors may also answer questions from journalists about their meeting presentations, but they should limit their discussion to explaining and clarifying the findings presented during the formal meeting presentation. Authors should not discuss any related manuscripts under consideration by a journal or accepted but not yet published and should not reveal the name of the journal to which their manuscript has been submitted. When authors talk with the media about their meeting presentations related to work that they plan to submit for subsequent publication in a journal, they should acknowledge that the results are preliminary and may change after the complete report undergoes peer review, editing, and publication in a journal.

When an author is presenting findings at a meeting that are also included in a manuscript that is under consideration or has been accepted by a journal but not yet published, the author should limit her or his remarks to the findings as presented at the meeting and should not reveal that the manuscript is under consideration by a specific journal (ie, should not name the journal). In this case, the author should inform the editor of plans to present the work at a meeting before the meeting occurs and should discuss options with the editor. Many journals offer options for expedited review and early online publication of important research articles to coincide with meeting presentation of the research (see 5.13.3, Embargo, and 5.13.4, Suggestions for Authors Interacting With the News Media). News media coverage (based on these interactions) about manuscripts that are accepted but not yet published or that are under consideration by a journal occurring before the journal embargo is lifted and without prior approval of the editor may be grounds for rejection of the manuscript by some journals.

Authors of manuscripts under consideration by a journal or accepted but not yet published, as well as representatives of the authors' institutions and funders, ordinarily should not participate in press conferences or extensive news interviews before publication of the peer-reviewed article. Thus, authors should not participate in press conferences at meetings separate from their scientific presentation or in-depth, extended news interviews, unless they have discussed this with the journal editor and have prior approval from the journal to which the full manuscript has been submitted.

As noted above, the journal editor and the author may plan to expedite review, revision, and publication to permit online publication of an important article to coincide with the date and time of the presentation of the findings during a scientific meeting (eg, with a late-breaking trial that is likely to have practice-changing implications). In these cases, news releases prepared by an author's institution or funder that summarize information to be published in a journal should be coordinated with the journal (see 5.13.5, News Releases). Proper planning is needed among all parties (journal, author, and meeting organizer) to ensure that findings are released in an orderly manner that does not create confusion for journalists or the public.

**5.13.1.2** **Release of Information Determined to Be of Urgent Public Need.** Contrary to what many authors and news reporters believe, few findings from scientific and medical research have such significant and urgently important implications for the public that the information should be released to the public before it has been peer reviewed, revised, and published by a journal. Calling such circumstances "exceptional," the ICMJE recommends that public health authorities should make such decisions and should be responsible for disseminating such information to health care professionals and the news media.[25] In such cases, the ICMJE notes, "If the author and the appropriate authorities wish to have a manuscript considered by a particular journal, the editor should be consulted before any public release. If editors acknowledge the need for immediate release, they should waive their policies limiting prepublication publicity."[21] However, an editor may recognize the public health urgency of releasing information contained in a manuscript under consideration without prompting from the authors or relevant authorities. In such a case, the editor should coordinate early release with the author. In situations in which there is an immediate public health need for the information, there should be no delay in its release. Journals should expedite the editorial and peer review process and speed the publication process to permit online publication as quickly as possible. Care should be taken that this is conducted in an orderly and consistent manner so as not to confuse journalists and the public.

**5.13.1.3** **Testimony Before Government Agencies.** An author's required testimony before a governmental agency or institution (eg, the US Congress or the US Food and Drug Administration) that includes information not yet published should not preclude consideration of that information in a manuscript under consideration or subsequently submitted for publication.[20] Authors and editors should discuss whether consideration and publication of a manuscript with information relevant to such testimony can be expedited to coincide with or be published before the testimony on a case-by-case basis.

**5.13.1.4** **Information in the Public Domain.** Reports of important information from national government or international agencies published and widely disseminated or easily accessible online (eg, an urgent health alert or web posting from the National Institutes of Health or the World Health Organization) should be considered selectively for publication in a peer-reviewed journal on a case-by-case basis.[20] In such a case, the editor needs to determine if the information would be useful to the journal's readers, if there is demonstrated need for an additional report (eg, additional important details or follow-up information is available), and if the initial alert did not already include the complete report. In addition, governmental legislation may require the public posting of guidelines or recommendations for public comment before a final version is released. In such cases, a journal editor should assess if additional peer review is needed and if publication in the journal is warranted.

**5.13.2** **Expedited Publication and Release of Information.** Many journals have policies to expedite the evaluation and publication of manuscripts deemed worthy of accelerated dissemination, including release of an article online ahead of an established publication schedule.[20] Editors should use consistent and orderly policies and procedures to identify manuscripts that contain such information; expedite the editorial, peer review, and publication process; coordinate timing with the authors; and, if feasible, notify and provide controlled advance access to journalists.

**5.13.3** **Embargo.** A news embargo is an agreement between journals and news reporters and their organizations not to report information contained in a manuscript that has been accepted but not yet published until a specified date and time in exchange for advance access to the information. Among medical journals, the embargo system may have been initiated by Morris Fishbein, MD, editor of *JAMA* between 1924 and 1949.[28]

As an example, the standard embargo date and time for a regular issue of *JAMA* is 11 AM eastern time on Tuesday (issue publication date). The JAMA Network journals also publish articles online first and online only, and there is a standard embargo for these articles as well. Credentialed and approved journalists are given early access to news releases and journal articles via a password-protected website for the news media during the embargo period (usually 2-5 days before publication date).[29] During this time, the embargo is intended to provide news reporters an equal amount of access and time to research and prepare their news stories. However, those news reports cannot be released until the embargo has lifted, which is the date and time of publication. The For the Media website also provides information about the journals' embargo policies and answers to frequently asked questions.

The news embargo has been criticized for being overly restrictive, delaying public access to information, and serving the self-interest of journals.[29] However, the embargo system is intended to create a level playing field for journalists to prepare accurate and complete news stories and to maintain consistency in the timing of release of scientific information to the public and help prevent confusion that may result from sporadic reporting on the same study at different dates and times. According to the ICMJE, such consistency of timing helps to minimize "economic chaos" surrounding those articles that contain information that may influence financial markets.[25] *JAMA* editors conducted a brief survey of journalists in 2017. Of the 404 respondents, 389 (96%) indicated wanting to continue the advanced embargoed release of journal content to the media, and 315 (81%) preferred the embargoed release to be 3 days in advance of publication (vs 1 or 2 days).

On occasion, a news reporter or organization may break an embargo and report on information from a peer-reviewed journal article before the embargo is lifted. In most cases, embargo breaks are unintentional (owing to miscommunication or misunderstanding) but on occasion are intentional to scoop competitors.[28,30,31] The rare intentional embargo break is a serious breach of trust and can result in the journal applying sanctions against the reporter and the news organization. Such sanctions may include barring the reporter, and perhaps the news organization, from receiving news releases and advance access to journal content and declining requests for interviews, access to authors, or other assistance. All embargo breaks, whether inadvertent or intentional, cause major problems for journals and journalists who have been abiding by the established embargo release time and may require early lifting of the embargo by the journal and modifying publishing plans scheduled by reporters and their media outlets.

**5.13.4** **Suggestions for Authors Interacting With the News Media.** The following recommendations are provided for interactions between authors and the news media.[20,25,32,33]

- Authors should abide by agreements with most journals to not publicize their work while their manuscript describing the work is under consideration or awaiting publication by a journal. If authors have any questions about release of such information, they should contact the journal's editorial office.[20,25]

- Authors presenting research at clinical and scientific meetings orally with slides or in posters may discuss their presentations with reporters but should refrain from distributing copies of their presentations, data, tables, or figures (see 5.3, Duplicate Publication and Submission).[20,25]

- Authors should inform editors of previous news coverage of their work at the time of manuscript submission (see 5.3, Duplicate Publication and Submission).[25]

- Authors of manuscripts under consideration by a journal or accepted but not yet published should not participate in press conferences or extended news interviews before publication of their findings in the journal unless this is an approved exception by the journal editor that is done in coordination with the journal.[20]

- Authors who receive requests from journalists for information about their research or other work reported in manuscripts that are under consideration but not yet accepted by a journal may indicate that the manuscript is under consideration but should not provide details or the name of the journal unless and until the manuscript is accepted (see 5.7.1, Confidentiality During Editorial Evaluation and Peer Review and After Publication).

- Authors should establish an understanding with a reporter before an interview about the journal's embargo policy[33] and should ask to review direct quotations for accuracy. Note: Authors should be cautious about making comments "off the record."

▪ For accepted manuscripts about to be published and those just published, authors should be as accessible to the news media as their schedules permit, keeping reporters' deadlines in mind and setting aside time to prepare for and give interviews.[32]

▪ During an interview, authors should take care to put the findings in context, appropriately represent the meaning and magnitude of the findings, and acknowledge study limitations and caveats. They should explain commonly used jargon and acronyms (and avoid their use if possible). They should provide easily understood statistics (eg, absolute risks for treatment and control groups) and avoid too many and exaggerated statistics (eg, relative changes without base rates, survival statistics to demonstrate benefit of screening). Authors also should avoid use of words that imply causation for findings of research that can only demonstrate association (eg, observational studies). In addition, they should avoid answering hypothetical questions and responding with "no comment" (it is better to provide an explanation for not being able to answer a specific question).[15,33-36]

▪ Authors should inform reporters and news organizations of errors in news stories and request published corrections if necessary and possible.[32]

▪ Authors who expect to be interviewed frequently by the news media should consider having training in providing informative and accurate interviews.[32]

In addition, journal editors should inform authors of accepted manuscripts of the journal's policies regarding release of information before publication and relations with the news media. For example, *JAMA* reminds authors of its policies on duplicate publication and news embargoes in acceptance letters, noting that authors and the news media should not release any information about the author's accepted article until the specified embargo date and time. This embargo does not preclude authors from participating in interviews with reporters who are preparing stories; it is meant to remind authors that any news stories that result from such interviews should not precede publication of the authors' articles in the journal.

Some journals notify authors of projected publication dates in their acceptance letters, and some journals include a notice of the publication date on the edited manuscript or page proof sent to authors for approval before publication. Editorial and publishing staff may also receive requests from authors asking about expected dates of publication. Staff and authors should not assume that such dates or their corresponding embargo dates are definite or final. Editors may rearrange the editorial content schedules of specific issues and online releases. When informing authors of the expected dates of publication for their accepted articles, editors should remind authors that publication dates may change.

If authors want to coordinate news coverage of their published articles through a press conference or news release, they should first contact the journal editor to ascertain the exact date of publication. Editors and publishers may want to help authors and representatives from their organizations coordinate press conferences and releases with the simultaneous publication of their articles. Editors and publishers can also help the news media prepare accurate reports by providing high-quality news releases, answering questions, providing access to the authors and other experts, and providing advanced access to journal articles.[21,22] This assistance should be contingent on agreement with and cooperation of the news media in timing their release of stories to coincide with the publication of the article. News releases, advance copies of journals, and journal articles released online in advance should indicate the date and time of the news embargo and be restricted to qualified news journalists and agencies that agree to honor the journal's embargo policy.

**5.13.5**  **News Releases.** Many journals issue news releases on selected articles determined by the editors to be of interest to the public. For example, experienced science writers prepare news releases for selected articles published in the JAMA Network journals, and these news releases are reviewed by the editors to ensure accuracy and objectivity. Some journals may also ask authors to review news releases to check for accuracy. News releases of journal editorial content should be under the authority of the editor, not the journal's publisher or owner (see 5.10, Editorial Freedom and Integrity).

News editors, writers, and producers receive hundreds of news releases a week. Thus, a news release must attract attention, but it also must conform to a familiar format and style. See **Box 5.13-1** for a guide to news release content and format and **Box 5.13-2** for sample news releases from the JAMA Network journals. Journalists are taught to present facts accurately, but they may not know how to interpret biomedical statistics or understand the specific context of new scientific information.[6,16] In news releases and news stories, research findings and statistics are often cited inaccurately or out of context to support an exaggerated medical claim.[2,5,8,10-15] To help prevent exaggerated or misleading claims, news releases must include accurate and clearly stated statistics[16,17,37,38] (see 19.1, Study Design and Statistics, The Manuscript: Presenting Study Design, Rationale, and Statistical Analysis). In addition, research findings must be placed in proper context and should include important background, summary of study methods, limitations of the methods, and information on study sponsorship and relevant conflicts of interests of authors (see 5.5, Conflicts of Interest). Care should be taken to provide balance (eg, citing a related editorial) and to avoid sensationalism (eg, use of terms such as *cure, miracle,* or *breakthrough*).[17] Examples of common problems to avoid in news releases are listed in **Box 5.13-3**.

**Box 5.13-1.** Guide for News Release Content and Format

- News releases should clearly indicate the name of the issuing organization (eg, journal, publisher, society, agency, institution, or company).

- The name, address, telephone number, and email and web address of the releasing organization should be prominently listed (eg, under the title "News Release" at the top of the release).

- The name, address, telephone number, and email address of the release contact person should be clearly identifiable.

- The release should be no longer than 200 to 600 words (1-2 pages in print or PDF). For print releases that exceed 1 page, the word *more* should appear at the bottom of the first page.

- The release can be structured and may include a representative table or figure (see example of a structured news release in Box 5.13-2).

- The time and date of the release and the embargo should appear prominently at the top of the release.

- An easily identifiable headline (eg, boldface or underlined) that provides the essence of the release should also appear at the top of the release.

- For most news releases, the location of the issuing organization of the release should appear in capital letters before the lead sentence. For journals that issue news releases about studies conducted elsewhere, this is not necessary (see Box 5.13-2).

- The lead sentence should contain the most important information. Details should be given in later paragraphs. The name of the journal in which the article appeared should be included in the lead sentence to help facilitate mention of the journal in the story as a source of the information.

- Authors of the article should be clearly identified with complete names, academic degrees, and affiliations; relevant conflicts of interest should be included in the news release or noted that these are included in the article.

- All sources of funding for the research or work should be identified in the news release or noted that these are included in the article.

- Releases should contain simple, declarative sentences and should avoid jargon and undefined abbreviations. All medical terms should be explained. Specify the details of complex interventions (eg, "counseling consisted of 10 weekly visits to dietitians") and translate meaning of exposure levels into ordinary activities (eg, "50 g of protein of processed meat is equivalent to 4 slices of bacon").

- All statistics and numbers should be properly explained and put in context.

- A complete citation and link to the article(s) cited in the news release should be included.

**Box 5.13-2.** Examples of News Releases[a]

**Unstructured Narrative News Release Example**

EMBARGOED FOR RELEASE: 11 A.M. (ET) TUESDAY, JULY 25, 2017

Media Advisory: To contact Ann C. McKee, M.D., email Gillian Smith (grsmith@bu.edu) or Pallas Wahl (pallas.wahl@va.gov).

**Related material:** The editorial "Advances and Gaps in Understanding Chronic Traumatic Encephalopathy" by Gil D. Rabinovici, M.D., of the University of California, San Francisco, also is available at the For the Media website.

**To place an electronic embedded link to this study in your story:** This link will be live at the embargo time: http://jamanetwork.com/journals/jama/fullarticle/10.1001/jama.2017.8334

*JAMA*

High Prevalence of Evidence of Chronic Traumatic Encephalopathy in Brains of Deceased Football Players

Chronic traumatic encephalopathy (CTE) was diagnosed post-mortem in a high proportion of former football players whose brains were donated for research, including 110 of 111 National Football League players, according to a study published by *JAMA*.

CTE is a progressive neurodegeneration associated with repetitive head trauma and players of American football may be at increased risk of long-term neurological conditions, particularly CTE.

Ann C. McKee, M.D., of the Boston University CTE Center and VA Boston Healthcare System, and colleagues conducted a study that examined the brains of 202 deceased former football players to determine neuropathological features of CTE through laboratory examination and clinical symptoms of CTE by talking to players' next of kin to collect detailed histories including on head trauma, athletic participation and military service.

Among the 202 football players (median age at death was 66), CTE was neuropathologically diagnosed in 177 players (87 percent) who had had an average of 15 years of football participation. The 177 players included: 3 of 14 high school players (21 percent); 48 of 53 college players (91 percent); 9 of 14 semiprofessional players (64 percent); 7 of 8 Canadian Football League players (88 percent); and 110 of 111 NFL players (99 percent).

Neuropathological severity of CTE was distributed across the highest level of play, with all three former high school players having mild pathology and the majority of former college (56 percent), semiprofessional (56 percent), and professional (86 percent) players having severe pathology. Among 27 participants with mild CTE pathology, 96 percent had behavioral or mood symptoms or both, 85 percent had cognitive symptoms, and 33 percent had signs of dementia. Among 84 participants with severe CTE pathology, 89 percent had behavioral or mood symptoms or both, 95 percent had cognitive symptoms, and 85 percent had signs of dementia.

"In a convenience sample of deceased football players who donated their brains for research, a high proportion had neuropathological evidence of CTE, suggesting that CTE may be related to prior participation in football," the article concludes. The authors acknowledge several other football-related factors may influence CTE risk and disease severity, including but not limited to age at first exposure to football, duration of play, player position and cumulative hits.

The study has several limitations, including that it is a skewed sample based on a brain donation program because public awareness of a possible link between repetitive head

(*continued*)

**Box 5.13-2.** Examples of News Releases (*continued*)

trauma and CTE may have motivated players and their families with symptoms and signs of brain injury to participate in this research. The authors urge caution in interpreting the high frequency of CTE in this study, stressing that estimates of how prevalent CTE may be cannot be concluded or implied.

For more details and to read the full study, please visit the For the Media website. (doi:10.1001/jama.2017.8334)

Editor's Note: Please see the article for additional information, including other authors, author contributions and affiliations, financial disclosures, funding and support, etc.

# # #

**For more information, contact JAMA Network Media Relations at 312-464-JAMA (5262) or email** mediarelations@jamanetwork.org.

---

**Structured News Release Example**

**Is Eating Fiber After Colorectal Cancer Diagnosis Associated With Lower Death Risk?**

*JAMA Oncology*

**EMBARGOED FOR RELEASE: 11 A.M. (ET), THURSDAY, NOVEMBER 2, 2017**

**Media advisory:** To contact corresponding author Andrew T. Chan, M.D., M.P.H., email to Katie Marquedant at Kmarquedant@mgh.harvard.edu. The full study is available on the For the Media website.

**Want to embed a link to this study in your story?** Links will be live at the embargo time http://jamanetwork.com/journals/jamaoncology/fullarticle/10.1001/jamaoncol.2017.3684

**Bottom Line:** Eating more fiber was associated with a lower risk of death overall and from colorectal cancer in patients with non-metastatic colorectal cancer.

**Why The Research Is Interesting:** Colorectal cancer is common and the number of people living with treated disease is estimated to grow with advances in diagnosis and treatment. Many cancer survivors look for self-care strategies, especially advice on what to eat. Fiber intake is thought to be protective against colorectal cancer. But whether fiber intake is associated with recurrent colorectal cancer and survival in patients already diagnosed and treated has not been examined.

**Who:** 1,575 health professionals with non-metastatic (stages 1 to 3) colorectal cancer who provided detailed diet information on food questionnaires.

**When:** Fiber consumption was measured beginning in the 1980s; deaths were measured until 2012; the study was conducted from December 2016 to August 2017.

**What (Study Measures):** Consumption of total fiber, different sources of fiber and whole grains from six months to four years after participants' colorectal cancer diagnosis (exposures); deaths from colorectal cancer specifically and any cause (outcomes).

**Box 5.13-2.** Examples of News Releases (*continued*)

How (Study Design): This is an observational study. In observational studies, researchers observe exposures and outcomes for patients as they occur naturally in clinical care or real life. Because researchers are not intervening for purposes of the study they cannot control natural differences that could explain study findings so they cannot prove a cause-and-effect relationship.

Authors: Andrew T. Chan, M.D., M.P.H., of Massachusetts General Hospital and Harvard Medical School, Boston, and coauthors

Results: During a median eight-year follow-up, a higher intake of fiber and whole grains after diagnosis of non-metastatic colorectal cancer was associated with a lower risk of death from that disease and other causes. Survival improved for patients who increased their fiber intake after diagnosis compared to those who did not.

Study Limitations: Information about fiber intake and sources was self-reported without adjustment for measurement error. Detailed treatment data for the patients were largely unavailable.

Study Conclusions: "Higher fiber intake after the diagnosis of non-metastatic CRC [colorectal cancer] is associated with lower CRC-specific and overall mortality. Increasing fiber consumption after diagnosis may confer additional benefits to patients with CRC."

Featured Image:

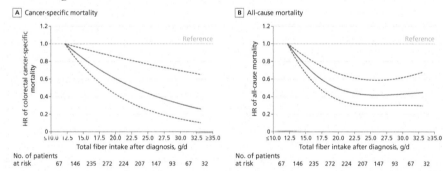

What The Image Shows: The image illustrates that overall and colorectal-cancer specific death appears to decline as total fiber intake increases after diagnosis.

For more details and to read the full study, please visit the For the Media website. (doi:10.1001/jamainternmed.2017.3684)

Editor's Note: The article contains conflict of interest and funding/support disclosures. Please see the article for additional information, including other authors, author contributions and affiliations, financial disclosures, funding and support, etc.

# # #

For more information, contact JAMA Network Media Relations at 312-464-JAMA (5262) or email mediarelations@jamanetwork.org.

ªNote: These news releases follow AP style, not AMA style.

**Box 5.13-3.** Common Problems to Avoid in News Releases of Scientific Studies

- **Unfamiliar mathematical and statistical terms and numbers** that are difficult to interpret should be avoided; do not confuse association and correlation with causation. See also HealthNewsReview's Tips for Understanding Studies.[17]

- **Results should be reported in context**, including locations and dates of the study, representativeness of the sample, and whether results are consistent with what is already known. Risks of events should be acknowledged to be common (eg, common cold) or rare (eg, being hit by lightning).[17,33]

- **Highlight cautions**, including limitations of the study.

- **If the results of a survey are reported**, the response rate should be provided along with a caveat that the results may not be generalizable if the response rate is low.

- **Key study facts:** Report duration and size of the study. If a news release mentions a specific sample that was studied or a specific number of cases, whether the number is large or small, information about the size of the total population from which the sample or cases were drawn should be included.

- **Causal language should be reserved** for reports of randomized clinical trials and laboratory studies and should be avoided for reports of observational studies that can only demonstrate association between findings and study variables, risks, exposures, or other factors.[34]

- **Avoid the word "significant" alone.** Statements about statistical significance should not be quoted from an article out of context or without an explanation.[20] Reporters and readers do not necessarily know the difference between statistical significance and clinical significance or importance. For example, quoting a statement that there was a trend toward a statistically significant association between a treatment and an outcome may give undue importance to a treatment that has no real clinical value. If statistical significance needs to be reported, include an explanation such as "the results are unlikely to be due to chance."

- **Absolute event rates should be reported.** Care should be taken to avoid confusing absolute and relative risks because relative risks are often erroneously translated to specific risks. For example, a decrease from 2.5% to 2.0% should not be reported as a 20% reduction in risk but could be reported as a 0.5% absolute risk reduction and 20% relative risk reduction. It may be helpful to report excess or decreased risk in terms of numbers per 1000 or 10 000. However, this must be done with caution. Percentages rather than frequencies (eg, number per 1000) may be more easily understood by the public. Rates may be difficult to understand, so in some cases it may be possible to translate rates into risks, and for time-to-event analyses, percentages for outcomes for each group at a specific time may be provided along with the median time to the event.[20,39]

- **Avoid reporting odds ratios**, especially for common outcomes, which may overstate a relative risk.[20,33,40]

- **Benefits and harms:** If reporting the results of a study about an intervention, event rates for benefits and harms should be reported equally and in a balanced manner.[33]

- **Check for accuracy.** Before news releases are distributed, they should be proofread and the content should be reviewed by a professional familiar with the article or report covered in the release or by the editor.

**Principal Author:** Annette Flanagin, RN, MA

## ACKNOWLEDGMENT

I thank the following for review and helpful comments: Howard Bauchner, MD, *JAMA* and JAMA Network; Deanna Bellandi, MPH, JAMA Network; Timothy Gray, PhD, JAMA Network; Iris Y. Lo, JAMA Network; and Lisa M. Schwartz, MD, MS, and Steven Woloshin, MD, MS, Center for Medicine and Media and The Dartmouth Institute for Health Policy and Clinical Practice, Lebanon, New Hampshire.

## ADDITIONAL INFORMATION

This work is dedicated to the memory of Lisa M. Schwartz, MD, MS, who conducted influential research on medicine and the media and was a champion for improved communication of medical evidence, bias, and public health risk.

## REFERENCES

1. Nelkin D. Journalism and science: the creative tension. In: *Health Risks and the Press*. Media Institute; 1989:53-71.
2. Moynihan R, Bero L, Ross-Degnan D, et al. Coverage by the news media of the benefits and risks of medications. *N Engl J Med*. 2000;342(22):1645-1650. doi:10.1056/NEJM200006013422206
3. Steinbrook R. Medical journals and medical reporting. *N Engl J Med*. 2000;342:1668-1671. doi:10.1056/NEJM200006013422212
4. Ankney RN, Moore RA, Heilman P. Newspaper coverage of medicine: a survey of editors and cardiac surgeons. *AMWA J*. 2001;16(1):23-32.
5. Schwartz LM, Woloshin S. News media coverage of screening mammography for women in their 40s and tamoxifen for primary prevention of breast cancer. *JAMA*. 2002;287(23):3136-3142. doi:10.1001/jama.287.23.3136
6. Voss M. Checking the pulse: midwestern reporters' opinions on their ability to report health care news. *Am J Public Health*. 2002;92(7):1158-1160.
7. Schwitzer G, Mudur G, Henry D, et al. What are the roles and responsibilities of the media in disseminating health information? *PLoS Med*. 2005;2(7):e215:0576-0582. doi:10.1371/journal.pmed.0020215
8. Motl SE, Timpe EM, Eichner SF. Evaluation of accuracy of health studies reported in mass media. *J Am Pharm Assoc*. 2005;45(6):720-725. doi:10.1331/1544345057740909670
9. Woloshin S, Schwartz LM. Media reporting on research presented at scientific meetings: more caution needed. *Med J Aust*. 2006;184(11):576-580.
10. Schwartz LM, Woloshin S, Andrews A, Stukel TA. Influence of medical journal press releases on the quality of associated newspaper coverage: retrospective cohort study. *BMJ*. 2012;344:d8164. doi:10.1136/bmj.d8164
11. Downing NS, Cheng T, Krumholz HM, Shah ND, Ross JS. Descriptions and interpretations of the ACCORD-Lipid Trial in the news and biomedical literature: a cross-sectional analysis. *JAMA Intern Med*. 2014;174(7):1176-1182. doi:10.1001/jamainternmed.2014.1371
12. Schwitzer G. A guide to reading health care news stories. *JAMA Intern Med*. 2014;174(7):1183-1186. doi:10.1001/jamainternmed.2014.1359
13. Kuriya B, Schneid EC, Bell CM. Quality of pharmaceutical industry press releases based on original research. *PLoS One*. 2008;3(7):e2828. doi:10.1371/journal.pone.0002828

14. Yavchitz A1, Boutron I, Bafeta A, et al. Misrepresentation of randomized controlled trials in press releases and news coverage: a cohort study. *PLoS Med.* 2012;9(9):e1001308. doi:10.1371/journal.pmed.1001308

15. Sumner P, Vivian-Griffiths S, Boivin J, Williams A, et al. The association between exaggeration in health related science news and academic press releases: retrospective observational study. *BMJ.* 2014;349:g7015. doi:10.1136/bmj.g7015

16. HealthNewsReview.org's 9th anniversary—that almost didn't happen. April 16, 2015. Accessed January 1, 2019. http://www.healthnewsreview.org/2015/04/healthnewsreview-orgs-9th-anniversary/

17. HealthNewsReview. Tips for understanding studies. Accessed January 1, 2019. http://www.healthnewsreview.org/toolkit/tips-for-understanding-studies/

18. Association of Health Care Journalists. Resources. Accessed January 1, 2019. https://healthjournalism.org/resources-jump.php

19. The Open Notebook. Accessed January 1, 2019. https://www.theopennotebook.com/

20. Fontanarosa PB, Flanagin A, DeAngelis CD. The Journal's policy regarding release of information to the public. *JAMA.* 2000;284(22):2929-2931. doi:10.1001/jama.284.22.2929

21. Butler D. "Publication by press conference" under fire. *Nature.* 1993;366(6450):6. doi:10.1038/366006a0

22. Schwartz LM, Woloshin S, Baczek L. Media coverage of scientific meetings: too much, too soon? *JAMA.* 2002;287(21):2859-2863. doi:10.1001/jama.287.21.2859

23. Kassirer JP, Angell M. The Ingelfinger rule revisited. *N Engl J Med.* 1991;325(19):1371-1373. doi:10.1056/NEJM199111073251910

24. Altman L. The Ingelfinger rule, embargoes, and journal peer review, part 1. *Lancet.* 1996;347(9012):1382-1386.

25. International Committee of Medical Journal Editors. Recommendations for the conduct, reporting, editing, and publication of scholarly work in medical journals. Updated December 2018. Accessed January 1, 2019. https://www.icmje.org/recommendations

26. Council of Science Editors. Responsibilities to the media. White Paper on Publication Ethics. Updated May 2018. Accessed January 1, 2019. https://www.councilscienceeditors.org/resource-library/editorial-policies/white-paper-on-publication-ethics/

27. World Association of Medical Editors. Recommendations on publication ethics policies for medical journals. Accessed January 1, 2019. http://wame.org/recommendations-on-publication-ethics-policies-for-medical-journals

28. Stacy J. The press embargo—friend or foe? *JAMA.* 1985;254(14):1965-1966. doi:10.1001/jama.1985.03360140123040

29. The JAMA Network. For the Media website. Accessed January 29, 2019. https://media.jamanetwork.com/

30. Fontanarosa PB, DeAngelis CD. The importance of the journal embargo. *JAMA.* 2002;288(6):748-750. doi:10.1001/jama.288.6.748

31. Godlee F. Breaking the embargo. *BMJ.* 2008;337:a2852. doi:10.1136/bmj.a2852

32. Rubin R, Rogers HL Jr. *Under the Microscope: The Relationship Between Physicians and the News Media.* Freedom Forum; 1993.

33. Stamm K, Williams JW, Noel PH, Rubin R. Helping journalists get it right: a physician's guide to improving health care reporting. *J Gen Intern Med.* 2003;18(2):138-145.

34. Editors of the Heart Journals. Statement on matching language to the type of evidence used in describing observational studies vs. randomized trials. *Eur Heart J.* 2013;34(1):20-21. doi:10.1093/eurheartj/ehs386

35. Malenka DJ, Baron JA, Johansen S, Wahrenberger JW, Ross JM. The framing effect of relative and absolute risk. *J Gen Intern Med.* 1993;8(10):543-548.

36. Cho H, Mariotto AB, Schwartz LM, Luo J, Woloshin S. When do changes in cancer survival mean progress? the insight from population incidence and mortality. *J Natl Cancer Inst Monogr.* 2014;(2014)49:187-197. doi:10.1093/jncimonographs/lgu014

37. Cohn V, Cope L. *News and Numbers: A Guide to Reporting Statistical Claims and Controversies in Health and Related Fields.* 2nd ed. Blackwell Publishing Professional; 2001.

38. Woloshin S, Schwartz LM. Press releases: translating research into news. *JAMA.* 2002;287(21):2856-2858. doi:10.1001/jama.287.21.2856

39. Woloshin S, Schwartz LM. Communicating data about the benefits and harms of treatment: a randomized trial. *Ann Intern Med.* 2011;155(2):87-96. doi:10.7326/0003-4819-155-2-201107190-00004

40. Schwartz LM, Woloshin S, Welch HG. Misunderstandings about the effects of race and sex on physicians' referrals for cardiac catheterization. *N Engl J Med.* 1999;341(4):279-283. doi:10.1056/NEJM199907223410411

# 6.0 Editorial Assessment and Processing

**6.0** **Editorial Assessment and Processing.** The principal goals of editing biomedical publications are to identify, select, improve, and disseminate scientific and clinical information that will advance the art and science of the discipline covered by the publication. For example, biomedical journals are a primary source for reporting research advances and for communicating information to improve medical care and public health. In addition to providing information to subscribers and other recipients of the journal, articles published in biomedical journals may be accessed and used by numerous other readers and constituencies, such as clinicians and researchers who seek information about particular topics; educators and opinion leaders who may use information from journal articles for teaching and informing colleagues; and members of the media, who frequently communicate information from research articles that involve medicine and health to the public.

However, perhaps the most important use of articles published in clinical biomedical journals is to provide valid and reliable information to physicians and other clinicians to promote the practice of evidence-based medicine, in which decisions about patient care are informed by acquiring, assessing, and applying relevant medical literature. These myriad uses of the biomedical literature illustrate the importance of journals having rigorous procedures for editorial assessment and processing to ensure the validity and improve the quality of published articles.

**6.1** **Editorial Assessment.** Editorial assessment of a manuscript ordinarily consists of 3 phases: initial editorial review, peer review, and editorial assessment and decision-making (**Figure 6.1-1**). During the initial editorial review, editors assess submitted manuscripts for overall quality and appropriateness for the readership of the journal. Manuscripts that do not pass this initial editorial review are rejected, whereas those that pass this initial evaluation proceed to the peer review phase. Peer review (see 6.1.2, Peer Review) involves evaluation of the manuscript by reviewers who have expertise in the topic and knowledge about the information reported in the manuscript and may include evaluation by reviewers with

**Figure 6.1-1.** Example of Editorial Assessment

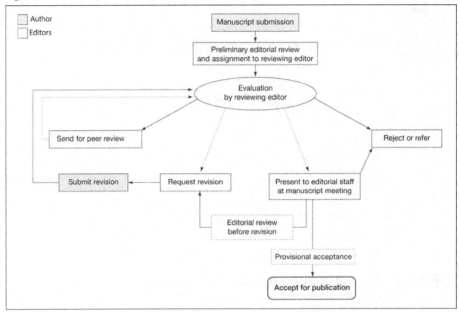

expertise in specific aspects of the manuscript, such as statistical reviewers. After completion of peer review, editors reassess the manuscript with consideration of the reviewers' comments and suggestions as part of editorial decision making. The integrity of the editorial assessment process requires strict confidentiality on the part of editors, journal staff, and peer reviewers and careful attention to possible biases and conflicts of interest of authors (see 5.7.1, Confidentiality During Editorial Evaluation and Peer Review and After Publication).

**6.1.1** **Manuscript Assessment Criteria.** Several criteria are central to the evaluation of manuscripts submitted for publication, including importance, validity, and quality. Assessment of *importance* involves determining whether the manuscript reports information that represents a scientific advance (recognizing that individual articles usually convey only small advances), has clinical relevance (if the journal is to be read and the information used by practicing clinicians), is sufficiently novel to add new scientific information to the field, and will likely be of interest to readers. An additional component of importance is *editorial priority*, a composite judgment made by the editor regarding the merits of a particular submission relative to the merits of other submissions under evaluation at the same time, weighed in the context of articles the journal has recently published, has scheduled for publication, or has under consideration.

Evaluation of *validity* of a research report involves critical assessment of the internal integrity of the manuscript to determine whether the research design and study execution support the findings, inferences, and interpretations reported in the manuscript. For original research reports, assessment of validity involves consideration of whether the design and methods are appropriate to answer the stated research questions; the research questions and the methods used to answer them are well described and rigorously conducted; the data analysis is appropriately performed; the conclusions are supported by the results; and patients or research participants were treated ethically (see 5.8, Protecting Research Participants' and Patients' Rights in Scientific Publication).

Assessment of *quality* of a research manuscript involves determining how well the authors present the information, such as overall organization and cohesiveness of the manuscript, clarity of the purpose of the study and description of the methods, logical and transparent reporting of data, including effective use of well-constructed tables and figures, appropriate and objective interpretation of the study findings, and inclusion of key and suitable references. Other aspects of quality assessment involve evaluating the quality of the writing and logical presentation of information and how well the authors follow the journal's guidelines or instructions for authors.

For research and review manuscripts (see 1.0, Types of Articles), writing quality and clarity may influence the evaluation by editors and peer reviewers even though the importance and quality of the research should be the main focus for assessment. Writing quality can be improved by manuscript editing (see 6.2.1, Manuscript Editing) but only if the research is described with sufficient clarity to permit basic understanding. Writing quality and presentation of information may be particularly important factors in the assessment of opinion articles, such as Viewpoints or invited opinion pieces, in which well-organized, well-argued, and well-written compelling manuscripts generally are more likely to receive higher priority for publication than poorly written manuscripts.

For research reports, the specific nature or direction of results should not ordinarily be a major factor in quality assessment. If a rigorously conducted investigation addresses an important clinical or scientific question, uses high-quality and rigorous methods, and has findings that are determined to be valid, the study results may be worth publishing regardless if "positive" (demonstrates an effect or an association) or "neutral" or "negative" (does not demonstrate an effect or association). Publication bias could result from a tendency for investigators not to submit or for editors not to accept manuscripts that do not report statistically significant positive results. However, depending on the topic being investigated, a well-conducted, adequately powered study that shows that a particular intervention is not effective may be as important as a study that reports a positive result.

For review articles and other reports that do not involve original research, editorial assessment involves determining the importance and relevance of the topic for the journal readership; the completeness, accuracy, timeliness, logical presentation, and, usually, clinical utility of the information presented; and the quality and rigor of the evidence provided to support recommendations, for example, for or against diagnostic testing or treatment.

**6.1.2** **Peer Review.** Peer review was first used for biomedical publications by the Royal Societies of London and Edinburgh in the 18th century but evolved haphazardly, was not used consistently until after World War II,[1,2] and has only come under scientific scrutiny since the 1980s.[3,4] Despite the routine use of peer review of manuscripts by scientific journals, the peer review process has been criticized for its reliance on human judgments that may be subject to biases and conflicts of interest. Moreover, until relatively recently, there was little empirical evaluation and documentation of the efficacy and value of the peer review process. However, with the advent of the International Congresses on Peer Review and Biomedical Publication in 1989[5] and subsequent congresses held every 4 years since then,[6] empirical research on editorial peer review and scientific publication has examined many aspects of these important practices, providing evidence-based information to better understand and improve the peer review process, the quality of research reporting, and the scientific publication process.

The essence of peer review for biomedical journals consists of asking experts, "How important and how good is this manuscript, and how can it be improved?" The involvement of expert consultants to advise editors about importance, validity, quality, and improvement of manuscripts has become a standard quality assessment measure in biomedical publication. Review of a manuscript by experts in the subject matter being reported is helpful to assess importance and quality of the work and to determine the context for the information being reported, such as whether study findings represent novel advances or are incremental additions to the scientific literature.

Peer reviewers should assess all components of a manuscript, including the title, abstract, and text of the manuscript, the references, the tables and figures, and all supplementary material. On the basis of this assessment, reviewers should provide an overall assessment of the manuscript, along with comments for the authors regarding the strengths and weaknesses of a manuscript, including specific methodologic or substantive issues that need to be addressed, as well as suggestions for improvement. Although specific criticisms and suggestions are much more valuable than summary judgments, reviewers also may be asked to provide an overall recommendation to the editor about suitability of the manuscript for publication in the journal. Although these suggestions are helpful, the comments and recommendations about publication from the peer reviewer consultants are considered advisory, and all decisions about rejection, revision, or acceptance are the responsibility of the journal editors (see 5.11.4, Editorial Responsibility for Peer Review).

**6.1.2.1** **Selection of Reviewers.** The selection of peer reviewers and the number of reviewers for evaluating a particular manuscript are matters of editorial judgment. In most cases, peer reviewers are usually experts who are not part of the journal staff or otherwise not associated with the journal, although members of the editorial staff or editorial board of the journal may serve as peer reviewers in areas of their expertise. The editor's knowledge of experts in a particular field often determines reviewer selection. Many journals maintain a database of reviewers indexed by areas of expertise, including information on review quality and turnaround time. The reference list of a manuscript may be a useful starting point for identifying potential peer reviewers who have been contributors to the literature on the same topic. A literature search by the editor can also be helpful in identifying potential reviewers.

Authors may suggest names of possible peer reviewers, and some journals encourage authors to make these suggestions, although some reviewers recommended by authors may provide more favorable reviews than reviewers selected by editors without suggestions from authors. At times, authors also may request that some persons not serve as reviewers for their manuscript, usually because of perceived bias. Editors should consider such requests and information, but the selection of peer reviewers is the responsibility of the editor, who must use judgment not only in selecting the reviewers but also in distinguishing a reviewer's valid praise or criticism from unwarranted bias for or against a particular manuscript. Reviewers are expected to disclose to the editor any conflicts of interest they may have regarding a topic or an author at the time they are invited to review the manuscript (see 5.5.6, Requirements for Peer Reviewers, and 5.11.4, Editorial Responsibility for Peer Review).

Evaluation of the scientific validity of original research reports usually requires peer review by reviewers with expertise in statistics, epidemiology, and research methodology to provide assessment of study design and research methods. For some journals, some statistical reviewers are members of the editorial staff or may serve as paid consultants. Epidemiologic and statistical review can be helpful in identifying weaknesses in study design and methods and in improving scientific reports for publication. Moreover, with the use of increasingly sophisticated research and statistical methods, having input from peer reviewers with specific methodologic expertise has become increasingly important in the assessment of the validity and quality of scientific reports.

**6.1.2.2** **Concealing of Author and Reviewer Identities.** Scientific journals usually adopt one of several models for conducting peer review that involve revealing or concealing the identities of authors and peer reviewers. Journal policies vary regarding whether author identities, reviewer identities, both, or neither are kept confidential or are revealed, and these practices should be indicated in the journal's information for authors (see 5.11.4, Editorial Responsibility for Peer Review).

Biomedical journals commonly use a single-blind (also called single-masked) review process in which authors' identities are revealed to reviewers, but the names of reviewers are not revealed to authors (see 5.7.1.1, Confidentiality Requirements During Blinded [Anonymous] Peer Review). This process recognizes the difficulty of concealing author identities, makes it easier for reviewers to detect certain forms of research irregularities (such as attempts at duplicate publication by the same authors), and may encourage more candid reviews because the reviewers know they are anonymous to the authors, who may be their professional colleagues. However, this single-blind approach may have some potential disadvantages. For instance, some reviewers might be influenced by knowing the identities and reputations of authors or their affiliations and therefore might not judge a manuscript solely on quality and importance.

Another approach involves a double-blind (also known as double-masked) peer review, in which neither the authors' nor the reviewers' identities are revealed. Authors who submit a manuscript to a journal that attempts to conceal author identities may be instructed to remove identifying information from all parts of the manuscript and to submit that information separately, such as author names, affiliations, and acknowledgments (including funding sources). Theoretically, the double-blind approach should contribute to a more objective evaluation of the manuscript because reviewers may be more likely to evaluate the manuscript based on quality, without being influenced by knowledge of the identities or affiliations of the authors. However, concealing author identities is not always successful because of self-referencing in the manuscript or reviewer knowledge of the authors' work. There is limited evidence to support the idea that reviewers who are unaware of authors' identities will provide more objective reviews (see 5.7.1.2, Confidentiality Requirements During Double-blind Peer Review).

A third approach used by some journals involves open (or open-identity) peer review, in which reviewers are aware of the identities of the authors, and authors are aware of the identities of those who reviewed their manuscript. Advocates of this approach to the manuscript review process support the importance of transparency in science and suggest that authors should know who is evaluating their work and that reviewers should stand by their critiques by signing them. In one study,[7] asking reviewers to consent to being identified to authors had no important effects on quality of reviews, recommendations regarding publication, or the time taken to review but increased the likelihood of reviewers declining to review (see 5.7.1.4, Open Review).

Regardless of the approach used for peer review, and despite its limitations, peer review has generally been considered "indispensable for the progress of biomedical science."[8] So far, convincing evidence has not demonstrated that a better alternative has emerged for the assessment and improvement of manuscripts submitted to biomedical and scientific journals.

**6.1.3**    **Editorial Decisions.** On the basis of the evaluation of the manuscript by the editors and, for manuscripts that have undergone peer review, consideration of the comments of the peer reviewers, submitted manuscripts are rejected, returned to authors with an invitation to submit a revised manuscript, or, on rare occasions, accepted without revision. For some journals, a substantial proportion of manuscripts are rejected on the basis of the initial editorial review and assessment, a smaller proportion are rejected after peer review, and an even smaller proportion proceed to revision and reevaluation.[9]

Although journals may have different approaches and models for editorial decision-making, the editor in chief has ultimate responsibility for all editorial decisions for rejection, revision, and acceptance of submitted manuscripts. For some journals, the editor in chief may delegate the responsibility to deputy editors or associate editors to make decisions about rejecting manuscripts after initial review and assessment, perhaps with a second opinion about the decision from another editor. Many journals may hold meetings (in person or by teleconference, videoconference, or internet communication) during which submitted manuscripts and their reviews, and also revised manuscripts, are presented and discussed among the editors before decisions are reached regarding proceeding with revision or acceptance for publication.

For manuscripts that are rejected without external peer review, editors may choose to provide brief comments that indicate the reason for the decision. For manuscripts that are rejected after peer review, the editors usually will provide the authors with comments from the peer reviewers and perhaps comments from the editors, so authors can consider this information as they revise the manuscript for submission to another journal.

Reports of original research and other major articles almost always undergo peer review, statistical review, and revision before acceptance for publication (see 1.0, Types of Articles), whereas manuscripts that express opinions, such as Viewpoints or Editorials, may be accepted after revision based on editorial review and evaluation.

**6.1.4** **Revisions.** If the editors decide to request a revision of a submitted manuscript, the authors should receive detailed recommendations from the editor about what is expected in the revision, instructions about how to improve the manuscript, and detailed comments from the peer reviewers. Guidance from the editor is particularly important if recommendations from the peer reviewers are discordant. In addition, at some journals, the editorial staff may conduct internal review of the manuscript and provide additional detailed comments regarding manuscript format, methods, data analysis, interpretation, presentation, and other issues for improving the manuscript. Authors are usually requested to submit a detailed response that addresses the comments, indicates how the revisions were completed, and provides reasons for any suggested revisions not undertaken when they return the revised manuscript. In most cases, it is advantageous for the authors to revise the manuscript promptly and thoroughly and to submit the revised manuscript within a relatively short time, perhaps 2 or 3 weeks.

However, authors should realize that a request for revision does not guarantee that the revised manuscript will be accepted for publication. Revised manuscripts are subject to editorial review and reevaluation and perhaps additional peer review. Important issues with the study methods or manuscript content may not become apparent until after revision. For some manuscripts, several rounds of review and revision may occur before a final decision is reached (see 5.11.6, Editorial Responsibility for Revision).

After submission of a revised manuscript that satisfactorily addresses the comments of the editors and reviewers, the editors will reevaluate the manuscript and make a decision about publication. Manuscripts often are accepted provisionally, contingent on authors fulfilling additional requested revisions or providing required items, such as completed authorship forms and copyright transfer statements.

**6.1.5** **Appealing an Editorial Decision.** If a manuscript is rejected, authors occasionally will appeal the decision and request reconsideration, most often because they perceive that the reviewers or the editor may have misjudged the importance of the submission. Journals should develop procedures for responding to these requests for appeal of editorial decisions. The editor in chief should be involved in the evaluation of the authors' request for reconsideration and the reasons for the request, with careful reassessment of the initial manuscript and the comments of the peer reviewers and detailed discussion with the editor who rendered the initial decision. In most cases, the initial editorial decision is upheld, unless the authors can provide objective and compelling grounds for reconsideration of the original decision, particularly if they can provide new data or new analyses, as opposed to differences of opinion about editorial priority (see 5.11.5, Editorial Responsibility for Rejection).

**6.1.6**     **Postpublication Review.** Postpublication review in peer-reviewed journals may include several potential mechanisms: letters to the editor about the published article that identify flaws, raise additional substantive concerns, or discuss additional important implications of the findings; online responses to published articles; efforts to replicate the work; and the reactions from clinicians applying the information in practice. Such evaluations are important for ensuring responsible scientific dialogue about published articles. Journals should encourage submission of letters to the editor raising issues and questions about published articles, and authors of the published article should be encouraged to prepare responses to those critiques. Publication of these scientific exchanges in the Letters section provides an avenue for postpublication review and discussion (see 5.11.8, Correspondence [Letters to the Editor]). Editors should also perform a quality review of each published issue of their journal to identify areas of content and format that can be corrected or improved in subsequent issues (see 5.11.14, Editorial Quality Review).

**6.1.7**     **Corrections.** As part of postpublication review, errors may be identified by authors or readers, editors, or other sources. Correction of errors is important to ensure the accuracy of the scientific record.[10] In most cases, corrections are minor and straightforward. The Correction notice is listed in the Table of Contents (in print, online, or both), and the Correction should be published in a specific section. For example, the JAMA Network journals publish Corrections at the end of the Letters section. Corrections should be indexed, with a reference and online link to the original article, thereby enabling online database services (such as MEDLINE) to link indexed articles with published corrections (see 5.11.8, Correspondence [Letters to the Editor], and 5.11.10, Corrections [Errata].) The erroneous information should be corrected in the online versions (HTML and PDF) of the published article, with the reason and date of the Correction prominently displayed. Corrections should also be linked from the article to the Correction on the journal's website and appended to the article PDF. If online-only corrections are made or if corrections are made online before the article appeared in print, the changes and date of the correction should be indicated in the electronic file. In some cases of pervasive error in a published article, such as when an error was inadvertent (eg, as may occur with incorrect coding of data), and the error resulted in incorrect data points throughout an article, yet the underlying science is still reliable and important, editors may consider retracting the article that contains the errors and publishing a corrected replacement article, with explanation from the authors.[11]

For journals that publish articles online first (eg, before republication in a print/online issue), corrections may be incorporated before the second publication in the print/online issue. The erroneous information should be corrected in all online versions (HTML and PDF) with the reason for and date of the correction prominently displayed.

For example, the JAMA Network journals include the following on page 1 of corrected articles in the PDF version: "Corrected on September 20, 2018."

In addition, in the Article Information at the end of the article, the following may be included:

"**Correction:** This article was corrected for errors in Table 1 on May 29, 2017."

Similarly prominent notes on the HTML version of the article and Correction notice should be displayed with reciprocal links. For example, the JAMA Network journals include the following at the top of a corrected article and Correction notice:

On the corrected article: "This article was corrected | View correction"

On the correction notice: "A correction has been published | View article"

**6.2**    **Editorial Processing.** Editorial processing refers to the processing of manuscripts after acceptance in preparation for publication. With the development of electronic document processing, the term *manuscript* has moved increasingly far from its handwritten origins to refer to a prepublication document, whether it happens to be a hard-copy proof or an electronic file. Manuscript submission, peer review, editing, processing, and tracking are now usually performed electronically. A major technical issue for many publishers is the need to efficiently process content for multiple publication outputs, such as print, web, reprints, and mobile apps. The use of electronic markup languages, such as XML, to provide coding for each content mode facilitates the conversions necessary for such multiple outputs (see 21.1.1, Editing With XML).

**6.2.1**    **Manuscript Editing.** After acceptance for publication, a manuscript undergoes copyediting, often referred to as *manuscript editing*. Extensive editing for clarity, accuracy, and internal consistency may be necessary for some manuscripts. The manuscript editor coordinates communication among the editor, author, and production staff. Manuscript editors incorporate suggestions made by senior journal editors; correct grammar, spelling, and usage; query ambiguities and inconsistencies; verify mathematical calculations; verify and correct reference citations; and edit to journal style. Tables, boxes, figures, and other elements (such as multimedia and video) are also edited for style (see 4.0, Tables, Figures, and Multimedia), accuracy, and consistency with the text. The manuscript editor sends the edited manuscript, with proposed additions and deletions clearly indicated (see 21.0, Editing, Proofreading, Tagging, and Display), as well as queries, along with a cover letter and the formatted figures and tables, to the author (and in some cases, to a scientific editor or editor in chief) for approval. After the author responds, the manuscript editor incorporates the author's changes. Any major substantive changes requested by the author (eg, inclusion of additional data or analyses, requests for addition of figures or tables, significant changes to wording) should be discussed with and approved by the editor in chief or the designated decision-making editor.

**6.2.2**    **Composition, Page Makeup, and Digital Content.** Once the modifications from the authors and journal editors have been incorporated into the manuscript file, the document is ready to be composed (ie, made into journal pages) or otherwise prepared for publication. In an electronic composition system, codes must be inserted for each element (eg, title, authors, abstract, headings, references, tables, figures) of an article according to journal style. Use of XML coding (tagging) of all elements and templates allows for automation of the composition of an article, whether for print/PDF, online, or multiple formats. This can be done automatically or for some journals with complicated designs for different article types, an electronic composition operator may need to use a mix of automated processes and manual placement of the text, tables, and art together in the electronic composition system to arrange all elements into pages according to design and typographic specifications. For print publication, the pages can be transmitted electronically to a printer. For online publication, XML-coded files are converted to an appropriate language (eg, HTML) or format (eg, PDF) following style sheets and templates for output to a website, app, or other platform (see also 21.0, Editing, Proofreading, Tagging, and Display).

**6.2.3** **Proofreading.** In a traditional publishing process, the proofreader checks the manuscript copy word for word against the composed copy, alerting the manuscript editor to any discrepancies (see 21.0, Editing, Proofreading, Tagging, and Display). In some systems the role of the proofreader has changed. The proofreader may look only for formatting issues, such as incorrect line breaks and problems that arose through improper coding (eg, spacing errors or incorrect font) or page makeup (eg, misplaced blocks of text or improper line justification). The manuscript editor, authors, and journal editors may perform the word-for-word reading once done by a proofreader. Revised page proofs can be generated and rechecked as needed. Content for online publication should also be reviewed for errors and missing elements before release.

**6.2.4** **Advertising.** At the same time as the manuscript editing and composition of articles for publication are proceeding, advertisements are scheduled for specific issues or online publication and possibly for specific positions in an issue (eg, back cover or facing the table of contents). Advertising sales and placement should be administratively separate from all editorial functions to ensure that there is no influence by an advertiser on any editorial decisions. Ideally, the editor in chief should have full and final authority for approving advertisements and enforcing advertising policies. Specific advertising and commercial content should not influence specific editorial decisions and content. For print journal issues, staff members responsible for issue makeup should ensure that there is no inadvertent link between advertisements and articles—for instance, that no advertisement for an antihypertension medication appears next to a research report on hypertension (see 5.12, Advertisements, Advertorials, Sponsorship, Supplements, Reprints, and e-Prints).

Online ads are not restricted by the physical limits of a printed page (see 5.12.6, Advertising and Sponsorship in Online Publications). Online publication has challenged the traditional print-based standards that separate advertising and editorial content. However, the general principles for protecting editorial integrity of print publications apply to advertising in online publications (see 5.12, Advertisements, Advertorials, Sponsorship, Supplements, Reprints, and e-Prints).

**6.2.5** **Issue Makeup and Review.** For journals that publish formal print issues, the production staff merges the editorial and the advertising content, numbers the pages, and produces a comprehensive list that shows the sequential order of pages with placement of editorial content, advertising content, and other material, such as filler pages. The journal editor or managing editor should determine the content of each issue by considering the balance of types of articles and thematic consistency (eg, there might be several articles on related topics). The made-up issue and table of contents are reviewed by the editorial and production staff, and final changes are incorporated. When final pages have been created, the electronic files can be printed. For print publication, proofs for each page may be prepared and returned to the journal for final review. When all pages have been approved, the issue is printed, bound, and mailed.

For journals that publish online-first releases of groups of articles or publish articles online as they are available, there may still be a need to review the online release package or online "issue." This review may include traditional review of PDFs of articles to be published online or review of the articles as they will appear online; this review also should include review of the online table of contents for these articles if one is to be released.

**6.2.6** **Reprints and e-Prints, Postpublication Copies of Articles, and Depositing Articles in an Approved Repository.** Some journals offer authors an option to purchase reprints or e-prints of their articles after publication. Reprints may also be sold to individuals, organizations, or companies interested in disseminating the article (see 5.6.9, Standards for Commercial Reprints and e-Prints).

Journals have different policies for permitting authors to post copies of their published articles in personal or institutional repositories. Many journals or publishers will deposit copies of published articles that report funded research in approved public repositories on behalf of authors for public access after a defined period (eg, 6 or 12 months) or for immediate access (eg, for author-pay open access). These options are based on the journal policies for authors, society members, public access, or open access. Journals should ensure that their policies on postpublication public access or open access are publicly available and transparent.

**Principal Authors:** Phil Fontanarosa, MD, MBA, Stacy Christiansen, MA, and Annette Flanagin, RN, MA

ACKNOWLEDGMENT

Thanks to the following for reviewing this chapter and providing comments: Helene Cole, formerly of *JAMA*; Carissa Gilman, MA, American Cancer Society, Atlanta, Georgia; Hope Lafferty, AM, ELS, Hope J. Lafferty Communications, Marfa, Texas; Trevor Lane, MA, DPhil, Edanz Group, Fukuoka, Japan; and Ana Marušić, MD, PhD, *Journal of Global Health*, and Department of Research in Biomedicine and Health, University of Split School of Medicine, Split, Croatia.

REFERENCES

1. Kronick DA. Peer review in 18th-century scientific journalism. *JAMA*. 1990;263(10):1321-1322. doi:10.1001/jama.1990.03440100021002
2. Burnham JC. The evolution of editorial peer review. *JAMA*. 1990;263(10):1323-1329. doi:10.1001/jama.1990.03440100023003
3. Godlee F, Jefferson T, eds. *Peer Review in Health Sciences*. BMJ Books; 1999:3-13.
4. Lock S. *A Difficult Balance: Editorial Peer Review in Medicine*. ISI Press; 1988.
5. Rennie D. Editorial peer review in biomedical publication: the First International Congress. *JAMA*. 1990;263(10):1317. doi:10.1001/jama.1990.03440100011001
6. International Congress on Peer Review and Scientific Publication. Accessed June 22, 2019. https://peerreviewcongress.org/index.html
7. Rooyen S, Godlee F, Evans S, et al. Effect of open peer review on quality of reviews and on reviewers' recommendations: a randomized trial. *BMJ*. 1999;318(7175):23-27. doi:10.1136/bmj.318.7175.23

8. Kassirer JP, Campion EW. Peer review: crude and understudied, but indispensable. *JAMA*. 1994;272(2):96-97. doi:10.1001/jama.1994.03520020022005

9. Bauchner H, Fontanarosa PB, Golub RM. To *JAMA* authors, reviewers, and readers—thank you. *JAMA*. 2018;319(13):1329-1330. doi:10.1001/jama.2018.3775

10. Christiansen S, Flanagin A. Correcting the medical literature: "to err is human, to correct divine". *JAMA*. 2017;318(9):804-805. doi:10.1001/jama.2017.11833

11. Heckers S, Bauchner H, Flanagin A. Retracting, replacing, and correcting the literature for pervasive error in which the results change but the underlying science is still reliable. *JAMA Psychiatry*. 2015;72(12):1170-1171. doi:10.1001/jamapsychiatry.2015.2278

# 7.0    Grammar

**7.0**    **Grammar.** A clear understanding of grammar is basic to good writing. Many excellent grammar books provide a detailed discussion of specific principles (see 23.3, Resources, General Style and Usage). In this section, the focus is on how to avoid common grammatical and writing errors. The content of this chapter is organized from the smallest parts of speech (eg, nouns and pronouns) to larger structures (eg, sentences and paragraphs).

**7.1**    **Nouns.** Nouns (words that name a person, place, thing, or idea) may serve as subjects or objects. Nouns are classified as common, proper, or collective.

Common nouns name something generic and are lowercased unless they appear at the beginning of a sentence or in a title.

| | |
|---|---|
| physician | hospital |
| day | phase |
| plan | journal |

Physicians and hospitals should work within the parameters of the plan.

Editors decide what to publish based on a variety of factors relevant to that journal.

*Title:* Addressing Physician Burnout: The Way Forward

Proper nouns name something specific and are always capitalized (see 10.3, Proper Nouns).

| | |
|---|---|
| Medicare | North America |
| Declaration of Helsinki | June |

Collective nouns name something abstract, something uncountable, or individuals treated as a group. Collective nouns are usually common nouns (see 7.5.5, Collective Nouns).

| | |
|---|---|
| faculty | evidence |
| society | committee |

The society has released new guidelines that detail the diagnosis and treatment of cardiomyopathy. (*But:* The Society of Critical Care Medicine published new sepsis guidelines this year.)

**7.1.1** **Nouns as Modifiers.** Although nouns can be used as modifiers, overuse of noun modifiers can lead to a lack of clarity. Purists may demand stricter rules on usage, but, as with the use of nouns as verbs (see 11.4, Back-formations), the process of linguistic change is inevitable, and grammatical rigor must be tempered by judgment and common sense.

| *Avoid* | *Preferred* |
|---|---|
| depression episode | depressive episode, episode of depression |
| elderly over-the-counter drug users | elderly patients using over-the-counter drugs |

In *The Careful Writer*, Bernstein[1] advises the use of no more than 2 polysyllabic noun modifiers per noun for the sake of clarity. However, long noun strings are sometimes difficult to avoid in scientific writing. If several of the attributive nouns are read as a unit, the use of more than 2 may not compromise clarity. Thus, noun strings may be more acceptable, for the sake of brevity, if the terms have been previously defined without noun strings. Some acceptable examples appear below.

| | |
|---|---|
| community hospital program | sudden infant death syndrome |
| risk factor surveillance system | nicotine replacement therapy |
| baseline CD4 cell counts | placebo pain medication |

| | |
|---|---|
| health care workers | autism spectrum disorder |
| proficiency testing program | HIV vaccine trial |
| clinical research organization | blood glucose concentration |
| tumor necrosis factor | physician claims database |
| community outreach groups | acute respiratory distress syndrome |

If there is a possibility of ambiguity, hyphens may be added for clarity (eg, large-vessel dissection) (see 8.3.1.1, Hyphen, Temporary Compounds).

An *appositive* is a noun or noun phrase that describes another noun or noun phrase.[2]

> Jonas Salk, developer of the first successful inactivated polio vaccine, was born in New York.

> Ipilimumab, a cytotoxic T-lymphocyte–associated antigen inhibitor, has been approved for the treatment of advanced melanoma.

Appositives are often set off by commas because they are considered nonrestrictive (ie, not essential to the meaning of the sentence). Sometimes, however, an appositive is restrictive and not flanked by commas (see 8.2.1, Comma).

> Christiaan Barnard, a South African heart surgeon, performed the first human-to-human heart transplant.

> South African heart surgeon Christiaan Barnard performed the first human-to-human heart transplant.

**7.1.2** **Modifying Gerunds.** When a noun or pronoun precedes a *gerund* (a verb form ending in *-ing* that is used as a noun), the noun or pronoun is possessive (see 8.7, Apostrophe).

> The toxicity of the drug was not a factor in the patient's dying so suddenly.

> The award recognized the researcher's planning as well as her performance.

Present participles (used adjectivally) should not be confused with gerunds. In the sentence below, the objective case (*them*) is correct.

> I watched them gathering in the auditorium.

If the possessive *their* were used instead of the objective *them*, the emphasis would be on the action (*gathering*).

> I supervised their gathering of the samples.

**7.1.3** **Subject-Complement Agreement.** Subjects and complements should agree in number.

> The boy can tie his own shoes.

> We asked trial participants to return their pill dispensers.

However, when the complement is shared by all constituents of the plural subject, that noun remains singular.

The authors were asked to revise their paper.

Most of the patients in the trial were asked to track their blood pressure.

**7.2  Pronouns.** Pronouns replace nouns. In this replacement, the antecedent must be clear, and the pronoun must agree with the antecedent in number and gender.

*Avoid:*  The authors unravel the process of gathering information about diethylstilbestrol and disseminating it. [Antecedent unclear; does *it* refer to information or to diethylstilbestrol?]

*Better:*  The authors unravel the process of gathering and disseminating information about diethylstilbestrol.

*Avoid:*  A questionnaire was given to each medical student and their spouses. [Disagreement of pronoun with referent in number; the referent is *each medical student* (singular), but the pronoun used is plural (*their spouses*).]

*Better:*  A questionnaire was given to the medical students and their spouses.
*or*
A questionnaire was given to each medical student and his or her spouse.

Note: The possessive pronoun *its* should not be confused with the contraction *it's* (short for *it is*) (see 8.7.2, Apostrophe, Possessive Pronouns).

*Possessive:*  The journal published its first issue last year.
*Contraction:*  It's not advised to take the medications together.

Note: Contractions are typically avoided in scientific writing.

**7.2.1  Personal Pronouns.** Use the correct case of personal pronouns: subjective case (the pronoun is the subject of the phrase or clause) or objective case (the pronoun is the object of the phrase or clause).

She was assigned to the active intervention group. (*She* is the subject.)

Collect all the samples and give them to her. (*Her* is the object.)

Your decision affects him and me. (Both *him* and *me* are objects.)

Do not substitute a reflexive pronoun, ending in *-self* or *-selves*, for a simple personal pronoun.

*Avoid:*  George, Patricia, and myself attended the lecture.
The author replied to the editor, illustrator, and myself.
*Better:*  George, Patricia, and I attended the lecture.
The author replied to the editor, illustrator, and me.

**7.2.1.1  *We*: Royal, Editorial, and First-Person Plural.** The pronoun *we* has several permutations, several of which are noted here. It is important that *we* not be ambiguous within a manuscript; for example, it should not be used to refer both to the authors of the paper and then to a larger group (such as all health care professionals) unless the distinction is clear.

The *royal we* is largely attributed to use by monarchs who used it to mean "God and I," and thus the ruler by divine right, or as the ruler and the ruled (the body politic).

> We are not amused. [attributed to Queen Victoria]

*We* is sometimes used when one is speaking for a group. This is called the *editorial we*.[2]

> We welcome submissions reporting original research as well as insightful opinion pieces.

The *editorial we* is also used by writers in an attempt to make the reader feel included.

> It is critical that we take an active and ongoing role in helping to optimize patients in this phase of survivorship.

> We need to determine the best way to encourage patients to modify their lifestyle.

In scientific writing, however, *we* should be reserved for the first-person plural subject, which is appropriate when writers are describing their work or their observations. Rewriting to exclude this form of *we* would promote the passive voice construction, which is less direct (see 7.4.1, Voice).

> Beginning in September 2010, we recruited serodifferent couples from 75 clinical sites in 14 European countries.

> We used the Breslow-Day test to examine differences in aspirin effect by site.

> We conducted a single-center randomized clinical trial of patients admitted to the intensive care unit for ARDS who required noninvasive ventilation.

**7.2.2    Relative Pronouns.** Relative pronouns (*who, whom, whose, that*, and *which*) introduce a qualifying clause.

**7.2.2.1    Who vs Whom.** *Who* is used as a subject and *whom* as an object. The examples below illustrate correct usage.

> Give the award to whomever you prefer. [Objective case: *whomever* is the object of the verb *prefer*.]

> Give the award to whoever will benefit most. [Subjective case: *whoever* is the subject of *will benefit*.]

> Whom did you consult? [Objective case: *whom* is the object of *consult*.]

> Who was the consultant on this case? [Subjective case: *who* is the subject of the sentence.]

> He is one of the patients whom Dr Rundle is treating. [Objective case: *whom* is the object of *is treating*.]

He is one of the patients who are receiving the placebo. [Subjective case: *who* is the subject of *are receiving*.]

**7.2.2.2**   *That* vs *Which*. Relative pronouns may be used in subordinate clauses to refer to previous nouns. The word *that* introduces a restrictive clause, one that is essential to the meaning of the noun it describes. The word *which* introduces a nonrestrictive clause, one that adds more information but is not essential to the meaning. Clauses that begin with *which* are preceded by commas. Two examples of correct usage follow.

A study on immune responses to insulin in children at risk for diabetes was published in the 2015 *JAMA* theme issue on child health, which contains articles on a range of similar topics. [*Nonrestrictive*; there was only one *JAMA* theme issue on child health in 2015.]

The issue of *JAMA* that contained the article on immune responses to insulin in children at risk for diabetes was the 2015 child health theme issue. [*Restrictive*; there are thousands of issues of *JAMA*.]

Following are examples of ambiguous or incorrect usage that highlight this grammatical problem.

*Incorrect:*   The high prevalence of antibodies to the 3 *Bartonella* species, which were examined in the present study, indicates that health care workers should be alert to possible infection with any of these organisms when treating intravenous drug users. [There are more than 3 species of *Bartonella*. Hence, the correct form here should be " . . . the 3 *Bartonella* species that were examined. . . ."]

*Ambiguous:*   Many reports have been based on series of patients from urology practices that may not fully reflect the entire spectrum of illness. [Do the patients or the practices not fully reflect the entire spectrum of illness? Also, do the reports involve all or only some urology practices?]

*Reworded:*   Many reports have been based on patients in urology practices, which may not fully reflect the entire spectrum of illness. [Urology practices in general do not capture the range of the disease.]

*or*

Many reports have been based on data from urology practices that may not fully reflect the entire spectrum of illness. [Some particular urology practices do not capture the range of the disease, but others might.]

Note: The omission of *that* to introduce a clause may cause difficulty in comprehension.

*Avoid:*   This morning he revealed evidence that calls the study's integrity into question has been verified.

*Better:*   This morning he revealed that evidence that calls the study's integrity into question has been verified.

The addition of *that* after *revealed* frees the reader from backtracking to uncover the meaning of the sentence above. The use of *that* to introduce a clause is particularly helpful when the second verb appears long after the first has been introduced (above, the interval between *revealed* and *has been verified*).

**7.2.3**   **Indefinite Pronouns.** Indefinite pronouns refer to nonspecific persons or things. Most indefinite pronouns express the idea of quantity and share properties of collective nouns (see 7.5.5, Collective Nouns).

**7.2.3.1**   **Pronoun-Verb Agreement.** Some indefinite pronouns (eg, *any, each, either, neither, one, no one, everyone, someone, anybody, nobody, somebody*) always take singular verbs; some (eg, *several, few, both, many*) always take plural verbs; and some (eg, *some, any, none, all, most*) may take either the singular or the plural, depending on the referents. In the last case, usually the best choice is to use the singular verb when the pronoun refers to a singular word and the plural verb when the pronoun refers to a plural word, even when the noun is omitted.

| | |
|---|---|
| *Singular referent:* | Some of her improvement is attributable to the increase in dosage. |
| *Plural referent:* | Some of his calculations are difficult to follow. |
| *Singular referent:* | Most of the manuscript was typed with a justified right-hand margin. |
| *Plural referent:* | Most of the manuscripts are edited electronically. |
| *Singular referent:* | Some of the manuscripts had merit, but none was of the caliber of last year's award winner. |
| *Plural referent:* | None of the demographic variables examined were found to be significant risk factors. |

**7.2.3.2**   **Pronoun-Pronoun Agreement.** The use of an indefinite pronoun as the antecedent of another pronoun can create confusion. ("Everyone should cite his sources"—whose sources are being cited?) Some writers may try to avoid gender bias by using distracting constructions, such as *s/he*, by consistently applying the same pronoun throughout (eg, *she*), or by using the formal-sounding *one* ("Everyone should cite one's sources").

There are several ways to deal with this potential problem. The examples below will not work in every situation; use judgment when writing or editing so as not to change the meaning of the sentence or overuse any device that could distract the reader.[2]

- Replace with a more concrete noun: Authors should cite their sources.

- Replace the second pronoun with an article: Everyone should cite the sources used.

- Change the verb to the imperative mood: Cite sources used *or* Cite your sources.

- Rewrite the sentence: All sources used should be cited.

- If permissible, use the "singular they": Everyone should cite their sources.

Like *The Chicago Manual of Style* and *AP Stylebook*, the *AMA Manual of Style* now permits the use of *they* as a singular pronoun when rewriting the sentence as plural would be awkward or unclear.[2,3] In addition, this construction can be useful in medical articles in which patient identifiability is a concern (eg, removal of gender-specific pronouns) (see 11.12.1, Inclusive Language, Sex/Gender).

**7.3** **Articles.** There are 2 types of articles—definite and indefinite—that function as adjectives and precede a noun or noun phrase. Which type to use depends on the context.

**7.3.1** **Definite Articles.** The definite article *the* describes a specific object. It can be used to describe both singular and plural nouns as well as both common and proper nouns (note that sometimes *the* is part of a proper name).

> The paper has been accepted.
>
> The journals are organized by issue number.
>
> Have you read the research reports in *The Lancet* this week?

**7.3.2** **Indefinite Articles.** The indefinite articles *a* and *an* indicate a nonspecific object. Their use is exclusively for singular items; nonspecific plural nouns drop the article.

> A paper has been accepted.
>
> Have you read an issue of the journal this week?
>
> Journals are organized by issue number.

**7.3.2.1** **Selecting *a* or *an*.** Deciding whether to use *a* or *an* depends on how the subsequent noun (or modifier) is pronounced aloud, regardless of spelling. "An" is always used before a vowel sound (but not necessarily always before an actual vowel) (see 11.11, Articles).

| | | |
|---|---|---|
| a eukaryote | an eye | |
| a histogram | an hour | |
| a laryngoscope | an LV anomaly | *But:* a LASIK procedure |
| a mammogram | an MMSE score | *But:* a MRSA outbreak |
| a neurologist | an NSAID | *But:* a NICU incubator |
| a one-way street | an otoscope | |
| a user | an ulcer | |
| a xenograft | an x-ray | |

**7.4** **Verbs.** Verbs express an action, an occurrence, or a mode of being. They have voice, mood, number, and tense (see 7.5, Subject-Verb Agreement).

**7.4.1** **Voice.** In the active voice, the subject does the acting; in the passive voice, the subject is acted on. In general, authors should use the active voice, except in instances in which the actor is unknown or the interest focuses on what is acted on (as in the following example of passive voice).

> A randomization list using variable blocks of 2, 4, or 6 was generated by an independent statistician. (*Compare*: An independent statistician generated a randomization list using variable blocks of 2, 4, or 6.)

If the actor is mentioned in the sentence, the active voice is preferred over the passive voice.

> *Passive:* Data were collected from 5000 patients by physicians.
>
> *Active:* Physicians collected data from 5000 patients.
>
> *Passive:* Baseline clinical features and a throat swab were obtained.
>
> *Active:* Study clinicians obtained baseline clinical features and a throat swab.
>
> *Passive:* Maintenance therapy and the clinical status of patients were evaluated every 6 months.
>
> *Active:* We evaluated maintenance therapy and the clinical status of patients every 6 months.

**7.4.2** **Mood.** Verbs may have 1 of 3 moods: (1) the indicative (the most common; used for ordinary objective statements), (2) the imperative (used for requesting or commanding), and (3) the subjunctive.

*Indicative verbs* are used to state a fact, opinion, or question.

> The surgeon entered the room.
>
> I think the study has serious flaws.
>
> Did you submit your paper?

*Imperative verbs* give direction or commands. They are often part of a "you understood" construction.

> Bring that wheelchair over here.
>
> Stop it.

*Subjunctive verbs* cause the most difficulty; they are used primarily for expressing a wish (I wish it were possible), a supposition (If I were to accept the position . . . ), or a condition that is uncertain or contrary to fact (If that were true . . . ; If I were younger . . . ). The subjunctive occurs in fairly formal situations and usually involves past (*were*) or present (*be*) forms.

| *Past form:* | If we were to begin treatment immediately, the patient's prognosis would be excellent. |
|---|---|
| *Present form:* | The patient insisted that she be treated immediately. |

**7.4.3**    **Tense.** Tense indicates the time relation of a verb: present (*I am*), past (*I was*), future (*I will be*), present perfect (*I have been*), past perfect (*I had been*), and future perfect (*I will have been*). It is important to choose the verb that expresses the time that is intended. It is equally important to maintain consistency of tense.

The present tense is used to express a general truth, a statement of fact, or something continuingly true.

> He discovered enzymes—RNA polymerases—that directly copy [not copied] the messages encoded in DNA.

For this reason, the present tense is often used to refer to recently published work, indicating that it is still valid.

> Kilgallen's assay results demonstrate the highest recorded sensitivity and specificity to date.

The present perfect tense illustrates actions completed in the past but connected with the present[1] or those still ongoing. It may be used to refer to a report published in the recent past that continues to have importance.

> Kaplan and Rose have described this phenomenon.

The past tense refers to a completed action. In a biomedical article the past tense is usually used to refer to the methods and results of the study being described:

> We measured each patient's blood pressure.

> Group 1 had a seropositivity rate of 50%.

The past tense is also used to refer to an article published months or years ago that is now primarily of historical value. Frequently a date will be used in such a reference.

> In their 1985 article, Northrup and Miller reported a high rate of mortality among children younger than 5 years.

In general, tense must be used consistently:

| *Incorrect:* | There were no adverse events reported in the control group, but there are 3 in the intervention group. |
|---|---|
| *Correct:* | There were no adverse events reported in the control group, but there were 3 in the intervention group. |

However, tense may vary within a single sentence, as dictated by context and judgment. For example, the past tense and the present tense may be used in the same sentence to place 2 things in temporal context:

> We determined which medications are used most frequently by this population.

> Although the previous report demonstrated a significant response, the follow-up study does not.

Even when tenses are mixed, however, consistency is still the rule:

*Incorrect:*   I found it difficult to accept Dr Smith's contention in chapter 3 that the new agonist has superior pharmacokinetic properties and was therefore more widely used.

*Correct:*   I found it difficult to accept Dr Smith's contention in chapter 3 that the new agonist has superior pharmacokinetic properties and is therefore more widely used.

**7.4.4**   **Double Negatives.** Two negatives used together in a sentence constitute a double negative. The use of a double negative to express a positive is acceptable, although it yields a weaker affirmative than the simpler positive and may be confusing:

Our results are not inconsistent with the prior hypothesis.

More direct incentives have produced substantial changes in behavior in the past, although not without adverse consequences.

Adverse effects were not uncommon in both groups.

However, it is not grammatically acceptable to use a double negative to emphasize the negative. In the following example, the double negative conveys the opposite of what is intended.

The results are not inconclusive.

A double negative is best avoided in scientific writing because it often causes the reader to go back and reread the sentence to make sure of the meaning.

**7.4.5**   **Split Infinitives and Verb Phrases.** Infinitives are the basic form of verbs. In English, they are always a 2-word construction that starts with *to* (to read, to write, to live). Although some may still advise the avoidance of split infinitives (usually by insertion of an adverb, such as in the phrase "to quickly understand"), this proscription—likely a holdover from Latin grammar, wherein the infinitive is a single word and cannot be split—has been relaxed. In some cases, moreover, clarity is better served by the split infinitive.

*Ambiguous:*   The authors planned to promote exercising vigorously. [Is it the exercising or the promotion of exercising that is vigorous?]

*Better:*   The authors planned to vigorously promote exercising.

*or*

The authors planned to promote vigorous exercise.

*Also:*   This examination was conducted to rapidly identify bleeding. [Changing the position of "rapidly" would alter the meaning of the sentence.]

**7.4.6**   **Contractions.** A contraction consists of 2 words combined by omitting 1 or more letters (eg, *can't, aren't*). An apostrophe shows where the omission has occurred. Contractions are usually avoided in formal writing.

**7.5**    **Subject-Verb Agreement.** The subject and verb must agree in number; use a singular subject with a singular verb and a plural subject with a plural verb. Unfortunately, this rule is often broken, especially in complex sentences.

**7.5.1**    **Intervening Phrase.** Plural nouns take plural verbs and singular nouns take singular verbs, even if a phrase ending in a plural noun follows a singular subject or if a phrase ending in a singular noun follows a plural subject.

> A review of all patients with grade 3 tumors was undertaken in the university hospital. [The subject in this sentence is *review*. Ignore all modifying prepositional phrases that follow a noun when determining verb agreement.]

> *Avoid:*    The patient, one of many study participants given access to state-of-the-art medical care from the university's clinical researchers, were followed up for more than a year. [The verb should be *was* followed up—the subject is *patient*.]

Sometimes the simplest solution is to rewrite it as 2 separate sentences:

> *Better:*    The patient was followed up for more than a year. She was one of many study participants given access to state-of-the-art medical care with the university's clinical researchers.

If the intervening phrase is introduced by *with, together with, as well as, along with, in addition to*, or similar constructions, the singular verb is preferred if the subject is singular because the intervening phrase does not affect the singularity of the subject.

> The editor, as well as the reviewers, believes that this article is ready for acceptance.

> The patient, together with her physician and her family, makes this decision.

> The patient, as well as her parents, was anxious. (*Better:* The patient and her parents were anxious.)

> The investigator, in addition to all participants, was expected to abide by the institution's safety guidelines.

In these instances, recasting the sentence may eliminate confusion.

> The patient, physician, and family members make this decision together.

**7.5.2**    **False Singulars.** A few plural nouns are used so often in the singular that they are often paired with a singular verb.

> The agenda has been set for our next meeting.

Frequently treated erroneously in this way are the plurals *bacteria, criteria, phenomena*, and *memoranda*. The distinction between singular and plural, however, should be retained; when the singular is intended, use *bacterium, criterion, phenomenon*, and *memorandum*.

The word *data* has engendered debate regarding singular vs plural presentation. The JAMA Network journals prefer to retain the use of the plural verb with *data* in all situations.

Very few data were [not very little data was] available to support our hypothesis.

The data show an association rather than causation, and other biases may have contributed directly or indirectly.

However, many resources now accept the use of *data* as singular.[4,5] In this usage, *data* is thought of as a collective noun and, when considered as a unit rather than as the individual items of data that compose it, it takes the singular verb.

The word *media* in the sense of communications media is becoming acceptable in this collective usage, although its use in this sense has not yet reached the acceptability that *agenda* has gained.[4,5] Most scientific journals retain the distinction between singular and plural.

The media give much attention to the managed care debate. [Here *media* refers to all types of news coverage.]

After publication, the article was widely cited on Twitter and other social media sites.

In the sense of laboratory culture or radiographic contrast, *medium* should be used for the singular and *media* for the plural.

Contrast medium is a dye injected into the vein to enhance visualization of organs, arteries, or veins during radiography.

(See 9.9, False Singulars.)

**7.5.3** **False Plurals.** Some nouns, by virtue of ending in a "plural" *-s* form, are mistakenly taken to be plurals even though they should be treated as singular and take a singular verb (eg, genetics, mathematics, measles, mumps, statistics) (see 9.9, False Singulars).

Genetics includes the study of heredity and variation of inherited characteristics.

Statistics is not my forte.

Measles was declared eliminated from the United States in 2000.

**7.5.4** **Parenthetical Plurals.** When *-s* or *-es* is added parenthetically to a word to express the possibility of a plural, the verb should be singular. However, in most instances it is preferable to avoid this construction and use the plural noun instead.

*Acceptable:* The risk factor(s) of each study participant was not always clear.

*Better:* The risk factors of the study participants were not always clear.

**7.5.5** **Collective Nouns.** A collective noun is one that names more than 1 person, place, or thing. When the group is regarded as a unit, the singular verb is the appropriate choice (see 9.2, Collective Nouns).

The couple has a practice in rural Montana. [*Couple* is considered a unit here and so takes the singular verb.]

Twenty percent of her time is spent on administration. [*Twenty percent* is thought of as a unit, not as 20 individual units, and so takes the singular verb.]

The paramedic crew responds to these emergency calls. [*Crew* is thought of as a unit here and so takes the singular verb.]

The National Institutes of Health (NIH) is evaluating grant applications for next year's funding. [The NIH comprises 27 institutes and centers, but in this case it is considered a single entity.]

When the individual members of the pair or group are emphasized, rather than the group as a whole, the plural verb is correct.

The couple are both family physicians. [*Couple* is thought of as the 2 individuals who compose the couple, not as a unit, and so takes the plural verb.]

Ten percent of the staff work flexible hours. [*Ten percent* is thought of as being composed of the individual members of the staff, not the staff as a unit, and so takes the plural verb.]

The surgical faculty were from all over the country. [*Faculty* here refers to the individual members of the faculty, rather than to the faculty as a group, and so takes the plural verb.]

The use of a phrase such as "the members of" may make this last example less jarring.

The members of the surgical faculty were from all over the country.

**7.5.6** **Compound Subject.** When 2 words or 2 groups of words, usually joined by *and* or *or*, are the subject of the sentence, either the singular or plural verb form may be appropriate, depending on whether the words joined are singular or plural and on the connector used.

**7.5.6.1** **Compound Subject Joined by *and*.** With a compound subject joined by *and*, a plural verb is usually correct.

The nurse and the physician are discussing my case.

A singular verb should be used if the 2 elements are thought of as a unit:

Dilation and curettage was suggested.

or refer to the same person or thing:

The first author and principal investigator takes responsibility for the data analysis.

**7.5.6.2** **Compound Subject Joined by *or* or *nor*.** With a compound subject joined by *or* or *nor*, the plural verb is correct if both elements are plural; if both elements are singular, the singular verb is correct. When one is singular and one is plural, the verb should agree with the noun closer to the verb.

*Both plural:*   Neither staphylococci nor streptococci were responsible for the infection.

*Both singular:*   Neither a false-positive result nor a false-negative result is definitive.

*Mixed:*   Neither the physicians nor the hospital was responsible for the loss.

**7.5.7** **Shift in Number of Subject and Resultant Subject-Verb Disagreement.** Elliptical constructions involve omission of the auxiliary verb because it is understood.

Her cholesterol levels were measured and her vital signs recorded.

The patient was examined and admitted.

This construction should not be used (ie, the auxiliary verb should not be omitted) if the number of the subject changes.

*Incorrect:*   Her tests were run and her chart updated.

*Correct:*   Her tests were run and her chart was updated.

*Incorrect:*   The diagnosis was made and physical therapy sessions begun.

*Correct:*   The diagnosis was made and physical therapy sessions were begun.

*or*

The diagnosis was made and physical therapy begun.

**7.5.8** **Subject and Predicate Noun Differ in Number.** A predicate noun is the complement of a subject; it identifies, describes, or renames the subject. When the subject and predicate noun differ in number, follow the number of the subject in selecting the singular or plural verb form.

*Incorrect:*   The most significant factor that affected the study results were interhospital variations in severity of illness.

*Correct:*   The most significant factor that affected the study results was interhospital variations in severity of illness.

Avoid this by rephrasing:

Study results were most affected by interhospital variations in severity of illness.

**7.5.9** ***Every* and *Many a*.** When *every* or *many a* is used before a word or series of words, use the singular verb form.

Many a clinician does not understand statistics. (*Better:* Many clinicians do not understand statistics.)

Every issue profiles a leader in medicine.

**7.5.10** ***One of Those*.** In clauses that follow *one of those*, either the plural or singular may be correct.

Dr Cotter is one of those researchers who prefer the library to the laboratory.

The nurse is one of those people who work tirelessly for others.

Unless one of those forms is completed, she cannot join the practice.

**7.5.11** **Number.** *The number* is singular and *a number of* is plural (see 7.5.5, Collective Nouns).

> The number that responded was surprising.

> A number of respondents were concerned about adverse effects.

The same is true for *the total* and *a total of.*

**7.6** **Modifiers.** A modifier describes another word or word group. Words, phrases (groups of words without a subject or predicate, usually introduced by a preposition or conjunction), and clauses (groups of words with a subject and verb within a compound or complex sentence) may all be modifiers. An adjective modifies a noun or a pronoun. An adverb modifies a verb, an adjective, another adverb, or a clause. Clauses or phrases may serve as adjectives or adverbs.

**7.6.1** **Misplaced Modifiers.** Misplaced modifiers result in failure to make clear what is being modified. Illogical or ambiguous placement of a word or phrase can usually be avoided by placing the modifying word or phrase close to the word it modifies.

> *Unclear:* Dr Young treated the patients using antidepressants. [Who used the antidepressants? Ambiguity makes 2 meanings possible.]
>
> *Better:* Dr Young treated the patients with antidepressants.
>
> *or*
>
> Dr Young treated the patients who were using antidepressants. [alternative meaning]
>
> *Unclear:* The patient was referred to a specialist with severe bipolar disorder. [Who had the bipolar disorder?]
>
> *Better:* The patient with severe bipolar disorder was referred to a specialist.

Likewise, sometimes it is necessary for clarity to place an adverb within a verb phrase. Note the shift in meaning when the adverb is moved outside the verb phrase.

> He had just called me.

> He had called just me.

Use of the word *only* as a modifier poses particular issues. *Only* should be placed immediately before the word or phrase it modifies for the meaning to be clear. The different meanings depend on placement in the examples below.

> Only medication can ease the pain.

> Medication only can ease the pain.

> Medication can only ease the pain.

> Medication can ease only the pain.

> Medication can ease the only pain.

> Medication can ease the pain only.

**7.6.2** **Verbal Phrase Danglers.** A participle is a verb form used as an adjective. A dangling participle implies an actor but fails to indicate correctly who or what that actor is. The following examples of dangling participles illustrate the problem.

*Avoid:* Working quickly, the study was completed early by my research team. [The participle appears to refer to *the study*; however, it is the *research team* that was working quickly.]

*Better:* My research team worked quickly and completed the study early.

*or*

The study was completed early because my research team worked quickly.

*Avoid:* Based on our experience, educational interventions are needed to foster higher-quality end-of-life care. [Are the educational interventions based on the authors' experience? No—it is the statement about the need for higher-quality end-of-life care that is based on the authors' experience.]

*Better:* We have found that educational interventions are needed to foster higher-quality end-of-life care.

*or*

Experience has shown that educational interventions are needed to foster higher-quality end-of-life care.

A gerund is a verb form used as a noun (see 7.1.2, Modifying Gerunds). Like the dangling participle, the dangling gerund implies an actor but does not specify who or what that actor is and sometimes may be confused with a participle modifying the wrong entity.

*Avoid:* Dietary therapy slows the return of hypertension after stopping long-term medical therapy. [This states that dietary therapy not only slows the return of hypertension but also stops medical therapy.]

*Better:* Dietary therapy slows the return of hypertension after cessation of long-term medical therapy.

*or*

After the patient discontinues long-term medical therapy, dietary therapy slows the return of hypertension.

*Avoid:* Before initiating an exercise program or engaging in heavy physical labor after a myocardial infarction, a physician should review the exercise program carefully. [A *physician* is erroneously implied to be the actor, the one initiating an exercise program or engaging in heavy physical labor.]

*Better:* Anyone about to initiate an exercise program or engage in heavy physical labor after a myocardial infarction should consult a physician.

**7.7** **Diction.** Diction, or word choice, is important for any writing to be understood by its intended audience. In scientific writing, concrete and specific language is preferred over the abstract and general.

Avoid:    The area under study provides new evidence for a solution.

Better:   Immunology provides new evidence for a solution.

Avoid:    An individual with a medical degree should examine this lesion.

Better:   A physician should examine this lesion.

**7.7.1**    **Homonyms.** *Homonyms* are words that sound alike but are spelled differently and have different meanings. They are easily confused, and computer spell-check programs are unable to differentiate them. Common examples include *affect/effect, accept/except, altar/alter, assistance/assistants, cite/site/sight, council/counsel, its/it's, patience/patients, peace/piece, peak/peek/pique, pleural/plural, principal/principle,* and *your/you're* (see 11.1, Correct and Preferred Usage of Common Words and Phrases).

**7.7.2**    **Idioms, Colloquialisms, and Slang.** Some language is best avoided in material written for a professional or academic audience.

*Idioms* are fixed expressions that cannot be understood literally (*kick the bucket, on a roll, put up with, pay attention*). In addition, some may have multiple meanings that can be understood only in context (*pass out, stand for*). Idioms are not governed by any rules, and each stands on its own. Be wary of using idioms, particularly for audiences that include readers whose first language is not English.

*Colloquialisms* (or casualisms[1]) are characteristic of informal, casual communication usually varying by geographic region (*ain't, anyways, cold turkey, flat line, OK, shell-shocked, tax hike*).

*Slang* includes informal, nonstandard terms whose meanings are not readily understood by all speakers of a language (eg, used by specific groups of people). Sometimes slang words are newly coined (*woke, rinky-dink, clickbait*), and sometimes they are created by applying new meanings to existing words (*bad, cool, random, sick, wicked*).

Colloquialisms and slang should be avoided except in special situations, such as "flavorful" prose or direct quotations.

> My sense is that part of the reason why Claude is able to survive is denial. He just says, flat out, "This ain't happening."

The technical terminology specific to various disciplines is considered *jargon* and should be avoided (see 11.5, Jargon).

**7.7.3**    **Euphemisms.** *Euphemisms* (from the Greek *eu,* meaning good, and *pheme,* meaning voice) are indirect terms used to express something unpleasant. Although such language is often necessary in social situations ("He passed away" or "The study animals were sacrificed"), directness is better in scientific writing ("The patient died" or "The study animals were killed") (see 11.5, Jargon).

**7.7.4**    **Clichés.** *Clichés* are worn-out expressions (*sleep like a log, dead as a doornail, first and foremost, crystal clear*). At one time they were clever metaphors, but overuse has left them lifeless, unable to conjure in the reader's mind the original image. Avoid clichés like the plague.

**7.8**    **Sentences.** A sentence must have, at minimum, a subject and a verb; it also usually contains modifiers.

**7.8.1** **Fragments.** Sentence fragments, which lack a subject or a verb, should not be used in scientific or technical writing (except within the structured abstract; see 2.5, Abstract). Writers of prose and poetry occasionally use sentence fragments intentionally, for effect.

> Her affect signaled depression. Utter depression.

In scientific writing, these fragments are likely to be unintentional and are inappropriate.

> *Incorrect:* The clinical spectrum of disease varying according to the population and age group under study.
>
> *Correct:* The clinical spectrum of disease varies according to the population and age group under study.

**7.8.2** **Run-ons.** *Run-on sentences* contain 2 (or more) independent clauses that run together without intervening punctuation or a coordinating conjunction. Run-on sentences are difficult to read and are not appropriate in scientific writing.

> *Incorrect:* A structured abstract is required see the instructions that follow.
>
> *Correct:* A structured abstract is required; see the instructions that follow.
>
> *Also:* A structured abstract is required, so see the instructions that follow.

**7.8.3** **Common Misperceptions About Sentence Beginnings and Endings.** There are a number of mistaken caveats about sentence beginning and ending words. Two of the most common are the use of conjunctions to begin a sentence and the use of prepositions to end a sentence.

**7.8.3.1** **Beginning a Sentence With a Conjunction.** The widely held belief that writers should not begin a sentence with a conjunction has no basis in formal English grammar.[2,4] In fact, it can be used (when used correctly) to good effect.

> A patient's last experience in life should not be one of fear. That hand gave me peace and hope, regardless of my outlook at the time. And maybe that is what we are missing when we educate generations of physicians about empathy and compassion.

> The committee's proposal to overhaul the payment model may help with the health plan's budget. But do you think the changes go far enough?

> Because there were few missing data, and in accordance with our statistical analysis plan, we did not conduct multiple imputation analyses.

**7.8.3.2** **Ending a Sentence With a Preposition.** There is also no grammatical basis for the admonition to avoid ending a sentence with a preposition.[2] Sometimes a sentence ending in a preposition simply sounds better and reads more clearly than one performing acrobatics to avoid the construction.

> These are the test results that I have been waiting for.
>
> vs
>
> These are the test results for which I have been waiting.

> The nurse assured the patient there was nothing to be frightened of.
>
> vs
>
> The nurse assured the patient there was nothing of which to be frightened.

**7.9**   **Parallel Construction.** *Parallel construction* is a series of like elements that can be used to build a sentence or emphasize a point. Each element used in a parallel construction has to match the others (eg, verb phrases, clauses, sentences).[2]

**7.9.1**   **Correlative Conjunctions.** Parallelism may rely on accepted cues (*either/or, neither/nor, not only/but also, both/and*). All elements of the parallelism that appear on one side of the coordinating conjunction should match corresponding elements on the other side.

> *Avoid:*     The compleat physician has not only mastered the science of medicine but also its art.
>
> *Correct:*     The compleat physician has mastered not only the science of medicine but also its art.
>
> *Better:*     The compleat physician has mastered both the science and the art of medicine.

> *Avoid:*     Poor drug efficacy may be caused by either lack of absorption or by increased clearance.
>
> *Correct:*     Poor drug efficacy may be caused either by lack of absorption or by increased clearance.
>
> *Also correct:*     Poor drug efficacy may be caused by either lack of absorption or increased clearance.

> *Avoid:*     Three patients did not either take their medication or took it incorrectly.
>
> *Correct:*     Three patients either did not take their medication or took it incorrectly.

Note: *Either/or* is used with only 2 comparators (use with more than 2 items is considered nonstandard).

> *Incorrect:*   This medication can be taken with either water, milk, or juice.
>
> *Correct:*   This medication can be taken with water, milk, or juice.

**7.9.2**   **Elliptical Comparisons.** The conjunction *than* often introduces an abridged expression (eg, "You are younger than I [am young].") Correct placement of *than* is important to avoid ambiguity.

> *Unclear:*   Women are more likely to take vitamins than men. [Are women more likely to consume vitamins than men are, or are women more likely to consume vitamins than they are to consume men?]
>
> *Better:*   Women are more likely than men to take vitamins.

**7.9.3**   **In Series or Comparisons.** Parallel construction may also present a series or make comparisons. In these usages, the elements of the series or of the comparison should be parallel structures (eg, nouns with nouns, prepositional phrases with prepositional phrases). (Note that it is not necessary to repeat auxiliary verbs in a correctly built parallel construction.)

> *Avoid:* Surgery, radiation therapy, and starting chemotherapy are possible therapeutic approaches.
>
> *Correct:* Surgery, radiation therapy, and chemotherapy are possible therapeutic approaches.

> *Avoid:* When an operation is designed to improve function rather than removal of an organ, surgical technique dictates outcome.
>
> *Correct:* When an operation is designed to improve the function of an organ rather than to remove the organ, surgical technique dictates outcome.

> *Avoid:* The new approach would have improved patient outcomes, would have shortened wait times, and would have saved money.
>
> *Better:* The new approach would have improved patient outcomes, shortened wait times, and saved money.

Note: Avoid the use of *nor* when the first negative is expressed by *not* or *no.*

> There were no negative effects on self-reported health status or [not *nor*] in measured clinical values.

**7.9.4** **Lists.** Parallel construction is also important in lists, whether run in or set off by bullets or some other device (see 8.2.2, Semicolon, and 18.5, Enumerations).

> After completing this CME exercise, readers should be able to
>
> ▪ identify the causal mechanism of the disease,
>
> ▪ describe the most common symptoms, and
>
> ▪ understand the limitations of pharmacologic treatment.

**7.10** **Paragraphs.** A *paragraph* is a cohesive group of sentences. It presents a thought or several related thoughts. Each paragraph should be long enough to stand alone but short enough to hold the reader's attention and then direct that attention to the next thought. Too many short paragraphs are jarring to the reader, whereas too many long paragraphs strain the reader's attention. Sentences within a single paragraph should use parallel structure and consistent tense as much as possible.

Transitions are words or phrases that signal a connection among ideas. Transitions build bridges between paragraphs (and between sentences) and help the text flow.[5]

> *To show addition:* also, furthermore, in addition, moreover
>
> *To show contrast:* however, yet, conversely, nevertheless, although
>
> *To show comparison:* similarly, likewise
>
> *To show results:* therefore, thus, as a result, consequently

*To show time sequence:* first (second, third, and so on), later, meanwhile, subsequently, while

*To summarize:* hence, in summary, finally

**7.11** **Grammar in Social Media.** Scientific articles often have a life beyond their formal full-text publication. Many publishers, institutions, and individuals post information about scientific content on various social media platforms, with Twitter and Facebook being 2 of the most popular. Because these posts have strict space limits (Twitter allows just 280 characters, including spaces) or expectations of brevity from social media followers, it is usually not possible, or even desirable, to strictly adhere to grammar, punctuation, and usage norms. However, some standards are necessary to ensure clarity.[6]

- Use proper capitalization; capital letters do not take up more characters than lowercase.

- Use basic punctuation to help ensure clarity.

- Avoid texting jargon, such as "U" for "you" or "L8" for "late"; these abbreviations are too colloquial and not widely understood.

- Contractions are appropriate, as are easily recognized symbols such as &, <, and =.

**Principal Author:** Stacy Christiansen, MA

### REFERENCES

1. Bernstein TM. *The Careful Writer: A Modern Guide to English Usage.* Free Press; 1998.
2. *The Chicago Manual of Style: The Essential Guide for Writers, Editors, and Publishers.* 17th ed. University of Chicago Press; 2017.
3. *The Associated Press Stylebook.* Associated Press; 2019.
4. Burchfield RW. *Fowler's Modern English Usage.* Rev 3rd ed. Oxford University Press; 2004.
5. *The American Heritage Dictionary of the English Language.* 5th ed. Houghton Mifflin Co; 2016.
6. Fogarty M. Grammar Girl's Strunk & Twite: an unofficial Twitter style guide. December 2009. Accessed December 9, 2018. http://www.quickanddirtytips.com/education/grammar/strunk-and-twite

### ADDITIONAL READINGS AND GENERAL REFERENCES

Fogarty M. *Grammar Girl's Quick and Dirty Tips for Better Writing.* Henry Holt & Co; 2008.

Follett W. *Modern American Usage: A Guide.* Wensberg E, ed. Hill & Wang; 1998.

Garner BA. *Garner's Modern American Usage.* 3rd ed. Oxford University Press; 2009.

Greenbaum S. *Oxford English Grammar.* Oxford University Press; 2011.

Lester M, Beason L. *The McGraw-Hill Handbook of English Grammar and Usage.* 2nd ed. McGraw-Hill; 2013.

Pinker S. *The Sense of Style: The Thinking Person's Guide to Writing in the 21st Century*. Viking; 2014.

Strunk W Jr, White EB. *The Elements of Style*. 3rd ed. Macmillan Publishing Co Inc; 1994.

The University of Chicago Press Editorial Staff. *But Can I Start a Sentence With "But"? Advice From the Chicago Style Q&A*. University of Chicago Press; 2016.

# 8.0 Punctuation

## 8.0 Punctuation.

> . . . *after journeying through the world of punctuation, and seeing what it can do, I am all the more convinced that we should fight like tigers to preserve our punctuation and we should start now.*
> Lynne Truss[1]

> *The popular image of the copy editor is of someone who favors rigid consistency. I don't usually think of myself that way. But, when pressed, I do find that I have strong views about commas.*
> Mary Norris[2]

**8.1** **Period, Question Mark, Exclamation Point.** Periods, question marks, and exclamation points are the 3 end-of-sentence punctuation marks.

**8.1.1** **Period.** Periods are the most common end-of-sentence punctuation mark. Use a period at the end of a declarative or imperative sentence and at the end of each table footnote and each figure legend or caption (but *not* at the end of figure or table titles).

> Advances in medical technology have saved many lives.

> Always listen carefully.

Indirect questions almost always take a period.

> She wondered why the peer review of her manuscript was taking so long.

> He wondered why there were no illustrations in the article.

See 8.1.2, Punctuation, Period, Question Mark, Exclamation Point, Question Mark, for advice on rhetorical questions and questions within unspoken dialogue.

**8.1.1.1** **Placement.** The period precedes ending quotation marks and reference citations.

> The child is rated in 7 areas, such as "accepts responsibility" and "interacts appropriately with peers."

> We followed the methods of Wilkes et al.[5]

The period follows a closing apostrophe:

> The intervention group's scores were better than previous patients'.

If a complete sentence is enclosed in parentheses or brackets, the period precedes the closing parenthesis or bracket.

> The serial comma can arouse strong feelings. (The serial comma is the one before the final *and* in a series of 3 or more items.)

However, see 8.5.1.3, Punctuation Marks With Parentheses, for examples where the punctuated statement is part of a sentence.

**8.1.1.2** **Lists.** Use a period after the arabic numeral when enumerating paragraphed items. The completed authorship form required by the journal included the following sections:

1. Authorship responsibility, criteria, and contributions
2. Confirmation of reporting conflicts of interest and funding
3. Acknowledgment statement

Lists may be run into the text or set off by numbers or bullets (see 18.5, Numbers and Percentages, Enumerations). However they appear, the question of end punctuation arises. Some simple guidelines:

- If the list consists of sentence fragments, use no end punctuation.
- If each listed item consists of 1 or more complete sentences, use end punctuation (eg, period or question mark) at the end of each sentence.
- If the list contains both (ie, sentence fragments and complete sentences), attempt to make all items parallel so that they may all be treated similarly.

The bulleted list below contains a mix of incomplete (first 2 bullets) and complete (last bullet) sentences.

Character and quality of pain were described as follows:

- Diffuse or multifocal, often waxes and wanes, and is frequently migratory

- Often accompanied by dysesthesia or paresthesia, described as "more neuropathic"

- Patients may note discomfort when they are touched or when wearing tight clothing

Make these consistent, as follows:

Character and quality of pain were described as follows:

- Diffuse or multifocal, often waxes and wanes, frequently migratory

- Often accompanied by dysesthesia or paresthesia, described as "more neuropathic"

- Producing discomfort when touched or when tight clothing is worn

If these items are all incomplete sentences or phrases, as those in the revised version are, then the decision about end punctuation is made simpler. However, although the items in the list, as incomplete sentences, do not require end punctuation, the final item *would* take a period if the items were treated as if they were in a single sentence:

Character and quality of pain were described as follows:

- diffuse or multifocal, often waxes and wanes, frequently migratory;

- often accompanied by dysesthesia or paresthesia, described as "more neuropathic"; and

- producing discomfort when touched or when tight clothing is worn.

These guidelines also apply to items in a table, box, or figure. They apply to items preceded by numbers or bullets and items that stand alone (see 18.5, Numbers and Percentages, Enumerations, for guidance on handling punctuation at the ends of items in bulleted or numbered enumerations and the Enumerations section in 8.2.2, Semicolon, for examples of ways to handle enumerations that are run into the text).

**8.1.1.3** **Decimals.** Use the period as a decimal indicator (see 18.7.1, Numbers and Percentages, Forms of Numbers, Decimals).

| | |
|---|---|
| $r = 0.75$ | .32 caliber |
| 0.1% | $P < .05$ |

**8.1.1.4** **When Not to Use a Period.** The JAMA Network journals do not use periods with honorifics (courtesy titles), scientific terms, or abbreviations (eg, St, Dr, Blvd) (*exceptions*: No. for "number" and St. when it is part of a person's surname, although no period is used with St or Ste in a city name, eg, St Louis, Missouri, or

Sault Ste Marie, Michigan) (see 2.2, Author Bylines and End-of-Text Signatures; 3.12.8, References to Books, Publishers; and 13.0, Abbreviations).

| | |
|---|---|
| Dr Bauchner | *JAMA* |
| Howard Bauchner, MD | Stacy L. Christiansen, MA |
| Howard C. Bauchner, MD | Ms Christiansen |
| *E coli* | Prof Hinders |
| St John's wort | ie |
| NIH | eg |
| HMR Publishing Co | vs |

**8.1.2** **Question Mark.** The primary use of the question mark is to end interrogative sentences.

> When did he go into private practice?

> Is it time to make mind-body approaches available for chronic low back pain?

Rhetorical questions posed as direct questions usually take a question mark.

> Are you serious?

Questions within unspoken dialogue also usually take a question mark.

> Why did I bother to attend this conference? she wondered.

**8.1.2.1** **In Dates.** Use the question mark to show doubt about specific dates.

> Hippocrates (460?-375 BCE) is often referred to as the Father of Medicine.

**8.1.2.2** **Placement.** When the question mark is part of the quoted or parenthetical material, place the question mark inside the end quotation mark (see 8.6.5, Quotation Marks, Placement), the closing parenthesis, or the end bracket.

> The patient asked her physician of 25 years, "Why are you retiring, Doctor?"

> The chapter on interpretation asks the question "Can I be wrong?"

> The mandate for health care reform (can we agree on this?) will change practice as we know it.

In declarative sentences that contain a question, place the question mark at the end of the interrogative statement.

> The patient asked, "What is 'average' pain?"

> The investigators asked the question "Have you ever injected drugs?" of every study participant.

Similarly, colons should not appear between the title and the subtitle when other punctuation follows the title.

> How Well Is the Affordable Care Act Doing? Reasons for Optimism

Note: The question mark, like the exclamation point (see 8.1.3.1, Punctuation, Period, Question Mark, Exclamation Point, Exclamation Point, Placement), is never combined with another question mark, exclamation point, period, semicolon, colon, or comma; thus, the need for a comma is obviated in the example below:

> The first section of the book, "What Medical Advances Made Open Heart Surgery Possible?" is certain to interest medical historians.

This situation is sometimes referred to as "dueling punctuation marks," and in this duel, the stronger mark wins.

An indirect question should not end with a question mark (see 8.1.1, Period, Question Mark, Exclamation Point, Period).

> She wondered why the article contained no illustrations.

**8.1.3**  **Exclamation Point.** Exclamation points indicate emotion, an outcry, or a forceful comment. Avoid their use except in direct quotations and in rare and special circumstances. They are not appropriate in scientific manuscripts and are more common in less formal articles, such as blog posts and informal essays, where added emphasis may be appropriate. If they are used, do not repeat the punctuation mark for emphasis.

> Beware!

> Although it may be referred to as the gold standard, nothing is perfect!

> I had almost given up hope of his recovery. He was terribly sick!

**8.1.3.1**  **Placement.** When it completes the emphasized material, the exclamation point goes inside the end quotation mark, parenthesis, or bracket. (The exclamation point, like the question mark [see 8.1.2.2, Period, Question Mark, Exclamation Point, Question Mark, Placement], is never combined with another exclamation point, question mark, period, semicolon, colon, or comma; thus, there is no comma in the first example below.)

> "Let the reader beware!" the editor warned.

> The frightened child cried, "I don't want my tonsils taken out!"

**8.1.3.2**  **Factorial.** In mathematical expressions, the exclamation point is used to indicate a factorial (see 20.6, Commonly Used Symbols).

$$5! = 5 \times 4 \times 3 \times 2 \times 1$$

**8.2**  **Comma, Semicolon, Colon.** Commas, semicolons, and colons can be used to indicate a break or pause in thought, to set off material, or to introduce a new but connected thought. Each of these punctuation marks has specific uses, and the strength of the break in thought determines which mark is appropriate.

**8.2.1**  **Comma.** Commas are the least forceful of the 3 marks. Although comma usage sometimes is subjective, there are definite rules for using commas. Follow these rules unless overriding considerations (such as clarity) require otherwise.

**8.2.1.1**  **Separating Groups of Words.** The comma is used to separate phrases, clauses, and groups of words and to clarify the grammatical structure and the intended meaning.

Use a comma after opening dependent clauses (whether restrictive or not) and long opening adverbial phrases.

> If the infection recurs within 2 weeks, an additional course of antibiotics should be given.

> When you have to pay for your own health care, does your consumption really become more efficient?

A comma is optional if the introductory phrase is short.

> In some patients midazolam produces paradoxic agitation.

Use commas to set off nonrestrictive subordinate clauses (see 7.2.2, Relative Pronouns) or nonrestrictive participial phrases.

> Ms Frederick, who had been waiting on hold for more than an hour, abandoned all hope of having her questions answered.

> The numbness, which had been apparent for 3 days, disappeared after drug therapy.

> The delegates, attaining consensus, passed the resolution.

But avoid setting off a phrase with commas where doing so would make the meaning ambiguous.

> *Avoid:* Although numerous investigators have called for measures to improve sight in nursing home residents, to our knowledge, none have attempted a study of the effect of a vision restoration-rehabilitation program on function and quality in this population.

In the example above, it is not clear whether the phrase "to our knowledge" applies to what precedes it or what follows it. Removing the comma after "to our knowledge" makes the meaning clear.

> *Better:* Although numerous investigators have called for measures to improve sight in nursing home residents, to our knowledge none have attempted a study of the effect of a vision restoration-rehabilitation program on function and quality in this population.

Use a comma to avoid ambiguous or awkward juxtaposition of words.

> Outside, the ambulance siren shrieked.

> Still, noting the trends and highlighting the lack of funding for achieving world health goals do not translate into more positive actions.

Use commas to set off appositives. Commas precede and follow the apposition.

> Two colleagues, John Smith and Amari Bhatnager, worked with me on this study.

> The battered child syndrome, a clinical condition in young children who have experienced serious physical abuse, is a frequent cause of permanent injury or even death.

**8.2.1.2** **Series.** In a simple coordinate series of 3 or more terms, separate the elements by commas (see 7.1.1, Nouns as Modifiers).

> Each patient was asked to complete a 21-item, 7-point, self-administered online questionnaire.

Use a comma before the conjunction that precedes the last term in a series to prevent ambiguity; this is often referred to as a *serial comma* or *Oxford comma*.

> Outcomes result from a complex interaction of medical care and genetic, environmental, and behavioral factors.

> The physician, the nurse, and the family could not convince the patient to take his medication daily.

> While in the hospital, these patients required neuroleptics, maximal observation, and seclusion.

However, a series of 3 or more modifiers should not be separated by commas when the modifiers are seen as 1 term or entity:

> The patient has chronic progressive multiple sclerosis.

> Gray matter magnetic resonance imaging was used to determine longitudinal brain atrophy.

Judgment and common sense are required in interpreting this rule. If the order of the adjectives can be rearranged without loss of meaning or clarity, use the comma.

> A physician's personal response to the patient and the patient's illness seems to violate the ideal of an objective, standardized, replicable view of the case.

> Practicing medicine is a unique, intricate, rewarding lattice of learning and relearning.

Note: When fewer than 3 modifiers are used, avoid adding a comma if the modifiers and the noun are read as one entity:

> We conducted a randomized placebo-controlled trial.

> Data from multicenter administrative databases were analyzed.

**8.2.1.3** **Names of Organizations.** When an enumeration occurs in the name of a company or organization, the comma is usually omitted before the ampersand or *and*. However, follow the punctuation used by the individual company or organization, except in references (see 3.12.8, References to Books, Publishers).

> Farrar, Straus and Giroux        Little, Brown and Company
>
> GlaxoSmithKline        Zeig, Tucker & Theisen
>
> Houghton Mifflin Harcourt

**8.2.1.4** ▪ **Setting Off *ie* and *eg*.** Use commas to set off *ie* and *eg* and the expanded equivalents, *that is* and *for example*.

> The use of standardized scores, eg, *z* scores, has no effect on statistical comparisons.

> The most important tests, that is, the white blood cell and platelet counts, were unduly delayed.

Note: If an independent clause follows these terms or their equivalents, precede the clause with a semicolon.

> Our double-blind study compared continuous with cyclic estrogen treatment; ie, estrogens for 4 weeks were compared with estrogens for 3 weeks followed by placebo for 1 week.

It may also be set off with parentheses.

> Our double-blind study compared continuous with cyclic estrogen treatment (ie, estrogens for 4 weeks were compared with estrogens for 3 weeks followed by placebo for 1 week).

**8.2.1.5** ▪ **Separating Clauses Joined by Conjunctions.** Use commas to separate independent clauses joined by coordinating conjunctions (*and, but, or, nor, for, yet, so*).

> Plasma lipid and lipoprotein concentrations were unchanged after low-intensity training, but high-intensity training resulted in a reduction in triglyceride levels.

> No subgroup of responders could be identified, and differences between centers were so great that no real comparison was possible.

If both clauses are short, the comma can be omitted.

> The test may be useful or it may be harmful.

> I have read the article and I am concerned about the data collection methods.

Unless the comma is needed for readability, do not insert a comma before the coordinating conjunction in a compound predicate.

> These facilities are beginning to resemble "minihospitals" and are losing their identity as freestanding ambulatory surgery centers.

Clauses introduced by *yet* or *so* and subordinating conjunctions (eg, *while, where, after, whereas*) are preceded by a comma (see 11.1, Correct and Preferred Usage of Common Words and Phrases).

> He taught medical students, performed careful research, and wrote thoughtful articles, yet was denied tenure.

> The United States spends more than $1000 per capita per year on paperwork related to health care, whereas Canada spends only approximately $300 per capita.

> One recent study found that low literacy was associated with worse mental health, whereas another concluded that literacy was not associated with depression.

If *yet* or *so* appear at the beginning of a sentence, they should not be followed by a comma.

> I have seen many cases of vertigo. Yet this one was particularly troubling.

**8.2.1.6** **Setting Off Parenthetical Expressions.** Use commas to set off parenthetical words, phrases, questions, and other expressions that interrupt the continuity of a sentence (eg, *therefore, moreover, on the other hand, of course, nevertheless, after all, consequently, however*) (see 8.8.1, Punctuation, Ellipses, Omission Within a Sentence).

> The real issue, after all, was how to fund the next study.

> Therefore, we were disappointed that the article did not include consideration of medical schools and their influence on the culture of medicine.

> What is needed, then, is collective empowerment of practitioners, guided by accountability to the public.

Note: In some cases, removal of the commas around parenthetical expressions changes the meaning of the sentence. In the example immediately above, *then* suggests a summing-up. Without these commas, *then* suggests time, ie, what comes next.

**8.2.1.7** **Setting Off Degrees and Titles.** Academic degrees and titles are set off by commas when they follow the name of a person. Although it is not incorrect to set off *Jr* and *Sr* by commas when they follow the name of a person, the JAMA Network journals do not use these commas.

> Berton Smith Jr, MD, and Priscilla Armstrong, MD, PhD, interpreted the radiographic findings in this study.

> Joyce Fredrickson-Smith, MD, PhD, vice-chancellor, attended the conference on health care reform.

**8.2.1.8** **Addresses.** In running text and affiliation footnotes, use commas to separate the elements in an address. Use commas after the city and state or country name. (Note: In US and Canadian addresses, commas are not used before the zip or postal code.)

> This year, the editorial board meeting will be held in conjunction with the annual meeting at the Westin Bonaventure Hotel and Suites, 404 S Figueroa St, Los Angeles, CA 90071.

> Dr Majeed may be reached at the Department of Primary Care and Public Health, Imperial College London, Reynolds Bldg, London W6 8RP, England.

> The study was conducted at The Wilmer Institute, Baltimore, Maryland, in 2010.

**8.2.1.9** **Dates.** In dates and similar expressions of time, use commas according to the following examples. Commas are not used when the month and year are given without the day or between a holiday and its year.

The first issue of *JAMA* was published on Saturday, July 14, 1883.

The patient's rhinoplasty was scheduled for August 19, 2014, at Strong Memorial Hospital, with postoperative evaluation on August 30.

The terrorist bombings in Boston, Massachusetts, in April 2013 led to further examination of preparedness for major disasters.

The publication offices were closed on New Year's Day 2013.

**8.2.1.10**   **Numbers.** In accordance with SI convention, separate digits with a thin space, not a comma, to indicate place values beyond thousands (see 17.4.3, Use of Numerals With Units, Number Spacing).

> 5034     12 345     615 478     9 473 209

As of September 2013, the Centers for Disease Control and Prevention estimated that 1 148 200 persons 13 years and older are living with HIV infection, and almost 1 in 5 (18.1%) are unaware of their infection.

A comma may be used to separate adjacent unrelated numerals if neither can be expressed easily in words, but it is preferable to reword the sentence or spell out one of the numbers.

> By December 2003, 929 985 cases of AIDS had been reported in the United States.

> *Better:*   By December 2003, a total of 929 985 cases of AIDS had been reported in the United States.

See 3.6, References, Citations, and 4.1.6, Tables, Punctuation.

**8.2.1.11**   **Units of Measure.** Do not use a comma between 2 or more measures whose units are the same dimension (eg, time or volume).

> 3 years 4 months 2 days old

> 3 lb 4 oz

> gestational age of 32 weeks 6 days or 32 6/7 weeks

**8.2.1.12**   **Placement.** The comma is placed inside quotation marks (see 8.6.5, Punctuation, Quotation Marks, Placement) and before superscript citation of references and footnote symbols.

> As a result of the "back-to-sleep campaigns," a call has been issued for a "back-to-the-bench" campaign.

> These missed opportunities occur during office visits,[6-9] health department appointments,[10-13] and hospitalizations.[16]

**8.2.1.13**   **To Indicate Omission.** The comma is used to indicate omission or avoid repeating a word when the sense is clear (see 7.5.7, Shift in Number of Subject and Resultant Subject-Verb Disagreement).

Four patients could not be studied: in 1, duration of treatment was too short; in 3, too long.

A plus indicates present; a minus, absent.

Commas are also used in titles of news items to replace *and* when space is limited.

Malaria Vaccine, Ebola Therapy Promising in Early Studies

**8.2.1.14** **Dialogue.** Commas are often used before direct dialogue or conversation is introduced (see 8.2.3.2, Punctuation, Comma, Semicolon, Colon, Colon, Introducing Quotations and Enumerations).

In the middle of the laboratory examination, a student asked, "Would it be OK to take a break?"

**8.2.2** **Semicolon.** Semicolons represent a more definite break in thought than commas. Generally, semicolons are used to separate 2 independent clauses. Often a comma will suffice if sentences are short, but when the main clauses are long and joined by coordinating conjunctions or conjunctive adverbs, especially if 1 of the clauses has internal punctuation, use a semicolon.

**8.2.2.1** **Separating Independent Clauses.** Use a semicolon to separate independent clauses in a compound sentence when no connective word is used. In most instances it is equally correct to use a period and create 2 sentences.

The conditions of 52% of the patients improved greatly; 4% of the patients withdrew from the study.

However, if clauses are short and similar in form, use a comma.

Seventy grafts were patent, 5 were occluded.

Use a semicolon between main clauses joined by a conjunctive adverb (eg, *also, besides, furthermore, hence, however, indeed, then, thus, yet*) or a coordinating conjunction *(and, but, for, nor, or, yet, so)* if one of the clauses has internal punctuation or is long.

The patient's fever had subsided; however, his condition was still critical.

The word *normal* is often used loosely; indeed, it is not easily defined.

Introduction to the knowledge, skills, and attitudes relevant to safety should begin in medical and nursing school; eg, the first 2 years of medical school may be the most appropriate to learn error science and principles of leadership.

**8.2.2.2** **Enumerations.** For clarity, use semicolons between items in a complex or lengthy enumeration within a sentence or in an enumeration that contains serial commas in at least 1 of the items listed. (In a simple series with little or no internal punctuation, even with multiword elements, use commas.) (See 18.5, Enumerations.)

A number of questions remain unresolved: (1) whether beverages that contain caffeine are an important factor in arrhythmogenesis; (2) whether such beverages can trigger arrhythmias de novo; and (3) whether their arrhythmogenic tendency is enhanced by the presence and extent of myocardial impairment.

Research questions examined the group's (1) origin, development, and operation; (2) influence; and (3) implications for modern practice.

The photomicrographic illustrations of the gross and microscopic features of normal skin, Spitz congenital and dysplastic nevi, lentigines, and melanoma demonstrated the complexity of pigmented lesions.

In less formal writing and where the last element of a series is also a series, commas are acceptable provided that clarity is preserved.

The statistician addressed limitations in case-control studies, cohort studies, and randomized, double-blind, controlled trials.

**8.2.3** **Colon.** The colon is the strongest of the 3 marks used to indicate a decided pause or break in thought. It separates 2 main clauses in which the second clause amplifies or explains the first.

This dictum is often believed to be in the Hippocratic Oath: First, do no harm.

See also last example in 8.2.3.2, Introducing Quotations or Enumerations.

**8.2.3.1** **When Not to Use a Colon.** Do not use a colon if the sentence is continuous without it.

You will need enthusiasm, organization, and a commitment to your beliefs.

*Incorrect*: You will need: enthusiasm, organization, and a commitment to your beliefs.

Avoid using a colon to separate a preposition from its object or to separate a verb (including *to be* in any of its manifestations) from its object or predicate nominative.

*Incorrect*: The point is: do not insert the catheter at this time.

*Better*: The point is to not insert the catheter at this time.

Do not use a colon immediately after *because* or forms of the verb *include*.

*Incorrect*: Symptoms of asthma include: wheezing, trouble breathing, chest tightness, and cough.

*Better*: Symptoms of asthma include the following: wheezing, trouble breathing, chest tightness, and cough.

*Still better*: Symptoms of asthma include wheezing, trouble breathing, chest tightness, and cough.

Do not use a colon between a title and subtitle when the title concludes with other punctuation (see 8.1.2.2, Question Mark, Placement, and 8.1.3.1, Exclamation Point, Placement).

**8.2.3.2** **Introducing Quotations or Enumerations.** Use a colon to introduce a formal or extended quotation. (If the sentence to follow is in quotation marks, the first word is capitalized.)

Harold Johnson, MD, chair of the committee, summarized: "The problems we face in developing a new vaccine are numerous, but foremost is isolating the antigen."

Use a colon to introduce an enumeration, especially after anticipatory phrasing such as *thus, as follows, the following.*

> The solution included the following components: phosphate buffer, double-distilled water, and a chelating agent.

> Laboratory studies yielded the following values: hemoglobin, 11.9 g/dL; erythrocyte sedimentation rate, 104 mm/h; calcium, 16.9 mg/dL; phosphorus, 5.6 mg/dL; and creatinine, 3 mg/dL.

> Phytoestrogens are subdivided into 3 main classes: isoflavones, lignans, and cumestrans.

If 2 or more grammatically independent statements follow the colon, they may be treated as complete sentences separated by periods, and the initial words may or may not be capitalized.

> The following procedure has been established for updating the journal's Instructions for Authors: (1) Update and review the Word file. (2) Style the Word document according to guidelines and send to the electronic media staff. (3) Insert links. (4) Proofread final version. (5) Code and post on the web.

**8.2.3.3** **Numbers.** Use a colon to separate chapter and verse numbers in biblical references, hours and minutes in expressions of time, and the elements of ratios when they are expressed as numbers or abbreviations. For ratios expressed as words, use the word *to* rather than a colon unless the term conventionally takes a hyphen (eg, "cost-benefit ratio"). In that case, follow the conventional usage and use a hyphen.

> The first mention of leprosy in the Old Testament is found in Exodus 4:6.

> Medication was given twice a day, at 8:30 AM and 8:30 PM.

> The chemicals were mixed in a 4:3 ratio.

> The study participants and controls were randomized in a 2:1 ratio.

> The ACTH:TSH ratio was elevated when the patient was first examined.

> The ratio of albumin to globulin was one of the outcome measures in the study.

> The student to instructor ratio was 7:1.

**8.2.3.4** **References.** In references, use a colon (1) between title and subtitle (unless the title ends with a question mark or an exclamation point); (2) for periodicals, between issue number and page numbers; and (3) after "doi" (see 3.0, References).

**8.3** **Hyphens and Dashes.** Hyphens and dashes are internal punctuation marks used for linkage and clarity of expression.

**8.3.1** **Hyphen.** The hyphen is a connector; it may join "what is similar and also what is disjunctive . . . it divides as well as marries."[3] The hyphen connects words, prefixes, and suffixes permanently or temporarily. Certain compound words always contain hyphens. Such hyphens are called *orthographic.* Examples are *merry-go-round,* *free-for-all, happy-go-lucky,* and *mother-in-law.* For temporary connections, hyphens help prevent ambiguity, clarify meaning, and indicate word breaks at the end of a line.

In general, hyphens should be used only as an aid to the reader's understanding, primarily to avoid ambiguity. For capitalization of hyphenated compounds in titles, subtitles, subheads, and table heads, see 10.2.2, Titles and Headings, Hyphenated Compounds.

**8.3.1.1** **Temporary Compounds.** Hyphenate temporary compounds according to current dictionary usage and the following rules:

Hyphenate a compound that contains a noun or an adverb (except for adverbs ending in *-ly*; see 8.3.1.6, When Not to Use Hyphens) and a participle that together serve as an adjective modifying the noun they precede (eg, angiotensin-converting enzyme). Do not use the hyphen if the compound follows the noun.

> breast-conserving surgery
>
> most-read work in the collection (*But*: The work was the most read in the collection.)
>
> It was a placebo-controlled trial. *(But*: The trial was placebo controlled.)
>
> This was a well-edited volume. *(But*: This volume was well edited.)
>
> The rash was a treatment-related adverse event. (*But*: The adverse event was treatment related.)

Hyphenate a compound adjectival phrase when it precedes the noun it modifies but not when it follows the noun. Hyphenation *before* the noun helps make the relationship of the words that precede the noun clearer and easier for a reader to understand.

> side-by-side placement (*But*: placed side by side)

Hyphenate an adjective-noun compound when it precedes and modifies another noun but not when it follows the noun. When such a compound follows the noun, the hyphenation is not required for easier understanding.

> low-quality suture material (*But*: suture material of low quality)
>
> highest-quality printing (*But*: printing of highest quality)
>
> low-density resolution (*But*: resolution of low density)
>
> high-altitude sickness *(But*: sickness at high altitude)
>
> very low-birth-weight children *(But*: children of very low birth weight)
>
> low-molecular-weight heparin *(But*: heparin of low molecular weight)
>
> very low-density lipoprotein *(But*: lipoprotein of very low density)
>
> foreign-body reaction (*But*: reaction to a foreign body)
>
> total-body imaging (*But*: imaging of the total body)
>
> total-breast radiation therapy (*But*: radiation therapy of the total breast)

Note: In most instances *middle-*, *high-*, and *low-* adjectival compounds are hyphenated.

For compound adjectival phrases, adverb-participle compounds, and adjective-noun compounds that have become commonplace and familiar in everyday usage, hyphenate these phrases or compounds whether they precede or follow the noun they modify.

> long-term therapy
> the commitment was long-term
>
> a middle-aged man
> he was already middle-aged
>
> the left-handed participants
> the participants who were left-handed
>
> cost-effective system
> a system that was cost-effective
>
> cafeteria-style dining
> the dining was cafeteria-style

However, for combinations representing colors, nouns plus adjectives, and nouns plus participles, hyphenate before but not after a noun. (Follow *The Chicago Manual of Style*, 17th edition, to verify.)

> up-to-date vaccinations
> the vaccinations were up to date
>
> state-of-the-art equipment
> equipment that was state of the art
>
> The author provided black-and-white illustrations.
> The author's illustrations were black and white.

Hyphenate a combination of 2 or more nouns used coordinately as a unit modifier when preceding the noun but not when following.

> the Binet-Simon test (*But*: the test of Binet and Simon)
>
> Beer-Lambert law (*But*: the law of Beer and Lambert)
>
> Charcot-Marie-Tooth disease (*But*: the disease described by Charcot, Marie, and Tooth)
>
> Hosmer-Lemeshow goodness-of-fit test (*But*: the goodness-of-fit test of Hosmer and Lemeshow)
>
> the patient-physician relationship (*But*: the relationship between the patient and the physician)

Presentation of ratios as numbers or abbreviations is an exception to this rule. In ratios presented as numbers or abbreviations, use a colon (see 8.2.3, Colon). For ratios presented as words, use the word *to* or, if the word combination has become accepted as a single term, such as *cost-benefit analysis,* a hyphen.

Hyphenate a combination of 2 or more nouns of equal participation used as a single noun (see 8.4.1, Forward Slash [Virgule, Solidus], Used to Express Equivalence or Duality).

William Carlos Williams was a physician-poet.

W. Somerset Maugham is considered a great physician-writer.

She is an obstetrician-gynecologist.

Many of *JAMA*'s contributors are physician-investigators.

This was a case-control study of sleep-wake problems.

The importance of having access to a cardioverter-defibrillator on the airplane was evident after this incident.

Provide the best health care for all, says the citizen-patient; but don't allow costs to rise, says the citizen-taxpayer.

The physician-patient may become impatient with treatment.

This was a 50-50 proposition.

The kidney-ureter-bladder abdominal radiograph showed normal bowel gas patterns.

Hyphenate the initials of an author with a hyphenated name when referred to parenthetically. For example, for parenthetical reference to author Horace Pendlebury-Davenport,

One of us (H.P.-D.) . . .

Hyphenate most compound nouns that contain a preposition. Follow the latest edition of *Merriam-Webster's Collegiate Dictionary*.

tie-in        tie-up        follow-up        hand-me-down        go-between

hand-me-downs        go-betweens

(*But*: onlooker, passerby, passersby, handout, workup, workups, makeup, upregulate, downregulate)

Hyphenate a compound in which a number is the first element and the compound precedes the noun it modifies (see 18.0, Numbers and Percentages).

18-factor blood chemistry analysis

7-fold increase

half-life

half-lives

3-dimensional (also 3-D)

2-way street

ninth-grade reading level

1-cm increments

Hyphenate 2 or more adjectives used coordinately or as conflicting terms whether they precede the noun or follow as a predicate adjective.

The false-positive test results were noted.
The test results were false-positive.

The patient was diagnosed as having relapsing-remitting multiple sclerosis.
The patient's multiple sclerosis was diagnosed as relapsing-remitting.

The patient's tonic-clonic seizures began in 2012.
In 2012, the patient began having seizures that were tonic-clonic.

We performed a double-blind study.
The test we used was double-blind.

Hyphenate color terms in which the 2 elements are of equal weight.

blue-gray eyes

blue-black lesions (lesions were blue-black)

bluish-gray lesions

Hyphenate compounds formed with the prefixes *all-*, *ex-*, and *self-* whether they precede or follow the noun.

all-powerful ruler                the patient's ex-husband

self-imposed dietary restrictions        self-reported intake

one's self-respect

Note: With the prefix *vice*, follow the latest edition of *Merriam-Webster's Collegiate Dictionary*, eg, vice-chancellor, vice-consul, *but* vice president, vice admiral.
Hyphenate compounds that contain the suffixes *-type, -elect,* and *-designate.*

Hodgkin-type lymphoma    president elect

Valsalva-type maneuver    secretary-designate

chair-elect

Hyphenate most contemporary adjectival *cross-* compounds (consult the latest edition of *Merriam-Webster's Collegiate Dictionary* for absolute accuracy; there are exceptions, eg, crossbred, crosshatched, crossover, crossmatch, cross section).

cross-reactive           cross-discipline training

cross-contamination      cross-coherence analysis

cross-tolerance reaction  cross-reference citation

Hyphenate adjectival compounds with *quasi*.

quasi-legislative group   quasi-analytic model

quasi-diplomatic efforts  quasi-experimental design

Most nouns that begin with *quasi* are not hyphenated but instead are set open (eg, quasi diplomat), although some are closed up (eg, quasicrystal, quasiparticle). Follow the latest edition of *Merriam-Webster's Collegiate Dictionary.*

Hyphenate some compounds in which the first element is a possessive. Consult the latest edition of *Merriam-Webster's Collegiate Dictionary.*

> bird's-eye view        bull's-eye
>
> crow's-feet          bird's-nest filter

Hyphenate all prefixes that precede a proper noun, a capitalized word, a number, or an abbreviation.

> pro-African initiatives
>
> pre-AIDS era
>
> post-2005 ruling

Note: There is increasing acceptance of the use of a stand-alone prefix with a hyphen in a form of ellipsis in which the prefix refers to the root of a subsequent word with an unhyphenated prefix.

> We found a need for pre- and postoperative examination.
>
> Patients were categorized as hyper- or hypotensive.
>
> This could be an in- or outpatient procedure.

The JAMA Network journals choose not to follow this trend and instead would use the following:

> We found a need for preoperative and postoperative examination.
>
> Patients were categorized as hypertensive or hypotensive.
>
> This could be an inpatient or outpatient procedure.

When 2 or more hyphenated compounds have a common base, omit the base in all but the last. In unhyphenated compounds written as 1 word, repeat the base.

> first-, second-, and third-grade students
>
> 10- and 15-year-old boys
>
> anterolateral and posterolateral aspects

Hyphenate compound numbers from 21 to 99 (cardinal and ordinal) when written out, as at the beginning of a sentence (see 18.1, Use of Numerals).

> Thirty-six patients were examined.
>
> Twenty-fifth through 75th percentile rankings were shown.
>
> One hundred thirty-two people were injured in the plane crash.

Hyphenate fractions used as nouns or adjectives.

Three-fourths of the questionnaires were returned.

A two-thirds majority was needed.

The flask was three-fourths full.

**8.3.1.2** **Clarity.** Use hyphens to avoid ambiguity. If a term could be misleading without a hyphen, hyphenate it. As with the use of commas to indicate pauses, the use of the hyphen to provide clarity may be subjective. What is clear to one person may be a source of ambiguity to another. Use the following guidelines and a healthy dose of common sense.

> a small-bowel constriction (constriction of the small bowel)
> a small bowel constriction (a small constriction of the bowel)
>
> a single-specialty center (a center devoted to a single specialty)
> a single specialty center (1 center devoted to a specialty)
>
> a large-bowel resection (resection of the large bowel) (*Better:* a colon resection)
> a large bowel resection (a large resection of the bowel)
>
> a solid-organ transplant program (a program for transplant of solid organs)
> a solid organ transplant program (a program for organ transplant that is solid, ie, well established) (*Better:* a well-established transplant program)
>
> It would be tough to conceive of a better smelling "machine" than a dog (dogs have a high ability to sniff out bombs).
> It would be tough to conceive of a better-smelling "machine" than a dog (dogs have a pleasing aroma).

Use a hyphen after a prefix when the unhyphenated word would have a different meaning.

> re-creation       re-press
>
> re-treat          re-present
>
> re-sort           re-formation
>
> re-sign           re-sent
>
> re-lease          un-ionized

Note: Do not hyphenate other forms of these words for which no ambiguity exists (eg, *retreatment, recreational*).

Occasionally, a hyphen is used after a prefix or before a suffix to avoid an awkward combination of letters, such as 2 of the same vowel or 3 of the same consonant (with exceptions noted in 8.3.1.6, When Not to Use Hyphens).

Follow the latest edition of *Merriam-Webster's Collegiate Dictionary* or *Dorland's* or *Stedman's* medical dictionaries.

| | |
|---|---|
| semi-independent | under-resourced |
| hull-less | co-dosed |
| ultra-atomic | meta-analysis |
| de-emphasize | multi-institutional |
| intra-abdominal | |
| bell-like | |
| anti-inflammatory | |

(Some exceptions to this rule include *microorganism, cooperation, reenter* [see 8.3.1.6, When Not to Use Hyphens].)

In complex modifying phrases that include suffixes or prefixes, combinations of hyphens and en dashes are sometimes used to avoid ambiguity (see 8.3.2.2, En Dash).

| | |
|---|---|
| non–self-governing | non–Q-wave myocardial infarction |
| non–group-specific blood | hematoxylin-eosin–stained biopsy specimens |
| non–brain-injured participants | |
| non–English-language journals | |

**8.3.1.3** **Expressing Ranges and Dimensions.** When expressing ranges or dimensions used as modifiers, use hyphens and spacing in accordance with the following examples in the left-hand column. The alternatives in the right-hand column show how to express dimensions when not used as modifiers.

| As modifier | Alternative |
|---|---|
| in a 10- to 14-day period | a period of 10 to 14 days |
| a 3 × 4-cm strip | a strip measuring 3 × 4 cm |
| a 5- to 10-mg dose | a dose of 5 to 10 mg |
| a 0.6-mg/kg dose | a dose of 0.6 mg/kg |
| in a 5-, 10-, or 15-mg dose | in a dose of 5, 10, or 15 mg |
| a 3-cm-diameter tube | a tube 3 cm in diameter |
| 5-mm-thick lesion | a lesion 5 mm thick |
| a 5-cm-wide strip | a strip 5 cm wide |

In the text, do not use hyphens to express ranges (see 18.4, Use of Digit Spans and Hyphens).

> The adverse events were experienced by 5% to 10% of the group.

Hyphens are, however, used for (1) ranges expressing fiscal years, academic years, life spans, or study spans, (2) ranges given in parentheses, and (3) in figures and tables.

> In subsequent national surveys, the prevalence of diabetes in the Chinese population was 2.5% in the 1994 survey and 5.5% in the 2000-2001 survey.

> The patients' median age was 56 years (range, 31-92 years).

Note that no hyphens are needed in cases of the following type:

> a case of mild to moderate hypertension

> the waist to hip ratio

> the cup to disc ratio

Do not use a hyphen to express ranges, even within parentheses or in a table, if one of the values in the span includes a minus sign (see 18.4, Use of Digit Spans and Hyphens).

> Change in body weight was −4.0 kg (95% CI, −5.8 to −2.3 kg).

**8.3.1.4** **Word Division.** Use hyphens to indicate division of a word at the end of a line (follow the latest edition of *Merriam-Webster's Collegiate Dictionary* or *Dorland's* or *Stedman's* medical dictionaries).

**8.3.1.5** **Division of URLs, Email Addresses, Karyotypes, Long Formulas.** Do not add a hyphen to URLs or email addresses that break at the end of a line.

For guidance on breaking long karyotypes, see 14.6.4.3.3, Human Chromosomes, Chromosome Rearrangements, Punctuation. For guidance on breaking long formulas, see 20.4, Long Formulas.

**8.3.1.6** **When Not to Use Hyphens.** Rules also exist for when not to use hyphens.

The following common prefixes are not joined by hyphens except when they precede a proper noun, or an abbreviation: *ante-, anti-, auto-, bi-, co-, contra-, counter-, de-, e-, eco-, extra-, infra-, inter-, intra-, micro-, mid-, multi-, non-, over-, pre-, post-, pro-, pseudo-, re-, semi-, sub-, super-, supra-, trans-, tri-, ultra-, un-, under-* (but see also 8.3.1.2, Punctuation, Hyphens and Dashes, Hyphen, Clarity). Note that *email* is treated as one word, without a hyphen. However, other words preceded by *e-* (eg, e-cigarette, e-commerce, e-prescribing, e-print) retain the hyphen.

> antimicrobial          coauthor
>
> autoimmune          codirects

| | |
|---|---|
| coexistence | nonresident |
| coidentity | overproduction |
| countermeasure | overrepresented |
| coworker | overtreatment |
| deidentify | postopearative |
| ecogenetic | posttraumatic |
| email | preexisting |
| interrater | reevaluation |
| midaxillary | repossess |
| midbrow | transsacral |
| multicenter | ultramicrotome |
| nonnegotiable | underrepresented |

Retain the hyphen if needed to avoid ambiguity or awkward spelling that could interfere with readability: co-opt, co-payment, co-twin, intra-aortic, non-breastfeeding.

Retain the hyphen when the term after the prefixes *anti-, neo-, pre-, post-,* and *mid-* is a proper noun or a number (see 8.3.1.1, Hyphen, Temporary Compounds), eg, mid-1900s, mid-Atlantic crossing.

The following suffixes are joined without a hyphen, with exceptions if the clarity would be obscured (see 8.3.1.1, Hyphen, Temporary Compounds): *-hood, -less, -like, -wise.*

| | |
|---|---|
| womanhood | shoeless |
| manhood | insulinlike |
| catatoniclike | probandwise concordance |

The suffix *-wide* is usually closed up (*worldwide, citywide*) unless it follows a proper noun (*Chicago-wide*) or a word of 3 or more syllables (*university-wide*). Editorial discretion may also dictate a hyphen in less common combinations to enhance readability (*genome-wide association studies, hospital-wide implementation*).

Some combinations of words are commonly read together as a unit. As such combinations come into common use, the hyphen tends to be omitted without a sacrifice of clarity. Use the latest editions of *Merriam-Webster's Collegiate Dictionary* and *Dorland's* and *Stedman's* medical dictionaries as guides to common usage (eg, *broad-spectrum antibiotics* is hyphenated in *Dorland's; open heart surgery, deep venous thrombosis,* and *small cell carcinoma* are not). For terms not found in these sources, use a reader's perspective and the context as guides. When no confusion is likely, leave open. If there is a possibility of confusion, hyphenate. A short list of examples that can usually be presented without hyphens is given here.

| | |
|---|---|
| amino acid levels | deep vein thrombosis |
| birth control methods | foreign body aspiration |
| bone marrow biopsy | fresh frozen plasma |

| | |
|---|---|
| health care system | patch test series |
| inner ear disorder | peer review process |
| lower extremity amputation | primary care physician |
| medical school students | public health official |
| multiple organ disease | small cell carcinoma |
| natural killer cell | soft tissue sarcoma |
| open access journal | tertiary care center |
| open heart surgery | |
| parallel furrow pattern | |

Do not hyphenate names of disease entities used as modifiers.

| | |
|---|---|
| basal cell carcinoma | connective tissue tumor |
| hyaline membrane disease | sickle cell trait |
| clam diggers' itch | grand mal seizures |

Do not use a hyphen after an adverb that ends in -*ly* even when used in a compound modifier preceding the word modified; in these cases, ambiguity is unlikely and the hyphen can be dispensed with.

Note: Do hyphenate terms such as early-onset Alzheimer disease. (*Early* merely happens to end in *ly* but is not an adverb created from another word.)

| | |
|---|---|
| the clearly stated purpose | clinically relevant variables |
| a highly developed species | biologically mediated therapy |
| clinically derived databases | previously published recommendations |

Do not hyphenate names of chemical compounds used as adjectives.

carbon dioxide laser

sodium chloride solution

tannic acid test

Most combinations of proper adjectives derived from geographic entities are not hyphenated when used as noun or adjective formations.

| | |
|---|---|
| South Americans | Pacific Rim countries |
| Southeast Asian countries | South American customs |
| African American | Latin Americans |
| Mexican American | |

(*But*: Scotch-Irish ancestry. Here the hyphen is used to indicate descent from Scottish settlers in Northern Ireland. Also sub-Saharan Africa. Here the hyphen connects the prefix *sub-* to the adjective *Saharan*.)

Do not hyphenate Latin expressions or non–English-language phrases used in an adjectival sense. Most of these are treated as separate words; a few are joined without a hyphen. Follow the latest edition of *Merriam-Webster's Collegiate Dictionary.*

| | |
|---|---|
| an a priori argument | antebellum South |
| per diem employees | in vivo specimens |
| prima facie evidence | carcinoma in situ |
| postmortem examination | café au lait spots |
| ex officio member | post hoc testing |

Note that when *post* is used as a combining adjectival form, as in *postmortem examination,* it is set closed up. When it is used as an adverb, as in *post hoc testing,* it is set as 2 separate words. This distinction is apparent in the examples below:

postpartum depression

depression that occurs post partum

Do not hyphenate modifiers in which a letter or number is the second element.

grade A eggs

study 1 protocol

type 1 diabetes

phase 2 study

**8.3.1.7** **Compound Official Titles.** Hyphenate combination positions of office but not compound designations as follows:

secretary-treasurer

acting secretary

honorary chair

editor in chief

(*But*: past vice president, executive vice president, past president)

For *then*, hyphenate and capitalize as in these examples.

This policy was enacted under the then-president.

This policy was enacted under then-President Obama.

**8.3.1.8** **Special Combinations.** Special combinations may or may not need the use of hyphens. Consult *Dorland's* or *Stedman's* medical dictionaries and the latest edition of *Merriam-Webster's Collegiate Dictionary.* Note that they may not always agree, and in these cases, a publication will need to indicate a preference to ensure internal consistency (see 14.0, Nomenclature, and 16.0, Greek Letters).

| | |
|---|---|
| B cell | B-cell helper |
| graft-vs-host disease | I beam (I-shaped beam) |
| T tube | T wave |

| | |
|---|---|
| β-blocker | Mann-Whitney test |
| J curve | T-shirt |
| T-cell marker | face-lift |
| brow-lift | prostate-specific antigen |
| f-stop or f-number | Z-plasty |
| white-coat hypertension | T square |
| S-100 protein | γ-globulin |
| C-reactive protein | *t* test |

**8.3.2** **Dashes.** Dashes, another form of internal punctuation, convey a particular meaning or emphasize and clarify a certain section of material within a sentence. Compared with parentheses, dashes may convey a less formal or more emphatic "aside."

There are 4 types of dashes, which differ in length: the *em* dash (the most common), the *en* dash, the *2-em* dash, and the *3-em* dash.

**8.3.2.1** **Em Dash.** Em dashes are used to indicate a marked or pronounced interruption or break in thought. It is best to use this mode sparingly; do not use an em dash when another punctuation mark (for instance, the comma or the colon) will suffice or to imply *namely, that is*, or *in other words*, when an explanation follows.

> He was young—in his early 50s—with a body ravaged by an incurable, highly aggressive prostate cancer.

> The *Amarin* decision—if it is neither modified nor reversed—may well put patients, and the evidence base for medical practice, at risk.

An em dash may be used to separate a referent from the subject of a clause that follows or precedes:

> Osler, Billings, Apgar—these were the physicians she tried to emulate.

> Direct-to-consumer laboratories have allowed patients to bypass the health care establishment, opening a door to our most personal data—DNA.

**8.3.2.2** **En Dash.** The en dash is longer than a hyphen but half the length of the em dash. The en dash shows relational distinction in a hyphenated or compound modifier, 1 element of which consists of 2 or more words or a hyphenated word, or when the word being modified is a compound.

| | |
|---|---|
| Winston-Salem–oriented group | reverse transcriptase–polymerase chain reaction |
| physician-lawyer–directed section | |
| anti–Norwalk virus | non–Q wave |
| non–critical access hospitals | phosphotungstic acid–hematoxylin stain |
| shock wave–facilitated intracoronary cell therapy | National Cancer Institute–funded research networks |

(*But*: National Cancer Institute [NCI]–funded research networks and NCI-funded research networks)

multiple sclerosis–like symptoms

decision tree–based analysis

post–World War I

non–small cell carcinoma

**8.3.2.3** **2-Em Dash.** The 2-em dash is used to indicate missing letters in a word.

The study was conducted at N—— Hospital, noted for its low autopsy rate.

**8.3.2.4** **3-Em Dash.** The 3-em dash is used to show 1 or more missing words.

Each participant was asked to fill in the blank in the following statement: "I usually sleep ——— hours per day."

I admire Dr ——— too much to expose him in this anecdote.

**8.4** **Forward Slash (Virgule, Solidus).** The forward slash is used to represent *per, and,* or *or* and to divide material (eg, numerator and denominator in fractions; month, day, and year in dates [only in tables and figures]; lines of poetry). It may also be used in URLs (see 2.0, Manuscript Preparation for Submission and Publication).

**8.4.1** **Used to Express Equivalence or Duality.** When 2 terms are of equal weight in an expression and *and* is implied between them to express this equivalence, the forward slash can be retained.

Developing skin cancer screening recommendations in the Hispanic/Latino population can be challenging.

The diagnosis and initial treatment/diagnostic planning were recorded.

There was an excess incidence of prostate cancer, thyroid cancer, and multiple myeloma in the rescue/recovery workers.

This is an and/or decision.

If the approval process raises concerns among the researchers or the ethics committee/institutional review board members, the author may want to explain the resolution of these issues.

When the question of duality arises in the he/she construction, change the slash construction when the sex or gender is to be specified; substitute the word *or* for the forward slash or, preferably, rephrase to be gender neutral.

Dr Kate Wolf and Dr Rob Cox agreed to serve on the nomenclature committee. Now I need to know whether he or she [not he/she] will lead the subcommittee on genetic nomenclature.

*Better*: Now I need to know which of them will lead the subcommittee.

If the sex is unspecified and does not matter, the slash construction is permissible.

This aspiration technique is one that any physician can master whether or not he/she has surgical expertise.

See also 7.2.3.2, Pronoun-Pronoun Agreement, regarding use of *they* as a singular pronoun when rewriting would be awkward or unclear.

Note: The trend is toward rephrasing such sentences and using the plural to avoid sexist language; eg, "This aspiration technique can be mastered by physicians whether or not they have surgical expertise." (See 11.12, Inclusive Language.)

Although the forward slash can be used to indicate alternative or combined states in the same person, such as Jekyll/Hyde personality, it is important that no ambiguity be present. If there is any likelihood of ambiguity, the sentence should be reworded or rephrased for clarity:

The study found that 86 (4.5%) were both perpetrators and survivors (originally "perpetrators/survivors").

**8.4.2** **Used to Mean *per*.** In the "per" construction, use a forward slash only when (1) the construction involves units of measure (including time) and (2) at least 1 element includes a specific numerical quantity and (3) the element immediately adjacent on each side is either a specific numerical quantity or a unit of measure. In such cases, the units of measure should be abbreviated in accordance with 13.12, Units of Measure (see 18.7.3, Reporting Proportions and Percentages).

The hemoglobin level was 14 g/dL.

The CD4+ cell count was 200/μL.

Blood volume was 80 mL/kg of body weight.

Respirations were 60/min; pulse rate was 98/min.

The drug dosage was 30 mg/d.

Annual screening in the reference group had an incremental cost-effectiveness of CaD $24 000 per quality-adjusted life-year (QALY); adding a smoking cessation program to screening could lower the incremental cost-effectiveness to CaD $52 000/QALY.

Do not use the forward slash in a "per" construction (1) when a prepositional phrase intervenes between the 2 units of measure, (2) when no specific numerical quantity is expressed, or (3) in nontechnical expressions.

4.5 mEq of potassium per liter
(*Avoid*: 4.5 mEq/L of potassium; instead reword: a potassium concentration of 4.5 mEq/L.)

expressed in milliliters per minute

2 days per year

An exception is often made in table footnotes to save space:

Cholesterol is expressed as mg/dL.

See also Table 4.1-10.

**8.4.3**    **In Dates.** Use the forward slash in dates only in tables and figures to save space (month/day/year) (see 4.1.6, Tables, Punctuation). Avoid this presentation of dates in the text.

**8.4.4**    **In Equations.** In equations that are set on the line and run into the text rather than centered and set off (see 20.2, Stacked vs Unstacked Fractions or Formulas), use the forward slash to separate numerator and denominator.

The stacked fraction $y = \dfrac{r_1 + r_2}{p_1 - p}$ is written as $y = (r_1 + r_2)/(p_1 - p_2)$ in this equation.

Note that when the slash is used for this purpose, parentheses and brackets must often be added to avoid ambiguity.

**8.4.5**    **Ratios.** Although a forward slash may be used to express a ratio (eg, the male/female [M/F] ratio was 2/1), the JAMA Network journals recommend use of a colon to express ratios that involve numbers or abbreviations (the Apo B:Apo A-I ratio was 2:1) and the word *to* to express ratios involving words (the male to female ratio) (see 8.2.3.3, Colon, Numbers).

**8.4.6**    **Phonetics, Poetry.** The forward slash is also used to set off phonemes and phonemic transcription and to divide run-in lines of poetry.

/d/ as in *dog*

. . . cold-breath'd earth!/Earth of the slumbering and liquid trees!/Earth of departed sunset—/Earth of the mountains misty-topt!

**8.5**    **Parentheses and Brackets.** Parentheses and brackets are internal punctuation marks used to set off material that is nonrestrictive or, as in the case of mathematical and chemical expressions, to alert the reader to the special functions occurring within. Note: Excessive use of parentheses and brackets can make text challenging to read and understand.

**8.5.1**    **Parentheses.**

**8.5.1.1**    **Supplementary Expressions.** Use parentheses to indicate supplementary explanations, identification, direction to the reader, or translation (see 8.3.2, Dashes, and 8.5.2, Brackets).

A known volume of fluid (100 mL) was injected.

The differences were not significant ($P = .06$).

One of us (B.O.G.) saw the patient in 2006.

Asymmetry of the upper part of the rib cage (patient 5) and pseudarthrosis of the first and second ribs (patient 8) were incidental anomalies (Table 3).

Of the 761 hospitalized patients, 171 (22.5%) were infants (younger than 1 year).

In this issue of the same journal (p 1037), a successful transplant is reported.

The 3 cusps of the aortic valve (the Mercedes-Benz sign) were clearly shown on the echocardiogram.

If there is a close relationship between the parenthetical material and the rest of the sentence, commas are preferred to parentheses.

The hemoglobin level, although in the reference range, was lower than expected.

If the relationship in thought after the expressions *namely, that is (ie),* and *for example (eg)* is incidental, use parentheses instead of commas.

He weighed the advice of several committee members (namely, Jones, Burke, and Easton) before making his proposal.

**8.5.1.2** **Back-to-Back Parentheses.** Back-to-back parentheses tend to be awkward. Sometimes they can be avoided by using a single set of parentheses and separating the items inside the parentheses with a semicolon.

The effect size was particularly high for respiratory tract infections (adjusted hazard ratio, 2.27; 95% CI, 1.32-3.91).

In other cases, however, combining back-to-back parentheses, although more streamlined, muddies the meaning.

Significantly more patients withdrew from the placebo group (n = 174) than from the chelation group (n = 115) (hazard ratio, 0.66; 95% CI, 0.41-0.85; *P* = .001). [Here, the back-to-back parentheses make it clear that the hazard ratio and *P* value apply to *both* groups, not just the chelation group.]

**8.5.1.3** **Punctuation Marks With Parentheses.** Use no punctuation before the opening parenthesis except in enumerations (see 8.2.3.2, Introducing Quotations or Enumerations).

Any punctuation mark can follow a closing parenthesis, but only the 3 end marks (the period, the question mark, and the exclamation point) may precede it when the parenthetical material interrupts the sentence. If a complete sentence is contained within parentheses, it is not necessary to have punctuation within the parentheses if it would noticeably interrupt the flow of the sentence. Note that with complete sentences (ie, if closing punctuation *is* used within the parentheses), the initial letter of the first word is capitalized.

The discussion on informed consent lasted 2 hours. (A final draft has yet to be written.) The discussion failed to resolve the question.

The discussion on informed consent lasted 2 hours (a final draft has yet to be written) and did not resolve the question.

After what seemed an eternity (It took 2 hours!), the discussion on informed consent ended.

When the parenthetical material includes special punctuation, such as an exclamation point or a question mark, or several statements, terminal punctuation is placed inside the closing parenthesis.

> Oscar Wilde once said (When? Where? Who knows? But I read it in a book once upon a time; hence, it must be true.) that "anyone who has never written a book is very learned."[4]

**8.5.1.4** **Identifying Numbers or Letters.** When an item identified by letter or number is referred to later by that letter or number only, enclose the letter or number in parentheses.

> You then follow (3), (5), and (6) to solve the puzzle.

If the category name is used instead, parentheses are not needed.

> Steps 1, 2, and 3 must be done slowly.

**8.5.1.5** **Enumerations.** For division of a short enumeration that is run in and indicated by numerals or lowercase italic letters, enclose the numerals or letters in parentheses (see 18.5, Enumerations.)

> The patient is to bring (1) all pill bottles, (2) past medical records, and (3) our questionnaire to the first office visit.

**8.5.1.6** **References in Text.** Use parentheses to enclose a full or partial reference given in the text (see 3.3, References Given in Text).

> A systematic review published in *JAMA Pediatrics* noted that, on any given day, 60% of young persons play video games (2013;167[6]:574-580).

**8.5.1.7** **In Legends or Captions.** In legends or captions, use parentheses to identify a case or patient and parts of a composite figure when appropriate (see 4.2.7, Titles, Legends, and Labels).

> Facial paralysis on the right side (patient 3).

> Long-term survival after early surgery vs initial medical management in the overall population (A) and in the propensity score–matched cohort (B).

> A, Axial T1 postcontrast image shows avid enhancement of nerve roots (patient 1). B, Sagittal T1 fat-saturated, postcontrast images of the lumbar spine show a rim-enhancing fluid collection in the dorsal epidural space (patient 2).

The date, if given, is similarly enclosed.

> Fracture of the left femur (patient 7, September 3, 2013).

For photomicrographs, give the magnification and the stain, if relevant, in parentheses (see 4.2.7, Titles, Legends, and Labels).

> Yellow arrowheads identify the prominent goblet cells in the intestinal metaplasia of Barrett esophagus (hematoxylin-eosin, original magnification ×20).

**8.5.1.8** **Trade Names.** If there is a reason to provide a trade name for a drug or for equipment, enclose the trade name in parentheses immediately after the first use of the nonproprietary name in the text and in the abstract (see 14.4.3, Drugs, Proprietary Names; 14.5, Equipment, Devices, and Reagents; and 5.6.15, Trademark).

> Treatment included oral administration of indomethacin (Indocin), 25 mg 3 times a day.

**8.5.1.9** **Abbreviations.** If used in the text, specialized abbreviations (as specified in 13.11, Clinical, Technical, and Other Common Terms) are enclosed in parentheses immediately after first mention of the term, which is spelled out in full.

> A data and safety monitoring board (DSMB) of investigators outside the university provided oversight.

> Abusive head trauma (ABT) of infants and young children has considerable morbidity and economic costs.

**8.5.1.10** **Explanatory Notes.** Explanatory notes, when incorporated into the text, are placed within parentheses. In such instances, terminal punctuation is used before the closing parenthesis, the sentence(s) within the parentheses being a complete thought but only parenthetical to the text.

**8.5.1.11** **Parenthetical Expressions Within a Parenthetical Expression.** Whenever a parenthetical expression is embedded within another, use brackets within parentheses.

> Antirejection therapy included parenteral antithymocyte globulin ([ATGAM], at a daily dosage of 15 mg/kg).

> *But*: In mathematical expressions, parentheses are placed *inside* brackets (see 8.5.2.2, Brackets, Within Parentheses).

**8.5.1.12** **Parenthetical Plurals.** Parentheses are sometimes used around the letters *s* and/or *es* to express the possibility of a plural when singular or plural could be meant (see 7.5.4, Subject-Verb Agreement, Parenthetical Plurals).

> The name(s) of the editor(s) of the book in reference 2 is unknown.

Note: If this construction is used, the verb should be singular, because the *s* is parenthetical. In general, try to avoid this construction or rephrase the sentence:

> We do not know the name(s) of the editor(s) of the book in reference 2.

**8.5.2** **Brackets.**

**8.5.2.1** **Insertions in Quotations.** Brackets are used to indicate editorial interpolation within a quotation and to enclose corrections, explanations, or comments in material that is quoted (see 8.6.1, Quotations; 8.8.6, Ellipses, Change in Capitalization; and 8.8.7, Ellipses, Omission of Ellipses).

"The following year [1947] was a turning point."

"Enough questions had arisen [these are not described] to warrant medical consultation."

Thompson stated, "Because of the patient's preferences, surgery was *absolutely* contraindicated [italics added]."

Note: Use *sic* (Latin for "thus" or "so") in brackets to indicate an error or peculiarity in the spelling or grammar of the preceding word in the original source of the quotation. As with apologetic quotation marks (see 8.6.8, Apologetic Quotation Marks), use *sic* with discretion.

"The plural [*sic*] cavity was filled with fluid."

"Breathing of the gas is often followed by extraordinary fits of extacy [*sic*]."

**8.5.2.2**  **Within Parentheses.** Use brackets to indicate parenthetical expressions within parenthetical expressions.

A nitrogen mustard (mechlorethamine hydrochloride [Mustargen]) was one of the drugs used.

In scientific text, one sometimes encounters complex parenthetical constructions, such as consecutive parentheses and brackets within parentheses.

Her platelet count was 100 000/mm$^3$ (100 × 10$^9$/L) (reference range, 150 000-450 000/mm$^3$ [150-450 × 10$^9$/L]).

Among the 3578 patients (2841 men [79.4%]) and 11 775 control group participants (91 845 men [78%]), all were diagnosed as having depression.

**8.5.2.3**  **In Formulas.** In mathematical formulas, parentheses are generally used for the innermost units. Parentheses are changed to brackets when the formula itself is parenthetical.

$$t = d(r_1 - r_2)$$

The equation suggested by this phenomenon *(t = d[r$_1$ − r$_2$])* can be applied in a variety of circumstances.

(See 20.2, Stacked vs Unstacked Fractions or Formulas.)

Make sure that every parenthetical or bracketed expression has an opening and closing parenthesis or bracket symbol. For chemicals, consult the most recent edition of *USP Dictionary of USAN and International Drug Names* for drug formulas and *The Merck Index* for chemical compounds to verify the correct use of parentheses and brackets.

An experimental drug (9-[(2-hydroxy-1-(hydroxymethyl)ethoxy methyl)]guanine) was used to treat the cytomegalovirus retinopathy in patients with AIDS.

If the older style of parentheses, braces, and brackets has been used by the author, retain it. The notation will be readily understood by the author's intended audience.

When a parenthetical or bracketed insertion in the text contains a mathematical formula in which parentheses or brackets appear, the characters within the formula should be left as given unless that would place 2 identical punctuation symbols (eg, 2 open parentheses) immediately adjacent to each other. To avoid adjacent identical characters, change parentheses to brackets or brackets to parentheses in the formula as needed, working from inside out, starting with parentheses, to brackets, to braces.

$$CV^2_t = [CV^2_b + (CV^2_a / NR)]/NS$$

In some instances, a better option might be to restructure the passage.

**8.6** **Quotation Marks.** Quotation marks are used to indicate material that is taken verbatim from another source.

**8.6.1** **Quotations.** Use quotation marks to enclose a direct quotation of limited length that is run into the text (see 8.6.14, Block Quotations).

> "The excitement of the brisk pace and glamorous environs that can characterize life in the big city seemingly could not compare with the simple glories of scenic northern New Mexico for Kenneth M. Adams, profiled in The Art of JAMA."

When the quotation marks enclose conversational dialogue, there is no limit to the length that may be set in run-in format.

In all quoted material, follow the wording, spelling, and punctuation of the original exactly. This rule does not apply when the quoted material, although part of a complete sentence in its original source, is now used as the start of a complete sentence. In this case, the lowercase letter in the quoted sentence would be replaced by a capital letter in brackets.

> "[L]ife in the big city seemingly could not compare with the simple glories of scenic northern New Mexico for Kenneth M. Adams, profiled in The Art of JAMA."

Similarly, in legal material any change in initial capital letters from quoted material should be indicated by placing the change in brackets (see 8.5.2.1, Brackets, Insertions in Quotations).

To indicate an omission in quoted material, use ellipses (see 8.8, Punctuation, Ellipses).

To indicate editorial interpolation in quoted material, use brackets (see 8.5.2.1, Brackets, Insertions in Quotations). Use [*sic*] after a misspelled word or an incorrect or apparently absurd statement in quoted material to indicate that this is an accurate rendition of the original source. However, when quoting material from another era that uses now obsolete spellings, use *sic* sparingly. Do not use *sic* with an exclamation point. (Note: The use of *sic* is not limited to quoted material; in other instances, it means that any unusual or bizarre appearance in the preceding word is intentional, not unintentional.) (See 8.5.2.1, Brackets, Insertions in Quotations.)

The author should always verify the quotation from the original source.

**8.6.2** **Dialogue.** With conversational dialogue, enclose the opening word and the final word in quotation marks.

> "Please don't schedule the surgery for a Tuesday."
>
> "OK, if that's inconvenient for you, I won't."

If a quotation is interrupted by attribution, punctuate as follows:

> "If there is no alternative," she said, "we can schedule the surgery for Tuesday."

**8.6.3** **Titles.** Within titles (including titles of articles, references, and tables), centered heads, and run-in sideheads, use double quotation marks.

> The "Sense" of Humor

**8.6.4** **Single Quotation Marks.** Use single quotation marks for quotations within quotations.

> He looked at us and said, "As my patients always told me, 'Be a good listener.'"

**8.6.5** **Placement.** Place closing quotation marks outside commas and periods, inside colons and semicolons. Place question marks, dashes, and exclamation points inside quotation marks only when they are part of the quoted material. If they apply to the whole statement, place them outside the quotation marks.

> Why bother to perform autopsies at all if the main finding is invariably "edema and congestion of the viscera"?
>
> The clinician continues to ask, "Why did he die?"
>
> "I'll lend you my stethoscope for clinic"—then she remembered the last time she had lent it and said, "On second thought, I'll be needing it myself."

Commas are not always needed before or after quoted material. For instance, in the following example commas are not necessary after "said" or to set off the quoted material.

> He said he had had his "fill of it all" and was "content" to leave the meeting.

**8.6.6** **Punctuation, Quotation Marks.** The opening quotation mark should be omitted when an article beginning with a stand-up or drop cap (dropped initial capital letter) also begins with a quotation. It is best, however, to avoid this construction in text.

> Doctors need some patients," a sage had said.

When excerpting long passages that consist of more than 1 paragraph, use opening double quotation marks before each paragraph and closing quotation marks only at the end of the final paragraph. However, if excerpted material runs several paragraphs, the material would be set as a block quotation (see 8.6.14, Block Quotations, and 8.8, Ellipses).

**8.6.7** **Coined Words, Slang, or Unfamiliar Terms.** Coined words, slang, unfamiliar terms, nicknames, and words or phrases used ironically or facetiously may be enclosed in quotation marks at first mention. Thereafter, omit quotation marks (see 21.9, Editing, Proofreading, Tagging, and Display).

> Diagnoses based on traditional Chinese medicine, such as "yin deficiency," may not jeopardize patients who have received a medical diagnosis before entering the study.

> There was a giant congenital nevus in the "bathing trunk" distribution.

> The second most common diagnosis before referral was "unknown."

> We further hope that, above all, those who have been fed only "docufiction" on this matter, as if it were truth, will cease to be misled.

> *Nelson Essentials of Pediatrics* is not a synopsis of or a companion to the *Nelson Textbook of Pediatrics,* although initially our associates dubbed it "Baby Nelson," "Half Nelson," and "Junior Nelson."[5]

> It has been said that shoes and latrines are the best "medicine" for ancylostomiasis (hookworm disease).

Do not use quotation marks when emphasizing a word, when using a non-English word, when mentioning a term as a term, or when defining a term. In these instances, italics are preferred (see 21.9, Editing, Proofreading, Tagging, and Display).

> The page number is called the *folio.*

> The eye associated with the greater reduction in hitting ability when dimmed by a filter was termed the *dominant eye* for motion stereopsis.

> *Pulsus paradoxus* is defined as an exaggeration of the physiologic inspiratory decrease in systolic blood pressure.

> The one and only Russian word we knew was *baleet* ("pain").

**8.6.8** **Apologetic Quotation Marks.** Quotation marks are sometimes used around words for special effect or to indicate irony. In most instances, however, they are unnecessary and should be avoided in scientific writing.

> *Avoid*: Funding for "big data" projects is increasing.

**8.6.9** **So-called.** A word or phrase following *so-called* should not be enclosed in quotation marks.

> The so-called harm principle holds that competent adults should have freedom of action unless they pose a risk to themselves or to the community.

**8.6.10** **Common Words Used in a Technical Sense.** Enclose in quotation marks common words used in a special technical sense when the context does not make the meaning clear (see 8.6.11, Definition or Translation of Non–English-Language Words).

> In many publications, "running feet" on left-hand pages face the "gutter" at the bottom of the page.

> "Coma vigil" (akinetic mutism) may be confused with conscious states.

**8.6.11** **Definition or Translation of Non–English-Language Words.** The literal translation of a non–English-language word or phrase is usually enclosed in quotation marks if it follows the word or phrase, whereas the simple definition of the word or phrase is not (see 12.2, Accent Marks [Diacritics]).

> Patients with hysteria may exhibit an attitude termed *la belle indifférence* ("beautiful indifference" or total unconcern) toward their condition.

**8.6.12** **Titles.** In the text, use quotation marks to enclose titles of short poems, essays, lectures, single episodes of a radio or television program, songs, the names of electronic files, parts of published works (eg, chapters, articles in a periodical), papers read at meetings, dissertations, and theses (see 10.5, Capitalization, Types and Sections of Articles, and 21.9.4, Specific Uses of Fonts and Styles, Italics).

**8.6.13** **Indirect Discourse, Discussions.** After indirect discourse, do not use quotation marks.

> The nurse said he would be discharged today.

> You foolish woman, I berate myself, as I resist this type of thinking every day.

Do not use quotation marks with yes or no.

> His answer to the question was no.

In interview or discussion formats when the name of the speaker is set off, do not use quotation marks.

> Dr Black: Now let us review the slides of the bone marrow biopsy.

> Dr Smith: The first slide reveals complete absence of granulocytic precursors.

**8.6.14** **Block Quotations.** Editorial judgment must be exercised to determine whether material quoted from texts or speeches is long enough to warrant setting it off in a block, ie, indented and without the quotation marks. Different modes of display (eg, print, online, optimized for mobile) should be considered when thinking about length. Paragraph indents are generally not used unless the quoted material is known to begin a paragraph. Space is often added both above and below quoted material that is indented. Block quotations are often preceded by a colon.

If a quotation appears within a block quote, use double quotation marks around the contained quotation, rather than setting it off in blocks, regardless of the length.

In Truss' *Eats, Shoots & Leaves*, she notes in the preface:

> One supporter of *Eats, Shoots & Leaves* wrote a 1,400-word column in *The Times* of London explaining (with glorious self-importance) that while his admiration for my purpose was "total," he disagreed with virtually everything I said.[1(pxix)]

## 8.7 Apostrophe.

**8.7.1** **To Show Possession.** Use the apostrophe to show the possessive case of proper nouns in accordance with the following examples (see 15.2, Eponyms, Nonpossessive Form):

Jones' bones (1 person named Jones)

the Joneses' bones (2 or more people named Jones)

If a singular or plural word does not end in *s*, add *'s* to form the possessive.

a child's wants

men's concerns

women's health

everyone's answer

If a proper noun or name ends in a silent *s, z,* or *x,* form the possessive by adding *'s.*

Theroux's *The Mosquito Coast*

Degas's work

If a noun ends in a nonsilent *s*, form the possessive by adding an apostrophe:

The scissors' point had been dulled over the years.

**8.7.2** **Possessive Pronouns.** Do not use *'s* with possessive pronouns: his, hers, ours, its, yours, theirs, whose.

The idea was hers.

Give the book its due.

Do not confuse the contraction of *it is* (*it's*) with the possessive *its*, eg, "It's an excellent resource. I have not seen its equal."

**8.7.3** **Possessive of Compound Terms.** Use *'s* after only the last word of a compound term.

father-in-law's health

someone else's problem

editor in chief's decision

secretary of health's ruling

the editors in chief's terms

**8.7.4** **Joint Possession.** When joint possession is being shown with an organization's or business firm's name, use the possessive form only in the last word of the noun or name.

US Food and Drug Administration's policy

Farrar, Straus and Giroux's books

Centers for Disease Control and Prevention's Task Force

Hammond and Horn's study

When possession is individual, each noun takes the possessive form.

We matched the infant's and mother's records.

Note: When one of the nouns takes a possessive pronoun, the other nouns take the possessive as well.

I presented the intern's and my workups.

**8.7.5** **Using Apostrophes to Form Plurals.** Do not use an apostrophe to indicate the plural of a name. Do not use an apostrophe in the name of an organization in which the qualifying term is used as an adjective or an attributive rather than a possessive. Of course, always follow the official name.

| | |
|---|---|
| Chicago Cubs | state parks rangers |
| Veterans Affairs | musicians union |
| Rainbow Babies Hospital | nurses station |

Use *'s* to indicate the plural of letters, signs, or symbols spoken as such or words referred to as words when *s* alone would be confusing. Note the italics with inflectional ending in roman type for words, letters, and numbers but not for symbols and signs.

He uses too many *and*'s.

The manuscript editor was mindful of the list of *do*'s and *don't*'s.

Mind your *p*'s and *q*'s.

There are 9 +'s on the page.

His *1*'s looked like *7*'s.

The 3 *A*'s of rhinoplasty: anatomy, aesthetics, and architecture

Do not use an apostrophe to form the plural of an all-capital abbreviation or of a numeral (including years) (see 9.6, Plurals, Abbreviations).

| | |
|---|---|
| ECGs | RBCs |
| EEGs | a woman in her 40s |
| IQs | during the late 1990s |
| WBCs | |

**8.7.6** **Units of Time and Money as Possessive Adjectives.** With units of time (minute, hour, day, month, year, and so on) used as possessive adjectives, an *'s* is added. (Note: For the plural units, add an ' after the *s*.) The same holds true for monetary terms:

| | |
|---|---|
| a day's wait | a few hours' time |
| an hour's delay | 6 months' gestation |
| 5 days' hard work | a dollar's worth |

**8.7.7** **Prime.** Do not use an apostrophe where a prime sign is intended (see 14.4.4, Nomenclature, Drugs, Chemical Names).

The methyl group was in the 5′ position.

**8.8** **Ellipses.** Ellipses are 3 spaced dots (. . .) generally used to indicate omission of 1 or more words, lines, paragraphs, or data from quoted material (this omission being the *ellipsis*). Excerpts from the following paragraph will be used to demonstrate the use of ellipses.

> Vilhelm Hammershøi (1864-1916) was a Danish artist best known for his somber, haunting interior scenes. A master of understatement, his best works are small interiors, often devoid of people. When human beings do appear, they often have their backs turned to the viewer and are apparently self-absorbed. Hammershøi's art transformed his apartment into a continuum of unsettling empty spaces where time seems suspended; his works are not still life paintings but are intended to convey a mood, often a melancholy stillness. He does so by limiting his palette to umber, sienna, brown, black, and white and by excluding warmer tones. Hammershøi's works are not naturalistic but, instead, reflect a mental climate without vitality and seem to speak to the loneliness and isolation of the individual.[6]

**8.8.1** **Omission Within a Sentence.** If the ellipsis occurs within a sentence, ellipses represent the omission.

> When human beings do appear, they . . . are apparently self-absorbed.

In some such instances, additional punctuation may be used on either side of the ellipses if it helps the sense of the sentence or better shows the omission.

> Hammershøi's works are not naturalistic but, instead,. . . seem to speak to the loneliness and isolation of the individual.

If the quotation *itself* contains ellipses, to make clear that the ellipses were part of the original a note to this effect should be included in brackets.

**8.8.2** **Omission at the End of a Sentence or Between Complete Sentences.** If the ellipsis occurs at the end of a complete sentence or between 2 complete sentences, ellipses follow the final punctuation mark, the final punctuation mark being set close to the word preceding it, even when this word is not the final word in that sentence in the original.

> Vilhelm Hammershøi (1864-1916) was a Danish artist best known for his somber, haunting interior scenes. . . . Hammershøi's art transformed his apartment into a continuum of unsettling empty spaces where time seems suspended. . . .

**8.8.3** **Grammatically Incomplete Expressions.** The sentence within which an ellipsis occurs should be a grammatically complete expression. However, ellipses with no period may be used at the end of a sentence fragment to indicate that it is purposely grammatically incomplete.

> Complete the sentence "When I retire, I plan to . . . " in 20 words or less.

**8.8.4** **Omissions in Verse.** Use 1 line of em-spaced dots to indicate omission of a full line or several consecutive lines of verse.

> Sometimes you say it's smaller. Today
>
> . . . . . . . . . . . . . . . . .
>
> you said it was a touch larger, and would change.
>
> Marc Straus, MD, "Autumn"

**8.8.5** **Omissions Between or at the Start of Paragraphs.** With material in which several paragraphs are being quoted and omissions of full paragraphs occur, a period and ellipses at the end of the paragraph preceding the omitted material are sufficient to indicate this omission.

> Indeed, it is no more than the just desert of Dr Theodore Schott and his late brother to attribute to them the credit of having introduced and elaborated a method capable of restoring most cases of heart disease to a state of complete compensation, after the failure of other means, such as digitalis. . . .

If the initial word(s) or the first sentence of the paragraph being quoted is omitted, begin that paragraph with a paragraph indention and ellipses to indicate that this is not the beginning of that paragraph.

> . . . it is no more than the just desert of Dr Theodore Schott and his late brother to attribute to them the credit of having introduced and elaborated a method capable of restoring most cases of heart disease to a state of complete compensation, after the failure of other means, such as digitalis. . . .

**8.8.6** **Change in Capitalization.** The first word after the end punctuation mark and the ellipses should use the original capitalization, particularly in legal and scholarly documents. This facilitates finding the material in the original source and avoids any change of meaning. If a change in the original capitalization is made, brackets should be used around the letter in question (see 8.5.2.1, Brackets, Insertions in Quotations, and 8.6.1, Quotation Marks, Quotations).

> [H]e shows a stark, rectangular grid lit by centers of rounded forms, brilliantly colored.

> In the cover story, the artist is described as using "[v]ivid oranges, reds, and purples, light greens, creamy violets, and color-flecked gold" to depict "a traditional subject."

**8.8.7** **Omission of Ellipses.** Ellipses are not necessary at the beginning and end of a quotation if the quoted material is a complete sentence from the original.

> In a 2016 The Art of JAMA piece, Jeanette M. Smith, MD, wrote, "In *Evening,* a woman who has witnessed the ebb and flow of many seasons sits in peaceful repose by a window."

Omit ellipses within a quotation when the omitted words occur at the same place as a bracketed editorial insertion (see 8.5.2.1, Brackets, Insertions in Quotations).

> "[Caillebotte] shows a stark, rectangular grid lit by centers of rounded forms, brilliantly colored."

When a quoted phrase is an incomplete sentence, readers understand that something precedes and follows; therefore, ellipses are not used.

> In *Place de L'Europe on a Rainy Day,* Caillebotte does not use "centers of rounded forms, brilliantly colored" but instead uses muted grays and purples to give the feel of the rain.

Ellipses are generally not needed when the first part of the sentence is deleted.

> Here Caillebotte "depicts a traditional subject in a manner far removed from the traditional. . . ."

**8.8.8** ▮ **Avoidance of Ellipses in Tables.** In tables, to avoid ambiguity, ellipses should not be used to indicate that no data were available or that a specific category of data is not applicable. Indicators such as NA (not available) or NR (not reported) should be used instead. Blank cells in a table also should be avoided unless the column heading does not apply to the entry or unless the entire section of the table does not contain data (see 4.1.4.5, Table Components, Field).

**Principal Author:** Cheryl Iverson, MA

## ACKNOWLEDGMENT

Thanks to the following for reviewing and providing substantial comments to improve the manuscript: Kevin Brown, JAMA Network; Barbara Gastel, MD, MPH, Texas A&M University, College City; Carissa A. Gilman, MA, American Cancer Society, Atlanta, Georgia; Hope J. Lafferty, AM, ELS, Hope J. Lafferty Communications, Marfa, Texas; Trevor Lane, MA, DPhil, Edanz Group, Fukuoka, Japan; Peter J. Olson, ELS, Sheridan Journal Services, Waterbury, Vermont; and Nicki Snoblin, NextWord Communications, Lake Bluff, Illinois.

## REFERENCES

1. Truss L. *Eats, Shoots & Leaves: The Zero Tolerance Approach to Punctuation.* Gotham Books; 2003:201.
2. Norris M. Holy writ: learning to love the house style. *New Yorker.* February 23 and March 2, 2015:78-90.
3. Shields C. Invention. In: *Dressing Up for the Carnival.* Penguin Putnam; 2000:151.
4. Ball P. *The Unauthorized Biography of a Local Doctor: Or From Infancy Through Puberty and On to Senility.* Exponent Publishers; 1993.
5. Behrman R, Kleigman R. *Nelson's Essentials of Pediatrics.* WB Saunders; 1990.
6. Harris JC. *Interior. With Piano and Woman in Black (Strandgade 30):* Vilhelm Hammershøi. *JAMA Psychiatry.* 2013;70(8):774-775. doi:10.1001/jamapsychiatry.2013.1999

# 9.0 Plurals

**9.0** **Plurals.**

**9.1** **How Plurals Are Formed.** The plurals of most nouns are formed by adding *s* or *es* (Table 9.1-1).

**Table 9.1-1.** Noun Plurals

| Singular | Plural |
| --- | --- |
| benefit | benefits |
| cervix | cervixes |
| correction | corrections |
| disease | diseases |
| guideline | guidelines |
| method | methods |
| inch | inches |

However, English is irregular enough that many exceptions exist (**Table 9.1-2**).

**Table 9.1-2.** Exceptions to Noun Plurals

| Singular | Plural |
| --- | --- |
| child | children |
| foot | feet |
| metastasis | metastases |
| louse | lice |
| offspring | offspring |
| sty | sties |
| tooth | teeth |
| woman | women |
| species | species |

**9.2** **Collective Nouns.** A *collective noun* denotes a group of individuals regarded as a unit. Collective nouns may take either singular or plural verbs, depending on whether the word refers to the group as a unit or to its members as individuals. In American English, most nouns naming a group regarded as a unit are treated as singular (see 7.5.5, Collective Nouns).

> Fifty percent of my time is spent on administration.
>
> Fifty percent of all physicians are included.
>
> At noon today the jury delivers its verdict.
>
> The team practices every Thursday.
>
> The committee decides who will receive tenure.

For a unit of measure, use a singular verb (see 17.0, Units of Measure).

> Five milliliters was injected.
>
> Two weeks of symptoms is common and should not be cause for alarm.
>
> Fifty million dollars was awarded to the discoverers of the vaccine.

**9.3** **Parenthetical Plurals.** When *s* or *es* is added parenthetically to a word to express the possibility of a plural, the verb should be singular. However, in most instances it is preferable to avoid this construction and use the plural noun instead (see 7.5.4, Parenthetical Plurals).

> *Acceptable:* The mechanism(s) of this disease process is still unclear.
>
> *Better:* The mechanisms of this disease process are still unclear.

**9.4** **Latin and Greek vs English.** There is a trend toward using English plurals rather than Latin or Greek, particularly for more common words (**Table 9.4-1**). However, in most cases the latest edition of *Merriam-Webster's Collegiate Dictionary* or *Dorland's* or *Stedman's* medical dictionary should be followed. Consistency within a manuscript is key.

**Table 9.4-1.** Preferred Plurals for Latin and Greek Words

| Singular | Preferred plural |
|---|---|
| alga | algae |
| amoeba | amoebas |
| appendix | appendixes *or* appendices [consult dictionary for specific usage] |
| cannula | cannulas |
| condyloma acuminatum | condylomata acuminata [with 2-word Latin plural, both parts become plural] |
| cranium | crania |
| esophagus | esophagi |

**Table 9.4-1.** Preferred Plurals for Latin and Greek Words (*continued*)

| Singular | Preferred plural |
|---|---|
| fistula | fistulas |
| formula | formulas |
| genus | genera |
| index | indexes *or* indices [consult dictionary for specific usage] |
| maxilla | maxillas |
| orbit | orbits |
| rhytid | rhytids |
| sequela | sequelae |
| vertebra | vertebrae |

**9.5** **Microorganisms.** When referring to the common vernacular plural of a genus, use roman lowercase letters (Table 9.5-1). For organisms that do not have a common plural, add the word *species* or *organisms* to the genus name to indicate a plural use (see 14.14, Organisms and Pathogens).

**Table 9.5-1.** Plural Noun Forms for Microorganisms

| Genus | Plural noun form |
|---|---|
| *Chlamydia* | chlamydiae |
| *Escherichia* | *Escherichia* organisms |
| *Mycobacterium* | mycobacteria |
| *Proteus* | *Proteus* species |
| *Pseudomonas* | pseudomonads |
| *Salmonella* | salmonellae |
| *Staphylococcus* | staphylococci |
| *Streptococcus* | streptococci |

**9.6** **Abbreviations.** For most all-capital abbreviations, the plural is formed by adding a lowercase *s*. Do not use an apostrophe before the *s* (see 8.7.5, Using Apostrophes to Form Plurals).

| | |
|---|---|
| CIs | ICUs |
| EEGs | ORs |
| HMOs | RBCs |

Note: When plural all-capital abbreviations are found in an all-capital setting, such as a heading, the plural *s* is still lowercase.

REFERRAL PATTERNS IN MIDWESTERN HMOs

**9.7**     **Plurals of Symbols, Letters, Numbers, and Years.** Use *'s* to indicate the plural of letters or symbols or for words referred to as words when *s* alone would be confusing. Note the use of italics with the inflectional ending in roman type for words and letters but not for symbols (see 8.7.5, Using Apostrophes to Form Plurals).

> All the capital *P*'s should be underlined.

> Please use +'s to indicate a positive result.

Note: If the symbol can be easily expressed using words, this is preferred:

> Please use plus signs to indicate a positive result.

Do not use an apostrophe to form the plural of numbers (including years).

> during the 1940s

> a man in his late 60s

**9.8**     **When Not to Use Plurals.** Do not pluralize nouns that cannot stand on their own as plurals.

> blood samples (not bloods)

> chemistry studies (not chemistries)

> serum samples (not sera)

> surgical procedures (not surgeries)

> urine tests (not urines)

**9.9**     **False Singulars.** Some nouns, because they end in a "plural" form, are mistaken for plurals, even though they should be treated as singular and take a singular verb.

> Measles is a deadly disease.

> Mathematics has always been her passion.

> Genetics is a rapidly changing field of study.

A few nouns are usually used in the plural form; however, the distinction between plural and singular should be retained where appropriate (**Table 9.9-1**) (see 7.5.3, False Plurals).

**Table 9.9-1.** False Singulars

| Plural | Singular |
|---|---|
| data[a] | datum |
| criteria | criterion |
| media[a] | medium |
| phenomena | phenomenon |

[a]Exception: when referring to *social media, news media*, or *the media*, use a singular verb. The same applies when referring to *big data* as a term for extremely large, often unstructured data sets that can be mined for business or social uses.

**Principal Author:** Brenda Gregoline, ELS

## ACKNOWLEDGMENT

I thank Barbara Gastel, MD, MPH, Texas A&M University, for review and comments.

# 10.0 Capitalization

## 10.0 Capitalization.

## 10.1 First Word of Sentences, Quotations, Titles, and Subtitles.
The first word of every complete sentence should be capitalized.

Capitalize the first word of a direct quotation (but see 8.6.1, Quotation Marks, Quotations).

> The speaker made the following observation: "There are limitations inherent to the use of rotational flaps."

Note: If the quotation is not a full sentence itself, a lowercase letter on the first word is preferable.

> The patient described her headache pain as feeling like "needles behind the eyes."

## 10.2 Titles and Headings.
Capitalize major words in titles, subtitles, and headings of books, journals, articles, musical compositions (including albums and songs), plays (stage and screen), radio and television programs, movies, paintings and other works of art, software programs, websites, blogs, electronic systems, trademarks, and names of ships, airplanes, spacecraft, awards, corporations, and monuments.

Do not capitalize a coordinating conjunction (*and, but, for, nor, or, so, yet*), an article, or a preposition of 3 or fewer letters, except when it is the first word in a title or subtitle. (For more on typeface rules in titles, see 21.5.9, Specific Uses of Fonts and Styles, Italics, and 8.6.3, Quotation Marks, Titles.)

| | |
|---|---|
| *The Collected Stories of Deborah Eisenberg* | the Android operating system |
| Tycho's song "Past Is Prologue" | the Lincoln Memorial |
| | PubMed |
| the Cochrane Database | *Double Indemnity* |
| *Girl With a White Dog* by Lucian Freud | *12 Years a Slave* (film) |
| | *Twelve Years a Slave* (book) |

Note: *The* may be dropped from titles if the syntax of the sentence improves without it.

This week's *Lancet* contains several articles on global health.

**10.2.1** **Titles of Medical Articles.** Titles of articles take initial capitals when they appear as titles in text but not when they appear in a reference list.

*Title:* Free Tissue Transfer for Head and Neck Reconstruction: A Contemporary Review

*Reference:* Cannady SB, Rosenthal EL, Knott PD, Fritz M, Wax M. Free tissue transfer for head and neck reconstruction: a contemporary review. *JAMA Facial Plast Surg.* 2014;16(5):367-373.

In titles and headings, capitalize 2-letter verbs, such as *go, do, am, is, be.* Note: In infinitives, "to" is not capitalized. Do not capitalize a coordinating conjunction, article, or preposition of 3 or fewer letters, except when it is the first word in the title or subtitle or part of a hyphenated term.

We Do Need to Treat Mild Hypertension

Opioid Prescribing for Chronic Pain: Not for the Faint of Heart

Association Between Hospital Conversions to For-Profit Status and Clinical and Economic Outcomes

Cardiovascular Risk Factors in Patients With Type 2 Diabetes

Predictors of In-Hospital Mortality in Trauma Patients

A Nomogram to Predict Long-term Survival After Resection for Intrahepatic Cholangiocarcinoma

Blisters and Erosions in a Neonate

Comparison of Laparoscopic vs Open Hepatectomy: Good Try, but We Still Have Selection Bias

For compound terms from languages other than English, capitalize all parts of the expression in the title.

Fluorescence In Situ Hybridization in Surgical Specimens of Lung Cancer

Perioperative Complications of Total En Bloc Spondylectomy

With a phrasal verb, such as "follow up," capitalize both parts in a title.

> Outcomes in Adolescents Followed Up Longitudinally After Injury Hospitalization

**10.2.2** **Hyphenated Compounds.** In titles, subtitles, and text headings, do not capitalize the second part of a hyphenated compound in the following instances:

If either part is a hyphenated prefix or suffix (see 8.3.1.1, Hyphen, Temporary Compounds)

> Nonsteroidal Anti-inflammatory Drugs for Ankylosing Spondylitis

If both parts together constitute a single word (consult the current edition of *Merriam-Webster's Collegiate Dictionary* or *Stedman's* or *Dorland's* medical dictionary)

> Reliability of Health Information Obtained Through Online Searches for Self-injury [compound words with the prefix *self-* are considered a single word]

> Short-term and Long-term Effects of Violent Media on Aggression in Children

> Follow-up Studies of Patients With Melanoma

> Full-time Coverage by Attending Physicians in a Pediatric Emergency Department

However, if a compound is temporary or if both parts carry equal weight, capitalize both words.

> Cost-Benefit Analysis

> Low-Level Activity

> Drug-Resistant Bacteria

> Obsessive-Compulsive Disorder

> Age-Related Macular Degeneration

In titles, subtitles, and text headings, capitalize the first letter of a word that follows a lowercase (but not a capital) Greek letter (see 16.2, Capitalization After a Greek Letter), a numeral (except when an abbreviated unit of measure that is never capitalized follows), a symbol, a stand-alone capital letter, or an italicized organic chemistry prefix, such as *trans-* or *cis-*.

> Effects of $\alpha_1$-Antitrypsin on Serine Proteinases During Inflammation

> Topical Treatment for Capillary Hemangioma of the Eyelid Using β-Blocker Solution

> Assessment of Plasma C-Reactive Protein as a Biomarker of Posttraumatic Stress Disorder Risk

**10.2.3** **Titles and Headings of Tables, Figures, or Boxes.** Capitalize each major word in the title of a table. In row headings (table stubs) and column headings, only the initial word should be capitalized. If a symbol, numeral, or lowercase Greek letter begins the stub, the word that follows should be capitalized.

**10.3**    **Proper Nouns.** Proper nouns are words used as names for unique individuals, events, objects, or places.

**10.3.1**    **Geographic Names.** Capitalize names of planets, cities, towns, counties, states, countries, continents, islands, airports, peninsulas, bodies of water, mountains and mountain ranges, streets, parks, forests, canyons, dams, and regions (current or historical).

| | |
|---|---|
| Abu Dhabi International Airport | Mangyshlak Peninsula |
| Arctic Ocean | Millennium Park |
| the Bay Area | Mexico City |
| Bernard Street | Norfolk, Virginia |
| Central America | Parambikulam Tiger Reserve |
| Cook County | Ryukyu Islands |
| El Paso | Saudi Arabia |
| Grand Canyon | the Silk Route |
| Hoover Dam | the West Coast |
| Lake Placid | West Nile virus |
| Maat Mons [on the planet Venus] | Woods Hole |

If a common noun that is part of a geographic name is capitalized in the singular, it is generally not capitalized in the plural.

Atlantic and Pacific oceans

Kennedy and Eisenhower expressways

Mississippi and Missouri rivers

Compass directions are not capitalized unless they are generally accepted terms for regions.

Walk east until you arrive at the lake.

There is no party like a West Coast party because a West Coast party does not stop.

His psychiatry practice is in northern Michigan.

In the Western World, cardiovascular disease is a major cause of mortality.

**10.3.2**    **Sociocultural Designations.** Capitalize names of languages, nationalities, racial categories, ethnicities, political parties, religions, and religious denominations. Do not capitalize political doctrines (conservative, progressive) or general forms of government (democracy, monarchy). Capitalize *Black* and *White* as a designation of race; avoid using in noun form (see 11.12.3, Race/Ethnicity).

| | |
|---|---|
| African American | Latina women |
| Alaska Native | Native American |
| Black individuals | Navajo |
| Chinese | Presbyterian |
| English language | Sanskrit |
| Indian American community | Spanish |
| Islam | Thai |
| of Italian heritage | White patients |

> **UPDATE:** In chapter 10.3.2, Sociocultural Designations, the examples of capitalizing racial categories was updated to reflect the decision to capitalize *Black* and *White* and to use them as modifiers, not as nouns. This change was made ***August XX, 2020.***

**10.3.3** **Events, Awards, and Legislation.** Capitalize the names of historical and special events, historical periods, and awards (but not common nouns that may follow the names).

| | |
|---|---|
| Civil War | Nobel Prize |
| Civil War era | Nobel Prize winner |
| Declaration of Helsinki | Special Olympics |
| Equal Rights Amendment | Title IX |
| Lasker Award | |

**10.3.4** **Eponyms and Words Derived From Proper Nouns.** With eponyms, capitalize the proper name but not the common noun that follows it (see 15.0, Eponyms).

| | |
|---|---|
| Breslow thickness | Papanicolaou test |
| Down syndrome | Trendelenburg position |

Most words derived from proper nouns are not capitalized. In general, follow the current edition of *Merriam-Webster's Collegiate Dictionary* or *Dorland's* or *Stedman's* medical dictionary.

| | |
|---|---|
| arabic numerals | mendelian |
| candidiasis | parkinsonism |
| darwinian | petri dish |
| india ink | roman numerals |

**10.3.5** **Proprietary Names.** Capitalize trademarks, proprietary names of drugs, and brand names of manufactured products and equipment. Do not capitalize generic names or descriptive terms. Do not include trademark and copyright symbols after proprietary and brand names (see 5.6.15.9, Use of Trademarked Names in Publication).

Each study patient was given 200 mg of diphenhydramine (Benadryl; McNeil Consumer Healthcare) as a sleep aid.

**10.3.6** **Organisms.** Capitalize the formal name of a genus when used in the singular, with or without a species name. Capitalize formal genus names but not traditional generic designations (eg, streptococci) or derived adjectives (streptococcal) (see 14.14.1.11, Collective Genus Terms). Do not capitalize the name of a species, variety, or subspecies. Do capitalize phylum, class, order, and family (see 14.14, Organisms and Pathogens). For capitalization of virus names, see 14.14.3, Virus Nomenclature.

**10.3.7** **Seasons, Deities, Holidays.** Do not capitalize the names of the seasons. Capitalize the names of specific deities and their manifestations.

| | |
|---|---|
| Allah | Jesus Christ |
| Ganesh | Nature |
| God or Goddess (when used in a monotheistic sense) | Shiva |
| | spring |
| the goddess Athena | winter |
| the Holy Spirit | Zeus |

Capitalize holidays and calendar events.

| | |
|---|---|
| Beltane | Mother's Day |
| Christmas | New Year's Eve |
| Eid al-Fitr | Passover |
| Fourth of July | Ramadan |
| Good Friday | Rosh Hashanah |
| Kwanzaa | Thanksgiving |
| Labor Day | World AIDS Day |

**10.3.8** **Tests.** The exact and complete titles of tests and subscales of tests should be capitalized. The word *test* is not usually capitalized except when it is part of the official name of the test. Always verify exact names of tests with the author or with reference sources.

| | |
|---|---|
| Cox-Stewart trend test | McNemar test |
| Fisher exact test | Mini-Mental State Examination |
| McCarthy Scales of Children's Abilities | Minnesota Multiphasic Personality Inventory |

**10.3.9** **Official Names.** Capitalize the official titles of organizations, businesses, conferences, congresses, institutions, and government agencies. Do not capitalize the conjunctions, articles, or prepositions of 3 or fewer letters contained within these names. For names of institutions, do not capitalize *the* unless it is part of the official title.

| | |
|---|---|
| Boka Restaurant Group | the International Subcommittee on Viral Nomenclature |
| Chicago Board of Education | Knox College |
| the Communist Party | MacArthur Foundation |
| Eighth International Congress on Peer Review and Biomedical Publication | Northwestern Memorial Hospital |
| | The Ohio State University |
| Federal Bureau of Investigation | Quaker Oats Corporation |
| | Society for Scholarly Publishing |
| House of Representatives | the US Navy |

*But:* the board of trustees, the boards of health, a state representative, the federal government, the navy

In running text, a singular form that is capitalized as part of the official name is usually not capitalized in the plural.

> She is chair of the Department of Pediatrics at the University of Wisconsin, Madison.

> Funding was received from the departments of pediatrics and neurology at the University of Wisconsin, Madison.

(See 2.3.3, Author Affiliations, for an example of capitalization of department titles in an affiliation.)

**10.3.10  Titles and Degrees of Persons.** Capitalize a person's title when it precedes the person's name but not when it follows the name.

> Program Chair Allison Hemmings is to be congratulated for our successful meeting.

> Allison Hemmings was named program chair at the 2015 annual meeting.

> Dr Colvin served as principal investigator.

> Principal Investigator Douglas Colvin, MD, directed the SIPR trial.

Capitalize academic degrees when abbreviated but not when written out.

> Sharita Evenson, MA

> Sharita Evenson received her master's degree from Vanderbilt University.

**10.4  Designators.** When used as specific designations within an article, with or without numerals, capitalize the singular and plural forms of the words *Table, Figure, Box* (as well as their online-only equivalents), and *Supplement*.

as seen in the Table

summarized in Table 4

the middle third of the
basilar artery (Figure 2)

a form of proximal subungual onychomycosis
(Figure)

eFigure 1 in the Supplement

listed in Box 1

Do not capitalize the following words, even when used as specific designators,
unless used as part of a heading or title:

| | |
|---|---|
| axis | month |
| case | notes |
| chapter | page |
| chromosome | paragraph |
| column | part |
| control | patient |
| day | phase |
| edition | schedule |
| experiment | section |
| factor | series |
| fraction | stage |
| grade | step |
| grant | type |
| group | volume |
| lead | wave |
| level | week |
| method | year |

*Exceptions:* Step I diet, Schedule II drug, Axis I of the *Diagnostic and
Statistical Manual of Mental Disorders* (Fifth Edition)

**10.5**    **Types and Sections of Articles.** General terms that refer to a type of article
or a section within an article should be set lowercase.

I strongly disagree with that editorial.

A structured abstract is required for all research papers.

However, when referring to a specific article or a section within a specific article,
capitalize the first letter of the category or section name.

In this Viewpoint, the authors critique the prevalent assumption that health
care expenditures are correlated with national estimates of life expectancy.

For a definition of other major opioids, see the Methods section.

**10.6** **Acronyms.** Do not capitalize the words from which an acronym is derived (see 13.0, Abbreviations).

> chronic obstructive pulmonary disease (COPD)

> fluorescence in situ hybridization (FISH)

Exception: When the words that form the acronym are proper names, use capitals as described in 10.3.9, Proper Nouns, Official Names:

> National Institute of Mental Health (NIMH)

When there has been a "stretch" to create a study name or a writing group name that is easy to say and somehow relates to the aim of the study but where the first letters of the major words do not match the acronym, do not use unusual capitalization to indicate how the study name was derived. Expanded study or group names use normal JAMA Network capitalization style.

> Clopidogrel in Unstable Angina to Prevent Recurrent Events (CURE)

> the STABILITY (Stabilization of Atherosclerotic Plaque by Initiation of Darapladib Therapy) Trial

**10.7** **Capitalized Electronic (Digital) Terms.** Use initial capitals with computer commands, functions, or features.

> Items in the Junk folder will be deleted after 90 days.

> Enter your search terms and press Go.

> Press Ctrl + Alt + Delete to bring up the Task Manager.

The words *internet* and *web* are not capitalized.
The word *email* takes a lowercase letter unless it is starting a sentence.

> Please submit any corrections via email.

> Email submissions are preferred.

Although email is no longer hyphenated, because it has become a commonly used word, newer compounds that start with "e-" retain the hyphen. In such words, the "e" is considered a prefix, and only the noun should be capitalized in a heading or at the start of a sentence.

> e-Commerce tracking is available for both web and app properties but first must be enabled at the view level.

> Estonia is aiming to become a global e-commerce superpower.

> e-Cigarettes and Future Battles in the Fight Against Smoking

> Minnesota health officials are planning to release results of the state's first-ever survey on the use of e-cigarettes.

**10.8** **URLs.** Website addresses (uniform resource locators [URLs]) are not case sensitive. As long as the underlying URL is valid, anyone clicking the link will be taken to the web page to which it points. However, there are times when a writer or publisher wishes to "expose" a URL in text. In that instance, URLs are normally presented as all lowercase.

https://www.ncbi.nlm.nih.gov/pubmed/

https://jamanetwork.com/journals/jamacardiology

https://www.amamanualofstyle.com/

This is true even when the URL contains an acronym that is normally capitalized.

The SEER database represents roughly 30% of the US population and uses data from 18 population-based registered cancer institutes (https://seer.cancer.gov).

Certain exceptions may apply when referring to websites by their name, rather than using the entire URL. For instance, the ClinicalTrials.gov website should be presented as shown, to help distinguish it from the journal *Clinical Trials* and because that presentation is a long-standing component of the trial registry's identity.

**10.9**    **Intercapped Compounds.** *Intercapped compounds* are words that contain capital letters within them. Proprietary and brand names with such intercapitalization should retain their spelling and format.

He sells antiques on eBay.

Figures should not be submitted as PowerPoint slides.

The official iMessage deregistration website lets you enter your telephone number, even if you no longer have an iPhone handy.

This type of article is not indexed in PubMed.

Avoid starting a sentence with one of these trade names if it begins with a lowercase letter. It is almost always preferable to reword the sentence so that it begins with a word that takes an initial capital letter, while retaining the preferred spelling of the trade name.

**Principal Author:** Brenda Gregoline, ELS

# 11.0 Correct and Preferred Usage

## 11.0 Correct and Preferred Usage.

> *Style, not least, adds beauty to the world. To a literate reader, a crisp sentence, an arresting metaphor, a witty aside, an elegant turn of phrase are among life's greatest pleasures. . . . [T]his thoroughly impractical virtue of good writing is where the practical effort of mastering good writing must begin.*
> Steven Pinker[1]

## 11.1 Correct and Preferred Usage of Common Words and Phrases.

Following simple rules for correct and preferred usage of common words and phrases is important in scientific communication because it increases clarity, provides consistency, and helps avoid miscommunication.

Note: All terms (and pairs of terms) are in alphabetical (not preferential) order.

**ability, capability, capacity**—These near-synonyms have slightly different meanings. *Ability* means an actual (as opposed to potential) skill, either mental or physical; it may be native or acquired. *Capability* is a unique fitness for a defined end; the word is sometimes used in place of *ability*, but its use in place of *capacity* is rarely correct. *Capacity* is the potential to exercise or develop a skill, usually mental; it is native as opposed to acquired.

> The ability to select candidates who will thrive and successfully complete a residency is especially critical for general surgery programs.

> The capacity of the patient to make medical decisions should be evaluated within the context of specific medical conditions.

In this study of the association between walking and future risk of dementia, findings are based on a sample of physically capable elderly men.

**abnormal, normal; negative, positive**—Examinations and laboratory tests and studies are not in themselves abnormal, normal, negative, or positive. These adjectives apply to observations, results, or findings (see 19.0, Study Design and Statistics). Avoid the use of *normal* and *abnormal* to describe persons' health status. Results of cultures and tests for specific reactions or microorganisms may be negative or positive. Other tests display a pattern of activity rather than a single feature, and in these a range of normal and abnormal results is possible. These tests include electroencephalograms and electrocardiograms and modes of imaging, such as isotopic scans, radiographic studies, and tomograms.

| | |
|---|---|
| *Incorrect:* | The physical examination was normal. |
| *Correct:* | Findings from the physical examination were normal. |
| *Incorrect:* | The throat culture was negative. |
| *Correct:* | The throat culture was negative for β-hemolytic streptococci. |
| *Incorrect:* | The electroencephalogram was positive. |
| *Correct:* | The electroencephalogram showed abnormalities in the temporal regions. |
| *Incorrect:* | Serologic tests for *Treponema pallidum* hemagglutination, which were previously negative, are now positive. |
| *Correct:* | Serologic test results for *Treponema pallidum* hemagglutination, which were previously negative, are now positive. |
| *Also correct:* | Serologic tests for *Treponema pallidum* hemagglutination, the results of which were previously negative, showed a titer of 1:80. |

See 11.10, Laboratory Values.

| | |
|---|---|
| *Exceptions:* | HIV-positive men |
| | seronegative women |
| | node-negative lung tumors |
| | gram-negative sepsis |
| | receptor-positive breast cancer |

**abort, terminate**—*Abort* means to stop a process prematurely. In pregnancy, *abortion* means the premature expulsion—spontaneous or induced—from the uterus of the products of conception. A pregnancy, not a fetus or a woman, may be aborted. The synonym *terminate*—to bring to an ending or a halt—may also be used.

**about, approximately, around**—Although each of these words is used to refer to a value that is estimated and therefore imprecise, whether it is acceptable to use them interchangeably depends in part on context and the level of accuracy being implied. When referring to an inexact value in casual conversation, *around, about*, and *approximately* are all acceptable. When referring to an inexact value in medical or other technical writing, *about* may very occasionally be used if one carefully assesses the context; *approximately* is nearly always the best choice. Also, *an estimated* may be better.

**accident, injury**—According to the National Center for Injury Prevention and Control of the US Centers for Disease Control and Prevention,[2] *accident* should not be used to refer to injuries from any cause. Although *accident* implies a random act that is unpredictable and unavoidable, epidemiologic studies and injury control programs indicate that injuries may be predictable and therefore preventable. The preferred terms refer either to the external cause (eg, injury from falls, injury from motor vehicle crashes, gunshot injury) or to the intentionality (*unintentional injury* for injuries resulting from acts that were not intended to cause harm and *violence* for any act in which harm was intended).[2]

*Accident* (and *accidental*) is considered by the public health community to be imprecise and should therefore be avoided. The injury-causing event can be described as noted above or with other terms, such as *motorcycle crash, shooting, drowning, collision, poisoning, suffocation, fall from stairs, burning, paintball injury.*

Note: Do not change *accident* if it is integral to the terminology being used, for example, an established injury classification system or as established terminology within a specific discipline (eg, Fatality Analysis Reporting System of the US National Highway Traffic Safety Administration, the World Health Organization's *International Classification of Diseases*, cerebrovascular accident).

**acute, chronic**—These terms should be used to describe symptoms, conditions, or diseases; they refer to duration, not severity. Avoid the use of *acute* and *chronic* to describe patients, parts of the body, treatment, or medication.

| | |
|---|---|
| *Avoid:* | chronic dialysis |
| | chronic heroin users |
| | acute administration of epinephrine |
| | chronic diagnosis |
| | chronic care |
| *Preferred:* | long-term dialysis (also maintenance dialysis) |
| | long-term heroin users |
| | immediate administration of epinephrine |
| | long-standing diagnosis of a chronic disease |
| | long-term care (see note below) |
| | chronic obstructive pulmonary disease |
| | acute kidney failure |
| | chronic kidney disease |
| | chronic arthritis |
| *Also:* | acute, severe cystitis |
| | acute, mild pruritus |

*Exception: Acute abdomen* is a specific serious intra-abdominal condition—for example, appendicitis—with pain, tenderness, and muscular rigidity and for which emergency surgery may be indicated.

A note on short- and long-term patient care: According to Kane and Kane,[3] "*acute care hospital* is preferred to *short-term care hospital. Long-term care* has come to include both an acute component (sometimes called *subacute care* or *postacute care*), which effectively provides the care formerly offered in hospitals, and the more traditional chronic component, which includes both medical and social services. As the name implies, subacute care has a shorter time frame and serves patients who are expected to recuperate or die, while the more chronic form provides more sustained supportive services."

**adapt, adopt**—To *adapt* means to modify or adjust to fit a particular circumstance or requirement. To *adopt* means to take by choice into a relationship.

> Despite health being vulnerable to the vagaries of climate, humans have adjusted their behavioral patterns and technologies to adapt to a diverse range of climates.

> Purchasers, plans, practitioners, and organizations that certify or license clinicians or accredit training programs should adopt systems for measuring, monitoring, and improving quality for psychosocial interventions.

**adherence, compliance**—Although these terms are often used as synonyms, there are differences. *Adherence* can be defined as the extent to which a patient's behavior (in terms of, for example, taking medication, following a diet, modifying habits, or attending clinics) coincides with medical or health advice. Use of the term *adherence* is intended to be nonjudgmental, a statement of fact rather than of blame of the prescriber, patient, or treatment.[4] *Noncompliance* has a negative connotation that may indicate a stigmatizing image of rule, enforcement, and control; dominance and submission; and deviance from expected social roles. Whether a patient chooses to adhere to a therapeutic regimen may depend on many aspects of his or her experience with the disease and the medical encounter itself.[5]

> Continued interaction with patients may provide an opportunity to identify barriers to medication adherence as well as a chance to suggest potential strategies to overcome them (eg, use of a pill box or cueing the taking of medications with a routine activity, such as toothbrushing).

*Possible exception:* A patient with a mental illness may be required to *comply* with court-ordered therapy.

**adverse effect, adverse event, adverse reaction, side effect**—*Side effect* is the secondary consequence of implementing an agent (usually a drug). The term is often used incorrectly when *adverse effect, adverse event*, or *adverse reaction* is intended. Because a side effect can be either beneficial or harmful, a specific term should be used.

> A recent study examined the incidence of serious and fatal adverse drug reactions in hospitalized patients.

> The beneficial side effects of aspirin include preventing myocardial infarctions and reducing the severity and damage from thrombotic strokes.

**affect, effect**—*Affect*, as a verb, means to have an influence on. *Effect*, as a verb, means to bring about or to cause. The 2 words cannot be used interchangeably.

> Ingesting massive doses of ascorbic acid may affect his recovery [influence the recovery in some way].

Ingesting massive doses of ascorbic acid may effect his recovery [produce the recovery].

*Affect*, as a noun, refers to immediate expressions of emotion (in contrast to *mood*, which refers to sustained emotional states). *Effect*, as a noun, means result. *Affect* is often used as part of psychiatric diagnostic terminology.

The patient's general lack of affect was considered an effect of recent trauma.

Note: In reports of research, use of the word *effect* should be limited to studies with designs that permit assessment of causal findings (eg, randomized trials, controlled laboratory experiments) and should not be used in reports of observational studies (eg, cohort, cross-sectional, case-control, case series, and meta-analysis) unless related to a statistical measurement such as effect size. See also **association, relationship** and 19.0, Study Design and Statistics.

**age, aged, school-age, school-aged, teenage, teenaged**—The adjectival form *aged*, not the noun *age*, should be used to designate a person's age. Similarly, *school-aged* and *teenaged* are preferred to *school-age* and *teenage*. However, a precise age or age range should be given whenever possible (see 11.7, Age and Sex Referents).

The patient, aged 75 years, had symptoms of mild cognitive impairment.

*Alternative:* The 75-year-old patient had symptoms of mild cognitive impairment.

The US Preventive Services Task Force recommends chlamydia and gonorrhea screening for all sexually active women younger than 25 years (including teenaged girls), even if they are not engaging in high-risk sexual behaviors.

Note: In some expressions regarding age, it is redundant to add *of age* after the number of months or years because it is implied in the adjectives *younger* and *older*.

Influenza vaccination is not recommended for infants younger than 6 months.

See 11.2.1, Redundant Words.

**aggravate, irritate**—When an existing condition is made worse, more serious, or more severe, it is *aggravated* (also *exacerbated*), not *irritated*. *Irritated* indicates reaction, often excessive (eg, inflammation) to a stimulus.

Symptoms of gastroesophageal reflux disease can be aggravated by certain foods, such as chocolate, citrus fruits, spicy and tomato-based foods, caffeine, and alcohol, or by eating just before going to bed.

Wool, chemicals, soaps, and other substances can irritate the skin and cause itching.

**alternate, alternative**—*Alternate* is an adjective, adverb, or verb and *alternative* is usually a noun. *Alternate* means "occurring in turn" and *alternative* means "another possibility."

Medications that interfere with testing should be stopped only if safe alternatives can be substituted.

The drugs should be taken on alternate days.

**although, though**—*Although* and *though* may be considered interchangeable. However, *although* is preferable as a complete conjunction because *though* in this construction is an "abbreviation" and thus may be less appropriate for formal prose. *Though* in the adverbial construction, meaning "however" or "nevertheless," is correct.

> Although the analysis was performed correctly, the terms of the investigation were too narrow to be interesting.

> Squamous cell skin cancer, though common, remains largely unreported and unstudied.

**ambiguous, equivocal**—The 2 words are close in meaning but distinct in usage. *Ambiguous* means able to be understood in more than one way, having more than one possible meaning, or not expressed or clearly understood. *Equivocal* is defined as having 2 or more possible interpretations or not easily explained or understood.

> The student was faulted for her ambiguous answer to a crucial question.

> Further assessment for the presence of human papillomavirus can clarify an equivocal result from Papanicolaou testing.

**among, between**—*Among* usually pertains to general collective relations and always in a group of more than 2. *Between* pertains to the relation or association of 1 item and 1 other item. For instance, a treaty may be made *between* 4 countries because each is defining a relationship with each of the others, but peace may exist *among* them.

> The patients shared the library books among themselves.

> Between the two of us, we are certain to find the common factor among the patients we have examined.

**analog, analogue**—Use *analog* when referring to items related to computers or electronic equipment. Use *analogue* when "something similar to something else" is meant or when referring to chemical compounds. Use *visual analog scale* (not *visual analogue scale*).

**apt, liable, likely**—*Apt* connotes a volition or habitual tendency and should not be used in regard to an inanimate object. *Apt* also means suited to a purpose. *Liable* connotes the possibility of risk or disadvantage. *Likely* merely implies probability and thus is more inclusive than *apt*.

> A child is apt to cry when frustrated.

> Patients receiving immunosuppressant drugs are liable to acquire fungal infections.

> The computer system is likely to crash if it is overloaded.

**article, manuscript, paper**—An unpublished study, report, or essay—that is, the document itself—may be referred to as a *manuscript* or *paper*. When published, it is an *article*.

> The authors thank Frank J. Kobler, PhD, for statistical review of the manuscript.

> Nancy MacClean, ELS(D), assisted with manuscript preparation.

The content of this article does not necessarily reflect the views or policies of the US Department of Health and Human Services.

The article by Carrozza and Sillke addresses the therapeutic options for a 69-year-old woman with disease of the left main coronary artery.

**as, because, since**—*As, because*, and *since* can all be used when "for the reason that" is meant. However, in this construction, *as* should be avoided when it could be construed to mean *while*.

| | |
|---|---|
| *Ambiguous:* | She could not answer her page as she was examining a critically ill patient. |
| *Better:* | She could not answer her page, as she was examining a critically ill patient [comma used]. |
| *Preferred:* | She could not answer her page because she was examining a critically ill patient. |

Similarly, *since* should be avoided when it could be construed to mean "from the time of" or "from the time that."

| | |
|---|---|
| *Ambiguous:* | She had not been able to answer her page since she was in the clinic. |
| *Preferred:* | She had not been able to answer her page because she was in the clinic. |

**association, relationship**—*Association* occurs between 2 or more variables in which the independent variable does not necessarily cause the other dependent variable(s). *Relationship* implies cause and effect, and in reports of research, the term should only be used for studies with designs that can demonstrate causality (eg, randomized clinical trials and controlled laboratory experiments) (see 19.5, Glossary of Statistical Terms).

To our knowledge, this is the first cohort study to analyze the association between a patient's expected prognosis and do-not-resuscitate decision-making.

There was an inverse relationship between cholesterol levels and coronary artery disease in the intervention group in this randomized clinical trial.

**assure, ensure, insure**—*Assure* means to provide positive information to a person or persons and implies the removal of doubt and suspense (*assure* the study's participants that their test results will be held in complete confidence). *Ensure* means to make sure or certain (ensure the statistical power of the study). *Insure* means to take precaution beforehand (insure his life).

The insurance company assured the families of workers the provision of adequate funds for a proper burial.

The journal editors can assure readers that research was conducted ethically by mandating that every relevant paper include a statement that an institutional review board reviewed the study protocol.

**because of, caused by, due to, owing to**—*Due to* and *caused by* are adjectival phrases, *owing to* and *because of* adverbial phrases. The use of *due to* in both situations can sometimes alter the meaning of a sentence.

One mechanism is the increase in macular inflammation due to retinal amyloid-β deposition.

*Meaning:* One mechanism is the increase in macular inflammation caused by retinal amyloid-β deposition

*Caused by* could be substituted for *due to*, and the meaning would be retained. *That is* could be inserted before *due to* without changing the meaning of the sentence.

Percentages have been rounded owing to missing data.

*Meaning:* Percentages have been rounded because of missing data.

*Because of* could be substituted for *owing to*, and the meaning would be retained. However, if *that are* is inserted before *owing to*, the meaning of the sentence changes.

*Clue to usage:* The phrase "coughs due to colds" is a good example of correct usage of *due to*. If "because of" sounds right, use it or "owing to." If "caused by" is intended, use it or "due to" (or possibly "attributable to").

**biopsy**—*Biopsy* refers to the removal and examination (usually microscopically) of tissue or cells from the living body. Use of *biopsy* as a verb was previously considered to be incorrect. However, such use has become common and acceptable.

*Acceptable:*   The lung mass was biopsied.

A biopsy of the lung mass was performed.

Lesions believed to be malignant were biopsied.

Observations are made of the biopsy specimen, not on the biopsy itself.

*Incorrect:*   Biopsy was normal.

*Correct:*   The results of the biopsy were normal.

The utility of standard biopsy in addition to targeted biopsy for prostate cancer was found to be limited.

Millions of breast biopsies are performed annually.

**blinding, masking**—The statistical term *blinding* (or *blinded review* or *assessment*) is the evaluation or categorization of an outcome in which the person assessing the outcome is unaware of the treatment assignment; blinding is used to avoid bias. The term is also used to refer to peer review, for example, single-blind review, where the reviewer can see the author's name and affiliation on the paper but the reviewer's identity is concealed, or double-blind review, where both reviewer and author identities are concealed. The equivalent term *masking* (or *masked review* or *assessment*) is preferred by some investigators and journals, particularly those in ophthalmology (see 5.7.1, Confidentiality During Editorial Evaluation and Peer Review and After Publication, and 19.5, Glossary of Statistical Terms).

**breastfeed, nurse**—When referring to human lactation, use *breastfeeding* (*breastfeed, breastfed*). This term is more specific than *nursing* and prevents any confusion with the profession of nursing.

**cadaver, donor**—When describing the source of human organs and tissues used for transplant, avoid *cadaver* (or *dead body*). Correct usage is *deceased donor* (or *recovered from deceased organ and tissue donors*). When referring to a deceased person whose body is to be used for anatomical dissection, *cadaver* is correct (*cadaveric* as an adjective).

**can, may, will**—Bernstein,[6] in his classic *The Careful Writer*, perhaps said it best: "Whatever the interchangeability of these words in spoken or informal English, the writer who is attentive to the proprieties will preserve the traditional distinction: *can* for ability or power to do something, *may* for permission to do it." When summing up findings, *will* is used to express futurity or inevitability; *may* suggests the possibility to do something.

> Use of the most common antibiotics in early life may increase the risk of autoimmunity in children at increased genetic risk.

> Use of the most common antibiotics in early life will increase the risk of autoimmunity in children at increased genetic risk.

> Improved air quality can promote molecular longevity from birth onward.

> Improved air quality will promote molecular longevity from birth onward.

**case, client, consumer, participant, patient, subject**—In biological research, a *case* is a particular instance of a disease. A *patient* is a particular person under medical care. A research *participant* (preferred to *subject*; see below) is a person with a particular characteristic or behavior or a person who undergoes an intervention as part of a scientific investigation. A control *participant* is a person who does not have at least some of the characteristics under study or does not receive the intervention but provides a basis of comparison with the case patient (see 19.0, Study Design and Statistics). In case-control studies, it is appropriate to refer to *cases, patients in the case group*, or *case patients* and *controls, participants in the control group*, or *control patients*.

Some consider *subject* (as in *study subject*) to be impersonal, even derogatory, as if the person in the study were in a subservient role. Similarly, the use of *case* is dehumanizing when referring to a specific person. For example,

> *Avoid:*  A 63-year-old case with type 2 diabetes . . .

> *Preferred:*  A 63-year-old patient with type 2 diabetes . . .

Note: Make the distinction between *person* and *patient*:

> Many persons in the United States have type 2 diabetes [persons with type 2 diabetes regardless of care].

> Many patients in the United States have type 2 diabetes [only persons under medical care].

A *case* is evaluated, documented, and reported. A *patient* is examined, undergoes testing, and is treated. A *research participant* is recruited, selected, sometimes exposed to experimental conditions, and observed. See also *diagnose, evaluate, examine, identify* and *follow, follow up, follow-up, observe.*

Note: In general, patients should not be referred to as *clients* or *consumers.* However, persons enrolled in substance use treatment programs, for example, or persons undergoing treatment at a dialysis center are sometimes referred to as *clients. Client* may also be used by social workers or psychologists and in some research settings where *patient* or *participant* is inappropriate. *Consumer*—one who consumes goods or services—has worked its way into the medical lexicon and may be appropriate in certain discussions. For instance, in the following example, *patient* would not fit the context:

> The internet has become an important mass medium for consumers seeking health information and health care services online.

**case-fatality rate, fatality; morbidity, morbidity rate; mortality, mortality rate—**
*Fatality* is the occurrence of death and *case-fatality rate* is the probability of death among people diagnosed as having a disease. The rate is calculated as the number of deaths during a specific period divided by the number of persons with the disease at the beginning of the period.[7] *Morbidity* is a diseased state, and *morbidity rate* is the frequency with which a disease appears in a population. *Mortality* is the number of deaths in a given time or place, and *mortality rate* is the death rate described by the following equation: [(Number of Deaths During Period) × (Period of Observation)]/ (Number of Individuals Observed)[7] (see 19.5, Glossary of Statistical Terms).

**catatonic, hysterical, manic, psychotic, schizophrenic—**Do not use these terms when referring to patients. It is dehumanizing to refer to a patient as "a schizophrenic." Use "a patient with schizophrenia" (see 11.12.6, Terms for Persons With Diseases, Disorders, or Disabilities).

**cerebrovascular accident, stroke, stroke syndrome—***Cerebrovascular accident* (abbreviated CVA) is an older but acceptable generic term synonymous with *stroke* and *stroke syndrome.* However, when using any of these terms, an author should also specify, if possible, the subtype(s) under discussion (eg, ischemic stroke, hemorrhagic stroke, and/or transient ischemic attack).

**cesarean delivery, cesarean section—**According to the American College of Obstetricians and Gynecologists Publications Department, the preferred terms are *cesarean delivery* or *cesarean birth.* Most etymologists believe that *cesarean* and *section* originated from the Latin verbs that both mean "to cut"; therefore, *cesarean section* is redundant.[8] Do not capitalize *cesarean.*

**chief complaint, chief concern—***Chief complaint* has been traditionally used by physicians when taking a patient's medical history. However, *chief concern* may be a better description because *complaint* may be construed as pejorative and confrontational. Also, patients report symptoms and concerns. Avoid "patient complaint."

**classic, classical—**In most scientific writing, the adjective *classic* generally means authentic, authoritative, or typical (the *classic* symptoms of myocardial infarction include angina, dyspnea, nausea, and diaphoresis). In contrast, *classical* refers to the humanities or the fine or historical arts (the elements of *classical* architecture can be applied in radically different architectural contexts than those for which they were developed).

> Primary liquid dysphasia is a classic symptom suggestive of achalasia.

> Darkening of the iris pigmentation and eyelash hypertrichosis are classic findings associated with the use of a prostaglandin analogue agent.

> The figure represents the aesthetic of the age: clear, beautiful, simple, and clean design, with a background of twirling leaves reminiscent of classical themes.

However, some disciplines (eg, genetics, immunology) use *classical* for specific terms:

> Classical lissencephaly may be caused by sequence variations of genes in chromosome bands 17p13.3 and Xq22.3-q23.

> The classical and alternative pathways of complement components are described in 14.8.3, Nomenclature, Complement.

> The authors suggest how to present results of data analysis under each of 3 statistical paradigms: classical frequentist, information-theoretic, and bayesian.

**clinician, practitioner**—Depending on context, these terms can be used to describe persons in the clinical practice of the health fields of medicine, nursing, psychology, dentistry, optometry, and podiatry, as distinguished from those specializing in laboratory science, research, policy, or theory, for example. When referring to a particular type of clinician or practitioner, it is preferable to use the more descriptive term (eg, physician, nurse, dentist, optometrist, podiatrist). The plural forms *clinicians* and *practitioners* may be appropriate to refer to a group of such professionals from different fields. Avoid use of the nonspecific term *provider.* See also *provider.*

**compare to, compare with**—One thing or person is usually compared *with* another when the aim is to examine similarities or differences in detail. An entity is compared *to* another when a single striking similarity (or dissimilarity) is observed or when a thing of one class is likened to one of another class, without analysis (ie, one entity is comparable to another).

> Patients in both active treatment groups had greater improvements from baseline in psychosocial functioning compared with patients receiving only routine medical care.

> Few medical discoveries can compare to the discovery of penicillin.

**compose, comprise**—*Comprise* means to be composed of or to include; it takes the active voice, whereas *compose* takes the passive voice. The whole is composed of its parts and comprises its parts.

> The chemotherapeutic regimen is composed of several toxic ingredients.

> The chemotherapeutic regimen comprises several toxic ingredients.

*Clue to usage:* Never use *of* with *comprise*.

A good alternative for *comprise* is to use "consist of" or "include."

**condition, disease, disorder**—Although these terms are frequently used interchangeably, differences between them exist and can assist in using them in more specific senses. *Condition* is perhaps the least specific, often denoting states of health considered normal or healthy but nevertheless posing implications for health care (eg, pregnancy). The term might also be used to indicate grades of health (eg, a patient might be described as in stable, serious, or critical condition). *Condition* indicates a state of health, whether well or ill. A condition conferring illness might further be classified as a disease or disorder; however, *condition* might be used in place of *disease* or *disorder* when a non–disease-specific term is indicated.

*Disease* is often used in a general sense when referring to conditions that affect a physical system (eg, cardiovascular disease) or a part of the body (eg, diseases of the eye). The term also may be used in specific senses; for example, a writer might refer in general terms to neurologic disease or cognitive impairment or in more specific terms to Alzheimer disease or dementia with Lewy bodies.

*Disorder*, in contrast, denotes a condition characterized by functional impairment without structural change. Although certain disorders or categories of disorders might be accompanied by specific signs and symptoms, their presence is not required for a condition to be termed a *disorder*.

**continual, continuous**—*Continual* means to recur at regular and frequent intervals. *Continuous* means to go on without pause or interruption.

> The patient with emphysema coughed continually.

> His labored breathing was eased by a continuous flow of oxygen through a nasal cannula.

**contrast, contrast agent, contrast material, contrast medium**—Distinguish between *contrast* (ie, blackness and whiteness on an image) and *contrast material* (or *contrast agent, contrast medium*) (ie, a compound administered to enhance portions of the anatomy on an image).

**criterion standard, gold standard**—*Criterion standard* is a test considered to be the diagnostic standard for a particular disease or condition, used as a basis of comparison for other (usually noninvasive) tests. A commonly used synonym, *gold standard*, is considered jargon by some in the methodological literature but not in the medical literature[9] (see 19.5, Glossary of Statistical Terms).

**diabetes**—The types of diabetes currently recognized by the American Diabetes Association are as follows:

| *Older Terms* | *Preferred Terms* |
| --- | --- |
| juvenile diabetes, juvenile-onset diabetes, or insulin-dependent diabetes | type 1 diabetes |
| maturity-onset diabetes, adult-onset diabetes, or non–insulin-dependent diabetes | type 2 diabetes |

*Prediabetes* refers to blood glucose levels that are higher than normal but not yet high enough to be diagnosed as diabetes. The term *prediabetes* is sometimes referred to as impaired glucose tolerance or impaired fasting glucose, depending on what test was used when it was detected.[10]

"Mellitus" need not be specified when referring to diabetes, even at first mention; the term *mellitus* has etymologic significance (and there are other, rarer, types of diabetes, such as insipidus), but mellitus need not be added.

| | |
|---|---|
| *Avoid*: chemical diabetes, borderline diabetes, or latent diabetes | *Preferred*: impaired glucose tolerance (nondiagnostic fasting blood glucose level, glucose tolerance abnormal) gestational diabetes |

For other specific types of diabetes, consult *Diabetes Care*.[11]

**diagnose, evaluate, examine, identify**—*Diagnose, evaluate*, and *identify* apply to conditions, syndromes, and diseases. Patients are *examined*. Patients may be *evaluated* for the possibility of a condition (eg, The patient was evaluated for possible cardiac disease). Although *diagnose* was formerly avoided when referring to a patient, it is now acceptable to say a patient "was diagnosed." See also **case, client, consumer, participant, patient, subject** and **management, treatment**.

The patient was diagnosed as having schizophrenia.

The patient was diagnosed with schizophrenia.

**die from, die of**—Persons die *of*, not *from*, specific diseases or disorders.

The patient died of complications of disseminated intravascular coagulation.

**dilate, dilation, dilatation**—According to the American College of Obstetricians and Gynecologists, *dilate* is a verb meaning to expand or open. *Dilation* means the act of dilating. *Dilatation* means the condition of being stretched or expanded.[8]

The patient's cervix dilated during a period of 12 hours.

The patient was treated with dilation and curettage.

After 4 hours of labor, cervical dilatation was 3 cm.

**disc, disk**—For ophthalmologic terms, use *disc* (eg, optic disc); for other anatomical terms, use *disk* (eg, lumbar disk).

**discomfit, discomfort, disconcert**—These words are commonly confused, perhaps because they begin with the same 5 letters and sound similar.

*Discomfit*, although occasionally still used in the sense of "to frustrate or thwart," is currently most often used to indicate mental, rather than physical, states, specifically in the sense of one's being perplexed or embarrassed (ie, *disconcerted*). *Discomfort* is most often used to indicate one's feeling physically or emotionally uncomfortable, resulting from the efforts of others, from personal excess, or from a condition or disease state. *Disconcert*, indicating perplexity or disturbed composure, is still occasionally used as a verb but currently is used much more frequently as an adjective.

The medical student felt discomfited by her palpable grief at the loss of a patient.

The excitement produced by the first meal since bariatric surgery may be followed by a feeling of abdominal discomfort.

I found the discussion to be premature and very disconcerting.

**discreet, discrete**—*Discreet* is defined as careful and circumspect in one's speech or actions, especially to avoid causing offense or to gain an advantage (ie, intentionally unobtrusive). *Discrete* means individually separate and distinct.

Working with sensitive patient information, physicians and other medical staff must be discreet.

Although the lesions are usually discrete, they can appear grouped and only rarely do they coalesce.

**disinterested, uninterested**—Although these 2 words are increasingly treated as synonyms in written and spoken language, their differences in meaning are sufficiently useful to be worth preserving. To be *disinterested* is to be unbiased or impartial and free from selfish motives; to be *uninterested* is to be unconcerned, indifferent, inattentive, or unbiased. A disinterested judge is admirable; an uninterested judge is not. As with many "word pairs," context is key:

She was uninterested in a career in basic research.

He was a disinterested observer of the complex procedure.

**doctor, physician**—*Doctor* is a more general term than *physician* because it includes persons who hold such degrees as PhD, DDS, EdD, DVM, and PharmD. Thus, the term *physician* should be used when referring specifically to a doctor of medicine, such as a person with an MD, MBBS, or a DO or equivalent degree. See also **clinician, practitioner** and **provider**, and 11.5, Jargon.

**dosage, dose**—A *dose* is the quantity to be administered at one time or the total quantity administered during a specified period. *Dosage* implies a regimen; it is the regulated administration of individual doses and is usually expressed as a quantity per unit of time.

The usual initial dosage of furosemide for adult hypertension is 80 mg/d, typically divided into doses of 40 mg twice a day. Dosage should then be adjusted according to the patient's response.

**effective, effectiveness; efficacious, efficacy**—*Efficacy* and *efficacious*, used especially in pharmacology and decision analysis, have to do with the ability of a medication or intervention (procedure, regimen, service) to produce the desired or intended effect under *ideal* conditions of use. The determination of efficacy is generally based on the results of a randomized clinical trial.

*Effective* and *effectiveness*, however, describe a measure of the extent to which an intervention produces the effect in *average* or *routine* conditions of use; a measure of the extent to which an intervention fulfills its objectives.

Few safe, effective weight-management drugs are currently available.

The researchers investigated the safety and efficacy of liraglutide vs placebo for weight management in adults with overweight or obesity and type 2 diabetes.

*Cost-effectiveness analysis* is the comparison of strategies to determine which provides the most clinical value for the cost.[12] *Comparative effectiveness research* is the conduct and synthesis of systematic research comparing different interventions and strategies to prevent, diagnose, treat, and monitor health conditions. The purpose of this research is to inform patients, health care professionals, and decision makers about which interventions are most effective for which patients under specific circumstances[13] (see 19.5, Glossary of Statistical Terms).

**eg, ie**—*eg* comes from the Latin *exempli gratia*: "for example" and *ie* comes from *id est*: "that is." Both should be followed by a comma.

> In this study, the general module of messages included information generally provided by secondary prevention programs, eg, on chest pain action plans, guidelines and risk factor targets, and medications and adherence.

> With 95% power and a 2-sided significance level of 5%, the study had statistical power to detect a significant odds ratio of 0.76 (ie, a 24% reduced risk) for individuals in the highest quartile of intake.

**elicit, illicit, solicit**—These words have distinctly different denotations, yet they are often confused or misused. In medical and scientific contexts, it is especially important to preserve the distinctions between them.

*Illicit*, denoting simply not permitted or unlawful (and sometimes used colloquially to indicate naughty, unseemly, or immoral), has limited use in medical writing. For example, written materials might convey the risks associated with the use of illicit drugs, discuss illicit relationships between researchers and industry, or report on the illicit trade in human body parts. Beyond such instances, the word is not often used in medical literature.

*Elicit*, however, means to call forth or draw out (as information or a response) or to draw forth or bring out (something latent or potential). The word occurs frequently in medical contexts. It might be used in both senses regarding a patient-physician encounter. For example, a physician evaluating a patient's pain will ask questions to elicit information about the characteristics of the pain (eg, location, nature, duration, exacerbating factors, severity). Having thus elicited information about a patient's pain, the physician then tries to elicit the real concern. In materials that cover the basic sciences and their clinical applications, *elicit* is perhaps most frequently used in the second sense. A writer might report that a new vaccine elicits a given immune response, describe pathological mechanisms that elicit organ damage, or present a theory of how a treatment might elicit changes in gene expression.

*Illicit* and *elicit* are easily distinguished from each other; *illicit* is always an adjective, whereas *elicit*—in current usage—is always a verb. It also can help to remember that *illicit* denotes illegal.

*Solicit* is most frequently used in medical contexts in the sense of to approach with a request or a plea. It is often used interchangeably with *elicit*. However, such use obscures an important distinction. The *Oxford Dictionary of American Usage and Style* states, "To solicit a response is to request it. To elicit a response is to get it."[14] Thus, the physician solicits information regarding the patient's pain and then performs a physical examination to elicit and evaluate actual pain. In medical contexts, the distinction has obvious implications for reports of survey studies and possibly for discussion of power calculations in reports of clinical trials.

**endemic, epidemic, hyperendemic, pandemic**—*Endemic* conditions or diseases are prevalent in a particular place or among a particular group. *Epidemic* conditions occur abruptly in a defined area and are (usually) temporary. A *hyperendemic* condition is one that has a high prevalence. A *pandemic* condition occurs abruptly throughout a wide geographic area, even worldwide, and is (usually) temporary.

> Cowpox is an orthopoxvirus infection endemic in European wild rodents but with a wide host range, including human beings.

> The Ebola epidemic sparked a much-needed course correction that favored strong health infrastructure.

> The researchers used remote sensing and geographic information system technology to identify individual high-risk residences in Westchester County, New York, where Lyme disease has been hyperendemic since 1982.

> Internationally, between 50 million and 100 million people died in the 1918-1919 influenza pandemic.

**erectile dysfunction, impotence**—*Erectile dysfunction* is the inability to develop and maintain an erection for satisfactory sexual intercourse or activity (in the absence of an ejaculatory disorder). *Erectile dysfunction* is the preferred term rather than the more commonly used term *impotence*.

**etc**—Use *etc* (or *and so on* or *and the like*) with discretion. Such terms are often superfluous and are used simply to extend a list of examples. When, in other instances, omission would be detrimental, substitute more specific phrasing, such as *and other methods* or *and other factors*. *Etc* may be used in a noninclusive listing when a complete list would be unwieldy *and* its content is obvious to the reader. The term is best avoided in scientific reports.

*Etc* is not followed by a period except when it is at the end of a sentence.

> Gelatin is made from animal ligaments, tendons, bones, etc, that have been boiled in water. Gelatin is often used in confectionery, ice cream, and other dairy products.

**fasted, fasting**—These terms are derivative forms (adjective and participle) of the noun and verb *fast* that are often used in the scientific literature.

| | |
|---|---|
| in the fasted and fed states | related to age, sex, oxygen deficiency, and short-term fasting |
| in the fasting and feeding conditions | |
| | effects of fasting and sex |
| in fasted rats | tests were performed with the patient in the fasting state |
| in the fasting mouse | |
| | patients had been fasting overnight |

**fellow, intern, internist, resident**—*Fellows* have completed their residency and can elect to complete further training in a specialty. *Interns* have graduated medical school and are in the first year of post–medical school training. Interns can only practice medicine within their training program. *Internists* are physicians specializing in internal medicine. *Residents* have completed their intern year and are still in training.

**fever, temperature**—*Fever* is a condition in which body temperature rises above that defined as normal. It is incorrect to say a person has a temperature if "fever" is intended. Everyone has a temperature, either normal or abnormal.

> *Incorrect:*   The patient has a fever of 39.5 °C.
>
> *Correct:*    The patient has a fever (temperature, 39.5 °C).
>
> *Correct:*    The patient is febrile (temperature, 39.5 °C).
>
> *Correct:*    The patient has an elevated temperature (39.5 °C).

**fewer, less**—*Fewer* and *less* are not interchangeable. Use *fewer* for number (individual persons or things that are countable) and *less* for volume, mass, and percentage/proportion (indicating degree or value).

> Fewer interventions may not always mean less care.

> The report suggests that fewer women are receiving screening mammograms.

Note: We spent less than $1000 (*not:* We spent fewer than $1000).

> There was less than 30% difference in outcomes.

> The outcome of interest occurred in less than 30% of the patients.

> They reported fewer data (*not:* They reported less data).

**follow, follow up, follow-up, observe**—Cases are *followed.* Patients are not *followed* but *observed.* However, either cases or patients may be *followed up* (eg, the maintenance of contact with or reexamination of a person or patient, especially after treatment). Their clinical course may be *followed.*

In a study, case or control participants may be *lost to follow-up* (eg, the investigators were unable to locate them to complete documentation on participants in the initial study groups) or *unavailable for follow-up* (eg, they could not be contacted or the investigators were unable to persuade them to complete the study).

> Patients with retained intracranial fragments have been followed up, and the sequelae of such fragments were analyzed. To date, 9 patients have been lost to follow-up.

**foreign-born**—This term may be considered derogatory and should not be used. It is preferable to say that a person was born outside the country of interest. For example, use non–US born or non–Canadian born.

> The best approach to testing among non–US-born residents is uncertain.

> We estimated the cost-effectiveness of testing and treatment for latent tuberculosis infection in residents born outside Canada.

**gender, sex**—*Sex* is defined as the classification of living things as male or female and is a "biological component, defined via the genetic complement of chromosomes, including cellular and molecular differences."[15]

*Gender* comprises "social, environmental, cultural, and behavioral factors and choices that influence a person's self-identity and health."[9] The term *gender* "includes gender identity (how individuals and groups perceive and present themselves), gender norms (unspoken rules in the family, workplace, institutional, or global culture that influence individual attitudes and behaviors), and gender relations (the relations between individuals of different gender identities)."[15]

The terms should not be used interchangeably. In reports of research, if demographic information about human participants is included, the term used should be indicated and defined and the method used to assess sex or gender should be described (eg, self-report, investigator observed, metadata in a database). In many instances, authors of articles in biomedical publications use the term *gender* when they intend the word *sex*. As noted by Clayton and Tannenbaum, "[W]hen sex is based on self-report, it will be incorrect in a very small percentage of individuals because some individuals will not be 46XX or 46XY. However, in most research studies, it is not possible to conduct detailed genetic evaluation to determine the genetic make-up of all participants."[15]

> A sex ratio of 1.06:1, the ratio of male to female births, has declined in the past decades.

> Many studies indicate that women are less likely than men to undergo cardiac procedures after an acute myocardial infarction, raising concerns of sexual bias in clinical care. However, no data exist about the relationship among patient sex, physician sex, and use of cardiac procedures.

> Responses to pain and pain therapies differ between men and women. Whether this difference is related to sex-based factors (physiological), gender-based factors (psychosocial), or both has not been determined.

> The survey of bias in the workplace asked women and men to self-report their gender.

*Transgender* means of, relating to, or being a person whose gender identity differs from the sex the person had or was identified as having at birth. *Cisgender* means of, relating to, or being a person whose gender identity corresponds with the sex the person had or was identified as having at birth.

Avoid using any *trans* term as a noun; the adjectival form is preferred (not *transman* or *transwoman* but *transgender man* and *transgender woman*).

> Surgeons are seeing an increase in consultations for surgical therapy to help transgender and gender-nonconforming individuals.

> The study examined the health status of gender minorities in the United States compared with cisgender peers.

See 11.7, Age and Sex Referents, the GLAAD Media Reference Guide-Transgender Issues website,[16] and the Gender Equity Resource Center website.[17]

**global, international**—*Global* relates to or involves the entire world; an equivalent term is *worldwide* (a global system of communication, global climate change, global health security).

> Spread of infection with Zika virus among pregnant women has become a global public health concern.

*International* affects 2 or more nations (international trade, international movement, international consortium).

> Researchers conducted an international survey, with respondents selected from Australia, China, France, the United Kingdom, and the United States.

*But:* global amnesia, global aphasia, global ischemia, global cognitive function, global pain relief, Global Assessment of Functioning Scale

**health care**—Express this term as 2 words. It is not necessary to hyphenate *health care* in its adjectival form (see 8.3, Punctuation, Hyphens and Dashes).

| | |
|---|---|
| health care professionals | health care organizations |
| health care system | health care reform |
| health care policy | health care insurance |

**historic, historical**—Although their meanings overlap and they are often used interchangeably, *historic* and *historical* have different usages. *Historic* means important or influential in history (a *historic* discovery). *Historical* is concerned with the events in history (a *historical* novel).

> This historical novel has had a historic impact.

> This article considers the historical effect of Medicare and Medicaid on mental health services and discusses this history as a basis for appraising the legislation now before the US Congress.

Note: The aspirant "h" in both *historic* and *historical* is not silent (see 7.3.2, Indefinite Articles, and 11.11, Articles).

**-ic, -ical**—*Merriam-Webster's Collegiate, Stedman's, Dorland's,* and *American Heritage* dictionaries are resources for determining the appropriate suffix for adjectives. In some cases, the "-ical" form is more remote from the word root and may have a meaning beyond that of the "-ic" form. Although, for example, "anatomic" may be used in the same sense as "anatomical," the latter is preferred as the adjectival form. The important guideline is that the use of terms must be consistent throughout an article or chapter, and preferably throughout the entire publication. Usually the "-al" may be omitted unless its absence changes the meaning of the word. Examples of such differences in meaning include

| | |
|---|---|
| biologic | biological |
| classic | classical |
| economic | economical |
| empiric | empirical |
| historic | historical |
| pathologic | pathological |
| periodic | periodical |
| physiologic | physiological. |

**immunize, inoculate, vaccinate**—*Immunize* means to induce or provide immunity by giving a vaccine, toxoids, or preformed antibodies. *Inoculate* means to introduce a serum, a vaccine, or an antigenic substance. *Vaccinate* refers to the act of administering a vaccine.

> To immunize the newborn of an HBsAg-positive woman against hepatitis B, the patient should be inoculated with both hepatitis B immunoglobulin and vaccine.

> All participants were inoculated intranasally with influenza A/Texas/36/91(H1N1) virus.

> Ten vaccinia-naive participants were vaccinated with undiluted smallpox vaccine.

> The World Health Organization is partnering with the United Nations Children's Fund to conduct a massive vaccination campaign in 7 countries to inoculate more than 20 million children against polio and other diseases.

**impaired, intoxicated**—These related terms are used in the United States to define impairment in driving performance attributable to the use of alcohol or drugs. For instance, in some jurisdictions, a blood or breath alcohol (ethanol) concentration of 0.08 g/dL is considered legal evidence of impairment for driving. By extension, some injury prevention researchers have considered this concentration of alcohol to be scientific evidence of impairment in other potentially hazardous activities. However, cognitive and other functions may be impaired at even lower concentrations of alcohol, particularly if other psychoactive drugs, including prescription drugs, have been taken. No specific blood or breath concentration of alcohol may be considered to be scientific evidence of intoxication or impairment for all persons in all settings and activities. Authors should explain, justify, and define the use of these terms, preferably in the Methods section of the manuscript.

**imply, infer**—To *imply* is to suggest or to indicate or express indirectly. To *infer* is to conclude or to draw conclusions from facts, statements, or indications.

> These results, though cross-sectional, imply that physical fitness is related to fewer coronary risk factors.

> Our study relied on cross-sectional data, restricting our ability to infer the causal directions underlying the observed associations.

Note: Inference is the process of passing from observations to generalizations, usually with calculated degrees of uncertainty.

> In the presence of missing data, mixed models can provide valid inferences under an assumption that data are missing at random.

See 19.5, Glossary of Statistical Terms (*inference*).

**incidence, prevalence**—*Incidence* refers to the number of new cases of disease among persons at risk that occur over time,[7] as contrasted with *prevalence*, which is the total number of persons with the disease at any given time.
See 19.5, Glossary of Statistical Terms.

**injecting, injection drug user; intravenous**—The terms *injecting drug user* and *injection drug user* are not necessarily the same as *intravenous drug user*. Injecting or injection drug users can inject drugs intravenously, intramuscularly, or subcutaneously. Do not substitute one term for the other. If *intravenous* is used, ascertain that the route of administration is through a vein. If *injecting* or *injection drug user* is used, specify the type of injection (eg, intravenous, intradermal) at first mention, unless all types are meant. If uncertain, query the author.

**in order to**—*In order* can often be removed from the phrase *in order to* without changing its meaning (see 11.2.1, Redundant Words). However, in some cases such a deletion may be awkward or change the meaning.

> *Avoid*: In order to meet the study sample size, participants were recruited from 3 centers.

> *Better*: To meet the study sample size, participants were recruited from 3 centers.

> Our students must have the learning opportunities that they need in order to acquire true understanding. [If "in order to" is removed, the syntax is disrupted ("need to acquire" would seem to apply to "opportunities"). The sentence might be reworded as "to be able to acquire" instead of "in order to acquire."]

**irregardless, regardless**—*Irregardless*—most likely a blend of *irrespective* and *regardless*—is incorrect regardless of usage.

**life expectancy, life span**—*Life expectancy* is the average period that a person may expect to live. *Life span* is the length of time a person lives.

**limited-income, low-income, resource-limited, resource-poor, transitional**—These adjectives are used to describe a nation, region, or group in which most of the population lives on far less money—with far fewer basic public services—than the population in wealthy countries. For the purposes of financing, debt relief, technical assistance and advisory services, and special initiatives, the World Bank also categorizes countries as *heavily indebted poor countries*, *middle-income countries*, *low-income countries under stress*, and *small states*. There is no universal, agreed-on criterion for describing a country in terms of its economic or human "development" and which countries fit these different categories, although there are different reference points, such as a nation's gross domestic product per capita or the limited nation's Human Development Index (HDI) compared with that of other nations.

Choice of an appropriate term will depend on context, and writers should choose respectful terms that reflect a specific country's economic and social situations.

Use of the terms *first world/third world* and *developed/developing* are not recommended as descriptors when comparing countries or regions. The term *third world* is pejorative and archaic. The term *developing* may seem like an acceptable alternative, but it too can be considered pejorative and insensitive to the many complexities of metrics used to measure economic, political, resource, and social factors. Best practice is to avoid such general terms and use specific terms that reflect what is being compared, such as low-income or high-income for an article comparing countries based on measures such as gross national product per capita.

**malignancy, malignant neoplasm, malignant tumor**—When referring to a specific tumor, use *malignant neoplasm* or *malignant tumor* rather than *malignancy*. *Malignancy* refers to the quality of being malignant.

> *Avoid:* Pancreatic cancer is a type of malignancy that eludes early detection.

*Preferred:*  Pancreatic cancer is a type of malignant neoplasm that eludes early detection.

Relatives of patients with carcinoma of unknown primary (CUP) are at increased risk of CUP and several other malignant neoplasms, including lung, pancreatic, and colon cancer.

**management, treatment**—To avoid dehumanizing usage, it is generally preferable to say that cases are *managed* and that patients are *cared for* or *treated*. However, constructions such as "the clinical management of the seriously ill patient" and "the management of patients with HIV infection" are acceptable when used to refer to a general treatment protocol. *Management* is especially applicable when the care of the patient does not involve specific interventions but may include, for example, watchful waiting (eg, for prostate cancer or mitral regurgitation). *Management* may also be used to refer to the monitoring or periodic evaluations of the patient.

**militate, mitigate**—These 2 words are not synonymous. *Militate* means to have weight or effect and is usually used with *against*. *Mitigate* means to moderate, abate, or alleviate.

The constraints of nationalism militate against state conformance with global health norms.

An increasing body of evidence presents the possibility of developing drugs to mitigate cognitive decline.

This review considered evidence related to mitigation of risk in the use of opioids for chronic pain.

**multivariable, multivariate; univariable, univariate**—*Multivariable* means many variables and refers to any statistical test that deals with 1 dependent variable and at least 2 independent variables. It may include nominal or continuous variables, but ordinal data must be converted to a nominal scale for analysis. *Multivariate analysis* is similar to multivariable analysis except that there is more than 1 dependent variable. The term *multivariate* is frequently incorrectly used in the scientific literature when multivariable analysis is meant. *Univariable analysis* refers to statistical tests involving only 1 dependent variable and no independent variables or may also apply to an analysis in which there are no independent variables. For *univariate*, the suffix "-ate" means to act on. Because no variable is acted on in a univariable analysis, *univariable* is a more appropriate term than *univariate* when there is only a single variable involved.

See 19.0, Study Design and Statistics.

**nauseous, nauseated**—These terms are often used interchangeably to mean feeling unwell, but they have distinctly different meanings. *Nauseous* refers to causing an illness or disgust, and *nauseated* refers to feeling ill or disgust.

The nauseous smell sickened several people in its vicinity.

The patient was nauseated after taking aspirin.

**-ology**—This suffix, derived from the Greek *logos*, meaning "word," "idea," or "thought," denotes *science of* or *study of*. Many terms with this suffix, like *morphology, histology, etiology,* and *symptomatology,* are general and abstract nouns and should not be used to describe individual and particular items. *Pathology* is an exception and can be used.

> *Avoid:*      Tumor registry data were supplemented by hospital record and histology in men aged 55 to 74 years with clinically localized prostate cancer.
>
> *Preferred:*      Tumor registry data were supplemented by hospital record and histologic examination findings in men aged 55 to 74 years with clinically localized prostate cancer.
>
> *Avoid:*      The buildup of infectious debris behind the tympanic membrane, along with inflammatory mediators, produces the symptomatology and signs of acute otitis media.
>
> *Preferred:*      The buildup of infectious debris behind the tympanic membrane, along with inflammatory mediators, produces the symptoms and signs of acute otitis media.

**on, upon**—In scientific articles, *upon* often simply means *on*, which is the preferred term.

**operate, operate on**—Surgeons *operate on* a patient or *perform an operation on* a patient. Similarly, patients are not *operated* but are *operated on*.

> *Incorrect:*      The operated group recovered quickly.
>
> *Correct:*      The surgical group recovered quickly.
>
> *Also correct:*      The group that underwent surgery recovered quickly.

**operation, surgical procedure, surgeries, surgery**—*Surgery* can mean surgical care, surgical treatment, or surgical therapy (ie, the care provided by a surgeon with the help of nurses and other personnel from the first consultation and examination, through the hospital stay, operation, and postoperative care, until the last follow-up visit is complete).

An *operation* is performed on a living body to repair damage or a defect or restore health; it is the *surgical procedure.*

*Surgery* is what a surgeon practices or a particular medical specialty. An *operation* is what a surgeon performs. In this context, there is no such word as *surgeries*. In the United Kingdom, *surgeries* are treatment rooms.[18]

**ophthalmologist, optician, optometrist**—*Ophthalmologists* are specialists in medical and surgical eye disease. *Opticians* are technical practitioners who design, fit, and dispense corrective lenses. *Optometrists* are health care professionals who provide primary vision care that ranges from sight testing and correction to the diagnosis, treatment, and management of vision changes.

**over, under**—Correct usage of these words depends on context.

> *Time:*      *Over* may mean either *more than* or *for* (*a period of*). In cases in which ambiguity might arise, *over* should be avoided and *more than* used.
>
> *Ambiguous:*      The cases were followed up over 4 years.
>
> *Preferred:*      The cases were followed up for more than 4 years.

| | |
|---|---|
| *Also:* | The cases were followed up for 4 years. |
| *Age:* | When referring to age groups, *over* and *under* should be replaced by the more precise *older than* and *younger than* (see also *age, aged, school-age, school-aged, teenage, teenaged*). |
| *Avoid:* | All participants in the study were over 65 years old. |
| *Preferred:* | All participants in the study were older than 65 years. |

Note: It is unnecessary and redundant to add *of age* after the number of years. When the terms *older* and *younger* are used, age is implied (see 11.2.1, Redundant Words).

**percent, percentage, percentage point, percentile**—See 18.7.2, Numbers and Percentages, Forms of Numbers, Percentages.

**persons, people**—Both terms are acceptable.

**place on, put on**—The phrase "to put [or to place] a patient on a drug" is jargon and should be avoided. Medications are *prescribed* or patients are *given* medications; therapy or therapeutic agents are started, administered, maintained, stopped, or discontinued.

| | |
|---|---|
| *Incorrect:* | If opioids are necessary, patients should be put on the lowest effective dose. |
| *Correct:* | If opioid therapy is necessary, patients should be prescribed the lowest effective dose. |
| *Correct:* | The patient with chronic pain was given the lowest possible dose of hydrocodone. |
| *Correct:* | A combination therapeutic regimen of hydrocodone bitartrate (5 mg) and acetaminophen (325 mg) was begun. |
| *Incorrect:* | The patient with newly diagnosed celiac disease was put on a gluten-free diet. |
| *Correct:* | The patient with newly diagnosed celiac disease was prescribed a gluten-free diet. |

**preventative, preventive**—As adjectives, *preventive* and its derivative *preventative* are equal in meaning. The shorter *preventive* is preferred.

**principal, principle**—These words sound the same but have very different meanings. *Principal* can be a noun or an adjective and has several definitions, including a loan amount that requires repayment, someone who has an important role, or something that is primary or pivotal. *Principle* is always a noun and only refers to a law or rule.

The patient was hospitalized with a principal diagnosis of chest pain.

The principal investigator observed the first 2 interventions.

The physician studied the principles of ethics of the American Medical Association.

**prostitute, sex worker**—Epidemiologic studies use the term *sex worker* (or *commercial sex worker*) to describe these persons of any gender, rather than the more derogatory *prostitute*.

**provider**—The term *provider* can mean a health care professional, a medical institution or organization, or a third-party payer. If the usage refers to 1 specific provider (eg, physician, hospital), use the specific name for that provider (eg, pediatrician, tertiary care hospital, managed care organization), rather than the general term *provider*. If the term connotes several providers, it can be used to avoid repeating lists of persons or institutions; however, the term(s) should always be defined at first mention.

> To protect the public health and safety during recovery operations after a hurricane, the Centers for Disease Control and Prevention has created guidelines of interest to health care providers (trauma surgeons, nurses, and psychologists), relief workers, and shelter operators.

The phrase *nonphysician provider* should be avoided because it is similarly imprecise and can refer to numerous health professionals licensed to provide a health care service. It is better to specify the type of professional (eg, nurse, pharmacist, dentist) or to use *health care professional* or *clinician*. If a phrase is needed to describe repeatedly and succinctly the many health care professionals who are not physicians, then *physician and other health care professionals* may be acceptable as long as the phrase is defined at first mention. This also applies to other professions (eg, avoid use of nonnurses, nonpharmacists, nondentists).

**psychiatrist, psychologist**—*Psychiatrists* are trained physicians who can prescribe medications and focus on medication management as a course of treatment. *Psychologists* cannot write prescriptions and focus on psychotherapy and treating patients with behavioral intervention.

**race, ethnicity**—These terms are not equivalent (see 11.12.3, Race/Ethnicity, for a discussion of usage).

**regime, regimen**—A *regime* is a form of government, a social system, or a period of rule (eg, a military regime). A *regimen* is a systematic schedule (involving, for example, diet, exercise, way of living, physical therapy, or medication) designed to improve or maintain the health of a patient.

> Resistant hypertension is the failure to reach goal blood pressure while adhering to full doses of an appropriate 3-drug regimen that includes a diuretic.

> A retrospective study compared mild-, moderate-, and high-intensity exercise regimens in patients with detectable hepatic fat.

**repeat, repeated**—*Repeat* is a noun or a verb and should not be used in place of the adjective *repeated*. *Repeated* implies repetition. For precision and clarity, the exact number should be given.

| | |
|---|---|
| *Incorrect:* | A repeat electrocardiogram was obtained. |
| *Possible but misleading:* | A repeated electrocardiogram was obtained. |
| *Preferred:* | A second electrocardiogram was obtained. |
| | The electrocardiogram was repeated. |
| | Two successive electrocardiograms showed no abnormalities. |

**respective, respectively**—These words indicate a one-to-one correspondence that may not otherwise be obvious between members of 2 series. When only 1 series, or none at all, is listed, the distinction is meaningless and should not be used.

*Incorrect:*   The 2 patients are 12 and 14 years old, respectively.

*Correct:*    Kate and Jake are 12 and 14 years old, respectively.

*Incorrect:*   The 2 patients' respective ages are 12 and 14 years.

*Correct:*    The 2 patients are 12 and 14 years old.

Low back pain, other muscular disorders, and neck pain rank first, third, and fourth, respectively, among the 30 leading diseases that contribute to years lived with disability in the United States.

**safe injection site, safer injection sites, supervised injection facility or site**—Use *supervised injection facility* or *site*.

**section, slice**—Use *section* to refer to a radiologic image; use *slice* to refer to a slice of tissue (eg, for histologic examination).

*But:* frozen-section biopsy

See also *cesarean delivery, cesarean section*.

**side effect**—See *adverse effect, adverse event, adverse reaction, side effect*.

**signs, symptoms**—*Signs* can be seen and read by other people. *Symptoms* can only be described by the person feeling them.

**substance abuse, substance use**—Never use the term *substance abuse*. Many consider it to be pejorative, but it is a clarity and accuracy issue as well. If what is meant is "use" ("The patient used heroin"), then "use" is sufficient. There is no difference between heroin "use" and heroin "abuse," so "abuse" adds no information. If what is meant is "The patient had depression and substance use disorder" (eg, both are medical illnesses), then saying "The patient had substance abuse" would be unclear and inaccurate (unless specifically referring to meeting the *DSM-IV* substance abuse definition). Use "substance use disorder" to mean uncontrolled use of a substance with recurrent consequences. Use "substance use" to mean the action of taking a substance without any conclusions about whether it has harmed the person or whether they have control over its use ("The patient used marijuana last night"). See 11.12.6, Terms for Persons With Diseases, Disorders, or Disabilities.

**suffer from, suffer with**—See 11.12.6, Terms for Persons With Diseases, Disorders, or Disabilities, for a discussion of usage.

**suggestive of, suspicious of**—To be *suggestive of* is to give a suggestion or to evoke. To be *suspicious of* is to distrust.

*Incorrect:*    The chest film was suspicious for tuberculosis.

*Correct:*     The chest film was suggestive of tuberculosis.

*Also correct:*   The chest film showed abnormalities suggestive of tuberculosis.

**supine, prone**—These terms are antonyms. *Supine* means lying on the back or with the face up. *Prone* means lying on the front of the body facing downward.

The patient was placed in supine position for thoracic surgery.

The patient was placed in a prone position for the spinal surgery.

**survivor, victim, victimization**—In scientific publications, avoid the use of the word *victim* when describing persons who experienced physical, domestic, sexual, or psychological violence, bullying, or a natural disaster. Similarly, avoid labeling (and thus equating) people with a disability or disease as victims (eg, AIDS victim, stroke victim; see 11.12.6, Terms for Persons With Diseases, Disorders, or Disabilities). The term *victimization* should likewise be avoided; instead, a term or phrase that describes the specific exposure should be used (eg, exposure to violence, experienced trauma, bullying, being bullied).

*Victim* may imply a state of helplessness.[19] Characterizing a person who has experienced abuse or other violence as a victim perpetuates the stereotype of a passive person who cannot recover from the experience or trauma. In such cases, *survivor* may be more appropriate (eg, rape survivor, tsunami survivor, survivor of torture).

Survivors of sexual assault often choose not to speak publicly about their experiences.

Refugees who reported experiencing violence had higher rates of anxiety than those who did not report such experience.

Children who were bullied and participated in the group counseling sessions reported lower scores for symptoms of depression compared with those who did not participate in the group counseling.

If a person who experienced such trauma has died, referring to them as a *victim* may be appropriate (victim of a landmine explosion or gunshot wound). *Victim* may also be used in the vernacular (victim of his own success).

**titrate, titration**—In therapeutics, *titrate* and *titration* refer to dosing schedules that start with a small dose and gradually are increased to the recommended or therapeutic dose. Patients are not titrated.

**toxic, toxicity**—*Toxic* means pertaining to or caused by a poison or toxin. Toxicity is the quality, state, or degree of being poisonous. A patient is not toxic. A patient does not have toxicity.

Dactinomycin is a toxic antineoplastic drug of the actinomycin group.

The drug had a toxic effect on the patient.

The patient had a toxic reaction to the drug.

The patient had a toxic appearance.

The toxicity of the drug must be considered.

*But:* toxic shock syndrome, toxic neuropathy, toxic epidermal necrolysis, toxic megacolon

**transplant, transplantation**—*Transplant* is both a noun (typically meaning the surgical operation itself but also increasingly referring to the overall field) and a transitive verb. Use *graft* (or *allograft, autograft, xenograft,* and so on, depending on the level of precision needed) as the general noun for the organ or tissue that is transplanted, or specify which organ or tissue (eg, liver, skin), rather than use the noun *transplant* in this context. *Transplantation* is traditionally the noun used to describe the overall field. Never use the plural *transplantations*.

|            |                                                                                  |
|-----------:|----------------------------------------------------------------------------------|
| *Incorrect:* | The patient was transplanted.                                                    |
|            | The surgeon transplanted the patient.                                            |
|            | The patient underwent a transplantation.                                         |
|            | Fifteen transplantations were performed.                                         |

|            |                                                                                  |
|-----------:|----------------------------------------------------------------------------------|
| *Correct:* | The patient underwent a transplant.                                              |
|            | The patient received a kidney allograft.                                         |
|            | The transplanted intestine functioned well.                                      |
|            | The surgeon transplanted the donor heart into a 4-year-old girl.                 |
|            | Fifteen transplants were performed.                                              |
|            | Dr Jones performed the first successful heart-lung transplant at our center.     |
|            | Cyclosporine has been used as monotherapy in pediatric liver transplantation [also, *transplant*]. |
|            | Islet transplantation [also, *transplant*] is now a clinical reality at our institution. |
|            | The researchers collected transplantation data.                                  |

For the adjectival form, use *transplant*, as well as *pretransplant* and *posttransplant* (not *pretransplantation* and *posttransplantation*).

|            |                                                                                  |
|-----------:|----------------------------------------------------------------------------------|
| *Avoid:* | The transplantation coordinator described the pretransplantation and posttransplantation data from her transplantation program. |
| *Preferred:* | The transplant coordinator described the pretransplant and posttransplant data from her transplant program. |

**ultrasonography, ultrasound**—These terms are not interchangeable. When referring to the imaging procedure, use *ultrasonography*. *Ultrasound* refers to the actual sound waves that penetrate the body during ultrasonography.

**use, usage, utility, utilize**—*Use* is almost always preferable to *utilize*, which has the specific meaning "to find a profitable or practical use for," suggesting the discovery of a new use for something. However, even where this meaning is intended, *use* would be acceptable.

We used correlation and hierarchical linear regression analyses.

Vitamin C helps the body use the iron present in the diet.

Some urban survivors utilized plastic garbage cans as "lifeboats" to escape flooding in the aftermath of Hurricane Katrina.

*Exception: Utilization review* and *utilization rate* are acceptable terms.

*Usage* refers to an acceptable, customary, or habitual practice or procedure, often linguistic in nature. For the broader sense in which there is no reference to a standard of practice, *use* is the correct noun form.

The correct usage of *compose* vs *comprise* was discussed earlier.

The style manual determines what the correct usage should be.

Some authors use the pretentious *usage* where *use* would be appropriate. As a rule of thumb, avoid *utilize* and be wary of *usage*. Use *use*.

Note: *Utility*—meaning fitness for some purpose, or usefulness—should never be changed to the noun *use*. Nor should the verb *employ* be routinely changed to *use*. Use *employ* to mean hire.

**vision, visual acuity**—*Vision* is a general term that describes the overall ability of the eye and brain to perceive the environment. *Visual acuity* is a specific measurement of one aspect of the sensation of vision assessed by an examiner.

A patient describing symptoms of his or her visual sensation would be describing the overall visual performance of the eye(s) and would use the term *vision*: "My vision is improved [or worse]."

A practitioner reporting the examination findings at one specific time would describe *visual acuity* (20/30, 20/15, etc). However, the practitioner might also refer to the general visual function as *vision*: "As the vitreous hemorrhage cleared, the vision improved and visual acuity returned to 20/20." It is possible to have normal visual acuity despite marked vision impairment (eg, when the peripheral visual field is abnormal).

## 11.2    Redundant, Expendable, and Incomparable Words and Phrases.

> *This parrot is no more. It has ceased to be. It's expired and gone to meet its maker. This is a late parrot. It's a stiff. Bereft of life, it rests in peace. If you hadn't nailed it to the perch, it would be pushing up the daisies. It's rung down the curtain and joined the choir invisible. This is an ex-parrot.*
> John Cleese, "Monty Python's Flying Circus"[20]

### 11.2.1    Redundant Words.

A redundancy is a term or phrase that unnecessarily repeats words or meanings. Below are some common redundancies that can usually be avoided (redundant words are *italicized*):

| | |
|---|---|
| *actual* fact | combine *together* |
| adequate *enough* | *completely* full [empty] |
| *added* bonus | consensus *of opinion* |
| *advance* planning | contemporaneous *in age* |
| aggregate *together* | continue *on* |
| *blatantly* obvious | could *potentially* |
| blend *together* | count [divide] *up* |
| brief *in duration* | covered *over* |
| browse *through* | *current* status quo |
| close *proximity* to | distinguishing *the difference* |
| collaborate *together* | each *individual* person |

eliminate *altogether*

empty *out*

end *result*

enter *into* (*exception:* enter into a contract)

*equally* as well as

estimated at *about*

*favorably* disposed

*fellow* colleagues

fewer *in number*

filled *to capacity*

*final* destination

*final* outcome

*first* discovered

*first and* foremost

*first* initiated

*free* gift

fuse *together*

*future* plans

*general* rule

*herein* we describe

*historic* milestone

interact *with each other*

interval *of time*

join *together*

*joint* cooperation

large [small, bulky] *in size*

lift *up*

*major* breakthrough

merge (mix) *together*

moment *in time*

near *to*

old adage

orbit *around*

*outward* appearances

*out* of [eg, 2 *out* of 12, *but:* out of bounds, out of place, out of the question, out of the jurisdiction, out of the woods]

outside *of*

oval [square, round, lenticular] *in shape*

own *personal* view

*past* history (experience)

period *of time, time* period, *point in* time

*personal* friend

pervade *throughout*

plan *ahead*

plan *in advance*

precedes *in time*

predict *in advance*

*prior* experience

reassessed *again*

red *in color*

revert *back*

rough [smooth] *in texture*

*skin* rash

software *programs*

soft [firm] *in consistency*

sour [sweet, bitter] *tasting*

split *up*

similar results were obtained *also* by

*still* continues

sum *total*

tender *to the touch*

*true* fact

*12* noon [midnight]

| | |
|---|---|
| *2* halves | *uniformly* consistent |
| whether *or not* [unless the intent is to give equal emphasis to the alternative] | younger [older] than 50 years *of age* |

**11.2.2** **Expendable Words and Circumlocution.** Some words and phrases can usually be omitted without affecting meaning, and omitting them often improves the readability of a sentence:

| | |
|---|---|
| as already stated | it was demonstrated that |
| in order to | it was found that |
| in other words | needless to say |
| it goes without saying | take steps to |
| it is important [interesting] to note | the fact that |
| it may be said that | the field of |
| it stands to reason that | to be sure |

*Quite, very*, and *rather* are often overused and misused and can be deleted in many instances (see 11.1, Correct and Preferred Usage, Correct and Preferred Usage of Common Words and Phrases).

Avoid roundabout and wordy expressions:

| *Avoid* | *Better* |
|---|---|
| an appreciable number of | many, several |
| an increased [decreased] number of | more [fewer] |
| as the result of | because |
| at this [that] point in time | now [then] |
| carry out | perform, conduct |
| commented to the effect that | said, stated |
| concerning the matter of | about |
| despite the fact that | although |
| draws to a close | ends |
| due to the fact that | because, due to |
| during the time that | while |
| fall off | decline, decrease |
| file a lawsuit against | sue |
| has the opportunity to | can |

| | |
|---|---|
| have an effect [impact] on | affect |
| in a situation in which | if |
| in close proximity to | near |
| in light of the fact that | because |
| in regard to, with regard to | about, regarding |
| in terms of | in, of, for |
| in the event that | if |
| in the vicinity of | near |
| in those areas where | where |
| look after | watch, care for |
| the majority of | most |
| produce an inhibitory effect that | inhibit |
| with the exception of | except |

**11.2.3** **Incomparable Words.** Some words are regarded as "absolute" adjectives, those not possessing a comparative or superlative form (eg, young, younger, youngest or loud, louder, loudest). Words considered incomparable that need no superlative or comparative modifier are listed below:

| | |
|---|---|
| absolute | omnipotent |
| ambiguous | original |
| complete [*but:* almost or nearly complete] | preeminent |
| | perfect [*but:* almost or nearly perfect] |
| comprehensive | |
| entire | preferable |
| equal | pregnant |
| eternal | supreme |
| expert | total |
| fatal [*but:* almost or nearly fatal] | ultimate |
| final | unique |
| full [*but:* half full, nearly full] | unanimous [*but:* almost or nearly unanimous] |
| infinite | |

Note: In general, superlatives should be avoided in scientific writing.

## 11.3     Spelling and Spacing Variations.

**ante mortem/antemortem**—Both forms are used depending on placement before or after the noun. *Ante mortem* means occurring before death and is used after the noun. *Antemortem* means before death and precedes a noun.

> The antemortem injuries were not the cause of death.

> The injuries were discovered ante mortem.

**bloodstream/blood stream**—*Bloodstream* is preferred.

**brainstem/brain stem**—*Brainstem* is preferred.

**caregiver/care giver**—*Caregiver* is preferred.

**caseload/case load**—*Caseload* is preferred.

**dataset/data set**—*Data set* is preferred.

**email/e-mail**—*Email (email)* is preferred.

**end point/endpoint**—*End point* is preferred

**fiberoptic(s)/fiber optic(s)**—*Fiberoptic(s)* is preferred.

**flowchart/flow chart**—*Flowchart* is preferred but use *flow diagram* over *flowdiagram*.

**gallbladder/gall bladder**—*Gallbladder* is preferred.

**healthcare/health care**—*Health care* is preferred.

**heartbeat/heart beat**—*Heartbeat* is preferred.

**needlestick/needle stick**—*Needlestick* is preferred.

**postmortem/post mortem**—Both forms are used depending on placement before or after the noun. *Postmortem* means after death and precedes a noun. *Post mortem* means occurring or performed after death or pertaining to the period after death and is used after a noun.

> A postmortem clot formed in the heart.

> The clot formed in the heart post mortem.

**postpartum/post partum**—Both forms are used depending on placement before or after the noun. *Postpartum* means after childbirth and precedes a noun. *Post partum* means occurring after childbirth with reference to the mother and is used after a noun.

> The new mother experienced postpartum depression.

> The new mother's depression began post partum.

**radiofrequency/radio frequency**—*Radiofrequency* is preferred.

**radioguided/radio guided**—*Radioguided* is preferred.

**skinfold/skin fold**—*Skinfold* is preferred.

**slitlamp/slit lamp**—*Slitlamp* is preferred.

**waveform/wave form**—*Waveform* is preferred.

**website/Web site**—*web* (lowercase "w") and *website* (1 word, lowercase "w") are preferred, but retain initial caps on the full name the World Wide Web.

**11.4**     **Back-formations.** The transformation of a noun into a verb is a back-formation, often seen in technical as well as informal writing. *Diagnose*, for example, is a mid–19th-century back-formation, from *diagnosis*. Back-formations in use include *dialyze* (from *dialysis*) and *anesthetize* (from anesthesia). A back-formation that is not widely accepted is *diurese* (from *diuresis*). Any use of back-formations should be checked in a dictionary.

| | |
|---|---|
| *Back-formation:* | The patient was diuresed. |
| *Preferred:* | The patient was given diuretics [or underwent diuresis]. |
| *Back-formation* | The individuals were cohortized. |
| *Preferred:* | The individuals were studied as a cohort. |
| *Also correct:* | The researchers used a cohort design. |
| *Back-formation:* | The patient was hysterectomized. |
| *Preferred:* | The patient had [or underwent] a hysterectomy. |

**11.5**     **Jargon.**

> *Many words have found their way into medical vocabularies with unusual meanings that are not recognized even by medical dictionaries. Such writings may be characterized as medical jargon or medical slang. When these words appear in medical manuscripts or in medical conversation, they are unintelligible to other scientists, particularly those of foreign countries; they are not translatable and are the mark of the careless and uncultured person.*
> **Morris Fishbein, MD**[21]

> *Jargon is . . . a language exquisitely precise, using terms in a highly specific sense. It is highly rational, addressed to the intellect and not the emotions; a technical language, intended for a particular group engaged in a particular activity. . . . Jargon has a specificity and precision of meaning, intelligible to a limited group but more or less baffling to other groups.*
> **Lester S. King, MD**[22]

Words and phrases that can be understood in conversation but are vague, confusing, or depersonalizing are generally inappropriate in formal scientific writing (see 7.7, Diction; 11.1, Correct and Preferred Usage of Common Words and Phrases; and 19.5, Glossary of Statistical Terms).

| Jargon | Preferred form |
|---|---|
| 4+ albuminuria | proteinuria (4+) |
| blood sugar | blood glucose |
| chart | medical record |
| chief complaint | chief concern |
| cocktail | mixture |
| congenital heart | congenital heart disease; congenital cardiac anomaly |
| emergency room | emergency department |
| exam | examination |
| flu | influenza |
| gastrointestinal infection | gastrointestinal tract infection *or* infection of the gastrointestinal tract |
| genitourinary infection | genitourinary tract infection *or* infection of the genitourinary tract |
| heart attack | myocardial infarction |
| hyperglycemia of 250 mg/dL | hyperglycemia (blood glucose level of 250 mg/dL) |
| jugular ligation | jugular vein ligation *or* ligation of the jugular vein |
| lab | laboratory |
| left heart failure | left ventricular failure [preferred, but query author]; left-sided heart failure |
| normal range | reference range |
| Pap smear | Papanicolaou test |
| the patient failed treatment | treatment failed |
| preemie | premature infant |
| preop/postop | preoperative/postoperative |
| prepped | prepared |
| psychiatric floor | psychiatric department, service, unit, ward |
| randomized patients | randomly assigned patients |

| respiratory infection | respiratory tract infection *or* infection of the respiratory tract |
| surgeries | operations or surgical procedures |
| symptomatology | symptoms [query author] |
| therapy of [a disease or condition] | therapy for |
| treatment for [a disease or condition] | treatment of |
| urinary infection | urinary tract infection *or* infection of the urinary tract |

The following terms and euphemisms should be changed to preferred forms:

| *Avoid* | *Use* |
| --- | --- |
| expired, passed, passed away, succumbed | died |
| sacrificed | killed; humanely killed; euthanized |

Avoid trivializing or dehumanizing disciplines or specialties. For example:

> *Osteopathic physician* and *osteopathic medicine*, not *osteopath* and *osteopathy*

> *Cardiologic consultant* or *cardiology consultation*, not *cardiology* [for the person]

> *Orthopedic surgeon*, not *orthopod*

Colloquialisms, idioms, and vulgarisms should be avoided in formal scientific writing. Exceptions may be made in editorials and informal articles.

**11.6** **Administration of Drugs.** When describing the administration of drugs, *buccal, cutaneous, dermal, inhalational, intra-articular, intracardiac, intramuscular, intrathecal, intravenous, intraventricular, intravitreal, nasal, ocular, oral, otic, parenteral, rectal, subconjunctival, subcutaneous, sublingual, topical, transdermal,* and *vaginal* are acceptable terms when these are the usual or intended routes of administration. Except for systemic chemotherapy, however, drugs are usually neither systemic nor local but are given for systemic or local effect.

> Some topical corticosteroid ointments produce systemic effects.

> Oral penicillin is often preferred to parenteral penicillin.

> Intravenously injected heroin may be contaminated.

*Exceptions:* Local anesthetics are a class of drug. Techniques for delivering anesthesia are general, local, and regional.

**11.7** **Age and Sex Referents.** Use specific terms to refer to a person's age.
*Neonates* or *newborns* are persons from birth to 1 month of age.

*Infants* are children aged 1 month to 1 year (12 months).

*Children* are persons aged 1 to 12 years. Sometimes, *children* may be used more broadly to encompass persons from birth to 12 years of age. They may also be referred to as *boys* or *girls*.

*Adolescents* are persons aged 13 through 17 years. They may also be referred to as *teenagers* or as *adolescent boys* or *adolescent girls*, depending on context.

*Adults* are persons 18 years or older and should be referred to as *men* or *women*. Persons 18 to 24 years of age may also be referred to as *young adults*.

Note: If the age of an individual patient is given, it may be expressed as a mixed fraction (eg, 6½ years) or as "6 years 6 months." However, when age is presented as a mean, use the decimal form: 6.5 years (see 19.4.1, Study Design and Statistics, Significant Digits and Rounding Numbers, Significant Digits).

Whenever possible, a patient should be referred to as a man, woman, boy, girl, or infant. Occasionally, however, a study group may comprise children and adults of both sexes. Then, the use of *male* and *female* as nouns is appropriate. *Male* and *female* are also appropriate adjectives.

See 11.12.4, Inclusive Language, Age.

**11.8**      **Anatomy.** Authors often err in referring to anatomical regions or structures as the "right heart," "left chest," "left neck," and "right brain." Generally, these terms can be corrected by inserting a phrase such as "part of the" or "side of the."

> right side of the heart, right atrium, right ventricle
>
> left side of the chest, left hemithorax
>
> left aspect of the neck
>
> right hemisphere
>
> ascending [not right] and descending [not left] colon

Where appropriate, use specific anatomical descriptors:

> proximal jejunum, distal esophagus, distal radius, distal ureter, femoral neck

The *upper extremity* comprises the arm (extending from the shoulder to the elbow), the forearm (from the elbow to the wrist), and the hand. The *lower extremity* comprises the thigh (extending from the hip to the knee), the leg (from the knee to the ankle), and the foot. Therefore, references to upper and lower arm and upper and lower leg are often redundant or ambiguous. When such references appear in a manuscript, the author should be queried.

**11.9**      **Clock Referents.** Occasionally, reference to a locus of insertion, position, or attitude is given in terms of a clock-face orientation, as seen by the viewer (see 18.1.4, Numbers and Percentages, Use of Numerals, Measures of Time).

> *Ambiguous:*      The foreign body was observed in the patient's left eye at 9 o'clock.
>
> *Use:*      The foreign body was observed in the patient's left eye at the 9-o'clock position.

Note: The terms *clockwise* and *counterclockwise* can also be confusing. The point of reference (eg, that of observer vs subject) should be specified if the usage is ambiguous.

**11.10** **Laboratory Values.** Usually, in reports of clinical or laboratory data, the substance per se is not reported; rather, a value is given that was obtained by measuring a substance or some function or constituent of it. For example, one does not report hemoglobin but hemoglobin level. Some other correct forms are as follows:

> agglutination *titer*
>
> antinuclear antibody *titer*
>
> creatinine *level*
>
> creatinine *clearance*
>
> differential white blood cell *count*
>
> erythrocyte sedimentation *rate*
>
> hemagglutination inhibition *titer*
>
> high-density lipoprotein *fraction*
>
> increase in antibody *level*
>
> increase in bilirubin *level*
>
> mean corpuscular *volume*
>
> platelet *count*
>
> prothrombin *time*
>
> pulse *rate*
>
> serum phosphorus *concentration*
>
> total serum cholesterol *value* or *level* or *concentration*
>
> 24-hour urine *output* or *volume*
>
> urinary placental growth factor *concentration*
>
> urinary protein *excretion*

In reports of findings from clinical examinations or laboratory values, data may be enumerated without repeating *value, level*, etc, in accordance with the following example:

> Laboratory values were as follows: white blood cell count, $19.5 \times 10^3/\mu L$; hemoglobin, 12.9 g/dL; hematocrit, 38.5; platelet count, 203; and international normalized ratio, 1.1.

**11.11** **Articles.** The article *a* is used before the aspirate *h* (eg, *a* historic occasion) and nonvocalic *y* (eg, *a* ubiquitous organism). Abbreviations and acronyms are preceded by *a* or *an* according to the *sound* following (eg, a UN resolution, an HMO plan) (see 13.8, Agencies, Organizations, Foundations, Funding Bodies, and Others and 7.0, Grammar).

| a hypothesis [*h* sound] | an ultraviolet source [*u* sound] |
|---|---|
| a WMA report [*d* sound] | a UV source [*y* sound] |
| a hematocrit [*h* sound] | an honorarium [*o* sound] |
| an MD degree [*e* sound] | an NIH grant [*e* sound] |
| a historic operation [*h* sound] | a historical reenactment [*h* sound] |

## 11.12 ▌ Inclusive Language.

*Any classification according to a singular identity
polarizes people in a particular way, but if we take note of
the fact that we have many different identities . . . we can
see that the polarization of one can be resisted by a fuller
picture. So knowledge and understanding are extremely
important to fight against singular polarization.*
Amartya Sen[23]

Avoid the use of language that imparts bias against persons or groups on the basis of gender or sex, race or ethnicity, age, physical or mental disability, or sexual orientation. Avoid generalizations (such as *minorities*) and stereotypes and be specific when choosing words to describe people.

Note: Avoid using "non-" (eg, "White and nonwhite participants"), which is a nonspecific "convenience" grouping and label. Such a category may be oversimplified and misleading, even incorrect. Occasionally, however, these are categorizations used for comparison in data analysis. In such cases, the author should be queried. *Multiracial* and *people of color* are sometimes used in part to address the heterogeneous ethnic background of many people.

### 11.12.1 Sex/Gender. *Sex* refers to the biological characteristics of males and females. *Gender* includes more than sex and serves as a cultural indicator of a person's personal and social identity. An important consideration when referring to sex is the level of specificity required: specify sex when it is relevant. In research articles, sex/gender should be reported and defined, and how sex/gender was assessed should be described.[15] In nonresearch reports, choose sex-neutral terms that avoid bias, suit the material under discussion, and do not intrude on the reader's attention (see 11.7, Age and Sex Referents).

| *Avoid* | *Preferred* |
|---|---|
| chairman, chairwoman | chair, chairperson [*but*: see note] |
| corpsman | medical aide, corps member (*corpsman* is used by the US Marine Corps and Texas A&M University Corps of Cadets, and it may refer to either a man or a woman) |
| fireman | firefighter |

| | |
|---|---|
| layman | layperson |
| mailman | letter carrier, mail carrier, postal worker |
| man, mankind | people, humans, humanity, humankind, human species [*but*: see note] |
| manmade | artificial, handmade, synthetic |
| manpower | employees, human resources, personnel, staffing, workforce, workers |
| mothering | parenting, nurturing, caregiving |
| policeman, policewoman | police officer |
| spokesman, spokeswoman | spokesperson |
| steward, stewardess | flight attendant |

Note: Use *man* or *men* when referring to a specific man or group of men and *woman* or *women* when referring to a specific woman or a group of women. Similarly, *chairman* or *spokesman* might be used if the person under discussion is a man and *chairwoman* or *spokeswoman* if the person is a woman. Any of these might be used in an official title, for example, Michele Smith, alderman of the 43rd Ward, City of Chicago.

Do not attempt to change all words with *man* to *person* (eg, *manhole*). If possible, choose a sex-neutral equivalent such as *sewer hole* or *utility access hole*.

Terms such as *physician, nurse*, and *scientist* are sex-neutral and do not require modification (eg, female physician, male nurse) unless the sex of the person or persons described is relevant to the discussion (eg, a study of only female physicians or male nurses).

> After completing internship, the physician specialized in emergency medicine and worked at several hospitals in California. She was selected as an astronaut candidate by NASA in 2007.

**11.12.1.1** **Presenting Data in Tables.** When reporting the sex of participants in a table, include both sexes, as defined in the study, regardless of ratio. Do not use "White" and "male" as the default. When reporting on racial and ethnic differences, be as specific as possible (even if these comprise a small percentage of participants). Define the participants who are in the "other" category (see 4.1.2, Organizing Information in Tables).

**11.12.2** **Personal Pronouns.** Avoid sex-specific pronouns in cases in which sex specificity is irrelevant. Do not use common-gender "pronouns" (eg, "s/he," "shem," "shim"). Reword the sentence to use a singular or plural non–sex-specific pronoun, neutral noun equivalent, or change of voice; or use "he or she" ("him or her," "his or her[s]," "they or their[s]"). The use of the "singular they" construction is permitted when rewriting would be awkward or unclear (see 7.2.3.2, Pronoun-Pronoun Agreement).

| Avoid | Preferred |
|---|---|
| The physician and his office staff can do much to alleviate a patient's nervousness. | Physicians and their office staff can do a lot to alleviate a patient's nervousness. [plural] |
| | The physician and the office staff can do a lot to alleviate a patient's nervousness. [neutral noun equivalent] |

**UPDATE:** In chapter 11.12.3, Race/Ethnicity, a paragraph was added to explain the decision to capitalize *Black* and *White* racial terms and to use them as modifiers, not as nouns. This change was made ***August XX, 2020.***

**11.12.3** **Race/Ethnicity.** *Race* is defined as "a category of humankind that shares certain distinctive physical traits."[24] *Ethnicity* relates to "groups of people classed according to common racial, national, tribal, religious, linguistic, or cultural origin or background."[24]

Similar to gender, race and ethnicity are cultural constructs, but they can have biological implications. Caution must be used when the race concept is described in health-related research. Some have argued that the race concept should be abandoned, based on the scientific evidence that human races do not exist per se. Others argue for retaining the term *race* but limiting its application to the social, as opposed to the biological, realm.

A person's genetic heritage can convey certain biological and therefore medically related predispositions (eg, cystic fibrosis in persons of Northern European descent, lactose intolerance in persons with Chinese or Japanese ancestry, Tay-Sachs disease in persons with Jewish Eastern European ancestry, sickle cell disease seen primarily in persons of West African descent).

Specifying the race or ethnicity of a person can provide information about the generalizability of the results of a specific study. However, because many people in ethnically diverse countries, such as the United States, Canada, and some European, South American, and Asian nations, have mixed heritage, a racial or ethnic distinction should not be considered absolute, and it is often based on a person's self-designation.

The JAMA Network journals include the following direction in their Instructions for Authors:

> Aggregate, deidentified demographic information (eg, age, sex, race/ethnicity, and socioeconomic indicators) should be reported for all research reports and systematic reviews along with all prespecified outcomes. All demographic variables assessed should be reported in the Methods section. All demographic information collected should be reported in the Results section, either in the main article and/or in an online supplement. If any demographic characteristics that were collected are not reported, this should be explained. Summary demographic information (eg, baseline characteristics of study participants) should be reported in the first line of the Results section of Abstracts.

An explanation of who classified individuals as to race, ethnicity, or both, the classifications used, and whether the options were defined by the investigator or the participant should be included in the Methods section. The reasons that race/ethnicity was assessed in the study also should be described in the Methods section. Race/ethnicity of the study population should be reported in the Results section.

## METHODS

### Study Population, Baseline Survey, and Resurvey

The design and methods of the China Kadoorie Biobank (CKB) study have been reported in detail elsewhere.[26,27] Overall, 512 891 adults aged 30 to 79 years were enrolled from June 25, 2004, through July 15, 2008, from 5 rural and 5 urban areas in China. The CKB participants were confirmed to be of Chinese ancestry based on findings of principal component analysis of genotyping data, where available. The baseline survey included a detailed questionnaire and physical measurements (including anthropometry and blood pressure).

## METHODS

### Self-reported Race

Individuals were categorized as African American or non–African American. Children's race was based on the parent's report.

## METHODS

### Study Populations

Three National Health and Nutrition Examination Survey (NHANES)[17] cross-sectional samples (2007-2008, 2009-2010, and 2011-2012) were used to characterize the ages (range, 8-80 years) at which self-reported African American (n=4973), white American (n=8886), and Mexican American (n=3888) populations transitioned between ideal blood pressure, prehypertension, and hypertension across the life course. This analysis began in September 2014 and was completed in November 2015. Participants who had a physical limitation on both arms (eg, rashes, casts, or edema) that prevented measurement of blood pressure were excluded. We also excluded non-Hispanic Asian, other Hispanic, and other race/ethnicity (including multiracial/multiethnic) because of small sample sizes. Demographic and health information collected in the study[17] followed appropriate procedures for written informed consent, and the study was approved by local institutional review boards.

Racial/ethnic terms should be capitalized, including *Black* and *White,* and should not be used in noun form, such as Blacks and Whites, instead preferring Black patients or White participants. There may be instances in which a particular context may merit exception to this guidance, for example, in cases for which capitalization could be perceived as inflammatory or otherwise inappropriate.

When mention of race or ethnicity is relevant to an understanding of scientific information, be sensitive to the designations that individuals or groups prefer. Be aware also that preferences may change and that individuals within a group may disagree about the most appropriate designation. For terms such as *White, Black*, and *African American,* manuscript editors should follow usage (although Caucasian is sometimes used to indicate White but is technically specific to people from the Caucasus region in Eurasia and thus should be avoided).

In the United States, the term *African American* may be preferred to *Black* (note, however, that this term should be allowed only for US citizens of African descent). A hyphen is not used in either the noun or adjectival form (see, 8.3.1.6, When Not to Use Hyphens).

In reference to persons indigenous to North America (and their descendants), *American Indian* is generally preferred to the broader term *Native American*, which is also acceptable but includes (by US government designation) Hawaiian, Samoan, Guamanian, and Alaskan natives. Whenever possible, specify the nation or peoples (eg, Navajo, Nez Perce, Iroquois, Inuit).

*Hispanic* and *Latino* are broad terms that may be used to designate Spanish-speaking persons as well as those descended from the Spanish-speaking people of Mexico, South and Central America, and the Caribbean. However, the terms are not interchangeable because *Latino* is understood by some to exclude those of Mexican or Caribbean ancestry. In either case, these terms should not be used in noun form, and when possible, a more specific term (eg, Mexican, Mexican American, Latin American, Cuban, Cuban American, Puerto Rican) should be used.

Similarly, Asian persons may wish to be described according to their country or geographic area of origin (eg, Chinese, Indian, Japanese, Sri Lankan). Note that *Asian* and *Asian American* (*Chinese, Chinese American*, and so on) are not equivalent or interchangeable.

**11.12.4** **Age.** Discrimination based on age (young or old) is ageism. Because terms like *seniors, elderly, the aged, aging dependents, old-old, young-old*, and similar "other-ing" terms connote a stereotype, avoid using them. Terms such as *older persons, older people, older adults, older patients, older individuals, persons 65 years and older*, or *the older population* are preferred. Use *older* adults, a term less likely to connote discrimination and negative stereotypes, when describing individuals 65 years old and older.
Note: In studies that involve human beings, age should always be given specifically (eg, "older people aged 75 to 84 years" or "children younger than 12 years") (see 11.7, Age and Sex Referents).
*Adultism* is a form of ageism in which children and adolescents are discounted.[25,26]

**11.12.5** **Socioeconomic Status.** Avoid labeling people with their socioeconomic status, such as *the poor* or *the unemployed*. Instead, terms such as *low income* and *no income* are preferred. See also **limited-income, low-income, resource-limited, resource poor, transitional**.

**11.12.6** **Terms for Persons With Diseases, Disorders, or Disabilities.** Avoid labeling (and thus equating) people with their disabilities or diseases (eg, the blind, schizophrenics, epileptics). Instead, put the person first. Avoid describing persons as *victims* or with other emotional terms that suggest helplessness (*afflicted with, suffering from, stricken with, maimed*). Avoid euphemistic descriptors, such as *physically challenged, special*, or *special needs*.

| Avoid | Preferred |
| --- | --- |
| AIDS victim, stroke victim | person with AIDS, person who has had a stroke |
| alcoholic, addict, user, abuser | she was addicted, people with opiate addiction, he misused drugs and alcohol |

| | |
|---|---|
| asthmatics | patient with asthma, asthma group |
| the blind, the visually impaired | blind people, those with visual impairment |
| confined (bound) to a wheelchair | uses a wheelchair |
| crippled, lame, deformed | physically disabled |
| the deaf | deaf persons, deaf adults, deaf culture or community |
| diabetics | persons with diabetes, study participants in the diabetes group |
| the disabled, the handicapped | persons with disability |
| disabled child, mentally ill person, retarded adult | child with a disability, person with mental illness, adult with intellectual disability |
| epileptic | person affected by epilepsy, patient with epilepsy |
| the infirm | patients with long-term illness |

Avoid metaphors that may be inappropriate or insensitive and do not translate well (blind to the truth, deaf to the request). For similar reasons, some publications avoid the term *double-blind* when referring to a study's methods.

Note: Some manuscripts use certain phrases many times, and changing, for example, "AIDS patients" to "persons with AIDS" at every occurrence may result in awkward and stilted text. In such cases, the adjectival form may be used, although this is not preferred.

**11.12.7** **Sexual Orientation.** Sexual orientation should be indicated in a manuscript only when scientifically relevant. The term *sexual preference* should be avoided because it implies a voluntary choice of sexual orientation not supported by the scientific literature. In some contexts, reference to specific sexual behaviors (eg, *men who have sex with men*) may be more relevant than *sexual orientation.*

The nouns *lesbians* and *gay men* are preferred to the broader term *homosexuals* when referring to specific groups. Avoid using *gay* or *gays* as a noun. *Heterosexual, homosexual, bisexual, asexual,* and *intersex* may be used as adjectives (eg, *heterosexual men*).

A member of a heterosexual or homosexual couple may be referred to as *spouse, companion, partner,* or *life partner. Same-sex couple* and *same-sex marriage* are appropriate terms.

See also *LGBTQAI* in 13.11 Clinical, Technical, and Other Common Terms, the GLAAD Reference Guide-Transgender Issues website,[16] and the Gender Equity Resource Center website.[17]

**Principal Authors:** Tracy Frey, BA, and Roxanne K. Young, ELS

## ACKNOWLEDGMENT

Thanks to the following for reviewing and providing comments to improve the manuscript: Helene M. Cole, MD, formerly of *JAMA*; Gabriel Dietz, MA, JAMA Network; Barbara Gastel, MD, MPH, Texas A&M University, College Station; Julie Gerke, ELS, IQVIA, Parsippany, New Jersey; Carissa Gilman, MA, American Cancer Society, Atlanta, Georgia; Emily A. Greenhow, *JAMA*; Trevor Lane, MA, DPhil, Edanz Group, Fukuoka, Japan; and Peter J. Olson, ELS, Sheridan Journal Services, Waterbury, Vermont.

## REFERENCES

1. Pinker S. *The Sense of Style: The Thinking Person's Guide to Writing in the 21st Century.* Penguin; 2014:9.
2. Centers for Disease Control and Prevention. Matrix of E-code groupings. Published August 10, 2011. Accessed June 22, 2019. https://www.cdc.gov/injury/wisqars/ecode_matrix.html
3. Kane RL, Kane RA. Long-term care. *JAMA.* 1995;273(21):1690-1691. doi:10.1001/jama.1995.03520450060030
4. McDonald HP, Garg AX, Haynes RB. Interventions to enhance patient adherence to medication prescriptions: scientific review. *JAMA.* 2002;288(22):2868-2879. doi:10.1001/jama.288.22.2868
5. Chren M. Doctor's orders: rethinking compliance in dermatology. *Arch Dermatol.* 2002;138(3):393-394. doi:10.1001/archderm.138.3.393
6. Bernstein TM. *The Careful Writer: A Modern Guide to English Usage.* Free Press; 1998.
7. Everitt BS. *The Cambridge Dictionary of Statistics in the Medical Sciences.* Cambridge University Press; 1995.
8. The American College of Obstetricians and Gynecologists. *A Guide to Writing for Obstetrics & Gynecology.* 4th ed. American College of Obstetricians and Gynecologists; 2007.
9. Porta M; International Epidemiological Association. *A Dictionary of Epidemiology.* 6th ed. Oxford University Press; 2014.
10. American Diabetes Association. Diagnosing diabetes and learning about prediabetes. Accessed June 22, 2019. https://www.diabetes.org/diabetes-basics/diagnosis
11. American Diabetes Association. Diagnosis and classification of diabetes mellitus. *Diabetes Care.* 2010;33(suppl 1):S62-S69. doi:10.2337/dc10-S062
12. Lang TA, Secic M. *How to Report Statistics in Medicine: Annotated Guide for Authors, Editors, and Reviewers.* 2nd ed. American College of Physicians; 2006.
13. National Information Center on Health Services Research and Health Care Technology. Comparative effectiveness research (CER). Accessed November 10, 2017. https://www.nlm.nih.gov/hsrinfo/cer.html
14. Garner BA. *The Oxford Dictionary of American Usage and Style.* Oxford University Press; 2002.

15. Clayton JA, Tannenbaum C. Reporting sex, gender, or both in clinical research? *JAMA*. 2016;316(18):1863-1864. doi:10.1001/jama.2016.16405

16. GLAAD Media Reference Guide-Transgender. Accessed October 29, 2019. https://www.glaad.org/reference/transgender

17. Gender Equity Resource Center (GenEq). Accessed October 29, 2019. https://geneq.berkeley.edu/lgbt_resources_definition_of_terms

18. Allen CJA. Surgeries. *Arch Surg*. 1996;131(2):128. doi:10.1001/archsurg.1996.01430140018003

19. Flanagin A. Re: violence and nursing. *J Professional Nurs*. 2000;16(4):252.

20. Cleese J, Chapman G. Dead parrot sketch. *Monty Python's Flying Circus*. Python Productions; 1969.

21. Words and phrases. In: Fishbein M. *Medical Writing: The Technic and the Art*. American Medical Association; 1938:48.

22. King LS. *Why Not Say It Clearly? Guide to Scientific Writing*. Little Brown & Co; 1978:146-147.

23. Amartya Sen on "Identity and Violence: The Illusion of Destiny" [transcript]. Live Q&As. *Washington Post*. June 12, 2006. Accessed December 3, 2018. https://www.washingtonpost.com/wp-dyn/content/discussion/2006/06/08/DI2006060800699.html

24. *Merriam-Webster's Collegiate Dictionary*. 11th ed. Merriam-Webster Inc; 2003. Accessed March 10, 2019. https://www.merriam-webster.com/

25. Orentlicher D. Rationing and the Americans with Disabilities Act. *JAMA*. 1994;271(4):308-314. doi:10.1001/jama.1994.03510280070036

26. US Department of Justice Civil Rights Division. Information and technical assistance on the Americans with Disabilities Act. Accessed June 22, 2019. https://www.ada.gov

# 12.0 Non-English Words, Phrases, and Accent Marks

**12.0** Non-English Words, Phrases, and Accent Marks.

**12.1** Non-English Words, Phrases, and Titles.

**12.1.1** **Use of Italics.** Some words and phrases derived from other languages have become part of standard English usage. If a word or phrase derived from another language has not become part of standard English usage, it should be italicized, and a definition may be given (particularly if the word or phrase is not likely to be understood from the context). Consult *Stedman's* and *Dorland's* medical dictionaries and the most recent edition of *Merriam-Webster's Collegiate Dictionary* for guidance.

> *Hwabyeong* (literally "anger illness" or "fire illness") is a Korean somatization disorder believed to be caused by a buildup of unresolved anger that disturbs the balance of the 5 bodily elements.

> From the 1860s onward, *raznochintsy* (people of miscellaneous ranks) provided most of the leaders for the Russian revolutionary movement.

> The Internal Revenue Service has set the per diem rates.

> By embracing the marginal, the unhealthy, and the deviant, the decadents attacked bourgeois life, which they perceived as the chief enemy of art.

Non-English street addresses, names of buildings, and names of organizations should not be italicized or translated.

> Send all correspondence to ABC Holding BV, Marijkestraat 11, NL-2518 BG Den Haag, The Hague, the Netherlands.

However, do use the English-language names for countries: "Italy" rather than "Italia," "Brazil" rather than "Brasil," etc.

**12.1.2** **Translation of Titles.** Non-English titles mentioned in the text may, at the author's discretion, appear in English translation only or in the original language. If the original title is used, an English translation should be given parenthetically, except in cases in which the work is considered well known. Both the English translation of the title (if given) and the non-English title should be italicized for books, journals, plays, long poems, works of art, television and radio programs, films, and musical compositions.

Bollywood superstar Amitabh Bachchan is back with a bigger and better seventh season of *Kaun Banega Crorepati* (*Who Wants to Be a Millionaire?*).

Charles Baudelaire published his book *Les Fleurs du Mal* (*Flowers of Evil*) on June 25, 1857, leading to his conviction on charges of blasphemy and obscenity.

The audience member collapsed and died during the last act of *Götterdämmerung*.

**12.1.3** **Capitalization and Punctuation.** Capitalize and punctuate non-English words and phrases according to that language's standard of correctness. For example, all nouns are capitalized in German: Die Sonne scheint und die Vögel singen (The sun is shining and the birds are singing). Follow language dictionaries and *The Chicago Manual of Style*.

**12.2** **Accent Marks (Diacritics).** An accent mark (*diacritic*) added to a letter indicates a phonetic value different from that of the unmarked letter. Many words once spelled with accent marks (eg, cooperate, preeminent, debride, Meniere disease) now are written and printed without them. Consult the most recent edition of *Merriam-Webster's Collegiate Dictionary* to resolve questions about whether a word should retain its accent.

In general, English words in common usage should be spelled without diacritical marks. Words from other languages not in common English usage should retain their accent marks. Accent marks should be clearly indicated on manuscript copy. Accent marks should always be retained in proper names.

Marc-André Bergeron

Ana Marušić

Mötley Crüe

Accent marks should also be retained in quotations.

When faced with writer's block, I am reminded of Valéry: En vérité, une feuille blanche/Nous déclare par le vide/Qu'il n'est rien de si beau/Que ce qui n'existe pas (In truth, a blank sheet/Declares by the void/That there is nothing as beautiful/As that which does not exist).

(Note: It is advisable to provide a translation when necessary for a reader to understand the context, as in the example above.)

Accent marks are often used to show pronunciation and syllabic emphasis.

centime (sän-tēm)

squamous (skwā-məs)

Table 12.2-1 gives examples of usage of accent marks.

**Table 12.2-1.** Examples of Accent Mark Usage

| Accent mark | Examples of usage |
|---|---|
| acute | école |
| breve | măr |
| cedilla | Behçet |
| circumflex | hôpital |
| dot | can be either underdot (mahāprāṇa) or overdot (marlė) |
| grave | bibliothèque |
| macron | Māori |
| ring | Anders Ångstrom |
| slash (sometimes called virgule) | Adam Bøving |
| tilde | Español |
| umlaut | Henoch-Schönlein purpura |
| wedge or haček | Louis Žabkar |

It is recommended that special characters that will be used online be rendered in Unicode because all newer browsers support it. Use of Unicode nearly guarantees that special characters and diacritical marks will be displayed correctly online.

**Principal Author:** Brenda Gregoline, ELS

## ACKNOWLEDGMENT

Thanks to Barbara Gastel, MD, MPH, Texas A&M University, College Station; Trevor Lane, MA, DPhil, Edanz Group, Fukuoka, Japan; Peter J. Olson, ELS, Sheridan Journal Services, Waterbury, Vermont; and Shannon Sparenga, MS, JAMA Network, for their review and suggestions on this chapter.

# 13.0 Abbreviations

## 13.0 Abbreviations.

*To the Editor.*—It seems to me that at the time that there are articles being considered (ABC), dutifully edited (DE), and found good (FG) for publication, an editor may show hesitation to interfere judiciously (HIJ), perhaps because he thinks his knowledge lacking (KL) compared with that of eminent members of national organizations (MNO), and, therefore, for the sake of peace, quiet, and restraint (PQR), he sets the text in unaltered version (STUV), thus failing to act the wise xenogogue (WX) and meekly accepting the yoke of zeitgeist (YZ).

$$\text{In summary: ABC + DE + FG (HIJ} - \text{KL cf MNO)} - \text{PQR}$$
$$\rightarrow \text{STUV} \neq \text{WX} - \text{YZ.}$$

Luke Harris, MD
Summit, New Jersey

*My initial instinct was to deny that allegation (DTA). But when I left "xenogogue" (XaG) alone editorially, forcing the reader to trace the word etymologically, I realized that I must plead guilty (PG). The letter is not merely delightful but instructive: Dr Harris has the courtesy to* spell out each word the first time used. *Other authors: please take note!*—ED.
*JAMA.* 1975;233(11):1166.

An *abbreviation* is a shortened form of a word or phrase that is used in place of the full word or name (eg, Dr for doctor, US for United States, dB for decibel).

An *acronym* is a word formed from the first letter(s) of one (or more) of the words in a phrase (eg, ANCOVA for analysis of covariance). Acronyms are pronounced as words (including such "hybrids" as DMARD for disease-modifying antirheumatic drug, EQUATOR [Network] for Enhancing the Quality and Transparency of Health Research).

An *initialism* is an abbreviation formed from initial letters and pronounced either as a word (eg, PAHO for Pan American Health Organization) or as a set of consecutive initials (eg, WHO for World Health Organization).

Overuse of abbreviations can be confusing and ambiguous for readers, especially those whose first language is not English or those outside a specific specialty or discipline. However, abbreviations are acceptable to use when the original word or words are repeated numerous times, are long and cumbersome to read, or cause the prose to be awkward.

Instructions for authors published in medical and scientific journals may include guidelines on the use of abbreviations. Authors, editors, manuscript editors, and others involved in preparing manuscripts should use good judgment, flexibility, and common sense when considering the use of abbreviations. Abbreviations that some consider universally known may be obscure to others. Author-invented abbreviations should be avoided. See specific entries in this section and in chapter 14, Nomenclature, for further guidance on correct use of abbreviations.

Note: The expanded form of an abbreviation is given in lowercase letters, unless the expansion contains a proper noun, is a formal name, or begins a sentence (capitalize first word only).

Do not use periods with honorifics or abbreviations (exceptions: "No." for "number" and " St." when it is part of a person's name [see 13.6, Names and Titles of Persons], although no period is used with "St" in a city name [eg, St Louis, Missouri]).

**13.1** **Academic Degrees and Honors.** Academic degrees are abbreviated in bylines and in the text when used with the full name of a person (see 13.6, Names and Titles of Persons). In some circumstances, however, use of the abbreviation alone is acceptable (eg, Krystal Goderitch is a doctor of medicine and also holds a PhD in biochemistry) (see 9.5, Abbreviations).

Generally, follow author preference for order of academic degrees if there is more than one.

Note: Do *not* use both an honorific and an academic degree with a person's name, for example, Claudia Achenbach, MD, PhD, *or* Dr Claudia Achenbach (*not* Dr Claudia Achenbach, MD, PhD).

Authors in the military, or retired from the military, should use their academic degrees rather than their military services and titles.

Authors should list their highest academic degree in the byline. Degrees below the master's level (eg, BS, BA), fellowship designations, or honorary degrees are generally not listed in bylines or elsewhere (see 2.2.3, Academic Degrees). However, if a bachelor's degree is the highest degree held, it may be listed. Exceptions are also made for specialized degrees, licenses, certifications, and credentials below the master's level in medical and health-related fields (see the following list). Any unusual degrees should be verified with the author.

| | |
|---|---|
| APRN | advanced practice registered nurse |
| ART | accredited record technician |
| BS | bachelor of science |
| BS, BCh, BC, CB, or ChB | bachelor of surgery |

| | |
|---|---|
| BSN | bachelor of science in nursing |
| CDE | certified diabetes educator |
| CGC | certified genetic counselor |
| CHES | certified health education specialist |
| CIH | certified industrial hygienist |
| CNM | certified nurse midwife |
| CNMT | certified nuclear medicine technologist |
| CNP | certified nurse practitioner |
| CNS | certified nurse specialist |
| CO | certified orthoptist |
| COMT | certified ophthalmic medical technologist |
| CPFT | certified pulmonary function technologist |
| CRNA | certified registered nurse anesthetist |
| CRT | certified respiratory therapist |
| CRTT | certified respiratory therapist technician |
| CTR | certified tumor registrar |
| DC | doctor of chiropractic |
| DCh or ChD | doctor of surgery |
| DDS | doctor of dental surgery |
| DHL | doctor of humane letters |
| DMD | doctor of dental medicine |
| DME | doctor of medical education |
| DMSc | doctor of medical science |
| DNE | doctor of nursing education |
| DNS or DNSc | doctor of nursing science |
| DO or OD | doctor of optometry |
| DO | doctor of osteopathic medicine |
| DPH or DrPH | doctor of public health; doctor of public hygiene |
| DPharm | doctor of pharmacy |
| DPM | doctor of podiatric medicine |
| DPT | doctor of physical therapy |
| DNP or DrNP | doctor of nursing practice |

| | |
|---|---|
| DrPH | doctor of public health |
| DSW | doctor of social work |
| DTM&H | diploma in tropical medicine and hygiene |
| DTPH | diploma in tropical pediatric hygiene |
| DVM, DMV, or VMD | doctor of veterinary medicine |
| DVMS | doctor of veterinary medicine and surgery |
| DVS or DVSc | doctor of veterinary science |
| | |
| EdD | doctor of education |
| ELS | editor in the life sciences |
| EMT | emergency medical technician |
| EMT-P | emergency medical technician-paramedic |
| | |
| GNP | gerontologic or geriatric nurse practitioner |
| | |
| JD | doctor of jurisprudence |
| | |
| LCP | licensed clinical psychologist |
| LCSW | licensed clinical social worker |
| LLB | bachelor of laws |
| LLD | doctor of laws |
| LLM | master of laws |
| LPN | licensed practical nurse |
| LVN | licensed visiting nurse; licensed vocational nurse |
| | |
| M(ASCP) | registered technologist in microbiology (American Society for Clinical Pathology) |
| MA or AM | master of arts |
| MB or BM | bachelor of medicine |
| MBA | master of business administration |
| MBBS or MB,BS | bachelor of medicine, bachelor of surgery |
| MD or DM | doctor of medicine |
| MDiv | master of divinity |
| ME | medical examiner |
| MEd | master of education |
| MFA | master of fine arts |

| | |
|---|---|
| MHA | master of hospital administration |
| MIDS | master of information and data science |
| MLS | master of library science |
| MMM | master of medical management |
| MN | master of nursing |
| MPA | master of public administration |
| MPH | master of public health |
| MPharm | master of pharmacy |
| MPhil | master of philosophy |
| MPPA | master of public policy administration |
| MRCP | member of the Royal College of Physicians |
| MRCS | member of the Royal College of Surgeons |
| MS, MSc, or SM | master of science |
| MS, SM, MCh, or MSurg | master of surgery |
| MSIS | master of information science |
| MSN | master of science in nursing |
| MSPH | master of science in public health |
| MStat | master of statistics |
| MSW | master of social welfare; master of social work |
| MT | medical technologist |
| MTA | medical technical assistant |
| MT(ASCP) | registered medical technologist (American Society for Clinical Pathology) |
| MUS | master in urban studies |
| ND | naturopathic doctor |
| NP | nurse practitioner |
| OT | occupational therapist |
| OTR | occupational therapist, registered |
| PA | physician assistant |
| PA-C | physician assistant, certified |
| PharmD, DP, or PD | doctor of pharmacy |

| | |
|---|---|
| PhD or DPhil | doctor of philosophy |
| PhG | graduate in pharmacy |
| PNP | pediatric nurse practitioner |
| PsyD | doctor of psychology |
| PT | physical therapist |
| | |
| RD | registered dietitian |
| RDN | registered dietitian nutritionist |
| RN | registered nurse |
| RNA | registered nurse anesthetist |
| RNC or RN,C | registered nurse, certified |
| RPFT | registered pulmonary function technologist |
| RPh | registered pharmacist |
| RPT | registered physical therapist |
| RRL | registered record librarian |
| RT | radiologic technologist; respiratory therapist |
| RTR | recreational therapist, registered |
| | |
| ScD, DSc, or DS | doctor of science |
| | |
| ThD or DTh | doctor of theology |

**13.2**    **US Military Services and Titles.** An abbreviation of a military service follows a name; an abbreviation of a military title (also called grade or rank) precedes a name (eg, Col Cornelia McNamara, USAF, MC, *not* Col Cornelia McNamara, MD). These abbreviations should not be used in bylines.

**13.2.1**    **US Military Services.**

US Army

| | |
|---|---|
| MC, USA | Medical Corps, US Army |
| ANC, USA | Army Nurse Corps, US Army |
| SP, USA | Specialist Corps, US Army |
| MSC, USA | Medical Service Corps, US Army |
| DC, USA | Dental Corps, US Army |
| VC, USA | Veterinary Corps, US Army |

Note: All the preceding designations also apply to the Army National Guard (ARNG) and US Army Reserve (USAR).

US Air Force

| | |
|---|---|
| USAF, MC | Medical Corps, US Air Force |
| USAF, NC | Nurse Corps, US Air Force |
| USAF, MSC | Medical Service Corps, US Air Force |
| USAF, DC | Dental Corps, US Air Force |
| USAF, BSC | Bio-Sciences Corps, US Air Force |

Note: All the preceding designations also apply to the Air National Guard (ANG) and US Air Force Reserve (USAFR). The US Air Force has no veterinary corps; veterinarians are in the Bio-Sciences Corps.

US Navy

| | |
|---|---|
| MC, USN | Medical Corps, US Navy |
| MSC, USN | Medical Service Corps, US Navy |
| NC, USN | Nurse Corps, US Navy |
| DC, USN | Dental Corps, US Navy |

Note: All the preceding designations also apply to the US Naval Reserve (USNR).

## 13.2.2    US Military Officer Titles (Grades and Ranks).

US Army

| | |
|---|---|
| General | GEN |
| Lieutenant General | LTG |
| Major General | MG |
| Brigadier General | BG |
| Colonel | COL |
| Lieutenant Colonel | LTC |
| Major | MAJ |
| Captain | CPT |
| First Lieutenant | 1LT |
| Second Lieutenant | 2LT |
| Chief Warrant Officer | CWO |
| Warrant Officer | WO |

US Navy and US Coast Guard

| | |
|---|---|
| Admiral | ADM |
| Vice Admiral | VADM |
| Rear Admiral | RADM |

| | |
|---|---|
| Captain | CAPT |
| Commander | CDR |
| Lieutenant Commander | LCDR |
| Lieutenant | LT |
| Lieutenant (Junior Grade) | LTJG |
| Ensign | ENS |
| Chief Warrant Officer | CWO |

Note: All medical professionals in the US Coast Guard (except physician assistants) are commissioned officers in the US Public Health Service (PHS). US Coast Guard chief warrant officers in medicine are designated CWO(Med). This also applies to the US Coast Guard Reserve.

US Air Force and US Marine Corps

| | |
|---|---|
| General | Gen |
| Lieutenant General | Lt Gen |
| Major General | Maj Gen |
| Brigadier General | Brig Gen |
| Colonel | Col |
| Lieutenant Colonel | Lt Col |
| Major | Maj |
| Captain | Capt |
| First Lieutenant | 1st Lt |
| Second Lieutenant | 2nd Lt |

Note: The US Marine Corps does not have its own medical organization. The medical care of the US Marine Corps is provided by the US Navy.

**13.3** **Days of the Week, Months, Eras.** Generally, days of the week and months are not abbreviated.

The manuscript was received at *JAMA*'s editorial offices in late December 2017 and accepted for publication on January 6, 2018, after expedited peer review, revision, and discussion among the editors. Because of the importance of its topic, the article was published 2 weeks later, on Tuesday, January 20, 2018.

In tables and figures, the following 3-letter abbreviations for days of the week and months may be used to conserve space (see 4.1, Tables, and 4.2, Figures):

| | |
|---|---|
| Monday | Mon |
| Tuesday | Tue |
| Wednesday | Wed |

| | |
|---|---|
| Thursday | Thu |
| Friday | Fri |
| Saturday | Sat |
| Sunday | Sun |
| January | Jan |
| February | Feb |
| March | Mar |
| April | Apr |
| May | May |
| June | Jun |
| July | Jul |
| August | Aug |
| September | Sep |
| October | Oct |
| November | Nov |
| December | Dec |

Occasionally, manuscripts may contain discussion of eras. Abbreviations for eras are set in small capitals with no punctuation. Numerals are used for years and words for the first through ninth centuries. The more commonly used era designations are AD (anno Domini [in the year of the Lord]), BC (before Christ), CE (common era), and BCE (before the common era). CE and BCE are equivalent to AD and BC, respectively. In formal usage, the abbreviation AD precedes the year number, and BC, CE, and BCE follow it.

> *Materia medica* is a Latin term for the body of collected knowledge about the therapeutic properties of any substance used for healing. The term derives from the title of a work by the ancient Greek physician Pedanius Dioscorides in the first century AD, *De materia medica* (*On Medical Material*).

> The prevalence of tuberculosis is thought to have increased greatly during the Middle Ages (roughly AD 500-1500), possibly because of the growth of towns across Europe.

> Cuneiform was probably invented by the Sumerians before 3000 BC.

> The plant source of colchicine, the autumn crocus (*Colchicum autumnale*), was described for the treatment of rheumatism and swelling in Egypt as early as 1500 BCE.

**13.4 Local Addresses.** Use abbreviations when *complete* local addresses are given:

> AMA Plaza is located on Wabash Avenue near the Chicago River.

> The JAMA Network editorial and publishing offices are located at 330 N Wabash Ave, Chicago, IL 60611.

In some cases, these designators may or may not be abbreviated, by convention:

Mount St Helens

Saint Louis University

Common abbreviations in addresses are shown below.

| | |
|---|---|
| Air Force Base | AFB |
| Army Post Office | APO |
| Avenue | Ave |
| Boulevard | Blvd |
| Building | Bldg |
| Circle | Cir |
| Court | Ct |
| Crescent | Cres |
| Drive | Dr |
| East | E |
| Fleet Post Office | FPO |
| Highway | Hwy |
| Lane | Ln |
| Mount | Mt |
| North | N |
| Northeast | NE |
| Northwest | NW |
| Parkway | Pkwy |
| Place | Pl |
| Post Office | PO |
| Road | Rd |
| Route | Rte |
| Rural Free Delivery | RFD |
| Rural Route | RR |
| Saint | St or Ste (eg, Sault Ste Marie [verify]) |
| South | S |
| Southeast | SE |
| Southwest | SW |
| Square | Sq |

| | |
|---|---|
| Street | St |
| Suite | Ste |
| Terrace | Terr |
| West | W |

Do not abbreviate the non-English counterparts of the above designators (eg, boulevard, avenue, place, Strasse, Platz).

14 boulevard Poissonnière

Hugstetter Strasse 55

When the plural form is used, do not abbreviate (eg, Broadway and Spring streets). When a street number is not given, do not abbreviate.

Bond University, Faculty of Health Sciences and Medicine, Centre for Research in Evidence Based Practice, University Drive, Gold Coast, Queensland 4229, Australia.

Do not abbreviate *room, department* (except in references; see 3.13.2, Government or Agency Reports), or *division*.

Do not use periods or commas with N, S, E, W, or their combinations.

There may be exceptions to these rules. For example, "One Magnificent Mile" and "One Gustave L. Levy Place" are not only addresses but also proper names of buildings or office centers. In these cases, it is appropriate to spell out address numbers that accompany designators such as "Place." In such cases, the editor or author should use common sense and verify unusual addresses.

**13.5** **Cities, States, Counties, Territories, Possessions, Provinces, Countries.**
At first mention, the name of a state, territory, possession, province, or country should be spelled out when it follows the name of a city. The JAMA Network journals do not add "United States" after the name of a US city and state. Journals differ in their preferences.

| | |
|---|---|
| Chicago, Illinois | Reykjavik, Iceland |
| Abu Dhabi, United Arab Emirates | London, England |
| | Brasilia, Brazil |
| Johannesburg, South Africa | |

Names of cities, states, counties, territories, possessions, provinces, and countries should be spelled out in full when they stand alone.

Names of states need not be repeated if listing more than one city name from that state.

The authors studied comparable groups of children in Chicago, Springfield, Rockford, and Peoria, all in Illinois.

Abbreviations such as "US" and "UK" may be used as modifiers (when they directly precede the word they modify) or as nouns and do not require expansion as long as the context is clear.

Use 2-letter abbreviations for US state and Canadian province names in addresses (with zip/postal codes) but not in the text. The US state and Canadian province names may also be abbreviated to save space in tables and figures.

The JAMA Network
330 N Wabash Ave
Chicago, IL 60611-5885

University of British Columbia
2329 West Mall
Vancouver, BC V6T 1Z4, Canada

| US state, territory, possession | US Postal Service abbreviation |
| --- | --- |
| Alabama | AL |
| Alaska | AK |
| American Samoa | AS |
| Arizona | AZ |
| Arkansas | AR |
| California | CA |
| Canal Zone | CZ |
| Colorado | CO |
| Connecticut | CT |
| Delaware | DE |
| District of Columbia | DC |
| Federated States of Micronesia | FM |
| Florida | FL |
| Georgia | GA |
| Guam | GU |
| Hawaii | HI |
| Idaho | ID |
| Illinois | IL |
| Indiana | IN |
| Iowa | IA |
| Kansas | KS |
| Kentucky | KY |
| Louisiana | LA |
| Maine | ME |

| | |
|---|---|
| Marshall Islands | MH |
| Maryland | MD |
| Massachusetts | MA |
| Michigan | MI |
| Minnesota | MN |
| Mississippi | MS |
| Missouri | MO |
| Montana | MT |
| Nebraska | NE |
| Nevada | NV |
| New Hampshire | NH |
| New Jersey | NJ |
| New Mexico | NM |
| New York | NY |
| North Carolina | NC |
| North Dakota | ND |
| Northern Mariana Islands | MP |
| Ohio | OH |
| Oklahoma | OK |
| Oregon | OR |
| Palau | PW |
| Pennsylvania | PA |
| Puerto Rico | PR |
| Rhode Island | RI |
| South Carolina | SC |
| South Dakota | SD |
| Tennessee | TN |
| Texas | TX |
| Utah | UT |
| Vermont | VT |
| Virginia | VA |
| Virgin Islands | VI |
| Washington | WA |

| West Virginia | WV |
|---|---|
| Wisconsin | WI |
| Wyoming | WY |

Canadian and Australian city names may be followed by the spelled-out province name in the text (eg, London, Ontario, Canada; Sydney, New South Wales, Australia) but are abbreviated in full postal addresses.

| Canadian province, territory | Canadian Postal Service abbreviation |
|---|---|
| Alberta | AB |
| British Columbia | BC |
| Manitoba | MB |
| New Brunswick | NB |
| Newfoundland and Labrador | NL |
| Northwest Territories | NT |
| Nova Scotia | NS |
| Nunavut | NU |
| Ontario | ON |
| Prince Edward Island | PE |
| Quebec | QC |
| Saskatchewan | SK |
| Yukon | YT |

At first mention in the text, the full name of the appropriate state or country should follow the name of a city whenever clarification of location is thought to be important for the reader, as in the following examples:

Katrina made its second landfall on August 29, 2005, as a category 3 hurricane with sustained winds of 200 km/h near Buras-Triumph, Louisiana.

The 21st International AIDS Conference was held in July 2016 in Durban, South Africa.

The province name may also be added for less well-known cities:

San Miguel, Hidalgo, Mexico

If the city, state, or country is clear from the context, as in the following examples, do not include it.

Studies were performed at the University of Michigan Medical School, Ann Arbor [unnecessary to add "Michigan"].

A cross-sectional survey assessing bicycle safety helmets was conducted in 3 Dutch primary schools in Breda, Maastricht, and Terneuzen [unnecessary to add "the Netherlands"].

Do not provide the state or country name in cases in which the entity is well known or such designation is irrelevant (eg, Chicago Blackhawks, Philadelphia chromosome, Glasgow sign, Uppsala virus, Lyme disease, *New York Times*).

Do not provide the location of an institution if it is clear that the location is not important (eg, "Using the Centers for Disease Control and Prevention criteria for AIDS . . . " or "Following the World Health Organization guidelines . . . ").

What does it matter that she was born in Boston or that after her parents had instilled in her the guiding principles of life, Harvard University had its turn?

In addition to the city name, provide the state name or country name in the author affiliation footnote and correspondence address.

*Affiliation Footnote:*

Division of Gastroenterology, Mayo Clinic, Rochester, Minnesota (McGill).

*Author Correspondence Address:*

Charles B. McGill, MD, Division of Gastroenterology, Mayo Clinic, Rochester, MN 55905 (mcgill@mayo.edu).

*Special Case:* "New York" may refer to either the city or the state. In the former case, the state name must be added:

New York State Psychiatric Institute, New York

New York University, New York, New York

When giving the location of an institution or organization whose formal name includes a city, do not insert the state or country within the name:

| | |
|---|---|
| *Correct:* | University of California, San Francisco, School of Medicine |
| *Correct:* | Stanford University School of Medicine in California |
| *Also correct:* | Stanford University School of Medicine, Stanford, California |
| *Not:* | Stanford University School of Medicine (California) |
| *And not:* | Stanford (California) University School of Medicine |
| *And not:* | Stanford University School of Medicine, California |

The style used in the latter correct examples may be applied in signature bylines:

| | |
|---|---|
| *Correct:* | Wilma Smith, MD<br>Stanford University School of Medicine<br>Stanford, California |
| *Not:* | Wilma Smith, MD<br>Stanford (California) University School of Medicine |

The following are examples of address style for many countries throughout the world (see 2.10.7, Corresponding Author Contact Information, and 13.4, Local Addresses).

Vivek Goal, MD, Department of Health Administration, McMurrich Bldg, 12 Queen's Park Cres W, Toronto, ON M5S 1A8, Canada.

Didier Blaise, MD, Unité de Transplantation et de Thérapie Cellulare, Institut Paoli-Calmettes, 232 Bd Ste Marguerite, 13273 Marseille CEDEX 09, France.

Mark P. Hehir, MD, Royal College of Surgeons in Ireland Unit, Department of Obstetrics and Gynaecology, Rotunda Hospital, Parnell Square, Dublin 1, Ireland.

Andrzej Szczeklik, PhD, Allergy and Immunology Clinic, Department of Medicine, Jagellonian University School of Medicine, ul Skawinska 8, 31-0666 Krakow, Poland.

Alain F. Broccard, MD, Division des Soins Intensifs, Département de Médecine, BH10-92, University Hospital (Centre hospitalier universitaire vaudois), CH-1011 Lausanne, Switzerland.

Aram S. A. van Brussel, MD, PhD, Internal Medicine, Gelre Hospital Apeldoorn, Albert Schweiterlaan 31, Apeldoorn, Utrecht 7334 DZ, the Netherlands.

Konstantinos I. Gourgoloulianis, MD, Pulmonary Department, Medical School, University of Thessaly, 22 Papakyriazi, Larissa 41222, Greece.

Ruben Terg, Unidad de Hepatologia, Hospital de Gastroenterologia Bonorino Udaondo, Escuela de Medicina, Universidad del Salvador, Avenida Caseros, 2061 (1264) Buenos Aires, Argentina.

Ditlev Fossen, MBBS, Department of Obstetrics and Gynecology, County Hospital of Oestfold (Sykenhuset Ostfold), 1603 Fredrikstad, Norway.

Hajime Fujimoto, MD, Third Department of Internal Medicine, Respiratory Division, Mie University School of Medicine, Edobashi 2-174, Tsu City, Mie 514-8507, Japan.

Kwang Hyun Kim, MD, Department of Otolaryngology–Head and Neck Surgery, Seoul National University, College of Medicine, 28 Tongon-Dong, Chongno-Gu, Seoul 110-744, Korea.

Colin L. Masters, MD, Department of Pathology, University of Melbourne, Parkville, VIC 3010, Australia.

Thomas Schwarz, MB, Division of Vascular Medicine, Department of Internal Medicine, University Hospital of Dresden Medical School, Fetscherstrasse 74, 01307 Dresden, Germany.

Antonio Torres, MD, PhD, Servei de Pneumologia, Hospital Clinic, C/Villarroel 170, 08036 Barcelona, Spain.

Lixing Lao, PhD, MB, School of Chinese Medicine, The University of Hong Kong, 10 Sassoon Rd, Pokfulam, Hong Kong.

David M. Fergusson, MStat, Christchurch Health and Development Study, Christchurch School of Medicine, 2 Riccarton Ave, Christchurch Central, Christchurch 8011, New Zealand.

Anand Job, MSc, Department of Otorhinolaryngology and Head and Neck Surgery, Unit 1, Christian Medical College, Vellore 632 004, India.

Andrew Farmer, DM, Nuffield Laboratory of Primary Care Health Sciences, University of Oxford, Oxford OX2 6AW, England.

Yasemin Giles, MD, Istanbul Tip Fakültesi, Genel Cerrahi ABD, Capa, Topkapi, Istanbul, Turkey 34390.

Shurong Zheng, MD, Department of Obstetrics and Gynecology, Peking University First Hospital, Beijing 100034, China.

Alfred Cuschieri, MD, Department of Surgery and Molecular Oncology, Ninewells Hospital and Medical School, University of Dundee, Dundee DD1 9SY, Scotland.

José Luis Soto-Hernandez, MD, Department of Infectious Diseases, Instituto Nacional de Neurología y Neurocirugia Manuel Valasco Suarez, Insurgentes Sur 3877, La Fama, Tlalpan CP 14269, Mexico.

J. Skordis, MBBS, Department of Public Health and Policy, London School of Hygiene and Tropical Medicine, Keppel Street, London WC1E 7HT, England.

Gar-Yang Chau, MD, MPH, Division of General Surgery, Department of Surgery, Taipei Veterans General Hospital, 201 Shih-Pai Rd, Section 2, Taipei, Taiwan 11217.

Luciana Tricai Cavalini, MD, PhD, Department of Health Information Technology, Rio de Janeiro State University, Av Prof Manoel de Abreu 444, Rio de Janeiro 20550-170, Brazil.

Guilia Ciccarese, MD, Department of Dermatology, IRCC Azienda Ospedaliera Universitaria San Martino–IST, DISSAL, Largo Rosanna Benzi 10, Genoa, 16132 Italy.

Matthieu LeGrand, MD, PhD, Department of Anesthesiology and Critical Care and Burn Unit, St Louis Hospital, Université Paris Diderot–Paris 7, rue Claude Vellefaux, 75010 Paris, France.

Anne-Marie Schjerning Olsen, MD, PhD, Department of Cardiology–Post 635, Copenhagen University Hospital, Gentofte, Niels Andersens Vej 65, 2900 Hellerup, Denmark.

Catterina Ferreccio, MD, MPH, Department of Public Health/Faculty of Medicine, Pontificia Universidad Católica de Chile, Marcoleta 434, Santiago, Chile.

**13.6** **Names and Titles of Persons.** Given (first) names should not be abbreviated in the text or in bylines except by using initials when so indicated by the author. The editor should verify the use of initials with the author. (Some publishers and journals prefer to use initials instead of given names in author bylines.)

Do not use Chas., Geo., Jos., Wm., etc, except when such abbreviations are part of the formal name of a company or organization that regularly uses such abbreviations (see 13.7, Commercial Firms). When an abbreviation is part of a person's name, retain the period after the abbreviation, eg, Oliver St. John Gogarty, MD; Frederick John de St. Vrain Schwankovsky.

Initials used in the text to indicate names of persons (eg, coauthors of an article) should be followed by periods and set close within parentheses. Note: This is one of the few instances in which periods are used with an abbreviation.

> Two authors (M.R.B. and C.D.-W.) independently screened the abstracts of the search results and independently assessed the remaining full-text articles for eligibility. Any disagreement was resolved with the help of the third author (D.C.B.).

A person who is not an author may also be included in the text, in which case the full name and academic degree are used.

> Although measurements of the various components were divided among 3 different examiners (R.Z., D.O.M., and Bert N. J. van Berckel, MD, PhD), each examiner measured the same components at each annual session.

*Senior* and *Junior* are abbreviated, without periods, when they are part of a name. The abbreviation follows the surname. A comma follows the abbreviation (but see 18.7.5, Roman Numerals, and 3.7, Authors). Note: These abbreviations are used only with the full name (never Dr Forsythe Jr).

> Peter M. Forsythe Jr, MD, performed his landmark research in collaboration with James Philips Sr, PhD, at the National Institute of Mental Health.

Names with roman numerals do not take a comma before the numeral.

> John Paul II
> Trey Riggs III, PharmD

Many titles of persons are abbreviated but only when they precede the full name (given name or initials and surname). Spell titles out when (1) used before a surname alone (except in some cases as described below), (2) used at the beginning of a sentence, and (3) used after a name (in this instance, the title should not be capitalized) (but see 13.2, US Military Services and Titles).

> Colonel Jonas
> Dr Jonas, colonel in the US Army
>
> Alderman Hopkins
> Brian Hopkins, alderman of the Second Ward of Chicago
>
> Associate Professor Panodolfino
> Maria Panodolfino, associate professor, Department of Infectious Diseases
>
> Father Doyle
> Fr Raymond G. Doyle
> Raymond G. Doyle, SJ
>
> Governor Brown
> Kate Brown, governor of Oregon

> Representative McDermott
> Jim McDermott, MD, representative from the state of Washington
>
> Senator Durbin (D, Illinois)
> Richard Durbin, US senator from Illinois
>
> Superintendent Smith
> Henry B. Smith, EdD, superintendent of schools
>
> President James K. Polk
> James K. Polk, president of the US

The following social titles are always abbreviated when preceding a surname, with or without first name or initials: Dr, Mr, Messrs, Mrs, Mmes, Ms, and Mss. Note that in most instances, the title Dr should be used only after the specific academic degree has been mentioned and only with the surname.

> Arthur L. Rudnick, MD, PhD, gave the opening address. At the close of the meeting, Dr Rudnick was named director of the committee on sports injuries.

The Reverend, Reverend, or Rev is used only when the first name or initials are given with the surname. When only the surname is given, use the Reverend Mr (or Ms or Dr), Mr (or Ms or Dr), or Father (Roman Catholic, sometimes Anglican). Never use the Reverend Brown, Reverend Brown, or Rev Brown.

> the Reverend Katharine M. Burke
>
> the Reverend Dr Burke

**13.7** **Commercial Firms.** In the text, use the name of a company exactly as the company uses it, but omit the period after any abbreviations used, such as *Co, Inc, Corp*, and *Ltd*. Do not abbreviate these terms if the company spells them out (eg, Apothecus Pharmaceutical Corporation).

However, to conserve space in references, abbreviate *Company, Corporation, Brothers, Incorporated, Limited*, and *and* (using an ampersand), without punctuation, even if the company expands them, and delete periods even with initials, in accordance with the following examples.

| Text style | Reference style |
| --- | --- |
| American Mensa, Ltd | American Mensa Ltd |
| Medsoftware, Inc | Medsoftware Inc |
| StataCorp LP | StataCorp |

**13.8** **Agencies, Organizations, Foundations, Funding Bodies, and Others.** Many organizations (eg, academies, associations, government agencies, research institutes) are known by abbreviations or acronyms rather than by their full names. Some of these organizations have identical abbreviations (eg, AHA for both American Heart Association and American Hospital Association). Therefore, to avoid confusion, the names of all organizations should be expanded at first mention in the text and other major elements of the manuscript, with the abbreviation following immediately in parentheses, in accordance with the guidelines offered in 13.11, Clinical, Technical, and Other Common Terms.

The article *the* is often used with abbreviated forms of agencies and organizations (eg, the UN, the AMA, the FDA); however, an article is not necessary with forms pronounced as words (eg, NASA [nas-ah], OSHA [oh-shuh], WAME [wa-mee]).

**13.9**    **Collaborative Groups.** Collaborative groups usually include study groups, multicenter trials, task forces, expert and ad hoc consensus groups, and periodic national and international health surveys. Such an entity's abbreviation should be provided in addition to its full name, even if it appears only once in a manuscript. Because some of these groups are better recognized by their acronyms than by their full names, the acronym can be placed first, with the expansion in parentheses, contrary to the order usually recommended.

To save space in titles, however, the acronym may be used alone if its expansion is provided early in the manuscript, for example, in the abstract and in the text. Alternatively, the acronym might be given in the manuscript's title and the expansion in its subtitle, or if space permits and both the expansion and the acronym convey separate and essential concepts, both could be given in the title or subtitle. The collaborative group name may be used as the byline (see 5.1.9, Group and Collaborative Authorship; 2.2, Author Bylines and End-of-Text Signatures; and 2.10, Acknowledgments [Article Information]).

| | |
|---|---|
| *Title:* | Lutein Plus Zeaxanthin and $\Omega3$ Fatty Acids for Age-Related Macular Degeneration |
| *Subtitle:* | The Age-Related Eye Disease Study 2 (AREDS2) |
| *Byline:* | The Age-Related Eye Disease Study 2 (AREDS2) Study Group |

When choosing the form in which collaborative group information is presented, consider the manuscript's context and audience, database searches, and ease of comprehension.

**13.10**    **Names of Journals.** Journal names should be abbreviated and italicized in reference listings. A journal name abbreviation is followed by a period, which denotes the close of the journal title group of bibliographic elements.

The following commonly referenced journals and their abbreviations are included as a subset limit (Core Clinical Journals) within PubMed. A list of those journal titles can be found at https://www.nlm.nih.gov/bsd/aim.html. Here, the Core Clinical Journal titles are presented as examples, along with their abbreviations. Note that single-word journal titles are not abbreviated.

| | |
|---|---|
| *Academic Medicine* | *Acad Med* |
| *AJR: American Journal of Roentgenology* | *AJR Am J Roentgenol* |
| *American Family Physician* | *Am Fam Physician* |
| *American Heart Journal* | *Am Heart J* |

| | |
|---|---|
| *American Journal of Cardiology* | *Am J Cardiol* |
| *American Journal of Clinical Nutrition* | *Am J Clin Nutr* |
| *American Journal of Clinical Pathology* | *Am J Clin Pathol* |
| *American Journal of Medicine* | *Am J Med* |
| *American Journal of the Medical Sciences* | *Am J Med Sci* |
| *American Journal of Nursing* | *Am J Nurs* |
| *American Journal of Obstetrics & Gynecology* | *Am J Obstet Gynecol* |
| *American Journal of Ophthalmology* | *Am J Ophthalmol* |
| *American Journal of Pathology* | *Am J Pathol* |
| *American Journal of Physical Medicine & Rehabilitation/Association of Academic Physiatrists* | *Am J Phys Med Rehabil* |
| *American Journal of Psychiatry* | *Am J Psychiatry* |
| *American Journal of Public Health* | *Am J Public Health* |
| *American Journal of Respiratory and Critical Care Medicine* | *Am J Respir Crit Care Med* |
| *American Journal of Surgery* | *Am J Surg* |
| *American Journal of Tropical Medicine and Hygiene* | *Am J Trop Med Hyg* |
| *Anaesthesia* | *Anaesthesia* |
| *Anesthesia & Analgesia* | *Anesth Analg* |
| *Anesthesiology* | *Anesthesiology* |
| *Annals of Emergency Medicine* | *Ann Emerg Med* |
| *Annals of Internal Medicine* | *Ann Intern Med* |
| *Annals of Otology, Rhinology, & Laryngology* | *Ann Otol Rhinol Laryngol* |
| *Annals of Surgery* | *Ann Surg* |
| *Annals of Thoracic Surgery* | *Ann Thorac Surg* |
| *Archives of Disease in Childhood* | *Arch Dis Child* |
| *Archives of Disease in Childhood: Fetal & Neonatal Edition* | *Arch Dis Child Fetal Neonatal Ed* |
| *Archives of Environmental & Occupational Health* | *Arch Environ Occup Health* |
| *Archives of Pathology & Laboratory Medicine* | *Arch Pathol Lab Med* |

| | |
|---|---|
| *Archives of Physical Medicine and Rehabilitation* | *Arch Phys Med Rehabil* |
| *Arthritis & Rheumatology* | *Arthritis Rheumatol* |
| *BJOG* | *BJOG* |
| *Blood* | *Blood* |
| *BMJ* | *BMJ* |
| *Brain: A Journal of Neurology* | *Brain* |
| *British Journal of Radiology* | *Br J Radiol* |
| *British Journal of Surgery* | *Br J Surg* |
| *CA: A Cancer Journal for Clinicians* | *CA Cancer J Clin* |
| *Cancer* | *Cancer* |
| *Chest* | *Chest* |
| *Circulation* | *Circulation* |
| *Clinical Orthopaedics and Related Research* | *Clin Orthop* |
| *Clinical Pediatrics* | *Clin Pediatr (Phila)* |
| *Clinical Pharmacology & Therapeutics* | *Clin Pharmacol Ther* |
| *Clinical Toxicology* | *Clin Toxicol* |
| *CMAJ* | *CMAJ* |
| *Critical Care Medicine* | *Crit Care Med* |
| *Current Problems in Surgery* | *Curr Probl Surg* |
| *Diabetes* | *Diabetes* |
| *Digestive Diseases and Sciences* | *Dig Dis Sci* |
| *Disease-a-Month* | *Dis Mon* |
| *Endocrinology* | *Endocrinology* |
| *Gastroenterology* | *Gastroenterology* |
| *Geriatrics* | *Geriatrics* |
| *Gut* | *Gut* |
| *H&HN: Hospitals & Health Networks* | *Hosp Health Netw* |
| *Heart* | *Heart* |
| *Heart & Lung: The Journal of Critical Care* | *Heart Lung* |
| *Hospital Practice* | *Hosp Pract* |
| *JAMA* | *JAMA* |

| | |
|---|---|
| *JAMA Cardiology* | *JAMA Cardiol* |
| *JAMA Dermatology* | *JAMA Dermatol* |
| *JAMA Internal Medicine* | *JAMA Intern Med* |
| *JAMA Network Open* | *JAMA Netw Open* |
| *JAMA Neurology* | *JAMA Neurol* |
| *JAMA Oncology* | *JAMA Oncol* |
| *JAMA Ophthalmology* | *JAMA Ophthalmol* |
| *JAMA Otolaryngology–Head & Neck Surgery* | *JAMA Otolaryngol* |
| *JAMA Pediatrics* | *JAMA Pediatr* |
| *JAMA Psychiatry* | *JAMA Psychiatry* |
| *JAMA Surgery* | *JAMA Surg* |
| *Journal of the Academy of Nutrition and Dietetics* | *J Acad Nutr Diet* |
| *Journal of Allergy and Clinical Immunology* | *J Allergy Clin Immunol* |
| *Journal of the American College of Cardiology* | *J Am Coll Cardiol* |
| *Journal of the American College of Surgeons* | *J Am Coll Surg* |
| *Journal of Bone & Joint Surgery: American Volume* | *J Bone Joint Surg Am* |
| *Journal of Clinical Endocrinology & Metabolism* | *J Clin Endocrinol Metab* |
| *Journal of Clinical Investigation* | *J Clin Invest* |
| *Journal of Clinical Pathology* | *J Clin Pathol* |
| *Journal of Family Practice* | *J Fam Pract* |
| *Journal of Immunology* | *J Immunol* |
| *Journal of Laryngology & Otology* | *J Laryngol Otol* |
| *Journal of Nervous and Mental Disease* | *J Nerv Ment Dis* |
| *Journal of Neurosurgery* | *J Neurosurg* |
| *Journal of Nursing Administration* | *J Nurs Adm* |
| *Journal of Oral and Maxillofacial Surgery* | *J Oral Maxillofac Surg* |
| *Journal of Pediatrics* | *J Pediatr* |
| *Journal of Thoracic and Cardiovascular Surgery* | *J Thorac Cardiovasc Surg* |

| | |
|---|---|
| *Journal of Trauma and Acute Care Surgery* | *J Trauma* |
| *Journal of Urology* | *J Urol* |
| *Journals of Gerontology: Series A, Biological Sciences & Medical Sciences* | *J Gerontol A Biol Sci Med Sci* |
| *Journals of Gerontology: Series B, Psychological Sciences & Social Sciences* | *J Gerontol B Psychol Sci Soc Sci* |
| *Lancet* | *Lancet* |
| *Mayo Clinic Proceedings* | *Mayo Clin Proc* |
| *Medical Clinics of North America* | *Med Clin North Am* |
| *Medical Letter on Drugs and Therapeutics* | *Med Lett Drugs Ther* |
| *Medicine: Analytical Reviews of General Medicine, Neurology,Psychiatry, Dermatology, and Pediatrics* | *Medicine (Baltimore)* |
| *Neurology* | *Neurology* |
| *New England Journal of Medicine* | *N Engl J Med* |
| *Nursing Clinics of North America* | *Nurs Clin North Am* |
| *Nursing Outlook* | *Nurs Outlook* |
| *Nursing Research* | *Nurs Res* |
| *Obstetrics & Gynecology* | *Obstet Gynecol* |
| *Orthopedic Clinics of North America* | *Orthop Clin North Am* |
| *Pediatric Clinics of North America* | *Pediatr Clin North Am* |
| *Pediatrics* | *Pediatrics* |
| *Physical Therapy* | *Phys Ther* |
| *Plastic and Reconstructive Surgery* | *Plast Reconstr Surg* |
| *Postgraduate Medicine* | *Postgrad Med* |
| *Progress in Cardiovascular Diseases* | *Prog Cardiovasc Dis* |
| *Public Health Reports* | *Public Health Rep* |
| *Radiologic Clinics of North America* | *Radiol Clin North Am* |
| *Radiology* | *Radiology* |
| *Southern Medical Journal* | *South Med J* |
| *Surgery* | *Surgery* |

| | |
|---|---|
| *Surgical Clinics of North America* | *Surg Clin North Am* |
| *Translational Research: Journal of Laboratory and Clinical Medicine* | *Translational Res* |
| *Urologic Clinics of North America* | *Urol Clin North Am* |

The National Library of Medicine's (NLM's) abbreviations are based on the American National Standard for Information Sciences—Abbreviation of Titles of Publications (ANSI Z39.5) (1985), as well as abbreviations formulated under earlier ANSI guidelines. Note that these abbreviations are capitalized and that articles, conjunctions, prepositions, punctuation, and diacritical marks are omitted in the abbreviated title form. Guidance for forming the abbreviated titles of journals indexed in PubMed can be found at https://www.nlm.nih.gov/tsd/cataloging/contructitleabbre.html.

The NLM's database can be searched using the journal title, the MEDLINE/PubMed title abbreviation, the PubMed ID (PMID) (NLM's unique journal identifier), the ISO (International Organization for Standardization) abbreviation, and the print and electronic International Standard Serial Numbers (pISSNs and eISSNs). The following list includes words commonly found in titles of journals and guidance on their abbreviation for reference lists. Note that some variations on a journal title word (eg, *Advanced, Advancement*, and *Advances*) use the same abbreviation (*Adv*).

| Word | Abbreviation (or word used) |
|---|---|
| Abnormal | Abnorm |
| Abuse | Abuse |
| Academia | Acad |
| Academy | Acad |
| Acoustical | Acoust |
| Actions | Actions |
| Acupuncture | Acupunct |
| Acute | Acute |
| Addiction (Addictions) | Addict |
| Additives | Addit |
| Administration | Adm |
| Adolescence | Adolescence |
| Adolescent | Adolesc |
| Advanced (Advancement, Advances) | Adv |
| Adverse | Adverse |

| | |
|---|---|
| Aesthetic | Aesthetic |
| Affairs | Aff |
| Affective | Affective |
| African | Afr |
| Age | Age |
| Ageing | Ageing |
| Agents | Agents |
| Aging | Aging |
| Air | Air |
| Alabama | Ala |
| Alaska | Alaska |
| Alcohol (Alcoholism) | Alcohol |
| Allergy | Allergy |
| Allied | Allied |
| America (American) | Am |
| Anaesthesia (Anaesthetists) | Anaesth |
| Anaesthetist | Anaesthetist |
| Analgesia | Analg |
| Anatomical (Anatomy) | Anat |
| Andrology | Androl |
| Anesthesia | Anesth |
| Anesthesiology | Anesthesiol |
| Angiology | Angiol |
| Angle | Angle |
| Animal | Anim |
| Ankle | Ankle |
| Annals | Ann |
| Annual | Annu |
| Anthropology | Anthropol |
| Antibiotics | Antibiot |
| Anticancer | Anticancer |
| Antigens | Antigens |

| | |
|---|---|
| Antimicrobial | Antimicrob |
| Antiviral | Antiviral |
| Apheresis | Apheresis |
| Appetite | Appetite |
| Applied | Appl |
| Archives | Arch |
| Argentina | Argent |
| Arizona | Ariz |
| Arkansas | Ark |
| Army | Army |
| Arteriosclerosis | Arterioscl |
| Artery | Artery |
| Arthritis | Arthritis |
| Artificial | Artif |
| Asian | Asian |
| Assessment | Assess |
| Association | Assoc |
| Asthma | Asthma |
| Audiology | Audiol |
| Audiovisual | Audiov |
| Auditory | Aud |
| Australia (Australian) | Aust |
| Autism | Autism |
| Autonomic | Auton |
| Avian | Avian |
| Aviation | Aviat |
| | |
| Bacteriology | Bacteriol |
| Bangladesh | Bangladesh |
| Basic | Basic |
| Behavior (Behavioral, Behaviors) | Behav |
| Biochemical (Biochemistry) | Biochem |
| Biocommunications | Biocomm |

| | |
|---|---|
| Biofeedback | Biofeedback |
| Biological (Biology) | Biol |
| Biomaterials | Biomater |
| Biomechanical | Biomech |
| Biomedical | Biomed |
| Biometrics | Biometrics |
| Biophysical (Biophysics) | Biophys |
| Bioscience | Biosci |
| Biosocial | Biosoc |
| Biosystems | Biosystems |
| Biotechnological (Biotechnology) | Biotechnol |
| Birth | Birth |
| Blood | Blood |
| Bone | Bone |
| Brain | Brain |
| Brazilian | Braz |
| Breast | Breast |
| British | Br |
| Bulletin | Bull |
| Burns | Burns |
| | |
| Calcified | Calcif |
| Calcium | Calcium |
| Canadian | Can |
| Cancer | Cancer |
| Carbohydrate | Carbohydr |
| Carcinogenesis | Carcinog |
| Cardiography | Cardiogr |
| Cardiology | Cardiol |
| Cardiovascular | Cardiovasc |
| Care | Care |
| Caries | Caries |
| Catheterization | Cathet |

| | |
|---|---|
| Cell (Cellular) | Cell |
| Cells | Cells |
| Central | Cent |
| Cephalagia | Cephalagia |
| Cerebral | Cereb |
| Ceylon | Ceylon |
| Chemical (Chemicals, Chemistry, Chemists) | Chem |
| Chemotherapy | Chemother |
| Chest | Chest |
| Child (Childhood, Children) | Child |
| Child's | Childs |
| Chinese | Chin |
| Chromatographic (Chromatography) | Chromatogr |
| Chronic | Chronic |
| Chronicle | Chron |
| Circulation (Circulatory) | Circ |
| Cleft | Cleft |
| Cleveland | Cleve |
| Clinic (Clinical, Clinics) | Clin |
| Cognition | Cogn |
| Collagen | Coll |
| College | Coll |
| Colon | Colon |
| Colorado | Colo |
| Communicable | Commun |
| Communication (Communications) | Commun |
| Community | Community |
| Comparative | Comp |
| Complement | Complement |
| Comprehensive | Compr |
| Computerized (Computers) | Comput |
| Connecticut | Conn |

| | |
|---|---|
| Connective | Connect |
| Consulting | Counsult |
| Contact | Contact |
| Contaminants (Contamination) | Contam |
| Contemporary | Contemp |
| Contributions | Contrib |
| Control (Controlled) | Control |
| Copenhagen | Copenh |
| Cornea | Cornea |
| Cornell | Cornell |
| Corps | Corps |
| Cortex | Cortex |
| Council | Counc |
| Craniofacial | Craniofac |
| Critical | Crit |
| Cryobiology | Cryobiol |
| Culture | Cult |
| Current (Currents) | Curr |
| Cutaneous | Cutan |
| Cutis | Cutis |
| Cybernetics | Cybern |
| Cyclic | Cyclic |
| Cytogenetics | Cytogenet |
| Cytology | Cytol |
| Cytometry | Cytometry |
| | |
| Dairy | Dairy |
| Danish | Dan |
| Deaf | Deaf |
| Defects | Defects |
| Deficiency | Defic |
| Delivery | Deliv |
| Demography | Demogr |

| | |
|---|---|
| Dental (Dentistry) | Dent |
| Dependencies | Dependencies |
| Dermatitis | Dermatitis |
| Dermatological (Dermatology) | Dermatol |
| Dermatopathology | Dermatopathol |
| Detection | Detect |
| Development | Dev |
| Devices | Devices |
| Diabetes | Diabetes |
| Diagnosis (Diagnostic) | Diagn |
| Dialysis | Dial |
| Diarrhoeal | Diarrhoeal |
| Dietetic | Diet |
| Differentiation | Differ |
| Digestion | Digestion |
| Digestive | Dig |
| Dimensions | Dimens |
| Directions (Directors) | Dir |
| Discussions | Discuss |
| Disease (Diseases) | Dis |
| Disorders | Disord |
| Disposition | Dispos |
| DNA | DNA |
| Drug | Drug |
| Drugs | Drugs |
| | |
| Ear | Ear |
| Early | Early |
| East African | East Afr |
| Economic | Econ |
| Ecotoxicology | Ecotoxicol |
| Educational | Educ |
| Egypt | Egypt |

| | |
|---|---|
| Electrocardiology | Electrocardiol |
| Electroencephalography | Electroencephalogr |
| Electromyography | Electromyogr |
| Electron | Electron |
| Electrotherapeutics | Electrother |
| Embryo | Embryo |
| Embryology | Embryol |
| Emergency | Emerg |
| Endocrine | Endocr |
| Endocrinological (Endocrinology) | Endocrinol |
| Endoscopy | Endosc |
| Engineering | Eng |
| Enteral | Enteral |
| Entomology | Entomol |
| Environmental | Environ |
| Enzyme | Enzyme |
| Enzymology | Enzymol |
| Epidemiologic (Epidemiology) | Epidemiol |
| Ergology | Ergol |
| Ergonomics | Ergonomics |
| Essays | Essays |
| Ethics | Ethics |
| Eugenics | Eugen |
| European | Eur |
| Evaluation | Eval |
| Exceptional | Except |
| Exercise | Exerc |
| Experimental | Exp |
| Eye | Eye |
| | |
| Factors | Factors |
| Family | Fam |
| Federation | Fed |

| | |
|---|---|
| Fertility | Fertil |
| Finnish | Finn |
| Fitness | Fitness |
| Florida | Fla |
| Food | Food |
| Foot | Foot |
| Forensic | Forensic |
| Foundation | Found |
| Function | Funct |
| Fundamental | Fundam |
| | |
| Gastroenterology | Gastroenterol |
| Gastrointestinal | Gastrointest |
| Gene | Gene |
| General | Gen |
| Genetic | Genet |
| Genetics | Genetics |
| Genitourinary | Genitourin |
| Geographical | Geogr |
| Georgia | Ga |
| Geriatric (Geriatrics) | Geriatr |
| Gerontologist | Gerontologist |
| Gerontology | Gerontol |
| Group | Group |
| Groups | Groups |
| Growth | Growth |
| Gut | Gut |
| Gynaecological (Gynaecology) | Gynaecol |
| Gynecologic (Gynecology) | Gynecol |
| | |
| Haematology | Haematol |
| Haemostasis | Haemost |
| Hastings Center | Hastings Cent |

| | |
|---|---|
| Hawaii | Hawaii |
| Head | Head |
| Headache | Headache |
| Health | Health |
| Hearing | Hear |
| Heart | Heart |
| Hematological (Hematology) | Hematol |
| Hemoglobin | Hemoglobin |
| Hemostasis | Hemost |
| Hepatology | Hepatol |
| Heredity | Hered |
| Hip | Hip |
| Histochemical (Histochemistry) | Histochem |
| Histology | Histol |
| Histopathology | Histopathol |
| History | Hist |
| Homosexuality | Homosex |
| Horizons | Horiz |
| Hormone (Hormones) | Horm |
| Hospital | Hosp |
| Hospitals | Hospitals |
| Human (Humans) | Hum |
| Hybridoma | Hybridoma |
| Hygiene | Hyg |
| Hypertension | Hypertens |
| Hypnosis | Hypn |
| Hypotheses | Hypotheses |
| | |
| Imaging | Imaging |
| Immunity | Immun |
| Immunoassay | Immunoassay |
| Immunobiology | Immunobiol |
| Immunogenetics | Immunogenet |

| | |
|---|---|
| Immunological (Immunology) | Immunol |
| Immunopharmacology | Immunopharmacol |
| Immunotherapy | Immunother |
| Implant | Implant |
| Including | Incl |
| India | India |
| Indian | Indian |
| Indiana | Indiana |
| Industrial | Ind |
| Infection (Infectious) | Infect |
| Inflammation | Inflamm |
| Informatics | Inform |
| Information | Inf |
| Inherited | Inherited |
| Injury | Inj |
| Inorganic | Inorg |
| Inquiry | Inquiry |
| Institutes | Inst |
| Instrumentation | Instrum |
| Insurance | Insur |
| Intellectual | Intellect |
| Intensive | Intensive |
| Interactions | Interact |
| Interferon | Interferon |
| Internal | Intern |
| International | Int |
| Internist | Internist |
| Interventional | Intervent |
| Intervirology | Intervirol |
| Intraocular | Intraocul |
| Invasion | Invasion |
| Invertebrate | Invertebr |

| | |
|---|---|
| Investigation (Investigations, Investigative) | Invest |
| Investigational | Investig |
| In Vitro | In Vitro |
| In Vivo | In Vivo |
| Iowa | Iowa |
| Irish | Ir |
| Isotopes | Isot |
| Isozymes | Isozymes |
| Israel | Isr |
| Issues | Issues |
| Istanbul | Istanbul |
| | |
| Japanese | Jpn |
| Joint | Joint |
| Journal | J |
| | |
| Kansas | Kans |
| Kentucky | Ky |
| Kidney | Kidney |
| Kinetics | Kinet |
| | |
| Laboratory | Lab |
| Language | Lang |
| Laparoendoscopic | Laparoendosc |
| Laryngology | Laryngol |
| Larynx | Larynx |
| Lasers | Lasers |
| Law | Law |
| Lectures | Lect |
| Legal | Leg |
| Leprosy | Lepr |
| Letters | Lett |
| Leukocyte | Leukoc |

| | |
|---|---|
| Leukotriene | Leukotriene |
| Leukotrienes | Leukotrienes |
| Library | Libr |
| Life | Life |
| Life-threatening | Life Threat |
| Lipid | Lipid |
| Lipids | Lipids |
| Literature | Lit |
| Louisiana | La |
| Lung | Lung |
| Lymphokine | Lymphokine |
| Lymphology | Lymphol |
| | |
| Madagascar | Madagascar |
| Magnesium | Magnesium |
| Magnetic | Magn |
| Main | Main |
| Making | Making |
| Malaysia | Malaysia |
| Management | Manage |
| Manipulative | Manipulative |
| Marital | Marital |
| Maritime | Marit |
| Maryland | Md |
| Mass | Mass |
| Mathematical | Math |
| Maxillofacial | Maxillofac |
| Measurement | Meas |
| Mechanisms | Mech |
| Media | Media |
| Medical (Medicine, Medicinal) | Med |
| Membrane | Membrane |
| Mental | Ment |

| | |
|---|---|
| Metabolic (Metabolism) | Metab |
| Metastasis | Metastasis |
| Methods | Methods |
| Mexico | Mex |
| Michigan | Mich |
| Microbial | Microb |
| Microbiological | Microbiol |
| Microcirculation | Microcirc |
| Microscopy | Microsc |
| Microvascular | Microvasc |
| Microwave | Microw |
| Military | Milit |
| Mineral | Miner |
| Minnesota | Minn |
| Mississippi | Miss |
| Missouri | Mo |
| Modification | Modif |
| Molecular | Mol |
| Monographs | Monogr |
| Morphology | Morphol |
| Motility | Motil |
| Muscle | Muscle |
| Mutagenesis | Mutagen |
| Mutation | Mutat |
| Mycobacterial | Mycobact |
| | |
| Narcotics | Narc |
| National | Natl |
| Natural (Nature) | Nat |
| Naval | Nav |
| Nebraska | Nebr |
| Neck | Neck |
| Neglect | Negl |

| | |
|---|---|
| Neonate | Neonate |
| Nephrology | Nephrol |
| Nephron | Nephron |
| Nervosa (Nervous) | Nerv |
| Netherlands | Neth |
| Neural | Neural |
| Neurobehavioral | Neurobehav |
| Neurobiology | Neurobiol |
| Neurochemistry | Neurochem |
| Neurocytology | Neurocytol |
| Neuroendocrinology | Neuroendocrinol |
| Neurogenetics | Neurogenet |
| Neuroimmunology | Neuroimmunol |
| Neurologic (Neurological, Neurology) | Neurol |
| Neuropathology | Neuropathol |
| Neuropediatrics | Neuropediatr |
| Neuropeptides | Neuropeptides |
| Neuropharmacology | Neuropharmacol |
| Neurophysiology | Neurophysiol |
| Neuropsychobiology | Neuropsychobiol |
| Neuropsychology | Neuropsychol |
| Neuropsychopharmacology | Neuropsychopharmacol |
| Neuroradiology | Neuroradiol |
| Neuroscience | Neurosci |
| Neurosurgery (Neurosurgical) | Neurosurg |
| Neurotoxicology | Neurotoxicol |
| Neurotrauma | Neurotrauma |
| New | N |
| New England | N Engl |
| New Jersey | N J |
| New Orleans | New Orleans |
| New York | N Y |

| | |
|---|---|
| New Zealand | N Z |
| North America | North Am |
| North Carolina | N C |
| Nose | Nose |
| Nuclear | Nucl |
| Nucleotide | Nucleotide |
| Nurse | Nurse |
| Nursing | Nurs |
| Nutrition (Nutritional) | Nutr |
| | |
| Obesity | Obes |
| Obstetric (Obstetrics) | Obstet |
| Occupational | Occup |
| Ocular | Ocul |
| Official | Off |
| Ohio | Ohio |
| Oklahoma | Okla |
| Oncology | Oncol |
| Ophthalmic | Ophthalmic |
| Ophthalmological (Ophthalmology) | Ophthalmol |
| Optical (Optics) | Opt |
| Optometric (Optometry) | Optom |
| Oral | Oral |
| Organization | Organ |
| Organs | Organs |
| Orthodontics | Orthod |
| Orthopaedic | Orthop |
| Orthopsychiatry | Orthopsychiatry |
| Orthotics | Orthot |
| Osaka | Osaka |
| Oslo | Oslo |
| Osteopathic | Osteopath |
| Otolaryngology | Otolaryngol |

| | |
|---|---|
| Otology | Otol |
| Otorhinolaryngology | Otorhinolaryngol |
| | |
| Pace | Pace |
| Paediatric (Paediatrics) | Paediatr |
| Palate | Palate |
| Panama | Panama |
| Pan American | Pan Am |
| Paper | Pap |
| Papua New Guinea | Papua New Guinea |
| Parasite | Parasite |
| Parasitology | Parasitol |
| Parenteral | Parenter |
| Pathology | Pathol |
| Pediatrician | Pediatrician |
| Pediatrics | Pediatr |
| Pennsylvania | Pa |
| Peptide (Peptides) | Pept |
| Perception | Perception |
| Perceptual | Percept |
| Perinatal | Perinat |
| Perinatology | Perinatol |
| Periodontal (Periodontology) | Periodont |
| Personality | Pers |
| Perspectives | Perspect |
| Pharmaceutical (Pharmacy) | Pharm |
| Pharmacokinetics | Parmacokinet |
| Pharmacology | Pharmacol |
| Pharmacopsychiatry | Pharmacopsychiatry |
| Pharmacotherapy | Pharmacother |
| Philosophical | Philos |
| Phosphorylation | Phosphorylation |
| Photobiology | Photobiol |

| | |
|---|---|
| Photochemistry | Photochem |
| Photodermatology | Photodermatol |
| Photography | Photogr |
| Physical (Physics) | Phys |
| Physician | Physician |
| Physicians | Physicians |
| Physiological (Physiology) | Physiol |
| Placenta | Placenta |
| Planning | Plann |
| Plastic | Plast |
| Podiatric | Podiatr |
| Podiatry | Podiatry |
| Poisoning | Poisoning |
| Policy | Policy |
| Politics | Polit |
| Pollution | Pollut |
| Population | Popul |
| Postgraduate | Postgrad |
| Poultry | Poult |
| Practice (Practitioners) | Pract |
| Pregnancy | Pregnancy |
| Prenatal | Prenat |
| Preparative | Prep |
| Prevention (Preventive) | Prev |
| Primary | Primary |
| Primatology | Primatol |
| Proceedings | Proc |
| Process | Process |
| Processes | Processes |
| Products | Prod |
| Programs | Programs |
| Progress | Prog |

| | |
|---|---|
| Prostaglandin | Prostaglandin |
| Prostaglandins | Prostaglandins |
| Prostate | Prostate |
| Prosthetic (Prosthetics) | Prosthet |
| Protein | Protein |
| Protozoology | Protozool |
| Psyche | Psyche |
| Psychiatric | Psychiatr |
| Psychiatry | Psychiatry |
| Psychoactive | Psychoactive |
| Psychoanalysis (Psychoanalytic) | Psychoanal |
| Psycholinguistic | Psycholinguist |
| Psychologist (Psychology) | Psychol |
| Psychoneuroendocrinology | Psychoneuroendocrinol |
| Psychopathology | Psychopathol |
| Psychopharmacology | Psychopharmacol |
| Psychophysiology | Psychophysiol |
| Psychosocial | Psychosoc |
| Psychosomatic (Psychosomatics) | Psychosom |
| Psychotherapy | Psychother |
| Public | Public |
| Puerto Rico | P R |
| | |
| Quantitative | Quant |
| Quarterly | Q |
| | |
| Radiation | Radiat |
| Radiography | Radiogr |
| Radioisotopes | Radioisotopes |
| Radiologists (Radiology) | Radiol |
| Rational | Ration |
| Reactions | React |
| Recombinant | Recomb |

| | |
|---|---|
| Reconstructive | Reconstr |
| Record | Rec |
| Rectum | Rectum |
| Regional | Reg |
| Regulation (Regulatory) | Regul |
| Rehabilitation | Rehabil |
| Renal | Renal |
| Report (Reports) | Rep |
| Reproduction (Reproductive) | Reprod |
| Research | Res |
| Residue | Residue |
| Resonance | Reson |
| Respiration (Respiratory) | Respir |
| Response | Response |
| Resuscitation | Resuscitation |
| Retardation | Retard |
| Retina | Retina |
| Review (Reviews) | Rev |
| Rheumatic (Rheumatism) | Rheum |
| Rheumatology | Rheumatol |
| Rhinology | Rhinol |
| Rhode Island | R I |
| | |
| Safety | Safety |
| Scandinavian | Scand |
| Scanning | Scan |
| Schizophrenia | Schizophr |
| School | Sch |
| Science (Sciences, Scientific) | Sci |
| Scottish | Scott |
| Security | Secur |
| Seminars | Semin |
| Series | Ser |

| | |
|---|---|
| Service | Serv |
| Sex (Sexual, Sexually) | Sex |
| Shock | Shock |
| Singapore | Singapore |
| Skeletal | Skeletal |
| Sleep | Sleep |
| Social (Societies, Society) | Soc |
| Sociological (Sociology) | Sociol |
| Somatic | Somatic |
| Somatosensory | Somatosens |
| South African | S Afr |
| South Carolina | S C |
| South Dakota | S D |
| Southeast | Southeast |
| Southern | South |
| Space | Space |
| Spectrometry | Spectrom |
| Speech | Speech |
| Spine | Spine |
| Sports | Sports |
| Stain | Stain |
| Standardization (Standards) | Stand |
| Statistical | Stat |
| Steroid | Steroid |
| Steroids | Steroids |
| Stockholm | Stockh |
| Strabismus | Strabismus |
| Stress | Stress |
| Stroke | Stroke |
| Structure | Struct |
| Studies | Stud |
| Subcellular | Subcell |

| | |
|---|---|
| Submicroscopic | Submicrosc |
| Substance | Subst |
| Suicide | Suicide |
| Superior | Super |
| Support | Support |
| Surgeon (Surgeons, Surgery, Surgical) | Surg |
| Swedish | Swed |
| Symposia (Symposium) | Symp |
| System (Systems) | Syst |
| | |
| Technical | Tech |
| Technology | Technol |
| Tennessee | Tenn |
| Teratogenesis | Teratogenesis |
| Teratology | Teratol |
| Thailand | Thai |
| Theoretical | Theor |
| Therapeutics (Therapies, Therapy) | Ther |
| Thermal | Therm |
| Thoracic | Thorac |
| Thorax | Thorax |
| Throat | Throat |
| Thrombosis | Thromb |
| Thromboxane | Thromboxane |
| Thymus | Thymus |
| Tissue | Tissue |
| Today | Today |
| Tokyo | Tokyo |
| Tomography | Tomogr |
| Topics | Top |
| Total | Total |
| Toxicologic (Toxicological, Toxicology) | Toxicol |
| Traditional | Tradit |

| | |
|---|---|
| Transactions | Trans |
| Transfer | Transfer |
| Transfusion | Transfusion |
| Transmission (Transmitted) | Transm |
| Transplant | Transplant |
| Transplantation | Transplantation |
| Traumatic | Trauma |
| Tropical | Trop |
| Tuberculosis | Tuberc |
| Tumor | Tumor |
| Tumour | Tumour |
| Tunis | Tunis |
| Turkish | Turk |
| | |
| Ulster | Ulster |
| Ultramicroscopy | Ultramicrosc |
| Ultrasonic | Ultrason |
| Ultrasonics | Ultrasonics |
| Ultrasound | Ultrasound |
| Ultrastructural (Ultrastructure) | Ultrastruct |
| Undersea | Undersea |
| Union | Union |
| Uremia | Uremia |
| | |
| Vision (Visual) | Vis |
| Vital | Vital |
| Vitamin (Vitamins) | Vitam |
| Vitaminology | Vitaminol |
| Vitro | Vitro |
| Vivo | Vivo |
| | |
| Welfare | Welfare |
| Western | West |

| | |
|---|---|
| West Indian | West Indian |
| West Virginia | W Va |
| Wildlife | Wildl |
| Wisconsin | Wis |
| Women | Women |
| Women's | Womens |
| | |
| Zoology | Zool |
| Zoonoses | Zoonoses |

**13.11** **Clinical, Technical, and Other Common Terms.** This compilation of clinical, technical, and other common terms and their abbreviations is not intended to be all-encompassing but is provided as a brief reference. There are many published listings of abbreviations, acronyms, and initialisms (see 23.0, Resources). If searching the internet, choose an authoritative source because abbreviations may vary from entity to entity.

Many entities share the same abbreviation (eg, AMA for the American Management Association, American Marketing Association, American Medical Association, Academy of Model Aeronautics, American Motorcycle Association, American Music Association, and Art Museum of the Americas). Thus, preciseness takes precedence over the urge to abbreviate.

In addition, some abbreviations encompass more than one grammatical variant (eg, noun, adjective) of a term. For example, ECG represents both electrocardiogram and electrocardiographic. It is unnecessary to redefine the abbreviation for each variation in usage within a body of work. Similarly, terms that have singular and plural forms (eg, NSAID and NSAIDs) are defined once, whichever form is mentioned first.

It is not necessary to reexpand an abbreviation after its components have been defined earlier in a manuscript. For example, if "acute myocardial infarction (AMI)" appears in a manuscript, later mentions of "MI" need not be expanded again. In addition, if "myocardial infarction (MI)" appears in a manuscript, a later mention of "acute myocardial infarction (AMI)" can be presented as "acute MI (AMI)."

Do not make abbreviations possessive at first mention, even if the expanded form is possessive at first mention. It is often preferable to reword the sentence.

> *Avoid:* The US Department of Health and Human Services' (HHS') strategic plan will be updated periodically to reflect the department's strategies, actions, and progress toward its goals.

> *Better:* The US Department of Health and Human Services (HHS) will update its strategic plan periodically to reflect the department's strategies, actions, and progress toward its goals.

Most terms should be expanded at first mention. However, considerations for when this general rule might be set aside include comprehensibility, recognition, and space, as well as avoidance of cumbersome expressions. It is often preferred to use the abbreviation instead of the expansion in a long title or subtitle, a letter to the editor, a short social media post, or an informal essay.

Use common sense in deciding whether to abbreviate the terms in the following list and other terms. For example, if "acute respiratory distress syndrome" appears only once or twice in an article, spell it out. If the article discusses acute respiratory distress syndrome and the term is used several times, expand the term at first mention with the abbreviation (ARDS) immediately following in parentheses. Abbreviate it thereafter, except at the beginning of a sentence (but see below). Some terms may be known better in their abbreviated form (eg, HIPAA), and abbreviating them at first mention (with the expanded form following in parentheses) may be appropriate.

It is preferred not to use abbreviations at the beginning of a sentence. Exceptions can be made if the expansion is especially cumbersome, such as a collaborative group or clinical trial name or other acronym pronounced as a word (NICE, DECAAF, AIDS, CLIA, UNICEF) or if the abbreviation appears so often in the text that it is easily understood.

> FDG-PET/CT imaging should be used to determine whether the next step should be biopsy or surgical resection [instead of "$^{18}$F-fludeoxyglucose–positron emission tomography/computed tomography (FDG-PET/CT) imaging should be used . . . "].

> US health care is in the midst of substantial change, potentially challenging the well-established self-governing structure of the medical profession and the professionalism of physicians [instead of "United States health care is in the midst of substantial change,. . . "].

> PICO (population, intervention, comparison, outcome) tables were constructed using evidence from a broad review of the literature.

Also, avoid introducing an abbreviation in a heading:

*Avoid:*
**Attention-Deficit/Hyperactivity Disorder (ADHD)**
Childhood disorders, such as ADHD, often persist into adolescence, when motor vehicle crash risk peaks.

*Preferred:*
**Attention-Deficit/Hyperactivity Disorder**
Childhood disorders, such as attention-deficit/hyperactivity disorder (ADHD), often persist into adolescence, when motor vehicle crash risk peaks.

Use an appropriate article (*a* or *an*) before an abbreviation according to the sound following the article (eg, a UN resolution, an ACE inhibitor) (see 7.3.2, Indefinite Articles, and 11.11, Articles).

Note: At a 2004 National Summit on Medical Abbreviations, The Joint Commission on Accreditation of Healthcare Organizations approved an official "do not use" list of abbreviations. This list applies to all medical orders and all medication-related documentation that are handwritten or on preprinted forms used in hospitals and other health care facilities and is designed to protect patients from potential harm. The Joint Commission's requirement does not necessarily apply to the use of abbreviations in the publication of articles in scientific journals. The Joint Commission's list is available at https://www.jointcommission.org/facts_about_do_not_use_list/.

### Common Abbreviations and Expansions

Abbreviations that do not require expansion are noted.

| Abbreviation | Expanded form |
| --- | --- |
| AAA | abdominal aortic aneurysm |
| ABC | avidin-biotin complex |
| ABG | arterial blood gas |
| ABI | ankle-brachial index |
| AC | alternating current |
| ACA | Patient Protection and Affordable Care Act |
| ACE | angiotensin-converting enzyme |
| ACEI | angiotensin-converting enzyme inhibitor |
| ACL | anterior cruciate ligament |
| ACLS | advanced cardiac life support |
| ACO | accountable care organization |
| ACS | acute coronary syndrome |
| ACTH | Use *corticotropin* (previously adrenocorticotropic hormone) |
| AD | Alzheimer disease |
| ADH | antidiuretic hormone |
| ADHD | attention-deficit/hyperactivity disorder |
| ADL | activities of daily living (but 1 ADL, 6 ADLs) |
| aDNA | ancient DNA |
| ADP | adenosine diphosphate |
| ADPase | adenosine diphosphatase |
| AED | automated external defibrillator; antiepileptic drug |
| AF | atrial fibrillation |
| AFP | $\alpha$-fetoprotein |
| AGREE | Appraisal of Guidelines for Research & Evaluation |

| | |
|---|---|
| AI | artificial intelligence |
| AIDS | acquired immunodeficiency syndrome (no need to expand) |
| AKA | above-the-knee [amputation] |
| ALL | acute lymphoblastic leukemia; acute lymphocytic leukemia |
| ALS | amyotrophic lateral sclerosis |
| ALT | alanine aminotransferase (previously SGPT) |
| AMI | acute myocardial infarction |
| AML | acute monocytic leukemia; acute myeloblastic leukemia; acute myelocytic leukemia |
| AMP | adenosine monophosphate |
| ANA | antinuclear antibody |
| ANCOVA | analysis of covariance |
| ANDA | abbreviated new drug application |
| ANLL | acute nonlymphocytic leukemia |
| ANOVA | analysis of variance |
| ANP | atrial natriuretic peptide |
| AOR | adjusted odds ratio |
| APACHE | Acute Physiology and Chronic Health Evaluation |
| APB | atrial premature beat |
| APC | atrial premature contraction |
| apo | apolipoprotein (apo AI, apoB, etc) |
| ARB | angiotensin receptor blocker (angiotensin subtypes I and II: AT1 and AT2) |
| ARC | AIDS-related complex (use *symptomatic HIV infection*) |
| ARDS | acute respiratory distress syndrome |
| ARMD | age-related macular degeneration |
| ARR | absolute risk reduction |
| ARRIVE | Animal Research: Reporting of In Vivo Experiments |
| ART | antiretroviral therapy |
| ASC | atypical squamous cell |
| ASC-US | atypical squamous cells of uncertain significance |
| ASCVD | atherosclerotic cardiovascular disease |
| ASD | atrial septal defect; autism spectrum disorder |
| AST | aspartate aminotransferase (previously SGOT) |

| | |
|---|---|
| ATP | adenosine triphosphate |
| ATPase | adenosine triphosphatase |
| AUC | area under the curve |
| AUD | alcohol use disorder |
| AUROC | area under the receiver operating characteristic curve |
| AVM | arteriovenous malformation |
| | |
| BAC | blood alcohol concentration |
| BAER | brainstem auditory evoked response |
| BAL | bronchoalveolar lavage |
| BCG | bacille Calmette-Guérin (but do not expand as a drug: BCG vaccine) |
| BCLS | basic cardiac life support |
| BDI | Beck Depression Inventory |
| bid | twice a day (do not use) |
| BKA | below-the-knee amputation |
| BMD | bone mineral density |
| BMI | body mass index |
| BMT | bone marrow transplantation |
| BNP | B-type natriuretic peptide; brain-type natriuretic peptide |
| BP | blood pressure |
| BPD | bronchopulmonary dysplasia |
| BPH | benign prostatic hyperplasia |
| BPRS | Brief Psychiatric Rating Scale |
| BSA | body surface area |
| BSE | bovine spongiform encephalopathy; breast self-examination |
| BUN | blood urea nitrogen (use *serum urea nitrogen*) |
| | |
| c, ca | circa (do not use) |
| C | complement (do not expand when used with a number, eg, C1, C2, . . . C9; see 14.8.3, Complement) |
| CABG | coronary artery bypass graft |

| | |
|---|---|
| CAC | coronary artery calcification; coronary artery calcium |
| CAD | coronary artery disease |
| CAHD | coronary artery heart disease |
| CAM | complementary and alternative medicine |
| cAMP | cyclic adenosine monophosphate |
| CARS | compensatory anti-inflammatory response syndrome |
| cART | combination (or combined) antiretroviral therapy |
| CBC | complete blood (add *cell*) count |
| CBT | cognitive behavior therapy |
| CCB | calcium channel blocker |
| CCTA | coronary computed tomographic angiography |
| CCU | cardiac care unit; critical care unit |
| CD | clusters of differentiation (use with a number, eg, CD4 cell; see 14.8.2, CD Cell Markers) |
| cDNA | complementary DNA |
| cfDNA | cell-free DNA or circulating free DNA |
| ctDNA | circulating tumor DNA |
| CEA | carcinoembryonic antigen; cost-effectiveness analysis |
| CEDEX | Courrier d'Entreprise à Distribution EXceptionnelle (special business mail) (no need to expand) |
| cEEG | continuous electroencephalogram |
| CEU | continuing education unit |
| cf | compare (from the Latin *confer*, to compare) (no need to expand) |
| CF | cystic fibrosis |
| CFS | chronic fatigue syndrome |
| CFT | complement fixation test |
| CFU | colony-forming unit |
| CGH | comparative genomic hybridization |
| cGMP | cyclic guanosine monophosphate |
| CHD | coronary heart disease; congenital heart disease |
| CHEERS | Consolidated Health Economic Evaluation Reporting Standards |
| CHF | congestive heart failure |

| | |
|---|---|
| CI | confidence interval (no need to expand) |
| CIED | cardiovascular implantable electronic device |
| CIN | cervical intraepithelial neoplasia |
| CIS | carcinoma in situ |
| CJD | Creutzfeldt-Jakob disease |
| CK | creatine kinase |
| CK-BB | creatine kinase BB (BB designates the isozyme) (largely replaced by troponin [Tn]) |
| CKD | chronic kidney disease |
| CK-MB | creatine kinase MB (largely replaced by troponin [Tn]) |
| CK-MM | creatine kinase MM (largely replaced by troponin [Tn]) |
| CL | confidence limit |
| CLABSI | central line–associated bloodstream infection |
| CLIA | Clinical Laboratory Improvement Amendments |
| CLL | chronic lymphocytic leukemia |
| CME | continuing medical education (no need to expand) |
| CMI | cell-mediated immunity |
| CMIT | carotid intima-media thickness |
| CML | chronic myelocytic leukemia |
| CMR | cardiac (or cardiovascular) magnetic resonance |
| CMV | cytomegalovirus |
| CNS | central nervous system |
| CONSORT | Consolidated Standards of Reporting Trials |
| COPD | chronic obstructive pulmonary disease |
| COREQ | Consolidated Criteria for Reporting Qualitative Research |
| COVID-19 | coronavirus disease 2019  (no need to expand) |
| COX-2 | cyclooxygenase 2 |
| CPAP | continuous positive airway pressure |
| CPD | continuing professional development |
| CPK | creatinine phosphokinase (use *creatine kinase*) |
| CPR | cardiopulmonary resuscitation |
| *CPT* | *Current Procedural Terminology* |

| | |
|---|---|
| CQI | continuous quality improvement |
| CRC | colorectal cancer |
| CRF | corticotropin-releasing factor |
| CRISPR | clustered regularly interspaced short palindromic repeats |
| cRNA | complementary RNA |
| CRP | C-reactive protein |
| CRT | chemoradiation therapy |
| CSF | cerebrospinal fluid; colony-stimulating factor |
| CT | computed tomographic; computed tomography |
| CUA | cost-utility analysis |
| CUD | cannabis use disorder |
| CVA | cerebrovascular accident (specify subtype: hemorrhagic stroke, ischemic stroke, and/or transient ischemic attack) |
| CVD | cardiovascular disease |
| CVS | chorionic villus sampling |
| DALY | disability-adjusted life-year |
| dAMP | deoxyadenosine monophosphate (deoxyadenylate) |
| D&C | dilation and curettage |
| DBS | deep brain stimulation |
| DC | direct current |
| DCIS | ductal carcinoma in situ |
| DDD | defined daily dose |
| DDT | dichlorodiphenyltrichloroethane (chlorophenothane) (no need to expand) |
| DE | dose equivalent |
| DECT | dual-energy computed tomography |
| DEV | duck embryo vaccine |
| DEXA | dual-energy x-ray absorptiometry |
| DFA | direct fluorescence assay |
| DFS | disease-free survival |
| dGMP | deoxyguanosine monophosphate (deoxyguanylate) |
| DIC | disseminated intravascular coagulation |
| DIF | direct immunofluorescence |

| | |
|---|---|
| DJD | degenerative joint disease |
| DMARD | disease-modifying antirheumatic drug |
| DNA | deoxyribonucleic acid (no need to expand) |
| DNase | deoxyribonuclease |
| DNR | do not resuscitate |
| DOB | date of birth |
| DOI | digital object identifier |
| DOT | directly observed therapy |
| DOTS | directly observed therapy, short course |
| dpi | dots per inch (no need to expand) |
| DRE | digital rectal examination |
| DRG | diagnosis related group |
| DS | duplex sonography |
| *DSM-III* | *Diagnostic and Statistical Manual of Mental Disorders* (Third Edition) |
| *DSM-III-R* | *Diagnostic and Statistical Manual of Mental Disorders* (Third Edition, Revised) |
| *DSM-IV* | *Diagnostic and Statistical Manual of Mental Disorders* (Fourth Edition) |
| *DSM-IV-TR* | *Diagnostic and Statistical Manual of Mental Disorders* (Fourth Edition, Text Revision) |
| *DSM-5* | *Diagnostic and Statistical Manual of Mental Disorders* (Fifth Edition) |
| DSMB | data and safety monitoring board |
| DT | delirium tremens |
| DTaP | diphtheria and tetanus toxoids and acellular pertussis [vaccine] |
| DTP | diphtheria-tetanus-pertussis [vaccine] |
| DVT | deep vein thrombosis |
| DXA | dual-energy x-ray absorptiometry |
| EBM | evidence-based medicine |
| EBP | evidence-based practice |
| EBV | Epstein-Barr virus |
| EC | ejection click |
| ECA | epidemiologic catchment area |

| | |
|---|---|
| ECG | electrocardiogram; electrocardiographic |
| ECMO | extracorporeal membrane oxygenation |
| ECT | electroconvulsive therapy |
| ED | effective dose; emergency department; erectile dysfunction |
| $ED_{50}$ | median effective dose |
| EDTA | ethylenediaminetetraacetic acid (no need to expand) |
| EEE | eastern equine encephalomyelitis |
| EEG | electroencephalogram; electroencephalographic |
| EF | ejection fraction |
| eg | for example (from the Latin *exempli gratia*; see 11.1, Correct and Preferred Usage of Common Words and Phrases) (no need to expand) |
| EGD | esophagogastroduodenoscopy |
| eGFR | estimated glomerular filtration rate |
| EHR | electronic health record |
| EIA | enzyme immunoassay |
| ELISA | enzyme-linked immunosorbent assay |
| EM | electron microscope; electron microscopic; electron microscopy |
| EMG | electromyogram; electromyographic |
| EMIT | enzyme-multiplied immunoassay technique |
| EMS | electrical muscle stimulation; emergency medical services; eosinophilia-myalgia syndrome |
| EMT | emergency medical technician |
| ENG | electronystagmogram; electronystagmographic |
| ENT | ear, nose, and throat |
| EPS | extrapyramidal symptoms |
| EOG | electro-oculogram; electro-oculographic |
| ERCP | endoscopic retrograde cholangiopancreatography |
| ERG | electroretinogram; electroretinographic |
| ESBL | extended-spectrum ß-lactamases |
| ESLD | end-stage liver disease |
| ESR | erythrocyte sedimentation rate |
| ESRD | end-stage renal disease |

**611**

| | |
|---|---|
| ESWL | extracorporeal shock wave lithotripsy |
| etc | et cetera (and so forth) (see 11.1, Correct and Preferred Usage of Common Words and Phrases) (no need to expand) |
| ETOH | ethyl alcohol |
| EVR | evoked visual response |
| EWAS | environment-wide association study; epigenome-wide association study |
| | |
| F | French (add *catheter*; use only with a number, eg, 12F catheter) |
| FA | fatty acid |
| FEF$_{25\%-75\%}$ | forced expiratory flow, midexpiratory phase (see 14.16, Pulmonary and Respiratory Terminology) |
| FEV | forced expiratory volume |
| FEV$_1$ | forced expiratory volume in the first second of expiration |
| FFP | fresh frozen plasma |
| FGM | female genital mutilation |
| FHR | fetal heart rate |
| F$_{IO_2}$ | fraction of inspired oxygen |
| FISH | fluorescence in situ hybridization |
| FLAIR | fluid-attenuated inversion recovery |
| fMRI | functional magnetic resonance imaging |
| FMT | fecal microbiota transplant |
| FSH | follicle-stimulating hormone |
| FTA | fluorescent treponemal antibody |
| FTA-ABS | fluorescent treponemal antibody absorption (add *test*) |
| FUO | fever of unknown origin |
| FVC | forced vital capacity |
| | |
| GABA | γ-aminobutyric acid |
| GAD | generalized anxiety disorder |
| GADPH | glyceraldehyde 3-phosphate dehydrogenase |
| GAF | Global Assessment of Functioning [Scale] |
| GCS | Glasgow Coma Scale |

| | |
|---|---|
| G-CSF | granulocyte colony-stimulating factor |
| GDP | guanosine diphosphate |
| GDS | Geriatric Depression Scale |
| GED | General Educational Development |
| GERD | gastroesophageal reflux disease |
| GFR | glomerular filtration rate |
| GH | growth hormone |
| GI | gastrointestinal |
| GIFT | gamete intrafallopian transfer |
| GIST | gastrointestinal stromal tumor |
| GLC | gas-liquid chromatography |
| GM-CSF | granulocyte-macrophage colony-stimulating factor |
| GMP | guanosine monophosphate (guanylate, guanylic acid) |
| GMRI | gated magnetic resonance imaging |
| GMT | geometric mean titer |
| GMT | Greenwich mean time (no need to expand) |
| GnRH | gonadotropin-releasing hormone (*gonadorelin* as diagnostic agent) |
| GRADE | Grading of Recommendations Assessment, Development, and Evaluation [criteria] |
| GU | genitourinary |
| GUI | graphical user interface |
| GVHD | graft-vs-host disease |
| GWA | genome-wide association |
| GWAS | genome-wide association study |
| | |
| H1N1 | hemagglutinin type 1 and neuraminidase type 1 |
| $H_2$ | histamine |
| HAART | highly active antiretroviral therapy |
| HALE | health-adjusted life expectancy |
| HAM-D | Hamilton Rating Scale for Depression (see also HDRS) |
| HAV | hepatitis A virus (see 14.14.3, Virus Nomenclature, and 14.14.4, Prions) |
| $HbA_{1c}$ | hemoglobin $A_{1c}$ |

| | |
|---|---|
| Hbco | carboxyhemoglobin |
| HBO | hyperbaric oxygen |
| Hbo$_2$ | oxyhemoglobin; oxygenated hemoglobin |
| HbS | sickle cell hemoglobin |
| HBsA | hepatitis B surface antigen (see 14.14.3, Virus Nomenclature, and 14.14.4, Prions) |
| HBSS | Hanks balanced salt solution |
| HBV | hepatitis B virus |
| hCG | human chorionic gonadotropin (do not abbreviate when used as a drug) |
| HCV | hepatitis C virus (see 14.14.3, Virus Nomenclature, and 14.14.4, Prions) |
| HDL | high-density lipoprotein |
| HDL-C | high-density lipoprotein cholesterol |
| HDRS | Hamilton Depression Rating Scale |
| HEV | hepatitis E virus |
| HF | heart failure |
| hGH | human growth hormone |
| HHV | human herpesvirus |
| Hib | *Haemophilus influenzae* type b [vaccine or disease] (see 14.14.2, Bacteria: Additional Terminology) |
| HIPAA | Health Insurance Portability and Accountability Act |
| HIV | human immunodeficiency virus (no need to expand) |
| HL | hearing level |
| HLA | human leukocyte antigen (use *HLA antigen*; see 14.8.5, HLA/Major Histocompatibility Complex System) |
| HMO | health maintenance organization |
| HMPV | human metapneumovirus |
| HPF | high-power field |
| HPLC | high-performance liquid chromatography |
| HPV | human papillomavirus (add hyphen to abbreviation when indicating type, eg, HPV-6) |
| HR | hazard ratio |
| HRQOL | health-related quality of life |

| | |
|---|---|
| HRT | hormone replacement therapy |
| hs-CRP | high-sensitivity (or highly sensitive) C-reactive protein |
| hs-cTn | high-sensitivity (or highly sensitive) cardiac troponin |
| HSIL | high-grade squamous intraepithelial lesion |
| HSV | herpes simplex virus |
| HT | hormone therapy |
| 5-HT | Use *serotonin* (also 5-hydroxytryptamine) |
| HTLV | human T-lymphotropic virus (use arabic numeral with specific type, eg, HTLV-1) |
| HUS | hemolytic uremic syndrome |
| | |
| IADL | instrumental activities of daily living (but: 1 IADL, 6 IADLs) |
| IBC | institutional biosafety committee |
| IBS | irritable bowel syndrome |
| ICC | intraclass correlation coefficient |
| ICD | implantable cardioverter-defibrillator |
| *ICD-9* | *International Classification of Diseases, Ninth Revision* |
| *ICD-9-CM* | *International Classification of Diseases, Ninth Revision, Clinical Modification* |
| *ICD-10* | *International Statistical Classification of Diseases, Tenth Revision* |
| *ICD-10-CM* | *International Classification of Diseases, Tenth Revision, Clinical Modification* |
| ICSI | intracytoplasmic sperm injection |
| ICU | intensive care unit |
| ID | infective dose |
| IDLE | indolent lesions of epithelial origin |
| IDU | injecting drug user; injection drug user |
| ie | that is (from the Latin *id est*; see 11.1, Correct and Preferred Usage of Common Words and Phrases) (no need to expand) |
| IFN | interferon (do not abbreviate when used as a drug; see 14.4.13.5, Interferons) |
| Ig | immunoglobulin (abbreviate only with specification of class, eg, IgA, IgG, IgM; see 14.8.6, Immunoglobulins) |

| | |
|---|---|
| IGF-1 | insulinlike growth factor 1 |
| IL | interleukin (abbreviate only when indicating a specific protein factor, eg, IL-2) (see 14.8.4, Cytokines) |
| IM | intramuscular; intramuscularly |
| IND | investigational new drug |
| INDA | investigational new drug application |
| INR | international normalized ratio |
| IOP | intraocular pressure |
| IPA | intimate partner abuse |
| IPV | intimate partner violence |
| IQ | intelligence quotient (no need to expand) |
| IQR | interquartile range |
| IRB | institutional review board |
| IRIS | immune reconstitution inflammatory syndrome |
| IRMA | immunoradiometric assay |
| IRS | immune reconstitution syndrome |
| ISBN | International Standard Book Number (no need to expand) |
| ISBN-A | actionable ISBN |
| ISG | immune serum globulin |
| ISSN | International Standard Serial Number (no need to expand) |
| ITI | intratubal insemination |
| ITP | idiopathic thrombocytopenic purpura |
| ITT | intent to treat; intention to treat |
| IUD | intrauterine device |
| IUGR | intrauterine growth retardation |
| IUI | intrauterine insemination |
| IV | intravenous; intravenously |
| IVF | in vitro fertilization |
| IVIG | intravenous immunoglobulin |
| IVP | intravenous pyelogram |
| IVUS | intravascular ultrasound |
| JCV | John Cunningham virus |
| JIA | juvenile idiopathic arthritis |

| | |
|---|---|
| JVP | jugular venous pulse |
| KUB | kidneys, ureter, bladder [plain abdominal radiograph] |
| KS | Kaposi sarcoma |
| LA | left atrium |
| LAD | left anterior descending coronary artery |
| LAO | left anterior oblique coronary artery |
| LASEK | laser epithelial keratomileusis |
| LASIK | laser in situ keratomileusis |
| LAV | lymphadenopathy-associated virus |
| LBBB | left bundle-branch block |
| LBP | lower back pain |
| LBW | low birth weight |
| LCA | left coronary artery |
| LCMV | lymphocytic choriomeningitis virus |
| LCR | locus control region |
| LCX, CX | left circumflex coronary artery |
| LD | lethal dose |
| $LD_{50}$ | median lethal dose |
| LDH | lactate dehydrogenase |
| LDL | low-density lipoprotein |
| LDL-C | low-density lipoprotein cholesterol |
| LGA | large for gestational age |
| LGBT | lesbian, gay, bisexual, transgender |
| LGBTQ | lesbian, gay, bisexual, transgender, queer; lesbian, gay, bisexual, transgender, questioning |
| LGBTQAI | lesbian, gay, bisexual, transgender, queer (or questioning), asexual (or allied), intersex |
| LH | luteinizing hormone |
| LHRH | luteinizing hormone–releasing hormone (*gonadorelin* as diagnostic agent) |
| LMIC | low- and middle-income countries |
| LMW | low molecular weight (usually refers to heparin, as in low-molecular-weight heparin [LMWH]) |

| | |
|---|---|
| LOC | loss of consciousness |
| LOCF | last observation carried forward |
| LOD | logarithm of odds |
| logMAR | logarithm of the minimum angle of resolution (no need to expand) |
| LOS | length of stay |
| LP | lumbar puncture |
| LR | likelihood ratio |
| LSD | lysergic acid diethylamide |
| LSIL | low-grade squamous intraepithelial lesion |
| LV | left ventricle; left ventricular |
| LVAD | left ventricular assist device |
| LVEDV | left ventricular end-diastolic volume |
| LVEF | left ventricular ejection fraction |
| LVH | left ventricular hypertrophy |
| LVOT | left ventricular outflow tract |
| | |
| *m-* | meta- (abbreviate only in chemical formulas or names) |
| MAOI | monoamine oxidase inhibitor |
| MAP | mean arterial pressure |
| MAPC | multipotent adult progenitor cell |
| MBC | minimum bactericidal concentration |
| MCH | mean corpuscular hemoglobin |
| MCHC | mean corpuscular hemoglobin concentration |
| MCI | mild cognitive impairment |
| MCV | mean corpuscular volume |
| MD | muscular dystrophy |
| MDR | multidrug-resistant |
| MDR-TB | multidrug-resistant tuberculosis |
| MEC | mean effective concentration |
| MEG | magnetoencephalographic magnetoencephalography |
| MELD | model for end-stage liver disease |
| MEM | minimal essential medium |

| MEN | multiple endocrine neoplasia (type 1: MEN-1; type 2: MEN-2; etc) |
| MERS | Middle Eastern respiratory syndrome |
| MeSH | Medical Subject Headings [of the US National Library of Medicine] |
| MET | metabolic equivalent task |
| MGUS | monoclonal gammopathy of uncertain significance |
| MHC | major histocompatibility complex |
| MI | mitral insufficiency; myocardial infarction |
| MIC | minimum inhibitory concentration |
| MICU | medical intensive care unit |
| MMPI | Minnesota Multiphasic Personality Inventory |
| MMR | measles-mumps-rubella [vaccine] |
| MMSE | Mini-Mental State Examination |
| MODS | multiple organ dysfunction syndrome |
| MODY | maturity-onset diabetes of the young (use *type 2 diabetes*) |
| MOOSE | Meta-analysis of Observational Studies in Epidemiology |
| MPI | myocardial perfusion imaging |
| MPS | Mortality Probability Score |
| MRA | magnetic resonance angiography |
| MRI | magnetic resonance imaging |
| mRNA | messenger RNA |
| MRSA | methicillin-resistant *Staphylococcus aureus* |
| MS | mitral stenosis; multiple sclerosis |
| MSA | metropolitan statistical area |
| MSET | multistage exercise test |
| MSM | male-male sexual contact; men who have sex with men |
| MVC | motor vehicle crash |
| MVP | mitral valve prolapse |
| NACT | neoadjuvant chemotherapy |
| NAD | nicotinamide adenine dinucleotide |
| NADP | nicotinamide adenine dinucleotide phosphate |
| NDA | new drug application |

| | |
|---|---|
| Nd:YAG | neodymium:yttrium-aluminum-garnet [laser] (no need to expand) |
| NEC | necrotizing enterocolitis |
| NET | neuroendocrine tumor |
| *NF* | *National Formulary* |
| NICU | neonatal intensive care unit |
| NK | natural killer (add *cells*) |
| NKTCL | natural killer/T-cell lymphoma |
| NLP | natural language processing |
| NMN | nicotinamide mononucleotide |
| NNH | number needed to harm |
| NNI | number needed to invite |
| NNS | number needed to screen |
| NNT | number needed to treat |
| NOS | not otherwise specified |
| npo | nothing by mouth (do not use) |
| NPV | negative predictive value |
| NRT | nicotine replacement therapy |
| NS | not significant (see 19.0, Study Design and Statistics) |
| NSAID | nonsteroidal anti-inflammatory drug |
| NSCLC | non–small cell lung cancer |
| NSTE | non–ST-segment elevation |
| NSTEMI | non–ST-segment elevation myocardial infarction |
| NT-proBNP | N-terminal pro–brain natriuretic peptide |
| | |
| *o-* | ortho- (abbreviate only in chemical formulas) |
| OC | oral contraceptive |
| OCD | obsessive-compulsive disorder |
| OCT | optical coherence tomography |
| OD | oculus dexter (right eye) (no need to expand) |
| OGTT | oral glucose tolerance test |
| OMIM | Online Mendelian Inheritance in Man (no need to expand) |
| OR | odds ratio |

| | |
|---|---|
| OS | oculus sinister (left eye) (no need to expand) |
| OSA | obstructive sleep apnea |
| OTC | over the counter |
| OU | oculus unitas (both eyes) or oculus uterque (each eye) (abbreviate only with a number) |
| OUD | opioid use disorder |
| | |
| *p-* | para- (abbreviate only in chemical formulas or names) |
| PA | pulmonary artery |
| PAC | premature atrial contraction; pulmonary artery catheter |
| PACU | postanesthesia care unit |
| PAD | peripheral artery disease |
| $Pa_{CO_2}$ | partial pressure of carbon dioxide, arterial (see 14.16, Nomenclature, Pulmonary and Respiratory Terminology) (no need to expand) |
| $Pa_{O_2}$ | partial pressure of oxygen, arterial (no need to expand) |
| $PA_{O_2}$ | partial pressure of oxygen in the alveoli |
| PAR | population attributable risk |
| PAS | periodic acid–Schiff |
| PAT | paroxysmal atrial tachycardia |
| PBS | phosphate-buffered saline |
| PCA | patient-controlled anesthesia |
| PCI | percutaneous coronary intervention |
| $P_{CO_2}$ | partial pressure of carbon dioxide (no need to expand) |
| PCP | *Pneumocystis jiroveci* pneumonia; primary care physician |
| PCR | polymerase chain reaction |
| PCS | postconcussion syndrome |
| PCW | pulmonary capillary wedge [pressure] |
| PD | Parkinson disease, peritoneal dialysis |
| PDA | patent ductus arteriosus |
| PDF | portable document format (no need to expand) |
| *PDR* | *Physicians' Desk Reference* |
| PE | pulmonary embolism |
| PEEP | positive end-expiratory pressure |

| | |
|---|---|
| PEG | percutaneous endoscopic gastrostomy; pneumoencephalographic; pneumoencephalography |
| PEP | postexposure prophylaxis |
| PET | positron emission tomographic; positron emission tomography |
| PFGE | pulsed-field gel electrophoresis |
| PFS | progression-free survival |
| PGF | placental growth factor |
| pH | negative logarithm of hydrogen ion concentration (no need to expand) |
| PICC | peripherally inserted central catheter |
| PICU | pediatric intensive care unit; pulmonary intensive care unit |
| PID | pelvic inflammatory disease |
| PKU | phenylketonuria |
| PMDD | premenstrual dysphoric disorder |
| PMID | PubMed identifier (no need to expand) |
| PML | progressive multifocal leukoencephalopathy |
| PMS | premenstrual syndrome |
| po | orally or by mouth (do not use) |
| $Po_2$ | partial pressure of oxygen (no need to expand) |
| POAG | primary open-angle glaucoma |
| POR | prevalence odds ratio |
| PPD | purified protein derivative (tuberculin) |
| PPE | personal protective equipment |
| PPI | proton pump inhibitor |
| PPO | preferred provider organization |
| PPROM | preterm premature rupture of membranes |
| PPV | positive predictive value |
| PRA | plasma renin activity |
| PRC | plasma renin concentration |
| PrEP | preexposure prophylaxis |
| PRISMA | Preferred Reporting Items for Systematic Reviews and Meta-Analyses |
| prn | as needed (do not use) |
| PROM | premature rupture of membranes |

| | |
|---|---|
| PSA | prostate-specific antigen |
| PSG | polysomnographic; polysomnography |
| Psqo$_2$ | subcutaneous tissue oxygen tension |
| PSRO | professional standards review organization |
| PSVT | paroxysmal supraventricular tachycardia |
| PT | physical therapy; prothrombin time |
| PTCA | percutaneous transluminal coronary angioplasty |
| PTS | posttraumatic stress |
| PTSD | posttraumatic stress disorder |
| PTT | partial thromboplastin time |
| PUD | peptic ulcer disease |
| PUFA | polyunsaturated fatty acid |
| PUVA | psoralen–UV-A |
| PVC | premature ventricular contraction |
| PVR | peripheral vascular resistance; pulmonary vascular resistance |
| PVS | persistent vegetative state |
| | |
| QA | quality assurance |
| QALE | quality-adjusted life expectancy |
| QALY | quality-adjusted life-year |
| QC | quality control |
| QCA | quantitative coronary angiography |
| qd | every day (do not use) |
| qh | each hour (do not use) |
| QI | quality improvement |
| qid | four times a day (do not use) |
| qod | every other day (do not use) |
| QOL | quality of life |
| qSOFA | quick Sequential Organ Failure Assessment |
| QUOROM | Quality of Reporting of Meta-analyses |
| | |
| RA | rheumatoid arthritis |
| RAST | radioallergosorbent test |
| RBBB | right bundle-branch block |

| | |
|---|---|
| RBC | red blood cell |
| RBRVS | resource-based relative value scale |
| RCA | right coronary artery |
| RCT | randomized clinical trial |
| RDA | recommended daily allowance; recommended dietary allowance |
| RDC | Research Diagnostic Criteria |
| rDNA | ribosomal DNA |
| RDoC | Research Domain Criteria |
| RDS | respiratory distress syndrome |
| REM | rapid eye movement |
| RFLP | restriction fragment length polymorphism |
| RFP | radiofrequency pulse |
| RFS | recurrence-free survival |
| rh | recombinant human |
| Rh | rhesus (of, related to, or being an Rh antibody, blood group, or factor) (no need to expand) |
| rhNGF | recombinant human nerve growth factor |
| RIA | radioimmunoassay |
| RIND | reversible ischemic neurological deficit |
| RNA | ribonucleic acid (no need to expand) |
| RNAi | RNA interference |
| ROC | receiver operating characteristic [curve] |
| ROM | read-only memory (no need to expand) |
| ROP | retinopathy of prematurity |
| RPR | rapid plasma reagin |
| RR | relative risk; risk ratio |
| RSV | respiratory syncytial virus |
| RT | radiation therapy; radiotherapy |
| RT-PCR | reverse transcriptase–polymerase chain reaction |
| RV | right ventricle; right ventricular |
| RVEF | right ventricular ejection fraction |
| RVOT | right ventricular outflow tract |

| | |
|---|---|
| SAD | seasonal affective disorder |
| SADS | Schedule for Affective Disorders and Schizophrenia; sudden arrhythmic death syndrome |
| SAE | serious adverse event |
| SAH | subarachnoid hemorrhage |
| SAPS | Simplified Acute Physiology Score |
| SARS | severe acute respiratory syndrome |
| SARS-CoV-2 | severe acute respiratory syndrome coronavirus 2 (no need to expand) |
| SAS | Statistical Analysis System (no need to expand) |
| SCID | severe combined immunodeficiency; Structured Clinical Interview for *DSM* (use with *DSM* edition number) |
| SD | standard deviation (no need to expand) |
| SE | standard error (no need to expand) |
| SEER | Surveillance, Epidemiology, and End Results |
| SEM | standard error of the mean (no need to expand) |
| SEM | scanning electron microscope; systolic ejection murmur |
| SES | socioeconomic status |
| SF-36 | 36-Item Short Form Health Survey |
| SGA | small for gestational age |
| SGML | standardized general markup language (no need to expand) |
| SGOT | serum glutamic-oxaloacetic transaminase (use *aspartate aminotransferase*) |
| SGPT | serum glutamic-pyruvic transaminase (use *alanine aminotransferase*) |
| SIADH | syndrome of inappropriate antidiuretic hormone secretion |
| SICU | surgical intensive care unit |
| SIDS | sudden infant death syndrome |
| SIL | squamous intraepithelial lesion |
| SIP | Sickness Impact Profile |
| siRNA | small interfering RNA |
| SIRS | systemic inflammatory response syndrome |
| SLE | systemic lupus erythematosus |
| SLN | sentinel lymph node |

SNP      single-nucleotide polymorphism (Note: Prefer SNV; see 14.6.1.1.1, Sequence Variations, Nucleotides.)

SNV      single-nucleotide variant

SOB      shortness of breath

SOFA      Sequential Organ Failure Assessment

SPECT      single-photon emission computed tomography

SPF      sun protection factor

SPIRIT      Standard Protocol Items: Recommendations for Interventional Trials

SPSS      Statistical Product and Service Solutions (formerly Statistical Package for the Social Sciences) (no need to expand)

SQUIRE      Standards for Quality Improvement Reporting Excellence

SRQR      Standards for Reporting Qualitative Research

SSC      standard saline citrate (no need to expand)

SSPE      sodium chloride, sodium phosphate, EDTA [buffer] (no need to expand)

SSPE      subacute sclerosing panencephalitis

SSRI      selective serotonin reuptake inhibitor

STARD      Standards for Reporting Diagnostic Accuracy

STD      sexually transmitted disease

STEM      science, technology, engineering, and math (or medicine)

STEMI      ST-segment elevation myocardial infarction

STI      sexually transmitted infection; structured treatment interruption

STM      science, technology, and medicine

STREGA      Strengthening the Reporting of Genetic Association Studies

STROBE      Strengthening the Reporting of Observational Studies in Epidemiology

SUD      substance use disorder

SUN      serum urea nitrogen

SUV      standardized uptake value

SVR      systemic vascular resistance

$t_{1/2}$      half-life

$T_3$      triiodothyronine

$T_4$      thyroxine

TAH      total abdominal hysterectomy

| | |
|---|---|
| TAHBSO | total abdominal hysterectomy with bilateral salpingo-oophorectomy |
| TAT | Thematic Apperception Test |
| TB | tuberculosis |
| TBI | traumatic brain injury |
| TBSA | total body surface area |
| TCA | tricyclic antidepressant |
| $TCD_{50}$ | median tissue culture dose |
| TDR-TB | totally drug-resistant tuberculosis |
| TE | echo time |
| THA | total hip arthroplasty |
| THR | total hip replacement |
| TI | inversion time |
| TIA | transient ischemic attack |
| TIBC | total iron-binding capacity |
| tid | three times a day (do not use) |
| TIL | tumor-infiltrating lymphocyte |
| TKR | total knee replacement |
| TLC | thin-layer chromatography; total lung capacity |
| TMJ | temporomandibular joint |
| TNF | tumor necrosis factor |
| TNM | tumor, node, metastasis (see 14.2.2, The TNM Staging System) (no need to expand) |
| TnT | troponin T |
| tPA | tissue plasminogen activator |
| TPN | total parenteral nutrition |
| TQM | total quality management |
| TR | repetition time |
| TRH | thyrotropin-releasing hormone (*protirelin* as diagnostic agent) |
| TRIPOD | Transparent Reporting of a Multivariable Prediction Model for Individual Prognosis or Diagnosis |
| tRNA | transfer RNA |
| TRP | tyrosine-related protein |
| TRUS | transrectal ultrasound |

| | |
|---|---|
| TSH | Use *thyrotropin* (previously thyroid-stimulating hormone) |
| TSS | toxic shock syndrome; toxic streptococcal syndrome |
| TTP | thrombotic thrombocytopenic purpura |
| TUD | tobacco use disorder |
| TUNEL | terminal deoxynucleotidal transferase–mediated biotin–deoxyuridine triphosphate nick-end labeling (use abbreviation first, with expansion immediately following in parentheses) |
| UHF | ultrahigh frequency |
| ul | uniformly labeled (use without expansion in parentheses; see 14.9.5, Isotopes, Uniform Labeling) |
| ULN | upper limit of normal |
| UNOS | United Network for Organ Sharing |
| URI | uniform resource identifier (no need to expand) |
| URL | uniform resource locator (no need to expand) |
| URN | uniform resource name (no need to expand) |
| URTI | upper respiratory tract infection |
| US | ultrasonography; ultrasound |
| USAN | United States Adopted Names |
| *USP* | *United States Pharmacopeia* |
| UTI | urinary tract infection |
| UV | ultraviolet (no need to expand) |
| UV-A | ultraviolet A (no need to expand) |
| UV-B | ultraviolet B (no need to expand) |
| UV-C | ultraviolet C (no need to expand) |
| VA | visual acuity |
| VAD | ventricular assist device |
| VAIN | vaginal intraepithelial neoplasia |
| VAP | ventilator-associated pneumonia |
| VAS | visual analog scale |
| VBAC | vaginal birth after cesarean |
| vCJD | variant Creutzfeldt-Jakob disease |
| VDRL | Venereal Disease Research Laboratory (add *test*) (no need to expand) |

| | |
|---|---|
| VEGF | vascular endothelial growth factor |
| VEP | visual evoked potential |
| VER | visual evoked response |
| VF | ventricular fibrillation |
| VHDL | very high-density lipoprotein |
| VHF | very high frequency; viral hemorrhagic fever |
| VLBW | very low birth weight |
| VLDL | very low-density lipoprotein |
| $\dot{V}_{O_2}$ | oxygen consumption per unit time |
| $\dot{V}_{O_2}$max | maximum oxygen consumption |
| VPB | ventricular premature beat |
| $\dot{V}$/Q | ventilation-perfusion [ratio or scan] |
| VRE | vancomycin-resistant *Enterococcus* |
| vs | versus (use *v* for legal references; see 3.16, US Legal References) (do not expand) |
| VSD | ventricular septal defect |
| VT | ventricular tachycardia |
| VTE | venous thromboembolism |
| VZV | varicella zoster virus |
| | |
| WAIS | Wechsler Adult Intelligence Scale |
| WBC | white blood cell |
| WEE | western equine encephalomyelitis |
| WISC-V | Wechsler Intelligence Scale for Children |
| | |
| XDR-TB | extensively drug-resistant tuberculosis |
| XML | extensible markup language (no need to expand) |
| XMRV | xenotropic murine leukemia virus–related virus |
| | |
| YLD | years living with disability |
| YPLL | years of potential life lost |
| | |
| ZES | Zollinger-Ellison syndrome |
| ZIFT | zygote intrafallopian transfer |
| zip | Zone Improvement Plan (do not expand: zip code) |

**13.12** **Units of Measure.** Quantitative values may be reported in conventional units or by using the International System of Units ("SI units" [Système International d'Unités]) (see 17.5.10, Laboratory Values, and 17.1, SI Units). JAMA Network journals report most analytes in conventional units.

Use the following abbreviations and symbols with a numerical quantity in accordance with guidelines in 17.0, Units of Measure. See especially 17.5, Conventional Units and SI Units in JAMA Network Journals; 17.5.10, Laboratory Values; and 8.4, Forward Slash [Virgule, Solidus]).

In rare instances, it may be appropriate to use *teaspoon, cup, pound, mile*, and so on in a scientific article when, for example, describing a survey in which such units may have been used in the original questionnaire. Conventional-unit equivalents may then be included parenthetically or in an explanatory footnote (as in a table or figure).

Note: Do not capitalize abbreviated units of measure (unless the abbreviation itself is always capitalized or contains capital letters).

Abbreviations listed in this section can be used without expansion except where noted otherwise. The abbreviations for measures of time (day, hour, millisecond, minute, month, second, week, and year) should be used only in a virgule construction and in tables and figures.

| Unit of measure | Abbreviation |
| --- | --- |
| acre | acre |
| ampere | A |
| angstrom | Convert to nanometers (1 A = 0.1 nm) |
| atmosphere, standard | atm |
| | |
| bar | bar |
| barn | b (expand at first mention) |
| base pair | bp (expand at first mention) |
| becquerel | Bq |
| billion electron volts | GeV (expand at first mention) |
| Bodansky unit | BU (expand at first mention) |
| British thermal unit | BTU |
| | |
| calorie | cal |
| candela | cd (expand at first mention) |
| Celsius | C (See policy about use of degree symbols in 18.1.5, Measures of Temperature.) |
| centigram | cg |
| centimeter | cm |
| centimeters of water | cm $H_2O$ |

| | |
|---|---|
| centimorgan | cM |
| centipoise | cP |
| coulomb | C (expand at first mention) |
| counts per minute | cpm |
| counts per second | cps |
| cubic centimeter | cm$^3$ (use milliliter for liquid and gas measure; avoid cc) |
| cubic foot | cu ft |
| cubic inch | cu in |
| cubic meter | m$^3$ |
| cubic micrometer | μm$^3$ |
| cubic millimeter | mm$^3$ (use microliter for liquid and gas measure) |
| cubic yard | cu yd |
| curie | Ci |
| cycles per second | Use hertz |
| dalton | Da |
| day | d (use only in virgule construction, tables, and figures) |
| decibel | dB |
| decigram | Convert to grams |
| deciliter | dL |
| decimeter | Convert to meters |
| diopter | D (expand at first mention) |
| disintegrations per minute | dpm (expand at first mention) |
| disintegrations per second | dps (expand at first mention) |
| dyne | dyne |
| electron volt | eV |
| electrostatic unit | ESU (expand at first mention) |
| equivalent | Eq |
| Fahrenheit | F (See policy about use of degree symbols in 18.1.5, Measures of Temperature.) |

| | |
|---|---|
| farad (electric capacitance) | F (expand at first mention) |
| femtogram | fg |
| femtoliter | fL |
| femtomole | fmol |
| fluid ounce | fl oz |
| foot | ft (convert to meters; query author) |
| | |
| gas volume | gas volume |
| gauss | G |
| gigabyte | GB |
| grain | grain |
| gram | g |
| gravity (acceleration due to) | *g* (use closed up to preceding number, eg, 200*g*) |
| gray | Gy |
| | |
| henry | H (expand at first mention) |
| hertz | Hz |
| horsepower | hp |
| hour | h (use only in virgule construction, tables, and figures) |
| | |
| immunizing unit | ImmU (expand at first mention) |
| inch | in |
| international benzoate unit | IBU (expand at first mention) |
| international unit | IU |
| | |
| joule | J |
| | |
| katal | kat (expand at first mention) |
| kelvin | K |
| kilobase | kb (expand at first mention) |
| kilobyte | kB |
| kilocalorie | kcal |
| kilocurie | kCi |

| | |
|---|---|
| kilodalton | kDa |
| kiloelectron volt | keV |
| kilogram | kg |
| kilohertz | kHz |
| kilojoule | kJ |
| kilometer | km |
| kilovolt | kV |
| kilovolt-ampere | kVA |
| kilovolt (constant potential) | kV(cp) (expand at first mention) |
| kilovolt (peak) | kV(p) (expand at first mention) |
| kilowatt | kW |
| King-Armstrong unit | King-Armstrong unit |
| knot | knot |
| | |
| liter | L |
| lumen | lumen |
| lux | lux |
| | |
| megabyte | MB |
| megacurie | MCi |
| megacycle | Mc |
| megahertz | MHz |
| megaunit | megaunit |
| megawatt | MW |
| meter | m |
| metric ton | metric ton |
| microampere | µA |
| microcurie | µCi |
| microfarad | µF (expand at first mention) |
| microgram | µg |
| microliter | µL |
| micrometer | µm |
| micromicrocurie | Use picocurie |
| micromicrogram | Use picogram |

| | |
|---|---|
| micromicrometer | Use picometer |
| micromolar | μM |
| micromole | μmol |
| micron | Use micrometer |
| micronormal | μN |
| microosmole | μOsm |
| microvolt | μV |
| microwatt | μW |
| mile | mile |
| miles per hour | mph |
| milliampere | mA |
| millicurie | mCi |
| millicuries destroyed | mCid (expand at first mention) |
| milliequivalent | mEq |
| millifarad | mF (expand at first mention) |
| milligram | mg |
| milligram-element | mg-el (expand at first mention) |
| milli–international unit | mIU |
| milliliter | mL |
| millimeter | mm |
| millimeters of mercury | mm Hg |
| millimeters of water | mm $H_2O$ |
| millimolar | mM |
| millimole | mmol |
| million electron volts | MeV |
| milliosmole | mOsm |
| millirem | mrem |
| milliroentgen | mR |
| millisecond | ms (use only in virgule construction, tables, and figures) |
| milliunit | mU |
| millivolt | mV |
| milliwatt | mW |
| minute (time) | min (use only in virgule construction, tables, and figures) |

| | |
|---|---|
| molar | M |
| mole | mol |
| month | mo (use only in virgule construction, tables, and figures) |
| morgan | M (expand at first mention) |
| megaunit | MU (expand at first mention) |
| mouse unit | MU (expand at first mention) |
| nanocurie | nCi |
| nanogram | ng |
| nanometer | nm |
| nanomolar | nM |
| nanomole | nmol |
| newton | N |
| normal (solution) | N |
| ohm | $\Omega$ |
| osmole | osm |
| ounce | oz |
| outflow (weight) | C (expand at first mention) |
| parts per million | ppm |
| pascal | Pa |
| picocurie | pCi |
| picogram | pg |
| picometer | pm |
| picomolar | pM |
| picomole | pmol |
| pint | pt |
| pound | lb (convert to milligrams, kilograms, or grams; query author) |
| pounds per square inch | psi |
| prism diopter | PD, $\Delta$ (expand at first mention) |
| quart | qt |

| | |
|---|---|
| rad | rad |
| radian | radian |
| rat unit | RU (expand at first mention) |
| revolutions per minute | rpm |
| roentgen | R |
| roentgen equivalents human (or mammal) | rem |
| roentgen equivalents physical | rep |
| Saybolt seconds universal | SSU (expand at first mention) |
| second | s (use only in virgule construction, tables, and figures) |
| siemens | S |
| sievert | Sv |
| sp g | specific gravity (use with a number, eg, sp g 13.6) |
| square centimeter | cm$^2$ |
| square foot | sq ft |
| square inch | sq in |
| square meter | m$^2$ |
| square millimeter | mm$^2$ |
| Svedberg flotation unit | Sf (expand at first mention) |
| terabyte | TB |
| tesla | T |
| torr | Use millimeters of mercury |
| tuberculin unit | TU |
| turbidity-reducing unit | TRU (expand at first mention) |
| unit | U |
| volt | V |
| volume | vol |
| volume per volume | vol/vol |
| volume percent | vol% |

| | |
|---|---|
| watt | W |
| week | wk (use only in virgule construction, tables, and figures) |
| weight | wt |
| weight per volume | wt/vol |
| weight per weight | wt/wt |
| | |
| yard | yd |
| year | y (use only in virgule construction, tables, and figures) |

**13.13** ▬▬ **Elements and Chemicals.** In general, the names of chemical elements and compounds should be expanded in the text at first mention and elsewhere in accordance with the guidelines for clinical and technical terms (see 14.4.4, Chemical Names, and 14.9, Isotopes). However, in some circumstances, it may be helpful or necessary to provide the chemical symbols or formulas in addition to the expansion if the compound under discussion is new or relatively unknown or if no nonproprietary term exists.

> 2,3,7,8-Tetrachlorodibenzo-p-dioxin (TCDD or dioxin) is often referred to as the most toxic synthetic chemical known. [Use "TCDD" or "dioxin" thereafter; TCDD is more specific because there is more than 1 form of dioxin.]

> 3,4-Methylenedioxymethamphetamine (MDMA, ecstasy), a synthetic analogue of 3,4-methylenedioxyamphetamine, has been the center of controversy over its potential for abuse vs its use as a psychotherapeutic agent. [Use "MDMA" or "ecstasy" thereafter, depending on the article's context.]

The following format may also be used:

> Isorhodeose (chemical name, 6-deoxy-D glucose [$CH_3(CHOH)_4CHO$]) is a sugar derived from cinchona bark. [Use "isorhodeose" thereafter.]

Names such as "sodium lauryl sulfate" are easier to express and understand (and typeset) than "$CH_3(CH_2)_{10}CH_2OSO_3Na$." Similarly, "oxygen" and "water" do not take up much more space than "$O_2$" and "$H_2O$" and hence should remain expanded throughout a manuscript, unless specific measurements (eg, gas exchange) are under discussion.

> The venous $CO_2$ pressure is always greater than arterial $CO_2$ pressure; specifically, $Pvco_2/Paco_2$ is greater than 1.0 except when $Po_2$ plus $Pco_2$ is measured. Nevertheless, the $CO_2$ levels should be carefully measured.

> Near the earth's surface, the atmosphere has a well-defined chemical composition, consisting of molecular nitrogen, molecular oxygen, and argon. It also contains small amounts of carbon dioxide and water vapor, along with trace quantities of methane, ammonia, nitrous oxide, hydrogen sulfide, helium, neon, krypton, xenon, and various other gases.

In the following example, *sodium* and *potassium* are not abbreviated.

Additional serum chemistry studies confirmed a serum sodium level of 131 mEq/L and a serum potassium level of 4.8 mEq/L.

In the text and elsewhere, the expansion of such symbols as $Na^+$ or $Ca^{2+}$ can be cumbersome because these symbols have a specific meaning for the reader. Usage should follow the context. For example, in narrative or nontechnical pieces, the flavor of the writing might be lost if the editor arbitrarily changed "$CO_2$" to "carbon dioxide" ("What's the patient's $CO_2$?").

When chemical symbols and formulas are used, they must be carefully marked for display and typesetting, especially when chemical bonds are expressed (see 20.0, Mathematical Composition). Three types of chemical bonds commonly seen in organic and biochemical compounds are single, double, and triple:

$$H_3 - CH_3 \qquad H_2C = CH_2 \qquad HC \equiv CH$$

mark single bond    mark double bond    mark triple bond

When deciding whether to expand or abbreviate element and chemical names, the editor and the author should consider guidelines for established terms; the manuscript's subject matter, technical level, and audience; and the context in which the term appears.

**13.14** **Radioactive Isotopes.** In general, the expanded forms for radioactive isotopes are preferred and are used in the JAMA Network journals, as described in 14.9, Isotopes, with exceptions noted for radioactive pharmaceuticals and certain chemical notations. The following list provides radioactive isotopes (and their symbols) used in medical diagnosis and therapy (see 14.9.2, Radiopharmaceuticals, and 14.9.3, Radiopharmaceutical Compounds Without Approved Names).

| Name | Symbol |
| --- | --- |
| americium | Am |
| aurum (gold) | Au |
| calcium | Ca |
| carbon | C |
| cesium | Cs |
| chromium | Cr |
| cobalt | Co |
| copper | Cu |
| fluorine | F |
| gadolinium | Gd |
| gallium | Ga |
| gold | Au |
| indium | In |
| iodine | I |

| | |
|---|---|
| iridium | Ir |
| iron | Fe |
| krypton | Kr |
| mercury | Hg |
| phosphorus | P |
| potassium | K |
| radium | Ra |
| radon | Rn |
| ruthenium | Ru |
| selenium | Se |
| sodium | Na |
| strontium | Sr |
| sulfur | S |
| technetium | Tc |
| thallium | Tl |
| xenon | Xe |
| ytterbium | Yb |

**Principal Author:** Brenda Gregoline, ELS

## ACKNOWLEDGMENT

Thanks to the following for their comments on this chapter: Barbara Gastel, MD, MPH, Texas A&M University, College Station; Trevor Lane, MA, DPhil, Edanz Group, Fukuoka, Japan; and Peter J. Olson, ELS, Sheridan Journal Services, Waterbury, Vermont.

# 14.0 Nomenclature

## 14.0  Nomenclature.

*Shakespeare has Romeo ask "What's in a name?" and answer "that which we call a rose by any other name would smell as sweet." Romeo was wrong, as he learned to his cost. Names matter.*[1]

This chapter is devoted to nomenclature: systematically formulated names for specific entities. Nomenclature is "the means of channelling the outputs of systematic research for general consumption"[2] and aims for international scope. Giangrande writes that international nomenclature efforts in coagulation "provide[d] an outstanding early example of international collaboration to resolve a scientific problem. This sort of co-operation is now commonplace, but was certainly not typical in [the post–World War II] period."[3(p710)] To facilitate worldwide access to the latest terms, large computerized databases have been created, but even computerized databases require consistent use of nomenclature.[4] Unique identifiers provide a home base for terms in large databases but are not practical for referring to entities throughout published articles and textbooks[5]—hence, names.

Biological nomenclature dates back at least to the 18th century and Linnaeus, the father of modern taxonomy. Since the mid-20th century, many biomedical disciplines have established committees to develop and promulgate official systems of nomenclature.

Accelerating knowledge in the mid-20th century, particularly from biochemistry and molecular biology, necessitated the standardized biomedical nomenclature systems, sometimes with striking results. In microbiology, with publication of the approved list of bacterial names in 1980,[6] the number of names of bacteria decreased by an order of magnitude, from approximately 30 000 to approximately 2000 (now estimated[7] to be <10 000). The CD (cluster of differentiation) nomenclature of cell-surface molecules is thought to have prevented mistakes in laboratory and clinical research.[8]

Those are some indications of the compelling need for systematic nomenclature, which requires the ongoing work of international groups. The development of nomenclature, however, faces challenges besides a multiplicity of names. There is tradition—"the ruins of previous systems"[9(p7)]—which investigators are often reluctant to give up. When disciplines converge—for instance, when the genetics of a physiologic system are delineated—preexisting systems of nomenclature may operate in parallel, and names proliferate.[4]

A system of nomenclature may face the test of sheer numbers. The count of assigned gene symbols has increased from several hundred[10,11] to more than

39 000.[12] Another challenge is to remain flexible. Those who deal with nomenclature accept it as a construct[13-16] and have noted the need to reflect new knowledge.[14,17] Biomedical classification is arbitrary and artificial, created by humans.[18,19] Nomenclature needs to evolve, "directed by insights in genome evolution and metagenomics but also by practical concerns."[7(pp264-265)]

Such flexibility, however, places a burden on clinicians, who must replace familiar names with new ones. Often, "colorful or descriptive names,"[8(p1245)] which are more easily retained,[20] give way to more efficient terms, such as the alphanumeric epithets of many systems.

Nomenclature systems may differ markedly in approach. Stability is an overriding principle of the codes of taxonomic nomenclature, which avoid name changes.[21] For instance, the bacteriologic code has a provision that a name may be rejected "whose application is likely to lead to accidents endangering health or life or both or of serious economic consequences."[22(p43)] For example, the name *Yersinia pseudotuberculosis* subsp *pestis* for the plague bacillus was rejected and the name *Y pestis* retained[22,23] because of concerns about public health hazards (owing to confusion of the name of the plague bacillus with that of the less virulent *Y pseudotuberculosis*[24,25]). In contrast, currency is an overriding principle of the official human gene nomenclature, with genes renamed to reflect new knowledge. (Of the approximately 260 gene symbols in the first Catalog of Gene Markers after introduction of the current system of gene nomenclature, more than half have been renamed.[11,26]) However, the principles of stability and currency are not mutually exclusive; for instance, the bacteriologic code requires name changes necessitated by revisions of taxonomy, and the human gene nomenclature acknowledges former names as aliases.

In medical nomenclature, the stylistic trend has been toward typographic simplicity, driven by computers. Terms lose hyphens, superscripts, subscripts, and spaces. However, such features have not been eliminated completely. For example, in 1950 standardized terms in pulmonary-respiratory medicine and physiology were put forth, and typographic features impossible on a typewriter were expressly retained, seen as indispensable components of a systematic and enlightening nomenclature.[17] Software is capable of generating unusual characters, and typographic simplification and electronic sophistication may cross paths before medical nomenclature loses its last defining flourishes.

An umbrella resource for biomedical terminology is the Unified Medical Language System (UMLS), a project of the National Library of Medicine (UMLS Knowledge Source Server [UMLSKS]). UMLS is intended to provide integrated terminology (including synonyms and relationships among terms) for use in electronic applications (eg, computer systems, electronic health records, online dictionaries).[27,28] A major component of UMLS is the Metathesaurus, a comprehensive repository of biomedical terms and their relationships. The Metathesaurus is accessible online at the UMLS Knowledge Source Server (https://www.nlm.nih.gov/research/umls/knowledge_sources/metathesaurus). That website offers concept and term searches that can be useful to medical authors and editors who seek explanations of particular terms, including their relationships to other terms (eg, human gene, protein, condition, and animal counterparts).[28]

In an ever-evolving health care system, it will be important to crosswalk research/genomic nomenclature with systems of medical coding, such as *International Classification of Disease, Tenth Revision, Clinical Modification (ICD-10-CM)*[29] and Systematized Nomenclature of Medicine (SNOMED)[30] with a high degree of specificity. Without the ability to do this, research and clinical care will be much more challenging in a future where genomic information is a part of the medical record.

Our purpose in the nomenclature chapter is not to explain how names should be devised (although we cite the sources of such rules) but rather which names should be used and how they should be styled. Official systems of nomenclature are not universally observed to the letter (literally or figuratively), but style that is consistent with official guidelines and within publications reduces ambiguity. Editors have the task of mediating between official systems and authors' actual usage. To that end, the goals of this chapter are to present style for terms in selected fields and to explain terms so that they are more easily dealt with.

Note: In this chapter, some style rules described elsewhere in this manual have been waived so as not to cause confusion regarding conventional presentation of terms (eg, in table cells, where normally initial caps would be used on each cell entry, lowercase is used unless the term is to be presented with an initial cap).

**Principal Author:** Cheryl Iverson, MA

## ACKNOWLEDGMENT

Thanks to W. Gregory Feero, MD, PhD, *JAMA*, and Maine-Dartmouth Family Medicine Residency, Augusta, Maine; Trevor Lane, MA, DPhil, Edanz Group, Fukuoka, Japan; Karen Boyd, formerly with the JAMA Network; and Philip Sefton, MS, ELS, *JAMA*, for reviewing and providing comments.

## REFERENCES

1. Wilczek F. What's in a scientific name? *Wall Street J.* May 27-28, 2017:C4.
2. Greuter W, Hawksworth DL. Preface. In: Greuter W, McNeill J, Farrie FR, et al. *International Code of Botanical Nomenclature (St Louis Code).* International Association for Plant Taxonomy; 2000. Updated June 28, 2018. Accessed July 23, 2019. https://archive.bgbm.org/iapt/nomenclature/code/SaintLouis/0000St.Luistitle.htm
3. Giangrande PL. Six characters in search of an author: the history of the nomenclature of coagulation factors. *Br J Haematol.* 2003;121(5):705-712. doi:10.1046/j.1365-2141.2003.04333.x
4. Cammack R. The biochemical nomenclature committees. *IUBMB Life.* 2000;50(3):159-161. doi:10.1080/152165400300001453
5. Beutler E, McKusick VA, Motulsky AG, Scriver CR, Hutchinson F. Mutation nomenclature: nicknames, systematic names, and unique identifiers. *Hum Mutat.* 1996;8(3):203-206. doi:10.1002/(SICI)1098-1004(1996)8:3<203::AID-HUMU1>3.0.CO;2-A
6. Skerman VBD, McGowan V, Sneath PHA. Approved lists of bacterial names. *Int J Syst Bacteriol.* 1980;30(1):225-420. doi:10.1099/00207713-30-1-225
7. Vandamme PAR. Taxonomy and classification of bacteria. In: Murray PR, ed. *Manual of Clinical Microbiology.* 11th ed. ASM Press; 2015:255-265.
8. Singer NG, Todd RF, Fox DA. Structures on the cell surface: update from the Fifth International Workshop on Human Leukocyte Differentiation Antigens. *Arthritis Rheum.* 1994;37(8):1245-1248. doi:10.1002/art.1780370820
9. Wildy P. *Classification and Nomenclature of Viruses: First Report of the International Committee on Nomenclature of Viruses.* S Karger AG; 1971:1-26. Melnick JL, ed. Monographs in Virology. Vol 5.

10. Shows TB, McAlpine PJ. The 1981 catalogue of assigned human genetic markers and report of the nomenclature committee. *Cytogenet Cell Genet.* 1982;32(1-4):221-245. doi:10.1159/000131702

11. Evans HJ, Hamerton JL, Klinger HP, McKusick VA. *Human Gene Mapping 5: Edinburgh Conference (1979): Fifth International Workshop on Human Gene Mapping.* S Karger; 1979.

12. HUGO Gene Nomenclature Committee website. Accessed May 18, 2018. https://www.genenames.org

13. Staley JT, Krieg NR. Bacterial classification, I: classification of procaryotic organisms: an overview. In: Krieg NR, Holt JF, eds. *Bergey's Manual of Systematic Bacteriology.* Vol 1. Williams & Wilkins; 1984:1-4.

14. Erzinclioglu YZ, Unwin DM. The stability of zoological nomenclature. *Nature.* 1986;320:687. doi:10.1038/321476b0

15. Lublin DM, Telen MJ. What is a blood group antigen? *Transfusion.* 1992;32(5):493. doi:10.1046/j.1537-2995.1992.32592327724.x

16. Lublin DM, Telen MJ. More about use of the term Drb. *Transfusion.* 1993;33(2):182. doi:10.1046/j.1537-2995.1993.33293158056.x

17. Pappenheimer JR, chairman; Comroe JH, Cournand A, Ferguson JKW, et al. Standardization of definitions and symbols in respiratory physiology. *Fed Proc.* 1950;9:602-605.

18. Madias JE. Killip and Forrester classifications: should they be abandoned, kept, reevaluated, or modified? *Chest.* 2000;117(5):1223-1226. doi:10.1378/chest.117.5.1223

19. Vandamme PAR. Taxonomy and classification of bacteria. In: Murray PR, Baron EJ, Jorgensen JH, Pfaller MA, Yolken RH, eds. *Manual of Clinical Microbiology.* 8th ed. ASM Press; 2003:271.

20. Flexner CW. In praise of descriptive nomenclature. *Lancet.* 1996;347(8993):68.

21. Jeffrey C. *Biological Nomenclature.* 3rd ed. Routledge Chapman & Hall; 1989.

22. Lapage SP, Sneath PHA, Lessel EF, Skerman VBD, Seeliger HPR, Clark WA; Sneath PHA, ed. *International Code of Nomenclature of Bacteria and Statutes of the Bacteriology and Applied Microbiology Section of the International Union of Microbiological Societies, 1990 Revision.* American Society for Microbiology; 1992.

23. Euzéby JP. List of prokaryotic names with standing in nomenclature: genus *Yersinia.* Accessed July 30, 2019. http://www.bacterio.net/yersinia.html

24. Williams JE. Proposal to reject the new combination *Yersinia pseudotuberculosis* subsp *pestis* for violation of the first principles of the International Code of Nomenclature of Bacteria: request for an opinion. *Int J Syst Bacteriol.* 1984;34(2):268-269. doi:10.1099/00207713-34-2-268

25. Judicial Commission of the International Committee on Systematic Bacteriology. Rejection of the name *Yersinia pseudotuberculosis* subsp. *pestis* (van Loghem) Bercovier et al. 1981 and conservation of the name *Yersinia pestis* (Lehmann and Neumann) van Loghem 1944 for the plague bacillus. *Int J Syst Bacteriol.* 1985;35(4):540. doi:10.1099/00207713-35-4-540

26. Gray KA, Seal RL, Tweedie S, Wright MW, Bruford EA. A review of the new HGNC gene family resource. *Hum Genomics.* February 2, 2016:10:6. doi:10.1186/540246-016-0062.6

27. US National Library of Medicine. Unified Medical Language System. Published July 29, 2009. Updated December 21, 2017. Accessed July 23, 2019. https://www.nlm.nih.gov/research/umls/about_umls.html

28. Bodenreider O. The Unified Medical Language System (UMLS): integrating bi-omedical terminology. *Nucleic Acids Res.* 2004;32(database issue):D267-D270. doi:10.1093/nar/gkh061

29. World Health Organization. *International Classification of Diseases, Tenth Revision, Clinical Modification (ICD-10-CM).* Updated August 18, 2017. Accessed May 18, 2018. https://www.cdc.gov/nchs/icd/icd10cm.htm

30. Overview of SNOMED CT. Published October 5, 2016. Updated October 14, 2016. Accessed July 23, 2019. https://www.nlm.nih.gov/healthit/snomedct/snomed_overview.html

## 14.1 Blood Groups, Platelet Antigens, and Granulocyte Antigens.

### 14.1.1 Blood Groups.
*Blood groups* in humans are characterized by erythrocyte (red blood cell) antigens with common immunologic properties. *Blood group systems* are series of such antigens encoded by a single gene or by a cluster of 2 or 3 closely linked homologous genes.[1-3]

The International Society of Blood Transfusion (ISBT) recognizes 346 antigen specificities and 36 blood group systems.[4-7] Other antigens may be assigned in the future but remain in officially designated series or collections. Some antigens are erythrocyte specific; others appear widely, but specifically, on cells of other organs and tissues.

The discovery of blood group antigens was prompted by hemolytic disease of the newborn and transfusion reactions, but many antigens have since been implicated in infection and other disease processes.[1,8] Erythrocytes are estimated to contain millions of antigen sites.[1]

#### 14.1.1.1 Traditional/Popular Nomenclature.
Traditional blood group system nomenclature is typically used in medical publications. "Until recently there was no attempt to be systematic. In the past, some blood groups were named after the individual . . . or animal . . . lacking the antigen. Others were named after the discoverers."[6(p509)] Some laboratories still use the traditional names, and some laboratories use other traditional nomenclature. Sometimes the same entity (eg, a particular erythrocyte antigen) can be expressed by more than one term. Authors and editors should generally follow the recommendations herein.

The principal elements named are blood group systems, antigens, phenotypes, genes, and alleles.

##### 14.1.1.1.1 Blood Group Systems.
Table 14.1-1 lists the blood group system names and symbols. (The column of derivations of names of blood group systems is provided for background interest.[1,2,6,9-17])

The ISBT prefers an all-capital style for blood group system symbols[4] (see 14.1.1.2, ISBT Name and Number).

The following are examples of usage:

ABO incompatibility

A cell

type AB recipient

type O donor

Hemolytic disease of the newborn occurs primarily from incompatibilities of the Rh, ABO, or Kell blood groups.

**Table 14.1-1.** Blood Group System Names and Symbols

| System name | System symbol | Derivation |
|---|---|---|
| ABO | ABO | Alphabetical (A and B); letter O may derive from "ohne" (German for *without*) |
| Chido/Rodgers | CH/RG | Names of antibody makers (Mrs Chido and Mr Rodgers) |
| Colton | CO | Name of antibody maker<br>Co$^a$ (from Calton [should have been Ca but handwriting on tube was misread as Colton]) |
| Cromer | CROM | Name of antibody maker (Mrs Cromer) |
| Diego | DI | Name of antibody maker (Mrs Diego) |
| Dombrock | DO | Named after proband |
| Duffy | FY | Name of antibody maker (Mr Duffy) |
| Forssman | FORS | Named after John Forssman, Swedish pathologist (Forssman antigen) |
| Gerbich | GE | Name of antibody maker (originally described by the "Yus-type" antibody) |
| Gill | GIL | Named after proband |
| Globoside | GLOB | Globoside synthetase |
| H | H | Concept ("heterogenetic") |
| I | I | Concept ("individuality") |
| Indian | IN | Geographic |
| John Milton Hagen | JMH | Initials of antibody maker |
| JR | JR | Rose Jacobs, name of antibody maker |
| Kell | KEL | Name of antibody maker (Kelleher) |
| Kidd | JK | Initials of infant of antibody maker (K already in use) |
| Knops | KN | Name of antibody maker (named after 1 of 3 siblings) |
| Kx | XK | Association with Kell and X chromosome |
| LAN | LAN | Langereis, name of antibody maker |
| Landsteiner-Wiener | LW | Names of investigators |
| Lewis | LE | Named after 1 of 2 original antibody makers |
| Lutheran | LU | Name of antibody maker (actually *Lutteran*[10] or *Luteran*[14]) |
| MNS | MNS | M, N: the word *immune*<br>S: location (Sydney, Australia)<br>U (an antigen of this system): universal |
| Ok | OK | Family name initials (Kobutso; letters reversed because "K$_o$" was in use) |
| P | P1 | Alphabetical |
| Raph | RAPH | Name of antibody maker |
| Rh | RH | Rhesus monkeys (antigens were LW antigens) |
| Rh-associated glycoprotein | RHAG | Rh-associated glycoprotein |
| Scianna | SC | Name of antibody maker (Scianna) |
| Xg | XG | X chromosome and location (Grand Rapids, Michigan) |
| Yt | YT | Name of antibody maker (Cartwright) |

**14.1.1.1.2** **Antigens.** Antigen terms use single or dual letters, often with a qualifier that is a letter (usually superscript) or number (subscript or typeset on the line).

A, $A_1$, $A_2$, $A_x$, B

$Cr^a$

$Fy^a$, $Fy^b$

He

$Jk^a$, $Jk^b$

K, k

$Kp^a$, $Kp^b$, Ku, $Js^a$, $Js^b$

K11, K12, K13, K14, Km

$Le^a$, $Le^b$, $Le^{bH}$, $ALe^b$, $BLe^b$

$Lu^a$, $Lu^b$

Lu3, Lu4, Lu5, Lu6

$P^1$

Sc1, Sc2

$Xg^a$

The Rh system historically has used 3 alternative schemes: the Wiener system, the Fisher-Race system, and the Rosenfield (numerical) system.[6] Although the first 2 models are not supported by genetic analysis, they are both used widely today because of their familiarity.[6(p516)] For an example of the 3 different systems for a single term, see below[6(p516)]:

Rh1 (Rosenfield)

D (Fisher-Race)

$Rh_0$ (Wiener)

**14.1.1.1.3** **Phenotypes.** In phenotypic expressions—terms that describe an individual's blood group or type—the presence or absence of an antigen is often indicated by a plus or minus sign:

*Antigen:*      M

*Phenotype:*     M+

M+N+S−s+ erythrocytes

M+N+S−s+ phenotype

Lowercase letters that were superscripts in the antigen terms are set on the line in parentheses in phenotypic terms.

| *Antigen:* | $Lu^b$ |
|---|---|
| *Phenotype:* | Lu(b+) |

More than 98% of the Western population is Lu(b+).

If the numerical terminology is used for the antigen, a colon is added in the phenotype.

| *Antigen:* | Sc1 |
|---|---|
| *Phenotype:* | Sc:1 |

the Sc:1,–2,3 phenotype

Other sample phenotypic terms include the following:

Fy(a–b+), Fy(a+b–), Fy(a–b–)

Jk(a–b+), Jk(a+b–), Jk(a+b+)

K+k–, Kp(a–b+), Js(a–b+)

Le(a–b+), Le(a+b–), Le(a–b–)

Lu(a–b+), Lu(a+b–), Lu(a+b+)

M+N+, M+,N–, M–N+, S+s+, S+s–, S–s+

$P_1$, $P_2$, $P_1^{\,k}$, $P_2^{\,k}$

Xg(a+), Xg(a–)

the silent phenotype Le(a–b–)

A superscript w can indicate a weak reaction:

$M+^w$

$K+^w$

Fy(a+$^w$)

The ABO system is an exception: its phenotypic terms do not feature plus or minus signs; A (not A+) indicates A erythrocyte antigens; O (not A– B–) indicates the absence of A and B antigens:

| *Groups:* | O, A, B, AB, $O_h$, $O_h^{\,A}$ |
|---|---|
| *Subgroups:* | $A_1$, $A_2$, $A_1B$, $A_2B$ |

$O_h^{\,A}$ individuals do not express the H determinant but have the *A* allele.

Terms for Rh phenotypes, which do not feature plus and minus signs, are also in use:

D-positive (Rh positive)

D-negative (Rh negative)

DccE, DCce

RH:1,2,3

$Rh_{null}$

Absence of C, c, E, and/or e antigens is indicated with 1 or 2 dashes[15]:

Dc− (1 dash)

D— (2 dashes)

Terms such as O+ ("O positive"), A+, and AB− are common parlance as shorthand for blood of the ABO system and its Rh specificity. However, in scientific articles, use standard terms that specifically indicate Rh status:

O Rh-positive

O Rh+

Note that this may be written either O Rh-positive or O Rh+.

An individual is considered Rh positive if his or her red blood cells express the D antigen. Conversely, Rh negative indicates the absence of the D antigen.[1(p2266),6(p516)] If the D antigen is present, the correct expression is Rh D-positive; if absent, Rh D-negative. Only if the specific Rh D status is being indicated is the word *positive* or *negative* preferred to the plus or minus sign.

group B, Rh D-negative

group A, Rh D-positive

In a blood group profile, elements from different systems may be separated by commas, as above, or, for more complex specificities, with semicolons:

The patient's blood was group B, Rh-positive, D+ C+ c+ E− e+; M+ N+ S− s+; $P_1$+; Le(a−b−); K− k+; Fy(a−b+); Jk(a+b−).[18(p846)]

Note that in phenotypic expressions commas do not appear within elements of the same blood group system:

*Use:* D+ C+ c+ E− e+

*Not:* D+, C+, c+, E−, e+

Commas may be dispensed with *between* blood groups in brief expressions:

K+Fy(a+)

**14.1.1.1.4** **Genes.** As with International Standard Gene Nomenclature (the Human Genome Organization [HUGO] recommendations; see 14.6.2, Human Gene Nomenclature), the ISBT gene terms are italicized. Traditional blood group gene symbols are often mixed uppercase and lowercase letters. However, symbols recommended by the ISBT, like those of HUGO, use all capital letters.

Table 14.1-2[3,4,6(pp510-511),8,19] lists gene symbols associated with blood group systems.

**Table 14.1-2.** Gene Symbols and Associated Blood Group Systems

| Traditional | ISBT | HUGO |
|---|---|---|
| ABO (ABO) | ABO | ABO |
| Chido/ Rodgers (CH/RG) | CH/RG | C4B, C4A |
| Colton (CO) | CO | AQP1 |
| Cromer (CROM) | CROM | CD55 |
| Diego (DI) | DI | SLC4A1 |
| Dombrock (DO) | DO | ART4 |
| Duffy (FY) | FY | DARC |
| Forssman (FORS) | GBGT1 | GBGT1 |
| Gerbich (GE) | GE | GYPC |
| Gill (GIL) | GIL | AQP3 |
| Globoside (GLOB) | GLOB | B3GALNT1 |
| H | H | FUT1 |
| I (I) | IGTN | GCNT2 |
| Indian (IN) | IN | CD44 |
| John Milton Hagen (JMH) | JMH | SEMA7A |
| JR (Junior) | ABCG2 | ABCG2 |
| Kell (KEL) | KEL | KEL |
| Kidd (JK) | JK | SLC14A1 |
| Knops (KN) | KN | CR1 |
| Kx (XK) | XK | XK |
| LAN (Langereis) | ABCB6 | ABCB6 |
| Landsteiner-Wiener (LW) | LW | ICAM4 |
| Lewis (LE) | LE | FUT3 |
| Lutheran (LU) | LU | B-CAM |
| MNS | MNS | GYPA, GYPB, GYPE |
| Ok (OK) | OK | BSG |
| P (P1) | P1 | P1 |
| Raph (RAPH) | RAPH | CD151 |
| Rh (RH) | RH | RHD, RHCE |
| Rh-associated glycoprotein (RHAG) | RHAG | RHAG |
| Scianna (SC) | SC | ERMAP |
| Xg (XG) | XG | XG |
| Yt (YT) (Cartwright) | YT | ACHE |

Abbreviations: ISBT, International Society of Blood Transfusion; HUGO, Human Genome Organization.

Gene symbols expressed according to ISBT[4] or HUGO[19] are preferred to traditional symbols.

Parenthetic synonyms are helpful:

*BSG* (formerly *Ok*), *OK* (*BSG, EMPRIN*)

*ERMAP* (also called *SC*), *SC* (*ERMAP*)

The Lutheran inhibitor gene is expressed as follows:

*In(Lu)* [traditional]

*INLU* [standard]

Do not confuse *In* with the traditional Indian blood group gene symbol *IN* (recommended symbol: *CD44*).

**14.1.1.1.5** **Alleles.** The italicized blood group symbol (eg, *BO, MNS, RH*) is used for alleles (which are also distinguished by an asterisk and number).[20] In the following example, compare the gene symbol and an allele term from the same blood group:

*SC\*1* [allele]

*ERMAP* [gene symbol]

Note that qualifiers that are subscripts in antigen terms are superscripts in allelic terms (eg, $A_1$ antigen, $A^1$ allele). The following are examples of genotypic terms.

*$A^1O$, $A^1A^1$, $A^1B$, OO*

*MN, MM, NN, MSNs*

*DCe/DCe ($R^1R^1$)*

*DcE/dce ($R^2r$)*

*dce/dce (rr)*

*D--/D--*

*$Lu^aLu^a$, $Lu^bLu^b$, $Lu^aLu^b$*

*Lele, LeLe, lele*

*$Fy^aFy^a$, $Fy^bFy^b$, FyFy*

*Kk, $Kp^b$,$Kp^b$, $Js^bJs^b$*

*$Jk^aJk^a$, $Jk^bJk^b$, $Jk^aJk^b$*

*$Xg^aXg^a$, $Xg^aXg$, XgXg*

*$Xg^aY$, XgY*

For expressing alleles, the ISBT gives an option: *$Fy^a$* or *FY\*01*. Mixing the 2 styles, however (eg, *FY\*A*), is not appropriate.[17]

**14.1.1.2** **ISBT Name and Number.** In the 1980s, the Working Party on Terminology for Red Cell Surface Antigens of the ISBT[3,8,21,22] developed an alphanumeric system of blood group notation (**Table 14.1-3**), intended to provide "a uniform nomenclature that

**Table 14.1-3.** The Alphanumeric System of Blood Group Notation

| System | | | Antigen No. within system | | | |
|---|---|---|---|---|---|---|
| Name | Symbol | No. | 001 | 002 | 003 | 004 |
| ABO | ABO | 001 | A | B | A,B | A1 |
| MNS | MNS | 002 | M | N | S | s |
| Rh | RH | 004 | D | C | E | c |
| Kx | XK | 019 | Kx | | | |

is both eye and machine readable and in keeping with the genetic basis of blood groups."[9(p273)] The system does not replace traditional terminology; rather, its terms correspond to traditional terms. It is also used to assign new terms as needed. In the ISBT terminology, each blood group system has a symbol, usually of 1 to 3 capital letters, and a system number of 3 digits. "Each blood group antigen is given an identification number consisting of six digits. The first three numbers represent the system to which the antigen has been assigned. The second three digits identify the antigen. Each system has an alphabetic symbol. For example, the ABO system is number 001, and the A antigen is the first antigen of that system; thus it has the ISBT number 001001 or ABO001. By convention, zeros may be omitted, and numbers are separated by a dot (i.e., the A antigen would be 1.1 or ABO1)."[6(p510)]

Sinistral (left-hand) zeros can be dropped from system and antigen terms, and system letter symbols can be used as part of the alphanumeric term. The following, for instance, are all acceptable for blood type AB:

AB

ABO:1,2,3

001:1,2,3

The following are acceptable terms for the antigen A,B:

A,B

ABO3

001003

Authors may use ISBT[4] terms in parentheses after traditional terms:

AB (1.3)

D (RH1)

Le$^a$ (007001)

The patient's red blood cells were negative for Cromer blood system antigens Cr$^a$ (CROM1) and Tc$^a$ (CROM2).

In systems that use plus and minus signs to express the presence and absence of particular antigens, phenotypic expressions in the numerical notation use a colon and numbers in place of letters, as in these examples:

LE:−1,2 [for Le(a−b+)]

FY:1,−2 [for FY(a+b−)]

Genotypic expressions are italicized:

*FY 1/2* or *FY\*1/2* (for *Fy$^a$Fy$^b$*)

Tables of blood group systems, symbols, antigens, and ISBT numbers are available at the ISBT Committee on Terminology for Red Cell Surface Antigens website.[4]

**14.1.2 Platelet-Specific Antigens.** The current system of human platelet antigen (HPA) nomenclature, adopted in 1990, is overseen by the Platelet Nomenclature Committee of the ISBT and the International Society on Thrombosis and Haemostasis.[23,24] As with blood groups, there are platelet antigen systems and specific antigens within those systems. The HPA nomenclature pertains to "all protein alloantigens expressed on the platelet membrane, except those coded by genes of the major histocompatibility complex (MHC)"[23] (see 14.8.5, HLA/Major Histocompatibility Complex). Currently, there are 6 HPA systems: HPA-1, HPA-2, HPA-3, HPA-4, HPA-5, and HPA-15.[24]

Complete tables of HPA terms are available at the Immuno Polymorphism Database (IPD-HPA) website.[24,25] To date, 33 platelet-specific antigens have been characterized. Currently, there are 27 HPA systems (HPA1-14 and HPA15-27).[7(pp453-455)] Sample terms are listed in **Table 14.1-4**.

**Table 14.1-4.** Sample Terms From Human Platelet Antigen (HPA) Nomenclature

| Term | Abbreviation |
| --- | --- |
| Antigen system | HPA-1 |
| Associated glycoprotein | GpIIIa |
| CD designation of glycoprotein | CD61 |
| Former names | Zw, P1A |
| Antigens | HPA-1a<br>HPA-1b |
| Former antigen names | Zw$^a$, P1$^{A1}$<br>Zw$^b$, P1$^{A2}$ |
| Gene | *ITGB3* |
| Alleles | *ITGB3\*001*<br>*ITGB3\*002* |
| Epitopes | HPA-1a<br>HPA-1b |
| Locuslink ID | 3690 |
| Ref_Seq | NM_000212 |
| Swiss-Prot | ITB3_Human |
| Nucleotide change | 176T>C |

**Table 14.1-5.** ISBT Rules for Well-Defined HNAs

| Antigen system | Antigen | Former name | Alleles |
|---|---|---|---|
| HNA-1 | HNA-1a | NA1 | *FCGR3B*1 (CD16)* |
| | HNA-1b | NA2 | *FCGR3B*2 (CD-16)* |
| | HNA-1c | SH | *FCGR3B*3 (CD-16)* |
| HNA-2 | HNA-2a | NB1 | *CD177*1* |
| HNA-3 | HNA-3a | 5b | *CTL2* |
| HNA-4 | HNA-4a | Mart[a] | *CD11B*1* |
| HNA-5 | HNA-5a | Ond[a] | *CD11A*1* |

Abbreviations: HNA, human neutrophil antigen; ISBT, International Society of Blood Transfusion.

For CD (clusters of differentiation) nomenclature, see 14.8.7, Lymphocytes. For gene and allele nomenclature, see 14.6.2, Human Gene Nomenclature. For database identifiers and nucleotide nomenclature, see 14.6.1, Nucleic Acids and Amino Acids.

**14.1.3**    **Granulocyte Antigens.** The Granulocyte Antigen Working Party of the ISBT has formulated rules for well-defined human neutrophil antigens,[26] as presented in **Table 14.1-5**, although at this writing they have not met with universal acceptance.[6(p540),27,28]

See 14.8.6, Immunoglobulins, for Fc receptor terminology and 14.8.7, Lymphocytes, for CD terminology.

**Principal Author:** Cheryl Iverson, MA

## ACKNOWLEDGMENT

Thanks to Emmanuel A. Fadeyi, MD, Wake Forest Baptist Medical Center, Winston-Salem, North Carolina, for reviewing and providing comments.

## REFERENCES

1. Reid ME. Erythrocyte antigens and antibodies. In: Kaushansky K, Lichtman MA, Beutler E, Kipps TJ, Seligsohn U, Prchal JT, eds. *Williams Hematology*. 8th ed. McGraw-Hill; 2011:2247-2268.
2. Schenkel-Brunner H. *Human Blood Groups: Chemical and Biochemical Basis of Antigen Specificity*. 2nd ed. Springer-Verlag; 2000.
3. Daniels GL, Fletcher A, Garraty G, et al. Blood group terminology 2004: from the International Society of Blood Transfusion Committee on Terminology for Red Cell Surface Antigens. *Vox Sang*. 2004;87(4):304-316. doi:10.1111/j.1423-0410.2004.00564.x
4. International Society of Blood Transfusion. Blood group terminology. Accessed July 23, 2019. https://www.isbtweb.org/working-parties/red-cell-immunogenetics-and-blood-group-terminology

5. Storry JR, Castilho L, Daniels G, et al. International Society of Blood Transfusion Working Party on red cell immunogenetics and blood group terminology: Berlin Report. *Vox Sang.* 2011;101(1):77-82. doi:10.1111/j.1423-0410.2010.01462.x

6. Smith JW, Arnold DM, Chan HHW, Heddle NM, Kelton JG. Red cell, platelet, and white cell antigens. In: Greer JP, Arber DA, Glader B, et al, eds. *Wintrobe's Clinical Hematology.* 13th ed. Lippincott Williams & Wilkins; 2014:509-546.

7. Fung MK, Grossman BJ, Hillyer CD, Westhoff CM, eds. *Technical Manual.* 18th ed. American Association of Blood Banks; 2014:453-455.

8. Dzieczkowski JS, Anderson KC. Transfusion biology and therapy. In: Longo DL, Fauci AS, Kasper DL, Hauser SL, Jameson JL, Loscalzo J, eds. *Harrison's Principles of Internal Medicine.* 18th ed. McGraw-Hill; 2012:951-957.

9. Daniels GL, Anstee DJ, Cartron JP, et al. Blood group terminology 1995: ISBT Working Party on Terminology for Red Cell Surface Antigens. *Vox Sang.* 1995;69(3):265-279. doi:10.1111/j.1423-0410.1995.tb02611.x

10. Garratty G, Dzik W, Issitt PD, Lublin DM, Reid ME, Zelinski T. Terminology for blood group antigens and genes—historical origins and guidelines in the new millennium. *Transfusion.* 2000;40(4):477-489.

11. Daniels GL, Anstee DJ, Cartron JP, et al. Reports and guidelines: International Society of Blood Transfusion Working Party on Terminology for Red Cell Surface Antigens. *Vox Sang.* 2001;80(3):193-196.

12. Daniels GL, Cartron JP, Fletcher A, et al. International Society of Blood Transfusion Committee on Terminology for Red Cell Surface Antigens: Vancouver Report. *Vox Sang.* 2003;84(3):244-247. doi:10.1046/j.1423-0410.2003.00282.x

13. The Blood Group Antigen Gene Mutation Database. Accessed July 31, 2019. ftp://ftp.ncbi.nlm.nih.gov/pub/mhc/rbc/Final Archive

14. SCARF: serum, cells & rare fluids exchange. Accessed July 31, 2019. ftp://ftp.ncbi.nlm.nih.gov/pub/mhc/mhc/Final%20Archive

15. Avent ND, Reid ME. The Rh blood group system: a review. *Blood.* 2000;95(2):375-387.

16. Storry JR, Olsson ML. The ABO blood group system revisited: a review and update. *Immunohematology.* 2009;25(2):48-74.

17. Reid ME, Lomas-Francis C, Olsson ML. *The Blood Group Antigen Facts Book.* 3rd ed. Academic Press; 2012.

18. Whitsett CF, Hare VW, Oxendine SM, Pierce JA. Autologous and allogeneic red cell survival studies in the presence of autoanti-AnWj. *Transfusion.* 1993;33(10):845-847.

19. Gene Search. HUGO Gene Nomenclature Committee. Accessed July 23, 2019. https://www.genenames.org/tools/search

20. Guidelines for ISBT Naming of Blood Group Alleles: Guidelines v2.0 110914. Accessed July 23, 2019. https://www.isbtweb.org/fileadmin/user_upload/files-2015/red%20cells/blood%20group%20allele%20terminology/ISBT%20Guidelines%20Naming%20Blood%20Group%20Alleles%20v2.0%20110914.pdf

21. Issitt PD, Moulds JJ. Blood group terminology suitable for use in electronic data processing equipment. *Transfusion.* 1992;32(7):677-682.

22. Daniels GL, Anstee DJ, Cartron JP, et al. Terminology for red cell surface antigens: ISBT Working Party Oslo Report. *Vox Sang.* 1999;77(1):52-57.

23. Metcalfe P, Watkins NA, Ouwehand WH, et al. Nomenclature of human platelet antigens. *Vox Sang.* 2003;85(3):240-245.

24. Robinson J, Halliwell JA, McWilliam H, Lopez R, Marsh SGE. IPD: the Immuno Polymorphism Database. *Nucleic Acids Res.* 2013;41(database issue):D1234-D1240. doi:10.1093/nar/gks1140

25. Immuno Polymorphism (IPD-HPA) Database. Accessed July 23, 2019. https://www.ebi.ac.uk/ipd/hpa/

26. Flesch BK; International Society of Blood Transfusion (ISBT) HNA Nomenclature Subcommittee. Human neutrophil antigens: a nomenclature based on new alleles and new antigens. *ISBT Sci Ser.* 2015;10:243-249.

27. Lalezari P. Nomenclature of neutrophil-specific antigens. *Transfusion.* 2002;42(11):1396-1397. doi:10.1046/j.1537-2995.2002.00255.x

28. Stroncek D, Bux J. Is it time to standardize granulocyte alloantigen nomenclature? *Transfusion.* 2002;42(4):393-395.

## 14.2 Cancer.

### 14.2.1 Cancer Stage.

Cancer stages are expressed with the use of capital roman numerals, with higher numbers indicating increasing extent of disease:

> stage I
>
> stage II
>
> stage III
>
> stage IV

The term "stage 0" usually indicates carcinoma in situ, with no spread of disease beyond the primary site.

Letter and numerical suffixes, usually set on the line, may be added to subdivide individual cancer stages, as in the following examples:

> stage 0a
>
> stage 0is
>
> stage IA
>
> stage IE
>
> stage IB2
>
> stage IIIE+S
>
> stage IVA
>
> stage IVB

Note: E indicates extralymphatic spread; S, splenic involvement (as seen in Hodgkin disease); is, in situ.

Histologic grades are expressed with arabic numerals (eg, grade 2). For some anatomical sites, grade 3 and grade 4 are combined into a single grade: grade 3-4 (for poorly differentiated to undifferentiated).[1(p13)]

### 14.2.2 The TNM Staging System.

The TNM (tumor, node, metastasis) staging system[1-8] is an internationally standardized system for the staging of cancer and is in its eighth decade of continuing formulation. The TNM classification is put forth by the American Joint Committee on Cancer (AJCC; https://cancerstaging.org) and the Union for International Cancer Control (UICC; https://www.uicc.org).[2] The AJCC's *Cancer Staging Manual*[1] and the UICC's *TNM Classification of Malignant Tumours*[3] present the stages of cancer as defined by TNM classifications. The TNM definitions and stage groupings are based on prognostic outcome. Information about TNM may be accessed at the UICC website. The TNM symbols follow.

- T: tumor (indicates size, extent, or depth of penetration of the primary tumor)

    T is followed by numerical or other suffixes set on the line, for example:

    TX: primary tumor cannot be assessed

    T0: no evidence of a primary tumor

    Tis: carcinoma in situ

    T1, T2, T3, T4: increasing size and/or local extent or other characteristics of the primary tumor

Note: The number following T does not refer to an absolute size. For example, for one type of tumor, T1 may indicate a size of 2 cm or less; for another, a depth (or thickness) of 0.75 mm or less; and for another, tumor confinement within the underlying mucosa.

- N: node (indicates the absence or presence and extent of regional lymph node involvement)

    NX: regional lymph nodes cannot be assessed

    N0: no regional lymph node metastasis

    N1, N2, N3: increasing metastatic involvement of regional lymph nodes according to criteria that vary for different anatomical sites

- M: metastasis (indicates absence or presence of distant metastasis)

    M0: no metastasis

    M1: distant metastasis

Note: MX (distant metastasis cannot be assessed) has been eliminated from the seventh edition of the TNM classification because "clinical assessment of metastasis can be based on physical examination alone."[3(p11)] This change will encourage the assignment of M0 and facilitate stage grouping.[6]

Site of metastasis may be indicated with parenthetic 3-letter abbreviations, for example, M1(PUL):

| | |
|---|---|
| ADR | adrenal glands |
| BRA | brain |
| HEP | hepatic |
| LYM | lymph nodes |
| MAR | bone marrow |
| OSS | osseous |

OTH     other

PER     peritoneum

PLE     pleura

PUL     pulmonary

SKI     skin

**14.2.2.1** **The TNM System and Cancer Staging.** Various combinations of the T, N, and M categories are used to define cancer stages (consult the AJCC[1] or UICC[2] manual for specifics). For example, a TNM stage grouping that defines stage I for many types of cancer is as follows:

T1N0M0

The combinations that define individual stages differ among anatomical sites, for example:

lung cancer, stage IIA       T1N1M0

pancreatic cancer, stage IIA    T3N0M0

More than one combination of the T, N, and M categories may constitute the definition of a single stage; for example, in a given cancer, stage III may be defined as T1N1M0 *or* T2N1M0 *or* T3N0M0 *or* T3N1M0.

**14.2.2.2** **Optional Descriptors.** Additional descriptors, although not part of the TNM staging system, may be used as adjuncts to the T, N, and M categories for defining the extent of disease; these are indicated by capital letters as follows:

certainty factor (C-factor)    C1, C2, C3, C4, C5

histopathologic grading      GX, G1, G2, G3, G4

lymphatic vessel invasion    LX, L0, L1

residual tumor             RX, R0, R1, R2

venous invasion           VX, V0, V1, V2

C-factor terms may be used together with T, N, and M categories (eg, T3C2, N2C1, M0C2).[3(p18)]

Lowercase prefixes to the T, N, M, and other symbols may be used to indicate the mode of determining criteria for tumor description and staging or other attributes (eg, cTNM, pT3) as follows:

a    autopsy T, N, or M classification or stage

c    clinical T, N, or M classification or stage

p    pathologic T, N, or M classification or stage

r    recurrent tumor T, N, or M classification or stage, when classified after a disease-free interval

y    classification during or after initial multimodality treatment

The T, N, M, and other symbols used in cancer staging may be followed by suffixes in addition to the common X, 0, and numerals, which further specify qualities, such as size, invasiveness, and extent of metastasis, eg:

| | | | | | |
|------|-------|-----|-----|---------|----------|
| Ta | T2a | M1a | N1a | pN1a | pN0 |
| Tis | T2(m) | M2a | N2a | pN1(mi) | pN0(i−) |
| T1b | T2(5) | | N2b | pN0(sn) | pN0(i+) |
| T1c | T3a | | N2c | pN3c | pN0(mol−) |
| T1a1 | | | | | pN0(mol+) |

Note: m indicates the presence of multiple primary tumors at a single site; mi, micrometastasis; sn, sentinel node status; i, isolated tumor cells; mol, isolated tumor cells demonstrated by nonmorphologic (eg, molecular) techniques.

Examples of such combined terms are as follows:

pN0(i−)(sn)

pT2cN1cM0

**14.2.2.3**    **Usage.** Terms such as *stage I cancer*, *TNM staging system*, and *T1N1M0* are widely recognized and may be used in articles without expansion. However, authors should specify the clinical and/or pathologic criteria that define any stage (optionally but preferably citing the staging system of the AJCC or UICC manual).

Use terms as given in **Table 14.2-1** (see 11.1, Correct and Preferred Usage of Common Words and Phrases [Case, Client, Consumer, Patient, Subject]).

For some sites, the histologic grade has been integrated into the staging system.

**Table 14.2-1.** Correct and Incorrect Usage of TNM Cancer Staging Terms

| Correct | Incorrect |
|---------|-----------|
| T category | T stage |
| N category | N stage |
| M category | M stage |
| stage III cancer, patient with stage III cancer | stage III patient |
| N1 lesions | N1 patients |
| patients with T1N0M0 tumor, T1N0M0 tumors, T1N0M0 cases | T1N0M0 patients |
| TXN0M0 classification | |

**14.2.2.4** **Other Staging Systems and the TNM System.** The AJCC-UICC TNM classification and stage grouping is not the only system used for staging cancer, and equivalency of the same stage number among different systems cannot be assumed. However, 2 cancer staging systems, the International Federation of Gynecology and Obstetrics (FIGO; http://www.figo.org) staging system for gynecologic cancers[9-11] and the Dukes stage system (expressed with letters: Dukes stages A through D) for colon and rectal cancers, have virtual equivalence with the AJCC-UICC stage. The AJCC-UICC system contains subsets of TNM classifications within stage groups that provide greater prognostic precision within each stage for colorectal cancer than does the Dukes system. The Dukes system has largely been replaced by the TNM system.[1(p143)]

FIGO stages are expressed similarly to TNM stages:

| | | | |
|---|---|---|---|
| stage I | stage II | stage III | stage IV |
| stage IA | stage IIA | stage IIIA | stage IVA |
| stage IA1 | stage IIA1 | stage IIIB | stage IVB |
| stage IA2 | stage IIA2 | | |
| stage IB | stage IIB | | |
| stage IB1 | | | |
| stage IB2 | | | |

**14.2.3** **Bethesda System for Cervical Cytology.** *The Bethesda System for Reporting Cervical Cytology*, dating to 1988, is a standardized, systematic means of reporting Papanicolaou test results.[12] Resources are the published handbook (the "blue book")[12] and the website (https://bethesda.soc.wisc.edu).[13]

Expand the following abbreviations at first mention, and punctuate as shown (**Table 14.2-2**).

In the following examples, unexpanded abbreviations are assumed to have been previously defined in the text:

> Low-grade squamous intraepithelial lesions (LSILs) have been described as a benign cytologic consequence of active human papillomavirus (HPV) replication. Several studies have reported that certain behavioral and biological risks exist for LSILs, suggesting that HPV alone is not sufficient for the development of LSILs.

> AIS (CP)

> ASC-H (CP)

> exfoliated endometrial cells (liquid-based preparation [LBP])

> atrophy (LBP)

> glandular cells post hysterectomy (CP)

**Table 14.2-2.** Bethesda System for Reporting Cervical Cytology Abbreviations

| Abbreviation | Expansion |
| --- | --- |
| AIS | adenocarcinoma in situ of endocervix |
| AGC | atypical glandular cell |
| ALTS | Atypical Squamous Cells of Undetermined Significance–Low-grade Squamous Intraepithelial Lesion (ASCUS/LSIL) Triage Study |
| ASC | atypical squamous cell |
| ASC | American Society of Cytopathology |
| ASCCP | American Society for Colposcopy and Cervical Pathology |
| ASC-H | atypical squamous cell, cannot exclude high-grade squamous intraepithelial lesion |
| ASCUS | atypical squamous cells of undetermined significance |
| BIRP | Bethesda Interobserver Reproducibility Project |
| BIRST | Bethesda Interobserver Reproducibility Study |
| CIN | cervical intraepithelial neoplasia |
| CIS | carcinoma in situ |
| CP | conventional preparation |
| EC/TZ | endocervical/transformation zone |
| HPV | human papillomavirus |
| HSIL | high-grade squamous intraepithelial lesion |
| IUD | intrauterine device or intrauterine contraceptive device |
| LBP | liquid-based preparation |
| LEEP | loop electrosurgical excision procedure |
| LMP | last menstrual period |
| LSIL | low-grade squamous intraepithelial lesion |
| LUS | lower uterine segment |
| MMMT | malignant mixed mesodermal tumor |
| N:C | nuclear to cytoplasmic ratio |
| NCI | National Cancer Institute, Bethesda, Maryland |
| NILM | negative for intraepithelial lesion or malignancy |
| NOS | not otherwise specified |
| SCUC | small cell undifferentiated carcinoma |
| SIL | squamous intraepithelial lesion |
| TBS | the Bethesda System |
| TCC | transitional cell carcinoma |
| T zone | transformation zone |
| VAIN | vaginal intraepithelial neoplasia |

Grades are expressed as follows:

CIN 1, CIN 2, CIN 3

VAIN 1, VAIN 2, VAIN 3

**14.2.4** **Multiple Endocrine Neoplasia.** Abbreviations for types of multiple endocrine neoplasia (MEN) feature arabic numerals and a space, as follows:

MEN 1

MEN 2

MEN 2A

MEN 2B

MEN 3

Gene terms are italicized with spaces closed up (see 14.6.2, Human Gene Nomenclature):

*MEN1*

*MEN2*

*MEN3*

**14.2.5** **Molecular Cancer Terminology.** See Table 14.10-2 in 14.10, Molecular Medicine. The style for the cell cycle is given in **Table 14.2-3**.

Miscellaneous molecular terms that are frequently seen are styled as detailed in **Table 14.2-4**[14,15] (see 14.6.3, Oncogenes and Tumor Suppressor Genes).

Note: Gene terms follow standard gene nomenclature style (see 14.6.2, Human Gene Nomenclature).

It is acceptable to use the terms *tumor mutation burden* and *mutation load* in oncology because in this situation, the changes are actually somatic de novo mutations.

**Table 14.2-3.** Cell Cycle Abbreviations

| Phase | Expansion or derivation |
| --- | --- |
| $G_1$ | growth 1 *or* gap 1 |
| S | synthesis (of DNA) |
| $G_2$ | growth 2 *or* gap 2 |
| M | mitosis |
| $G_0$ | quiescent state |
| R point | restriction point |

**Table 14.2-4.** Miscellaneous Molecular Terms

| Gene symbol | Protein (alias[a]) | Derivation | Variant examples |
| --- | --- | --- | --- |
| ACTN1, ACTN2, ACTN3 | ACTN1, ACTN2, ACTN3 | α-actinin | |
| BCL2 | BCL2 | B-cell lymphoma | bcl-2 |
| BCLX | BCLX (CAK[a]) | cyclin-activating enzyme (cyclin H/CDK7) | bcl-X |
| CTNNB1 | CTNNB1 | | β-catenin |
| CDC2 | CDC2 | cell division cycle | |
| CDK2 | CDK2 | cyclin-dependent kinase | cdk2 |
| | CDKI | CDK inhibitor | |
| | cyclin/CDK complex | | cyclin B/CDK1, cyclin D/CDK4/CDK6 |
| | G protein | GTP-binding regulatory protein | |
| CDKN2A | CDKN2A (INK4[a]) | inhibitors of CDK4 | p16$^{Ink4}$ (p16) |
| CDKN1A | CDKN1A (p21[a]) | | |
| TP53 | TP53 (p53[a]) | | |
| RB1 | RB1 | retinoblastoma protein | |
| TGFB | TGF-β | tumor (or transforming) growth factor | |
| TNF | TNF | tumor necrosis growth factor | |

[a]Although these gene symbol aliases or "nicknames" may still be used by some, use of the approved gene symbol, not the alias, is strongly preferred. Use of the approved gene symbol will minimize confusion and make it possible to provide links to genome databases for online versions of the article and to facilitate data retrieval in a number of databases. If an author insists on using an alias, provide the alias parenthetically after the approved gene symbol at first mention in the text and abstract. This practice will link the two and provide a learning experience for those not yet familiar with the approved gene symbol.

Principal Author: Cheryl Iverson, MA

ACKNOWLEDGMENT

Thanks to Boris C. Pasche, MD, PhD, Wake Forest Baptist Medical Center, Winston-Salem, North Carolina; Mary L. Disis, MD, *JAMA Oncology,* and University of Washington, Seattle; Carissa A. Gilman, MA, American Cancer Society, Atlanta, Georgia; and John J. McFadden, MA, JAMA Network, for reviewing and providing comments.

REFERENCES

1. Edge SB, Byrd DR, Compton CC, Fritz AG, Greene FL, Trotti A III, eds; American Joint Committee on Cancer. *AJCC Cancer Staging Manual.* 7th ed. Springer; 2010.
2. International Union Against Cancer/Union Internationale Contre le Cancer website. Accessed March 20, 2019. https://www.uicc.org

3. Sobin LH, Gospodarowicz MK, Wittekind C, eds; International Union Against Cancer. *TNM Classification of Malignant Tumours.* 7th ed. Wiley-Blackwell; 2009.

4. Wittekind C, Compton CC, Brierley J, Sobin LH, eds. *TNM Supplement: A Commentary on Uniform Use.* 4th ed. Wiley-Blackwell; 2012.

5. Gospodarowicz MK, O'Sullivan B, Sobin LH, eds. *Prognostic Factors in Cancer.* 3rd ed. Wiley-Liss; 2006.

6. Sobin LH, Compton CC. *TNM Seventh Edition*: what's new, what's changed. *Cancer.* 2010;116(22):5336-5339. doi:10.1002/cncr.25537

7. Greene FL, Sobin LH. A worldwide approach to the TNM staging system: collaborative efforts of the AJCC and UICC. *J Surg Oncol.* 2009;99(5):269-272. doi:10.1002/jso.21237

8. Gospodarowicz MK, Miller D, Groome PA, Greene FL, Logan PA, Sobin LH; UICC TNM Project. The process for continuous improvement of the TNM classification. *Cancer.* 2004;100(1):1-5. doi:10.1002/cncr.11898

9. Benedet JL, Bender H, Johnes H III, Pecorelli S; the FIGO Committee on Gynecologic Oncology. FIGO staging classifications and clinical practice guidelines in the management of gynecologic cancers. *Int J Gynaecol Obstet.* 2000;70(2):209-262. doi:10.1016/S0020-7292(00)90001-8

10. Kim HS, Song YS. International Federation of Gynecology and Obstetrics (FIGO) staging system revised: what should be considered critically for gynecologic cancer? *J Gynecol Oncol.* 2009;20(3):135-136. doi:10.3802/jgo.2009.20.3.135

11. International Federation of Gynecology and Obstetrics. Accessed March 20, 2019. https://www.figo.org

12. Nayar R, Wilbur D, eds. *The Bethesda System for Reporting Cervical Cytology: Definitions, Criteria, and Explanatory Notes.* 3rd ed. Springer; 2015. Accessed February 23, 2017. https://www.springer.com/us/book/9783319110738

13. Solomon D, Davey D, Kurman R. The 2001 Bethesda System: terminology for reporting results of cervical cytology. *JAMA.* 2002;287(16):2114-2119. doi:10.1001/jama.287.16.2114

14. HUGO Gene Nomenclature Committee. FAQ about gene nomenclature. Accessed March 19, 2019. https://www.genenames.org/help/faq/

15. Nayar R, Wilbur DC. The Pap test and Bethesda 2014. *Acta Cytol.* 2015;59(2).121-132. doi:10.1159/000381842

**14.3  Cardiology.** Several areas of cardiology use simple letter terms and alphanumeric terms that do not need to be expanded at first mention.

**14.3.1  Electrocardiographic Terms.** International standardization of electrocardiographic nomenclature dates back to the mid-20th century.[1-4] The preferred abbreviation for electrocardiogram and electrocardiographic is ECG, not EKG. In the following examples of ECG terms, note the use of capitals, lowercase letters, subscripts, and hyphens.

**14.3.1.1  Leads.** Leads (recording electrodes) are designated in **Table 14.3-1**.

**14.3.1.2  Deflections.** The main deflections of the ECG (**Figure 14.3-1**) are named in alphabetical sequence (P, Q, R, S, T, U), a usage that dates back to the inventor, Willem Einthoven.[2] Other deflections use initial letters of the entity being described.

**Table 14.3-1.** Types and Names of Electrocardiographic Leads

| Types of leads | Names |
|---|---|
| standard (bipolar) leads | I, II, III |
| augmented limb leads/unipolar extremity leads (a, augmented; V, voltage; R, right arm; L, left arm; F, foot) | aVR, aVL, aVF |
| inverted aVR lead | −aVR |
| (unipolar) precordial (chest) leads | $V_1$, $V_2$, $V_3$, $V_4$, $V_5$, $V_6$, $V_7$, $V_8$, $V_9$ (eg, leads $V_3$ through $V_6$ [*not* $V_3$-$V_6$ or $V_{3-6}$]) |
| right precordial leads | $V_1R$, $V_2R$, $V_3R$, $V_4R$, $V_5R$, $V_6R$ |
| modified chest lead using $V_1$ | $MCL_1$ |

Capital letters are used to describe generic ECG deflections.

Improper paper speed during ECG recording will spuriously alter the QRS configuration [*not* qrs configuration].

In reference to an individual ECG tracing, or in descriptions of some specific ECG patterns, capital letters may indicate larger waves and lowercase letters smaller waves; in practice, this most often applies to the Q, R, and S waves.

Pathologic Q waves occur in myocardial infarction.

The q wave in aVF and the Rr′ pattern in lead $V_3$ in this patient's ECG were considered normal findings.

An rSR′ complex in the anterior chest leads and qRs in the left chest leads may indicate right bundle-branch block.

As a guide, hyphens usually do not link deflection terms in the same PQRSTU complex (eg, QT) but link deflections in different waves (eg, R-R), with the

**Figure 14.3-1.** Electrographic Deflections (Schematic)

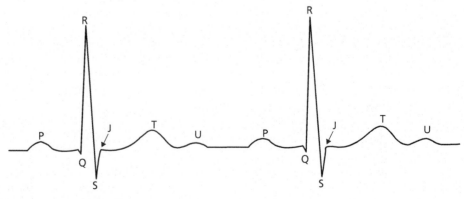

exception of ST-T. The following are examples of terms descriptive of deflections and patterns in ECG tracings:

delta wave (preferred over Δ wave; a slurred upstroke in the QRS complex that is associated with a short PR interval)

F wave (atrial flutter wave)

f wave (atrial fibrillation wave)

J point, J junction (junction of QRS complex and ST segment)

J-ST axis, vector

LQTS (long QT syndrome)

NSTEMI (non–ST-segment elevation myocardial infarction)

NSTE ACS (non–ST-segment elevation acute coronary syndrome)

P wave, axis, etc

PR interval, segment, etc (*not* P-R)

Q wave, q wave

qR complex

QR-type complex

QRS complex (usually a combination of Q, R, and S waves), QRS configurations (if the QRS complex lacks an R wave, it is called a QS complex; if the QRS complex lacks a Q wave, it is called an RS complex)

QRS-T complex

QS wave, qs wave

QT interval, prolongation, etc (*not* Q-T)

QTc (corrected QT interval)

R wave, r wave, R′ wave, r′ wave

R-on-T

R-R interval

rS, RS, Rs complex, configuration, etc

R/S (ratio)

rSR′ pattern

S wave, s wave

S′ wave, s′ wave

ST segment, depression, axis, etc (*not* S-T)

ST-segment abnormality

ST-T segment, elevation, changes, axis, etc (*not* S-T-T)

STEMI (ST-segment elevation myocardial infarction)

T wave, axis, etc

Ta wave (atrial repolarization)

TQ segment

U wave

When terms such as the foregoing are used as modifiers, use a hyphen before the modifying noun (see 8.3, Hyphens and Dashes).

P-wave duration

Q-wave irregularity

non–Q-wave myocardial infarction

ST-segment depression (*not* S-T)

The following symbols are used in connection with ECGs obtained from patients with pacemakers:

A      atrial stimulus

V      ventricular stimulus

AV      interval from atrial stimulus to succeeding ventricular stimulus

AR      interval from atrial stimulus to conducted spontaneous ventricular depolarization

PV      interval from spontaneous atrial depolarization to succeeding "atrial-synchronous" ventricular stimulus

Lead and tracing terms may be combined to describe pattern and location together.

| | |
|---|---|
| $R_I$ | R wave in lead I |
| RaVL | R wave in aVL |
| $S_{III}$ | S wave in lead III |
| $_RV_3$ | R wave in $V_3$ |
| $S_1Q_3T_3$ pattern | prominence of S wave in lead I, Q wave in lead III, and T-wave inversion in lead III |
| $SV_1 + RV_5$ | sum of voltages of S wave in $V_1$ and R wave in $V_5$ |

The P axis, QRS axis, ST axis, and T axis are specified with a plus or minus sign followed by the number of degrees in arabic numerals (eg, +60°, −30°).

**14.3.2**    **Electrograms.** Electrogram (EGM) terms pertain to invasive electrophysiologic recording of cardiac impulse conduction. Expand these terms at first mention.

| | |
|---|---|
| AH interval | atrial-His interval |
| His | His potential |
| HV interval | His-ventricular interval |

**14.3.3** **Heart Sounds.** The 4 heart sounds and 4 components are commonly abbreviated in discussions of cardiac auscultatory findings; numerical subscripts are used.

$S_1$ first heart sound
  $M_1$ mitral valve component

  $T_1$ tricuspid valve component

$S_2$ second heart sound
  $A_2$ aortic valve component

  $P_2$ pulmonic valve component

$S_3$ third heart sound
  The presence of an audible $S_3$ was consistent with the patient's ventricular aneurysm.

$S_4$ fourth heart sound
  An audible $S_4$ may be due to a variety of cardiac and systemic conditions.

Sound names may be written out in full when discussed generically.

Third heart sounds are suggestive of congestive heart failure, but an $S_3$ gallop may be a normal finding in children and young adults.

*or*

The $S_3$ is suggestive of congestive heart failure, but an $S_3$ gallop may be a normal finding in children and young adults.

For plurals, follow the term with "sounds" or another noun.

$S_3$ sounds [*not* $S_3$s] may be normal or pathologic.

$S_3$ gallops may be a normal finding in children and young adults.

**14.3.4** **Murmurs.** Murmurs are graded from soft (lower grade) to loud (higher grade). Murmur grades are written in arabic numerals. Systolic murmurs may be graded from 1 to 6 (see Freeman and Levine[5]) and diastolic from 1 to 4. Murmurs may also be presented by means of a virgule construction to indicate highest grade, as in the following examples:

grade 2 systolic murmur

grade 1 diastolic murmur

grade 4/6 systolic murmur

grade 2/4 diastolic murmur

The patient had a grade 3 systolic murmur radiating to the axilla consistent with the diagnosis of mitral valve regurgitation.

**14.3.5** **Jugular Venous Pulse.** The jugular venous pulse (JVP) contours are expressed with italic single letters and roman words:

*a* wave (atrial)

*x* descent

$z$ point

$c$ wave

$x'$ descent

$v$ wave (ventricular)

$y$ descent (*or* $y$ trough)

$h$ wave

Examples are as follows:

prominent $a$ wave

giant $a$ wave

steep $x$ descent

increased $v$ wave

abrupt $y$ descent

**14.3.6** **Echocardiography.** The names of major echocardiographic methods are listed below. Expand any abbreviations at first mention.

2-dimensional echocardiography (2DE)

3-dimensional echocardiography (3DE)

4-dimensional echocardiography (4DE)

adenosine stress echocardiography

cardiac catheter echocardiography

color Doppler echocardiography

color flow Doppler echocardiography

continuous-wave Doppler echocardiography (CW Doppler)

contrast echocardiography

dipyridamole stress echocardiography

dobutamine stress echocardiography

Doppler echocardiography

Doppler flow imaging

exercise echocardiography

intravascular ultrasonography (IVUS)

pharmacologic stress echocardiography

pulsed Doppler echocardiography

spectral Doppler echocardiography

standard transthoracic echocardiography[6] (a combination of 2-dimensional echocardiography, M-mode [motion mode], and Doppler flow imaging)

echocardiography, M-mode [motion mode], and Doppler flow imaging

stress echocardiography

transesophageal echocardiography (TEE)

The following commonly used echocardiographic indexes should also be expanded at first mention:

| | |
|---|---|
| AVA | aortic valve area |
| EF | ejection fraction |
| EPSS | E point septal separation |
| FAC | fractional area change |
| FS | fractional shortening |
| IVS, IVST | interventricular septal thickness |
| LVID | left ventricular internal dimension |
| MVA | mitral valve area |
| PHT | pressure half-time |
| PW, PWT | posterior wall thickness |
| RVID | right ventricular internal dimension |
| SAM | systolic anterior motion of the mitral valve |
| d or ed | end diastole |
| s or es | end systole |

Terms are combined as in the following examples:

| | |
|---|---|
| IVSd | interventricular septal thickness at diastole |
| IVSs | interventricular septal thickness at systole |
| LVIDd | left ventricular internal diameter at diastole |
| LVIDed | left ventricular internal diameter at the end of diastole |
| LVIDes | left ventricular internal diameter at the end of systole |
| LVIDs | left ventricular internal dimension at systole |
| LVPWd | left ventricular posterior wall dimension at diastole |
| LVPWs | left ventricular posterior wall dimension at systole |
| RVIDd | right ventricular internal dimension at diastole |

Ejection fraction (EF) is expressed as a percentage (eg, 60%) (see 18.0, Numbers and Percentages).

**14.3.7** **Pacemaker Codes.** The capabilities and operation of cardiac pacemakers are described by 3- to 5-letter codes.[7,8]

> DDIR pacing
>
> VVI pacemaker

The code system for antibradycardia pacemakers endorsed by the North American Society of Pacing and Electrophysiology (NASPE) and the British Pacing and Electrophysiology Group (BPEG) is known as the NASPE/BPEG Generic Code or NBG Code. Although the code need not be expanded when mentioned in passing, it is good practice to describe pacing modes in prose at first mention, for example, "dual-chamber, adaptive-rate (DDDR) pacing." The NBG Code was revised in 2001 to apply to antibradycardia, adaptive rate, and multisite pacing.[9,10]

In **Table 14.3-2**, positions I through V refer to the first through fifth letters of the NBG Code. The character for "none" is the letter O, not the numeral 0. In practice, the first 3 positions are always given; the fourth and fifth are added when necessary to provide additional information.

**14.3.8** **Implanted Cardioverter-Defibrillators.** A similar code, known as the NASPE/ BPEG Defibrillator Code or NBD Code,[11] exists for implanted cardioverter/ defibrillators (ICDs), as defined in **Table 14.3-3**. Examples are as follows:

> DDH defibrillator
>
> VOEO defibrillator

There is also a Short Form of the NBD Code intended only for use in conversation:

| ICD-B | ICD with antibradycardia pacing as well as shock |
| ICD-T | ICD with antitachycardia pacing as well as shock and antibradycardia pacing |
| ICD-S | ICD with shock capability only |

**Table 14.3-2.** Revised North American Society of Pacing and Electrophysiology (NASPE)/British Pacing and Electrophysiology Group (BPEG) Generic Code for Antibradycardia Pacing[a]

| Position | I | II | III | IV | V |
|---|---|---|---|---|---|
| Category | Chamber(s) paced | Chamber(s) sensed | Response to sensing | Rate modulation | Multisite pacing |
| | O = none | O = none | O = none | O = none | O = none |
| | A = atrium | A = atrium | T = triggered | R = rate modulation | A = atrium |
| | V = ventricle | V = ventricle | I = inhibited | | V = ventricle |
| | D = dual (A+V) | D = dual (A + V) | D = dual (T + I) | | D = dual (A + V) |
| Manufacturers' designation only | S = single (A or V) | S = single (A or V) | | | |

[a]Reproduced with permission from Bernstein et al.[9]

**Table 14.3-3.** Revised NASPE/BPEG Generic Code for Defibrillators[a]

| Position I (shock chamber) | Position II (antitachycardia pacing chamber) | Position III (tachycardia detection) | Position IV (antibradycardia pacing chamber) |
|---|---|---|---|
| O = none | O = none | E = electrocardiogram | O = none |
| A = atrium | A = atrium | H = hemodynamic | A = atrium |
| V = ventricle | V = ventricle | | V = ventricle |
| D = dual (A + V) | D = dual (A + V) | | D = dual (A + V) |

[a]Reproduced with permission from Bernstein et al.[11]

The foregoing terms can each represent a variety of devices; for instance, ICD-S could indicate VO, VOE, VOEO, DOH, or DOHV. The same devices may also be represented by more than 1 term; for instance, ICD-B may also represent VO and VOE, among other devices. Therefore, only the Long Form is used in writing. As in the case of the NBG Code, at first mention of an ICD it is good practice to include a prose description and the NBD Code designation.

For maximum conciseness and completeness in ICD labeling and record keeping, the first 3 positions of the NBD Code are given, followed after a hyphen by the first 4 positions of the NBG Code. Thus, VAE-DDDR refers to an ICD providing ventricular shock, atrial antitachycardia pacing, EGM sensing for tachycardia detection, and dual-chamber, adaptive-rate antibradycardia pacing.

**14.3.9 Pacemaker-Lead Code.** The NASPE/BPEG Pacemaker-Lead Code (NBL Code)[12] is detailed in **Table 14.3-4**.

Typically, all 4 positions are mentioned (eg, UPSO, BAPS).

Cardiac resynchronization therapy (CRT) devices, also known as biventricular devices, have additional functions and can be combined with implantable cardioverter-defibrillators, such as ICD/CRT, or can be stand-alone CRT devices.

**14.3.10 Heart Disease Classifications and Scoring Systems.** Several classifications and scoring systems pertinent to heart disease are in use (**Table 14.3-5**).

**Table 14.3-4.** Revised North American Society of Pacing and Electrophysiology (NASPE)/British Pacing and Electrophysiology Group (BPEG) Pacemaker-Lead Code[a]

| I (Electrode configuration) | II (Fixation mechanism) | III (Insulation material) | IV (Drug elution) |
|---|---|---|---|
| U = unipolar | A = active | P = polyurethane | S = steroid |
| B = bipolar | P = passive | S = silicone rubber | N = nonsteroid |
| M = multipolar | O = none | D = dual (P + S) | O = none |

[a]Reproduced with permission from Bernstein and Parsonnet.[12]

**Table 14.3-5.** Heart Disease Classifications

| Classification | Applies to | Classes | Example |
|---|---|---|---|
| Braunwald[13] | unstable angina | I-III<br>IA-IIIC | Braunwald class I<br>Braunwald class IIIB |
| Canadian Cardiovascular Society (CCS)[14,15] | exertional angina | I-IV | CCS class II |
| $CHA_2DS_2$-VASc score[16] | atrial fibrillation stroke risk | Score of 0, low risk; ≥2, high risk; maximum score, 10 | $CHA_2 DS_2$-VASc Score ≥2 |
| Forrester[17-19] | cardiac function after myocardial infarction | I-IV | Forrester class I |
| Global Registry of Acute Coronary Events (GRACE)[20,21] | acute coronary events | ST-segment–elevation myocardial infarction; non–ST-segment–elevation myocardial infarction; unstable angina | GRACE variables include ST-segment elevation and patient age |
| Killip[19, 22,23] | cardiac status after myocardial infarction | I-IV | Killip class I heart failure |
| New York Heart Association (NYHA)[24] | cardiac disease and functional capacity | I-IV | NYHA class I |
| Thrombolysis in Myocardial Infarction (TIMI)[25] (eg, TIMI Risk Score, TIMI Grade Flow) | acute coronary syndrome | Score of 0-1, lowest risk; 6-7, highest risk | TIMI score 0-1 |

The classes are assessed in various ways, for instance, by physical examination (Killip), hemodynamic measurement (Forrester), and patient history (NYHA). The detailed meanings of each class are beyond the scope of this book, but several style points may be noted:

- Severity increases from lower to higher numbers and letters.

- There is no automatic correspondence among classes (eg, Killip class I is not equivalent to NYHA class I).

- The numerals for the classes, unlike those for the scores, are designators and are not quantitative or semiquantitative. Therefore, roman numerals are appropriate for those, whereas arabic numerals are used for the scores. The scores are a sum of points for various components.

> *Avoid:*      Forrester class >2
>
> *Preferred:*  Forrester class above II
>
>                    class greater than Forrester II
>
>                    Forrester classes III and IV

▪ Authors should describe their classification criteria, for instance:

> Killip class on admission was determined as the following: patients whose disease was considered class I were free of rales and a third heart sound; patients whose disease was class II had rales up to 50% of each lung field regardless of the presence of the third heart sound. . . (adapted from Neskovic et al[26]).

> We suggest that cases of unstable angina class IIIB now be subdivided into troponin-positive and troponin-negative subgroups. . . (adapted from Hamm and Braunwald[27][p120]).

**14.3.11** **Coronary Artery Angiographic Classifications.** Guidelines are available for nomenclature of coronary artery segments,[28] used in coronary artery catheterization and thrombolysis in myocardial infarction flow (TIMI flow).

The TIMI flow is expressed as grade 0, grade 1, grade 2, or grade 3, from lowest flow (or severest lesion) to highest flow.[27]

**14.3.12** **Cellular and Molecular Cardiology.**

**14.3.12.1** **Cardiac Muscle.** These descriptive terms do not require expansion:

| | |
|---|---|
| A band | actin-myosin overlap |
| H band | Hensen (discoverer) |
| M line | mesophragma |
| T tubules | tubulus transversus |
| Z line | *Zückung* (German: "contraction") |

Expand these terms at first mention:

| | |
|---|---|
| TnC | troponin C (binds calcium) |
| TnI | troponin I (inhibits actin-myosin interactions) |
| TnT | troponin T (binds to tropomyosin) |
| cTnC | troponin C, cardiac form |
| cTnI | troponin I, cardiac form |
| cTnT | troponin T, cardiac form |
| hsTn | high-sensitivity troponin |

**14.3.12.2** **Lipoproteins and Related Terms.** Expand the following lipoproteins and related terms at first mention:

| | |
|---|---|
| acyl CoA | acyl coenzyme A |
| HDL | high-density lipoprotein |
| $HDL_1$ | HDL variant |

| | |
|---|---|
| HDL$_2$ | HDL subfraction 2 |
| HDL$_3$ | HDL subfraction 3 |
| HDL-C | HDL cholesterol |
| HDL-R | HDL receptor |
| HMG-CoA | 3-hydroxy-3-methylglutaryl coenzyme A |
| IDL | intermediate-density lipoprotein |
| IDL-C | IDL cholesterol |
| IDL-R | IDL receptor |
| LDL | low-density lipoprotein |
| LDL-C | LDL cholesterol |
| LDL-P | LDL particle number |
| LDL-R | LDL receptor |
| Lp(a) | lipoprotein a |
| *LPL* | lipoprotein lipase gene (see 14.6.2, Human Gene Nomenclature) |
| LPL$_{188}$ | sequence variation in LPL at codon 188 (see 14.6.1, Nucleic Acids and Amino Acids) |
| LPL$_{Asn29Ser}$ | substitution in LPL of serine at asparagine residue 29 |
| LP-X | lipoprotein X |
| LRP$_1$ | LDL-R–related protein |
| LRP$_2$ | LDL-R–related protein 2 |
| VHDL | very high-density lipoprotein |
| VLDL-C | VLDL cholesterol |
| VLDL-R | VLDL receptor |

Expand *apo* as *apolipoprotein* at first mention of terms such as the following:

| | | | | | |
|---|---|---|---|---|---|
| apo AI | apo B$_{48}$ | apo CI | apoD | apoE | apoJ |
| apo AII | apo B$_{100}$ | apo CII | apo E2 | | |
| apo AIII | apo CIII | apo E3 | | | |
| apo AIV | | | | | |
| apo(a) | | | | | |
| apo AI$_{Milano}$ | | | | | |
| apo AI$_{Arg173Cys}$ | (substitution of cysteine at arginine 173 residue) (see 14.6.1, Nucleic Acids and Amino Acids) | | | | |

**14.3.12.3** **Miscellaneous Cellular and Biochemical Terms.** If an expansion is given, use at first mention. Otherwise, terms may be used without expansion.

| | |
|---|---|
| athero-ELAM | endothelial leukocyte adhesion molecule involved in atherosclerosis |
| BNP | B-type natriuretic peptide |
| CK-MB | creatine kinase, myocardial (largely considered obsolete as a test for myocardial infarction; replaced by troponin [Tn]) |
| NOS | nitric oxide synthase |
| NOS1 | neuronal NOS (named in order of discovery, also nNOS |
| NOS2 | also iNOS (inducible NOS) |
| NOS3 | also eNOS, ecNOS (endothelial constitutive isoform of NOS) |
| P cell | nodal cells of the sinus node |
| tPA | tissue plasminogen activator |

**Principal Author:** Cheryl Iverson, MA

### ACKNOWLEDGMENT

Thanks to the following for reviewing and providing comments: Philip Greenland, MD, *JAMA*, and Northwestern University, Chicago, Illinois; Eric D. Peterson, MD, MPH, *JAMA*, and Duke University School of Medicine, Durham, North Carolina; Rita F. Redberg, MD, MSc, *JAMA Internal Medicine*, and Women's Cardiovascular Services, University of California, San Francisco; Rochelle C. Lodder, formerly with JAMA Network; and Philip Sefton, MS, ELS, *JAMA*. Thanks also to David Song, JAMA Network, for obtaining permissions.

### REFERENCES

1. Barnes AR, Pardee HEB, White PD, Wilson FN, Wolferth CC; Committee of the American Heart Association for the Standardization of Precordial Leads. Standardization of precordial leads: supplementary report. *Am Heart J.* 1938;15(2):235-239.
2. Barnes AR, Katz LN, Levine SA, Pardee HEB, White PD, Wilson FN. Report of the Committee of the American Heart Association on the Standardization of Electrocardiographic Nomenclature. *Am Heart J.* 1943;25(4):528-534.
3. Barnes AR, Pardee HEB, White PD, Wilson FN, Wolferth CC. Second supplementary report by the Committee of the American Heart Association for the Standardization of Precordial Leads. *Am Heart J.* 1943;25(4):535-538.
4. Wilson FN, Kossmann CE, Burch GE, et al. Recommendations for standardization of electrocardiographic and vectorcardiographic leads. *Circulation.* 1954;10(4):564-573.
5. Freeman AR, Levine SA. The clinical significance of the systolic murmur: a study of 1000 consecutive "non-cardiac" cases. *Ann Intern Med.* 1933;6(11):1371-1385.

6. Mann DL, Zipes DP, Libby P, Bonow RO. *Braunwald's Heart Disease: A Textbook of Cardiovascular Medicine*. 10th ed. Elsevier Saunders; 2014.

7. Bernstein AD, Camm AJ, Fletcher RD, et al. The NASPE/BPEG Generic Pacemaker Code for antibradyarrhythmia and adaptive-rate pacing and antitachyarrhythmia devices. *Pacing Clin Electrophysiol*. 1987;10(4, pt1):794-799. doi:10.1111/j.1540-8159.1987.tb06035.x

8. Parsonnet V, Furman S, Smyth NPD. Implantable cardiac pacemakers status report and resource guideline: Pacemaker Study Group. *Circulation*. 1974;50(4):A21-A35.

9. Bernstein AD, Daubert J-C, Fletcher RD, et al. The revised NASPE/BPEG generic code for antibradycardia, adaptive-rate, and multisite pacing. *PACE*. 2002;25(2):260-264. doi:10.1046/j.1460-9592.2002.00260.x

10. Bernstein AD, Camm AJ, Furman S, Parsonnet V. The NASPE/BPEG codes: use, misuse, and evolution. *Pacing Clin Electrophysiol*. 2001;24(5):787-788. doi:10.1046/j.1460-9592.2001.00787.x

11. Bernstein AD, Camm AJ, Fisher JD, et al. North American Society of Pacing and Electrophysiology Policy Statement: the NASPE/BPEG Defibrillator Code. *Pacing Clin Electrophysiol*. 1993;16(9):1776-1780. doi:10.1111/j.1540-8159.1993.tb01809.x

12. Bernstein AD, Parsonnet V. The NASPE/BPEG pacemaker-lead code (NBL Code). *Pacing Clin Electrophysiol*. 1996;19(11, pt 1):1535-1536. doi:10.1111/j.1540-8159.1996.tb03177.x

13. Braunwald E. Unstable angina: a classification. *Circulation*. 1989;80(2):410-414. doi:10.1161/01.CIR.80.2.410

14. Campeau L. Grading of angina pectoris. *Circulation*. 1976;54(3):522-523. doi:10.1161/01.CIR.54.3.522.b

15. Campeau L. The Canadian Cardiovascular Society grading of angina pectoris revisited 30 years later. *Can J Cardiol*. 2002;18(4):371-379.

16. Lip GYK, Nieuwlaat R, Pisters R, Lane DA, Crijns HGM. Refining clinical risk stratification for predicting stroke and thromboembolism in atrial-fibrillation using a novel risk factor-based approach: the Euro Heart Survey on Atrial Fibrillation. *Chest*. 2010;137(2):263-272. doi:10.1378/chest.09-1584

17. Forrester JS, Diamond G, Chatterjee K, Swan HJC. Medical therapy of acute myocardial infarction by application of hemodynamic subsets (first of two parts). *N Engl J Med*. 1976;295(24):1356-1362. doi:10.1056/NEJM197612092952406

18. Forrester JS, Diamond GA, Swan HJC. Correlative classification of clinical and hemodynamic function after acute myocardial infarction. *Am J Cardiol*. 1977;39(2):137-145. doi:10.1016/S0002-9149(77)80182-3

19. Madias JE. Killip and Forrester classifications: should they be abandoned, kept, reevaluated, or modified? *Chest*. 2000;117(5):1223-1226. doi:10.1378/chest.117.5.1223

20. Granger CB, Goldberg RJ, Dabbous OH, et al; Global Registry of Acute Coronary Events Investigators. Predictors of hospital mortality in the Global Registry of Acute Coronary Events. *Arch Intern Med*. 2003;163(19):2345–2353. doi:10.1001/archinte.163.19.2345

21. Fox KA, Dabbous OH, Goldberg RJ, et al. Prediction of risk of death and myocardial infarction in the six months after presentation with acute coronary syndrome: prospective multinational observational study (GRACE). *BMJ*. 2006;333(7578):1091. doi:10.1136/bmj.38985.646481.55

22. Killip T, Kimball JT. Treatment of myocardial infarction in a coronary care unit: a two year experience with 250 patients. *Am J Cardiol*. 1967;20(4):457-464. doi:10.1016/0002-9149(67)90023-9

23. Werns SW, Bates ER. The enduring value of Killip classification. *Am Heart J.* 1999;137(2):213-215. doi:10.1053/hj.1999.v137.93200
24. Dolgin A; Criteria Committee of the New York Heart Association. *Nomenclature and Criteria for Diagnosis of Diseases of the Heart and Great Vessels.* 9th ed. Little Brown & Co; 1994:254.
25. Antman EM, Cohen M, Bernink PJ, et al. The TIMI risk score for unstable angina/non-ST elevation MI: a method for prognostication and therapeutic decision making. *JAMA.* 2000;284(7):835-842. doi:10.1001/jama.284.7.835
26. Neskovic AN, Otasevic P, Bojic M, Popovic AD. Association of Killip class on admission and left ventricular dilatation after myocardial infarction: a closer look into an old clinical classification. *Am Heart J.* 1999;137(2):361-367. doi:10.1053/hj.1999.v137.89744
27. Hamm CW, Braunwald E. A classification of unstable angina revisited. *Circulation.* 2000;102(1):118-122. doi:10.1161/01.CIR.102.1.118
28. Scanlon PJ, Faxon DP, Audet AM, et al. ACC/AHA guidelines for coronary angiography: a report of the American College of Cardiology/American Heart Association Task Force on Practice Guidelines (Committee on Coronary Angiography). *J Am Coll Cardiol.* 1999;33(6):1756-1824. doi:10.1016/S0735-1097(99)00126-6

**14.4** ■ **Drugs.** Physicians and other health care professionals, patients, researchers, manufacturers, and the public may refer to drugs by several names, including the nonproprietary name (often referred to as the generic name) and at least 1 proprietary (brand) or trademark name selected by the manufacturer of the drug. Other drug identifiers include chemical names, trivial (unofficial) names, and code designations.[1] However, only 1 drug name, the nonproprietary name, is coined to ensure consistent usage and no duplication with other drugs. Once a drug has been assigned a nonproprietary name, the nonproprietary name should always be used to refer to the drug (see 14.4.2, Nonproprietary Names).

The nonproprietary name is established through nomenclature agencies, such as the United States Adopted Names (USAN) Council (https://www.ama-assn.org/about-us/usan-council), which work with the World Health Organization (WHO) to establish a single nonproprietary name. According to the WHO, "the existence of an international nomenclature for pharmaceutical substances, in the form of INN [international nonproprietary name], is important for the clear identification, safe prescription and dispensing of medicines to patients, and for communication and exchange of information among health professionals and scientists worldwide."[2] The nonproprietary names of drugs that are to be marketed within the US must be approved by the USAN Council. The nomenclature rules provided in 14.4.13, Nomenclature for Biological Products, are established by the USAN Council.

The pharmaceutical naming system of the WHO has been in operation since 1953. When a drug is being considered for possible approval, the sponsoring manufacturer must file an INN application with the WHO Essential Drugs and Medicines team of Quality Safety and Medicines Policy or with one of the drug nomenclature councils, such as USAN or Japanese Adopted Names (JAN). The European Union does not have a separate council but requires that the INN be used for drugs marketed within the European Union. These organizations work in conjunction with the WHO to approve a nonproprietary name identical to the

INN.[3] Manufacturers in countries without a nomenclature agency can request an INN from the WHO directly or apply in a country that has a nomenclature agency.[1]

**14.4.1** **The Drug Development and Approval Process.** This brief summary of the drug development process is provided to help define the origins of different names used to identify drugs.

Drugs intended for clinical use undergo several phases of development before they can be considered for human use. Animal studies are performed initially to assess pharmacologic and toxicologic effects. While clinical studies are being conducted, animal studies may continue to assess effects on reproduction, teratogenicity, and carcinogenicity.[4(pp7-11)]

To perform clinical studies in the US, the developer or manufacturer must obtain an investigational new drug (IND) approval from the US Food and Drug Administration (FDA).[4(pp7-11)] Once an IND application has been filed, the company must apply to the USAN Council for a nonproprietary name. Until a nonproprietary name has been approved, the developers of a drug may refer to it by the code name. The code designation is usually alphanumeric, with letters to refer to the institution or manufacturer that assigns the code designation for the drug and numbers to refer to the chemical compound.[1(pp17-18)]

Drug developers should adhere to the Declaration of Helsinki[5] and obtain institutional review board approval and patient informed consent to perform drug studies in humans. Phase 1 studies generally are conducted in 20 to 100 healthy volunteers to assess safety, biological effects, metabolism, kinetics, and drug interactions.[4(pp8-9),6] Phase 2 studies usually are conducted in up to several hundred people who have the disease or condition to establish the therapeutic efficacy of a drug for its proposed indication and to study dose range, kinetics, and metabolism.[4(pp8-9),6] Phase 3 studies typically are randomized clinical trials that assess a drug's safety and efficacy in a large sample of patients (generally 2000-3000).[4(pp8-9)] The patients selected have the condition(s) for which the drug is thought to be effective and for which the manufacturer wishes to obtain approval. The 3 phases of clinical testing take 2 to 10 years (average, 5.6 years).[4(pp8-9)] Phase 4 occurs once the drug or device has been approved by the FDA, during the postmarketing safety monitoring period.[6]

In the US, a drug cannot be marketed or prescribed (other than for specific exceptions) until it has been approved by the FDA. The FDA approves *labeling* for the drug for specific indications for which the FDA determines that sufficient evidence of effectiveness has been provided. Approved labeling defines the indications for which the drug can be *marketed*. The FDA does not approve indications for which a drug may be *prescribed* because a company may not study all possible conditions for which a drug may be effective. In what is known as *off-label prescribing*, physicians may prescribe a marketed drug for indications for which it does not have FDA approval for labeling or marketing. The approved labeling is included in prescribing information, marketing materials, and the National Library of Medicine's DailyMed.[7]

Because the number of patients tested before a drug is approved is insufficient to identify rare adverse events, some countries require physicians to report adverse events experienced by patients, and some manufacturers may be required to systematically monitor drug adverse events after approval in a process known as *postmarketing surveillance*. Physicians and other health care professionals in the US should report adverse drug events to the voluntary reporting system MedWatch (https://www.fda.gov/safety/medwatch) or to the pharmaceutical manufacturer, which is obligated to file reports with the FDA. The United Kingdom, Canada, New Zealand, Denmark, and Sweden have legally mandated adverse event reporting systems.[4] The Instructions for Authors for the JAMA Network journals advise as follows: "Authors submitting manuscripts or letters to the editor regarding adverse drug or medical device reactions, reportable diseases, etc, should also report this information to the relevant government agency."[8] In addition, the WHO maintains the WHO Collaborating Centre for International Drug Monitoring in Uppsala, Sweden. There are 123 official member countries and 28 associate member countries.[9] In 2015, this group launched Vigimed, a "web-based forum for those working at national centres in the WHO Programme to enable them to have easy access to safety concerns in other countries, to check regulatory status, and to expedite the sharing of drug information."[9]

**14.4.2** **Nonproprietary Names.** The nonproprietary name (eg, INN or USAN) identifies a specific pharmaceutical substance or active pharmaceutical ingredient. The nonproprietary name is in the public domain and can be used without restriction. It is sometimes referred to colloquially as the *generic name*.[3] However, the terms *generic* and *nonproprietary* are not synonymous. Generic drugs are nontrademarked formulations of a drug that can be manufactured once a drug is no longer under patent restrictions. Generic drugs should be referred to by their nonproprietary name, just as proprietary drugs are.

The nonproprietary name reflects the chemistry, pharmacologic action, and therapeutic use through its stem. Herbal supplements (see 14.4.15, Herbal and Dietary Supplements), homeopathic products, mixtures, drugs in common use for decades (eg, morphine, codeine), and those with trivial chemical names (eg, acetic acid) do not receive nonproprietary names. The INN Expert Group, with representatives from national nomenclature committees worldwide (including the USAN Council), agree to a name that is then published as a proposed INN. During a 4-month comment period, any person can comment on or object to the proposed INN. If no objection is raised, the drug name is published as a recommended INN. New INNs are published in *WHO Drug Information* in English, French, and Spanish (http://www.who.int/druginformation). A cumulative INN list is published, which also includes INNs in Russian. More than 10 000 INNs have been designated as of 2014; 150 to 200 are added each year.[2]

**14.4.2.1** **Stems.** In addition to having a distinct sound and spelling to avoid confusion with other names, both the INN and USAN include a "stem" that designates the drug as a member of a family of related drugs, indicating that the drug has similar pharmacologic properties.[2]

The stem is usually a suffix common to a particular drug class that is incorporated into new drug names to indicate a chemical and/or pharmacologic relationship to older drugs.[10] For example:

> $H_2$-receptor antagonists: cimetidine, ranitidine, lupitidine (*-tidine* is the stem)

> Tyrosine kinase inhibitors: canertinib, imatinib, mubritinib (*-tinib* is the stem)

β-Blockers: propranolol, timolol, atenolol (-*olol* is the stem)

Combined α- and β-blockers: labetalol, medroxalol (-*alol* is the stem)

For some classes of drugs, the position of the stem varies within the drug name. For the group of antiviral drugs (not necessarily having common pharmacologic properties), the stem may be *vir-*, *-vir-*, or *-vir*:

ganciclovir, enviradene, viroxime, alvircept, delavirdine

Approved stems are provided on the USAN website[10] and in the *USP Dictionary*.[1(pp1959-1969)]

The goal of the WHO INN system is to have a single INN for each drug used throughout the world. However, if the substance was in existence before the coordination of nomenclature by WHO, nonproprietary names may differ among countries. For example, *acetaminophen* is the USAN for the same drug that has the BAN and INN name *paracetamol*.[1(pp37)] The USAN *albuterol* has a JAN of *salbutamol* (not to be confused with *salmeterol*, a longer-acting β-adrenergic agonist).[1(p56)] For these few drugs for which nonproprietary names differ by country, the nonproprietary name used depends on the primary audience, although the European Union has required that nonproprietary names that differ from the INN will be phased out over time. In cases in which international recognition is essential (eg, adverse drug reactions), both names should be given at first mention.

Acetaminophen (paracetamol) was recommended in the practice guidelines.

The existence of more than 1 nonproprietary name is also important when performing searches on drugs in journals or databases; all nonproprietary names for a particular drug should be used for a complete search. The *USP Dictionary*[1] lists the INN and nonproprietary names by nomenclature agency, if they differ.

**14.4.2.2** **Orphan Drugs.** Drugs that may be used to treat relatively rare diseases but that otherwise are believed to have limited marketability are termed *orphan drugs*.[11] When a drug is designated an orphan drug by the FDA, the name it receives is not necessarily the name it will receive if it is approved or licensed for marketing.[1(p15)] A list of orphan drugs is available at https://rarediseases.info.nih.gov/diseases/fda-orphan-drugs

**14.4.2.3** **Changes in Nonproprietary Names.** Nonproprietary names may be changed if they are deemed to be confusing or could result in medication errors or if they are proven to infringe on trademark. For example, the antineoplastic compound mithramycin became plicamycin to avoid confusing mithramycin with the similar-sounding antineoplastic mitomycin and its proprietary name Mutamycin. The nomenclature committees have procedures for applying to change the nonproprietary name.

**14.4.3** **Proprietary Names.** The manufacturer's name for a drug (or other product) is called a *proprietary name* or *brand name*.[1(p17)] Proprietary names use initial capitals, with a few exceptions (eg, pHisoHex). In scientific publications, the trademark symbol (™) or the registered trademark symbol (®) is not recommended because capitalization indicates the proprietary nature of the name (see 5.6.15, Trademark). The International Trademark Association has information about specific trademarks and may be reached at https://www.inta.org or International Trademark Association, 655 Third Ave, 10th Floor, New York, NY 10017 or International Trademark Association Europe, 14B rue de la Science, 1040 Brussels, Belgium (see 5.6.15, Trademarks).

Proprietary names for drugs often differ among countries (eg, nifedipine initially was marketed as Procardia in the US and Adalat in Europe). Most US proprietary names are listed in the *USP Dictionary*[1] and are cross-referenced to their USAN name. Unlike the nonproprietary name, the proprietary name does not undergo a coordinated international effort to provide consistent naming. One example is albuterol, a $\beta_2$-adrenergic receptor agonist used for the relief of bronchospasm. It has been marketed by GlaxoSmithKline as Ventolin, Ventoline, Ventilan, Aerolin, or Ventorin, depending on the market; by Cipla as Asthalin and Asthavent; by Schering as Proventil; by Teva as Proair and Novo-Salbutamol HFA (Canada), Salamol, or Airomir; by Beximco (Bangladesh) as AZMZAOL; by Ad-din Pharma as Ventosol; and by Alphapharm as Asmol. Even when the same brand name does not refer to different drugs in different countries, a drug is often marketed under different brand names in different countries. Therefore, because the medical literature is read internationally and confusion about the intended drug could lead to patient harm, the nonproprietary name should always be used and the proprietary name should almost never be used in the medical literature.

The exceptions to this rule are reports of adverse events that might be unique to a specific product formulation or comparison of a generic formulation of a drug with the drug that was first approved. When both the nonproprietary and proprietary names are used in text, the nonproprietary name should appear first, with the proprietary name capitalized and in parentheses. Use of the proprietary name should be limited in these cases to only essential mention. Because proprietary drugs and manufacturers are listed in the *USP Dictionary of USAN and International Drug Names*[1] and other sources, the manufacturer does not need to be listed after the proprietary name.

> The lot of penicillin G potassium (Pentids) was inspected and found to meet the industry production standards.

Proprietary names may be used in questionnaires when the individuals responding may be unfamiliar with the nonproprietary name or when the specific proprietary product is important; in these cases, the exact wording of the question should be maintained, but the nonproprietary name should still be provided.

> Parents were asked, "Have you ever given your child Tylenol [acetaminophen, paracetamol] or products containing Tylenol?"

Herbal supplements and "natural" products generally do not have nonproprietary names. Whenever possible, the nonproprietary name (as listed in the *USP Dictionary*, for example) should be used. For some proprietary formulations that comprise a blend of ingredients, however, the proprietary name may be the only way to refer to the formulation (see 14.4.15, Herbal and Dietary Supplements).

> The authors used mass spectrometry to analyze samples from a bottle of Niagra Actra-R$_x$ and a bottle of Actra-R$_x$ (Body Basics) for the presence of sildenafil.

**14.4.4** **Chemical Names.** The chemical name describes a drug in terms of its chemical structure.[1(pp15-16)] Chemical names are provided in the American Chemical Society's *Chemical Abstracts* (https://www.cas.org/) and can be listed in 1 of 2 ways; the first reflects the way in which *Chemical Abstracts* indexes inverted chemical names:

> hydrazinecarboxyimidamide, 2-[-(2,6-dichlorophenoxy)ethyl]-, sulfate, (2:1)

The second is the uninverted form:

> 2-[-(2,6-dichlorophenoxy)ethyl] hydrazinecarboxyimidamide sulfate, (2:1)

Both forms follow the recommendations of the International Union of Pure and Applied Chemistry and the International Union of Biochemistry and Molecular Biology. Each chemical is also designated a registry number with the Chemical Abstract Society (https://www.cas.org). This number is included in the *USP Dictionary*[1] listing for the drug. Chemical names and registry numbers are rarely used in medical publications, and nonproprietary names are preferred.[1(pp15-16)]

**14.4.5** **Code Designations.** A code designation is a temporary designation assigned to a product by the institution or manufacturer and may be used to refer to a drug under development before a nonproprietary name has been assigned. Codes may be numeric, alphabetic, or alphanumeric; letters in alphanumeric codes designate the institution or manufacturer assigning the code designation of the drug and are followed by numbers to designate the chemical compound.[1(pp17-18)]

Once a nonproprietary name has been assigned, code designations become obsolete and are rarely used in medical publications. If both the code and the nonproprietary name are provided, such as in discussion of the history of a drug, the nonproprietary name should be used preferentially and the code name may be added in parentheses.

> A new drug for the treatment of heart failure, consisting of sacubitril and valsartan (Entresto; formerly known as LCZ696), was approved by the FDA in 2015.

> Edoxaban (formerly known as DU-176) was approved by the FDA in early 2015.

> Zidovudine (BW A509U) first became known as azidothymidine (commonly known as AZT) during testing and eventually was marketed as Retrovir.

**14.4.6** **Trivial Names.** Drugs occasionally become known by an unofficial trivial name, a term that does not give any indication as to the class of drug or chemical structure (eg, aspirin, caffeine, epinephrine). The trivial name should be used in biomedical publications only to reproduce the exact language used as part of a study (eg, in a questionnaire), for historical reasons, or rarely when readers may be unfamiliar with the nonproprietary name. When reproducing the exact language used in a study, the nonpropietary name should be provided in brackets after the term used in the study.

> The participants were asked, "Have you ever taken AZT [zidovudine]?" Participants who said they had taken zidovudine were classified as having had prior exposure to antiretroviral agents.

When names other than the nonproprietary name are used for historical reasons or because readers are unfamiliar with the nonproprietary name, the nonproprietary name should be used preferentially and the alternative name provided in parentheses.

> Semustine (NSC-95441) has been referred to in the scientific literature by its trivial name, methyl-CCNU, a contraction of its chemical name, 1-(2-chloroethyl)-3-(4-methylcyclohexyl)-1-nitrosourea.

**14.4.7** **Drugs With Inactive Components.** Many drugs contain a pharmacologically inactive component (eg, a base, salt, or ester) that is not responsible for the drug's mechanism of action but lends stability or other properties to the drug. Drugs with both an active and inactive component generally require a 2-part name that provides the active and inactive portion of the drug. Inorganic salts and simple organic acids are named in the order cation-anion (eg, sodium chloride, magnesium citrate). For more complex organic compounds, the active component is named first (eg, oxacillin sodium).[1(p904)]

Pharmacologically inactive components are generally salts, esters, and complexes. Sodium, potassium, chloride, hydrochloride, sulfate, mesylate, and fumarate are common components of salts.

> acyclovir sodium
>
> midazolam hydrochloride
>
> benztropine mesylate
>
> morphine sulfate

Quaternary ammonium salts usually are designated by a 2-part name and have the suffix *-ium* on the first word of the name.

> alcuronium chloride
>
> aclidinium bromide

Salts and esters are frequently designated by 2 words, with the second word ending in *-ate*. Three-word names are used for compounds that are both salts and esters.

> clomegestone acetate [ester]
>
> hydrocortisone valerate [ester]
>
> testosterone cypionate [ester]
>
> methylprednisolone sodium phosphate [salt and ester]
>
> roxatidine acetate hydrochloride [ester and salt]

Complexes of 2 or more components may include a term ending in *-ex* to indicate a complex.

> bisacodyl tannex
>
> nicotine polacrilex
>
> codeine polystirex

Chemical names are often too complex for general use. In such cases, shorter nonproprietary names may be created. For example, for the drug erythromycin acistrate, *acistrate* refers to the 2′-acetate (ester) and octadecanoate (salt). For the drug erythromycin estolate, *estolate* refers to the double salt propanoate and dodecyl sulfate.[1(p480)]

In the past, some INNs included inactive components as part of their name (eg, levothyroxine sodium). The WHO modified this policy so that the INN refers to only the active component of the drug (oxacillin, ibufenac). The name that includes the salt (oxacillin sodium, ibufenac sodium) is referred to as the *modified INN* (INNM). However, for drugs originally named for the full entity, such as levothyroxine sodium, the shorter (active entity only) name, for example, levothyroxine, is considered the INNM.[2] Through the USAN Program, names are provided for both forms of the drug substance: the parent species (active moiety) and the salt form. This is done because the drug may be formulated and dosages calculated in either form or both forms in the future.

When a drug is referred to as a general category, the nonproprietary name for the drug can be used without providing the inactive moiety.

> The β-blockers most selective for $β_1$ activity are bisoprolol and metoprolol; acebutolol, carvedilol, and nebivolol are somewhat selective. All lose their selectivity when given at higher doses.

However, if a specific drug is discussed for a specific use, particularly when more than 1 formulation is available, the inactive moiety should be included with the drug name.

> The patient was given erythromycin ethylsuccinate, 400 mg by mouth every 6 hours.

The inactive component should not be used when referring to an organism's sensitivity to an antibiotic or to allergic reactions to drugs.

> The strain of *Streptococcus pneumoniae* isolated by the laboratory was highly resistant to penicillin.

> The patient's plasma lithium level at 8 AM was 2.0 mEq/L.

> The woman developed urticaria after taking erythromycin.

**14.4.8** **Stereoisomers.** Some molecules may occur with identical atoms in the same sequence but with different spatial arrangements. These are referred to as *stereoisomers*. A stereoisomer that is nonsuperimposable on its mirror image is *chiral*, and an atom with 4 different substituents is a *chiral center*; the 2 mirror images are *enantiomers*.[12] An equal mixture of the 2 enantiomers is *racemic*. Generally, only 1 enantiomer is biologically active, as in the case of ibuprofen. In some cases, one enantiomer may be biologically beneficial, whereas the other enantiomer is harmful. For example, one enantiomer of thalidomide is a beneficial drug, whereas the other enantiomer causes birth defects when taken by pregnant women. The enantiomers may be designated by their optical activity, typically by using a polarimeter. The enantiomer that rotates plane-polarized light to the left is *levorotatory* (from Latin *laevus*, meaning left).[12] This is shown in the name with the prefix (−), for example, (−)-thalidomide, which has replaced the now-obsolete designation l-. The enantiomer that rotates plane-polarized light to the right is *dex-trorotatory* (from Latin *dexter*, meaning right), shown in the name with the prefix (+), for example, (+)-thalidomide, replacing the now-obsolete designation d-. A racemic mixture has the prefix (±), which replaces the now-obsolete designation dl-, for example, (±)-thalidomide.

Molecules may also be designated by their spatial configuration. The enantiomers can be labeled with the prefix D- or L-, depending on the arrangement of the substituents of the chiral center in relation to those of glyceraldehyde; this system is typically used to label biomolecules, such as amino acids and carbohydrates. Conversely, the enantiomers may be labeled with the prefixes (*R*)- or (*S*)-, which refer to the priority given to the orientation of groups of atoms that surround the chiral center according to the Cahn-Ingold-Prelog priority rules, with (*R*)- if the rank by atomic number is clockwise and (*S*)- if it is counterclockwise; these designations are especially useful for describing compounds with multiple asymmetric centers. Note that the (+)/(−), D-/L-, and (*R*)-/(*S*)- naming systems are unrelated (eg, an L-labeled compound can be dextrorotatory).[12]

(S)-(−)-verapamil

(R)-(+)-secobarbital

D-lactic acid

For racemic mixtures, *rac-* or *race-* is added to the name of the compound (eg, racepinephrine). For the levorotatory form, the (*S*)- enantiomer may use the *lev-* or *levo-* prefix (eg, levamisole, levdobutamine), whereas the (*R*)- enantiomer may use the *ar-* prefix. For the dextrorotatory form, the (*S*)- enantiomer may use the *es-* prefix (eg, escitalopram), whereas the (*R*)- isomer uses the *dex-* or *dextro-* prefix (eg, dexibuprofin, dextroamphetamine, dexamisole).[12]

**14.4.9 Combination Products.** For combination products (mixtures), the names of the active ingredients should be provided. The proprietary name of the combination may be given in parentheses if necessary to clarify the product to which the article refers.

pseudoephedrine hydrochloride and triprolidine hydrochloride (Actifed)

povidone and hydroxyethylcellulose (Adsorbotear)

If the list of active ingredients is too long to use when referring to the combination product, the active ingredients should be listed at first mention and an abbreviation or the proprietary name used thereafter.

The patient reported having taken several doses of Vanex-HD, a liquid suspension of hydrocodone bitartrate, 10 mg, phenylephrine hydrochloride, 30 mg, and chlorpheniramine maleate, 12 mg, per 30 mL, the previous day.

The patient had been given an artificial tear product that contained hydroxyethylcellulose, 0.42%, and povidone, 1.67% (Adsorbotear).

Only the active ingredients must be listed. However, in some circumstances it may be necessary to include all ingredients, including preservatives, if sensitivity to an ingredient may be important.

> The patient reported red, itchy eyes after using an artificial tear product that contained hydroxyethylcellulose and povidone with edetate disodium and thimerosal as preservatives (Adsorbotear).

The USP may provide a pharmacy equivalent name (PEN)[1(pp14-15)] to refer to a combination product, such as co-triamterzide for the combination of triamterene and hydrochlorothiazide. However, PEN terms are not official USP titles and should be used only if they are familiar and clear to readers. Because co-triamterzide is unlikely to be familiar to most readers, the following approach can be used:

> Participants were given a capsule that contained a combination of 25 mg of hydrochlorothiazide and 50 mg of triamterene each day at 8 AM. Those not able to tolerate hydrochlorothiazide-triamterene were given 50 mg of metoprolol at 8 AM.

> Trimethoprim-sulfamethoxazole (80 mg of trimethoprim and 400 mg of sulfamethoxazole) administered once daily effectively prevented reinfection in 93% of patients.

**14.4.10** **Drug Preparation Names That Include a Percentage.** Some drug names, such as those used in topical preparations, include the percentage of active drug contained in the preparation. In these cases, the percentage should be listed after the drug name.

> The patient was treated with adapalene, 1%.

> Metronidazole lotion, 0.75%, was applied twice a day.

**14.4.11** **Multiple-Drug Regimens.** Regimens that include multiple drugs may be referred to by an abbreviation after the nonproprietary names of the drugs have been provided at first mention (see 14.4.12, Drug Abbreviations, and 13.11, Clinical, Technical, and Other Common Terms). Drug regimens used in oncology frequently are referred to by abbreviations of combinations of antineoplastic agents, but often the abbreviations are not derived from the nonproprietary names. For example, the letter *O* in MOPP is derived from Oncovin, the proprietary name for vincristine sulfate, and the *A* in ABVD is derived from Adriamycin, the proprietary name for doxorubicin hydrochloride. Proprietary names may be provided in parentheses after the nonproprietary names to clarify the origin of the abbreviation.

> The MOPP (methotrexate, vincristine sulfate [Oncovin], prednisone, and procarbazine hydrochloride) regimen has been replaced by ABVD (doxorubicin hydrochloride [Adriamycin], bleomycin sulfate, vinblastine sulfate, and dacarbazine) for the treatment of Hodgkin disease.

**14.4.12** **Drug Abbreviations.** Some drugs have commonly used abbreviations, such as INH for isoniazid and TMP for trimethoprim. However, abbreviations may be used inconsistently, be confused with other terms, or be unfamiliar to some readers. Because of the potential for harm from erroneous interpretation of abbreviated drug names, abbreviations should not be used except in rare instances (eg, trimethoprim-sulfamethoxazole may not fit in a table heading and may need to be abbreviated, eg, TMP-SMX; in that case the expansion should be provided in a table footnote).

**14.4.13** **Nomenclature for Biological Products.** Several categories of drugs are identical to or derived from biological products. Some hormones given as drugs, for example, require special mention because the drug name differs from the name used for the endogenous substance. Other categories of biologicals are derived from specific guidelines developed by the USAN Council, outlined below.

Using the appropriate name can help clarify that the substance referred to is a drug, although for less familiar drug names it may be necessary to include the endogenous hormone name in parentheses to clarify the action of the drug for readers. (For more information on appropriate abbreviations for hormones, see 13.11, Clinical, Technical, and Other Common Terms). The following information is based on the *USP Dictionary*.[1]

**14.4.13.1** **Hypothalamic Hormones.** The suffix *-relin* denotes prehormones or hormone-release stimulating peptides, and the suffix *-relix* denotes hormone-release inhibiting peptides (Table 14.4-1). For example,

> After venipuncture, protirelin (synthetic thyrotropin-releasing hormone) was injected.

**Table 14.4-1.** Nomenclature for Hypothalamic Hormones

| Native substance | Diagnostic/therapeutic agent |
|---|---|
| thyrotropin-releasing hormone (TRH) | protirelin |
| luteinizing hormone–releasing factor (or gonadotropin-releasing factor) | buserelin acetate, gonadorelin acetate (or hydrochloride), histrelin, lutrelin acetate, nafarelin acetate |
| growth hormone–releasing factor (GHRF) | somatorelin |
| growth hormone release–inhibiting factor (somatostatin, GHRIF) | detirelix acetate |

**14.4.13.2** **Growth Hormone.** The *som-* prefix is used for growth hormone derivatives (Table 14.4-2).

**Table 14.4-2.** Growth Hormone Nomenclature

| Native substance | Diagnostic/therapeutic agent |
|---|---|
| growth hormone | somatrem (methionyl human growth hormone) |
|  | somidobove, sometribove, somagrebove (bovine somatotropin derivatives) |
|  | somalapor, somenopor, sometripor, somfasepor (bovine somatotropin derivatives) |

**14.4.13.3** **Thyroid Hormones.** Abbreviations for thyroxine and triiodothyronine are provided in parentheses and may be used after the name is expanded at first mention (Table 14.4-3).

**Table 14.4-3.** Thyroid Hormone Nomenclature

| Description | Therapeutic agent INN |
| --- | --- |
| levorotatory thyroxine (T$_4$) | levothyroxine sodium |
| triiodothyronine (T$_3$) | liothyronine sodium |
| dextrorotatory triiodothyronine | dextrothyroxine sodium |
| mixture of liothyronine sodium and levothyroxine sodium | liotrix sodium |

**14.4.13.4** **Insulin.** Insulin terms can be a source of clinically important confusion, particularly with regard to insulin concentrations and types. Insulin concentrations are as follows (not necessary to expand at first mention):

U100 contains 100 U of insulin per milliliter (the most commonly used concentration).

U40 contains 40 U of insulin per milliliter.

U500 contains 500 U of insulin per milliliter.

Insulin types include those that may be administered intravenously, subcutaneously, or intramuscularly (injections) and those that may be administered only subcutaneously or intramuscularly (suspensions). Another form of insulin may be inhaled.

Insulin is prepared with the use of recombinant DNA technology (referred to as human insulin because the source is human DNA) or as a synthetic modification of porcine insulin. Proprietary names are provided below because they are often used to refer to the potentially confusing various types of insulin preparations. For clarity and conciseness, use of proprietary terms in addition to the nonproprietary terms may be necessary in some cases. The following lists are not comprehensive but are intended to provide examples of the nonproprietary names that should be used and their corresponding proprietary names.

**14.4.13.4.1** **Injections.** Preferred terms and proprietary names for common injections are given in Table 14.4-4.

**14.4.13.4.2** **Suspensions.** Insulin is available in single suspensions and combinations of injections and suspensions. Preferred terms and proprietary names for common suspensions and combinations of injections and suspensions are given in Table 14.4-5.

**14.4.13.5** **Interferons.** Interferon is defined as "proteins formed by the interaction of animal cells with viruses, capable of conferring resistance to virus infection in animal cells"[1(p597)] (see 14.8, Immunology).

**Table 14.4-4.** Injection Nomenclature

| Preferred term | Proprietary name |
|---|---|
| human insulin injection | Humulin R, Novolin R (also known as regular, or R, insulin), Humulin NPH, Novolin NPH, Apidra (nonproprietary name, insulin glulisine) |
| insulin lispro injection | Humalog |
| insulin aspart injection | Novolog |
| insulin glargine injection | Lantus (this can only be administered subcutaneously) |

**Table 14.4-5.** Nomenclature for Suspensions and Combinations of Suspensions and Injections

| Preferred term | Proprietary name |
|---|---|
| insulin zinc suspension, prompt | Semilente |
| insulin zinc suspension | Lente |
| human insulin extended zinc suspension | Ultralente |
| insulin isophane suspension | NPH [neutral protamine Hagedorn][a] |
| 70% human isophane suspension/30% human insulin injection | Humulin 70/30 |
| 70% insulin aspart protamine suspension/30% insulin aspart injection | Novolog Mix 70/30 |
| 75% insulin lispro protamine suspension/25% insulin lispro injection | Humalog Mix 75/25 |
| 50% insulin isophane suspension/50% human insulin injection | Humulin 50/50 |
| inhaled insulin | Afrezza |

[a]NPH is the single exception to expressing drugs as abbreviations and can be used in its abbreviated form.

The 3 main types used for therapy are as follows:

> interferon alfa (formerly leukocyte or lymphoblastoid interferon)
>
> interferon beta (formerly fibroblast interferon)
>
> interferon gamma (formerly immune interferon)

Subcategories are designated by a numeral and a lowercase letter. The lowercase letter after the number differentiates one manufacturer's interferon from another's. Examples of pure interferons are as follows:

> interferon alfa-2a
>
> interferon alfa-2b
>
> interferon beta-1a
>
> interferon beta-1b
>
> interferon gamma-la

For naturally occurring mixtures of interferons, a lowercase *n* precedes the numeral:

> interferon alfa-n1
>
> interferon alfa-n3

See 14.8.4.6, Interferons, for abbreviations for these interferons.

**14.4.13.6** **Interleukins.** There are 12 interleukin derivatives (**Table 14.4-6**). All except interleukin 3 end in *-kin* (eg, aldesleukin). Interleukin 3 is designated by the *-plestim* stem (eg, daniplestim) and is a pleiotropic colony-stimulating factor (see 14.4.13.7, Colony-Stimulating Factors).

See 14.8.4.5, Interleukins, for abbreviations of these interleukins.

**Table 14.4-6.** Interleukin Derivatives

| Stem | Interleukin |
|------|-------------|
| *-nakin* | interleukin 1 derivatives |
| *-onakin* | interleukin 1α derivatives |
| *-benakin* | interleukin 1β derivatives |
| *-leukin* | interleukin 2 derivatives |
| *-trakin* | interleukin 4 derivatives |
| *-penkin* | interleukin 5 derivatives |
| *-exakin* | interleukin 6 derivatives |
| *-eptakin* | interleukin 7 derivatives |
| *-octakin* | interleukin 8 derivatives |
| *-nonakin* | interleukin 9 derivatives |
| *-decakin* | interleukin 10 derivatives |
| *-elvekin* | interleukin 11 derivatives |
| *-dodekin* | interleukin 12 derivatives |

**14.4.13.7** **Colony-Stimulating Factors.** Therapeutic recombinant colony-stimulating factors are named according to the following guidelines[1(pp1955-1973)] (see 14.8, Immunology).

The suffix *-grastim* is used for granulocyte colony-stimulating factors (G-CSFs):

> lenograstim
>
> filgrastim

The suffix *-gramostim* is used for granulocyte-macrophage colony-stimulating factors (GM-CSFs):

> molgramostim
>
> regramostim
>
> sargramostim

The suffix -*mostim* is used for macrophage colony-stimulating factors (M-CSF):

mirimostim

The suffix -*plestim* is used for interleukin 3 (IL-3) factors, which are classified as pleiotropic colony-stimulating factors:

muplestim

daniplestim

The suffix -*distim* is used for conjugates of 2 different types of colony-stimulating factors:

milodistim

The suffix -*cestim* is used for stem cell-stimulating factors:
ancestim

**14.4.13.8** **Erythropoietins.** The word *epoetin* is used to describe erythropoietin preparations that have an amino acid sequence that is identical to that of the endogenous cytokine. The words *alfa, beta*, and *gamma* are added to designate preparations with different composition and carbohydrate moieties.[1(p1706)]

epoetin alfa

epoetin beta

epoetin gamma

**14.4.13.9** **Monoclonal Antibodies.** Therapeutic monoclonal antibodies and fragments are designated by the suffix -*mab*. Monoclonal antibodies are derived from animals and humans, and the nomenclature is based on the source of the antibody (mouse, rat, hamster, primate, or human) and the disease target or antibody subclass. Some examples of monoclonal antibodies are abciximab, adalimumab, daclixumab, infliximab, ipilimumab, and satumomab pendetide.[1]

The following letters are used to identify the source of the monoclonal antibody:

u       human

e       hamster

o       mouse

i       primate

a       rat

xi      chimera

zu      humanized

These identifiers precede the -*mab* suffix stem, for example:

-*umab*       human

-*omab*       mouse

-*ximab*      chimeric

-*zumab*      humanized

The general disease state subclass is also incorporated into the name by use of a code syllable.

| | |
|---|---|
| —*v(i)*- | viral |
| *b(a)*- | bacterial |
| *-l(i)*- | immune |

Key elements are combined in the following sequence: the letters that represent the target disease state, the source of the product, and the monoclonal root *-mab* used as a suffix (eg, bi*ciromab*, sa*tumomab*) (Table 14.4-7). When a target or disease stem is combined with the source stem for chimeric monoclonal antibody, the last consonant of the target or disease syllable is dropped to facilitate pronunciation.

**Table 14.4-7.** Monoclonal Antibody Nomenclature

| Target | Source | -mab Stem | USAN |
|---|---|---|---|
| -*cir*- | -*xi* | -*mab* | abciximab |
| -*lim*- | -*zu* | -*mab* | daclizumab |

**14.4.13.10** **Radiolabeled or Conjugated Products.** Some products are radiolabeled or conjugated to other chemicals, such as toxins. Such conjugates are identified by a separate, second word or other acceptable chemical designation. For monoclonal antibodies conjugated to a toxin, the "*-tox*" stem indicates the toxin (eg, zolimomab *aritox*, in which the designation *aritox* was selected to identify ricin A-chain). For radiolabeled products, the isotope, element symbol, and isotope number precede the monoclonal antibody[1] (see 14.9.2, Radiopharmaceuticals).

technetium Tc 99m biciromab

indium In 111 altumomab pentetate

A separate term is also used to designate a linker or chelator that conjugates the monoclonal antibody to a toxin or isotope or for pegylated (having polyethylene glycol, or PEG, attached) monoclonal antibodies.[1(p1707)]

telimomab aritox

indium In 111 satumomab pendetide

enlimomab pegol

**14.4.14** **Vitamins and Related Compounds.** The familiar letter names of most vitamins generally refer to the substances as found in food and in vivo. With the exception of vitamins A, E, and B complex, the nonproprietary names for vitamins given therapeutically differ from their in vivo names. (To enhance clarity for readers, the equivalent vitamin name may also be provided.) Various types of carotenoids (alpha and beta carotene and beta cryptoxanthin) may be converted to vitamin A within the body, so the specific agent that is administered should be provided.

The native form of vitamin A is most often supplied as retinol acetate. Other forms of vitamin A may be administered topically (eg, retinoic acid). Vitamin E refers to a group of tocopherol compounds, and the specific chemical names should be provided (eg, alpha tocopherol, gamma tocopherol, delta tocopherol, or mixed tocopherols). The specific stereoisomers and whether the product is natural or synthetic should be provided where relevant (eg, DL-alpha tocopherol acetate). For vitamin B complex, the specific components included in the B complex should be provided. **Table 14.4-8** provides examples of USAN drug names equivalent to their vitamin names.[1]

**Table 14.4-8.** USAN Drug Names and Equivalent Vitamin Names

| Native vitamin | Drug name |
| --- | --- |
| vitamin $B_1$ | thiamine hydrochloride |
| vitamin $B_1$ mononitrate | thiamine mononitrate |
| vitamin $B_2$ | riboflavin |
| vitamin $B_6$ | pyridoxine hydrochloride |
| vitamin $B_8$ | adenosine phosphate |
| vitamin $B_{12}$ | cyanocobalamin |
| vitamin C | ascorbic acid |
| vitamin D | cholecalciferol |
| vitamin $D_1$ | dihydrotachysterol |
| vitamin $D_2$ | ergocalciferol |
| vitamin G | riboflavin |
| vitamin $K_1$ | phytonadione |
| vitamin $P_4$ | troxerutin |

**14.4.15** **Herbal and Dietary Supplements.** Herbal and dietary supplements do not receive nonproprietary names, and they are not regulated as drugs in many countries, including the US (as mandated by the Dietary Supplement Health and Education Act, passed in 1994[13]). The US Congress has defined a dietary supplement as

> a product taken by mouth that contains a "dietary ingredient" intended to supplement the diet. The "dietary ingredients" in these products may include: vitamins, minerals, herbs or other botanicals, amino acids, and substances such as enzymes, organ tissues, glandulars, and metabolites. Dietary supplements can also be extracts or concentrates, and may be found in many forms such as tablets, capsules, softgels, gelcaps, liquids, or powders. They can also be in other forms, such as a bar, but if they are, information on their label must not represent the product as a conventional food or a sole item of a meal or diet. Whatever their form may be, [Dietary Supplement Health and Education Act] places dietary supplements in a special category under the general umbrella

of "foods," not drugs, and requires that every supplement be labeled a dietary supplement.[13,14]

Components of dietary supplements may be pharmacologically active, so accurate and specific nomenclature is essential. As noted above, dietary supplements are often mixtures of several ingredients, and quantities of each may be proprietary. Such a mixture makes standard nomenclature policy difficult to establish. Whenever possible, a nonproprietary name should be used to refer to a dietary supplement. However, if the dietary supplement is a mixture of many components, either an abbreviation derived from the components or the proprietary name must be used (see 14.4.9, Combination Products).

> Metabolife 356 (Metabolife International Inc) was a dietary supplement that contained 19 labeled ingredients, including ephedra and caffeine (hereinafter abbreviated as DSEC), and is no longer manufactured.

The *USP Dictionary*,[1] *Physicians' Desk Reference for Nonprescription Drugs and Dietary Supplements*,[15] *Physicians' Desk Reference for Herbal Medicines*,[16] *The Complete German Commission E Monographs: Therapeutic Guide to Herbal Medicine*,[17] and *The ABC Guide to Herbs*[18] are useful resources for naming herbals and dietary supplements. If these resources are not productive, the web can be helpful in identifying substances as well, although of course the accuracy of the source should be considered.

Herbal medicines generally can be named according to their botanical genus and species, although the lack of regulation in some countries makes consistent nomenclature a challenge. A review of regulation of herbal medicines worldwide has been completed by WHO.[19-21] Monitoring of herbal medicines remains challenging.[22] In countries in which botanicals are not regulated, the specific herbal and manufacturer, wherever relevant, should be included because different manufacturing techniques result in different biological activity. According to WHO,

> [I]t is not unusual for a common name to be used for two or more different species. Unless the names of herbal plants follow an international system of plant nomenclature, the potential for confusion when exchanging information is enormous. The information attached to a name is thus crucial. As an example, because common names are often used, heliotrope (*Heliotropium europaeum*)—containing potent hepatotoxins—is often confused with garden heliotrope (*Valeriana officinalis*), which is used as a sedative and muscle relaxant. Identification of the herbal preparation by the Latin binomial system, in addition to the common name, is therefore essential.[21]

Thus, whenever possible, herbals derived from a specific plant should be named according to the botanical name (eg, *Ginkgo biloba, Echinacea purpurea*) to ensure that the correct entity is identified. When the plant is referred to, the genus and species may be abbreviated after being spelled out at first mention.

> The main pharmacologic substances with immunostimulant activity in experimental and clinical studies are purified polysaccharides that can be extracted only in small quantity from pressed *Echinacea purpurea*.

Given our laboratory findings, the symptoms we have described may be attributed to an overdose of *Illicium verum,* contamination with *Illicium anisatum,* or a combination of both.

Kava is derived from the dried root of the pepper plant *Piper methysticum.* Kava has gained widespread popularity as an anxiolytic and sedative.

Extracts from St John's wort, also known by its Latin botanical name, *Hypericum perforatum,* have been studied extensively for the treatment of depression in adults, with mixed results.

One day before taking *Ginkgo biloba* or placebo and again at the end of the 6-week double-blind period (while still taking *G biloba* and within 3 days of the end of the study), participants underwent neuropsychological evaluation, including tests of learning, memory, attention and concentration, and expressive language.

In some cases, the vernacular name is not the genus or species and should be provided as well to ensure that the reader understands which plant is intended.

*Hypericum perforatum* (St John's wort) is a popular herbal product used to treat depression, but it has been implicated in drug interactions.

When referring to a specific product or formulation, as in a study, the specific proprietary name and manufacturer should be listed because formulations vary by manufacturing technique.

Participants were randomly assigned to 1 of 2 conditions: *Ginkgo biloba* (Ginkoba) or placebo control (1:1 ratio).

A marketed enteric-coated preparation (Tegra) that contains 5 mg of steam-distilled garlic (*Allium sativum*) oil bound to a matrix of beta cyclodextrin and matching placebos, whose coating tasted like garlic, was used.

Guggulipid, which is an extract from the plant *Commiphora mukul* (guggul), contains numerous other substances besides the small amounts of guggulsterones purported to be the active ingredients.

**Principal Author:** Cheryl Iverson, MA

## ACKNOWLEDGMENT

Thanks to Stephanie C. Shubat, MS, USAN Program, American Medical Association, Chicago, Illinois; Anne Rentoumis Cappola, MD, ScD, *JAMA*, and Smilow Center for Translational Research, Philadelphia, Pennsylvania; and Karen Leslie Boyd, formerly with JAMA Network, for reviewing and providing comments.

## REFERENCES

1. *USP Dictionary of USAN and International Drug Names.* 53rd ed. US Pharmacopoeia; 2017.
2. Guidance on INN. World Health Organization. 1997. Accessed July 23, 2019. https://www.who.int/medicines/services/inn/innguidance/en/

3. Lists of recommended and proposed INNs. World Health Organization. Last updated 2018. Accessed July 23, 2019. https://www.who.int/medicines/publications/druginformation/innlists/en/

4. Rivera SM, Gilman AG. Drug intervention and the pharmaceutical industry. In: Brunton LL, ed; Chabner BA, Knollmann BC, assoc eds. *Goodman & Gilman's The Pharmacological Basis of Therapeutics*. 12th ed. McGraw-Hill Book Co; 2011:3-16.

5. World Medical Association. Declaration of Helsinki: ethical principles for medical research involving human subjects. *JAMA*. 2013;310(20):2191-2194. doi:10.1001/JAMA.2013.281053

6. US Food and Drug Administration. The drug development process. Last updated January 4, 2018. Accessed July 23, 2019. https://www.fda.gov/patients/learn-about-drug-and-device-approvals/drug-development-process

7. National Library of Medicine. DailyMed. Posted December 19, 2017. Accessed May 30, 2018. https://dailymed.nlm.nih.gov/dailymed/index.cfm

8. JAMA Instructions for Authors. Last updated July 15, 2019. Accessed July 23, 2019. http://jama.jamanetwork.com/journals/jama/pages/instructions-for-authors

9. Introduction to the WHO Programme for International Drug Monitoring. World Health Organization. Last updated 2016. Accessed May 30, 2018. http://www.who.int/medicines/areas/quality_safety/safety_efficacy/en/

10. Approved stems. USAN. Updated July 2018. Accessed March 1, 2019. https://www.ama-assn.org/about/united-states-adopted-names/united-states-adopted-names-approved-stems

11. Orphan Drug Act, Pub L No. 97-414. 1983. Accessed July 23, 2019. https://www.fda.gov/media/99546/download

12. Voet D, Voet JG, Pratt CW. *Fundamentals of Biochemistry*. 4th ed. John Wiley & Sons Inc; 2012:86-88.

13. National Institutes of Health, Office of Dietary Supplements. Dietary Supplement Health and Education Act of 1994. US Food and Drug Administration, Accessed July 23, 2019. https://ods.od.nih.gov/About/DSHEA_Wording.aspx

14. US Food and Drug Administration. Dietary supplements. Updated July 22, 2019. Accessed July 23, 2019. https://www.fda.gov/food/dietary-supplements/

15. *PDR for Nonprescription Drugs and Dietary Supplements*. 34th ed. PDR Network; 2013.

16. *PDR for Herbal Medicines*. 4th ed. Thomson Healthcare; 2007.

17. American Botanical Council; Blumenthal M, Busse WR, Klein S, et al, eds. *The Complete German Commission E Monographs: Therapeutic Guide to Herbal Medicines*. Lippincott Williams & Wilkins; 1998.

18. Blumenthal M, ed. *The ABC Guide to Herbs*. American Botanical Council; 2003.

19. World Health Organization. Regulatory situation of herbal medicines: a worldwide review. Accessed July 23, 2019. https://apps.who.int/iris/handle/10665/63801

20. WHO Traditional Medicine Strategy 2002-2005. Accessed July 31, 2019. http://www.wpro.who.int/health_technology/book_who_traditional_medicine_strategy_2002_2005.pdf

21. Farah MH. Consumer protection and herbal remedies. *WHO Drug Inf*. 1998;12(3):141-142. Accessed August 5, 2019. https://apps.who.int/medicinedocs/index/assoc/s14169e/s14169e.pdf

22. Ekor M. The growing use of herbal medicines: issues relating to adverse reactions and challenges in monitoring safety. *Front Pharmacol.* 2014;4:177. doi:10.3389/fphar.2013.00177

### ADDITIONAL READINGS AND GENERAL REFERENCES

PDR (Presaribers Digital Reference). Accessed July 23, 2019. https://www.pdr.net

*WHO Drug Information.* Updated February 2019. Accessed March 20, 2019. https://www.who.int/medicines/publications/druginformation/en/

## 14.5 Equipment, Devices, Reagents, and Software.

### 14.5.1 Equipment, Devices, and Reagents.

Nonproprietary names or descriptive phrasing is preferred to proprietary names for devices, equipment, and reagents, particularly in the context of general statements and interchangeable items (eg, urinary catheters, intravenous catheters, pumps). However, if several brands of the same product are being compared or if the use of proprietary names is necessary for clarity or to replicate the study, proprietary names should be given at first mention along with the nonproprietary name. In such cases, the name of the manufacturer or supplier is also important, and authors should include this information in parentheses after the name or description. Authors should provide this information for any reagents, antibodies, enzymes, or probes used in investigations. Because the location of the manufacturer is easy to look up online, this information is no longer required.

The following are examples in which specific information is required:

> Dual-lumen cannulas avoid this problem by being inserted through a single neck vein. The Avalon (Maquet Cardiovascular) is inserted through the right internal jugular or subclavian vein with the tip ending in the inferior vena cava. The Protek Duo (CardiacAssist Inc) is inserted through the right internal jugular vein and ends in the proximal pulmonary artery.

> The incisions were closed with running 3-0 polyglactin sutures (Vicryl; Ethicon Inc).

> The cells were further incubated with goat antimouse Alexa 488 (Molecular Probes), washed, fixed, and analyzed using a confocal microscope.

> The face mask group was managed with a single-limb noninvasive ventilator (Philips Respironics V60).

> Bacterial cells were centrifuged at 5000$g$ for 10 minutes, and the pellet was suspended in 5 volumes of Bacterial PE (G-Biosciences).

The following are examples of more general references that do not require specific descriptions or information on the manufacturer:

> Currently, treatment by Nd:YAG laser is the accepted method to surgically open the opacified posterior capsule.

> Topical treatments for erosive pustular dermatosis of the scalp include corticosteroids and retinoids.

> Participants were randomly assigned to reduce their smoking by 75% with the help of their choice of short-acting nicotine replacement therapy products (gum, nasal spray, lozenges) or nicotine patches.

As with drugs and isotopes, proprietary names should be capitalized; the registered trademark symbol is not used.

If a device is described as "modified," the modification should be explained or an explanatory reference cited.

> On the basis of the procedural measurements of relative visceral vessels, clock position, and distance, we selected a 38 X 77 TX2 graft (Cook Medical LLC) that was modified[6] and implanted within a few hours of the patient's transfer.

If equipment or apparatus is provided free of charge by the manufacturer, this fact should be included in the acknowledgment (see 2.10.10, Funding/Support; 5.2.1, Acknowledging Support, Assistance, and Contributions of Those Who Are Not Authors; and 5.5.3, Reporting Funding, Sponsorship, and Other Support).

**14.5.2** **Software.** For statistical software, the proprietary name should always be given.

> The data were analyzed with QMass MR 7.2 (Medis Inc) and Diagnosoft 2.71 (Diagnosoft Inc).

> All prediction and survival analyses were performed using SAS statistical software, version 9.3 (SAS Institute Inc); Kaplan-Meier curves were plotted using R, version 3.1.3 (R Foundation for Statistical Computing).

> Analyses were conducted using Stata, release 12 (StataCorp LP) and Joinpoint, version 4.2 (National Cancer Institute) statistical software.

> Investigators used advanced 3-dimensional reconstruction imaging software (Aquarius WS) to obtain accurate measurements of the relative origins of the visceral arteries.

**Principal Author:** Cheryl Iverson, MA

### ACKNOWLEDGMENT

Thanks to Karen Leslie Boyd, formerly with JAMA Network, for reviewing and providing comments.

**14.6** **Genetics.**

**14.6.1** **Nucleic Acids and Amino Acids.** Standards for molecular nomenclature are set jointly by the International Union of Biochemistry and Molecular Biology (IUBMB) and the International Union of Pure and Applied Chemistry (IUPAC).[1] The recommendations in this section are based on conventions put forth by the IUBMB-IUPAC Joint Commission on Biochemical Nomenclature and the Nomenclature Committee of the IUBMB.[2]

**14.6.1.1** **DNA.** The nucleic acids DNA and RNA are nucleotide polymers. DNA is the molecule forming the substrate for the genetic code and is contained in the chromosomes of higher organisms. It is made up of (1) molecules called *bases*, (2) the sugar 2-deoxyribose, and (3) phosphate groups. The DNA bases fall into 2 classes: pyrimidines (including cytosine and thymine) and purines (including adenine and guanine).

Structurally, DNA in the nucleus of a living cell is a double-stranded, antiparallel helical polymer of deoxyribose linked by phosphate groups; 1 of 4 bases projects from each sugar molecule of the sugar-phosphate chain. A base-sugar unit is a *nucleoside*. A base-sugar-phosphate unit is a *nucleotide* (**Figure 14.6-1**).

The carbons in the sugar moiety are numbered with prime symbols, not apostrophes (eg, 3′ carbon, 5′ carbon). Sometimes chemical moieties are specified in connection with the 3′ and 5′ ends:

3′ hydroxyl end (3′ OH end)

5′ phosphate (5′ P) end

5′ OH end

(See 13.13, Elements and Chemicals.)

The phosphates that join the DNA nucleotides link the 3′ carbon of one deoxyribose to the 5′ carbon of the next deoxyribose. The end of the DNA strand with an unattached 5′ carbon is known as the 5′ end (or terminal) and the end with an unattached 3′ carbon as the 3′ end (or terminal) (**Figure 14.6-2**) (see 13.13, Elements and Chemicals).

The carbons and nitrogens of the bases are numbered 1 through 6 (pyrimidines) or 1 through 9 (purines), and the carbons of deoxyribose are designated by numbers with prime symbols 1′ through 5′ (**Figure 14.6-3**).

This section presents nomenclature for nucleotides of DNA, especially nomenclature used for DNA sequences (ie, nucleotide polymers). For nomenclature of nucleotides as DNA precursors and energy molecules, see 14.6.1.3, Nucleotides as Precursors and Energy Molecules.

A 1-letter designation represents each base, nucleoside, or nucleotide (**Table 14.6-1**). The letters are commonly used without expansion.

**Figure 14.6-1.** Nucleosides and Nucleotides: General Structure

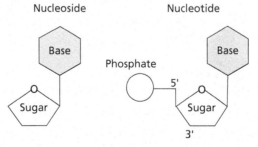

**Figure 14.6-2.** DNA Double Helix

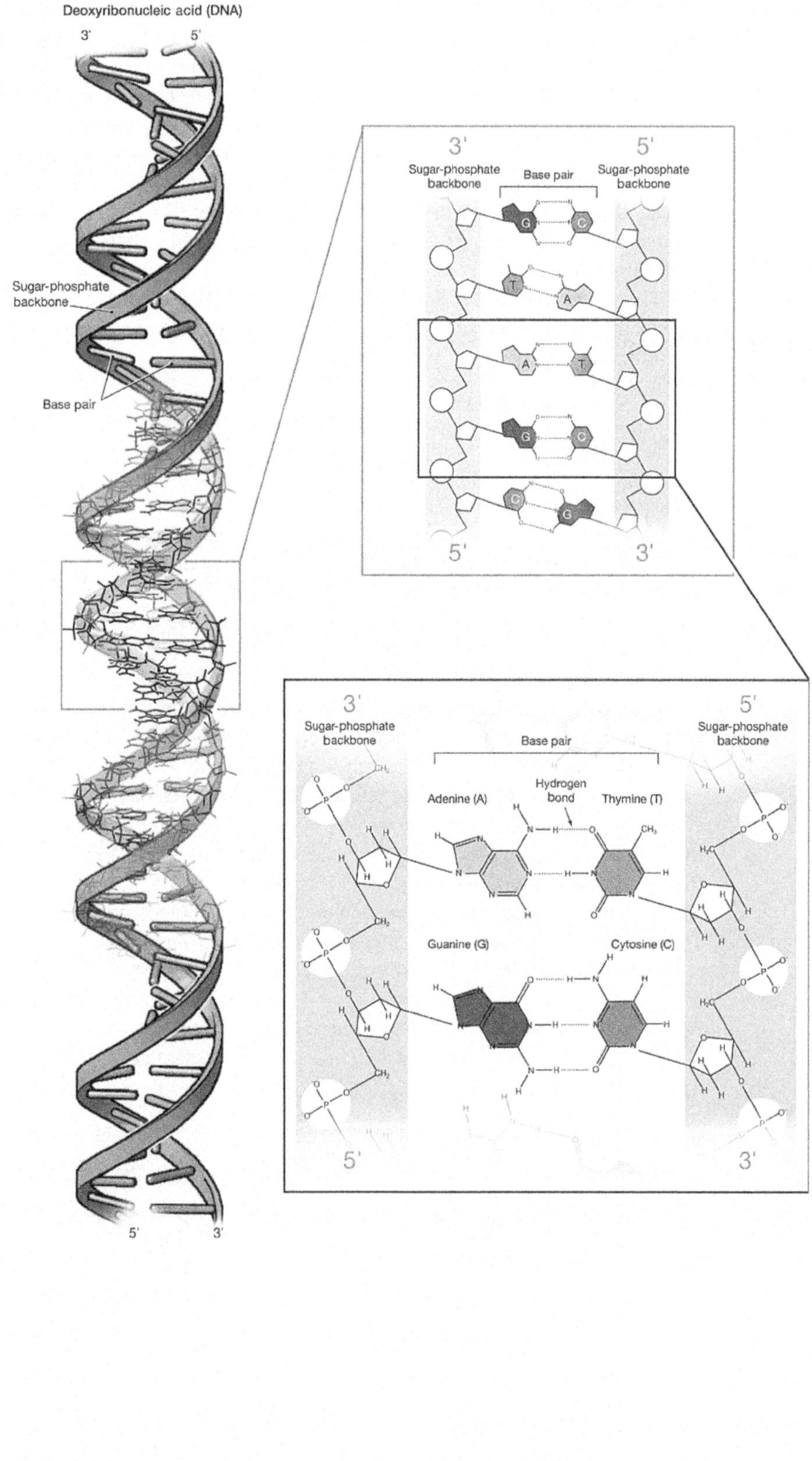

Deoxyribonucleic acid (DNA)

**Table 14.6-1.** Abbreviations for DNA Nucleotides

| Abbreviation | Base | Nucleoside; nucleotide[a] residue in DNA | Molecular class |
|---|---|---|---|
| A | adenine | deoxyadenosine | purine |
| C | cytosine | deoxycytidine | pyrimidine |
| G | guanine | deoxyguanosine | purine |
| T | thymine | deoxythymidine | pyrimidine |

[a]The technical name for nucleotides is nucleoside phosphates.

The chemical structure of bases is illustrated in **Figure** 14.6-3.

**Figure 14.6-3.** DNA Bases: Chemical Structure

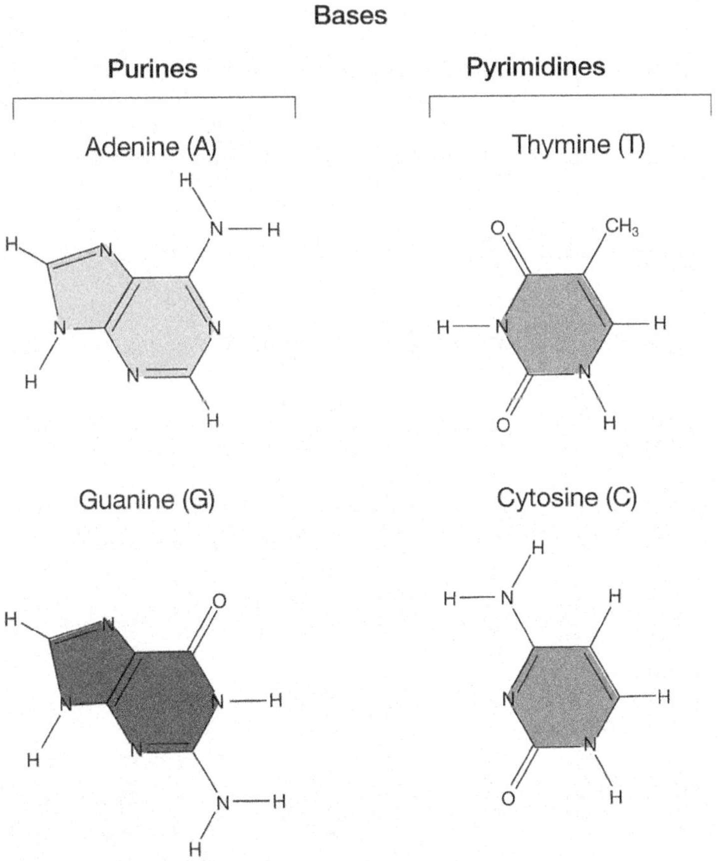

Bases

When a base (or nucleoside or nucleotide) is described that cannot be firmly identified as A, C, G, or T, it is most commonly reported as N (uncertain). Other single-letter designators that reflect biochemical properties may be used, but because these designations are not as well known as A, C, G, T, and N, it is best to define them (Table 14.6-2).

Various forms of DNA are commonly abbreviated as follows; expand at first use:

bDNA        branched DNA

cDNA        complementary DNA, coding DNA

dsDNA       double-stranded DNA

gDNA        genomic DNA

hn-cDNA     heteronuclear cDNA (heterogeneous nuclear cDNA)

mtDNA       mitochondrial DNA

nDNA        nuclear DNA

rDNA        ribosomal DNA

scDNA       single-copy DNA

ssDNA       single-stranded DNA

There are several classes of DNA helixes, which differ in the direction of rotation and the tightness of the spiral (number of base pairs per turn):

A-DNA (alternate DNA)

B-DNA (balanced DNA)

C-DNA (9 base pairs [bp] per turn of spiral)

D-DNA (8 base pairs [bp] per turn of spiral)

Z-DNA (zigzag)

In eukaryotic cells, DNA is bound with special proteins associated with chromosomes (see 14.6.4, Human Chromosomes). This DNA-protein complex is known as *chromatin*. DNA in chromatin is organized into structures called *nucleosomes* by proteins known as *histones*. The 5 classes of histones are as follows:

H1 (linker histone)

H2A (core histone)

H2B (core histone)

H3 (core histone)

H4 (core histone)

Almost all native DNA exists in the form of a double helix, in which 2 DNA polymers are paired, linked by hydrogen bonds between individual bases on each chain. Because of the biochemical structure of the nucleotides, A always pairs with T and C with G (Figure 14.6-2). Such pairs may be indicated as follows:

**Table 14.6-2.** Examples of Other Single-Letter Designators for Bases[a]

| Symbol | Stands for | Derivation |
|--------|-----------|------------|
| R | G or A | *pu*rine |
| Y | T or C | p*y*rimidine |
| M | A or C | a*m*ino |
| K | G or T | *k*eto |
| S | G or C | *s*trong interaction (3 hydrogen bonds) |
| W | A or T | *w*eak interaction (2 hydrogen bonds) |
| H | A or C or T | not G (H follows G in the alphabet) |
| B | G or T or C | not A (B follows A in the alphabet) |
| V | G or C or A | not T (V follows T in the alphabet; U is not used because it stands for uracil in RNA [see 14.6.1.2, RNA]) |
| D | G or A or T | not C (D follows C in the alphabet) |
| N | G or A or T or C | *any* |

[a]Adapted with permission from Moss.[2] Copyright IUBMB.

$$A \cdot T, A = T$$

$$C \cdot G, C \equiv G$$

Mispairings (which may occur as a consequence of a variant or sequence variation) may be shown in the same way:

$$C \cdot T$$

Unpaired DNA sequences are quantified by means of the terms *base* (a single base), *kilobase* (kb, a thousand bases), and *megabase* (Mb, a million bases) (see 13.12, Units of Measure). Paired DNA sequences use the terms *base pairs* (bp), *kilobase pairs* (kb), *megabase pairs* (Mb), and *gigabase pairs* (Gb). (Do not use "kbp" or "Mbp.") For example:

a 20-base fragment

a 235-bp repeat sequence

a 27-bp region

a 47-kb vector genome

1 Mb of DNA

The size of the human haploid genome is approximately $3 \times 10^9$ bp.

Sometimes the number of nucleotides in a DNA molecule is indicated using the suffix "mer":

20mer    (20 nucleotides)

24mer    (24 nucleotides)

(This formation is based on the terms *dimer, trimer, tetramer,* etc.) It is sometimes referred to as kmer or k-mer (eg, a kmer of length 20 rather than 20mer).

A DNA sequence might be depicted as follows, with standard notation of DNA sequences from 5' to 3':

GGATCC means 5' GGATCC 3'

Unknown bases may be depicted by using N (see Table 14.6-2):

GNCGANNG

Instead of N, a lowercase n or a hyphen may be used for visual clarity:

GnCGAnnG

*or*

G-CGA--G

A double-stranded sequence that consists of a strand of DNA and its complement would be as follows:

GTCGACTG

CAGCTGAC

To show correct pairing between the bases in the 2 strands, sequences need to be aligned properly. In the sequence above, the first base pair is G · C, the next is T · A, etc. Note how the first G is directly above the first C, the first T above the first A, etc.

By convention in printed sequences, for single strands, the 5' end is at the left and the 3' end at the right; thus, a sequence such as the following

CCCATCTCACTTAGCTCCAATG

would be assumed to have this directionality:

5'-CCCATCTCACTTAGCTCCAATG-3'

The complementary strands of DNA have opposite directionality; by convention, the top strand reads from the 5' end to the 3' end, whereas its complementary strand appears below it with the 3' end on the left. The 5' strand is the *sense strand* or *coding strand* or *positive strand.* The 3' strand is the *antisense strand* or *noncoding strand.* (Note that it is the noncoding strand that actually gets transcribed.) In the example

CCCATCTCACTTAGCTCCAATG

GGGTAGAGTGAATCGAGGTTAC

this directionality is implied:

5'-CCCATCTCACTTAGCTCCAATG-3' (sense strand, coding strand)

3'-GGGTAGAGTGAATCGAGGTTAC-5' (antisense strand, noncoding strand)

Text should specify which strand, sense or antisense, is displayed. The sense strand "is the strand generally reported in the scientific literature or in databases."[3(p25)]

A codon is a sequence of 3 nucleotides in a DNA molecule that (ultimately) codes for an amino acid (see below), biosynthetic message, or signal (eg, start transcription, stop transcription). Codons are also referred to as codon triplets. Examples are as follows:

CAT    ATC    ATT

The genetic code—typically a list or table of all the codons and the amino acids they each encode—is widely reproduced (eg, in medical dictionaries and textbooks and on the internet).

Promoter sequences are DNA sequences that define where the transcription of a gene by RNA polymerase begins. They include the following:

CAT box (CCAAT)

CG island, CpG island (CG-rich sequence)

GC box (GGGCGGG consensus sequence)

5′ UTR (5′ untranslated region) (5′ is defined below)

TATA box

Enhancers are short (50- to 1500-bp) regions of DNA that can be bound by proteins (activators) to increase the likelihood that transcription of a particular gene will occur. The κ light chain enhancer (κ enhancer), for example, contains the sequence GGGACTTTCC.

Sequences of repeating single nucleotides are named as follows:

polyA

polyC

polyG

polyT

*Example*: polyA tail

or, optionally, with lowercase d (within parentheses) for deoxyribose:

poly(dT)

Repeating single-nucleotide pairs (in double-stranded DNA) are similarly named:

poly(dA-dT)

poly(dG-dC)

The phosphate groups linking the nucleotides are sometimes indicated with a lowercase p:

pGpApApTpTpC

CpG island

Methylated bases may be shown with a superscript lowercase m, which refers to the nucleotide residue to the right:

GAT$^{m}$CC

Sequences of repeating nucleotides, also known as tandem repeats, are indicated as follows (n stands for number of repeats):

(TTAGGG)$_n$

(GT)$_n$

(CGG)$_n$

Within a long sequence, the first repeat may be designated n, the next p, the next q, etc:

(TAGA)$_n$ATGGATAGATTA(GATG)$_p$AA(TAGA)$_q$

The number of repeats may be specified:

(GATG)$_2$

(TAGA)$_{12}$

Long sequences pose special typesetting problems. Such sequences should be depicted as separate figures, rather than within text or tables, whenever possible.

For DNA, it must be made clear whether the sequence is single-stranded or double-stranded. A double-stranded sequence such as that of the following example

CCCATCTCACTTAGCTCCAATG

GGGTAGAGTGAATCGAGGTTAC

might be mistaken for a single-stranded sequence and set as such:

CCCATCTCACTTAGCTCCAATGGGGTAGAGTGAATCGAGGTTAC

Conversely, mistaking a single-stranded sequence for a double-stranded sequence and typesetting accordingly should also be avoided.

Always maintain alignment in 2-stranded sequences—take care that the following

CCCATCTCACTTAGCTCCAATG

GGGTAGAGTGAATCGAGGTTAC

does not become this:

CCCATCTCACTTAGCTCCAATG

GGGTAGAGTGAATCGAGGTTAC

Numbering and spacing may be used as visual aids in presenting sequences. A space every 3 bases indicates the codon triplets:

. . . GCA GAG GAC CTG CAG GTG GGG . . .

DNA sequences for protein-coding regions in most eukaryotic cells contain both exons (coding sequences of triplets) and introns (intervening noncoding sequences). An intron occurs within the sequence (examples from Cooper[4[p273]]):

intron: GTGAG . . . GGCAG

sequence in preceding example with intron included:

```
. . . GCA GAG GAC CTG CAG G GTGAG . . . GGCAG TG GGG . . .
```

Another way to display introns amid exons is to use lowercase letters for introns and uppercase letters for exons. There is a space on either side of the intron, and the next exon continues in the same frame or phase as before, to resume the correct codon sequence:

```
...GCA GAG GAC CTG CAG G gtgag...ggcag TG GGG...
```

In longer DNA sequences, spaces every 5 or 10 bases are customary visual aids:

```
GAATT CCTGA CCTCA GGTGA TCTGC CCGCC TCGGC CTCCC AAAGT GCTGG
GAATTCCTGA CCTCAGGTGA TCTGCCCGCC TCGGCCTCCC AAAGTGCTGG
```

Several types of numbering are further aids. In the following example (from Cooper,[4(p133)] "lowercase letters indicate uncertainty in the base call"), numbers on the left specify the number of the first base on that line:

```
  1   5'-GAATTCCTGA CCTCAGGTGA TCTGCCCGCC TCGGCCTCCC AAAGTGCTGG

 51      GATTTACAGG CATGAGGCAC CACACCTGGC CAGTTGCTTA GCTCTCTAAG

101      TCTTATTTGC TTTACTTACA AAATGGAGAT ACAACCTTAT AGAACATTCG

151      ACATATACTA GGTTTCCATG AACAGCAGCC AGATCTCAAC TATATAGGGA

201      CCAGTGAGAA ACCAATCTCA GGTAGCTGAT GATGGGCAAa GGgATGGGgA

251      CTGATATGCC cNNNNNGACG ATTCGAGTGA CAAGCTACTA TGTACCTCAG

301      CTTTtCATCT tGATCTTCAC CACCCATGGg TAGGTGTCAC TGAAaTT-3'
```

Alternatively, numbers may appear above bases of special interest:

```
     6                                     39
GAATTCCTGA CCTCAGGTGA TCTGCCCGCC TCGGCCTCCC AAAGTGCTGG
```

When the base number is large, the right-most digit should be directly over the base being designated:

```
                         21 857
21 831  ACATATACTA GGTTTCCATG AACAGCAGCC AGATCTCAAC TATATAGGGA
```

When a long sequence is run within text, use a hyphen at the right-hand end of the line to indicate the bond linking successive nucleotides:

```
GATTTACAGGCATGAGGCACCACACCTGGCCAGTTGCTTAGCTCTCTAAGTC-

TTATTGCTTTACTTACAAAATGGAGATACAACCTTATAGACATTCG
```

A hyphen is not necessary if spacing is used, as long as the break between groups occurs at the end of the line. The DNA sequence may be displayed as follows:

```
5'-CCT GGG

CAA AGC AAG GTA GG-3'
```

Recognition sequences are sections of a sequence recognized by proteins such as restriction enzymes, which cleave DNA in specific locations (see 14.6.1.4, Nucleic Acid Technology). To indicate sites of cleavage, virgules or carets may be used:

*single-stranded:*

CATCGTG

C/TCGTG

*double-stranded:*

CGWCG^

^GCWGC

CGWCG/

/GCWGC

Other conventions should be defined, in parentheses for text or in legends for tables and figures.[5] For example:

CACNN↓NNGTG (↓ indicates cleavage at identical position in both strands)

**14.6.1.1.1** **Sequence Variations, Nucleotides.** Recommendations for sequence variation (mutation) nomenclature have been one of the major activities of the HUGO Mutation Database Initiative, now the Human Genome Variation Society (HGVS).[6] Members devised the nomenclature after extensive community discussion.[7-12] Authors should consult the Recommendations page of the HGVS website for the latest recommendations,[6] the HGVS Simple section of the HGVS website,[13] and the 2016 update.[14] Basic style points are as follows (see 14.6.1.5.1, Sequence Variations, Amino Acids):

- For sequence variations described at the nucleotide level, the nucleotide number precedes the capital-letter nucleotide abbreviation.

    12345A>T

- Numbers at the *end* of the term, if any, do not stand for the nucleotide number but rather indicate numbers of nucleotides involved in the change or, in the case of repeated sequences, numbers of repeats.

    c.54GCA[21]      [an allele of 21 GCA repeats]

- The nucleotide number should be preceded by g plus dot (g.) for gDNA (genomic), c plus dot (c.) for cDNA (complementary or coding), n plus dot (n.) for noncoding, r plus dot (r.) for RNA, m plus dot (m.) for mitochondrial, or p plus dot (p.) for protein.

- The symbol > is used for substitutions. The following abbreviations are used: ins, insertion; del, deletion; indel, insertion and deletion; dup, duplication; inv, inversion; con, conversion; and t, translocation. An underscore character separates a range of affected nucleotide residues.

    c.4375C>T [C nucleotide at position 4375 changed to a T]

    c.4375_4379del [nucleotides from positions 4375 to 4379 (GATT) are missing (deleted)]

- One set of brackets is used for 2 variations in a single allele, and 2 sets with a semicolon are used for 2 variations in paired alleles.

    [76C>T;283G>C] [2 variants on 1 molecule]

    [76C>T];[283G>C] [the same 2 variants on 2 different molecules]

▪ Nucleotide numbers may be positive or negative.

▪ The HGVS recommends avoiding the terms *mutation* and *polymorphism*, preferring instead the terms *sequence variant, sequence variation, alteration,* or *allelic variant*. In view of this recommendation, single-nucleotide variation (SNV) is now more frequently being used instead of SNP (single-nucleotide polymorphism) and may become standard in the future. To aid readers' understanding during this transition, at first mention SNV may be used, with SNP in parentheses:

"SNV (formerly SNP)"

Note the examples in **Table 14.6-3**. In general medical publications, textual explanations should accompany the shorthand terms at first mention.

When a gene symbol is used with a sequence variation term, only the gene symbol is italicized (see 14.6.2, Human Gene Nomenclature).

*ADRB1* 1165C>G (not: *ADRB1 1165C>G)*

Note: Sequence variants are often indicated by using virgules, but this is not recommended.[12]

| *Avoid:* | 1721G/A |
|---|---|
| *Preferred:* | 1721G, 1721A |
| *Avoid:* | 2417A/G |
| *Preferred:* | 2417A>G |

In practice, means other than the symbol > are commonly used to indicate substitutions. Of the following, the JAMA Network journals prefer the arrow:

1691G→A

1691G-A

1691GtoA

1691G-to-A

Any symbol for substitution is better than no symbol; otherwise the expression may be misinterpreted as indicating a dinucleotide at the site. For instance, 1691GA would imply a change involving the dinucleotide GA (1691G and 1692A).

When genotype is being expressed in terms of nucleotides (eg, sequence variants), italics and other punctuation for the nucleotides are not needed (see 14.6.2, Human Gene Nomenclature):

*MTHFR* 677 CC and TT genotypes

For nucleotide numbering of a cDNA reference sequence, nucleotide +1 is the A of the ATG initiator codon. The first nucleotide immediately 5′ (upstream) of the ATG initiator codon is −1. So for the sequence 5′AGC CTG ATG GAC CTC 3′ the G immediately 5′ of the ATG is −1, and A is +1. The nucleotide 3′ of the translation stop codon is *1. For nucleotides in introns, those at the 5′ end of the intron are numbered with a "plus" relative to the last base of the immediately preceding exon, whereas those at the 3′ end are numbered with a "minus" relative to the first base of the immediate downstream exon. For example:

**Table 14.6-3.** Examples of Sequence Variation Nomenclature

| Term | Explanation |
|---|---|
| 1691G>A | G-to-A substitution at nucleotide 1691 |
| 253Y>N | pyrimidine at position 253 replaced by another base |
| [76A>C;83G>C] | 2 substitutions in single allele (Note: Variations in same allele are indicated by brackets.) |
| [76A>C] + [87delG] | substitution and deletion in paired alleles |
| [76A>C (+) 83G>C] | 2 sequence changes in 1 individual, alleles unknown |
| 977_978insA | A inserted between nucleotides 977 and 978 |
| 186_187insC | C inserted between nucleotides 186 and 187 |
| 926_927insAAAAAAAAAAA | insertion of 11 A's between nucleotides 926 and 927 |
| 185_186delAG | deletion of A and G between nucleotides 185 and 186 |
| 617_618delT | deletion of T between nucleotides 617 and 618 |
| 188_199del11 | 11-bp deletion between nucleotides 188 and 199 |
| 1294_1334del40 | 40-bp deletion between nucleotides 1294 and 1334 |
| c.5delA | A deleted at position 5 (cDNA) |
| c.5_7delAGG | AGG deleted at positions 5 through 7 (cDNA) |
| g.5_123del | nucleotides deleted from positions 5 through 123 (gDNA) |
| g.7dup | duplication of a T at position g.7 in the sequence ACTTACTGCC to ACTTACTTGCC |
| 1007fs | frameshift mutation at codon 1007 |
| 112_117delinsTG | |
| 112_117delAGGTCAinsTG | deletion from nucleotide 112 through 117 and insertion of TG |
| 112_117>TG | |
| 203_506inv | |
| 203_506inv304 | 304 nucleotides inverted from positions 203 through 506 |
| 167(GT)6-22 | 6 to 22 GT repeats starting at position 167 |
| g.167(GT)8 | 8 GT repeats starting at position 167 (gDNA) |
| c.827_XYZ:233del | Examples[7] with hypothetical gene symbol *XYZ* incorporated (but not italicized) (see 14.6.2, Human Gene Nomenclature) |
| c.827_oXYZ:233del | o: opposite (antisense[a]) strand |

Abbreviations: bp, base pair; cDNA, complementary or coding DNA; gDNA, genomic DNA.

[a]A DNA molecule consists of 2 strands; one is the sense strand and one is the antisense strand. The sense strand (also called *coding strand, plus strand*, or *nontemplate strand*) contains codons and is the same as mRNA except that thymine in DNA is replaced by uracil in RNA. The antisense strand (also called *noncoding strand, minus strand*, or *template strand*) contains noncodons and acts as a template for the synthesis of mRNA. Therefore, the antisense strand is complementary to the sense strand and mRNA.[15]

c.77+2T     cDNA, nucleotide 77 of preceding exon, position 2 in intron, T residue

c.78-1G     cDNA, nucleotide 78 of next exon, position 1 in intron, G residue

Nucleotide numbering of a DNA reference sequence is arbitrary (ie, there is no defined starting point as in cDNA). Therefore, authors should describe their numbering scheme. No plus signs or minus signs are used with gDNA reference sequences.

Listing both the official and the traditional names next to each other in the variant summary will help authors and readers become more familiar with the official (preferred) terms.

*Preferred (Official):*     c.88+2T>G

*Replaces (Traditional):*     IVS#+2T>G

Promoter variants (promoter sequence variants) have been commonly expressed with terms such as

−765G>A

which implies nucleotide numbering in terms of a cDNA reference sequence. However, authors are advised to instead (or additionally) describe the variant in relation to a gDNA reference sequence (see 14.6.1.1.2, Unique Identifiers).[14]

L01531.1:g.1561C>T

Terms with a capital delta have been used to indicate exonic deletions. For example:

Δ ex 1a-15

Δ ex 1a-12

Δ ex 3

**14.6.1.1.2**   **Unique Identifiers.** Official recommendations include mentioning a sequence variant's unique identifier, for instance, a number assigned by a locus-specific curator or the OMIM number.[16] Allelic variants are designated by the 6-digit OMIM number, followed by a decimal point and a unique 4-digit variant number. The asterisk that precedes the number indicates that it is a gene (see 14.6.2.1, OMIM, for an explanation of OMIM numbering system and symbols). For a list of locus-specific database curators, see the HGVS website under Nomenclature for the Description of Sequence Variants.[6] For example:

1311C>T (OMIM *305900.0018)

880C>T (OMIM *600681.0002)

**14.6.1.1.3**   **Database Identifiers for Genomic Sequences.** Several databases record genomic sequence information:

*Nucleotides:*

GenBank (https://www.ncbi.nlm.nih.gov/genbank)

RefSeq (https://www.ncbi.nlm.nih.gov/refseq/)

EMBL (European Molecular Biology Laboratory) (https://www.embl.de)

DDBJ (DNA Data Bank of Japan) (https://www.ddbj.nig.ac.jp)

International HapMap Project (https://www.genome.gov/10001688/international-hapmap-project)

*Proteins:*

RCSB Protein Data Bank (https://www.rcsb.org/)

Protein database (https://www.ncbi.nlm.nih.gov/protein)

UniProt Knowledgebase (https://www.uniprot.org)

UniProtKB/Swiss-Prot (web.expasy.org/docs/swiss-prot_guideline.html)

PIR-PSD (Protein Information Resource: Protein Sequence Database) (https://proteininformationresource.org/pirwww/dbinfo/pir_psd.shtml)

For a review of databases in molecular biology, including several of the foregoing, see the 2018 Database Issue of the journal *Nucleic Acids Research*.[17]

Accession numbers are assigned when researchers submit unique sequences to any one of the databases. In published articles, accession numbers are useful in indicating specific sequences:

Founder effects were investigated using 2 previously undescribed, highly polymorphic microsatellite markers that flank presenilin 1. The first is a GT repeat at position 33117 (GenBank AF109907). The second is a CA repeat at position 23 000 of this same sequence.[18]

Accession numbers should include the version (eg, .1, .2) if possible[6]:

NM_000130.1

NM_000130.2

L01538.1

The following example shows variation expressed with the accession number[7]:

NM_004006.1:c.3G>T

For unambiguous identification, both version number *and* accession number should be used.[6] Common formatting for nucleotide data was determined in 1988 by representatives of GenBank, EMBL (European Molecular Biology Laboratory), and DDBJ (DNA Data Bank of Japan), forming the International Nucleotide Sequence Database Collaboration.[19]

**14.6.1.2** **RNA.** Functionally associated with DNA is RNA. It contains the 3 bases adenine (A), cytosine (C), and guanine (G) but differs from DNA in having the base uracil (U) instead of thymine (T) and the sugar ribose rather than deoxyribose. The corresponding nucleosides are adenosine, cytidine, guanosine, and uridine.

An example of an RNA sequence is as follows:

5′-UUAGCACGUGCUAA-3′

Examples of RNA codons are as follows:

CAU    UUG    AUU

Expand these common abbreviations at first use:

| | |
|---|---|
| cRNA | complementary RNA |
| dsRNA | double-stranded RNA |
| gRNA | genomic RNA |
| hnRNA | heteronuclear RNA (heterogeneous RNA) |
| mRNA | messenger RNA |
| miRNA | microRNA |
| mtRNA | mitochondrial RNA |
| nRNA | nuclear RNA |
| RNAi | RNA interference |
| rRNA | ribosomal RNA |
| siRNA | short interfering RNA |
| snRNA | small nuclear RNA |
| tRNA | transfer RNA |

Types of tRNA may be further specified; follow typographic style closely (these need not be expanded after the initial expansion of tRNA):

| | |
|---|---|
| $tRNA^{Met}$ | tRNA specific for methionine |
| $Met\text{-}tRNA^{Met}$ | methionyl-tRNA |
| $tRNA^{fMet}$ | tRNA specific for formylmethionine |
| $fMet\text{-}tRNA^{fMet}$ *or* $fMet\text{-}tRNA_f$ | $N$-formylmethionyl-tRNA |
| $tRNA^{Ala}$ | tRNA specific for alanine |
| $tRNA^{Val}$ | tRNA specific for valine |

The 3-dimensional structure of tRNA has several different arms, which allow it to recognize a codon on mRNA and deliver the appropriate amino acid during protein synthesis:

AA (amino acid) arm

DHU (dihydrouridine) arm

anticodon arm

T$\psi$C arm ($\psi$ for the unusual base pseudouridine)

**14.6.1.2.1** RNA Sequence Variations. Style for abbreviated sequence variation terms described at the RNA level is essentially the same as for DNA (see 14.6.1.1.1, Sequence Variations, Nucleotides). The main exception is that the RNA nucleotide abbreviations are lowercase. The prefix r. is used to signify RNA[12] but is not required.

> 78a>u
>
> r.76a>c

RNA sequences are quantified by use of the same units as for DNA (ie, base, bp, kb, and Mb) (see 13.12, Units of Measure):

> 240-bp dsRNA
>
> 10-25 RNA bases
>
> a 7.5-kb RNA probe

**14.6.1.3** Nucleotides as Precursors and Energy Molecules. The nucleotides of DNA and RNA are also important individually as the precursors of DNA and RNA and as energy molecules. They may bind 1, 2, or 3 phosphate molecules, giving rise to compounds with the following abbreviations (see 13.11, Clinical, Technical, and Other Common Terms) or alternative shorthand.

**14.6.1.3.1** Ribonucleotides. See Table 14.6-4 for examples of terms and their abbreviations.

**Table 14.6-4.** Examples of Terms and Abbreviations for Ribonucleotides

| Terms | Abbreviation | Alternative shorthand |
|---|---|---|
| adenosine monophosphate, adenylic acid | AMP | pA |
| adenosine diphosphate | ADP | ppA |
| adenosine triphosphate | ATP | pppA |
| cytidine monophosphate, cytidylic acid | CMP | pC |
| cytidine diphosphate | CDP | ppC |
| cytidine triphosphate | CTP | pppC |
| guanosine monophosphate, guanylic acid | GMP | pG |
| guanosine diphosphate | GDP | ppG |
| guanosine triphosphate | GTP | pppG |
| uridine monophosphate, uridylic acid | UMP | pU |
| uridine diphosphate | UDP | ppU |
| uridine triphosphate | UTP | pppU |

**14.6.1.3.2** Deoxyribonucleotides. See **Table 14.6-5** for examples of terms and abbreviations for deoxyribonucleotides.

**Table 14.6-5.** Examples of Terms and Abbreviations for Deoxyribonucleotides

| Term | Abbreviation | Alternative shorthand[a] |
|---|---|---|
| deoxyadenosine monophosphate, deoxyadenylic acid | dAMP | pdA |
| deoxyadenosine diphosphate | dADP | |
| deoxyadenosine triphosphate | dATP | |
| deoxycytidine monophosphate, deoxycytidylic acid | dCMP | pdC |
| deoxycytidine diphosphate | dCDP | |
| deoxycytidine triphosphate | dCTP | |
| deoxyguanosine monophosphate, deoxyguanylic acid | dGMP | pdG |
| deoxyguanosine diphosphate | dGDP | |
| deoxyguanosine triphosphate | dGTP | |
| deoxythymosine monophosphate, deoxythymidylic acid | dTMP | pdT |
| deoxythymosine diphosphate | dTDP | |
| deoxythymosine triphosphate | dTTP | |

[a]Terms such as ppdA and pppdA are, by analogy with ribonucleotide shorthand, feasible but not commonly found.

In the foregoing examples, monophosphates are assumed to be phosphorylated at the 5′ position, and the more specific term may be used:

5′-AMP

The additional phosphate groups of diphosphates and triphosphates are linked sequentially to the first phosphate group. Other phosphate positions and variations may be specified as follows:

2′-UMP

3′-UMP          Up

3′,5′-ADP          pAp

3′,5′-AMP          cAMP (cyclic AMP)

Note that the p follows the capital letter when 3′-phosphate is indicated.

**14.6.1.4**  **Nucleic Acid Technology.** Laboratory methods of analyzing DNA make use of special DNA sequences, which include the following:

RFLPs          restriction fragment length polymorphisms

SNPs          single-nucleotide polymorphisms (pronounced "snips") (note that SNVs is now preferred; see 14.6.1.1.1, Sequence Variations, Nucleotides)

| SNVs  | single-nucleotide variants       |
|-------|----------------------------------|
| STRs  | short tandem repeats             |
| STRPs | STR polymorphisms                |
| STSs  | sequence tagged sites            |
| VNTRs | variable number of tandem repeats |

Note: Satellite DNA repeats, microsatellite (repeating sequences of 1-9 bp) repeats (or markers), and minisatellite (repeating sequences of 10-100 bp) repeats[20] (or markers) are distinct types of tandem repeat sequences.

An SNV sequence may be preceded by rs (for reference SNV ID) or ss (for submitted SVP ID), used for accession numbers assigned by the National Center for Biotechnology Information:

rs1002138(-)

**14.6.1.4.1** **The Reference Genome.** The publication of the draft human genome sequence in 2001 heralded the beginning of the current era of genomic medicine.[21] Since that time, rapid advances in technology have facilitated increasingly accurate and inexpensive methods for interrogating the genomes of humans and model organisms for research and clinical care.

Current sequencing technologies do not sequence chromosomes from end to end. Rather, in a massively parallel process, genomic DNA is fragmented, sequenced, and reassembled for purposes of representation of a nearly complete genome.[22] In some applications only the protein coding regions of the genome are sequenced (exome sequencing), but increasingly it is feasible to sequence the entire genome for research or clinical purposes.

Of importance, a genome assembly and a genome are not the same thing. "A genome is the physical entity that defines an organism. An assembly is not a physical object; it is the collection of all sequences used to represent the genome of an organism."[22] Assemblies can be of varying degrees of completeness; for example, some regions of the human genome remain refractory to sequencing or assembly with current technologies. Informaticians and geneticists are continually striving to refine the accuracy of these assemblies known as reference genomes. As sequencing and assembly technologies continue to evolve, so does the notion of a reference assembly. The sequences in the human reference genome assembly do not represent the genome of a single individual but are mosaics constructed from the DNA of many anonymous individuals. Contributions from one individual comprise approximately 70% of the assembly sequence, although more than 50 individuals are represented in GRCh38.[23] The human reference genome assembly or build[23] (currently GRCh38) acts as the coordinate system for the human genome and the features annotated on it and is often the representation used for comparisons with other human genomes for diagnosis or research. Initially produced by the Human Genome Project, it is now maintained by the Genome Reference Consortium. However, other genomes may also be used as a reference in comparative analyses (eg, a parent's genome vs an offspring's genome). In publication, the most reliable means to define a genome assembly is by its unique GenBank (INSDC: http://insdc.org/)[24] accession number (eg, GRCh38 = GCA_000001405.15). If an assembly has not been deposited in GenBank, typically, at a minimum, an identifier for the sample from which the assembly is derived is provided (eg, INSDC BioSample accession [eg, SAMN06710886] or other identifier [eg, Coriell: NA10874]). Publications may include names for genome assemblies along with accession numbers or sample identifiers (eg, HuRef = GCA_000002125.2) (see 14.6.1.1.3, Database Identifiers for Genomic Sequences). Note: Use care with the term *reference*. Although the Human Genome Project produced the first notion of a human reference genome assembly, there are several ongoing efforts to create high-quality genome assemblies that could serve as population-specific reference assemblies.[25] None of these have yet been formally recognized by the global research community as a reference, but "it may be possible that the future human 'reference' genome is a panel of assemblies, rather than a single assembly" (Valerie Schneider, PhD, staff scientist, National Center for Biotechnology Information, written communication, May 2, 2017). There are also multiple efforts under way to use graph formats (rather than the traditional linear sequence format) to create references that represent population-level variation.[26]

For patients with disorders that have a primarily genetic origin, massively parallel sequencing of the total complement of an individual's DNA (genome sequencing) has proven to be a powerful diagnostic approach. Genome-scale sequencing can be performed on DNA from white blood cells or on buccal cells from saliva. In sequence analysis, each individual's genome contains millions of sites where his or her DNA differs from a reference sequence. Clinical interpretation requires assessing whether any of these variants are associated with disease.[27] See **Figure 14.6-4** for the analysis processing sequence.

**14.6.1.4.2** **Methods of Analysis.** Methods of analysis include the following:

| | |
|---|---|
| ASO | allele-specific oligonucleotide probes |
| DGGE | denaturing gradient gel electrophoresis |
| EMSA | electrophoretic mobility shift assay |
| FISH | fluorescence in situ hybridization |
| OSH | oligonucleotide-specific hybridization |
| PCR | polymerase chain reaction |
| PTT | protein truncation test |
| RT-PCR | reverse transcriptase–polymerase chain reaction |
| SKY | spectral karyotyping, a type of fluorescence in situ hybridization |
| SSCP | single-stranded conformational polymorphism |

**14.6.1.4.3** **Blotting.** The first blotting technique, used for identifying specific DNA sequences in gDNA isolated in vitro by means of nucleic acid probes, was named Southern blotting for its originator, Edwin Southern. Similar techniques have since been named (with droll intent) for compass directions and include Northern blotting (RNA identified; nucleic acid probe), Western blotting (protein identified; antibody probe), Southwestern blotting (DNA protein identified; DNA probe), and

**Figure 14.6-4.** Informatic and Human Analysis Required for Finding Rare Pathogenic Variants in a Human Genome

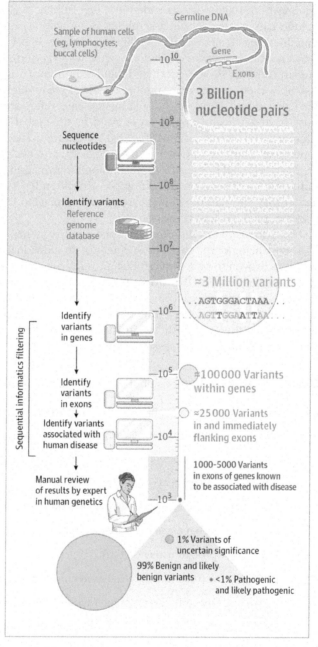

Genetic variants are informatically filtered to remove those with very low likelihood of pathogenicity (eg, variants known to be benign or present at very high frequency in the general population). This informatic processing incorporates annotations of individual variants (eg, population allele frequencies, prior literature reports, computational predictions of functional effect) for use in manual analysis. Reproduced from Evans et al.[27]

Far Western blotting (protein-protein interaction identified; protein probe).[28,29] Recombinant DNA is DNA created by combining isolated DNA sequences of interest. Among the tools used in this process are cloning vectors, such as plasmids, phages (see 14.14.3, Virus Nomenclature, and 14.4.4, Prions), and hybrids of these, cosmids, and phagemids. Additional tools are bacterial artificial chromosomes (BACs) and yeast artificial chromosomes (YACs).

Basic explanations of these entities are available in medical dictionaries and textbooks. A few that present special nomenclature problems are described here.

**14.6.1.4.4** **Cloning Vectors.** Plasmids are typically named with a lowercase p followed by a letter or alphanumeric designation; spacing may vary:

pBR322

pJS97

pUC

pUC18

pSPORT

pSPORT 2

Phage cloning vectors are named for the phages. For example:

phage λ:      λgt10, λgt11, λgt22A

M13 phage:   M13KO7, M13mp

**14.6.1.4.5** **Restriction Enzymes.** Restriction enzymes (or restriction endonucleases) are special enzymes that cleave DNA at specific sites. They are named for the organism from which they are isolated, usually a bacterial species or strain. An authoritative source of information is REBASE.[5] As originally proposed,[30] their names consist of a 3-letter term, italicized and beginning with a capital letter, taken from the organism of origin, for example:

*Hpa* for *Haemophilus parainfluenzae*

followed by a roman numeral, which is a series number, for example:

*Hpa*I

*Hpa*II

In some cases, the series number is preceded by a capital or lowercase letter (roman, not italic), an arabic numeral, or a number and letter combination, which refers to the strain of bacterium; there are no spaces between any of these elements of the term:

*Eco*RI

*Hin*fI

*Sau*96I

*Sau*3AI

Many variations in the form of the names of these enzymes have appeared (eg, *Hin* d III, *Hin* dIII, *Hind* III, *Hind* III). It is currently recommended that italics and spacing be given as noted in the preceding paragraph to differentiate the species name, strain designation, and enzyme series number. **Table 14.6-6** gives examples of commonly used restriction enzymes.

**Table 14.6-6.** Examples of Commonly Used Restriction Enzymes and the Organism of Origin

| Enzyme name | Organism of origin |
|---|---|
| *Acc*I | *Acinetobacter calcoaceticus* |
| *Alu*I | *Arthrobacter luteus* |
| *Alw*NI | *Acinetobacter lwoffii* N |
| *Bam*HI | *Bacillus amyloliquefaciens* H |
| *Bcl*I | *Bacillus caldolyticus* |
| *Bst*EII | *Bacillus stearothermophilus* ET |
| *Bst*XI | *Bacillus stearothermophilus* X |
| I-*Ceu*I | *Chlamydomonas eugametos* |
| *Dpn*I | *Streptococcus* (diplococcus) *pneumoniae* M |
| *Eco*RI | *Escherichia coli* RY13 |
| *Eco*RII | *Escherichia coli* R245 |
| *Hae*II | *Haemophilus aegyptius* |
| *Hinc*II | *Haemophilus influenzae* Rc |
| *Hind*III | *Haemophilus influenzae* Rd |
| *Hinf*I | *Haemophilus influenzae* Rf |
| *Mse*I | *Micrococcus* species |
| *Msp*I | *Moraxella* species |
| *Ple*I | *Pseudomonas lemoignei* |
| *Pml*I | *Pseudomonas maltophilia* |
| *Pst*I | *Providencia stuartii* |
| *Sau*3AI | *Staphylococcus aureus* 3A |
| *Sau*96I | *Staphylococcus aureus* PS96 |
| *Sma*I | *Serratia marcescens* |
| *Sst*I | *Streptomyces stanford* |
| *Taq*I | *Thermus aquaticus* YT-1 |
| *Xba*I | *Xanthomonas badrii* |
| *Xho*I | *Xanthomonas holicola* |

Prefixes may further specify type of enzyme action, for example:

I-*Ceu*I        I: intron-coded endonuclease        *Chlamydomonas eugametos*

M.*Mly*I       M: methylase                                    *Micrococcus lylae*

N.*Mly*I       N: nicking enzyme

Restriction enzyme names are often seen as modifiers, for example:

a *Bam*HI fragment

an *Eco*RI site

For information on recognition sequences, see 14.6.1.1, DNA.

**14.6.1.4.6**  **Modifying Enzymes.** Enzymes exist that synthesize DNA and RNA (polymerases), cleave DNA (nucleases), join nucleic acid fragments (ligases), methylate nucleotides (methylases), and synthesize DNA from RNA (reverse transcriptases) (see 14.10.3, Enzyme Nomenclature). Those in laboratory use come from living systems, often from the same organisms that furnish restriction enzymes. Because the names may be similar, it is essential to specify the type of enzyme so that there is no confusion, for example:

*Alu*I methylase

*Pfu* DNA polymerase (*Pyrococcus furiosus*)

*Taq*I methylase

*Taq* DNA ligase

Modifying enzyme names are often seen as modifiers, for example:

a *Taq*I RFLP

In the following enzyme terms, T plus numeral refers to the related phage (see 14.14.3, Virus Nomenclature, and 14.4.4, Prions):

T7 DNA polymerase

T4 DNA polymerase

T4 polynucleotide kinase

T4 RNA ligase

**14.6.1.4.7**  **DNA Families.** Some sequences belonging to non–protein-coding regions of the genome can also be classified by their base content. Non–protein-coding DNA includes that which is transcribed into functional noncoding RNA molecules (eg, transfer RNA, ribosomal RNA, and regulatory RNA, such as microRNA), as well as families of repetitive sequence, some of which include transposons and retrotransposons. Families include the following:

*Collective term*: SINEs (short interspersed nuclear elements)

*Example: Alu* family (named for *Alu*I; see 14.6.1.4.5, Restriction Enzymes)

*Category*: Interspersed

*Collective term:* LINEs (long interspersed nuclear elements)

*Example:* L1 family (from LINE 1 family)

*Category:* Tandem

**14.6.1.5** **Amino Acids.** Twenty amino acids are encoded by triplet base codons in DNA and constituents of proteins. Each has 1 or more distinct codons in DNA (eg, GCU, GCC, GCA, and GCG code for alanine).

Table 14.6-7 gives the amino acids of proteins and their preferred 3- and single-letter symbols. Although these amino acids have systematic names (eg, alanine is 2-aminopropanoic acid), the trivial names are the most widely recognized and used. The single-letter symbols are usually used for longer sequences; otherwise, the 3-letter symbols are preferred. Do not mix single-letter and 3-letter amino acid symbols. In publications for a general audience, it may be helpful to define the single-letter symbols (eg, in a key) and to expand the 3-letter symbols at first mention as well.

The symbols Asp and Glu apply equally to the anions aspartate and glutamate, respectively, the forms that exist under most physiological conditions.

Other amino acids are also well known by their trivial names and have 3-letter codes. These, however, should always be expanded at first mention, as the example of cystine, whose 3-letter code is the same as that of cysteine, bears out:

| | |
|---|---|
| citrulline | Cit |
| cystine | Cys |
| homocysteine | Hcy |
| homoserine | Hse |
| hydroxyproline | Hyp |
| ornithine | Orn |
| thyroxine | Thx |

The side chains of amino acids are known as R groups, and the letter R is used in molecular formulas when indicating a nonspecified side chain, as in this general formula for an amino acid:

$$H_2N-\underset{R}{\overset{COOH}{\underset{|}{\overset{|}{C}}}}-H$$

**Table 14.6-7.** Amino Acids of Proteins and Their 3- and Single-Letter Symbols

| Amino acid | 3-Letter symbol | Single-letter symbol |
| --- | --- | --- |
| alanine | Ala | A |
| arginine | Arg | R |
| asparagine | Asn | N |
| aspartic acid | Asp | D |
| asparagine or aspartic acid | Asx | B |
| cysteine | Cys | C |
| glutamic acid | Glu | E |
| glutamic acid or glutamine | Glx | Z |
| glutamine | Gln | Q |
| glycine | Gly | G |
| histidine | His | H |
| isoleucine | Ile | I |
| leucine | Leu | L |
| lysine | Lys | K |
| methionine | Met | M |
| phenylalanine | Phe | F |
| proline | Pro | P |
| serine | Ser | S |
| threonine | Thr | T |
| tryptophan | Trp | W |
| tyrosine | Tyr | Y |
| vallne | Val | V |
| unspecified amino acid | Xaa | X |

Do not confuse the R with the single-letter abbreviation for arginine (see Table 14.6-7).

Peptide bonds are bonds between the α-carboxyl group of one amino acid and the α-amino group of the next. Long peptide sequences are the backbones of proteins. A peptide sequence might be indicated as follows, with hyphens representing peptide bonds:

Gly-Ile-Val-Glu-Gln-Cys-Cys-Ala-Ser-Val-Cys-Ser-Leu-Tyr

By convention in such a sequence, the amino end of the peptide (the end of the peptide whose amino acid has a free amino group, also known as the N terminal) is on the left and the carboxyl end (the end of the peptide whose amino acid has a free carboxyl group, also known as the C terminal) is on the right. The symbols

NH$_2$ and COOH may be included in the representation of the peptide sequence, as follows:

NH$_2$-Gly-Ile-Val-Glu-Gln-Cys-Cys-Ala-Ser-Val-Cys-Ser-Leu-Tyr-COOH

The same left-to-right convention applies to sequences using single letters. The above sequence using single letters would be as follows:

GIVEQCCASVCSLY

When the NH$_2$ group appears on the right of a sequence, it has a meaning other than amino end. For instance, in the following sequence, Val-NH$_2$ indicates the amide derivative of valine:

His-Phe-Arg-Lys-Pro-Val-NH$_2$

To indicate bonds other than the peptide bonds described above, lines, rather than hyphens, are used:

Glu └ Cys-Gly     Glu

or └

─ Cys-Gly (glutathione)

Cys-Tyr-Ile-Gln-Asn-Cys-Pro-Leu-Gly-NH2 (oxytocin)

(Adapted with permission from Moss.[2] Copyright IUPAC and IUBMB.)

For a multiline peptide sequence in running text, use a hyphen at the right end of one line to indicate a break and at the start of the next line to indicate the peptide bond:

Ala-Ser-Tyr-Phe-Ser-

-Gly-Pro-Gly-Trp-Arg

or, in figures, use a line:

Ala-Ser-Tyr-Phe-Ser ─┐

└─ Gly-Pro-Gly-Trp-Arg

(Adapted with permission from Moss.[2] Copyright IUPAC and IUBMB.)

In special cases, such as cyclic compounds (illustrated here by gramicidin S), the bond from C-2 to N-2 can be shown with arrows, as follows:

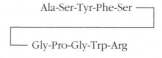

(gramicidin S)

(Adapted with permission from Moss.[2] Copyright IUPAC and IUBMB.)

As with nucleic acid sequences, alignment is important in protein sequences. In the following examples, the amino acid residues must remain aligned with the nucleic acid triplets:

```
MetSerIleGlnHis              Met-Ser-Ile-Gln-His

AGTATGAGTATTCAACAT    or   AGT ATG AGT ATT CAA CAT

TCATACTCATAAGTTGTA         TCA TAC TCA TAA GTT GTA
```

(Adapted with permission from Moss.[2] Copyright IUPAC and IUBMB.)

An amino acid term plus number refers to the amino acid by codon number (when known) or by protein residue. For example:

Arg506

**14.6.1.5.1** **Sequence Variations, Amino Acids.** HGVS has expressed a preference for the 3-letter amino acid abbreviation to be used in shorthand descriptions of sequence variations in proteins because several amino acids start with the same initial letter (eg, Ala, Arg, Asn, Asp). The use of only 1 letter could lead to ambiguity or confusion. The 1-letter style still may be seen but is not recommended. For sequence variations described at the protein level, recommended style for abbreviated terms is similar to that for nucleotides (see 14.6.1.1.1, Sequence Variations, Nucleotides, and 14.6.2, Human Gene Nomenclature). Note, as indicated in **Table 14.6-8**, that the amino acid abbreviation begins the term, preceding the position number (in contrast to nucleotide sequence variant terms, in which the residue number precedes the residue abbreviation). Explanation of such terms at first mention is recommended. Use of the prefix p. (protein) is another recent recommendation.

X is officially recommended as the symbol for the stop codon, but it can also be the single-letter abbreviation for unspecified or unknown amino acid. Therefore, when an amino acid sequence expressed with single letters that includes X is used, the X should be explained in the text.

When an amino acid sequence variation is used with a gene symbol, italicize only the gene symbol:

*ADRB1* Arg389Gly (not: *ADRB1 Arg389Gly* )

(See 14.6.2, Human Gene Nomenclature.)

Note: Residue numbering begins at the translation initiator methionine, +1.

For further details on expressing sequence variations in proteins, consult the HGVS recommendations.[6]

**Table 14.6-8.** Sequence Variations in Proteins and Their 3- and Single-Letter Descriptions

| 3-Letter style | Single-letter style | Explanation |
|---|---|---|
| Arg506Gln | R506Q | arginine at residue 506 replaced by glutamine |
| Leu10ins | L10ins | leucine inserted at position 10 |
| Leu141del | L141del | leucine deleted at position 141 |
| Gln318X *or* Gln318ter | G318X | glutamine at 318 changed to stop codon (X or ter) |
| p.Trp26Cys | p.W26C | tryptophan at residue 26 replaced by cysteine |

**Principal Author:** Cheryl Iverson, MA

## ACKNOWLEDGMENT

Thanks to the following for reviewing and providing comments: W. Gregory Feero, MD, PhD, *JAMA*, and Maine-Dartmouth Family Medicine Residency, Augusta; Valerie Schneider, PhD, National Center for Biotechnology Information, Bethesda, Maryland; Trevor Lane, MA, DPhil, Edanz Group, Fukuoka, Japan; and John J. McFadden, MA, JAMA Network. Thanks also to David Song, JAMA Network, for obtaining permissions.

## REFERENCES

1. Cammack R. The biochemical nomenclature committees. *IUBMB Life.* 2000;50(3):159-161. doi:10.1080/152165400300001453

2. Moss GP. International Union of Biochemistry and Molecular Biology recommendations on biochemical & organic nomenclature, symbols & terminology, etc. Updated May 21, 2018. Accessed June 25, 2018. https://www.qmul.ac.uk/sbcs/iubmb/

3. Nussbaum RL, McInnes RR, Willard HF. *Thompson & Thompson Genetics in Medicine.* 8th ed. Elsevier; 2016.

4. Cooper NG. *The Human Genome Project: Deciphering the Blueprint of Heredity.* University Science Books; 1994.

5. Roberts RJ, Vincze T, Posfai J, Macelis D. REBASE: a database for DNA restriction and modification: enzymes, genes and genomes. *Nucleic Acids Res.* 2010;38(database issue):D234-D236. Accessed July 31, 2019. https://www.ncbi.nlm.gov/pmc/articles/PMC2808884

6. Human Genome Variation Society website. Updated May 17, 2018. Accessed July 31, 2019. http://www.hgvs.org

7. den Dunnen JT, Antonarakis SE. Mutation nomenclature extensions and suggestions to describe complex mutations: a discussion. *Hum Mutat.* 2000;15(1):7-12. doi:10.1002/(SICI)1098-1004(200001)15:1<7::AID-HUMU4>3.0.CO;2-N

8. Antonarakis SE; Nomenclature Working Group. Recommendations for a nomenclature system for human gene mutations. *Hum Mutat.* 1998;11(1):1-3. doi:10.1002/(SICI)1098-1004(1998)11:1<1::AID-HUMU1>3.0.CO;2-O

9. Beutler E, McKusick VA, Motulsky AG, Scriver CR, Hutchinson F. Mutation nomenclature: nicknames, systematic names, and unique identifiers. *Hum Mutat.* 1996;8(3):203-206. doi:10.1002/(SICI)1098-1004(1996)8:3<203::AID-HUMU1>3.0.CO;2-A

10. Ad Hoc Committee on Mutation Nomenclature. Update on nomenclature for human gene mutations. *Hum Mutat.* 1996;8(3):197-202. doi:10.1002/humu.1380080302

11. Beaudet AL, Tsui L-C. A suggested nomenclature for designing mutations. *Hum Mutat.* 1993;2(4):245-248. doi:10.1002/humu.1380020402

12. den Dunnen JT, Antonarakis E. Nomenclature for the description of human sequence variations. *Hum Genet.* 2001;109(1):121-124. doi:10.1007/s004390100505

13. Sequence variant nomenclature. HGVS Simple. Accessed June 25, 2018. http://varomen.ghvs.org/bg-material/simple/

14. den Dunnen JT, Dalgleish R, Maglott DR, et al; Human Genome Variation Society (HGVS) and Human Genome Organization (HUGO). HGVS recommendations for the description of sequence variants: 2016 update. *Hum Mutat.* 2016;37(6):564-569. doi:10.1002/humu.22981

15. Major Differences. Accessed March 17, 2019. http://www.majordifferences. com/2015/01/difference-between-sense-and-antisense.html

16. Online Mendelian Inheritance in Man (OMIM). National Center for Biotechnology Information website. Updated daily. Accessed July 31, 2019. https://www.ncbi.nlm.nih.gov/omim

17. Rigden DJ, Fernández XM. The 2018 *Nucleic Acids Research* database issue and the online molecular biology database collection. *Nucleic Acids Res.* doi:10.1093/nar/gkx1235

18. Athan ES, Williamson J, Ciappa A, et al. A founder mutation in presenilin 1 causing early-onset Alzheimer disease in unrelated Caribbean Hispanic families. *JAMA.* 2001;286(18):2257-2263. doi:10.1001/jama.286.18.2257

19. About INSDC. International Nucleotide Sequence Database Collaboration website. Accessed July 31, 2019. www.insdc.org/about

20. Difference between minisatellite and microsatellite. July 14, 2017. Accessed July 31, 2019. https://www.differencebetween.com/difference-between-minisatellite-and-vs-microsatellite

21. Pasche B. Whole-genome sequencing: a step closer to personalized medicine. *JAMA.* 2011;305(15):1596-1597. doi:10.1001/JAMA.2011.484

22. Schneider V, Church D. Genome Reference Consortium. In: *The NCBI Handbook.* 2nd ed. National Center for Biotechnology Information; 2013.

23. Schneider VA, Graves-Lindsay T, Howe K, et al. Evaluation of GRCh38 and de novo haploid genome assemblies demonstrates the enduring quality of the reference assembly. *Genome Res.* 2017;27(5):849-864. doi:10.1101/gr.213611.116

24. International Nucleotide Sequence Database Collaboration (INSCD). Accessed July 31, 2019. http://www.insdc.org

25. McDonnell Genome Institute. Reference genome improvement. Accessed July 24, 2017. https://www.genome.wustl.edu/items/reference-genome-improvement/

26. Novak AM, Hickey G, Garrison E, et al. Genome graphs. Accessed July 24, 2017. doi:10.1101/101378

27. Evans JP, Powell BC, Berg JS. Finding the rare pathogenic variants in a human genome. *JAMA.* 2017;317(18):1904-1905. doi:10.1001/jama.2017.0432

28. Nicholas MW, Nelson K. North, South, or East? blotting techniques. *J Invest Dermatol.* 2013;133(7):e10. doi:10.1038/jid.2013.216

29. Wu Y, Li Q, Chen X-Z. Detecting protein-protein interaction by Far Western blotting. *Nat Protoc.* 2007;2(12):3278-3284. doi:10.1038/nprot.2007.459

30. Smith HO, Nathans D. A suggested nomenclature for bacterial host modification and restriction systems and their enzymes. *J Mol Biol.* 1973;81(3):419-423. doi:10.1016/0022-2836(73)90152-6

**14.6.2** **Human Gene Nomenclature.** The International System for Human Gene Nomenclature (ISGN), a system for gene symbols, was inaugurated in 1979[1,2] and has been continually updated. The history of naming genes and proteins is littered with redundancy because investigators often make discoveries separately and choose a name without following any sort of naming convention. Hence, the literature, especially literature more than a decade old, can be confusing because the same gene may have multiple names. Standardization helps both research and clinical care. The Human Gene Mapping Nomenclature Committee (HGNC), which developed the ISGN, put forth a "one human genome–one gene language" principle:

> Certainly there exists a genetic and molecular basis for a single human gene language without dialects. All human nuclear genes as we know them follow the same genetic, molecular, and evolutionary principles. . . .Thus it is

reasonable and logical to develop a standard and consolidated gene nomenclature system rather than have a human gene language based on different gene systems.[3(p12)]

The HGNC is 1 of 7 committees of the Human Genome Organisation (HUGO) and is "responsible for gene name validation."[4(p115)] Gene names and symbols are assigned by the HGNC.[5,6] To date, the HGNC has assigned more than 42 000 gene names.

■ *Gene Symbols:* A gene symbol is a short term, typically 3 to 7 characters long, that conveys in abbreviated form the name or other attribute of a gene. Human gene symbols usually consist of uppercase letters and may also contain (but never begin with) arabic numerals. Approved gene symbols do not contain Greek letters, roman numerals, superscripts, or subscripts and, usually, contain no punctuation. Gene symbols should be italicized, per official recommendations.[7] Italicizing is a useful way to make clear that a gene, and not a similarly named entity such as a condition or product of the gene, is being discussed. Italics are not necessary in published catalogs of gene symbols.[7] For style rules for gene symbols, see **Table 14.6-9.**

Approved symbols may represent other entities, such as chromosomal regions, certain syndromes, genes whose existence is inferred (supported by linkage analysis or association with known markers), cloned DNA segments, pseudogenes, and DNA fragments.

Within larger terms, only the gene symbol is italicized:

*ADRB2* 46G>A (*not: ADRB2 46G>A*)

*ADRB2* Gly16Arg (*not: ADRB2 Gly16Arg*)

(For an explanation of 46G>A and Gly16Arg, see 14.6.1, Nucleic Acids and Amino Acids.)

Authors are encouraged to use the most up-to-date gene symbol, which may be verified at the HGNC database (www.genenames.org),[5] previously known as Entrez Gene.[8] One area of growth in the HGNC database has been the increase in the number of gene families: to date, the database includes more than 1100 families, "with 51% of the protein coding genes within [the] database associated to at least one family."[6] The HGNC symbols and names are seen as a standard and are used in all the major databases that concentrate on human genes and proteins, for example, UniProt and NCBI Gene, as well as disease and phenotype resources, including Online Locus Reference Genomic (LRG),[9] a manually curated record that contains stable, and thus unversioned, reference sequences designed specifically for reporting sequence variants with clinical implications,[6] and Online Mendelian Inheritance in Man (OMIM).

**14.6.2.1** **OMIM.** Online Mendelian Inheritance in Man (OMIM) is a continually updated catalog of human genes and genetic disorders and traits, with focus on the molecular relationship between genetic variation and phenotypic expression.[10,11]

When a specific syndrome is mentioned, it is helpful to include the OMIM number (see 14.6.1.1.2, Unique Identifiers):

bronchomalacia (OMIM 211450)

DiGeorge syndrome (OMIM #188400)

Each entry is given a unique 6-digit number. Allelic variants are designated by the OMIM number of the entry, followed by a decimal point and a unique 4-digit variant number. For example:

> Allelic variants in the factor IX gene (OMIM 300746) are numbers 300746.0001-300746.0101.

Symbols precede many OMIM numbers. These are explained in the OMIM frequently asked questions (FAQ) site,[12] as follows:

- An asterisk before an entry number indicates a gene.

- A number symbol (#) indicates that it is a descriptive entry, usually of a phenotype, and does not represent a unique locus.

- A plus sign, the entry contains the description of a gene of known sequence and a phenotype.

- A percent sign, the entry describes a confirmed mendelian phenotype or phenotype locus for which the underlying molecular basis is not known.

- No symbol, description of a phenotype for which the mendelian basis, although suspected, has not been clearly established or the separateness of the phenotype from that in another entry is unclear.

- A caret (^), the entry no longer exists because it was removed from the database or moved to another entry.

Consistent use of the approved gene symbol provides advantages when searching for information in multiple databases.[13]

- *Gene Names:* Genes are usually named for the molecular product of the gene, the function of the gene, or the condition associated with the gene, if known. Gene names are not italicized. As shown in Table 14.6-9, the approved gene names, available in the above-mentioned databases, expand Greek letters and do not use subscripts (so that, for instance, in searching for a term with $\alpha$ online, one would type "alpha"). Descriptions based on the approved gene names but styled according to the journal in question (eg, using Greek letters and subscripts) or omitting some terms from the full name are permissible in general medical journals.

| approved gene name: | the alpha-fetoprotein gene |
|---|---|
| description: | the $\alpha$-fetoprotein gene |

| approved gene name: | the gene for beta-2-microglobulin |
|---|---|
| description: | the gene for $\beta_2$-microglobulin |

A number of conventions are followed when gene symbols and names are officially designated. Related genes are often assigned symbols by sequentially numbering a stem, the root symbol for the gene family:

*ABC*: root symbol

genes: *ABCA1, ABCG4,* etc

**Table 14.6-9.** Examples of Style Rules for Gene Symbols

| Gene description | Approved gene name | Approved gene symbol | Rule illustrated |
|---|---|---|---|
| α-fetoprotein | alpha fetoprotein | AFP | Greek letter changed to Latin letter (but not moved to end of symbol; exception to recommendation) |
| α-galactosidase | galactosidase alpha | GLA | Greek letter changed to Latin letter and moved to end of symbol |
| β₁-galactosidase | galactosidase beta 1 | GLB1 | Greek letter changed to Latin letter and moved with numeral to end of term; no subscripts or punctuation |
| β₂-microglobulin | beta-2-microglobulin | B2M | Greek letter changed to Latin letter; no subscripts or punctuation |
| coagulation factor VIII | coagulation factor VIII | F8 | roman numeral changed to arabic numeral |
| heterogeneous nuclear ribonucleoprotein A2/B1 | heterogeneous nuclear ribonucleoprotein A2/B1 | HNRNPA2B1 | no punctuation marks or spaces |
| MCF.2 cell line–derived transforming sequence | MCF.2 cell line derived transforming sequence | MCF2 | no punctuation marks |
| 5′-nucleotidase, cytosolic | 5′, 3′-nucleotidase, cytosolic | NT5C | number moved from the start of symbol; no punctuation |
| 5S RNA, cluster 1 | RNA, 5S ribosomal 1 | RNA5S1 | first character is always a letter, not a number; @ sign indicates gene cluster in chromosomal region |
| thromboxane A₂ receptor | thromboxane A2 receptor | TBXA2R | no superscripts or subscripts |

> *TNF*: root symbol
>
> genes: *TNF, TNFAIP1, TNFAIP2, TNFAIP3,* etc

Other conventions involve stereotypic abbreviations; for example, *CR* will usually signify a chromosome region. (However, a given letter or letter combination does not always signify conventional usage. For instance, *L* at or near the end of a symbol often, but not always, indicates "like.") In **Table 14.6-10**, the conventions in column 1 reflect HGNC recommendations.[5] (Note: DNA sequences are available from GenBank.)

Gene symbols can be used without expansion, with the identifying OMIM (see 14.6.2.1, OMIM) or GenBank (see 14.6.2.2, GenBank) number given parenthetically, as in the following examples:

> Most of these trials included patients with metastatic colorectal cancer or assessed only *KRAS* (OMIM 190070) exon 2 variants.

> The *HSD3B1* gene (OMIM 109715) encodes for the enzyme 3β-hydroxysteroid dehydrogenase-1 (3βHSD1), which catalyzes adrenal androgen precursors into dihydrotestosterone (DHT), the most potent androgen.

> Sequencing the *APTX* gene (OMIM 606350) was performed on request for cases of cerebellar ataxia with hypoalbumunemia and/or early-onset

**Table 14.6-10.** Examples of Conventions for Gene Names and Gene Symbols

| Convention illustrated | Gene symbol | Gene description |
|---|---|---|
| @: gene family or cluster; *RN*, RNA | *RN5S1@* | RNA, 5S ribosomal 1q42 cluster |
| *AP*: associated protein | *BRAP* | BRCA1-associated protein |
| *AS*: antisense | *IGF2-AS* | IGF2 antisense RNA (no longer used: insulinlike growth factor 2, antisense) |
| *BP*: binding protein | *IL18BP* | interleukin 18 binding protein |
| C: catalytic | *G6PC* | glucose 6-phosphatase, catalytic (glycogen storage disease type I, von Gierke disease) |
| *CASP* (stem), sequentially numbered | *CASP1, CASP2, CASP3,* etc | caspase 1, 2, 3, etc, apoptosis-related cysteine protease |
| *CF* (formerly); name modified after discovery of gene product | *CFTR* | cystic fibrosis transmembrane conductance regulator |
| *CR*: chromosome region | *ANCR* | Angelman syndrome chromosome region |
| *CR*: chromosome region | *DCR* | Down syndrome chromosome region |
| D: DNA; *19*, chromosome 19; S: (unique DNA) segment; E: expressed | *TOMM40 (D19S1177E* is an alias; the official term should be preferred) | translocase of outer mitochondrial membrane 40 homolog (yeast) (no longer used; DNA: segment sequence) |
| D: domain-containing | *BRD1* | bromodomain containing 1 |
| F: series letter; *X*, X chromosome | *F81A* (no longer used: *DXS522E*) | coagulation factor VIII–associated 1 (no longer used: DNA segment sequence) |
| F: series letter, *X*, X chromosome | *FRAXF* | fragile site, folic acid type, rare, fra(X)(q28) F |
| *FAM*: family with sequence similarity | *ULK4P1* (no longer used: *FAM7A1*) | ULK4 pseudogene (no longer used; family with sequence similarity 7, member A1) |
| *FRA*: fragile site; *10*, chromosome 10; G: series letter | *FRA10G* | fragile site, aphidicolin type, common, fra(10)(q11.2) (see 14.6.4, Human Chromosomes) |
| *6GPD*: glucose-6-phosphate dehydrogenase (named for gene product) | *6GPD* | glucose-6-phosphate dehydrogenase |
| *HBA*: hemoglobin subunit alpha (named for gene product) | *HBA1* | hemoglobin subunit alpha 1 |
| *HCL*: hair color (named for characteristic) | *HCL1* | hair color 1 (brown) |
| *HLA* (punctuation exception for HLA genes) | *HLA-A* | major histocompatibility complex, class 1, A |
| *HOX*: "homeobox" gene family | *HOXA7* | homeobox A7 |
| *IL*: interleukin | *IL2RA* (no longer used: *IDDM10*) | interleukin 2 receptor subunit alpha (no longer used: insulin-dependent diabetes mellitus 10) |
| *INS*: insulin (named for gene product) | *INS* | Insulin |
| *IP*: interacting protein | *SCHIP1* | schwannomin interacting protein 1 |

(*continued*)

**Table 14.6-10.** Examples of Conventions for Gene Names and Gene Symbols (*continued*)

| Convention illustrated | Gene symbol | Gene description |
|---|---|---|
| *L*: "like" sequence | *G6PDL* | glucose-6-phosphate dehydrogenase–like |
| *L* (in this case, *L* at the end does not signify "like"); named for condition | *CDL1* | Cornelia de Lange syndrome 1 |
| *LG*: ligand | *CAMLG* | calcium modulating ligand |
| *LOH*: loss of heterozygosity | *LINC00312* (no longer used: *LOH3CR2A*) | long intergenic non–protein coding RNA 312 (no longer used: loss of heterozygosity 3, chromosomal region 2, gene A) |
| *M*: mitochondrial; *RP*, ribosomal protein | *MRPL57* (previously *MRP63*) | mitochondrial ribosomal protein L57 |
| *MAG*: melanoma antigen (named for condition and gene product) | *MAGEA2* | melanoma antigen, family member A2 |
| *MT*: mitochondrial | *MT7SDNA* | mitochondrially encoded 7S DNA |
| *MT*: mitochondrial, used with hyphen (punctuation exception) | *MT-RNR1* | mitochondrially encoded 12S RNA |
| *MY*: myosin | *MYH14* (no longer used: *DFNA4*) | myosin, heavy chain 14, nonmuscle (no longer used: deafness, autosomal dominant 4) |
| *N*: inhibitor | *CDKN1B* | cyclin-dependent kinase inhibitor 1B |
| *orf* (lowercase exception for open reading frame) | *TMEM258* (no longer used: *C11orf10*) | transmembrane protein 258 (no longer used: chromosome 11 open reading frame 10) |
| *P*: "pseudogene" | *HBAP1* | hemoglobin subunit alpha pseudogene 1 |
| *P*: does not always signify "pseudogene" | *HIVEP2* | human immunodeficiency virus 1 enhancer binding protein 2 |
| *PD*: programmed cell death (named for function) | *PD-1* | programmed cell death 1 protein |
| *PD-L*: programmed cell death ligand (named for function) | *PD-L1* | programmed cell death 1 ligand 1 |
| *PDL-L*: programmed cell death ligand (named for function) | *PD-L2* | programmed cell death 1 ligand 2 |
| *R*: receptor | *INSR* | insulin receptor |
| *R*: receptor; *L*: like | *INSRL* | insulin receptor–like |
| *REN*: renin (named for gene product) | *REN* | renin |
| *REN*: renin (named for gene product); *BP*, binding protein | *RENBP* | renin binding protein |
| *RG*: regulator | *TCIRG1* | T-cell, immune regulator 1, ATPase, H+ transporting, lysosomal V0 subunit A3 |
| *TTR* | *TTR* (transthyretin) (no longer used: *CTS1*) | transthyretin (no longer used: carpal tunnel syndrome 1) |
| *TUB*: tubulin (named for gene product) | *TUBAC3* | tubulin alpha 3C$a_2$ tubulin |
| *ZNF*: zinc finger protein | *ZNF160* | zinc finger protein 160 |

cerebellar ataxia combined with peripheral neuropathy and/or cerebellar atrophy using brain magnetic resonance imaging.

Autosomal dominant cerebellar ataxias are most often caused by CAG repeat expansions in *ATXN1* (OMIM 601556), *ATXN2* (OMIM 601517), *ATXN3* (OMIM 607047), *CACNA1A* (OMIM 601011), *ATXN7* (OMIM 607640), *TBP* (OMIM 600075), or *ATN1* (OMIM 607462).

Patients with stage IV melanoma and established *BRAF* (GenBank NM_004333.5) or *NRAS* (GenBank NM_002524.4) variants treated with pembrolizumab or nivolumab alone or in combination between July 3, 2014, and May 24, 2016, were included.

**14.6.2.2** **GenBank.** GenBank[14] is the National Institutes of Health genetic sequence database, an annotated collection of all publicly available DNA sequences. It is part of the International Nucleotide Sequence Database Collaboration, which includes 3 organizations: the DNA DataBank of Japan, the European Nucleotide Archive, and GenBank at the National Center for Biotechnology Information. These organizations exchange data daily, and a new release is issued every 2 months.

When a gene name or symbol has been changed, both the new and former names (the latter known as the previous name) are available in gene databases.[5,6,8] Authors should use the most up-to-date name. The previous symbol may be included parenthetically at first mention:

*CYP2A6* (previously *CYP2A3*)

*SOD1* (previously *ALS* and *ALS1*)

*ERBB2* (previously *HER2/neu*)

**14.6.2.3** **Glossary of Genomic Terms.** To help clinicians understand the latest developments in genetics so that they can make the most informed decisions for their patients, in 2017 *JAMA* began a series entitled Genomics and Precision Health. Associated with this ongoing series is a glossary of genomics terms. This may be accessed at https://sites.jamanetwork.com/genetics/#glossary.[15]

**14.6.2.4** **Writing About Genes: Italicizing Gene Symbols.** Observing the rule of italicizing gene symbols makes clear whether the writer is referring to a gene or to another entity that might be confused with a gene.

In any discussion of a gene, it is recommended that the approved gene symbol be mentioned at some point, preferably in the title and abstract if relevant. However, the gene symbol need not be mentioned every time the writer refers to the gene. Authors may refer to genes (or gene loci) by their official gene names or other descriptive expression. Any of these is acceptable, depending on context and syntax. Of names, descriptions, and symbols, only the gene symbol is italicized. Examples are given in **Table 14.6-11**.

In the foregoing examples, the gene names and descriptions are readily distinguishable from the gene symbols. Sometimes, however, the gene symbol may be easily confused with the abbreviation for the product or condition associated with the gene unless the gene symbol is italicized. See, for instance, **Table 14.6-12**.

**Table 14.6-11.** Examples of Expressions of Gene Symbols

| Gene symbol | Gene description | Acceptable expression |
|---|---|---|
| *BRCA1* | breast cancer 1, early-onset gene | the breast and ovarian cancer susceptibility gene |
| *CFTR* | cystic fibrosis transmembrane conductance regulator gene | the cystic fibrosis locus |
| *F8* | coagulation factor VIII, procoagulant component (hemophilia A) gene | the factor VIII locus |
| *F8* | coagulation factor VIII, procoagulant component (hemophilia A) gene | the hemophilia A locus |
| *SYN1* | synapsin I gene | the gene for synapsin I |
| *TP53* | tumor protein p53 (Li-Fraumeni syndrome) gene | the *TP53* gene (p53 is the alias term; the official term should be preferred to the alias) |

**Table 14.6-12.** Examples of Potentially Confusing Nongene Terms

| Gene | Potentially confusing nongene term |
|---|---|
| *ABO* | ABO blood group system (see 14.1, Blood Groups, Platelet Antigens, and Granulocyte Antigens) |
| *APOE* | apoE (apolipoprotein E) |
| *EPO* | erythropoietin (Epo) |
| *GRIFIN* | GRIFIN protein (galectin-related interfiber protein) |
| *HLA-A, HLA-B,* etc | HLA-A, HLA-B, etc (see 14.8.5, HLA/Major Histocompatibility Complex) |
| *MS* | multiple sclerosis (MS) |
| many hormone genes (eg, *CRH, GHRH, GNRHR, PTH, TRH*) | hormone name abbreviations (eg, CRH, GHRH, GNRH receptor, PTH, TRH) |

In other expressions, italics distinguish different meanings:

| | |
|---|---|
| *HD* | gene for huntingtin (protein), Huntington disease gene |
| HD | Huntington disease |
| person with HD | person with Huntington disease |
| *TH* variant | variant of the *TH* gene |
| TH deficiency | deficiency of the enzyme TH |

Therefore, it is best to make clear by italicizing gene symbols and through context whether the gene or another entity is being discussed.

Gene symbols do not immediately follow the term in the gene name that they might seem to abbreviate but rather should relate to the word *gene*, usually following it:

> the guanylate cyclase 2D gene, *GUCY2D* (*Not:* the guanylate cyclase 2D [*GUCY2D*] gene)

> the Huntington disease gene, *HD*

> the tyrosine hydroxylase gene, *TH*

> The cystic fibrosis transmembrane conductance regulator gene, *CFTR,* is implicated in cystic fibrosis.

In the following examples, both gene aliases and approved symbols are used; however, authors are encouraged to use the approved name (see 13.11, Clinical, Technical, and Other Common Terms):

> the retinal guanylate cyclase 2D (GUCY2D) gene, *GUCY2D*

> the retinal guanylate cyclase 2D (RetGC1) gene, *GUCY2D* (*Not:* the guanylate cyclase 2D [*GUCY2D*] gene)

In discussions of variants, the gene symbol remains italicized; specific variants, however, are *not* italicized (see 14.6.1, Nucleic Acids and Amino Acids):

> *ADRB2* 46G>A

> variant of the *GUCY2D* gene

> variant of *GUCY2D*

> *GUCY2D* variant

> The objective of this study was to describe the phenotype in 4 families with dominantly inherited cone-rod dystrophy, 1 with an R838C variant and 1 with an R838H variant in the guanylate cyclase 2D gene (*GUCY2D*) encoding retinal guanylate cyclase 1.

> *LRP5*$_{v171}$: valine substitution at codon 171 of the *LRP5* gene

In gene mapping, when the order of genes along the chromosome is known, the genes are listed from short-arm end (pter) to the centromere (cen) or long-arm end (qter) (see 14.6.4, Human Chromosomes).

> pter-*ENO1-PGM1-AMY1*-cen

In gene mapping, when the order of genes along the chromosome is not known, the genes are listed alphabetically and parentheses are used:

> pter-*PGD-AK2-(ACTA,APOA2,REN)*-qter

**Table 14.6-13** presents some examples of gene names and symbols from fields covered elsewhere in this chapter.

**Table 14.6-13.** Gene Names and Symbols From Fields Covered Elsewhere in This Chapter

| Approved gene symbol | Gene description |
| --- | --- |
| **14.1, Blood Groups, Platelet Antigens, and Granulocyte Antigens** | |
| *A4GALT* | α-1,4-galactosyltransferase (P blood group) |
| *ABO* | ABO blood group (transferase A, α-1-3-*N*-acetylgalactosaminyltransferase; transferase B, α-1-3-galactosyltransferase) |
| *ACHE* | acetylcholinesterase (Cartwright blood group) |
| *ACKR1* (was atypical *DARC*) | chemokine receptor 1 (Duffy blood group) |
| *AQP1* (was *CO*) | aquaporin 1 (Colton blood group) |
| *ART4* (was *DO*) | ADP-ribosyltransferase 4 (Dombrock blood group) |
| *BCAM* (was *LU*) | basic cell adhesion molecule (Lutheran blood group) |
| *BSG* | basigin (OK blood group) |
| *C4A* | complement 4A (Rodgers blood group) |
| *C4B* | complement 4B (Chido blood group) |
| *CD44* | CD44 molecule (Indian blood group) |
| *CD151* (was *MER2*) | CD151 molecule (Raph blood group) |
| *CR1* | complement C3b/C4b receptor 1 (Knops blood group) |
| *CD55* (was *DAF*) | CD55 molecule (Cromer blood group) |
| *ERMAP* (was *SC*) | erythroblast membrane-associated protein (Scianna blood group) |
| *FUT1* | fucosyltransferase 1 (H blood group) |
| *FUT3* | fucosyltransferase 3 (Lewis blood group) |
| *GYPA* | glycophorin A (MNS blood group) |
| *GYPB* | glycophorin B (MNS blood group) |
| *GYPC* | glycophorin C (Gerbich blood group) |
| *GYPE* | glycophorin E |
| *ICAM4* | intercellular adhesion molecule 4 (Landsteiner-Wiener blood group) |
| *KEL* | Kell blood group |
| *P1* | P blood group (P1 antigen) |
| *RHCE* | Rh blood group, CcEe antigens |
| *RHD* | Rh blood group, D antigen |
| *SLC4A1* | solute carrier family 4, member 1 (Diego blood group) |
| *SLC14A1* | solute carrier family 14, member 1 (Kidd blood group) |

**Table 14.6-13.** Gene Names and Symbols From Fields Covered Elsewhere in This Chapter (*continued*)

**14.1, Blood Groups, Platelet Antigens, and Granulocyte Antigens**

| | |
|---|---|
| *XG* | Xg blood group |
| *XK* | Kell blood group precursor (McLeod phenotype) |

**14.2, Cancer (See 14.6.3, Oncogenes and Tumor Suppressor Genes)**

| | |
|---|---|
| *ACTN1* | $\alpha_1$-actinin, actin alpha 1 |
| *ACTN2* | $\alpha_2$-actinin, actin alpha 2 |
| *BCL2* | B-cell/CLL lymphoma 2 |
| *BCL7A* | BCL tumor suppressor 7A |
| *CCND1* (formerly *BCL1*) | cyclin D1 |
| *CDC2* | cell division cycle 2, $G_1$ to S and $G_2$ to M |
| *CDK2* | cyclin-dependent kinase 2 |
| *CDKN1A* | cyclin-dependent kinase inhibitor 1A |
| *CTNNB1* | catenin beta 1 |
| *MEN1* | menin 1 |
| *RB1* | RB transcriptional copressor 1 |
| *RET* (formerly *MEN2A, MEN2B*) | ret proto-oncogene |
| *TGFA* | transforming growth factor alpha |
| *TGFB1* | transforming growth factor beta 1 |
| *TNF* | tumor necrosis factor receptor superfamily |
| *TNFRSF1A* | TNF receptor superfamily member 1A |
| *TP53* | tumor protein p53 |

**14.3, Cardiology**

| | |
|---|---|
| *ANK2* (formerly *LQT4*) | ankyrin 2 |
| *APOA1* | apolipoprotein AI |
| *APOB* | apolipoprotein B |
| *APOC2* | apolipoprotein C2 |
| *APOD* | apolipoprotein D |
| *APOE* | apolipoprotein E |
| *GPR1* | G protein–coupled receptor 1 |
| *HDLBP* | high-density lipoprotein-binding protein |
| *KCNH2* (formerly *LQT2*) | potassium voltage-gated channel, subfamily H, member 2 |
| *KCNQ1* (formerly *LQT*) | potassium voltage-gated channel subfamily Q member 1 |
| *LDLR* | low-density lipoprotein receptor |
| *LPL* | lipoprotein lipase |

(*continued*)

**Table 14.6-13.** Gene Names and Symbols From Fields Covered Elsewhere in This Chapter (*continued*)

**14.3, Cardiology**

| | |
|---|---|
| *NOS1* | nitric oxide synthase 1 |
| *NOS2* | nitric oxide synthase 2 |
| *NOS2P2* | nitric oxide synthase 2 pseudogene 2 |
| *NOS2P1* | nitric oxide synthase 2 pseudogene 1 |
| *NOS3* | nitric oxide synthase 3 |
| *PLAT* | plasminogen activator, tissue type |
| *SCN5A* (formerly *LQT3*) | sodium voltage-gated channel alpha subunit 5 |
| *TNNC1* | troponin C1, slow skeletal and cardiac type |
| *TNNC2* | troponin C2, fast skeletal type |
| *TNNI1* | troponin I1, slow skeletal type |
| *TNNI2* | troponin I2, fast skeletal type |
| *TNNI3* | troponin I3, cardiac type |
| *TNNT1* | troponin T1, slow skeletal type |
| *TNNT2* | troponin T2, cardiac type |
| *TNNT3* | troponin T3, fast skeletal type |
| *VLDLR* | very-low-density lipoprotein receptor |

**14.7, Hemostasis**

| | |
|---|---|
| *A2M* | $\alpha_2$-macroglobulin |
| *CALM1* | calmodulin 1 |
| *CCL5* | chemokine (C-C motif), ligand 5 |
| *CLEC3B* (was *TNA*) | C-type lectin domain family 3, member B |
| *F2* | coagulation factor II (thrombin) |
| *F2R* | coagulation factor II thrombin receptor |
| *F2RL1* | F2R-like trypsin receptor 1 |
| *F3* | coagulation factor III, tissue factor |
| *F5* | coagulation factor V |
| *F7* | coagulation factor VII |
| *F7R* | coagulation factor VII regulator |
| *F8* | coagulation factor VIII |
| *F8A1* | coagulation factor VIII associated 1 |
| *F9* | coagulation factor IX |
| *F10* | coagulation factor X |
| *F11* | coagulation factor XI |

**Table 14.6-13.** Gene Names and Symbols From Fields Covered Elsewhere in This Chapter (*continued*)

**14.7, Hemostasis**

| | |
|---|---|
| *F12* | coagulation factor XII |
| *F13A1* | coagulation factor XIII, A chain |
| *F13A2* | coagulation factor XIII, A2 polypeptide |
| *F13B* | coagulation factor XIII, B chain |
| *FGA* | fibrinogen, α chain |
| *FGB* | fibrinogen, β chain |
| *FGG* | fibrinogen, γ chain |
| *FGL1* | fibrinogenlike 1 |
| *FGL2* | fibrinogenlike 2 |
| *GP5* | glycoprotein V (platelet) |
| *GP6* | glycoprotein VI (platelet) |
| *GP9* | glycoprotein IX (platelet) |
| *GP1BA* | glycoprotein Ib, (platelet), alpha subunit |
| *ICAM1* | intercellular adhesion molecule 1 |
| *ICAM2* | intercellular adhesion molecule 2 |
| *ITGA1* | $α_1$-integrin integrin subunit alpha 1 |
| *ITGA2* | $α_2$-integrin integrin subunit alpha 2 |
| *ITGA2B* | integrin subunit alpha 2B |
| *ITGA3* | $α_3$-integrin integrin subunit alpha 3 |
| *ITGA6* | $α_6$-integrin integrin subunit alpha 6 |
| *ITGAV* | vitronectin, α polypeptide, antigen V |
| *ITGB1* | integrin subunit beta 1 |
| *ITGB3* | integrin subunit beta 3 |
| *ITPKA* | Inositol-triphosphate 3-kinase A |
| *KLKB1* | kallikrein B1 |
| *KNG1* | kininogen 1 |
| *NOS3* | nitric oxide synthase 3 |
| *PDGFA* | platelet-derived growth factor subunit A |
| *PDGFC* | platelet-derived growth factor C |
| *PDGFRA* | platelet-derived growth factor receptor alpha |
| *PDGFRL* | platelet-derived growth factor receptor-like |
| *PECAM1* | platelet and endothelial cell adhesion molecule 1 |

(*continued*)

**Table 14.6-13.** Gene Names and Symbols From Fields Covered Elsewhere in This Chapter (*continued*)

**14.7, Hemostasis**

| | |
|---|---|
| *PLAT* | plasminogen activator, tissue type |
| *PLAU* | plasminogen activator, urokinase |
| *PLAUR* | plasminogen activator, urokinase receptor |
| *PLG* | plasminogen |
| *PLGLA1* | plasminogenlike A |
| *PLGLB1* | plasminogenlike B1 |
| *PPBP* | proplatelet basic protein |
| *PROC* | protein C |
| *PROS1* | protein S |
| *PROSP* | protein S pseudogene |
| *PROZ* | protein Z, vitamin K–dependent plasma glycoprotein |
| *PTGDR* | prostaglandin $D_2$ receptor |
| *PTGDS* | prostaglandin $D_2$ synthase |
| *PTGFR* | prostaglandin F receptor |
| *PTGFRN* | prostaglandin $F_2$ receptor inhibitor |
| *PTGIR* | prostaglandin $I_2$ (prostacyclin) receptor |
| *PTGIS* | prostaglandin $I_2$ synthase |
| *PTGS1* | prostaglandin-endoperoxide synthase 1 |
| *SELE* | selectin E |
| *SELP* | selectin P |
| *SERPINA1* | serpin family A, member 1 |
| *SERPINC1* | serpin family C, member 1 |
| *SERPINE1* | serpin family E, member 1 |
| *SERPINF2* | serpin family F, member 2 |
| *TBXA2R* | thromboxane $A_2$ receptor |
| *TBXAS1* | thromboxane A synthase 1 |
| *TFPI* | transferrin pseudogene 1 |
| *TFPI2* | tissue factor pathway inhibitor 2 |
| *THBD* | thrombomodulin |
| *VCAM1* | vascular cell adhesion molecule 1 |
| *VWF* | von Willebrand factor |
| *VWFP* | von Willebrand factor pseudogene 1 |

**Table 14.6-13.** Gene Names and Symbols From Fields Covered Elsewhere in This Chapter (*continued*)

**14.8, Immunology**

**14.8.1, Chemokines**

| | |
|---|---|
| *CCL1* | C-C motif chemokine ligand 1 |
| *CX3CL1* | C-X3-C motif chemokine ligand 1 |
| *CXCL1* | C-X-C motif chemokine ligand 1 |
| *PF4* | platelet factor 4 |
| *XCL1* | X-C motif chemokine ligand 1 |

**14.8.2, CD Cell Markers**

| | |
|---|---|
| *CD14* | CD14 molecule |
| *CD19* | CD19 molecule |
| *CD1A* | CD1a molecule |
| *CD3D* | CD3D molecule |
| *CD46* | CD46 molecule |
| *CD55* | CD55 molecule (Cromer blood group) |
| *CD6* | CD6 molecule |
| *CD79A* | CD79A molecule |
| *CD97* | CD97 molecule |
| *CR1* | complement C3b/C4b receptor type 1 (Knops blood group) |
| *FCGR3A* | Fc fragment of IgG receptor IIIa |
| *ICAM3* | intracellular adhesion molecule 3 |
| *MME* | membrane metalloendopeptidase |

**14.8.3, Complement**

| | |
|---|---|
| *C1QA* | complement C1q A chain |
| *C1QB* | complement C1q B chain |
| *C1QBP* | complement C1q binding protein |
| *C1R* | complement C1r |
| *C1S* | complement C1s |
| *C2* | complement C2 |
| *C3* | complement C3 |
| *C4A* | complement C4a (Rodgers blood group) |
| *C4B* | complement C4b (Chido blood group) |
| *C4BPA* | complement component 4, binding protein alpha |
| *C5* | complement component C5 |

(*continued*)

**Table 14.6-13.** Gene Names and Symbols From Fields Covered Elsewhere in This Chapter (*continued*)

**14.8, Immunology**

| | |
|---|---|
| C5AR1 | complement C5a receptor 1 |
| C6 | complement C6 |
| C7 | complement C7 |
| C8A | complement C8, alpha chain |
| C8B | complement C8, beta chain |
| C9 | complement C9 |
| CD55 (was DAF) | CD55 molecule (Cromer blood group) |
| CFH | complement factor H |
| CFP | complement factor properdin |

**14.8.4, Cytokines**

| | |
|---|---|
| CRLF1 | cytokine receptorlike factor 1 |
| CRLF2 | cytokine receptorlike factor 2 |
| CSF1 | colony-stimulating factor 1 |
| CSF2 | colony-stimulating factor 2 |
| CSF3 | colony-stimulating factor 3 |
| CSF3R | colony-stimulating factor 3 receptor |
| EPO | erythropoietin |
| EPOR | erythropoietin receptor |
| GH1 | growth hormone 1 |
| GH2 | growth hormone 2 |
| GHR | growth hormone receptor |
| IFNA1 | interferon alpha 1 |
| IFNA2 | interferon alpha 2 |
| IFNB1 | interferon beta 1 |
| IFNG | interferon gamma |
| IFNW1 | interferon omega 1 |
| IL1A | interleukin 1 alpha |
| IL1B | interleukin 1 beta |
| IL1R1 | interleukin 1 receptor type 1 |
| IL1R2 | interleukin 1 receptor type 2 |
| IL1RAP | interleukin 1 receptor accessory protein |
| IL1RN | interleukin 1 receptor antagonist |
| IL2 | interleukin 2 |

**Table 14.6-13.** Gene Names and Symbols From Fields Covered Elsewhere in This Chapter (*continued*)

**14.8, Immunology**

| | |
|---|---|
| *LEP* | leptin |
| *LEPR* | leptin receptor |
| *PRL* | prolactin |
| *SOCS1* | suppressor of cytokine signaling 1 |
| *TGFA* | transforming growth factor alpha |
| *TGFB1* | transforming growth factor beta 1 |
| *THPO* | thrombopoietin |
| *TNF* | tumor necrosis factor |

**14.8.5, HLA/Major Histocompatibility Complex**

| | |
|---|---|
| *HLA-A* | HLA-A, major histocompatibility complex, class I, A |
| *HLA-B* | HLA-B, major histocompatibility complex, class I, B |
| *HLA-C* | HLA-C, major histocompatibility complex, class I, C |
| *HLA-DMA* | major histocompatibility complex, class II, DM alpha |
| *HLA-DMB* | major histocompatibility complex, class II, DM beta |
| *HLA-DOA* | major histocompatibility complex, class II, DO alpha |
| *HLA-DOB* | major histocompatibility complex, class II, DO beta |
| *HLA-DPA1* | major histocompatibility complex, class II, DP alpha |
| *HLA-DQA1* | major histocompatibility complex, class II, DQ alpha |
| *HLA-DQB1* | major histocompatibility complex, class II, DQ beta |
| *HLA-DRA* | major histocompatibility complex, class II, DR alpha |
| *HLA-DRB1* | major histocompatibility complex, class II, DR beta 1 |
| *HLA-E* | major histocompatibility complex, class I, E |
| *HLA-F* | major histocompatibility complex, class I, F |
| *HLA-G* | major histocompatibility complex, class I, G |
| *HLA-H* | major histocompatibility complex, class I, H |
| *HLA-J* | major histocompatibility complex, class I, J |

**14.8.6, Immunoglobulins**

| | |
|---|---|
| *IGHA1* | immunoglobulin heavy constant alpha 1 |
| *IGHA2* | immunoglobulin heavy constant alpha 2 |
| *IGHD* | immunoglobulin heavy constant delta |
| *IGHD1-1* | immunoglobulin heavy diversity 1-1 |
| *IGHE* | immunoglobulin heavy constant epsilon |
| *IGHG1* | immunoglobulin heavy constant gamma 1 |

(*continued*)

**Table 14.6-13.** Gene Names and Symbols From Fields Covered Elsewhere in This Chapter (*continued*)

**14.8, Immunology**

| | |
|---|---|
| *IGHG2* | immunoglobulin heavy constant gamma 2 |
| *IGHG3* | immunoglobulin heavy constant gamma 3 |
| *IGHG4* | immunoglobulin heavy constant gamma 4 |
| *IGHJ1* | immunoglobulin heavy joining 1 |
| *IGHM* | immunoglobulin heavy constant mu |
| *IGHV1-2* | immunoglobulin heavy variable 1-2 |
| *IGHV1-18* | immunoglobulin heavy variable 1-18 |
| *IGKC* | immunoglobulin kappa constant |
| *IGKJ2* | immunoglobulin kappa joining 2 |
| *IGKV1-5* | immunoglobulin kappa variable 1-5 |
| *IGLC1* | immunoglobulin lambda constant 1 |
| *IGLJ1* | immunoglobulin lambda joining 1 |
| *IGLV10-54* | immunoglobulin lambda variable 10-54 |

**14.8.7, Lymphocytes**

| | |
|---|---|
| *TRAC* | T-cell receptor alpha constant |
| *TRBC1* | T-cell receptor beta constant 1 |
| *TRBC2* | T-cell receptor beta constant 2 |
| *TRBV10-3* | T-cell receptor beta variable 10-3 |
| *TRGC1* | T- cell receptor gamma constant 1 |
| *TRGJ1* | T-cell receptor gamma joining 1 |
| *TRGJ2* | T-cell receptor gamma joining 2 |
| *TRDC* | T-cell receptor delta constant |

**14.10, Molecular Medicine**

| | |
|---|---|
| *APBA1* | amyloid-β precursor protein binding family A, member 1 |
| *ADIPOQ* | adiponectin, C1Q, and collagen domain containing |
| *ADIPOR1* | adiponectin receptor 1 |
| *ADIPOR2* | adiponectin receptor 2 |
| *ACSL1* | acyl-CoA synthetase long-chain family member 1 |
| *ADAMTS1* | ADAM metallopeptidase with thrombospondin type 1 motif 1 |
| *AHCY* | adenosylhomocysteine |
| *AMD1* | adenosylmethionine decarboxylase 1 |
| *AKT1* | AKT serine/threonine kinase 1 |
| *ATP1A1* | ATPase, Na+/K+ transporting subunit, alpha 1 polypeptide |

**Table 14.6-13.** Gene Names and Symbols From Fields Covered Elsewhere in This Chapter (*continued*)

**14.10, Molecular Medicine**

| | |
|---|---|
| *BPGM* | bisphosphoglycerate mutase |
| *CALM1* | calmodulin 1 |
| *CCAR1* | cell division cycle and apoptosis regulator 1 |
| *CCPG1* | cell cycle progression 1 |
| *CDK20* | cyclin dependent kinase |
| *CDC2* | cyclin dependent kinase 2 |
| *CDK2* | cyclin-dependent kinase 2 |
| *CDK7* | cyclin-dependent kinase 7 |
| *CDKN1A* | cyclin-dependent kinase inhibitor 1A |
| *CDKN1C* | cyclin-dependent kinase inhibitor 1C |
| *CDKN2A* | cyclin-dependent kinase inhibitor 2A |
| *COASY* | coenzyme A (CoA) synthetase |
| *COX4I1* | cytochrome c oxidase subunit 4I1 |
| *COX5B* | cytochrome c oxidase subunit 5b |
| *CRP* | C-reactive protein |
| *CYP1A2* | cytochrome P450 family 1, subfamily A, member 2 |
| *DHFR* | dihydrofolate reductase |
| *DKK1* | dickkopf WNT signaling pathway, inhibitor 1 |
| *ERBB2* | erb-b2 receptor tyrosine kinase 2 |
| *FBP1* | fructose bisphosphatase 1 |
| *FDX1* | ferredoxin 1 |
| *FDX2* | ferredoxin 2 |
| *FHIT* | fragile histidine triad |
| *GNA12* | G protein subunit alpha 12 |
| *GNG2* | G protein subunit gamma 2 |
| *GALNT1* | polypeptide *N*-acetylgalactosaminyltransferase 1 |
| *G6PD* | glucose-6-phosphate dehydrogenase |
| *B3GALT1* | beta-1,3-galactosyltransferase |
| *CDKN2A* | cyclin-dependent kinase inhibitor 2A |
| *GFI1* | growth factor independent 1 transcriptional repressor |
| *GRB2* | growth factor receptor-bound protein 2 |
| *GRIN1* | glutamate ionotropic receptor, *N*-methyl-ᴅ-aspartate (NMDA) type, subunit 1 |

(*continued*)

**Table 14.6-13.** Gene Names and Symbols From Fields Covered Elsewhere in This Chapter (*continued*)

**14.10, Molecular Medicine**

| | |
|---|---|
| *HBA1* | hemoglobin type, subunit alpha 1 |
| *HBB* | hemoglobin subunit beta |
| *HMGCS1* | 3-hydroxy-3-methylglutaryl CoA synthase 1 |
| *IGF1* | insulinlike growth factor 1 |
| *IGF1R* | insulinlike growth factor 1 receptor (IGF-R1) |
| *IKBKB* | inhibitor of nuclear factor kappa B kinase, subunit beta |
| *ITPKA* | inositol-triphosphate 3-kinase A |
| *MNAT1* | CDK activating kinase assembly factor |
| *MB* | myoglobin |
| *MCM2* | minichromosome maintenance complex, component 2 |
| *NMNAT1* | nicotinamide nucleotide adenyltransferase 1 |
| *NPY* | neuropeptide Y |
| *NPPA* | natriuretic peptide |
| *OGDH* | oxoglutarate dehydrogenase |
| *INPP5J* | inositol polyphosphate-5-phosphatase J |
| *PYY* | peptide YY |
| *RBBP4* | RB binding protein 4 |
| *RNASE1* | ribonuclease A family member 1 pancreatic |
| *SFPQ* | splicing factor proline and glutamine rich |
| *SNCA* | synuclein alpha |
| *TAF1* | TATA-box binding protein associated factor 1 |
| *TBP* | TATA-box binding protein |
| *THPO* | thrombopoietin |
| *TNFSF11* | TNF superfamily member 11 |
| *TP53* | tumor protein p53 |
| *UCP1* | uncoupling protein 1 |
| *WNT1* | Wnt family member 1 |

**14.11, Neurology**

| | |
|---|---|
| *ASIC2* | acid sensing ion channel subunit 2 |
| *ACHE* | acetylcholinesterase (Cartwright blood group) |
| *ADORA1* | adenosine A1 receptor |
| *ADRA1A* | adrenoreceptor alpha 1A |
| *ADRB1* | adrenoreceptor beta 1 |
| *BDNF* | brain-derived neurotrophic factor |

**Table 14.6-13.** Gene Names and Symbols From Fields Covered Elsewhere in This Chapter (*continued*)

**14.11, Neurology**

| | |
|---|---|
| *CACNA1A* | calcium voltage-gated channel subunit alpha 1A |
| *CHRM1* | cholinergic receptor, muscarinic 1 |
| *CHRNA1* | cholinergic receptor, nicotinic, alpha 1 subunit |
| *CNTF* | ciliary neurotrophic factor |
| *COMT* | catechol-O-methyltransferase |
| *DRD1* | dopamine receptor D1 |
| *EGF* | epidermal growth factor |
| *GABBR1* | gamma-aminobutyric acid type B receptor subunit 1 |
| *GDNF* | glial cell line–derived neurotrophic factor |
| *GRIA1* | glutamate inotropic receptor AMPA type, subunit 1 |
| *GRIN1* | glutamate ionotropic receptor, NMDA type, subunit 1 |
| *HRH1* | histamine receptor H1 |
| *HTR1A* | 5-hydroxytryptamine receptor 1A |
| *ITPKA* | inositol triphosphate 3-kinase A |
| *KCNJ3* | potassium voltage-gated channel, subfamily J, member 3 |
| *MAOA* | monoamine oxidase A |
| *NGF* | nerve growth factor |
| *NGFR* | nerve growth factor receptor |
| *NMB* | neuromedin B |
| *NOS1* | nitric oxide synthase 1 |
| *NPY* | neuropeptide Y |
| *NPY1R* | neuropeptide Y receptor Y1 |
| *NRTN* | neurturin |
| *NTF3* | neurotrophin 3 |
| *NTS* | neurotensin |
| *NTSR1* | neurotensin receptor 1 |
| *OPRD1* | opioid receptor delta 1 |
| *OPRK1* | opioid receptor kappa 1 |
| *OPRM1* | opioid receptor mu 1 |
| *SIGMAR1* | sigma nonopioid intracellular receptor 1 |
| *PCP2* | Purkinje cell protein 2 |
| *SLC1A1* | solute carrier family 1, member 1 |
| *SLC18A1* | solute carrier family 18, member A1 |

(*continued*)

**Table 14.6-13.** Gene Names and Symbols From Fields Covered Elsewhere in This Chapter (*continued*)

| 14.11, Neurology | |
| --- | --- |
| *SNAP25* | synaptosomal-associated protein, 25 kDa |
| *SNCA* | synuclein alpha |
| *TAC1* | tachykinin, precursor 1 |
| *TAC3* | tachykinin 3 |
| *TRPA1* | transient receptor potential cation channel, subfamily A, member 1 |
| *TSNARE1* | t-SNARE domain containing 1 (see 14.11, Neurology, for expansion) |
| *VAMP1* | vesicle-associated membrane protein 1 |
| **14.14.3 and 14.14.4, Virus and Prion Nomenclature** | |
| *AAVS1* | adeno-associated virus integration site 1 |
| *BNIP1* | BLC2 interacting protein 1 |
| *CR2* | complement component C3d receptor 2 |
| *CXADR* | CXADR, Ig-like cell adhesion molecule |
| *CXB3S* | coxsackie virus B3 sensitivity |
| *E11S* | ECHO virus (serotypes 4, 6, 11, 19) sensitivity |
| *GPR183* | G protein–coupled receptor 183 |
| *EBVM1* | Epstein-Barr virus modification site 1 |
| *EBVS1* | Epstein-Barr virus integration site 1 |
| *HAVCR1* | hepatitis A virus cellular receptor 1 |
| *RSF1* | remodeling and spacing factor 1 |
| *LAMTOR5* | late endosomal/lysosomal adaptor, MAPK and MTOR activator 5 |
| *HCVS* | human coronavirus sensitivity |
| *CCNT1* | cyclin T1 |
| *HPV6AI1* | human papillomavirus (type 6a) integration site 1 |
| *FOXN2* | forkhead box N2 |
| *HV1S* | herpes simplex virus type 1 sensitivity |
| *ICAM1* | intercellular adhesion molecule 1 |
| *MX1* | MX dynam-like GTPase 1 |
| *PVR* | poliovirus receptor |
| *PRND* | prion-like protein doppel |
| *PRNP* | prion protein |
| *PRNPIP* | prion protein interacting protein |
| *PRNT* | prion locus lncRNA, testis expressed |

**14.6.2.5** **Alleles.** Alleles denote alternative forms of a gene. Alleles are often characterized by particular variant sequences (mutations). For variant sequence nomenclature see 14.6.1, Sequence Variations, Nucleotides.

Because alleles are alternative forms of a particular gene, they are expressed by means of both the gene name or symbol and an appendage that indicates the specific allele.

Classically, allele symbols consist of the gene symbol plus an asterisk plus the italicized allele designation.[7] For example:

*HBB\*S*     *S* allele of the *HBB* gene

As with gene terms, Greek letters are changed to Latin letters in allele terms:

*APOE\*E4*     allele producing the ε4 type of apolipoprotein E

See HGNC guidelines for Greek to Latin alphabet conversion.[16] If clear in context, the allele symbol may be used in a shorthand form that omits the gene symbol and includes only the asterisk and the allele designation that follows. For example:

*\*S*

*\*E4*

In the case of alleles of the major histocompatibility locus, which are not italicized (see 14.8.5, HLA/Major Histocompatibility Complex), each HLA allele name has a unique number corresponding to up to 4 sets of digits separated by colons.[17] The digits before the first colon describe the type (this often corresponds to the serologic antigen carried by an allotype). The next set of digits list the subtype (numbers are assigned in the order in which DNA sequences have been determined). A portion of the gene name is usually included in the shortened form:

Full name: HLA-DRB1:03:01

Shortened form: DRB1:03:01

In practice, common or trivial names for alleles, which take various forms, are used. The same allele is often expressed in different ways that diverge from the recommended nomenclature. For example:

*s:* short allele of serotonin transporter gene (*SLC6A4*)

*l:* long allele of *SLC6A4*

As another example of common allele names, the following expressions are all used for *APOE\*E4;* follow author preference:

ε4 allele

epsilon 4 allele

E4 allele

*APOE\*4*

apo e4

*APOEE4*

**14.6.2.5.1** Genotype and Phenotype Terminology. The genotype comprises the set of alleles in an individual. Because individuals almost always have 2 of each autosome (nonsex chromosome) (see 14.6.4, Human Chromosomes), individuals have 2 alleles (which may be the same alleles or 2 different alleles) for each autosomal gene.

The simplest genotype term for an individual would describe 1 gene and consist of the names of 2 alleles. Larger genotypes would contain 2 or more allele symbol pairs.

As originally formulated in ISGN, allele groupings may be indicated by placement above and below a horizontal line or on the line. As seen in the following examples (from Shows et al[2,3]), such placement, as well as order, spacing, and punctuation marks (virgules [/], semicolons, spaces, and commas), has specific meanings.

Alleles of the same gene are indicated by placement above and below a horizontal line or with a virgule:

$$\frac{ADA^*1}{ADA^*2} \quad or \quad ADA^*1/ADA^*2$$

In theoretical discussions when a single letter is substituted for the allele symbol, the line or virgule may be dispensed with:

*AA*

*Aa*

*aa*

*ss*

*ll*

*sl*

Semicolons separate pairs of alleles at unlinked loci:

$$\frac{ADA^*1}{ADA^*2}; \quad \frac{ADH1^*1}{ADH1^*1}; \quad \frac{AMY1^*A}{AMY1^*B}$$

*or*

ADA*1/ADA*2; ADH1*1/ADH1*1; AMY1*A/AMY1*B

*or*

ADA*1/*2; ADH*1/*1; AMY1*A/*B

A single space separates alleles together on the same chromosome from alleles together on another chromosome (phase [assignment of alleles of genes on the same or different chromosomal copy] known):

$$\frac{AMY1^*A \ PGM1^*2}{AMY1^*B \ PGM1^*1}$$

*or*

AMY1*A PGM1*2/AMY1*B PGM1*1

*Commas* indicate that alleles above and below the line (or on either side of the virgule) are on the same chromosome pair but not on which chromosome of the pair specifically (phase unknown):

$$\frac{PGM1{*}1}{PGM1{*}2}, \quad \frac{AMY1{*}A}{AMY1{*}B}$$

*or*

*PGM1\*1/PGM1\*2, AMY1\*A/AMY1\*B*

A special form for hemizygous males is

*G6PD\*A/Y*

When genotype is being expressed in terms of nucleotides (eg, a polymorphism), italics and other punctuation are not needed (see 14.6.1, Nucleic Acids and Amino Acids):

*MTHFR* 677 TT genotype

CC genotype

the "long/short" (5HTTLPR) polymorphism in *SLC6A4*

(LPR: length polymorphism region)

When the subject is being described in terms of the 2 possible amino acids at 1 position in the protein owing to a single-nucleotide variation (formerly single-nucleotide polymorphism) (nonsynonymous mutation), the corresponding amino acids are separated by a virgule (see 14.6.1, Nucleic Acids and Amino Acids):

Val/Val      (homozygous)

Met/Val      (heterozygous)

Met/Met      (homozygous)

Such terms should be explained at first mention with the amino acid terms expanded:

the common methionine/valine (Met/Val) polymorphism at codon 129

The virgule is not needed in expressions such as the following:

$\alpha_1$-antitrypsin MZ heterozygotes

individuals with the ZZ phenotype

The phenotype is the collection of traits in an individual that result from his or her genotype. Genotypes usually contain pairs of symbols, whereas phenotypes contain single symbols. When phenotypes are expressed in terms of the specific alleles, the phenotype term derives from the genotype term, but no italics are used, and, instead of asterisks, spaces are used.[18]

Genotype: *ADA\*1/ADA\*1*

Phenotype: ADA 1

Genotype: *ADA\*1/ADA\*2*

Phenotype: ADA 1, 2

Genotype: *C2\*C/C2\*QO*

Phenotype: C2 C, QO

The normal allele of a gene is identified by adding \*N. Adding \*D or \*R to a gene symbol designates a dominant or recessive allele, respectively.

Genotype: *CFTR\*N/CFTR\*R*

Phenotype: CFTR N

**Principal Author:** Cheryl Iverson, MA

## ACKNOWLEDGMENT

Thanks to the following for reviewing and providing comments: W. Gregory Feero, MD, PhD, *JAMA*, and Maine-Dartmouth Family Medicine Residency, Augusta; Trevor Lane, MA, DPhil, Edanz Group, Fukuoka, Japan; and John J. McFadden, MA, JAMA Network.

## REFERENCES

1. Klinger HP. Progress in nomenclature and symbols for cytogenetics and somatic-cell genetics. *Ann Intern Med.* 1979;91(3):487-488. doi:10.7326/0003-4819-91-3-487

2. Shows TB, Alper CA, Bootsma D, et al. International system for human gene nomenclature (1979). *Cytogenet Cell Genet.* 1979;25(1-4):96-116. doi:10.1159/000131404

3. Shows TB, McAlpine PJ, Boucheix C, et al. Guidelines for human gene nomenclature: an international system for human gene nomenclature (ISGN, HGM9). *Cytogenet Cell Genet.* 1987;46(1-4):11-28. doi:10.1159/000132471

4. Rangel P, Giovannetti J. *Genomes and Databases on the Internet: A Practical Guide to Functions and Applications.* Horizon Scientific Press; 2002.

5. HUGO Gene Nomenclature Committee. Accessed July 31, 2019. https://www.genenames.org/

6. Gray KA, Yates B, Seal RL, Wright MW, Bruford EA. Genenames.org: the HGNC resources in 2015. *Nucleic Acids Res.* 2015;43(database issue):D1079-D1085. doi:10.1093/nar/gku1071

7. Wain HM, Bruford EA, Lovering RC, Lush MJ, Wright MW, Povey S. Guidelines for human gene nomenclature (2002). *Genomics.* 2002;79(4):464-470. doi:10.1006/geno.2002.6748

8. Entrez Gene. Accessed January 9, 2018. https://www.ncbi.nlm.nih.gov/gene

9. Locus Reference Genomic (LRG). Accessed July 23, 2019. https://www.lrg-sequence.org

10. Hamosh A, Scott AF, Amberger JS, Bocchini CA, McKusick VA. Online Mendelian Inheritance in Man (OMIM), a knowledge base of human genes and genetic disorders. *Nucl Acids Res.* 2005;33(database issue):D514-D517. doi:10.1093/nar/gki033

11. Online Mendelian Inheritance in Man (OMIM). Updated July 22, 2019. Accessed July 23, 2019. https://omim.org

12. OMIM Frequently Asked Questions. Accessed July 23, 2019. https://omim.org/help/faq

13. HGNC. FAQs about gene nomenclatures. Accessed January 9, 2018. https://www.genenames.org/help/faq/

14. GenBank. Updated November 2017. Accessed July 23, 2019. https://www.ncbi.nlm.nih.gov/genbank/

15. Glossary of genetic terms. Accessed July 31, 2019. https://sites.jamanetwork.com/genetics/#glossary

16. HGNC guidelines. Table 1: Greek to Latin alphabet conversion. Accessed July 23, 2019. https://www.genenames.org/about/guidelines

17. Nomenclature for factors of the HLA system. Updated June 7, 2018. Accessed July 23, 2019. https://www.hla.alleles.org/nomenclature/naming.html

18. Pasternak JJ. *An Introduction to Human Molecular Genetics: Mechanisms of Inherited Disease*. 2nd ed. Published January 27, 2005. Accessed June 13, 2018. http://www.wiley.com/WileyCDA/WileyTitle/product_Cd0471474266.html

**14.6.3** ▎ **Oncogenes and Tumor Suppressor Genes.** Oncogenes and tumor suppressor genes are 2 of the main types of genes that play a central role in cancer. "An important difference between oncogenes and tumor suppressor genes is that oncogenes result from the *activation* (turning on) of proto-oncogenes, but tumor suppressor genes cause cancer when they are *inactivated* (turned off)."[1]

**14.6.3.1** ▎ **Oncogenes.** An oncogene is a "mutated gene that contributes to the development of a cancer. In their normal, unmutated state, oncogenes are called proto-oncogenes, and they play a role in the regulation of cell division."[2] Oncogenes were discovered and characterized in viruses and animal experimental systems. These genes exist widely outside the systems in which they were discovered, and their normal cellular homologues are important in cell division and differentiation.

Human oncogenes should be expressed according to the style for human gene symbols (see 14.6.2, Human Gene Nomenclature). Mouse oncogenes (and other nonhuman oncogenes) should be expressed according to style for mouse gene symbols (see 14.6.5, Nonhuman Genetic Terms). Retroviral oncogenes are expressed in a style typical of microbial genes (see 14.6.5, Nonhuman Genetic Terms), namely, 3 letters, italicized, lowercase. The protein products of the oncogenes (oncoproteins) typically use the same abbreviation as the oncogene but in roman type. In humans, the protein is all capitals; in mice, the protein has an initial capital. Some examples of human, mouse, and retroviral oncogenes appear in **Table 14.6-14**.

Examples of use are as follows:

> ras activation and inactivation

> protein derived from the *ras* gene, ras, functions as a signaling molecule

Commonly, the oncogene term contains a prefix that indicates the source or location of the gene: v- for virus or c- for the oncogene's cellular or chromosomal counterpart. The c- form is also known as a proto-oncogene and in standard gene nomenclature (see 14.6.2, Human Gene Nomenclature) is given in all capitals, as in the Human Gene Homologues column of Table 14.6-14 and the following examples. Note that the v and the c are set roman.

**Table 14.6-14.** Human, Mouse, and Retroviral Oncogenes

| Retroviral oncogenes | Human gene homologue(s); mouse gene homologue(s) | Human protein product(s); mouse protein product(s); retroviral oncoprotein | Viral origin |
|---|---|---|---|
| *abl* | Human: *ABL1, ABL2*<br>Mouse: *Abl1, Abl2* | Human: ABL1, ABL2<br>Mouse: Abl1, Abl2<br>Retroviral: abl | Abelson murine leukemia |
| *bcl-2* | Human: *BCL2*<br>Mouse: *Bcl2* | Human: BCL2<br>Mouse: Bcl2<br>Retroviral: bcl | B-cell CLL/lymphoma 2 |
| *erb*[a] | Human: *ERBB2, ERBB3, ERBB4*<br>Mouse: *Erbb2, Erbb3, Erbb4* | Human: ERBB2, ERBB3, ERBB4<br>Mouse: Erbb2, Erbb3, Erbb4<br>Retroviral: erb | avian erythroblastic leukemia |
| *ets* | Human: *ETS1, ETS2*<br>Mouse: *Ets1, Ets2* | Human: ETS1, ETS2<br>Mouse: Ets1, Ets2<br>Retroviral: ets | avian erythroblastosis |
| *fes* | Human: *FES*<br>Mouse: *Fes* | Human: FES<br>Mouse: Fes<br>Retroviral: fes | Gardner-Arnstein feline sarcoma |
| *fms* | Human: *CSF1R* (formerly *FMS*)<br>Mouse: *Csf1r* (formerly *Fms*) | colony stimulating factor 1 receptor (CSF1R) | McDonough feline sarcoma |
| *fos* | Human: *FOS, FOSB*<br>Mouse: *Fos, Fosb* | Human: FOS, FOSB<br>Mouse: Fos, Fosb<br>Retroviral: fos | FBJ murine osteogenic sarcoma |
| *jun* | Human: *JUN, JUNB, JUND*<br>Mouse: *Jun, Junb, Jund* | Human: JUN, JUNB, JUND<br>Mouse: Jun, Junb, Jund<br>Retroviral: jun | avian sarcoma 17 |
| *kit* | Human: *KIT*<br>Mouse: *Kit* | Human: KIT<br>Mouse: Kit<br>Retroviral: kit | Hardy-Zuckerman feline sarcoma |
| *mos* | Human: *MOS*<br>Mouse: *Mos* | Human: MOS<br>Mouse: Mos<br>Retroviral: mos | Moloney sarcoma |
| *myb* | Human: *MYB*<br>Mouse: *Myb* | Human: MYB<br>Mouse: Myb<br>Retroviral: myb | avian myeloblastosis |
| *myc* | Human: *MYC*<br>Mouse: *Myc* | Human: MYC<br>Mouse: Myc<br>Retroviral: myc | avian myelocytomatosis |

**Table 14.6-14.** Human, Mouse, and Retroviral Oncogenes (*continued*)

| Retroviral oncogenes | Human gene homologue(s); mouse gene homologue(s) | Human protein product(s); mouse protein product(s); retroviral oncoprotein | Viral origin |
|---|---|---|---|
| *raf* | Human: *RAF1, ARAF, BRAF* <br> Mouse: *Raf1, Araf, Braf* | Human: RAF1, ARAF1, BRAF <br> Mouse: Raf1, Araf, Braf <br> Retroviral: raf | 3611 murine leukemia |
| *ras* | Human: family with many human homologues, eg, *HRAS, NRAS, RAB9A, RRAS, RRAS2* <br> Mouse: *Hras1, Nras, Rab9, Rras, Rras2* | Human: HRAS1, NRAS, RAB9A, RRAS, RRAS2 <br> Mouse: Rab9a, Rras, Rras2, Hras, Nras, Rab9 <br> Retroviral: ras | retrovirus-associated DNA sequence |
| *sis* | Human: *PDGFB* <br> Mouse: *Pdgfb* | Human: PDGFB (platelet-derived growth factor, B chain) <br> Mouse: Pdgfb <br> Retroviral: sis | simian sarcoma |
| *src* | Human: *SRC* <br> Mouse: *Src* | Human: SRC <br> Mouse: Src <br> Retroviral: src | Rous sarcoma |

[a]See 14.6.3.1.1, *ERBB2* and *HER2/neu*.

| | |
|---|---|
| c-*abl* (*ABL1*) | c-*mos* (*MOS*) |
| v-*abl* | v-*mos* |

The protein product may be similarly prefixed:

| | |
|---|---|
| c-abl | c-mos |
| v-abl | v-mos |

Additional prefixes may further identify oncogenes. Note that these prefixes are set roman and are hyphenated. Examples of expansions of some prefixes are given below, but it should not be inferred that the gene in question is associated only with the tumor for which it is named:

| | |
|---|---|
| B-*lym* | B-cell lymphoma |
| L-*myc* | small cell lung carcinoma |
| N-*myc* | neuroblastoma |
| H-*ras* | Harvey rat sarcoma |
| K-*ras* | Kirsten rat sarcoma |
| N-*ras* | neuroblastoma |

For example:

> The K-*ras* variant assay is more sensitive than the conventional histologic diagnosis in detecting minute cancer invasion around the superior mesenteric artery.

Numbers or letters designate genes in a series. For example:

> K-*ras*-2
>
> H-*ras*-1
>
> *erb*-b2

**14.6.3.1.1** *ERBB2* **and** *HER2/neu.* The oncogene known as *HER2/neu,* which stimulates the growth of breast cancer, is actually *ERBB2. HER2* (from human epidermal growth factor receptor 2) and *neu* are the same as *ERBB2* and are current aliases for *ERBB2.*[3] Because the term *HER2/neu* is widely used and recognized, it may be included in parentheses after the first mention of *ERBB2.*

> *ERBB2* (formerly *HER2* or *HER2/neu*)

**14.6.3.1.2** **Fusion Oncogenes and Oncoproteins.** The result of fusion of an oncogene and another gene is known as a *fusion oncogene.* The product of a fusion oncogene is a fusion oncoprotein. Terms for fusion oncogenes and their products may use traditional oncogene format or standard human gene format, as in the examples in **Table 14.6-15.**

Example of use in text:

> The BCR-ABL fusion oncoprotein is the key driver of pathogenesis in most cases of chronic myelogenous leukemia.

**14.6.3.2** **Tumor Suppressor Genes.** Tumor suppressor genes are "normal genes that slow down cell division, repair DNA mistakes, or tell cells when to die. . . .When tumor suppressor genes don't work properly, cells can grow out of control, which can lead to cancer."[1] Examples are given in **Table 14.6-16.**

**Table 14.6-15.** Examples of Terms for Fusion Oncogenes and Their Products

| Fusion oncogene | Fusion oncoprotein | Expansion[4] |
|---|---|---|
| *bcr-abl* | BCR-ABL | fusion of the *BCR* and *ABL* genes |
| *c-fos/c-jun* | C-FOS/C-JUN | protein product of FOS and JUN proto-oncogenes |
| *gag-onc* | GAG-ONC | general term for fusion proteins of viral *gag* (group-specific antigen) gene and oncogene |
| *gag-jun* | GAG-JUN | general term for fusion proteins of viral *gag* (group-specific antigen) gene and oncogene, with JUN representing a specific oncogene |
| *PML-RARA* | PML-RARα | promyelocytic leukemia–retinoic acid receptor α |

**Table 14.6-16.** Examples of Tumor Suppressor Genes and Their Products

| Gene | Gene product (alias[a]) | Expansion |
|---|---|---|
| CDKN1A | CDKN1A (p21[a]) | cyclin-dependent kinase (CDK) inhibitor 1A |
| CDKN1B | CDKN1B (p27[a]) | CDK inhibitor 1B |
| CDKN1C | CDKN1C (p57[a]) | CDK inhibitor 1C |
| DCC | DCC, a transmembrane receptor protein | deleted in colorectal carcinoma |
| GLTSCR1 | | glioma tumor suppressor candidate region gene 1 |
| NF1 | neurofibromin 1 | |
| RB1 | Rb protein | retinoblastoma 1 |
| TP53 | TP53 (p53[a]) | a 53-kd protein |
| WT1 | a zinc finger protein | Wilms tumor 1 (also called Wilms tumor protein) |

[a]Although these gene symbol aliases or nicknames may still be used by some, use of the approved gene symbol, not the alias, is strongly preferred. Such use will minimize confusion and make it possible to provide links to genome databases for online versions of the article and to facilitate data retrieval in a number of databases. If an author insists on using an alias, provide the alias parenthetically after the approved gene symbol at first mention in text and abstract. This practice will link the two and provide a learning experience for those not yet familiar with the approved gene symbol.

**Principal Author:** Cheryl Iverson, MA

### ACKNOWLEDGMENT

Thanks to the following for reviewing and providing comments: W. Gregory Feero, MD, PhD, *JAMA*, and Maine-Dartmouth Family Medicine Residency, Augusta, Maine; Trevor Lane, MA, DPhil, Edanz Group, Fukuoka, Japan; and John J. McFadden, MA, JAMA Network.

### REFERENCES

1. American Cancer Society. Oncogenes and tumor suppressor genes. Last revised June 25, 2014. Accessed July 31, 2019. https://www.cancer.org/cancer/cancercauses/geneticsandcancer/genesandcancer/genes-and-cancer-oncogenes-tumor-suppressor-genes.html
2. National Human Research Gene Institute Talking Glossary of Genetic Terms. Accessed June 6, 2018. https://genome.gov/glossary
3. V-ERB-B2 avian erythroblastic leukemia viral oncogene homolog 2; ERBB2. OMIM. Updated September 27, 2016. Accessed July 31, 2019. https://omim.org/entry/164870
4. NCI Dictionary of Cancer Terms. Accessed June 6, 2018. https://www.cancer.gov/publications/dictionaries/cancer-terms?cdrid=561237

**14.6.4**    **Human Chromosomes.** Chromosomes are structures in the cell nucleus that contain short and long arms, joined at the centromere. They are composed of chromatin (chromatin is made up of DNA, RNA, and proteins) that carries genetic information (definition after Nussbaum et al[1] and Turnpenny and Ellard[2]). Structural variation of chromosomes has traditionally been studied from the perspective of direct visualization of bands, using staining techniques. However, sophisticated fluorescent technologies, such as FISH (fluorescence in situ hybridization),[3] are now widely in use to probe for structural variations (eg, deletions, duplications, and large-scale copy number variants, as well as insertions, inversions, and translocations)[4] (see 14.6.4.4, In Situ Hybridization), leading to important gains in medical diagnosis and research, as well as gene ordering and mapping. Microarray technologies are increasingly being used to detect microdeletions, inversions, deletions, and so on. Sequencing technologies are making gains as well in being able to detect structural variation. Regardless of the development of these technologies, the essential purpose of cytogenetics remains the same: to study genomic organization and the structure, function, and evolution of chromosomes.

Translocations involve a segment of one chromosome being transferred to a nonhomologous chromosome or to a new site on the same chromosome. They are often associated with negative consequences, such as cancer.[5]

Structural variation in cancer is different from that seen in germline variation and is clearly related to pathogenesis in some cancers (eg, Philadelphia chromosome; see 14.6.4.5, Marker Chromosomes, Derivative Chromosomes, and the Philadelphia Chromosome).

Formalized standard nomenclature for human chromosomes dates from 1960 and, since 1978, has been known as the International System for Human Cytogenetic Nomenclature (ISCN).

Material in this section is based on recommendations in *ISCN 2016*.[6]

Human chromosomes are numbered from largest to smallest from 1 to 22. There are 2 additional chromosomes, X and Y. The numbered chromosomes are known as autosomes, and X and Y as the sex chromosomes. Chromosomes can also be grouped based on similar size and centromere position, as follows[6(p8)]:

| | |
|---|---|
| Group A | chromosomes 1-3 |
| Group B | chromosomes 4, 5 |
| Group C | chromosomes 6-12, X |
| Group D | chromosomes 13-15 |
| Group E | chromosomes 16-18 |
| Group F | chromosomes 19, 20 |
| Group G | chromosomes 21, 22, Y |

A chromosome may be referred to by number or by group:

chromosome 14

a group D chromosome

**14.6.4.1** **Chromosome Bands.** Chromosome bands are elicited by multiple staining methods; a band is "a part of a chromosome clearly distinguishable from adjacent parts by virtue of its lighter or darker staining intensity."[6(p9-10)] Banding pattern terms in the left-hand column of the following list need not be expanded. Their technique or purpose is shown to the right of the banding pattern.

| | |
|---|---|
| Q-banding, Q-bands | quinacrine |
| G-banding, G-bands | Giemsa |
| R-banding, R-bands | reverse Giemsa |
| C-banding, C-bands | constitutive heterochromatin |
| T-banding, T-bands | telomeric |
| NORs | nucleolus organizing regions |

Banding technique codes of several letters provide more information about the banding method. These abbreviations must be expanded, but the letters in the list above (Q, G, R, C, T, NOR) within those terms need not be expanded:

| | |
|---|---|
| QF | Q bands by fluorescence |
| QFQ | Q bands by fluorescence using quinacrine |
| CBG | C bands by barium hydroxide using Giemsa stain |
| Ag-NOR | NOR staining, silver nitrate technique |

**Figure 14.6-5** shows a chromosome illustrating bands and subbands at different levels of resolution.

The short arm is designated by p, for *petit,* and the long arm by the next letter of the alphabet, q.[6(p11)] Arm designations follow the chromosome number:

| | |
|---|---|
| 17p | short arm of chromosome 17 |
| 3q | long arm of chromosome 3 |
| Xq | long arm of the X chromosome |

Expressions such as those on the left need not be expanded. It is incorrect to refer to chromosome arms as chromosomes:

| | |
|---|---|
| *Acceptable:* | chromosome arm 17p |
| | short arm of 17 |
| | 17p |
| *Not Acceptable:* | chromosome 17p |

Regions are determined by major chromosome band landmarks. Chromosome arms contain 1 to 4 regions, numbered outward from the centromere. The region number follows the p or the q:

| | |
|---|---|
| 4q3 | region 3 of long arm of chromosome 4 |

The regions are divided into bands, also numbered outward from the centromere. Bands have subdivisions or subbands (these are seen only when the chromosomes are extended). The band number follows the region number, and the subband number follows a period after the band number. When a subband is further subdivided, the sub-subband number follows the subband number without

**Figure 14.6-5**  Frequently Altered Chromosome Territories With Significant Associations to Other Territories in the Discovery Set (37 Associations)[a]

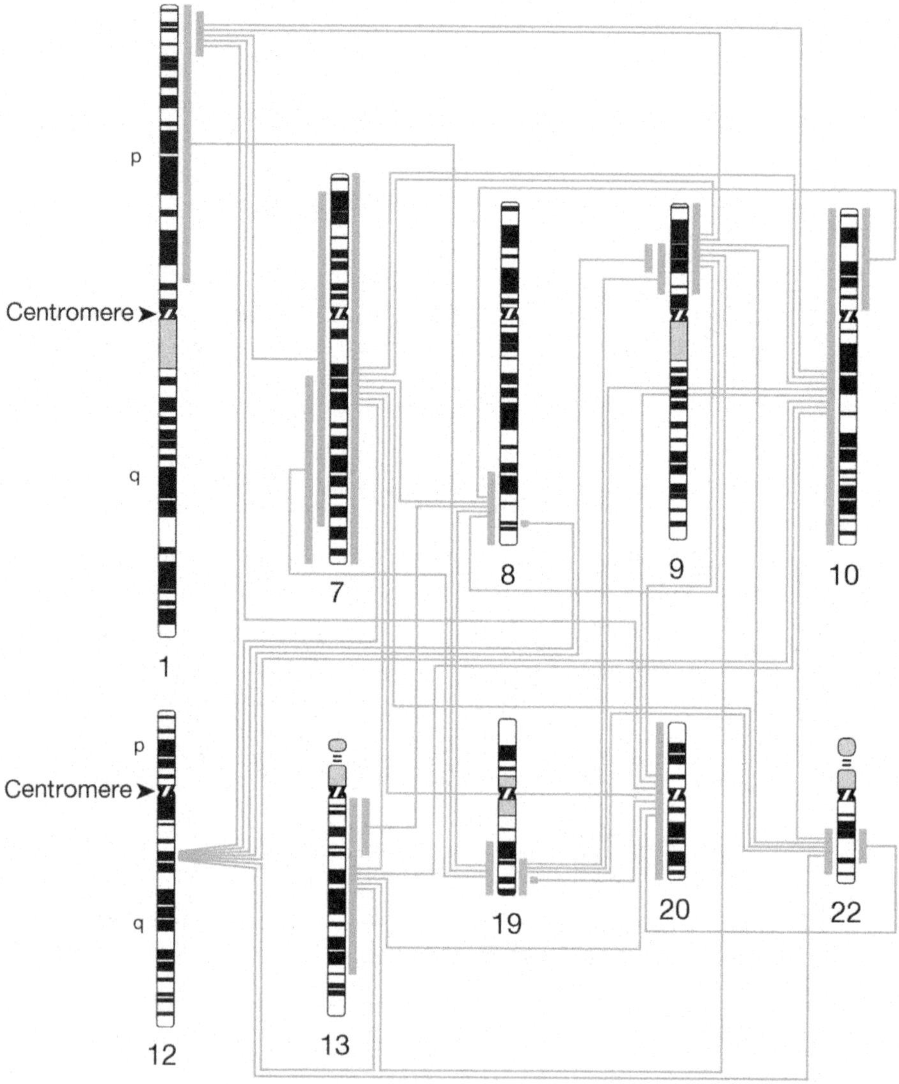

[a]From Bredel et al.[7]

a period or other intervening punctuation. A generic formula for the order shown (with punctuation or no punctuation indicated) is chromosome,arm,region[no punctuation]band[no punctuation].subband[no punctuation]sub-subband. Some examples illustrate this:

| | |
|---|---|
| 11q23 | chromosome 11, long arm, band 23 (region 2, band 3) |
| 11q23.3 | band in above subdivided, resulting in subband 23.3 |
| 20p11.23 | chromosome 20, short arm, sub-subband 11.23 (region 1, band 1, subband 2, sub-subband 3) |

It is correct usage to refer to the previous expressions as "band 11q23," "band 11q23.3," and "band 20p11.23."

The centromere is designated band 10, as in the following:

p10     (portion of centromere facing short arm)

q10     (portion of centromere facing long arm)

Visualization of genomic information by chromosome region in humans and other organisms is available at the National Center for Biotechnology Information Genome Data Viewer.[8]

**14.6.4.2**   **Karyotype.** *Karyotype* is the chromosome complement of an individual, tissue, or cell line. Karyotype is expressed as the number of chromosomes in a cell, including the sex chromosomes, a description of the sex chromosome composition, and, whenever applicable, any chromosome abnormality.

The *karyogram* and the *idiogram* are graphic representations of karyotype. The karyogram is "a systemized array of the chromosomes"[6(p7)] that has been prepared using methods such as photomicrography. An idiogram is a "diagrammatic representation of a karyotype."[6(p7)]

In karyotype expressions, the sex chromosomes, which should always be specified, are separated from the chromosome number by a comma, without an intervening space, as in the following examples:

46,XX     46 chromosomes (2 each of chromosomes 1-22 and 2 X chromosomes in human female karyotype)

46,XY     46 chromosomes (2 each of chromosomes 1-22, 1 X and 1 Y in human male karyotype)

45,X      45 chromosomes (2 each of chromosomes 1-22 and 1 X chromosome) (Turner syndrome)

47,XXY    47 chromosomes (2 each of chromosomes 1-22, 2 X chromosomes, and 1 Y chromosome) (Klinefelter syndrome)

47,XYY    47 chromosomes (2 each of chromosomes 1-22, 1 X chromosome, and 2 Y chromosomes)

69,XXX    69 chromosomes (3 each of chromosomes 1-22 and 3 X chromosomes)

A virgule (forward slash) is used to indicate more than 1 karyotype in an individual, tumor, cell line, and so on:

45,X/46,XX

Descriptions of autosomal chromosome abnormalities are presented after the sex chromosomes and listed in numerical order regardless of aberration type, separated from the sex chromosomes by a comma. For instance, the karyotype of a person with trisomy 21 (Down syndrome) with an extra chromosome 21 is specified as follows:

47,XX,+21

*or*

47,XY,+21

A karyotype description may contain both constitutional and acquired elements. For instance, the karyotype of a tumor cell from a person with trisomy 21 could show both the constitutional anomaly and an acquired neoplastic anomaly (eg, an acquired extra chromosome 8) and would be expressed as follows:

48,XX,+8,+21c

The lowercase c specifies that the trisomy 21 is constitutional, as distinguished from the acquired trisomy 8.

An individual with more than 1 karyotypic clone may have a *mosaic* (single-cell origin) karyotype or a *chimera* (multicell origin) karyotype, which should be specified with a 3-letter abbreviation at first mention of the karyotype. For example:

mos 45,X/46,XY

chi 46,XX/46,XY

Brackets indicate the number of cells observed in a clone:

chi 46,XX[25]/46,XY[10]

A double slash (virgule, forward slash), used in chimeras that result from bone marrow transplants, separates recipient and donor cell lines. Recipient karyotype precedes the double slash, donor karyotype follows the double slash, and either or both may be specified. For example:

46,XY[3]//

//46,XX[17]

46,XY[3]//46,XX[17]

Three cells from the male recipient were identified, along with 17 cells from the female donor.

For details on order in such expressions, consult *ISCN 2016*.[6]

Meiotic karyotypes may begin with a term such as MI and contain a haploid or near-haploid number of chromosomes and may (if the sex chromosomes are associated) or may not (if the sex chromosomes are separate) have a comma between X and Y:

MI,23,XY

MI,24,X,Y

**14.6.4.3** **Chromosome Rearrangements.** The abbreviations and symbols in Table 14.6-17 are used in descriptions of chromosomes, including chromosome rearrangements. The symbols in the list of chromosomes from *ISCN 2016* are part of an efficient shorthand that describes the exact changes in a karyotype that contains rearranged chromosomes. In publications that range beyond the field of cytogenetics, the symbols should always be defined.

**Table 14.6-17.** Chromosome Rearrangement Abbreviations and Symbols[a]

| Abbreviation | Explanation |
| --- | --- |
| AI | first meiotic anaphase |
| AII | second meiotic anaphase |
| ace | acentric fragment |
| add | additional material of unknown origin |
| arr | microarray |
| b | break |
| c | constitutional anomaly |
| cen | centromere |
| cgh | comparative genomic hybridization |
| chi | chimera |
| chr | chromosome |
| cht | chromatid |
| cp | composite karyotype |
| cx | complex rearrangements |
| del | deletion |
| der | derivative chromosome |
| dia | diakinesis |
| dic | dicentric |
| dim | diminished |
| dip | diplotene |
| dis | distal |
| dit | dictyotene |
| dmin | double minute |
| dn (de novo) | chromosome abnormality not inherited |
| dup | duplication |
| E | exchange |
| end | endoreduplication |
| enh | enhanced |
| fem | female |
| fis | centric fission |
| fra | fragile site |
| G | gap |

(*continued*)

**Table 14.6-17.** Chromosome Rearrangement Abbreviations and Symbols (*continued*)

| Abbreviation | Explanation |
| --- | --- |
| H | heterochromatin, constitutive |
| hsr | homogeneously staining region |
| I | isochromosome |
| idem | stemline karyotype in a subclone |
| ider | isoderivative chromosome |
| idic | isodicentric chromosome |
| inc | incomplete karyotype |
| ins | insertion |
| inv | inversion or inverted |
| ish | in situ hybridization |
| lep | leptotene |
| MI | first meiotic metaphase |
| MII | second meiotic metaphase |
| mal | male |
| mar | marker chromosome |
| mat | maternal origin |
| med | medial |
| min | minute acentric fragment |
| mos | mosaic |
| neo | neocentromere |
| nuc | nuclear or interphase |
| oom | oogonial metaphase |
| or | alternative interpretation |
| P | short arm of chromosome |
| PI | first meiotic prophase |
| pac | pachytene |
| pat | paternal origin |
| pcc | premature chromosome condensation |
| pcd | premature centromere division |
| prx | proximal |
| ps | satellited short arm of chromosome |
| psu | pseudo- |
| pvz | pulverization |

**Table 14.6-17.** Chromosome Rearrangement Abbreviations and Symbols (*continued*)

| Abbreviation | Explanation |
|---|---|
| q | long arm of chromosome |
| qdp | quadruplication |
| qr | quadriradial |
| qs | satellited long arm of chromosome |
| r | ring chromosome |
| rea | rearrangement |
| rec | recombinant chromosome |
| rev | reverse, including comparative genomic |
| rob | robertsonian translocation |
| roman numerals | |
| I | univalent structure |
| II | bivalent structure |
| III | trivalent structure |
| IV | quadrivalent structure |
| s | satellite |
| sce | sister chromatid exchange |
| sdl | sideline |
| SI | stemline |
| spm | spermatogonial metaphase |
| stk | satellite stalk |
| subtel | subtelomeric region |
| t | translocation |
| tas | telomeric association |
| ter | terminal end of chromosome or telomere |
| tr | triradial |
| trc | tricentric chromosome |
| trp | triplication |
| upd | uniparental disomy |
| var | variant or variable region |
| xma | chiasma(ta) |
| zyg | zygotene |
| : | break, in detailed system |

(*continued*)

**Table 14.6-17.** Chromosome Rearrangement Abbreviations and Symbols (*continued*)

| Abbreviation | Explanation |
|---|---|
| :: | break and reunion, in detailed system |
| ; | separates altered chromosomes and break points in structural rearrangements involving 2 or more chromosomes; separates probes on different derivative chromosomes |
| → | from-to, in detailed system |
| + | additional normal or abnormal chromosomes; increase in length; locus present on a specific chromosome |
| − | loss; decrease in length; locus absent from a specific chromosome |
| ~ | intervals and boundaries of a chromosome segment or number of chromosomes, fragments, or markers |
| <> | angle brackets for ploidy |
| [] | square brackets for number of cells or genome build |
| = | number of chiasmata |
| × | multiple copies of rearranged chromosomes |
| ? | questionable identification of a chromosome or chromosome structure |
| / | separates clones or contiguous probes |
| // | separates chimeric clones |

ªAdapted from McGowan-Jordan et al,[6] with permission of S Karger AG.

Single-letter abbreviations combined with other abbreviations are set closed up:

    chte      chromatid exchange

Three-letter symbols combined are set with a space:

    cht del    chromatid deletion

    psu dic    pseudodicentric

Chromosome rearrangement terms can be written using a short system or short form. Complex abnormalities are designated by the more specific detailed system or long form. The detailed form uses symbols such as arrows to describe individual derivative chromosomes that result from complex rearrangements (even the short system can result in a complex expression). For example:

    *Short:* 46,XY,t(2;5)(q21;q31)

    *Long:* 46,XY,t(2;5)(2pter→2q21::5q31→5qter;5pter→5q31::2q21→2qter)

The complete nomenclature, formulated for consistency in the description of chromosomal rearrangements, is detailed in *ISCN 2016*.[6] The following sections contain terms that illustrate some of the basic principles of the ISCN. Terms such as these may stand alone or may be part of longer expressions such as those previously listed.

**14.6.4.3.1** **Order.** For aberrations that involve more than 1 chromosome, the sex chromosome appears first, then other chromosomes in numerical order (or, less commonly, in group order if only the group is specified).

> t(X;13)(q27;q12)   translocation involving bands Xq27 and 13q12

For 2 breaks in the same chromosome, the short arm precedes the long arm, and there is no internal punctuation:

> inv(2)(p21q31)   inversion in chromosome 2

Exceptions to numerical order convey special conditions; for example, when a piece of one chromosome is inserted into another (3-break rearrangement), the recipient chromosome precedes the donor:

> ins(5;2)(p14;q21q31)   insertion of portion of long arm of chromosome 2 into short arm of chromosome 5

**14.6.4.3.2** **Plus and Minus Signs.** A plus sign *preceding* a chromosome indicates addition of the entire chromosome:

> +14   entire chromosome 14 gained

A plus sign *following* p or q and the chromosome number indicates an addition to that chromosome:

> 14p+   addition to 14p

Such a term is ambiguous; it might refer to one of many possible specific additions to 14p of an individual karyotype, to an unknown addition to 14p, or to additions to 14p in general. A term such as 14p+ may be used after context has been provided. In the case of karyotype descriptions, this means using more specific terms that incorporate symbols, such as add, der, and ins:

> Shorter Term: 14p+   Karyotype term: add(14)(p13)
>
> Shorter Term: 14q+   Karyotype term: add(14)(q32)

For example:

> The 14q+ cytogenetic abnormality was found to be add(14)(q32).

A minus sign *preceding* a chromosome signifies loss of the *entire* chromosome:

> –5   all of chromosome 5 missing

A minus sign *following* a chromosome arm signifies loss *from* that arm, but this should be reserved for text, whereas more specific notation is used in karyotype descriptions. For example:

> **Text**   **Karyotype**
>
> 5q–   del(5)(q13q31)

A deletion of the entire long arm of a chromosome should not be expressed in text with a minus sign.

del(5q)   (*not* 5q–)

Use more specific terms in karyotypes.

**14.6.4.3.3** Punctuation.

■ *Parentheses:* The number of the affected chromosome follows the rearrangement symbol in parentheses:

inv(2)   inversion in chromosome 2

Details of the aberration follow in a second set of parentheses:

inv(2)(p13p24)   inversion in chromosome 2 involving bands 13 and 24 of the short arm

■ *Semicolon:* In structural rearrangements that involve 2 or more chromosomes, a semicolon is used:

t(2;5)(q21;q31)   translocation involving breaks at 2q21 and 5q31

■ *Comma:* Commas separate the chromosome number, sex chromosomes, and each term describing an abnormality:

46,XX,r(18)(p11q22)   female karyotype with ring chromosome 18 with ends joined at bands p11 and q22

**14.6.4.3.4** Underlining. In different clones within the same karyotype, an underline (underscore) distinguishes homologous aberrations of the same chromosome (eg, 2 homologous chromosome 1s):

46,XX,der(1)t(1;3)(p34;q21)/46,XX,der(<u>1</u>)t(<u>1</u>;3)(p34;q21)

In manuscripts, authors should indicate that the underline is intended, so that it will not be set as italics, per typographic convention, in the published version.

**14.6.4.3.5** *Or.* The word *or* indicates "alternative interpretations of an aberration"[6(p48)] or alternative results (for instance, breaks that appear in consecutive bands using different techniques):

add(19)(p13 or q13)

add(10)(q22 or q23)

**14.6.4.3.6** Spacing. As seen in previous examples, there is no spacing between the elements of a karyotype description (except after mos and chi, between 2 or more 3-letter abbreviations [eg, cht del, rev ish enh], and before and after "or").

**14.6.4.3.7** Long Karyotypes. Multiline karyotypes carry over from 1 line of text to the next with no punctuation other than that of the original expression (eg, no hyphen at the end of the first line), as in the following tumor karyotype:

46,XX,t(8;21)(q22;q22)[12]/45,idem,–X[19]/46,idem,

–X,+8[5]/47,idem,–X,+8,+9[8]

**14.6.4.4** **In Situ Hybridization.** Style for terms that describe karyotypes identified by means of this technique alone or along with cytogenetic analysis (traditional karyotyping techniques) is similar to that described above (see 14.6.1, Nucleic Acids and Amino Acids). Some symbol meanings may differ. **Table 14.6-18** is adapted from *ISCN 2016.*[6]

Examples are as follows:

46,XY.ish del(22)(q11.2q11.2)(D22S75–)

47,XY,+mar.ish der(8)(D8Z1+)

(D22S75 refers to the probe for the DNA segment sequence *D22S75;* see 14.6.2, Human Gene Nomenclature.)

**Table 14.6-18.** In Situ Hybridization Abbreviations and Symbols[a]

| Term | Explanation |
|------|-------------|
| amp | amplified signal |
| arr | microarray |
| cgh | comparative genomic hybridization |
| con | connected signals |
| dim | diminished |
| enh | enhanced |
| fib ish | extended chromatin/DNA fiber in situ hybridization |
| ish | in situ hybridization |
| nuc ish | nuclear or interphase in situ hybridization |
| pcp | partial chromosome paint |
| rev ish | reverse in situ hybridization |
| sep | separated signals |
| subtel | subtelomeric region |
| wcp | whole chromosome paint |
| ; | separates altered chromosomes and break points in structural arrangements that involve >1 chromosome; separates probes on different derivative chromosomes |
| . | [period] separates various techniques |
| + | additional normal or abnormal chromosomes; increase in length; locus present on a specific chromosome |
| ++ | 2 hybridization signals or hybridization regions on a specific chromosome |
| – | loss; decrease in length; locus absent from a specific chromosome |
| × | multiple copies of rearranged chromosomes; aberrant polyploidy clones in neoplasias; precedes number of signals seen; multiple copies of a chromosome or chromosomal region |

[a]Adapted from McGowan-Jordan et al,[6] with permission of S Karger AG.

**14.6.4.5**  **Marker Chromosomes, Derivative Chromosomes, and the Philadelphia Chromosome.**
A *marker chromosome* "is a structurally abnormal chromosome that cannot be un-
ambiguously identified or characterized by conventional banding cytogenetics"[6(p70)]
and might be included in a karyotype as shown below:

> 47,XX,+mar

A structurally abnormal chromosome in which any part can be recognized is considered a *derivative chromosome*, defined as "a structurally rearranged chromosome generated either by a rearrangement involving two or more chromosomes or
by multiple aberrations within a single chromosome."[6(p60)]

A derivative chromosome is specified in parentheses, followed by the aberrations
involved in the generation of the derivative chromosome. The aberrations are not
separated by a comma. For instance,

> der(1)t(1;3)(p32;q21)t(1;11)(q25;q13)

signifies a derivative chromosome 1 generated by 2 translocations, one involving
the short arm with a break point in 1p32 and the other involving the long arm with
a breakpoint in 1q25.

For example, *Philadelphia chromosome* is the name given to a particular derivative chromosome found in chronic myelogenous leukemia and some types of
acute leukemia. The Philadelphia chromosome can be abbreviated as Ph chromosome or, if clear in context, Ph. Appendages, as in Ph[1], Ph1, Ph$_1$, or Ph′, are
not necessary, and Ph is the preferred form. The Ph chromosome is the derivative
chromosome 22 that results from the translocation t(9;22)(q34;q11.2) and may be
described as follows:

> der(22)t(9;22)(q34;q11.2)

The Ph chromosome is the result of a rearrangement that juxtaposes the oncogene *ABL* with the breakpoint cluster region gene *BCR* (see 14.6.2, Human Gene
Nomenclature, and 14.6.3, Oncogenes and Tumor Suppressor Genes).

**Principal Author:** Cheryl Iverson, MA

ACKNOWLEDGMENT

Thanks to the following for reviewing and providing comments: W. Gregory Feero,
MD, PhD, *JAMA*, and Maine-Dartmouth Family Medicine Residency, Augusta;
Trevor Lane, MA, DPhil, Edanz Group, Fukuoka, Japan; and John J. McFadden,
MA, JAMA Network. Thanks also to David Song, JAMA Network, for obtaining
permissions.

REFERENCES

1. Nussbaum RL, McInnes RR, Willard HF. *Thompson & Thompson Genetics in
   Medicine*. 8th ed. Saunders; 2016.
2. Turnpenny PD, Ellard S. *Emery's Elements of Medical Genetics*. 14th ed. Churchill
   Livingstone; 2012.
3. Riegel M. Human molecular cytogenetics: from cells to nucleotides. *Genet Mol Biol*.
   March 2014:37(suppl 1):194-209.

4. Feuk L, Carson AR, Scherer SW. Structural variation in the human genome. *Nat Rev Genet.* 2006;7(2):85-97. doi:10.1038/nrg1767

5. O'Connor C. Human chromosome translations and cancer. *Nature Educ.* 2008;1(1):56.

6. McGowan-Jordan J, Simons A, Schmid M, eds. *ISCN 2016: An International System for Human Cytogenetic Nomenclature (2016).* S Karger AG; 2016.

7. Bredel M, Scholtens DM, Harsh GR, et al. A network model of a cooperative genetic landscape in brain tumors. *JAMA.* 2009;302(3):261-275. doi:10.1001/jama.2009.99

8. Genome Data Viewer. Accessed July 31, 2019. https://www.ncbi.nlm.nih.gov/genome/gdv/

**14.6.5** **Nonhuman Genetic Terms.** Comparative genome analysis has shown that eukaryote species share genes to a great extent.[1] Therefore, similar or identical names designate the same gene across species whenever possible. Italicization of gene symbols is uniformly observed.

**14.6.5.1** **Vertebrates.** Animal gene symbols resemble human gene symbols (see 14.6.2, Human Gene Nomenclature).[2,3] However, unlike human gene symbols, animal gene symbols typically use or include lowercase letters and punctuation marks.

Gene terms for the laboratory mouse *(Mus musculus domesticus)* and laboratory rat *(Rattus norvegicus)*, often seen in medical publications because of the common use of those species in investigating diseases that affect humans, are prototypic of such style.

**14.6.5.1.1** **Mouse and Rat Gene Nomenclature.** Mouse and rat gene nomenclature guidelines were unified in 2003 by the International Committee on Standardized Genetic Nomenclature for Mice and Rat Genome and Nomenclature Committee.[4]

Mouse and rat gene symbols resemble human symbols in several respects.[4,5] They are descriptive, short (typically 3-5 characters), and italicized. Symbols begin with letters not numbers. They contain roman letters in place of Greek letters and arabic numerals in place of roman numerals.

Mouse and rat gene symbols differ from human symbols in the use of lowercase letters. Symbols usually contain an initial capital. Capital letters within a mouse gene symbol may indicate the laboratory code (see 14.6.5.1.4, Laboratory Codes) or code for another species/vector. A symbol with all lowercase letters (ie, no initial capital) indicates a recessive trait. Mouse and rat gene symbols may contain hyphens and other punctuation.

The central source for mouse gene terms is the Mouse Genome Database,[6] and for rats, RATMAP: Rat Genome Database[3] (**Box 14.6-1**). Gene names and symbols may be verified by means of the search features at those sites.

Style rules and conventions for mouse and rat gene symbols are given in **Tables 14.6-19** through **14.6-21**. (Note: The gene descriptions in the tables that follow are based on but not identical to the approved gene names available in the Mouse Genome Informatics database,[7] which are more complete and do not use Greek letters and other typographic variants. For instance, in searching for a term with $\alpha$ online, one would type "alpha.") Note that a given letter or letter combination often but not always signifies conventional usage. For instance, *l* at

**Box 14.6-1.** Resources/Websites for Nonhuman Species

| Website (reference) | URL | Description |
|---|---|---|
| ArkDb[2] | Now closed. See Hu et al[2] | General genomics and proteomics databases: resources for human, goat, mouse, deer, rat, and horse genomes |
| RATMAP: Rat Genome Database[3] | https://rgd.mcw.edu/ | Genetic, genomic, phenotype, and disease data generated from rat research; also provides access to corresponding human and mouse data for cross-species comparisons |
| MGI: Mouse Genome Informatics[6] | www.informatics.jax.org | Official names for mouse genes, alleles, and strains |
| FlyBase[10] | http://flybase.org | Database of *Drosophila* genes and genomes |
| WormBase[12] | https://www.wormbase.org/ | Genetics, genomics, and biology of *Caenorhabditis elegans* and related nematodes |
| OMIA[13] | https://omia.org/ | Catalog/compendium of inherited disorders, other traits, and genes in animal species other than human, mouse, and rat |
| SGD[15] | https://www.yeastgenome.org/nomenclature-conventions | Comprehensive integrated biological information for the budding yeast *Saccharomyces cerevisiae* |
| Entrez Genomes[18] | https://www.ncbi.nlm.nih.gov/genome | More than 3000 completely sequenced organisms, including Archaea, bacteria, eukaryotes, viruses, viroids, and plasmids |
| Maize Genetics and Genomics Database[21] | https://maisegdb.org/ | Federally funded informatics service to researchers focused on the crop and plant and model organism *Zea mays* |
| Rice Genome Annotation Project[22] | rice.plantbiology.msu.edu/ | National Science Foundation–sponsored database that provides sequence and annotations for the rice genome |
| SoyBase and the Soybean Breeder's Toolbox[23] | https://soybase.org/ | Repository for genetics, genomics, and related data sources for the soybean |

**Table 14.6-19.** Style Rules for Mouse Gene Symbols and Comparison With Human Gene Symbols (Examples)

| Mouse gene symbol | Mouse gene description | Rule illustrated | Human gene symbol (when known) |
|---|---|---|---|
| a | nonagouti | lowercase initial capital because named for mutant recessive trait | ASIP |
| Afp | α-fetoprotein | initial capital, otherwise lowercase, Greek letter changed to roman | AFP |
| B2m | β₂-microglobulin | no subscript | B2M |
| Gla | α-galactosidase | Greek letter changed to roman and moved to end of symbol | GLA |
| Gt(ROSA)26Sor | gene trap, ROSA 26, Philippe Soriano[a] | parentheses may be used | |
| Rn4.5s | 4.5S RNA | period permissible | |
| Rn5s | 5S RNA | symbol does not begin with number | RN5S1@ (@ signifies gene family; see 14.6.2, Human Gene Nomenclature) |

[a]The eponymous naming of genes is not uncommon.

**Table 14.6-20.** Examples of Mouse Gene Symbols Compared With Human Gene Symbols

| Mouse gene symbol | Mouse gene description | Convention illustrated | Human gene symbol (when available) |
|---|---|---|---|
| Brca1 | breast cancer 1 | same as human symbol except for case | BRCA1 |
| Cafq1 | caffeine metabolism QTL 1 | q: quantitative locus | |
| C4bp-ps1 | complement component 4 binding protein, pseudogene 1 | -ps: pseudogene | C4BPB |
| D10Mit1 | DNA segment, Chr 10, Massachusetts Institute of Technology 1 | symbol for DNA segment identified only in the mouse; includes laboratory code (see 14.6.5.1.4, Laboratory Codes) | |
| D17H21S56 | DNA segment, Chr 17, human D21S56 | H21 indicates DNA segment resides on human chromosome 21 | D21S56 |
| G6pdx | glucose-6-phosphate dehydrogenase X-linked | similar but not identical to human gene symbol | G6PD |
| Gna-rs1 | guanine nucleotide binding protein, related sequence 1 | -rs: related sequence | GNL1 |
| Gtl10 | gene trap locus 10 | Gt: gene trap | |

(continued)

**Table 14.6-20.** Examples of Mouse Gene Symbols Compared With Human Gene Symbols (*continued*)

| Mouse gene symbol | Mouse gene description | Convention illustrated | Human gene symbol (when available) |
|---|---|---|---|
| Gt(ROSA)26Sor | gene trap ROSA 26, Philippe Soriano | vector in parentheses; laboratory code indicated (see 14.6.5.1.4, Laboratory Codes) | |
| H2-Aa | histocompatibility 2, class II antigen A, α | | HLA-DQA1 |
| Hbb | hemoglobin β-chain complex | same as human symbol except for case | HBB |
| Hc9 | heterochromatin, Chr 9 | Hc: heterochromatin | |
| Hras1 | Harvey rat sarcoma virus oncogene 1 | see 14.6.3, Oncogenes and Tumor Suppressor Genes | HRAS |
| Ighmbp2 (formerly nmd) | immunoglobulin heavy chain μ binding protein 2 (formerly neuromuscular degeneration) | name change with new information about gene | IGHMBP2 |
| l17Wis9 | lethal, Chr 17, University of Wisconsin 9 | initial l: lethal | |
| Lamb1-1 | β₁ laminin, subunit 1 | hyphen separates 2 adjacent numbers | LAMB1 |
| Lzp-s | P lysozyme structural | s: structural | |
| mt-Rnr1 | 12S RNA, mitochondrial | mt: mitochondrial | MT-RNR1 |
| Mcptl | mast cell protease–like | l: like | |
| Nidd1, Nidd2, Nidd3, Nidd4 | non–insulin-dependent diabetes mellitus 1, 2, 3, 4 | same stem (root) for gene families | |
| Nup160 | nucleoporin 160 | name change (formerly Gtl1-13) | NUP160 |
| Rnr13 | rRNA, chromosome 13 cluster | | |
| Tcrb | T-cell receptor β-chain | | TRB@ (formerly TCRB; @ signifies gene family or cluster; see 14.6.2, Human Gene Nomenclature) |
| Tel10p | telomeric sequence, Chr 10, centromere end | Tel: telomere; 10: Chr 10; p: short arm | |
| Tg(APOE)1Vln | transgene insertion 1, Fred Van Leuven | Tg: transgene; parenthetic material: inserted gene, in this case the human gene APOE; Vln: founder or "laboratory of" designation | |

**Table 14.6-21.** Conventions for Mouse Gene Symbols Identified in Collaborative Sequencing Efforts (Examples)[a]

| Mouse gene symbol | Mouse gene description | Convention illustrated | Human gene symbol (when available) |
|---|---|---|---|
| *0610005C13Rik* | RIKEN cDNA 0610005C13 gene | RIKEN symbol assigned to sequence that does not match known genes in other species; *Rik:* RIKEN Institute, Japan | |
| *Cdc42ep3* | CDC42 effector protein (rho GTPase binding) 3; formerly *3200001F04Rik* | RIKEN symbol changed when gene identified in another organism | *CDC42EP3* |
| *BC023055* | cDNA sequence BC023055 | *BC* indicates sequence from Mammalian Gene Collection of the National Institutes of Health | *C10orf83* |
| *Aldob* | aldolase 2, B isoform, formerly *BC016435* | Mammalian Gene Collection symbol changed when gene identified in another organism | *ALDOB* |
| *AF179933* | cDNA sequence AF179933 | GenBank symbol for genes with no other information available in other organisms or sequencing efforts | |
| *Ppt2* | palmitoyl-protein thioesterase 2, formerly *AA672937* and *0610007M19Rik* | GenBank sequence ID withdrawn when gene identified in other organism | *PPT2* |

[a]See Database Identifiers for Genomic Sequences in 14.6.1, Nucleic Acids and Amino Acids.

or near the end of a symbol often, but not always, indicates "like." Mammalian Orthology Markers (OrthoMaM),[8] a database of orthologous mammalian markers, allows comparative searches of more than 40 vertebrate species. It can be queried to better understand the evolutionary dynamics of genes.

**14.6.5.1.2** **Mouse Alleles.** A mouse allele symbol consists of a mouse gene term often, but not always, with a superscript. As with mouse gene terms, mouse allele terms are italicized. Allele symbols can be verified within the records of a mouse gene:

- Search for the gene symbol at http://www.informatics.jax.org/marker

- Select the link for the gene symbol that has been located

- Under Phenotypes, select Phenotypic Diseases

Conventions and rules for mouse allele symbols are shown in **Table 14.6-22.**
In a phenotype expression, a superscript plus sign indicates wild type, for example,

$$Nf1^{tm1Fcr}/Nf1^{+}$$

which indicates a phenotype with a variant neurofibromatosis allele (targeted sequence variation 1, Fredrick Cancer Research and Development Center) and the wild-type neurofibromatosis allele.

**Table 14.6-22.** Rules and Conventions for Mouse Allele Terms (Examples)

| Allele symbol | Allele name | Convention or rule illustrated |
|---|---|---|
| *abn* | abnormal | recessive trait, thus begins with lowercase; because there is no superscript indicating an allelic term, use context to clarify |
| *Dbf* | doublefoot | dominant trait, thus begins with capital; because there is no superscript indicating an allelic term, use context to clarify |
| *Dnahc11$^{iv}$* | situs inversus viscerum allele of dynein, axon, heavy chain 11 gene | allele superscript designation is lowercase (recessive) |
| *Ins2$^{Akita}$* | Akita allele of insulin 2 gene | allele superscript designation has initial capital (dominant) |
| *Lama2$^{dy-2J}$* | dystrophia muscularis allele, Jackson 2, of α$_2$-laminin gene (second allele discovered at the Jackson Laboratory) | laboratory code included in superscript (see 14.6.5.1.4, Laboratory Codes); hyphens used |
| *Matp$^{Uw-dbr}$* | underwhite dominant brown alleles of membrane-associated transporter protein gene | multiple alleles separated by hyphen in superscript |

**14.6.5.1.3** **Mouse Chromosomes.** Chromosome nomenclature is similar for mice and humans (see 14.6.4, Human Chromosomes). However, in mice, rearrangement terms are capitalized. The following listing and subsequent examples are from the International Committee on Standardized Genetic Nomenclature for Mice[4]:

| | |
|---|---|
| Cen | centromere |
| Del | deletion |
| Df | deficiency |
| Dp | duplication |
| Hc | pericentric heterochromatin |
| Hsr | homogeneous staining region |
| In | inversion |
| Is | insertion |
| MatDf | maternal deficiency |
| MatDi | maternal disomy |
| MatDp | maternal duplication |
| Ms | monosomy |
| Ns | nullisomy |
| PatDf | paternal deficiency |

| PatDi | paternal disomy |
|-------|-----------------|
| PatDp | paternal duplication |
| Rb | robertsonian translocation |
| T | translocation |
| Tc | transchromosomal |
| Tel | telomere |
| Tet | tetrasomy |
| Tg | transgenic insertion |
| Tp | transposition |
| Ts | trisomy |
| UpDf | uniparental deficiency |
| UpDi | uniparental disomy |
| UpDp | uniparental duplication |

As with human chromosomes, lowercase p represents the short arm and lowercase q the long arm. When specific chromosomes are referred to, the word *Chromosome* is capitalized (and abbreviated Chr after first mention), for example:

Human chromosome 1 shows extensive homology to several mouse chromosomes, especially Chromosome (Chr) 4 and Chr 1.

Chromosome anomaly symbols usually include a unique laboratory code (see 14.6.5.1.4, Laboratory Codes) and a series number, for example:

In5Rk    fifth inversion found by Roderick

T37H    37th translocation found at Harwell

Chromosome number appears in parentheses:

In(2)5Rk    inversion in Chr 2

Semicolons separate numbers of chromosomes involved in translocations:

T(4;X)37H    translocation involving Chr 4 and Chr X

Periods indicate the centromere in robertsonian translocations:

Rb(9.19)163H    robertsonian translocation that involves Chr 9 and Chr 19

In insertions, the donor chromosome number comes first:

Is(7;1)40H    insertion from Chr 7 to Chr 1

For further rules and conventions for chromosomes, see the Chromosome Nomenclature section of the Mouse Genome Informatics website.[4]

**14.6.5.1.4** **Laboratory Codes.** Laboratory registration codes appear as 1- to 5-letter symbols in animal genetic terms, including chromosomal, DNA locus, and mouse strain nomenclature (see below). Such codes help identify specific colonies, useful in genetic studies that can extend over many generations. Laboratory codes are registered with the Institute of Laboratory Animal Research at the National Academy of Sciences in Washington, DC.[9] These codes uniquely identify an investigator, laboratory, or institution that produces or maintains an animal strain. Laboratory codes have initial capitals and appear without expansion. Examples are as follows:

| | |
|---|---|
| Arb | Arthritis and Rheumatism Branch, National Institute of Arthritis and Musculoskeletal and Skin Diseases |
| Ddd | University of Durham, Drug Dependence Group |
| J | The Jackson Laboratory |
| Jr | John Rapp |
| Kyo | Kyoto University |
| Maar | Silvère van Maarel Leiden University Medical Center |
| McW | Medical College of Wisconsin |
| N | National Institutes of Health |
| Ty | Benjamin A. Taylor, The Jackson Laboratory |
| Wil | Jean Wilson, University of Texas |

**14.6.5.1.5** **Mouse Strains.** Mouse strain names[6] are registered at the Mouse Genome Informatics website. Mouse strain names are available at the International Committee Standardized Genetic Nomenclature for Mice database.[4] (Rat strain names are registered at the Rat Genome Database.[3])

Mouse strain names consist of capital letters or combinations of capital letters and numbers:

A

BXH

CBA

C57BL

FVB

HDA32

A few earlier strains have names that are entirely numeric, for example:

129

A substrain is indicated by a term following the strain name after a virgule, usually the laboratory registration codes (see above), for example:

129/J

A/J

atherosclerosis in CBA/J mice

FVB/N mice used as controls

A serial number may precede the laboratory code, such as the 10 before the J in this example:

C57BL/610J

(Note: The 6 belongs to the substrain name.)
Exceptions to the initial capital after the virgule exist in the case of 2 well-known strains (not substrains) of mouse:

BALB/c

C57BR/cd

Many standard laboratory mouse strains are derived from crosses dating back to the early 20th century or even older lines, and the names reflect abbreviations for characteristics:

A      albino

BALB   Bagg, albino

DBA    dilute, brown, nonagouti

However, mouse strain names are not expanded.
Strain names may be abbreviated using approved abbreviations, for example:

B      C57BL

C      BALB/c

Note that some abbreviations are the same as some names of different strains (eg, the strain C and the abbreviation C), so context must clarify. Additional abbreviations are available at the International Committee on Standardized Genetic Nomenclature for Mice and Rat Genome and Nomenclature Committee.[4]

Abbreviations and the letter X are used to indicate recombinant inbred strains (female parental strain first), for example:

CXB    BALB/c x C57BL

Capital F followed by a number in parentheses may appear after a strain designation to indicate the number of inbred generations:

F(20)   20 inbred generations

For further guidelines on mouse strain nomenclature, see the Mouse Genome Informatics website.[4]

**14.6.5.2** **Invertebrates.**

**14.6.5.2.1** *Drosophila melanogaster.* Gene symbols for the fruit fly *Drosophila melanogaster* are generally capital and lowercase and, for recessive phenotypes, all lowercase. This convention is also observed for gene names. Gene symbols may include punctuation.[10] Nomenclature rules and symbol search are available at FlyBase[10] (Box 14.6-1). Examples are as follows:

*Ppi*     Preproinsulinlike

*SerT*    Serotonin transporter

        *su(Hw)*          Suppressor of Hairy wing

        *tRNA:S7:23Ea*    Transfer RNA:ser7:23Ea (ser7: seventh isoform of serine; 23E: map position)

As with mouse alleles, *Drosophila* alleles are indicated with superscripts:

        *Hn$^r$, Hn$^{r2}$* (Henna gene, eye color–defective alleles)

**14.6.5.2.2** *Caenorhabditis elegans.* The gene symbols for this nematode (roundworm) (Box 14.6-1) consist of 3 lowercase letters, a hyphen, an arabic numeral (sometimes a decimal), and, sometimes, a roman numeral after a space[11,12]:

        *dpy-1*

        *dpy-5 I*

        *let-37 X*

        *sir-2.1*

Parentheses indicate sequence variation in the gene:

        *let-37(mn138)*

Sequence variation symbols consist of 1- or 2-letter terms plus a number:

        *mn138*

A characteristic of a variant may be indicated by a 2-letter ending set in roman type:

        *bc17*ts (ts: temperature sensitive)

**14.6.5.3** **Online Mendelian Inheritance in Animals.** Online Mendelian Inheritance in Animals (OMIA) (Box 14-6.1) is the counterpart to Online Mendelian Inheritance in Man (OMIM; see 14.6.2, Human Gene Nomenclature)[13,14] and includes a database of inherited disorders, other traits, and genes in animal species other than humans, mice, and rats.

**14.6.5.4** **Microorganism Gene Nomenclature.**

**14.6.5.4.1** **Yeasts.** Gene symbols for the fungus *Saccharomyces cerevisiae* (Box 14-6.1) consist of 3 capital letters plus a number (or, occasionally, a number-letter) ending,[15] for example:

        *ACT1*     actin

        *CDC25*   adenylate cyclase regulatory protein

        *COX5A*   cytochrome c oxidase chain Va

This represents a change from earlier style in which all-lowercase symbols were used for loci named for recessive variants and all-capital symbols for loci named for dominant variants. Allele symbols still follow the case convention (ie, capital for dominant, lowercase for recessive).

**14.6.5.4.2** **Bacterial Gene Nomenclature.** Gene terms typically consist of an italicized lower-case 3-letter abbreviation often with an uppercase locus designator. The phenotype or encoded entity (eg, enzyme) is in all roman letters with an initial capital.[16,17] See examples below.

| | |
|---|---|
| *araA* | AraA (L-arabinose isomerase) |
| *asr* | Asr (acid shock protein) |
| *imp* (formerly *ostA*) | OstA (organic solvent intolerance; imp: increased membrane permeability) |
| *katE* | KatE (catalase) |
| *sodA* | SodA (superoxide dismutase, manganese) |
| *sodB* | SodB (superoxide dismutase, iron) |

The genetic nomenclature for bacteriophages is different from that for bacteria; there may be a separate convention for each phage.[17]

A number of bacterial genome databases are available on the internet. The National Center for Biotechnology Information sponsors Entrez Genomes[18] (select Gene, then search for the gene in question) (Box 14.6-1).

Alleles are designated with a number after the uppercase letter or following a hyphen, when not assigned to a locus. Wild-type alleles are designated with a superscript plus sign, mutant phenotypes with a superscript minus sign:

*ara$^+$*

*araA1*

*ara-23*

*sodA1*

**14.6.5.4.3** **Retroviral Gene Nomenclature.** HIV and other retroviruses contain 3 main structural genes and a number of regulatory genes[19] (see 14.6.3, Oncogenes and Tumor Suppressor Genes):

*Structural:*

| | |
|---|---|
| *env* | envelope gene |
| *gag* | group-specific core antigen gene |
| *pol* | polymerase gene |

*Regulatory:*

| | |
|---|---|
| *nef* | negative factor |
| *rev* | regulator of viral protein expression |
| *tat* | transactivator of viral transcription |
| *vif* | viral infectivity |

> *vpr*    viral protein R
>
> *vpu*    viral protein U
>
> *vpx*    viral protein X

Compare typographic style (**Table 14.6-23**) of gene names and their products (p stands for protein, gp for glycoprotein).

**14.6.5.4.4** **Plant Genetics.** Plants are extremely important food sources, and genetic alteration of plants is increasingly used to confer disease and pest resistance as well as to enhance the nutritional value of food crops. Such genetically modified organisms in food sources have generated controversy and relate to biomedicine. Included below are a few guidelines for 3 common food sources for which complete genome sequence data are available: corn (maize), rice, and soybeans.

- **Corn:** The name and symbol of the gene should be lowercase and italic, eg, *defective kernel12, dek12*. Note: There is no hyphen between the gene name and the numerical suffix.[21]

- **Rice:** A transcription unit, equivalent to a gene or locus, uses the naming scheme x.tyyyy, where x refers to the pseudomolecule assembly identifier and yyyy to the distinct identifier of the transcription unit.[22]

- **Soybeans:** The full locus identifier can be used as part of each gene name, or a locus name can be provided separately to describe a set of genes, for example:

    We studied Glyma.01g123450 in genotype, assembly, and annotation version Glyma.Wm82.a2.v1.
    Thereafter, the shorter locus name, Glyma.01g123450, may be used.[23]

**Table 14.6-23.** Some Examples of Typographic Style of Gene Names and Their Products

| Gene | Gene product (protein or polypeptide) | Protein products (examples)[a] |
|------|----------------------------------------|-------------------------------|
| *env* | Env | gp41, gp120 |
| *gag* | Gag | p6, p7, p17, p24 |
| *pol* | Pol | p12, p32, p66/51 |
| *nef* | Nef | p27 |
| *rev* | Rev | p19 |
| *tat* | Tat | p14 |
| *vif* | Vif | p24 |
| *vpr* | Vpr | p15 |
| *vpu* | Vpu | p16 |
| *vpx* | Vpx | p14 |

[a]A helpful resource for protein nomenclature is UniProt,[20] a central resource for functional information on proteins, including amino acid sequence, protein name or description, taxonomic data, and citation information.

**Principal Author:** Cheryl Iverson, MA

## ACKNOWLEDGMENT

Thanks to the following for reviewing and providing comments: W. Gregory Feero, MD, PhD, *JAMA*, and Maine-Dartmouth Family Medicine Residency, Augusta; Trevor Lane, MA, DPhil, Edanz Group, Fukuoka, Japan; and Garth D. Ehrlich, PhD, Center for Advanced Microbial Processing, Drexel University College of Medicine, Philadelphia, Pennsylvania.

## REFERENCES

1. Gene Ontology Consortium. Accessed June 7, 2018. http://www.geneontology.org/
2. Hu J, Mungall C, Law A, et al. The ARKdb: genome databases for farmed and other animals. *Nucleic Acids Res*. 2001;29(1):106-110. doi:10.1093/nar/29.1.106
3. RatMapGroup. RATMAP: Rat Genome Database. Accessed June 7, 2018. https://rgd.mcw.edu/
4. International Committee on Standardized Genetic Nomenclature for Mice and Rat Genome and Nomenclature Committee. Guidelines for nomenclature of mouse and rat strains. Revised January 2016. Accessed July 31, 2019. www.informatics.jax.org/mgihome/nomen/strains.shtml
5. Maltais LJ, Blake JA, Chu T, Lutz CM, Eppig JT, Jackson I. Rules and guidelines for mouse gene, allele, and mutation nomenclature: a condensed version. *Genomics*. 2002;79(4):471-474. doi:10.1006/geno.2002.6747
6. Jackson Laboratory. MGI: Mouse Genome Informatics. Updated May 29, 2018. Accessed July 31, 2019. www.informatics.jax.org
7. Mouse Genome Informatics. Mammalian Orthology Query Form. Accessed August 5, 2019. http://www.informatix.jax.org
8. The OrthoMaM (Orthologous Mammalian Markers) database. April 2015. Accessed August 5, 2019. http://www.orthomam.univ-montp2.fr/orthomam/html/index.php
9. ILAR: Institute for Laboratory Animal Research. International Laboratory Code Registry. Accessed August 5, 2019. http://dels.nas.edu/global/ilar/Lab-Codes
10. FlyBase: a database of *Drosophila* genes & genomes. Released May 3, 2018. Accessed July 31, 2019. http://flybase.org
11. *C elegans* genetic nomenclature basics. Last modified March 5, 2014. Accessed August 5, 2019. http://home.sandiego.edu/~cloerlab/nomenclature.html
12. WormBase. Last edited June 4, 2018. Accessed July 31, 2019. https://www.wormbase.org
13. Nicholas F. Online Mendelian Inheritance in Animals (OMIA). Updated May 31, 2018. Accessed July 31, 2019. http://omia.org/
14. Rangel P, Giovannetti J. *Genomes and Databases on the Internet: A Practical Guide to Functions and Applications*. Horizon Scientific Press; 2002.
15. SGD gene nomenclature conventions. Accessed July 31, 2019. https://www.yeastgenome.org/nomenclature-conventions
16. Demerec M, Adelberg EA, Clark AJ, Hartman PE. A proposal for a uniform nomenclature in bacterial genetics. *Genetics*. 1966;54(1):61-76.
17. *Journal of Bacteriology* instructions to authors. Updated January 2019. Accessed August 5, 2019. https://jb.asm.org/sites/additional-assets/JB-ITA.pdf
18. National Center for Biotechnology Information (NCBI). Entrez Genomes. Accessed July 31, 2019. https://www.ncbi.nlm.nih.gov/genome

19. Collins DR, Collins KL. HIV-1 accessory proteins adapt cellular adaptors to facilitate immune evasion. *PLoS Pathogens*. Published January 23, 2014. doi:10.1371/journal.ppat.1003851

20. UniProt. Updated 2018. Accessed June 7, 2018. www.uniprot.org

21. Maize Genetics and Genomics Database. Updated May 8, 2018. Accessed July 31, 2019. https://www.maizegdb.org/

22. Rice Genome Annotation Project. Accessed July 31, 2019. rice.plantbiology.msu.edu/

23. Soybase and the Soybean Breeder's Toolbox. Accessed July 31, 2019. https://soybase.org/

**14.6.6**   **Pedigrees.** Pedigree format recommendations are established by the Pedigree Standardization Task Force (now called the Pedigree Standardization Work Group) of the National Society of Genetic Counselors[1,2] (see 5.8.3, Rights in Published Reports of Genetic Studies). The 2008 update recommends including on the pedigree the reason for referral (eg, abnormal findings on ultrasonography, family history of cancer).

A square represents a male individual; a circle, a female individual; and a diamond, an individual whose sex is not specified, a person with a congenital disorder of sex development, or a person who is transgender (**Figure 14.6-6**).[2]

Shading indicates an affected individual (**Figure 14.6-7**). Partitions with different shading should be used for individuals with more than one condition. Define all shading in a legend or key.

Multiple individuals are indicated by a number inside the shape (**Figure 14.6-8**). For unknown number, a roman "n" is preferred to a question mark.

A slash mark (**Figure 14.6-9**) indicates a deceased individual.

A pregnancy is indicated with a capital "P" inside the shape (**Figure 14.6-10**). Symbols would not be shaded unless the pregnancy was affected.

The proband (the first affected family member who seeks medical attention) is indicated by a capital "P" with an arrow outside the shape (**Figure 14.6-11**).

The consultand (person seeking medical attention) is indicated with an arrow (**Figure 14.6-12**).

Textual information appears below the individual symbol (**Figure 14.6-13**). Preferred order is age information, evaluation, and pedigree number.

An obligate carrier (ie, unaffected individual inferred by pedigree analysis to carry a trait) is indicated with a central dot (**Figure 14.6-14**).

**Figure 14.6-6.**  Shapes Used to Represent an Individual in a Pedigree

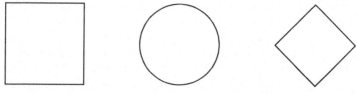

Square indicates male; circle, female; and diamond, individual whose sex is not specified, a person with a congenital disorder of sex development, or a person who is transgender.

**Figure 14.6-7.** Use of Shading in a Pedigree

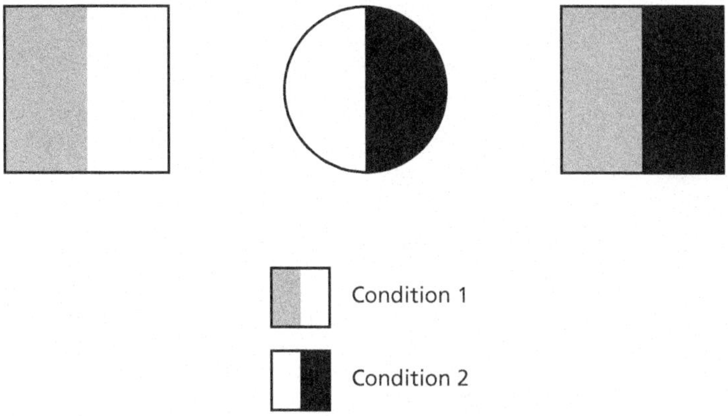

Condition 1
Condition 2

**Figure 14.6-8.** Indication of Number of Individuals in a Pedigree

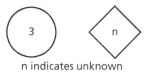

3
n
n indicates unknown

**Figure 14.6-9.** Indication of a Deceased Individual in a Pedigree

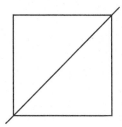

**Figure 14.6-10.** Indication of a Pregnancy in a Pedigree

P
P
P

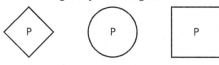

**Figure 14.6-11.** Indication of the Proband in a Pedigree

P
P

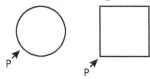

**Figure 14.6-12.** Indication of the Consultand (Person Seeking Medical Attention) in a Pedigree

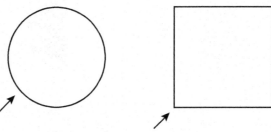

**Figure 14.6-13.** Indication of Textual Information About an Individual in a Pedigree

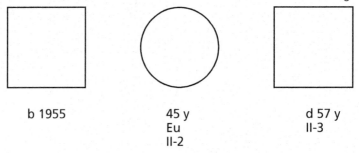

b 1955           45 y           d 57 y
Eu           II-3
II-2

Eu: uninformed evaluation

**Figure 14.6-14.** Indication of an Obligate Carrier (Unaffected Individual Inferred by Pedigree Analysis to Carry a Trait) in a Pedigree

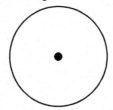

**Figure 14.6-15.** Indication of a Pregnancy Not Carried to Term in a Pedigree

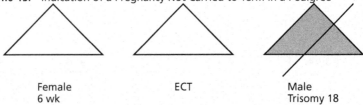

Female           ECT           Male
6 wk                           Trisomy 18

ECT indicates ectopic pregnancy. A slash indicates termination of pregnancy.

**Figure 14.6-16.** Indication of Stillborn Individuals in a Pedigree

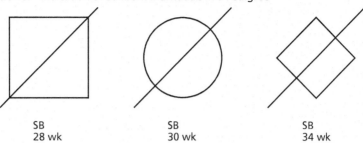

A small triangle indicates a pregnancy not carried to term (**Figure 14.6-15**). Sex, if known, is indicated with text. (Sex is often unknown, especially with miscarriages.) Shading is used as described above for affected individuals. The symbol should be shaded only if the cause of the abnormality is known, and the abnormality should be defined in the key or under the symbol.

Stillborn individuals use full-sized shapes with SB in the caption (**Figure 14.6-16**).

Partner relationships are indicated by a straight, horizontal line (**Figure 14.6-17**). It is preferred that the male partner be shown on the left.

A vertical line (the line of descent) indicates the offspring (**Figure 14.6-18**).

Siblings should appear in order of birth (oldest to the left), connected by lines as shown in **Figure 14.6-19**.

Offspring are indicated by vertical lines (**Figure 14.6-20**). Use of a shorter line to indicate a pregnancy not carried to term is no longer recommended because it is made redundant graphically by the use of a triangle for pregnancies not carried to term.

An ended relationship is indicated by a double slash (**Figure 14.6-21**).

Consanguinity (kinship because of common ancestry) is indicated by a double line (**Figure 14.6-22**), and the relationship should be noted (eg, first cousins, second cousins).

Two diagonal lines indicate twins; 3, triplets (**Figure 14.6-23**). A horizontal bar specifies monozygotic; no horizontal bar, dizygotic; and a question mark, unknown.

No offspring is indicated by perpendicular lines; infertility, by perpendicular lines with a double horizontal line (**Figure 14.6-24**).

**Figure 14.6-17.** Indication of Partner Relationships in a Pedigree

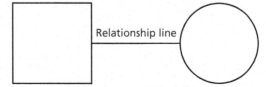

**Figure 14.6-18.** Indication of the Line of Descent in a Pedigree

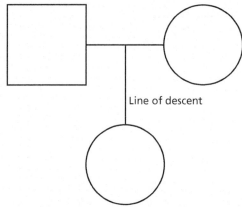

Line of descent

**Figure 14.6-19.** Indication of Siblings in a Pedigree

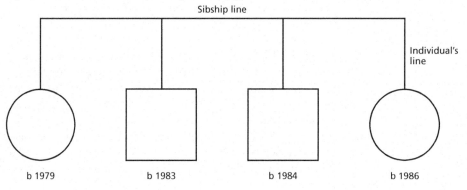

Sibship line

Individual's line

b 1979          b 1983          b 1984          b 1986

**Figure 14.6-20.** Indication of Offspring in a Pedigree

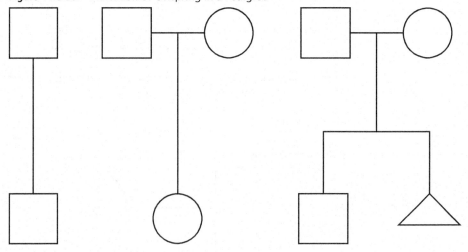

**Figure 14.6-21.** Indication of an Ended Relationship in a Pedigree

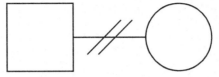

**Figure 14.6-22.** Indication of Consanguinity in a Pedigree
First cousins

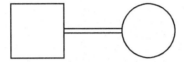

**Figure 14.6-23.** Indication of Twins or Triplets in a Pedigree

Monozygotic twins · Dizygotic twins · Zygosity unknown

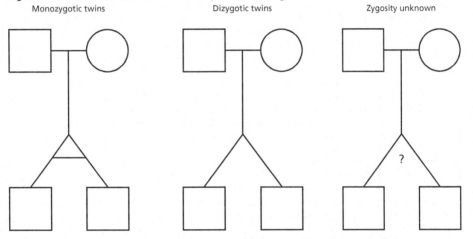

A horizontal bar specifies monozygotic; no horizontal bar, dizygotic; and a question mark, unknown.

**Figure 14.6-24.** Indication of No Offspring or of Infertility in a Pedigree

No offspring by choice or reason unknown · Infertility

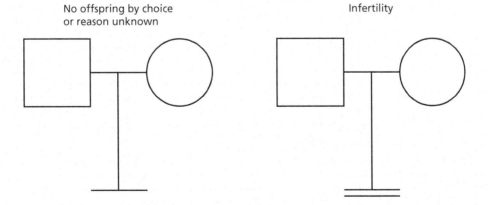

**Figure 14.6-25.** Indication of an Adopted Individual and of Legal Parentage in a Pedigree

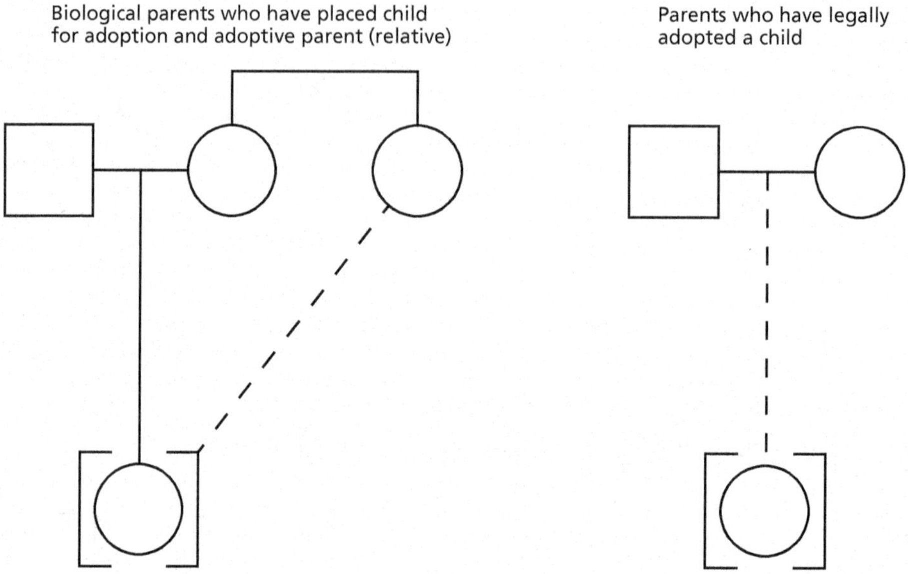

Biological parents who have placed child
for adoption and adoptive parent (relative)

Parents who have legally
adopted a child

Brackets indicate an adopted individual and dashed lines legal parentage, for example, adoptive parent (**Figure 14.6-25**).

In pedigrees that show relationships defined by assisted reproductive technologies (**Figure 14.6-26**), D indicates donor (sperm or ovum) and S, surrogate carrier of the pregnancy.

Diagonal lines indicate other parental relationships (**Figure 14.6-27**).

Haplotypes may be indicated with shaded rectangles below the individual (**Figure 14.6-28**). Meaning should be clarified by means of a key.

In a complete pedigree (**Figure 14.6-29**), generations are indicated on the left by roman numerals. See Bennett[3] for more examples of complete pedigrees.

**14.6.6.1**  **Deidentification of Pedigrees.** As noted in 5.8.3, Rights in Published Reports of Genetic Studies, the rules for ethical approval of studies, obtaining informed consent, and protecting patients' rights to privacy in scientific publication also apply to genetic studies of family pedigrees. If appropriate consent cannot be obtained from those identified in pedigree charts, nonessential identifying information can be removed or not presented. However, data should not be altered or "scrambled" in an attempt to protect the identities of individuals or family members, although relevant information may be masked. As noted in 5.8.3, Rights in Published Reports of Genetic Studies, for example, in pedigree charts, diamonds or another sex-neutral symbol can be used instead of squares or circles if the sex of family

**Figure 14.6-26.** Indication of Relationships That Are Defined by Assisted Reproductive Techniques in a Pedigree

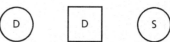

D indicates donor (sperm or ovum)
and S, surrogate carrier of the pregnancy.

**Figure 14.6-27.** Indication of Other Parental Relationships in a Pedigree

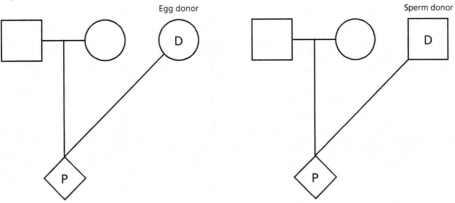

**Figure 14.6-28.** Indication of Haplotypes in a Pedigree

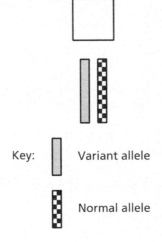

**Figure 14.6-29.** Example of a Complete Pedigree, With Generations Indicated on the Left by Roman Numerals

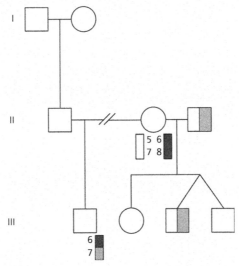

members is not essential to the report (eg, if the disease or condition is known not to be sex linked), or sections of pedigrees may be excluded from pedigree charts or not described in detail if appropriate consent could not be obtained, as long as such omissions are noted.

**Principal Author:** Cheryl Iverson, MA

## ACKNOWLEDGMENT

Thanks to the following for reviewing and providing comments: Robin L. Bennett, MS, CGC, Division of Medical Genetics, University of Washington, Seattle; Trevor Lane, MA, DPhil, Edanz Group, Fukuoka, Japan; and John J. McFadden, MA JAMA Network. Thanks also to Karen Bucher, *JAMA*, for preparing the illustrations.

## REFERENCES

1. Bennett RL, Steinhause KA, Uhrich SB, et al. Recommendations for standardized human pedigree nomenclature. *Am J Hum Genet.* 1995;56(3):745-752. Also published in *J Genet Counseling.* 1995;4(4):267-279.
2. Bennett RL, French KS, Resta RG, Doyle DL. Standardized human pedigree nomenclature: update and assessment of the recommendations of the National Society of Genetic Counselors. *J Genet Counseling.* 2008;17:424-433. doi:10.1007/s10897-008-9169-9
3. Bennett RL. Handy reference tables of pedigree nomenclature. In: *The Practical Guide to the Genetic Family History.* Wiley-Liss Inc; 1999.

**14.7** **Hemostasis.** Hemostasis consists of platelet plug formation (primary hemostasis)[1] and blood coagulation (secondary hemostasis, coagulation, clotting). Hemostasis and its control involve complex interactions of numerous procoagulants and anticoagulants. Description of hemostatic processes depends on consistent use of terms.

**14.7.1** **Primary Hemostasis (Initiation).** Note the typography of the terms listed in Table 14.7-1, which are found in descriptions of platelet hemostasis[2-4] (use parenthetical abbreviated terms in accordance with 13.11, Clinical, Technical, and Other Common Terms).

See 14.1.2, Granulocyte Antigens and Platelet-Specific Antigens.

**14.7.2** **Endothelial Factors.** Structures and products of endothelial cells—the cells lining blood vessels—maintain blood fluidity by preventing excessive clotting and prevent bleeding by promoting clotting. The endothelium-associated terms listed in Table 14.7-2 are presented as a guide to style.

Three glycoprotein complexes are synonymous with 3 integrins and take part in hemostasis:

| Glycoprotein | Integrin |
|---|---|
| GpIa-IIa | $\alpha_2\beta_1$ |
| GpIc-IIa | $\alpha_6\beta_1$ |
| GpIIb-IIIa | $\alpha_{IIb}\beta_3$ |

**Table 14.7-1.** Platelet Hemostasis Terms and Abbreviations

| Term | Abbreviation |
| --- | --- |
| α-granules | |
| arachidonic acid | AA |
| ATP P2X1 receptor | P2X1 |
| β-thromboglobulin | βTG *or* BTG |
| calcium-calmodulin complex | Ca-CaM *or* Ca-CM |
| cyclooxygenase | COX |
| diacylglycerol | DAG |
| G proteins (proteins that hydrolyze guanosine triphosphate) | |
| glycoprotein Ia/IIa complex | GpIa-IIa |
| glycoprotein Ib/IX complex | GpIb-IX |
| glycoprotein Ib/IX/V complex | GpIb-IX-V |
| glycoprotein IIb/IIIa complex | GpIIb-IIIa |
| glycoprotein IV (CD36; see 14.8.7, Lymphocytes) | GpIV |
| glycoprotein VI | GpVI |
| inositol triphosphate | $IP_3$ |
| myosin light chain | MLC |
| myosin light chain kinase | MLCK |
| myosin light chain, phosphorylated | $MLC\text{-}PO_4$ |
| phosphatidylinositol 4,5-biphosphate | $PIP_2$ |
| phosphodiesterase 3A | PDE3A |
| phospholipase $A_2$ | $PLA_2$ |
| phospholipase C | PLC |
| platelet activating factor | PAF |
| platelet-derived growth factor | PDGF |
| platelet factor 3 | PF3 |
| platelet factor 4 | PF4 |
| platelet ADP P2T adenylate cyclase receptor | $P2T_{AC}$ |
| platelet ADP P2X1 receptor | P2X1 |
| platelet ADP P2Y1 receptor | P2Y1 |
| platelet ADP P2Y12 receptor | P2Y12 |
| prostacyclin, prostaglandin $I_2$ | $PGI_2$ |
| prostaglandin $D_2$ | $PGD_2$ |

(*continued*)

**Table 14.7-1.** Platelet Hemostasis Terms and Abbreviations (*continued*)

| Term | Abbreviation |
|---|---|
| 6-keto prostaglandin $F_1\alpha$ | 6-keto $PGF_1\alpha$ |
| prostaglandin $G_2$ | $PGG_2$ |
| prostaglandin $H_2$ | $PGH_2$ |
| protein p47 | p47 |
| protein p47, phosphorylated | p47[phox] |
| protein kinase C | PKC |
| thromboxane $A_2$ | $TXA_2$ |
| thromboxane $B_2$ | $TXB_2$ |
| von Willebrand factor (see 14.7.3.6, von Willebrand Factor) | VWF |

**Table 14.7-2.** Endothelium-Associated Terms and Abbreviations

| Class and term | Abbreviation |
|---|---|
| cellular (or cell) adhesion molecules | CAMs |
|    intercellular adhesion molecule 1 | ICAM-1 |
|    intercellular adhesion molecule 2 | ICAM-2 |
|    platelet-endothelial cellular adhesion molecule | PECAM |
|    vascular cellular adhesion molecule 1 | VCAM-1 |
| cytokines (see 14.8.4, Cytokines) | |
|    gro (growth-stimulating factor) | GSF |
|    RANTES (regulated on activation, normal T-expressed, and secreted[5(p1638)]) | |
| integrins | |
|    $\alpha_1\beta_1$ integrin | |
|    $\alpha_2\beta_3$ integrin | |
|    $\alpha_3\beta_1$ integrin | |
|    $\alpha_6\beta_1$ integrin | |
|    $\alpha_v\beta_1$ integrin | |
|    $\alpha_v\beta_3$ integrin | |
| miscellaneous | |
|    nitric oxide | NO |
|    endothelial (or epithelial) nitric oxide synthase | eNOS (also NOS3) |
|    endothelial cell–associated ADPase (CD39; see 14.8.7, Lymphocytes) | |

**Table 14.7-2.** Endothelium-Associated Terms and Abbreviations (*continued*)

| Class and term | Abbreviation |
| --- | --- |
| prostacyclin, prostaglandin I$_2$ | PGI$_2$ |
| E-selectin | |
| L-selectin | |
| P-selectin | |
| tissue plasminogen activator (see 14.7.4, Inhibition of Coagulation and Fibrinolysis) | tPA |
| urokinase or urinary-type plasminogen activator (see 14.7.4, Inhibition of Coagulation and Fibrinolysis) | uPA |

**14.7.3** **Secondary Hemostasis (Amplification and Propagation).** Blood coagulation (secondary hemostasis[1]) is the phase of clot formation dependent on plasma coagulation factors (also known as clotting factors).

**14.7.3.1** **Pathways.** The laboratory evaluation of plasma factor–dependent coagulation has been divided into 2 pathways (systems, phases). The following terms and synonyms are used:

| Term | Synonym |
| --- | --- |
| intrinsic pathway | contact system–initiated pathway |
| extrinsic pathway | tissue factor–mediated or tissue factor–dependent pathway |

**14.7.3.2** **Clotting Factors.** An international system of nomenclature, formulated from 1954 through 1963,[6,7] clarified clotting factor terminology. A major update to the standard nomenclature was published by Blomback et al[8] in the early 1990s.[9]

A number of clotting factors were named for the patients whose disorders led to their discovery.

Roman numerals are used to designate most of the major plasma coagulation factors. These designations when formulated were seen as having advantages over eponyms and functional names for comprehension by readers of non-Western languages.[7] "The sequence of numbers in current terminology is . . . based on the historical order in which the coagulation factors were discovered."[7(p710)]

Table 14.7-3 gives roman numeral designations, descriptive names, and synonyms for the plasma coagulation factors. If a term other than the preferred term is used, the preferred term should be given in parentheses at the first mention of a factor. Common abbreviations appear here, but their use should conform to guidelines in 13.11, Clinical, Technical, and Other Common Terms. (The term *factor VI*, originally designating activated factor V, is not used.)

A lowercase *a* designates the activated form of a factor (eg, IXa).

**Table 14.7-3.** Roman Numeral Designations, Descriptive Names, and Synonyms for the Plasma Coagulation Factors

| Factor No. | Descriptive name | Synonym(s) |
|---|---|---|
| (factor I)[a] | fibrinogen[b] | |
| factor II | prothrombin[b] | prethrombin |
| (factor III)[a] | tissue factor[b] | thromboplastin<br>tissue thromboplastin<br>tissue extract |
| (factor IV)[a] | calcium[b] | calcium ion<br>Ca$^{2+}$ |
| factor V[b] | proaccelerin | (labile factor)<br>(accelerator globulin [AcG]) |
| factor VII[b] | proconvertin | (stable factor)<br>(serum prothrombin conversion accelerator [SPCA]) |
| factor VIII[b] | antihemophilic factor (AHF) | antihemophilic globulin (AHG)<br>antihemophilic factor A |
| factor IX[b] | plasma thromboplastin component (PTC) | Christmas factor<br>antihemophilic factor B |
| factor X[b] | Stuart factor | Prower factor<br>Stuart-Prower factor |
| factor XI[b] | plasma thromboplastin antecedent (PTA) | (antihemophilic factor C) |
| factor XII[b] | Hageman factor | activation factor<br>contact factor<br>(glass factor) |
| factor XIII[b] | fibrin-stabilizing factor (FSF) | (Laki-Lorand factor [LLF])<br>(fibrinase)<br>(protransglutaminase) |
| | prekallikrein[b] | Fletcher factor |
| | high-molecular-weight kininogen (HMW kininogen, HMWK, HK)[b] | Fitzgerald factor |

[a]Terms in parentheses are rarely used.
[b]Preferred term.

In diagrams of coagulation pathways, activation is indicated with a solid arrow:

X ⟶ Xa

and action on another factor, with a dashed arrow:

XIIa ------▶ XI

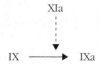

Examples of additional terms related to secondary hemostasis are as follows:

Term	Abbreviation
γ-glutamyl carboxylic acid residues	Gla residues
tissue factor/VIIa complex	TF-VIIa complex
or	
VIIa/tissue factor complex	VIIa-TF complex
active factor XII fragment	XIIf

14.7.3.3 **Clotting Factor Variants.** Some specific variants or abnormal forms have been named for locations where they were discovered, as follows:

factor V Cambridge

factor V Leyden [*sic*]

factor X San Antonio

fibrinogen Paris

protein C Vermont

prothrombin Barcelona

prothrombin Himi I

prothrombin Himi II

Clotting factor variants that have been characterized molecularly are specified by means of terms that indicate the molecular change (ie, nucleotide or amino acid alteration).[10] The abbreviations ins (insertion), del (deletion), In (intron), Ex (exon), ter (termination codon), MAF (maximum allele frequency), LD (linkage disequilibrium), and SNV (single nucleotide variation; formerly SNP [single-nucleotide polymorphism]) are used within such terms.[10] See 14.6.1.1.1, Sequence Variation, Nucleotides for a more detailed description of such notation. Examples are as follows:

factor VIII Arg1689Cys	*or*	VIII R1689C
factor VIII Glu1987ter	*or*	VIII G1987ter
factor VIII Ex24-25del		

A shorthand expression is permissible after the term is first defined:

The factor II resulting from the 20210G→A variant (mutation) in the prothrombin gene (factor II A^{20210}) . . .

14.7.3.4 **Thrombin.** The protein thrombin is the end result of the coagulation factor cascade. Related terms include the following:

α-thrombin

β-thrombin

γ-thrombin

thrombin A loop, B loop, C loop, E loop, γ loop

β-thromboglobulin

**14.7.3.5** **Hemophilias and Thrombophilias.** Hemophilias are bleeding disorders. Hemophilia A is associated with factor VIII deficiency, hemophilia B with factor IX deficiency, hemophilia C with factor XI deficiency, and von Willebrand disease with von Willebrand factor deficiency. (Factor IX was originally named Christmas factor, after a patient's surname. Hemophilia B is known as Christmas disease and was reported in the Christmas 1952 issue of the *BMJ*.[6,7]) Examples of subtypes include hemophilia A, CRM(+) variant (CRM: cross-reacting material), hemophilia B Leyden [*sic*], and hemophilia Bm.

Thrombophilias are excessive clot-forming disorders. One variety occurs with factor V Leyden.

See 14.7.3.3, Clotting Factor Variants, for molecularly based nomenclature.

**14.7.3.6** **von Willebrand Factor.** Because factor VIII, involved in coagulation, and von Willebrand factor (VWF), involved in platelet adhesion, form a noncovalent bi-molecular complex, they were originally difficult to distinguish biochemically and immunologically. Original nomenclature reflected this difficulty; for instance, what was first referred to as factor VIII–related antigen (abbreviated VIIIR:Ag) was found to be the factor that is deficient in von Willebrand disease.

Factor VIII and VWF, although functionally associated, are physiologically, genetically, and clinically distinct. In 1985 the International Committee on Coagulation and Thrombosis put forth preferred terms that were meant (1) to distinguish factor VIII from VWF and (2) to clarify exactly which entity was being specified (**Table 14.7-4**). The committee noted that it is acceptable to use the term *VIII-VWF* for the biomolecular complex but not for either single component.[11,12]

The terms in column 1 of Table 14.7-4 are not only preferred but also familiar exactly as shown to those conversant with the field. However, for most audiences, authors should clarify the preferred term by including the synonym or an explanation (eg, column 4, "Meaning") at first mention.

**14.7.3.7** **von Willebrand Disease.** Variants of von Willebrand disease[13-16] include, but are not limited to, the following:

| Type | Sample molecular variants |
|---|---|
| type 1 | VWF Arg854Gln, VWF Cys1149Arg |
| type 2A | VWF Ile865Thr, VWF Arg834Trp |
| type 2B | VWF Trp550Cys, VWF Arg545Cys |
| type 2M | has at least 28 variants |
| type 2N | VWF Thr28Met |
| type 3 | VWF Arg1659ter, VWF Arg2635ter |

**Table 14.7-4.** Factor VIII and von Willebrand Factor Terms

| Preferred | Synonym | Old (avoid) | Meaning |
|---|---|---|---|
| factor VIII | antihemophilic factor (AHF) | VIII:C | factor VIII protein |
| VIII:Ag | factor VIII antigen | VIII:CAg | factor VIII antigen |
| VIII:c | | | factor VIII coagulant activity |
| VWF | von Willebrand factor | VIIIR:Ag VIII/vWF AHF-like protein | von Willebrand factor protein |
| VWF:Ag | | VIIIR:Ag | von Willebrand factor antigen |
| VWF:CB | | | collagen-binding |
| ristocetin cofactor (RCoF) | | VIIIR:RCoF VIII:R:RCo VIIIR:vWF | von Willebrand factor function (ie, platelet aggregation-promoting property of VWF in the presence of the drug ristocetin) |

Nomenclature for sequence variants (mutations and polymorphisms) of the *VWF* gene is indicated according to 14.6.1.1.1, Sequence Variation, Nucleotides, or as in the following examples[17]:

| | |
|---|---|
| 1234G>A | adenine substituted for guanine at position 1234 in *VWF* cDNA sequence |
| g1234G>A | as above, in complete *VWF* sequence |
| 1234insN | nucleotide insertion after nucleotide 1234 in *VWF* cDNA sequence |
| R123G | glycine substitute for arginine at position 123 in pre-pro VWF sequence |
| R123del | arginine deletion at position 123 in pre-pro VWF sequence |
| 1234A/G | adenine/guanine polymorphism at position 1234 in *VWF* cDNA |

## 14.7.4 ▍ Inhibition of Coagulation and Fibrinolysis

**14.7.4.1 ▍ Inhibition of Coagulation.** The sample terms listed in **Table 14.7-5** are included for reference. Expand at first mention in accordance with 13.11, Clinical, Technical, and Other Common Terms.

Note: Protein C was named for an investigator's chromatographic fraction C in which it was discovered. The S in protein S refers to Seattle, where it was discovered. Protein S is not the same as S protein (see 14.8.3, Complement).

**Table 14.7-5.** Coagulation Terms and Abbreviations

| Term | Abbreviation |
|---|---|
| $\alpha_1$-antitrypsin | AAT |
| $\alpha_2$-macroglobulin | AMG |
| antithrombin III | ATIII |
| $\alpha$-ATIII isoform | $\alpha$-ATIII |
| $\beta$-ATIII isoform | $\beta$-ATIII |
| ATIII/heparin complex | Do not abbreviate |
| C1 inhibitor | C1 INH (see 14.8.3, Complement) |
| heparin cofactor II | Do not abbreviate |
| lupus coagulation inhibitor (also called lupus anticoagulant) | LCI |
| protein C | Do not abbreviate |
| activated protein C | APC |
| protein S | Do not abbreviate |
| protein Z | Do not abbreviate |
| serpin (serine protease inhibitor) | Do not abbreviate |
| tissue factor pathway inhibitor | TFPI |

**14.7.4.2** **Fibrinolysis (Fibrin Degradation, Clot Degradation, Thrombolysis).** The sample terms listed in Table 14.7-6 represent entities that are involved in fibrinolysis or its inhibition. Expand at first mention in accordance with 13.11, Clinical, Technical, and Other Common Terms.

**14.7.4.3** **Tests of Coagulation.** Two among several tests of coagulation are the prothrombin time (PT) and the partial thromboplastin time (PTT). When the more common activated partial thromboplastin time (aPTT) is used instead of the PTT, this should be specified.

Traditionally, the prothrombin ratio (PTR) had been reported as a ratio of the patient's PT to the mean laboratory control PT. Reporting the PTR has been refined by use of a modified PTR, the international normalized ratio (INR).[18-20] In accordance with a 1985 policy statement of the International Committee on Thrombosis and Haemostasis and the International Committee for Standardization in Haematology,[18] authors are encouraged to report the INR if at all possible. Unlike conversions between conventional and SI units (see 17.1, SI Units), there is no simple conversion factor from the PTR to the INR because the international sensitivity index (ISI) of the thromboplastin used in the actual assay performed must be known. The INR is calculated as shown:

$$INR = PTR^{ISI}$$

**Table 14.7-6.** Fibrinolysis Terms and Abbreviations

| Term | Abbreviation |
|---|---|
| $α_2$-plasmin inhibitor, $α_2$-antiplasmin | $α_2$PI |
| aminocaproic acid (Amicar) | ACA |
| ε-aminocaproic acid | EACA |
| dimerized plasmin fragment D | D-dimer |
| fibrin degradation products or fibrin split products | FDP or FSP |
| Glu-plasminogen (see 14.6.1, Nucleic Acids and Amino Acids) | Do not abbreviate |
| Lys-plasminogen (see 14.6.1, Nucleic Acids and Amino Acids) | Do not abbreviate |
| a plasminogen activator inhibitor | PAI-1 |
| protein C inhibitor | PAI-3 |
| thrombin-activated fibrinolytic inhibitor | TAFI |
| tissue plasminogen activator (when a specific therapeutic formulation of tPA is intended, use the USAN term; see 14.4, Drugs) | tPA |
| tissue plasminogen activator receptor | tPAR |
| urokinase or urinary-type plasminogen activator | uPA |
| urokinase or urinary-type plasminogen activator receptor | uPAR |

Authors should specify the exact method by which their results were initially reported by the laboratory performing the assay and the method of conversion, if any, used on the original results.

**Principal Author:** Cheryl Iverson, MA

## ACKNOWLEDGMENT

Thanks to David Green, MD, PhD, Feinberg School of Medicine of Northwestern University, Chicago, Illinois, for reviewing and providing comments.

## REFERENCES

1. Monroe DM, Hoffman M. What does it take to make the perfect clot? *Arterioscler Thromb Vasc Biol.* 2006;26(1):41-48. doi:10.1161/01.ATV.0000193624.28251.83
2. Marder VJ, Aird WC, Bennett JS, Schulman S, White GC II, eds. *Hemostasis and Thrombosis: Basic Principles and Clinical Practice.* 6th ed. Lippincott Williams & Wilkins; 2013.
3. *Dorland's Illustrated Medical Dictionary.* 32nd ed. WB Saunders; 2012.
4. Konkle B. Bleeding and thrombosis. In: Longo DL, Kasper DL, Jameson JL, Fauci AS, Hauser SL, Loscalzo J, eds. *Harrison's Principles of Internal Medicine.* 18th ed. McGraw-Hill; 2012:457-464.
5. *Stedman's Medical Dictionary.* 28th ed. Lippincott Williams & Wilkins; 2006.

6. Owen CA Jr. *A History of Blood Coagulation*. Mayo Foundation for Education and Research; 2001.

7. Giangrande PL. Six characters in search of an author: the history of the nomenclature of coagulation factors. *Br J Haematol*. 2003;121(5):703-712. doi:10.1046/j.1365-2141.2003.04333.x

8. Blomback M, Abildgaard U, van den Besselaar AM, et al. Nomenclature of quantities and units in thrombosis and haemostasis (recommendation 1993): a collaborative project of the Scientific and Standardization Committee of the International Society on Thrombosis and Haemostasis (ISTH/SSC) and the Commission/Committee on Quantities and Units (in Clinical Chemistry) of the International Union of Pure and Applied Chemistry–International Federation of Clinical Chemistry (IUPAC-IFCC/CQU[CC]). *Thromb Haemost*. 1994;71(3):375-394.

9. The International Society on Thrombosis and Haemostasis website. Accessed July 31, 2019. https://www.isth.org

10. Peake I, Tuddenham E. A standard nomenclature for factor VIII and factor IX gene mutations and associated amino acid alterations: on behalf of the ISTH SSC Subcommittee on Factor VIII and Factor IX. *Thromb Haemost*. 1994;72(3):475-476.

11. Marder VJ, Mannucci PM, Firkin BG, Hoyer LW, Meyer D. Standard nomenclature for factor VIII and von Willebrand factor: a recommendation by the International Committee on Thrombosis and Haemostasis. *Thromb Haemost*. 1985;54(4):871-872.

12. Marder VJ, Roberts HR. Proposed symbols for factor VIII and von Willebrand factor. *Ann Intern Med*. 1986;105(4):627. doi:10.7326/0003-4819-105-4-627_1

13. von Willebrand Factor Variant database. Accessed July 31, 2019. www.vwf.group.shef.ac.uk/variant.html

14. Sadler JE, Budde U, Eikenboom JCJ, et al; Working Party on von Willebrand Disease Classification. Update on the pathophysiology and classification of von Willebrand disease: a report of the Subcommittee on von Willebrand Factor. *J Thromb Haemost*. 2006;4(10):2103-2114. doi:10.1111/j.1538-7836.2006.02146.x

15. OMIM: Online Mendelian Inheritance in Man. Updated May 15, 2018. Accessed May 16, 2018. https://www.ncbi.nlm.nih.gov/omim

16. Hampshire DJ, Goodeve AC. The International Society on Thrombosis and Haemostasis von Willebrand Disease database: an update. *Semin Thromb Hemost*. 2011;37(5):470-479. doi:10.1055/s-0031-1281031

17. Goodeve AC, Eikenboom JCJ, Ginsburg D, et al. A standard nomenclature for von Willebrand factor gene mutations and polymorphisms on behalf of the ISIH SSC Subcommittee on von Willebrand Factor. *Thromb Haemost*. 2001;85(5):929-931.

18. International Committee for Standardization in Haematology, International Committee on Thrombosis and Haemostasis: ICSH/ICTH recommendations for reporting prothrombin time in oral anticoagulant control. *Thromb Haemost*. 1985;53(1):155-156.

19. Hirsh J, Dalen JE, Deykin D, Poller L. Oral anticoagulants: mechanism of action, clinical effectiveness, and optimal therapeutic range. *Chest*. 1992;102(suppl 4):312S-326S.

20. Hirsh J, Poller L. The international normalized ratio: a guide to understanding and correcting its problems. *Arch Intern Med*. 1994;154(3):282-288. doi:10.1001/archinte.1994.00420030084008

## 14.8 ▌ **Immunology.**

### 14.8.1 ▌ **Chemokines.** Chemokines comprise a family of more than 40 low-molecular-weight cytokines (see 14.8.4, Cytokines) with important roles in the immune system and functions beyond it.[1-6] The name *chemokine,* a contraction of "chemotactic cytokine," reflects the common property, by which they were originally identified, of promoting leukocyte chemotaxis.

Chemokines are defined by structure, not function, and are classified into 4 subfamilies based on their cysteine (C) residues and other amino acid (X) residues (see 14.6.1, Nucleic Acids and Amino Acids):

CXC     1 amino acid residue between the 2 *N*-terminal cysteines

CC       *N*-terminal cysteines adjacent

XC       cysteines 1 and 3 not present

CX3C    3 amino acids between the cysteine residues

The group names are roots followed by the letter L and a number (eg, CXCL1).[4(p146)] Examples of specific chemokines, by subfamily, are given in **Table 14.8-1**.

Expanded common names of the chemokines are often unwieldy and uninformative and so are rarely used, although use of the abbreviations persists. Terms such as those in Table 14.8-1 for chemokine, chemokine subfamily, and chemokine receptor do not need to be expanded, but context should be provided at first mention:

the CXC chemokine family

the chemokine CXCL1

chemokine receptor CXCR2

### 14.8.2 ▌ **CD Cell Markers.** CDs (clusters of differentiation) are a system for identifying cellular surface markers, a number of which define lymphocyte subsets (see 14.8.7, Nomenclature, Lymphocytes).[7-12] The system and its nomenclature were formalized in a 1982 international workshop. Originally, CD terms specified the monoclonal antibodies (mAbs) that clustered statistically in their reactivities to target cells. More recently, the CD terms apply to the cellular molecules themselves. The CDs, which now number nearly 400 (and may eventually number in the thousands[12]), are defined at the Human Cell Differentiation Molecules workshops (formerly Human Leukocyte Differentiation Antigen Workshops). Workshops involve "multiple laboratories examining coded panels of antibodies [with] multilaboratory blind analysis and statistical evaluation of the results."[11(p226)] Although reactivity and cellular expression originally were key in identifying CDs, gene-based molecular relatedness has become an important determinant.[11,12] See the Human Cell Differentiation Molecules website for updates on the most recent workshop and conference, including confirmed, validated antibodies and newly assigned CDs.[13]

Some CDs are known most commonly by their CD designation. Other molecules have been assigned CD numbers retroactively; although they will be referred to

**Table 14.8-1.** Examples of Specific Chemokines by Subfamily

| Subfamily name | Synonym | Examples[5] Systematic name | Common names and abbreviation | Receptors |
|---|---|---|---|---|
| CXC | α class | CXCL1 | growth-related oncogene α (GRO-α), melanoma growth stimulatory activity protein (MGSA) | CXCR2 |
| | | CXCL4 | platelet factor 4 (see 14.7, Hemostasis) | NA |
| | | CXCL5 | epithelial cell–derived neutrophil attractant 78 (ENA-78) | CXCR2 |
| | | CXCL6 | granulocyte chemoattractant protein 2 (GCP-2) | CXCR1, CXCR2 |
| | | CXCL8 | interleukin 8 (IL-8) (see 14.8.4, Cytokines) | CXCR1, CXCR2 |
| | | CXCL14 | chemokine isolated from breast and kidney tissue (BRAK), bolekine | NA |
| CC | β class | CCL1 | inducible 309 (I-309) | CCR8 |
| | | CCL3 | macrophage inflammatory protein 1a or 1α (MIP-1α) | CCR1, CCR5 |
| | | CCL5 | regulated on activation of normal T cells expressed and secreted (RANTES) | CCR1, CCR3, CCR5 (also called CD195; see 14.8.2, CD Cell Markers) |
| | | CCL7 | monocyte chemoattractant (or chemotactic) protein 3 (MCP-3) | CCR1, CCR2, CCR3 |
| | | CCL21 | secondary lymphoid tissue chemokine (SLC), chemokine β-9 (CKβ-9), exodus 2, 6Ckine | CCR7 (also called CDw107; see 14.8.2, CD Cell Markers) |
| XC | γ class | XCL1 | lymphotactin, activation-induced, T-cell–derived, and chemokine-related (ATAC), single cysteine motif 1α (SCM-1α) | XCR1 |
| | | XCL2 | single cysteine motif 1β (SCM-1β) | XCR1 |
| CX3C | δ class | CX3CL1 | fractalkine | CX3CR1 |

Abbreviation: NA, not applicable.

by their common names, it is useful for authors to include the CD designations.[11] Terms related to CDs do not need to be expanded. See the examples in **Table 14.8-2**.

A lowercase w (for "workshop") signifies a provisional cluster (which is likely to become final, and have the w dropped, in an upcoming workshop[11]):

CDw186

**Table 14.8-2.** Examples of Terms Related to Clusters of Differentiation

| CD terms | Other name(s)[13,14] |
|---|---|
| CD1a | CD1, CD1A |
| CD3d | CD3D, CD3-delta, T3D |
| CD4 | NA (see 14.8.7, Lymphocytes) |
| CD6 | TP120 |
| CD8a | CD8A, CD8, p32 (see 14.8.7, Lymphocytes) |
| CD10 | membrane metalloendopeptidase (MME), CALLA (common acute lymphoblastic leukemia antigen), CD10, neprilysin (NEP), enkephalinase |
| CD16a | FCGR3A (an Fc receptor; see 14.8.6, Immunoglobulins), FCG3, FCGR3, CD16 |
| CD35 | complement receptor type 1 (CR1; see 14.8.3, Complement), C3BR, CD35 |
| CD41 | glycoprotein IIb (see 14.1.2, Platelet-Specific Antigens), GP2B, GPIIb, CD41B |
| CD44R | CD44 variant, CD44v1-10 |
| CD46 | membrane cofactor protein (MCP; see 14.8.3.3, Complement Regulators), MGC26544 |
| CD50 | intracellular adhesion molecule 3 (ICAM-3) |
| CD55 | delay accelerating factor (DAF; see 14.8.3, Complement) |
| CD62P | CD62, PSEL (P selectin), granule membrane protein 140 (GMP-140), GRMP |
| CD79a | Igα (see 14.8.6, Immunoglobulins); MB-1 |
| CD97 | TM7LN1 |
| CD107a | lysosomal-associated membrane protein 1 (LAMP-1), CD107A |
| CD120a | tumor necrosis factor receptor (TNF-R) type 1, TNFR |
| CD139 | NA |
| CD195 | CCR5 (see 14.8.1, Chemokines) |
| CD213a2 | IL-13Ra2 (see 14.8.4, Cytokines) |
| CD220 | NA |
| CD235a | glycophorin a (GPA) |
| CD240CE | Rh blood group, CcEe antigens (see 14.1.1, Blood Groups) |

Abbreviation: NA, not available.

The new designation of CDw128a is CD181.

Complexes of more than 1 CD molecule are indicated with a virgule:

CD11a/CD18 (leukocyte functional antigen 1 [LFA-1])

CD11b/CD18 (CR3 or C3bi receptor; see 14.8.3, Complement)

CD49c/CD29

The CD nomenclature displaced previous terms, for example, CD8 for T8 or OKT8, CD4 for T4 or OKT4, CD5 for Leu-1, Lyt-1, and CD5 for T1.

For therapeutic monoclonal antibody nomenclature, see 14.4, Drugs.

**14.8.3** **Complement.** The term *complement* refers to a group of serum proteins activated sequentially and rapidly in a cascade that produces molecules providing resistance to pathogens.[15] The system was named in 1899 for its complementarity with antibodies in destroying microbes.[15]

Current nomenclature derives largely from the 1968 World Health Organization Bulletin "Nomenclature of Complement,"[16] with subsequent modifications as mechanisms of action were further elucidated.

Three complement activation pathways are recognized: the classical pathway (activation by antibody), the alternative pathway (despite the name, the more phylogenetically ancient), and the lectin pathway. They culminate in a common terminal pathway. Components of the classical and terminal pathways are designated with a C and a number, reflective of the order of discovery of the component rather than the reaction sequence. (The prime, as in C′, has been discontinued.) Letters and abbreviations other than C typify the components of the other pathways. Complement component terms need not be expanded:

| | |
|---|---|
| Classical | C1, C4, C2 |
| Alternative | factors D, B, P (P for properdin ["destruction-bringing"[14]]) |
| Lectin or MB lectin | mannose-binding lectin (MBL), MBL-associated serine protease 1 (MASP-1), MASP-2, MASP-3 |
| Terminal | C5, C6, C7, C8, C9 |
| | C3 (common to all pathways) |

**14.8.3.1** **Fragments.** Appended lowercase letters indicate complement fragments. Usually, a lowercase b indicates the larger, active (membrane-binding) fragment and a lowercase a, the smaller, release fragment (released on cleavage of the parent molecule). However, C2 is inconsistent: C2a is the larger active fragment and C2b the smaller release fragment. Other letters represent fragments of b fragments.

| | | | | | |
|---|---|---|---|---|---|
| C3a | C3b | C3c | C3d | Cdg | C3f |
| C4a | C4b | C4c | C4d | | |
| C5a | C5b | | | | |
| Bb | | | | | |

**14.8.3.2** **Subunits.** The subunits of C1 are as follows:

C1q    C1r    C1s

Various notations that combine the C1 subunits convey the stoichiometry (relative quantities of subunits) of the complex; all such styles are acceptable:

$(C1r)_2$

$C1r_2C1s_2$

$C1qC1r_2C1s_2$

$C1qr_2s_2$

C1s-C1r-C1r-C1s

Isotypes of C4 have capital letters appended:

C4A          C4B

Protein chains have Greek letters appended:

C8$\alpha$

C8$\beta$

C8$\gamma$

C3$\alpha$ is the $\alpha$ chain of C3.

Cleavage of C3$\alpha$ produces C3a and C3b.

An i signifies inactive forms:

iC3 or C3i

iC3b

Complement components that form a complex are written in a series without spaces:

C4b2a3b

C4bC2

Sometimes a hyphen is used to indicate a series:

C5b67 or C5b-7

C5-9

An asterisk shows nascent or metastable state:

C4b*

C3b*

C5b*

C5b-7*

Convertase complexes are linked complement fragments that activate other complement components. For example, the convertase that activates C3 is known as C3 convertase. As in the following examples, the convertases have different compositions, depending on which complement pathway generated them:

C3 convertase    Classical pathway, C4b2a; alternative pathways, C3bBb, C3bBbP, C3(H$_2$O)Bb(Mg$^{2+}$)

C5 convertase    Classical pathway, C4b2a3b; alternative pathways, C3bBbC3b, (C3b)2Bb

Note: Occasionally, authors have changed the designation of the activated moiety of C2 from C2a to C2b, to be consistent with other complement components.[17,18(p8)] A tipoff to the change is the designation of classical pathway C3 convertase as C4b2b.

**14.8.3.3** **Complement Regulators.** Complement regulators include those listed in **Table 14.8-3**.

**14.8.3.4** **Complement Receptors.** Complement receptors include those listed in **Table 14.8-4**.

**14.8.4** **Cytokines.** Cytokines are proteins or glycoproteins produced after stimulation (such as activation of immune cells) that act at short distances in low concentrations

**Table 14.8-3.** Examples of Complement Regulators

| Name | Other terms |
|---|---|
| C1 inhibitor (C1-INH)[a] | C1 esterase inhibitor, C1 esterase INH |
| C3 membrane proteinases | NA |
| C4 binding protein (C4bp) | NA |
| carboxypeptidases | NA |
| CD59 | membrane inhibitor of reactive lysis (MIRL), membrane attack complex–inhibitory factor (MACIF), homologous restriction factor 20 (HRF20), P18, protectin |
| decorin | NA |
| delay accelerating factor (DAF) | CD55 |
| factor H | formerly β$_1$H |
| factor I [letter I, not roman numeral "one"] | NA |
| factor H–like protein (FHL-1) | NA |
| membrane cofactor protein (MCP) | CD46 |
| S protein[a] | vitronectin |
| SP-40,40 | clusterin |

Abbreviation: NA, not applicable.
[a]Not the same as protein S (see 14.7.4, Inhibition of Coagulation and Fibrinolysis).

**Table 14.8-4.** Examples of Complement Receptors

| Name | Other terms |
|---|---|
| complement receptor type 1 (CR1) | C3b receptor, CD35 |
| CR2 | C3d receptor, CD21, CD21S (short isoform), CD21L (long isoform) |
| CR3 | Mac-1, CD11b/CD18 |
| CR4 | p150/95, CD11c/CD18 |
| C3aR | NA |
| C4aR | NA |
| C5aR | CD88 |
| cC1qR | collectin receptor; c prefix: collagen region of C1q |
| gC1qR | g prefix: globular head portion of C1q |
| C1qR$_p$ | NA |
| factor H receptor (fH-R) | NA |

Abbreviation: NA, not applicable.

to produce various effects, such as immune and inflammatory reactions, repair processes, and cell growth and differentiation.[4,6,19-22] Like hormones, cytokines are growth factors. Each cytokine has multiple effects and overlaps with other cytokines, including structurally dissimilar ones, in those effects. The multiple effects (pleiotropy) are explained by the presence of cytokine receptors on a wide variety of cells and the overlap (redundancy) by structural similarities of the intracellular portions of cytokine receptors.[23]

Cytokines were originally named by function. Because of their multiple and overlapping functions,[19] the interleukin nomenclature[24,25] was proposed to simplify terminology of this major class of cytokines and, it was hoped, subsequent regulatory immune system proteins. The more recent grouping of cytokines by receptor families and signaling pathways, however, does not necessarily correspond to previous groupings (eg, the interleukins fall into more than one family).

**14.8.4.1** **Cytokine Families and Subfamilies.** Molecular similarity of cytokine receptors has resulted in their grouping into families and subfamilies[23]:

> chemokine families (see 14.8.1, Chemokines)
>
> colony-stimulating factor (CSF)
>
> interleukin 1/toll-like receptors (IL-1/TLR)
>
> platelet-derived growth factor family (PDGF)
>
> receptor tyrosine kinases
>
> transforming growth factor β (TGF-β) receptor serine kinase family
>
> tumor necrosis factor (TNF)

type 1 (hematopoietins)

$\beta_c$-utilizing (common cytokine receptor β chain)

$\gamma_c$-utilizing (common cytokine receptor γ chain)

gp130-utilizing

heterodimeric

homodimeric

type 2 (interferons; IL-10 family receptors)

heterodimeric

Cytokine signaling pathways are associated with families and subfamilies (**Table 14.8-5**).

The pathway terms need not be expanded, but context should be clear at first mention:

the Jak1 signaling pathway

**14.8.4.2** **Chemokines.** See 14.8.1, Chemokines.

**14.8.4.3** **Colony-Stimulating Factors.** Colony-stimulating factors (CSFs) stimulate growth and differentiation of 1 or more blood cell types (neutrophils, eosinophils, monocytes/macrophages). Terms often, but not always, include the letters SF (eg, interleukins 3, 4, and 5—IL-3, IL-4, IL-5—which are also CSFs). Expand such terms at first mention:

| | |
|---|---|
| granulocyte-macrophage colony-stimulating factor | GM-CSF |
| granulocyte colony-stimulating factor | G-CSF |
| macrophage colony-stimulating factor | M-CSF |

**14.8.4.4** **Hormones.** These hormones are also considered cytokines:

| | |
|---|---|
| erythropoeitin | Epo |
| growth hormone | GH |
| leptin | |
| prolactin | PrL |
| thrombopoietin | Tpo |

**14.8.4.5** **Interleukins.** A subset of cytokines were designated as interleukins in 1978 for "their ability to act as communication signals between different populations of leukocytes."[24(p2929)] The interleukins have other biological effects as well. Their nomenclature was formalized in 1991.[25] They are designated by number in order of discovery (eg, interleukin 1, interleukin 18, interleukin 29) but in general have no structural or functional association with one another. Although most have now been recognized as members of larger cytokine families, they retain their original designations. Specific interleukins are mentioned most commonly in their abbreviated form (note hyphen):

**Table 14.8-5.** Cytokine Signaling Pathways and Associated Families

| Cytokine signaling pathways | Expansion or origin of term | Associated cytokine family |
| --- | --- | --- |
| caspases | | TNF |
| FADD | Fas-associated death domain | TNF |
| FAST-1 | forkhead activin signal transducer | TGF-β receptor serine kinase family |
| IRAK | IL-1 receptor–associated kinase | IL-1/TLR |
| Jak1 | Janus kinase 1 | type 1 |
| Jak2 | Janus kinase 2 | type 1 |
| Jak3 | Janus kinase 3 | type 1 |
| MyD88 | myeloid differentiation marker | IL-1/TLR |
| NF-κB | nuclear factor–κB | IL-1/TLR |
| Ras/Raf/MAPK | ras protein, raf protein (see 14.6.3, Oncogenes and Tumor Suppressor Genes), mitogen-activated protein kinases | type 1, receptor tyrosine kinases |
| SARA | SMAD anchor for receptor activation | TGF-β receptor serine kinase family |
| SMADs | mothers against decapentaplegic (dpp) signaling (MAD) in *Drosophila* and *Sma* genes from *Caenorhabditis elegans*[26] | TGF-β receptor serine kinase family |
| STAT1 | signal transducer and activator of transcription 1 | type 1 |
| STAT2 | | type 1 |
| STAT3 | | type 1 |
| STAT4 | | type 1 |
| STAT5 | | type 1 |
| STAT5a | | type 1 |
| STAT5b | | type 1 |
| STAT6 | | type 1 |
| TAK1 | TGF-β–associated kinase | TGF-β receptor serine kinase family |
| TRADD | TNF receptor–associated death domain | TNF |
| TRAFs | TNF-α receptor–associated factors | TNF |
| TRAF6 | | IL-1/TLR |
| Tyk2 | tyrosine kinase 2 | type 1 |

IL-1

IL-18

IL-29

The IL-1 family includes 2 forms of IL-1:

IL-1α

IL-1β

and the IL-1 receptor antagonist:

IL-1ra

Receptors for interleukins are designated, at minimum, with the interleukin name plus a capital R:

IL-2R

IL-4R

Receptor names designating subtypes may be even more specific:

IL-1RI

IL-1RII

Greek letters are used for subunits (chains) of the same receptor:

| | |
|---|---|
| IL-2Rα | IL-2Rβ |
| IL-6Rα | IL-6Rβ |
| IL-12Rβ1 | IL-12Rβ2 |

Terms for interleukins from different species should be expanded at first mention:

| | |
|---|---|
| human IL-2 | hIL-2 |
| mouse IL-4 | mIL-4 |
| viral IL-10 | vIL-10 |

For terminology for therapeutic interleukins, see 14.4.13, Nomenclature for Biological Products.

**14.8.4.6** **Interferons.** Interferons (IFNs) are another group of cytokines, originally discovered (and named) because of their interference with viral replication.
The type I IFNs, also known as *antiviral interferons,* are as follows:

IFN-α

IFN-β

IFN-λ1 (IL-29)

IFN-λ2 (IL-28A)

IFN-λ (IL-28B)

IFN-κ

IFN-ω

IFN-τ

Type II IFN, also known as *immune interferon,* is

IFN-γ

For terminology for therapeutic interferons, see 14.4.13, Nomenclature for Biological Products.

**14.8.4.7** **Other Cytokines.** Other cytokines and their abbreviations include the following:

| | |
|---|---|
| cardiotrophin 1 | CT-1 |
| ciliary neurotrophic factor | CNTF |
| endothelial growth factor | EGF |
| fibroblast growth factor | FGF |
| FLT-3/FLT-2 ligand | FL |
| high-mobility group box chromosomal protein 1 | HMGB-1 |
| leukemia inhibitory factor | LIF |
| lymphotoxin α | LTα |
| oncostatin M | OSM |
| receptor activator of NF-κB ligand | RANKL |
| stem cell factor | SCF, c-kit ligand |
| transforming growth factor β | TGF-β, TGF-β1, TGF-β2, TGF-β3 |
| tumor necrosis factor α | Use tumor necrosis factor, TNF |
| tumor necrosis factor β | Use lymphotoxin |
| vascular endothelial growth factor | VEGF |

**14.8.5** **HLA/Major Histocompatibility Complex.** Antigens of what is known as the HLA system appear on virtually all nucleated cells of human tissues and on platelets. Just as red blood cell antigens determine blood type (see 14.1, Blood Groups, Platelet Antigens, and Granulocyte Antigens), HLA antigens determine tissue type.

HLA antigens were discovered to be determinants of the success of tissue transplantation (histocompatibility, *histo-* meaning "relating to tissue"). They were subsequently found to be critical for activating many immune responses, and certain HLA antigens are associated with particular diseases. Because of the great variation among individuals in these antigens (polymorphism), they have been used in forensic identification.

There are approximately 21 main polymorphic genes of interest in the HLA system that are encoded within a region of the short arm of chromosome 6 known as the *major histocompatibility complex* (MHC). More than 10 000 variants have been identified.[27] The magnitude of this polymorphism distinguishes the HLA system from other gene families and has resulted in a detailed system for naming alleles and antigens.

Although HLA alleles were originally classified based on serologic and cellular assays, the current classification is based on DNA sequencing. Accordingly, in 1987, new nomenclature for these alleles consistent with the International System for Human Gene Nomenclature (see 14.6.2, Human Gene Nomenclature) was built onto the original nomenclature.[28,29] A prime goal was for the nomenclature to reflect the association between serologically defined antigen specificities and those defined by DNA technology.[30] With a large growth in the number of new alleles identified by DNA sequencing, many new alleles lack known serologic counterparts.[31]

**14.8.5.1** **Nomenclature.** Nomenclature of the HLA system, first formalized in 1967,[32] is determined by the World Health Organization Nomenclature Committee for Factors of the HLA System. Full reports on HLA nomenclature, which present officially recognized antigens and alleles, appear annually, with monthly updates, in the journals *Human Immunology, HLA* (formerly *Tissue Antigens*), and *International Journal of Immunogenetics*; on the website of the Anthony Nolan Research Institute (https://www.anthonynolan.org/clinicians-and-researchers/anthony-nolan-research-institute); and at the IMGT/HLA Sequence database.[27]

**14.8.5.1.1** **HLA.** The abbreviation HLA has come to signify *human leukocyte antigen(s)*. The original term was *HL-A*, the A being a simple letter designation, not an abbreviation for "antigen."[30] The term *HLA* applies to the locus of the human genome (MHC) that encodes specific HLA proteins and to the encoded proteins themselves. The term *MHC* is more generic, applicable to HLA molecules and their animal counterparts.

**14.8.5.1.2** **HLA Class I (MHC Class I Antigens).** The components of MHC class I molecules include the following:

- A polymorphic membrane-linked $\alpha$ chain or heavy chain, encoded within the MHC, comprising 3 domains: $\alpha_1$, $\alpha_2$, and $\alpha_3$

- A soluble invariant light chain called $\beta$-microglobulin ($\beta_2$m); encoded on chromosome 15, not within the MHC locus

- A short peptide, typically 8 to 11 amino acids long, that is variable in sequence

There are 3 genes encoding MHC class I–like heavy chain that also associate with $\beta_2$m:

class I genes: *HLA-A*   *HLA-B*   *HLA-C*

There are 3 additional genes encoding class I–like heavy chain that also associate with $\beta_2$m:

nonclassical (or class Ib): *HLA-E*   *HLA-F*   *HLA-G*

**14.8.5.1.3** **HLA Class II (MHC Class II Antigens).** The components of an MHC class II molecule include the following:

- A polymorphic membrane-linked α chain with 2 domains: $α_1$ and $α_2$

- A polymorphic membrane–linked β chain with 2 domains: $β_1$ and $β_2$

- A peptide, typically approximately 13 to 17 amino acids long, that is variable in sequence

The α and β chains of class I and class II molecules are not identical, despite the similar naming conventions, but rather are distinct proteins. Both the α chain and the β chain of MHC class II molecules are encoded within the MHC. There are 3 pairs of human MHC class II genes:

> class II genes:    *HLA-DR*    *HLA-DQ*    *HLA-DP*

**14.8.5.1.4** **Serologically Defined HLA Antigens.** Historically, antigen specificities of HLA class I molecules were defined serologically and indicated with numbers following the gene (major) locus letter(s), for example:

> HLA-A1    HLA-B27    HLA-DR1

A w (for "workshop") is used for serotype distinctions:

> HLA-Bw4 and Bw6 distinguish distinct serotypes of HLA-B heavy chains

> HLA-Cw1, HLA-Cw2, HLA-Cw3, etc, denote distinct serotypes

The term *cross-reactive group* (CREG) refers to serologically related groups of antigens. The abbreviation should be expanded at first mention. Note the following sample terms:

> the HLA-A1 cross-reactive group (CREG)

> the HLA-A2 CREG

> the B5 cross-reactive group HLA-B51, B52, and B53

> B7 CREG

Phrases such as the following may be used:

> HLA-A, HLA-B, and HLA-C associations, which can denote disease associations with the presence of particular HLA class I genotypes

> possible associations with HLA-B18, HLA-A2, and HLA-DQB1, which can denote disease associations with the presence of particular HLA class I or class II serotypes

> testing for HLA-A (A2, A26) and HLA-B (B35, B44), which denotes testing for particular HLA class I serotypes

> high prevalence of HLA-A1 (63%) and HLA-B8 (42%), which indicates frequencies of particular HLA class I serotypes within a test group

frequencies of HLA-A2 and A29, which refer to frequencies of indicated HLA class I serotypes within a test group

**14.8.5.1.5** **HLA Haplotypes.** The HLA haplotype is the set of HLA alleles on a given chromosome. Each person possesses 2 such haplotypes, 1 from each parent. Because of the high degree of polymorphism of the HLA class I and class II genes in the population, there are typically 2 different alleles of each of the class I and class II genes in an individual. When HLA typing is performed serologically, antigen specificities of the individual's phenotype are presented as follows:

| | |
|---|---|
| A3, A23, B51, B7, Cw2, Cw5, DR7, DR11 | all antigens listed collectively |
| A23, B7, Cw5, DR7/A3, B51, Cw2, DR11 | virgule separates antigens of one chromosome from those of other chromosome |
| A3, A23, B51, B7, Cw2, Cw5, DR11,- | hyphen indicates undetermined antigen |
| A1, B8, Cw4, DR17(3)/A2, B27, Cw5,- | DR for this haplotype not typed or untypable |
| A1, B8, Cw4, DR17(3)/A2, B27, Cw5, DR17(3) | 2 identical DR specificities |

Shorter haplotype expressions are shown below:

HLA-Cw6–bearing haplotype

the A1-B8-DR3 haplotypes

DRB1, DQA1, and DQB1 haplotypes

A25 B18 BFS DR11 haplotype

**14.8.5.1.6** **Other Histocompatibility Loci.** HLA antigens represent only some of the products of the MHC. Others, also important in immunity, are as follows:

*Class I loci*

MIC (MHC class I–related chain)

variants: MICA, MICB, MICC, MICD, MICE

*Class II loci*

*TAP* (transporter associated with antigen processing) and *TAPBP* are genes involved in the intracellular assembly of MHC class I molecules

*TAP1* and *TAP2* encode subunits of the TAP transporter

PSMB (proteosome-related sequence)

specificities: PSMB8 (formerly LMP7), PSMB9 (formerly LMP2), which encode interferon γ–inducible subunits of the proteasome, a proteolytic complex relevant to antigen presentation by HLA class I molecules

DM

*DMA* and *DMB*, encoding subunits of HLA-DM, important for the intracellular assembly of HLA class II molecules

DO

DOA and DOB, encoding subunits of HLA-DO, important for the intracellular assembly of HLA class I molecules

*Class III loci* (loci for 4 components of complement; see 14.8.3, Complement):

C2

C4 (2 genes: *C4A* and *C4B*)

Bf (B factor, properdin)

A haplotype of complement types is called a *complotype,* for example:

BfS, C2C, C4AQO, C4B1

(QO designates a deficiency.)

**14.8.5.1.7** **Genetic and Allele Nomenclature.** Use italics to distinguish HLA genes or gene loci from protein products (eg, *HLA-A, HLA-DRB1*) (see 14.6.2, Human Gene Nomenclature). The hyphen is retained in HLA gene expressions, an exception permitted in official gene nomenclature. Terms with asterisks indicate that HLA typing has been performed by molecular techniques. Terms with 2 digits (eg, A*02) indicate antigen typing with known serologic equivalent. Terms with 4 digits (eg, A*02:01) represent alleles. In contrast to other alleles, HLA alleles are usually not italicized. Authors should make clear from context whether the gene or its product is being discussed.

**Table 14.8-6,** adapted from Marsh,[33] summarizes nomenclature for HLA designations.

For the HLA-D region, the gene name includes a letter for the chain that the gene codes for (A for α, B for β), often followed by a number for the chain gene (*not* the domain number, as described in the previous section on class I and class II molecules). For instance,

*DRB1*     gene for first DR β chain

*DQA1*     gene for first DQ α chain

The HLA prefix (including the hyphen) may be dropped from allele designations in series after first mention, eg:

comparative frequencies of HLA-DRB1*14, DQA1*03, DQA1*05, DQA1*01, DQB1*06

(*not:* HLA-DRB1*14 , -DQA1*03, -DQA1*05, -DQA1*01, -DQB1*06)

The conjunction *and* may be used to separate haplotypes but is not used before the final element in any single haplotype:

HLA-B38, DRB1*04:02, DRB4*01:01, DQB1*02:01, DQB1*03:02 (*not* and DQB1*03:02)

**Table 14.8-6.** Nomenclature for HLA Designations

| | |
|---|---|
| HLA | HLA region, prefix for an *HLA* gene |
| HLA-DRB1 *or HLA-DRB1 or DRB1* | A particular HLA locus, ie, DRB1 (B refers to the β-chain locus) |
| HLA-DRB1*13 | A group of alleles that encode the DR13 antigen (antigen conferring DR13 specificity) |
| HLA-DRB1*13:01:02[a] | An allele that differs by a synonymous variation from DRB1*13:01:01 |
| HLA-DRB1*13:01:01:02 | An allele that contains a variation outside the coding region from DRB1*13:01:01:01 |
| HLA-DRB1*13:01 | A specific HLA allele |
| HLA-A*24:09N | A null (N) allele, an allele that is not expressed |
| HLA-A*30:14L | An allele encoding a protein with significantly reduced or low (L) cell surface expression |
| HLA-A*24:02:01:02L | An allele encoding a protein with significantly reduced or low cell surface expression, where the variation is found outside the coding region |
| HLA-B*44:02:01:02S | An allele encoding a protein expressed as a secreted (S) molecule only |
| | cytoplasm (C)[b] |
| | aberrant (A) expression[b] |
| HLA-A*32:11Q | An allele that has a variation previously shown to have a significant effect on cell surface expression but where this has not been confirmed and its expression remains questionable (Q) |

[a]Change from previous nomenclature: fifth digit only (2) for synonymous variation. Former term: HLA-DRB1*13:01:2.
[b]As of March 2017, no alleles have been named with the C or A suffixes.[33]

HLA-B38, DRB1*04:02, DRB4*01:01, DQB1*02:01, DQB1*03:02 and HLA-B*07:02, DRB1*16:01, DRB5*02, DQB1*05:02 haplotypes

The portion of the term before the asterisk may be dropped in a series, provided it would be the same in each term:

DRB4*01:01:01:01, *01:03:01:02N, *01:03:02, *01:03:03, *01:05

Commas signify *and* and virgules (forward slashes) signify *or*.[34]

Thus, commas indicate corresponding alleles from chromosome pairs (see 14.8.5.1.5, HLA Haplotypes), eg:

Donor: A*01, 02; B*08, 44; DRB1*01, 03; DRB3

Recipient: A*02, 11; B*40, 15; DRB1*09, 11; DRB3, DRB4

Virgules (forward slashes) indicate an ambiguous result in HLA typing, eg, the term A*02:01/02:03/02:05 means that A*02:01 or A*02:03 or A*02:05 is present.

Multiple alleles can encode serologically defined antigens. Also, alleles not defined serologically may have no known associated antigenic specificity. Examples of specificities and allele names are shown below.

| | |
|---|---|
| A203 | A*02:03 |
| B78 | B*78:01, B*78:02:01, B*78:02:02 |
| B65(14) | B*14:02 |
| B50(21) | B*50:01 |
| DR53 | DRB4 (various, eg, DRB4*01:02, *01:03:03) |
| none | the E alleles (E*01:01, 01:02, etc) |
| none | the F allele F*01:01 |
| none | the G alleles (G*01:01:01, 01:01:02, etc) |

HLA pseudogenes (see 14.6.2, Human Gene Nomenclature) resemble and are located near the HLA loci but are not transcribed to produce functional products. The class I pseudogenes end in letters after *G*, and the class II pseudogenes end in numbers after *1*:

*HLA-H*    *HLA-J*    *HLA-K*    *HLA-L*    *HLA-N*

*HLA-S*    *HLA-X*    *HLA-Z*


*HLA-DRB2*    *HLA-DRB6*    *HLA-DRB8*    *HLA-DRB9*

*HLA-DQA2*    *HLA-DQB2*    *HLA-DQB3*    *HLA-DPA2*    *HLA-DPB2*

**14.8.5.2** **Animals.** In animals, major histocompatibility locus is abbreviated Mhc, using uppercase and lowercase.

The names for the Mhc in other animals[35] usually correspond to the expression HLA for humans (but not always, eg, the prototypical mouse locus, H-2). In this convention, the name is based on a common name or species name combined with LA (leukocyte antigen):

| | |
|---|---|
| cat | FLA |
| dog | DLA |
| domestic cattle | BoLA |
| domestic fowl | B |
| guinea pig | GPLA |
| horse | EqLA |
| mole rat | Smh |
| mouse | H-2 |

**Table 14.8-7.** Examples of Common Animal Terms

| Common animal name | Species designation | Mhc term | Former LA term |
|---|---|---|---|
| chimpanzee | *Pan troglodytes* | MhcPatr | ChLA |
| gorilla | *Gorilla gorilla* | MhcGogo | GoLA |
| orangutan | *Pongo pygmaeus* | MhcPopy | OrLA |
| rhesus macaque | *Macaca mulatta* | MhcMamu | RhLA |

| | |
|---|---|
| pig | SLA |
| rabbit | RLA |
| rat | RT1 |

Primate researchers use an alternative style based on the genus and species name (see 14.14, Organisms and Pathogens), which substitutes Mhc for LA.[35] Note the examples in **Table 14.8-7.**

**14.8.6**    **Immunoglobulins.** Immunoglobulins are the Y-shaped glycoproteins on the surface of B cells (see 14.8.7.1, B Lymphocytes) that can be secreted as antibodies in response to an antigenic stimulus (any molecule or composition of molecules from pathogens: bacterium, virus, parasite, or from transplanted organ that are recognized by immunoglobulin). Secreted antibodies can bind specifically to their antigens and in some cases can neutralize pathogens. The immunoglobulins were first recognized by serum electrophoresis and, because they were localized to the electrophoretic gamma zone, were originally referred to as γ-globulins.[36-40]

Each immunoglobulin monomer contains 2 heavy chains and 2 light chains connected by disulfide bonds and abbreviated as follows:

H        L

Each H chain and L chain, in turn, contains both constant and variable regions, abbreviated as follows:

C        V

$V_H$        variable region of heavy chain

$V_L$        variable region of light chain

$C_H$        constant region of heavy chain

$C_L$        constant region of light chain

Heavy chains have 1 variable ($V_H$) and 3 or 4 constant ($C_H$) domains that are abbreviated as follows:

$C_H1$    $C_H2$    $C_H3$    $C_H4$

Light chains have 1 variable ($V_L$) and 1 constant ($C_L$) domain.

**14.8.6.1** **Immunoglobulin Antigen-Binding Site.** The $V_H$ and the $V_L$ domains of the immunoglobulin's heavy and light chains have variable amino acid sequences, and together constitute the immunoglobulin antigen-binding site (Fab), also called immunoglobulin variable region (V).

There are 3 specific hypervariable regions within the variable regions of an immunoglobulin H or L chain that are known as complementarity-determining regions (CDRs) and are named as follows:

CDR1    CDR2    CDR3

Heavy- and light-chain CDRs are termed HDCR1, etc, and LDCR1, etc, respectively. Four relatively invariable regions between hypervariable regions are called framework regions and are designated as follows:

FR1    FR2    FR3    FR4

**14.8.6.2** **Immunoglobulin Constant Regions** The $C_H$ and $C_L$ domains of the carboxyl terminal of an immunoglobulin's heavy and light chains have an amino acid sequence that does not vary within a given class or subclass of immunoglobulin and are called immunoglobulin constant (C) regions. The carboxyl-terminal tail $C_H$ regions of 2 immunoglobulin heavy chains are called the immunoglobulin Fc region.[36(p2673)]

Enzyme cleavage and antibody engineering result in fragments of the immunoglobulin molecule with specific names. Expansion of these terms is not necessary.

| | |
|---|---|
| Fab | antigen-binding fragment |
| Fab′ | Fab with part of hinge region (flexible amino acid stretch in the central part of the IgG and IgA heavy chains, which links these 2 chains by disulfide bonds) |
| F(ab′)$_2$ | 2 linked Fab′ fragments |
| Fabc | |
| Fb | constant part of Fab fragment |
| Fc | crystallizable fragment |
| pFc′ | fragment that includes Fc that is formed by pepsin cleavage; the remaining fragment is F(ab′)$_2$ |
| Fd | portion of the heavy chain that is included in Fab fragment |
| Fv | variable part of Fab fragment |
| scFv | single-chain Fv, not Ab fragment; a fusion protein of $V_H$ and $V_H$ connected with a short peptide linker |

**14.8.6.3** **Heavy Chains.** There are 5 different classes of immunoglobulins that differ in the sequence and structure of their heavy-chain constant regions ($C_H$). The type of heavy chain identifies the class (isotype) of immunoglobulin. Heavy chains are named with the Greek letter that corresponds to the class of immunoglobulin.

These are listed below from the most to the least abundant antibodies in human serum[41,42]:

$\gamma$      IgG

$\alpha$      IgA

$\mu$      IgM

$\gamma$      IgD

$\varepsilon$      IgE

IgG and IgA subclasses and corresponding heavy chains are as follows:

$\gamma1$      IgG1

$\gamma2$      IgG2

$\gamma3$      IgG3

$\gamma4$      IgG4

$\alpha1$      IgA1

$\alpha2$      IgA2

$C_H$ domains may be specified according to isotype. For example,

$$C_\varepsilon 2 \quad C_\mu 4 \quad C_\alpha 3 \quad C_\gamma 3$$

The 2 transmembrane accessory proteins associated with surface immunoglobulins on some immune cells should not be confused with terms for immunoglobulin classes or heavy chains:

Ig$\alpha$ (immunoglobulin-associated $\alpha$, CD79a; this is not IgA or the $\alpha$ heavy chain)

Ig$\beta$ (immunoglobulin-associated $\beta$, CD79b)

**14.8.6.4**    **Light Chains.** There are 2 types of light chain (named for initials of the discoverers' surnames[43]):

$\kappa$      $\lambda$

Both types of light chain are associated with all 5 immunoglobulin classes; that is, an immunoglobulin molecule of any type might have $\kappa$ or $\lambda$ light chains (but not both types in the same molecule). In humans, there are 6 classes (isotypes) of $\lambda$ chain:

$$\lambda1 \quad \lambda2 \quad \lambda3 \quad \lambda4 \quad \lambda5 \quad \lambda6$$

$C_L$ and $V_L$ regions may be specified by light chain type, as follows:

$C_\kappa$      $C_\lambda$

$V_\kappa$      $V_\lambda$

Serologic markers and their associated chains are indicated with roman letters and a lowercase m:

| | |
|---|---|
| G1m | $\gamma 1$ |
| G2m | $\gamma 2$ |
| G3m | $\gamma 3$ |
| A2m, A2m(1), A2m(2)[44] | $\alpha 2$ |
| Em | $\varepsilon$ |
| Km | $\kappa$ |

**14.8.6.5** **Other Immunoglobulin Components.** The secretory forms of IgM and IgA contain an additional polypeptide, the J chain (not to be confused with the joining or J segments of the immunoglobulin gene loci; see 14.8.6.9, Immunoglobulin Genetics).

Secreted IgA also contains a secretory component, SC.

**14.8.6.6** **Molecular Formulas.** Different immunoglobulin isotypes could be secreted as monomers (IgG, IgA, IgE, IgD), dimers (IgA), or pentamers (IgM). The formulas below indicate the number of polypeptide chains that constitute an immunoglobulin molecule:

| | |
|---|---|
| $\gamma_2 L_2$ | IgG monomer with 2 $\gamma$ chains and 2 light chains |
| $\alpha_2 L_2$ | IgA monomer with 2 $\alpha$ chains and 2 light chains |
| $(\alpha_2 L_2)_2 SCJ$ | IgA dimer with 4 $\alpha$ chains, 4 light chains, an SC, and a J chain |
| $(\mu_2 L_2)_5$ | IgM pentamer with 10 $\mu$ chains and 10 light chains |
| $(\mu_2 L_2)_5 J$ | IgM pentamer with 10 $\mu$ chains, 10 light chains, and a J chain |
| $\delta_2 \kappa_2$ | IgD monomer with 2 $\delta$ chains and 2 $\kappa$ light chains |
| $\varepsilon_2 \lambda_2$ | IgE monomer with 2 $\varepsilon$ chains and 2 $\lambda$ light chains |

**14.8.6.7** **Ig Prefixes.** The following are examples of terms combining Ig and a single-letter prefix. It is best to expand these terms at first mention (especially those with the letters m or s, each of which has more than 1 meaning):

| | |
|---|---|
| mIgM | monomeric IgM |
| mIgM | membrane-bound IgM |
| pIg | polymeric immunoglobulin |
| pIgA | polymerized IgA |
| pIgR | receptor for polymeric immunoglobulin |
| sIg | surface immunoglobulin |
| sIgM | surface IgM |
| sIgA | secretory IgA |

**14.8.6.8**   **Fc Fragments and Fc Receptors.** Immunoglobulins bind to the Fc receptors expressed on the accessory cells via their FC regions and modulate functions of the cells. Fc fragments may be specified by the heavy chain class from which they arise[45]:

| | | | |
|---|---|---|---|
| Fcγ1 | Fcγ2 | Fcγ3 | Fcγ4 |
| Fcα1 | Fcα2 | | |
| Fcμ | | | |
| Fcδ | | | |
| Fcε | | | |

Receptors for the Fc portion of immunoglobulin molecules are named as follows (cell surface marker identities, if applicable, are shown in parentheses; see 14.8.2, CD Cell Markers):

| | | |
|---|---|---|
| IgG receptors: | FcγRI | (CD64) |
| | FcγRII | (CD32) |
| | FcγRIIIA | (CD16a) |
| | FcγRIIIB | (CD16b) |
| IgA receptor: | FcαR | (CD89) |
| IgM receptor: | FcμR | |
| IgE receptors: | FcεRI | |
| | FcεRII | (CD23) |

**14.8.6.9**   **Immunoglobulin Genetics.** Immunoglobulin H-chain and L-chain gene loci consist of families of gene segments, sequentially arrayed along the chromosome, with each set of segments containing alternative versions of the immunoglobulin V region. The 2 types of gene segment that encode the L-chain V region are called variable (V) and joining (J) gene segments. The H-chain locus includes an additional set of diversity (D) gene segments that lies between the arrays of V and J gene segments. These gene segments encoding the L-chain variable region can be referred to as follows:

$$V_L \quad J_L \quad C_H \text{ (or } V_\kappa \quad V_\lambda \quad J_\kappa)$$

These gene segments encoding the H-chain variable region can be referred to as follows:

$$V_H \quad D_H \quad J_H$$

Downstream of the gene segments encoding immunoglobulin variable region, there are segements of genes encoding constant immunoglobulin region. Heavy chain constant region gene segments contain regions encoding various classes (isotypes) of immunoglobulins and can be referred to as follows (the subscript number refers to the isotype subtype):

$$C_{\gamma 2} \quad C_{\mu} \quad C_{\alpha 2}$$

Subgroups (various nonallelic forms) of V, D, J, and C gene segments are specified numerically (subscript numbers refer to the class of Ig, online numbers refer to the subgroup), as follows:

$$V_{\kappa}1 \quad V_{\lambda}3 \quad D_{H}1 \quad D_{H}3 \quad J_{\kappa}2 \quad J_{H}1 \quad C_{\alpha 2}5 \quad C_{\lambda 1}1 \quad C_{\lambda}2$$

A superscript plus sign may be used to indicate expression of a specific segment, eg, by a particular B lymphocyte (see 14.8.7, Lymphocytes):

$$V_{\kappa}3^{+}$$

The V, D, and J gene segments are brought together by DNA rearrangement. Descriptive terms for this process include the following:

| | |
|---|---|
| V/J exon, segment, region, gene, recombination | in L-chain genes |
| V/D/J exon, segment, region, gene, recombination | in H-chain genes |
| V/(D)/J | L- and/or H-chain genes |
| VDJ, V/D/J, V-D-J, variable-diversity-joining | alternative terms |

A leader segment (L), which codes for a leader (L) peptide, precedes each V segment.

Note the following potential sources of confusion:

V, D, and J segments code for the variable (V) region of an immunoglobulin protein.

J segment does not refer to the J chain of the secretory forms of IgA and IgM (see 14.8.6.5, Other Immunologic Components).

L (leader) gene segment and L (light) immunoglobulin chain are different entities. (Subscript L's, as in various terms in this section, typically refer to the light chain.)

**14.8.6.10** **Official Gene Terminology.** Official gene symbols for specific genes of the types discussed above are presented in **Table 14.8-8** (see 14.6.2, Human Gene Nomenclature). Follow author usage.

**14.8.6.11** **Alleles.** Alleles are indicated with an asterisk and number following the gene name:

IGHA1*01

IGHD*02

IGHD1-7*01

IGLJ1*01

IGLV2-11*01

**Table 14.8-8.** Examples of Official Gene Symbols and Immunogenetic Terms

| Official gene symbol | Immunogenetic term |
| --- | --- |
| IGHA1 | $C_\alpha 1$ |
| IGHD | $C_\delta$ |
| IGHD1-1 | member of $D_H 1$ subgroup |
| IGHE | $C_\varepsilon$ |
| IGHG1 | $C_\gamma 1$ |
| IGHJ1 | $J_H 1$ |
| IGHV@ | $V_H$ |
| IGHV1-2 | member of $V_H 1$ subgroup |
| IGKC | $C_\kappa$ |
| IGKJ@ | $J_\kappa$ |
| IGKJ2 | $J_\kappa 2$ |
| IGKV@ | $V_\kappa$ |
| IGKV1-5 | member of $V_\kappa 1$ subgroup |
| IGLC@ | $C_\lambda$ |
| IGLC1 | $C_\lambda 1$ |
| IGLJ@ | $J_\lambda$ |
| IGLJ1 | $J_\lambda 1$ |
| IGLV@ | $V_\lambda$ |
| IGLV1-36 | member of $V_\lambda 1$ subgroup |

For more detailed molecular information about immunoglobulin genetics, consult the International ImMunoGeneTics database.[46]

**14.8.7** **Lymphocytes.** Lymphocytes are the cells that carry out antigen-specific immune responses.[47-49] The 2 main types are the T lymphocyte and the B lymphocyte, also called the T cell and the B cell. A hyphen does not appear in these terms, unless they are used adjectivally. The terms are not customarily expanded.

| | | |
| --- | --- | --- |
| T lymphocyte | T cell | T-cell lymphoma |
| B lymphocyte | B cell | B-cell signaling |

Historically, the letters T and B reflected the anatomic sites of maturation of the 2 groups of cells, the thymus and the bursa of Fabricius, respectively. (The bursa of Fabricius is a specialized organ in birds.) Because in human adults B cells mature in the bone marrow, the letter B is sometimes taken as signifying *bone marrow.*

A third group of lymphocytes is known as natural killer cells, abbreviated NK cells.

**14.8.7.1** **B Lymphocytes.** In the context of B-lymphocyte development, the prefixes pre- and pro- are encountered; note hyphenation:

> pro-B cell
>
> pre-B cell

B-cell subsets are named in various ways, eg:

> CD5$^+$ B cells
>
> B1 B cells
>
> MZ B cells

B-cell antigen receptors (BCRs) are membrane complexes of membrane immunoglobulins and the molecules Igα and Igβ (see 14.8.6, Immunoglobulins).

**14.8.7.2** **T Lymphocytes.** The main types of T lymphocyte are as follows (expand at first mention):

> helper T cells:  $T_H$ cells
>
> cytotoxic T cells:  $T_C$ cells, also called cytotoxic lymphocytes (CTL)

Most helper T cells express the cell marker CD4, and most cytotoxic T cells express the cell marker CD8 (see 14.8.2, CD Cell Markers), giving rise to the following terms:

> CD4 T cells  CD8 T cells

When presence or absence of a marker on a T cell is emphasized, superscript plus or minus signs are used. Presence and absence of the CD4 and CD8 markers are often indicated by the terms *positive* and *negative* (eg, double-positive lymphocytes), as shown in **Table 14.8-9.**

Because other cells (eg, monocytes) may express CD4, authors should use terms more specific than "CD4 cells," unless context has made clear which cells are referred to, eg:

> CD4 lymphocyte count (*not* CD4 cell count)

Subtypes of helper T cells are as follows:

> $T_H0$  $T_H1$  $T_H2$
>
> $T_H17$  Treg

The theoretical helper T precursor to these subtypes is abbreviated:

> $T_HP$

**Table 14.8-9.** Examples Indicating Presence or Absence of CD4 or CD8 Markers

| | | |
|---|---|---|
| CD4+ | | |
| CD4− | | |
| CD4+CD8− | single positive | a CD4 cell |
| CD4−CD8+ | single positive | a CD8 cell |
| CD4−CD8− | double negative | |
| CD2+CD4−CD8− | double negative | |
| CD4+CD8+ | double positive | |
| CD2+CD4+CD8− | single positive | a CD4 cell |
| CD2+CD4−CD8+ | single positive | a CD8 cell |
| CD3+CD4+CD8− | single positive | a CD4 cell |
| CD3+CD4−CD8+ | single positive | a CD8 cell |

**14.8.7.3** **T-Cell Receptors.** T-cell receptors (TCRs) are protein complexes on the surface of T cells.[50] The T-cell receptor–CD3 complex (abbreviated TCR-CD3) is a structure that recognizes antigen. Its subunits, or chains, are designated by Greek letters:

α chain

β chain

γ chain

δ chain

ε chain

ζ chain

η chain

(Do not confuse these chains with the components of MHC or Ig molecules, although there is some homology among them; see 14.8.5, HLA/Major Histocompatibility Complex, and 14.8.6, Immunoglobulins.)

The α and β chains are also referred to as follows:

TCRα and TCRβ

Linked α and β chains and linked γ and δ chains result in these terms:

| | |
|---|---|
| αβ dimer | γδ dimer |
| αβ heterodimer | γδ heterodimer |
| αβ receptor | γδ receptor |

$\alpha\beta$ cell $\qquad\qquad$ $\gamma\delta$ cell

$\alpha\beta$ T cell $\qquad\qquad$ $\gamma\delta$ T cell

T $\alpha\beta$ $\qquad\qquad$ T $\gamma\delta$

CD8$\alpha\beta$

The $\gamma$, $\delta$, $\epsilon$, $\zeta$, and $\eta$ chains constitute the CD3 complex. The CD3 chains are also referred to individually and as dimers:

CD3$\gamma$ $\qquad$ CD3$\delta$ $\qquad$ CD3$\epsilon$ $\qquad$ CD3$\zeta$ $\qquad$ CD3$\eta$

CD3$\gamma\epsilon$ $\qquad$ CD3$\delta\epsilon$ $\qquad$ CD3$\zeta\zeta$ $\qquad$ CD3$\zeta\eta$

There are 2 subtypes of the $\gamma$ chain:

$\gamma$1 $\qquad$ $\gamma$2

The TCR protein has variable (V) and constant (C) regions or domains. The gene for TCR$\alpha$ is made up of variable (V), joining (J), and constant (C) segments, as is the $\beta$ chain, which also has a diversity (D) segment. (These are analogous to the segments of the immunoglobulin genes; see 14.8.6, Immunoglobulins.) These segments may also be referred to as follows:

$V_\alpha$ $\quad$ $V_\beta$ $\quad$ $J_\alpha$ $\quad$ $J_\beta$ $\quad$ $D_\beta$ $\quad$ $C_\alpha$ $\quad$ $C_\beta$

Subgroups (various nonallelic forms) of the V, D, or J segments are specified numerically, eg:

$V_\alpha$2 $\qquad$ $J_\beta$7

T-cell expression of a particular segment may be indicated by using a superscript plus sign:

$V_\beta 2^+$

**14.8.7.4** **T-Cell Receptor Gene Terminology.** Because the V, D, and J gene segments together encode the variable (V) region of the protein, it is unusual to refer to D or J regions of the protein.[50]

The V, D, and J gene segments are brought together by DNA rearrangement. Descriptive terms include the following:

| | |
|---|---|
| V/J exon, segment, region, gene, recombination | for $\alpha$ or $\gamma$ chain genes |
| V/D/J exon, segment, region, gene, recombination | for $\beta$ or $\delta$ chains |
| V/(D)/J | of $\alpha$ and $\gamma$ or $\beta$ and $\delta$ chains |
| VDJ, V/D/J,V-D-J, variable-diversity-joining | alternative terms |

**14.8.7.5** **Official Gene Terminology.** Official gene symbols for specific genes of the types discussed above are presented in 14.6.2, Human Gene Nomenclature. The TCR genes begin with *TR* and use roman letters that correspond to the Greek letters of the TCR component chains, and they contain V, C, D, and J corresponding to the above terms. Like other immune genes, they may contain hyphens:

> *TRAC*    *TRBC*    *TRBV10-3*    *TRGC1*    *TRGJ*    *TRDC*

**14.8.7.6** **Alleles.** Alleles are indicated with an asterisk and number following the gene name:

TRBV7-1*01

**Principal Author:** Cheryl Iverson, MA

## ACKNOWLEDGMENT

Thanks to Preeti Malani, MD, MSJ, *JAMA*, and Department of Internal Medicine, University of Michigan, Ann Arbor; Irina Grigorova, PhD (Immunoglobulins and B Cells), Department of Microbiology and Immunology, University of Michigan, Ann Arbor; Malini Raghavan, PhD (HLA Antigens), Department of Microbiology and Immunology, University of Michigan, Ann Arbor; and Cheong-Hee Chang, PhD (T Lymphocytes), Department of Microbiology and Immunology, University of Michigan, Ann Arbor, for reviewing and providing comments.

## REFERENCES

1. IUIS/WHO Subcommittee on Chemokine Nomenclature. Chemokine/chemokine receptor nomenclature. *J Interferon Cytokine Res.* 2002;22(10):1067-1068. doi:10.1089/107999002760624305

2. Zlotnik A, Yoshie O. Chemokines: a new classification system and their role in immunity. *Immunity.* 2000;12(2):121-127. doi:10.1016/S1074-7613(00)80165-X

3. Murphy PM. Chemokines. In: Paul WE, ed. *Fundamental Immunology.* 7th ed. Lippincott Williams & Wilkins; 2013:681-707.

4. Rich RR, Fleisher T, Shearer WT, Schroeder HW Jr, Frew AJ, Weygand CM, eds. *Clinical Immunology: Principles and Practice.* 4th ed. WB Saunders; 2013.

5. Thomson AW, Lotze MT. *The Cytokine Handbook.* 4th ed. Academic Press; 2003.

6. Cytokine Family Database (dbCFC). Published August 3, 2010. Accessed October 18, 2019. http://cmbi.bjmu.edu.cn/cmbdata/cgf/CGF_Database/cytokine.medic. kumamoto-u.ac.jp/default.htm

7. Bernard A, Boumsell L. The clusters of differentiation (CD) defined by the First International Workshop on Human Leukocyte Differentiation Antigens. *Hum Immunol.* 1984;11(1):1-10. doi:10.1016/0198-8859(84)90051-X

8. Bernard A, Bernstein I, Boumsell L, et al. Differentiation human leukocyte antigens: a proposed nomenclature. *Immunol Today.* 1984;5(6):158-159. doi:10.1016/0167-5699(84)90002-1

9. IUIS/WHO Subcommittee on CD Nomenclature. Nomenclature for clusters of differentiation (CD) of antigens defined on human leukocyte populations. *Bull World Health Organ.* 1984;62(5):809-811.

10. Singer NG, Todd RF, Fox DA. Structures on the cell surface: update from the Fifth International Workshop on Human Leukocyte Differentiation Antigens. *Arthritis Rheum.* 1994;37(8):1245-1248. doi:10.1002/art.1780370820

11. Zola H. The CD nomenclature: a brief historical summary of the CD nomenclature, why it exists and how CDs are defined. *J Biol Regul Homeost Agents.* 1999;13(4):226-228.

12. Zola H, Swart B. The human leucocyte differentiation antigens (HLDA) workshops: the evolving role of antibodies in research, diagnosis and therapy. *Cell Res.* 2005;15(9):691-694. doi:10.1038/sj.cr.7290338

13. HCDM: Human Cell Differentiation Molecules website. Accessed July 31, 2019. http://www.hcdm.org

14. HUGO Nomenclature Committee. Gene family: CD molecules. Accessed July 31, 2019. https://www.genenames.org/cgi-bin/genefamilies/set/471

15. Morgan BP. Complement. In: Paul WE, ed. *Fundamental Immunology.* 7th ed. Lippincott Williams & Wilkins; 2013:863-890.

16. World Health Organization. Nomenclature of complement. *Bull World Health Organ.* 1968;39(6):935-938.

17. Letendre P. Complement: to be or not to be? *Transfusion.* 1990;30(5):478-479. doi:10.1046/j.1537-2995.1990.30590296388.x

18. Playfair JHL, Lydyard PM. *Medical Immunology Made Memorable.* 2nd ed. Churchill Livingstone; 2000.

19. Oppenheim JJ, Feldmann M. Introduction to the role of cytokines in innate host defense and adaptive immunity. In: Durum SK, Hirano T, Vilcek J, Nicola NA, eds. *Cytokine Reference: A Compendium of Cytokines and Other Mediators of Host Defense.* Academic Press; 2001:3-20.

20. Leonard WJ. Type I cytokines and interferons, and their receptors. In: Paul WE, ed. *Fundamental Immunology.* 7th ed. Lippincott Williams & Wilkins; 2013:601-638.

21. Ware CF. Tumor necrosis factor–related cytokines in immunity. In: Paul WE, ed. *Fundamental Immunology.* 7th ed. Lippincott Williams & Wilkins; 2013:659-680.

22. O'Shea JJ, Gadina M, Siegel R. Cytokines and cytokine receptors. In: Rich RR, Fleisher TA, Shearer WT, Schroeder HW Jr, Frew AJ, Weygand CM, eds. *Clinical Immunology: Principles and Practice.* 4th ed. WB Saunders; 2013:108-135.

23. Fitzgerald KA, O'Neill LAJ, Gearing AJH, Callard RE. *The Cytokine FactsBook.* 2nd ed. Academic Press; 2001.

24. Aarden LA, Brunner TK, Cerottini J-C, et al. Revised nomenclature for antigen-nonspecific T cell proliferation and helper factors. *J Immunol.* 1979;123(6):2928-2929.

25. Paul WE, Kishimoto T, Melchers F, et al. Nomenclature for secreted regulatory proteins of the immune system (interleukins). *Clin Exp Immunol.* 1992;88(2):367. doi:10.1111/j.1365-2249.1992.tb03089.x

26. Lagna G, Hata A, Hemmati-Brivanlou A, Massague J. Partnership between DPC4 and SMAD proteins in TGF-beta signalling pathways. *Nature.* 1996;383(6603):832-836. doi:10.1038/383832a0

27. Robinson J, Halliwell JA, Hayhurst JD, Flicek P, Parham P, Marsh SG. The IPD and IMGT/HLA database: allele variant databases. *Nucl Acids Res.* 2015;43(database issue):D423-D431. doi:10.1098/nar/gku1161

28. Bodmer WF, Albert E, Bodmer JG, et al. Nomenclature for factors of the HLA system, 1987. *Hum Immunol.* 1989;26(1):3-14.

29. Mickelson E. A brief history of the International Histocompatibility Workshops. Accessed May 16, 2018. https://ihiws.org/workshop-history/

30. Bodmer WF. HLA 1991. In: Tsuji K, Aizawa M, Sasazuki S, eds. *HLA 1991: Proceedings of the Eleventh International Histocompatibility Workshop and Conference Held in Yokohama, Japan, 6-13 November, 1991.* Oxford University Press; 1992:7-16.

31. Marsh SGE. Nomenclature for factors of the HLA system, update June 2017. *Int J Immunogenet.* 2017;44(5):243-250. doi:10.1111/iji.12331

32. Bodmer JG. Nomenclature 1991 foreword. *Hum Immunol.* 1992;34(1):2-3. doi:10.1016/0198-8859(92)90078-2

33. Marsh SGE. Nomenclature for factors of the HLA system. Updated April 4, 2017. Accessed January 30, 2018. http://hla.alleles.org/nomenclature/index.html

34. Tiercy J-M, Marsh SGE, Schreuder GMT, Albert E, Fischer G, Wassmuth R. Guidelines for nomenclature usage in HLA reports: ambiguities and conversion to serotypes. *Eur J Immunogenet.* 2002;29(3):273-274. doi:10.1046/j.1365-2370.2002.00336.x

35. Klein J, Bontrop RE, Dawkins RL, et al. Nomenclature for the major histo-compatibility complexes of different species: a proposal. *Immunogenetics.* 1990;31(4):217-219. doi:10.1007/BF00204890

36. Haynes BF, Soderberg KA, Fauci AS. Introduction to the immune system. In: Longo DL, Kasper DL, Jameson JL, Fauci AS, Hauser SL, Loscalzo J, eds. *Harrison's Principles of Internal Medicine.* 18th ed. McGraw-Hill; 2012:2650-2685.

37. Schroeder HW Jr, Wald D, Greenspan NS. Immunoglobulins: structure and function. In: Paul WE, ed. *Fundamental Immunology.* 7th ed. Lippincott Williams & Wilkins; 2013:129-149.

38. Nairn R, Helbert M. *Immunology for Medical Students.* 2nd ed. Mosby; 2007.

39. Lefranc M-P, Lefranc G. *The Immunoglobulin FactsBook.* Academic Press; 2001.

40. Parslow TG. Immunoglobulins and immunoglobulin genes. In: Parslow TG, Stites DP, Terr AI, Imboden JB, eds. *Medical Immunology.* 10th ed. Lange Medical Books/McGraw-Hill; 2001:95-114.

41. Kao NL. How immunoglobulins were named. *Ann Intern Med.* 1992;117(5):445. doi:10.7326/0003-4819-117-5-445_2

42. Black CA. A brief history of the discovery of the immunoglobulins and the origin of the modern immunoglobulin nomenclature. *Immunol Cell Biol.* 1997;75(1):65-68. doi:10.1038/icb.1997.10

43. Recommendations for the nomenclature of human immunoglobulins. *Biochemistry.* 1972;11(18):3311-3312. doi:10.1021/bi00768a001

44. IUIS/WHO Subcommittee on IgA Nomenclature. Nomenclature of immunoglob-ulin A and other proteins of the mucosal immune system. *J Immunol Methods.* 1999;223(2):263-264. Also: *Eur J Immunol.* 1999;29(3):1057-1058.

45. IUIS Subcommittee on Nomenclature. Nomenclature of the Fc receptors. *Bull World Health Organ.* 1989;67(4):449-450.

46. Lefranc M-P, Giudicelli V, Duroux P, et al. IMGT, the International ImMunoGeneTics Information System 25 years on. *Nucl Acids Res.* 2015;43(D1):D413-D422. doi:10.1093/nar/gku1056

47. Parslow TG. Lymphocytes and lymphoid tissues. In: Parslow TG, Stites DP, Terr AI, Imboden JB, eds. *Medical Immunology.* 10th ed. Lange Medical Books/McGraw-Hill; 2001:40-60.

48. DeFranco AL. B-cell development and the humoral immune response. In: Parslow TG, Stites DP, Terr AI, Imboden JB, eds. *Medical Immunology.* 10th ed. Lange Medical Books/McGraw-Hill; 2001:115-130.

49. Imboden JB, Seaman WE. T lymphocytes and natural killer cells. In: Parslow TG, Stites DP, Terr AI, Imboden JB, eds. *Medical Immunology.* 10th ed. Lange Medical Books/McGraw-Hill; 2001:131-147.

50. LeFranc M-P, LeFranc G. *The T Cell Receptor FactsBook.* Academic Press; 2001.

**14.9** **Isotopes.** Isotopes may be referred to in the medical literature alone or as a component of a radiopharmaceutical administered for therapeutic or diagnostic purposes. The nomenclature for the isotopes incorporated in radiopharmaceuticals follows the international nonproprietary name (INN) drug nomenclature and therefore differs from that of isotopes that occur in elements alone.

**14.9.1** **Elements.** An isotope referred to as an element rather than as part of the name of a chemical compound may be described at first mention by providing the name of the element spelled out followed by the isotope number in the same typeface and type size (no hyphen, subscript, or superscript is used). The element abbreviation may be listed in parentheses at first mention and used thereafter in the article, with the isotope number preceding the element symbol as a superscript.

> Of the 13 known isotopes of iodine, only iodine 128 ($^{128}$I) is not radioactive. The investigators used $^{128}$I to avoid the difficulty and expense of disposing of radioactive waste.

The symbol representing a single element should not be used as an abbreviation for a compound (eg, do not abbreviate the compound gallium citrate Ga 67 as $^{67}$Ga).

**14.9.2** **Radiopharmaceuticals.** The nomenclature for the isotopes incorporated in radiopharmaceuticals follows US adopted name (USAN, the US nomenclature agency) or INN (the international nomenclature agency) style. The *USP Dictionary of USAN and International Drug Names*[1] publishes USAN and INN, with USAN appearing in boldface type and INN in roman type. All USANs are reviewed by the INN Committee. The INN agent (if not intended to be marketed in the US) may not have a USAN. Almost all nomenclature is the same between the 2 groups. The single difference is stylistic. In INN style, the order is (1) name of the drug that contains the radioactive element, (2) isotope number, (3) element symbol, and (4) carrier name, if there is one. In USAN style, the order is (1) name of the drug that contains the radioactive element, (2) element symbol, (3) isotope number, and (4) carrier name, if there is one. In both, the isotope number appears as a superscript. The JAMA Network journals follow the INN style.

Because the nonproprietary name comprises all these components, the complete name should be provided at first mention unless the radiopharmaceuticals being referred to are a general category. Subsequently, a shorter term may be used, such as *iodinated albumin* or *gallium scan*.

Although the nonproprietary name for the radiopharmaceutical may appear to contain redundant information, maintaining consistent terms is important for clarity. For example, technetium Tc 99m is contained in more than 40 nonproprietary radiopharmaceuticals, from technetium Tc 99m albumin to technetium Tc 99m teboroxime.[1] The isotope number appears in the same type (not superscript) as the rest of the drug name, and it is not preceded by a hyphen. A few commonly used drugs appear below. For drugs not listed here, consult the most recent edition of the *USP Dictionary*.[1]

> cyanocobalamin Co 60
>
> fibrinogen I 125

> fludeoxyglucose F 18
>
> indium In 111 altumomab pentetate
>
> indium In 111 satumomab pendetide
>
> iodohippurate sodium I 131
>
> sodium iodide I 125
>
> technetium Tc 99m sestamibi
>
> Strontium chloride Sr 89 can be used to treat pain from skeletal metastases.
>
> In an earlier study, 50 patients underwent lung imaging with technetium Tc 99m sulfur colloid.
>
> The patient underwent an exercise stress test with injection of thallous chloride Tl 201 (thallium stress test).
>
> Placement of seeds labeled with radioactive iodine I 125 ($^{125}$I) did not interfere with lymphoscintigraphy or intraoperative identification of sentinel lymph nodes. The $^{125}$I seeds were used in 10 patients in this 12-patient study.

In a discussion that does not refer to administration of a specific drug, the more general term may be used.

> For a patient recuperating from a myocardial infarction who wishes to begin an exercise program, a treadmill test with or without thallium imaging may be useful to determine whether the patient is at high risk for recurrent ischemia.

At the beginning of a sentence, the name rather than the element symbol should be used (even if the abbreviation has been previously used).

> The patient was treated with sodium iodide I 131 after she was diagnosed with hyperthyroidism. Iodine 131 levels were then monitored by measuring the amount of radioactivity in the patient's urine.

**14.9.3**   **Radiopharmaceutical Compounds Without Approved Names.** Compounds may be combined with radioisotopes for research purposes. Such compounds would not receive an INN if no commercial use is intended. In lieu of an INN, standard chemical nomenclature should be followed (see 14.9.1, Elements, or consult the *CRC Handbook of Chemistry and Physics*[2] for more information).

After first mention, the name of the substance can be abbreviated. Use the superscript form of the isotope number to the left of the element symbol. Enclose the isotope symbol in brackets and close up with the compound name if the nonradioactive isotope of the element is normally part of the compound.

> glucose labeled with radioactive carbon ($^{14}$C) [or glucose tagged with carbon 14]
>
> [$^{14}$C]glucose (not glucose C 14)

Use no brackets and separate the element and compound name with a hyphen if the compound does not normally contain the isotope element.

amikacin labeled with iodine 125

$^{125}$I-amikacin

If uncertain as to whether the isotope element is normally part of a compound, consult the *USP Dictionary*[1] for drugs and *The Merck Index*[3] for other compounds.

**14.9.4** **Radiopharmaceutical Proprietary Names.** In proprietary names of radiopharmaceuticals, isotope numbers may appear in the same position as in the approved nonproprietary names, but they are usually joined to the rest of the name by a hyphen and are not necessarily preceded by the element symbol. Follow the *USP Dictionary*[1] or the usage of individual manufacturers.

| Proprietary | Nonproprietary (preferred) |
|---|---|
| Iodotope I-131 | sodium iodide I 131 |
| Glofil-125 | iothalamate sodium I 125 |

**14.9.5** **Uniform Labeling.** The abbreviation *ul* (for *uniformly labeled*) may be used without expansion in parentheses:

[$^{14}$C]glucose (ul)

Similarly, terms such as *carrier-free, no carrier added*, and *carrier added* may be used. In general medical publications, these terms should be explained at first mention because not all readers will be familiar with them.

**14.9.6** **Hydrogen Isotopes.** Two isotopes of hydrogen have their own specific names, deuterium and tritium, which should be used instead of hydrogen 2 and hydrogen 3, respectively. In text, the specific names are also preferred to the symbols $^2$H or D (for deuterium, which is stable) and $^3$H (for tritium, which is radioactive). The 2 forms of heavy water, $D_2O$ and $^3H_2O$, should be referred to by the approved nonproprietary names deuterium oxide and tritiated water, respectively.

**14.9.7** **Metastable Isotopes.** The abbreviation *m*, as in krypton Kr 81m or technetium Tc 99m, stands for *metastable*. The abbreviation should never be deleted because the term without the *m* designates a different radionuclide isomer.

**Principal Author:** Cheryl Iverson, MA

## ACKNOWLEDGMENT

Thanks to Stephanie C. Shubat, MS, USAN Program, American Medical Association, Chicago, Illinois, for reviewing and providing comments.

## REFERENCES

1. *USP Dictionary of USAN and International Drug Names*. 53rd ed. US Pharmacopoeia; 2017.
2. Haynes WM, ed. *CRC Handbook of Chemistry and Physics*. 95th ed. CRC Press; 2014.
3. O'Neil MJ, ed. *The Merck Index: An Encyclopedia of Chemicals, Drugs, & Biologicals*. 15th ed. Royal Society of Chemistry Publishing; 2013.

**14.10**   **Molecular Medicine.** Molecules and their interactions underlie every area of medicine. Many classes of molecules are described according to rules or conventions, some of which are covered in other sections of this chapter. The Joint Commission on Biochemical Nomenclature formulates nomenclature policy for classes of biochemicals.[1] The Joint Commission on Biochemical Nomenclature enzyme nomenclature is described in 14.10.3, Enzyme Nomenclature.[2] The US National Center for Biotechnology Information is a searchable information resource on molecular biology with links to databases.[3]

This section provides information on various molecular terms, including expansions, derivations, typography, and usage information (but not rules for naming molecules). It is meant to assist the editor or reader encountering an unfamiliar term and to guide the author in using such terms. For terms not described herein, helpful sources include the Medical Subject Headings database of the National Library of Medicine,[4] medical texts and dictionaries, and internet searches. For a review of molecular biology databases, see the 2016 Database Issue of *Nucleic Acids Research*.[5]

**14.10.1**   **Molecular Terminology: Other Sections of Chapter 14.** The following sections of chapter 14 have subsections on molecular terms: 14.2, Cancer; 14.3, Cardiology; and 14.11, Neurology. The following sections of chapter 14 substantially deal with molecular terminology: 14.1, Blood Groups, Platelet Antigens, and Granulocyte Antigens; 14.6, Genetics; 14.7, Hemostasis; and 14.8, Immunology.

Table **14.10-1** gives molecular terms associated with subjects covered elsewhere in this chapter.

**14.10.2**   **Molecular Terms: Considerations and Examples.** Molecular terms often are more familiar in unexpanded form; their expansions may be obscure. Molecular terms often mix numbers, letters, and cases. They may be abbreviations or abbreviations within abbreviations (for instance, see TAF and subsequent entries in **Table 14.10-2**). Molecular terms differ from standard abbreviations, which typically are uppercase initialisms (eg, PVC for premature ventricular contraction). In contrast, many molecular terms are (or incorporate) contractions of single words, using all lowercase letters or mixing capital and lowercase letters (eg, apo for apolipoprotein; Hb for hemoglobin).

Letter prefixes (including Greek letters) and numeric prefixes are linked to the main term by hyphens.

$\alpha_1$-antitrypsin

$\beta$-catenin

$\lambda$-tubulin

glucose 6-phosphate

However, these terms are not hyphenated:

$\alpha$ helix

$\beta$ sheet

**Table 14.10-1.** Molecular Terms and Chapter Section Numbers

| Entity | Section |
| --- | --- |
| amino acids | 14.6.1, Nucleic Acids and Amino Acids |
| antitrypsins, antithrombins | 14.7.4, Inhibition of Coagulation and Fibrinolysis |
| apolipoproteins | 14.3.12, Cellular and Molecular Cardiology |
| bacterial strains and proteins | 14.14.2, Bacteria: Additional Terminology |
| blood gas terminology (eg, Pao$_2$) | 14.16, Pulmonary and Respiratory Terminology |
| cancer molecules | 14.2.5, Molecular Cancer Terminology<br>14.6.3, Oncogenes and Tumor Suppressor Genes |
| cellular adhesion molecules | 14.7.2, Endothelial Factors<br>14.8, Immunology |
| chemokines | 14.8, Immunology |
| chromosomes | 14.6.4, Human Chromosomes |
| cloning vectors | 14.6.1, Nucleic Acids and Amino Acids |
| clotting factors | 14.7.3, Secondary Hemostasis (Amplification and Propagation) |
| clusters of differentiation (CDs) | 14.8, Immunology<br>14.1.2, Platelet-Specific Antigens |
| codons | 14.6.1, Nucleic Acids and Amino Acids |
| colony-stimulating factors | 14.8, Immunology |
| complement | 14.8, Immunology |
| creatine kinases | 14.3.12, Cellular and Molecular Cardiology |
| cytokines | 14.8, Immunology |
| D-dimer | 14.7.4, Inhibition of Coagulation and Fibrinolysis |
| DNA | 14.6.1, Nucleic Acids and Amino Acids |
| genes | 14.6.2, Human Gene Nomenclature<br>14.6.3, Oncogenes and Tumor Suppressor Genes<br>14.6.5, Nonhuman Genetic Terms |
| glycoproteins | 14.1.2, Platelet-Specific Antigens<br>14.7.1, Primary Hemostasis (Initiation)<br>14.7.2, Endothelial Factors |
| guanine nucleotides | 14.3.12, Cellular and Molecular Cardiology<br>14.6.1, Nucleic Acids and Amino Acids |
| hemostatic molecules | 14.7.1, Primary Hemostasis (Initiation) |
| hepatitis antigens and antibodies | 14.14.3, Virus Nomenclature |
| histones | 14.6.1, Nucleic Acids and Amino Acids |
| HLA antigens | 14.8, Immunology |
| immunoglobulins | 14.8, Immunology |

(continued)

**Table 14.10-1.** Molecular Terms and Chapter Section Numbers (*continued*)

| Entity | Section |
| --- | --- |
| influenza types and strains | 14.14.3, Virus Nomenclature |
| integrins | 14.7.2, Endothelial Factors |
| interferon | 14.8, Immunology |
| interleukins | 14.8, Immunology |
| ion channels | 14.11.5, Molecular Neuroscience |
| lipoproteins | 14.3.12, Cellular and Molecular Cardiology |
| muscle cell components | 14.3.12, Cellular and Molecular Cardiology |
| myosin chains | 14.7.1, Primary Hemostasis (Initiation) |
| neurotransmitters and receptors | 14.11.5, Molecular Neuroscience |
| nitric oxide synthase | 14.3.12, Cellular and Molecular Cardiology<br>14.7.2, Endothelial Factors |
| nodal cells | 14.3.12, Cellular and Molecular Cardiology |
| nucleic acid technology (eg, polymerase chain reaction [PCR], single-nucleotide variations [SNVs] (formerly single-nucleotide polymorphisms [SNPs]), short tandem repeats [STRs]) | 14.6.1, Nucleic Acids and Amino Acids |
| nucleosides, nucleotides | 14.6.1, Nucleic Acids and Amino Acids |
| phages | 14.14.3, Virus Nomenclature |
| phospholipase | 14.7.1, Primary Hemostasis (Initiation) |
| plasminogen activators | 14.3.12, Cellular and Molecular Cardiology<br>14.7.2, Endothelial Factors |
| platelet-activating factors | 14.7.1, Primary Hemostasis (Initiation) |
| prions | 14.14.3, Virus Nomenclature |
| prostaglandins | 14.7.1, Primary Hemostasis (Initiation) |
| restriction enzymes | 14.6.1, Nucleic Acids and Amino Acids |
| retrovirus gene terms | 14.6.3, Oncogenes and Tumor Suppressor Genes<br>14.6.5, Nonhuman Genetic Terms |
| RNA | 14.6.1, Nucleic Acids and Amino Acids |
| serotonin | 14.11.5, Molecular Neuroscience |
| thromboxanes | 14.7.1, Primary Hemostasis (Initiation) |
| troponins | 14.3.12, Cellular and Molecular Cardiology |
| variations | 14.6.1, Nucleic Acids and Amino Acids |
| von Willebrand factor | 14.7.3, Secondary Hemostasis (Amplification and Propagation) |

Hyphens are added in adjectival usages:

    β-pleated sheet

    glucose-6-phosphate dehydrogenase

Hyphens are used as follows in numbers that interrupt a word:

    propan-1,2-diol (propanol)

    flavan-3-ol

For letter or number suffixes, hyphens typically are not used with expanded terms but are handled in various ways with abbreviated terms:

    interleukin 1 (IL-1)

    phosphodiesterase 3A (PDE3A)

    6-keto prostaglandin $F_{1\alpha}$ (6-keto $PGF_{1\alpha}$)

The chemical prefixes L (levo) and D (dextro) are small capitals when referring to biomolecules, such as amino acids and carbohydrates, in the D/L system of configuration.

    L-folinic acid

    D-glutaraldehyde

Element symbols in chemical names, such as $S$ (sulfur) and $N$ (nitrogen), are italicized. Other capital letters are not italicized.

    $N$-acetyl-D-glucosamine

    cytochrome P450

    N-terminal, C-terminal

    D-dimer

A subscript letter indicates a modifier of the main term.

    $P_i$ (inorganic phosphate)

Plus signs and minus signs that indicate charges are set superscript. Numerals that indicate quantities of an element within a molecule are set subscript. Numerals that indicate a charge are set superscript.

    $HCO_3^-$

    $Fe^{3+}$

Although proteins may often be expressed as p plus a numeral signifying the atomic weight in kilodaltons (eg, p53, a 53-kDa protein), p53 is an alias or nickname and should be replaced with the official symbol, TP53 (see Table 14.10-2 and 14.6.3.2, Tumor Suppressor Genes). Affixes, such as superscripts, further specify the protein (important because different proteins may have the same weight) (Table 14.10-2). Although the gene symbols for such proteins are often given as the same term italicized (eg, the tumor suppressor gene *p53*), the correct gene symbols should be used (eg, in humans *TP53*, in mice, *Tp53*). Use the search feature at the HUGO Gene Nomenclature Committee website[6] (see 14.6, Genetics).

The term *stem cell* has the general meaning of a precursor, pluripotent, or progenitor cell. Research articles should specify the type(s) of stem cell referred to, for example, *adult, bone marrow, embryonic, germline, hematopoietic, mesenchymal, neural, peripheral blood, somatic, umbilical cord–derived, unrestricted somatic,* and so forth. (The preceding terms are not all mutually exclusive.)

Terms in Table 14.10-2 are included as a reference. Some context or explanation of such terms is desirable at first mention, but, in contrast to abbreviations (see 13.0, Abbreviations), first mention need not be a literal expansion and the term may be stated as an appositive rather than in parentheses:

> the cyclin-dependent kinase CDK2

When an abbreviation is used in the Suggested Usage at First Mention column in Table 14.10-2, it is assumed that in the article the abbreviated term has already been introduced and defined or expanded; for example, if INK4 (an alias [not the official symbol] for CDKN2A) is defined as "inhibitors of CDK4" at first mention, it is assumed that CDK4 was previously defined or expanded. Providing more information is often helpful. For instance, at first mention, CDKN1A (alias [not the official symbol]: p21) may be referred to as "cyclin-dependent kinase (CDK) inhibitor 1A" or given additional context (see Table 14.10-2 for further explanation of these terms).

**14.10.3** **Enzyme Nomenclature.** Enzyme nomenclature was formalized in the 1950s.[2] It is formulated by the International Union of Biochemistry (IUB) and the International Union of Pure and Applied Chemistry (IUPAC), more specifically, the Nomenclature Committee of the International Union of Biochemistry and Molecular Biology (NC-IUBMB) and the IUPAC-IUB Joint Commission on Biochemical Nomenclature, and "is probably the single largest task of the committee."[2]

Supplements of new enzymes are published annually. A complete list is available online.[8] This list is searchable and includes the recommended name and number of each enzyme. Officially assigned names and numbers for enzymes are available at the Enzyme Nomenclature database,[2] along with rules for enzyme nomenclature.

There are 3 types of enzyme names: recommended name (common, working, or trivial name), systematic name, and Enzyme Commission (EC) number. The recommended name is the name by which the enzyme is commonly known. The systematic name incorporates the reaction the enzyme catalyzes. The EC number is a unique identifier assigned to each enzyme.

Because systematic names can be unwieldy and recommended names are well known, recommended names are used in general medical publications. For unambiguous identification, the EC number, the systematic name, or both may be included at first mention.

The parts of the EC number are as follows:

> class
>
> subclass
>
> sub-subclass
>
> serial number within sub-subclass

**Table 14.10-2.** Molecular Terms and Explanations

| Official term (alias[a]) | Explanation | Suggested usage at first mention |
|---|---|---|
| Aβ peptide, Aβ42 | amyloid-β peptide | amyloid-β peptide (Aβ), $A\beta_{42}$ peptide, *or* 42-residue form of Aβ |
| Aβ*56 | 56-kDa Aβ fragment | 56-kDa Aβ fragment |
| Ach | acetylcholine | acetylcholine |
| Acrp30 (*or* adiponectin) | adipocyte-complement–related 30-kDa protein | the protein Acrp30 *or* adiponectin |
| acyl-CoA | acyl derivatives of coenzyme A | acyl coenzyme A |
| acyl-*S*-CoA | sulfonated acyl-CoA | sulfonated acyl–coenzyme A |
| ADAMTS[7] | a disintegrin like and metalloprotease domain (reprolysin-type) with thrombospondin type 1 motifs | ADAMTS protease |
| specific ADAMTS, eg, ADAMTS-13 | ADAMTS-13; trivial name von Willebrand factor (VWF) protease (see 14.7, Hemostasis) | ADAMTS-13 *and/or* vWFc protease |
| adoHcy | *S*-adenosylhomocysteine | *S*-adenosylhomocysteine |
| ado-Met (also SAM) | *S*-adenosylmethionine | *S*-adenosylmethionine |
| Akt kinase | a serine-threonine kinase, also known as protein kinase B, related to *akt* oncogene (origin: AKT retrovirus isolated from AKR mouse thymoma) | Akt protein kinase |
| allo-SCT | allogeneic stem cell transplant | allogeneic stem cell transplant |
| ATCase | aspartate transcarbamoylase | aspartate transcarbamoylase |
| ATPase | adenosine triphosphatase | adenosine triphosphatase |
| BNP | brain (*or* b-type) natriuretic peptide | brain (*or* b-type) natriuretic peptide |
| 1,3-BPG | 1,3-bisphosphoglycerate | 1,3-bisphosphoglycerate |
| CAK (*or* cyclin H/CDK7) | CDK-activating enzyme | the CDK-activating enzyme (CAK) cyclin H/CDK7 |
| CaM | calmodulin | calmodulin |
| CDK2, CDK3, CDK7, etc | cyclin-dependent kinases | the cyclin-dependent kinase CDK2, etc |
| CDKI | CDK inhibitors (see INK4 below) | CDK inhibitors |
| CoA | coenzyme A | coenzyme A |
| COX-1, COX-2 | cyclooxygenases 1 and 2 | cyclooxygenase 1 (COX-1), cyclooxygenase 2 (COX-2) |
| C-reactive protein | protein reactive to pneumococcal cell wall C polysaccharide | C-reactive protein (CRP) |

*(continued)*

**Table 14.10-2.** Molecular Terms and Explanations (*continued*)

| Official term (alias[a]) | Explanation | Suggested usage at first mention |
|---|---|---|
| cyclin D/CDK4/CDK6, cyclin E/CDK2 | cyclin-CDK complexes | the cyclin D/CDK4/CDK6 complex; the cyclin E/CDK2 complex |
| CYP1A2, CYP2C9, CYP2C19, CYP2D6, CYP3A4 | isoforms of cytochrome P450 enzymes (also cytochrome P450 isozymes) (P: pigment; 450: 450-nm absorbance) | various, eg, cytochrome P450 1A2 isozyme (CYP1A2); cytochrome P450 3A4 isozyme (CYP3A4 *or* P450 3A4 *or* 3A4) |
| Dkk-1 | dickkopf-1 | the inhibitor protein Dkk-1 |
| $F_0$ (subscript is zero, not capital O) | portion of mitochondrial ATP synthase (F: energy-coupling factor) | context, eg, $F_0$ portion of mitochondrial ATP synthase, proton channel portion of ATP synthase, etc |
| $F_0F_1$ | complex portion of mitochondrial ATP synthase | context, eg, $F_0F_1$ mitochondrial ATP synthase, $F_0F_1$ complex, etc |
| $F_1$ | portion of mitochondrial ATP synthase | context, eg, $F_1$ portion of mitochondrial ATP synthase, catalytic portion of ATP synthase |
| F1P, F6P | fructose 1-phosphate, fructose 6-phosphate | fructose 1-phosphate, fructose 6-phosphate |
| FAD | flavin adenine dinucleotide | flavin adenine dinucleotide |
| $FADH_2$ | reduced (hydrogenated) FAD | $FADH_2$ *or* reduced (*or* hydrogenated) FAD |
| FBPase-1, FBPase-2 | fructose 1,6-bisphosphatase, fructose 2,6-bisphosphatase | fructose 1,6-bisphosphatase, fructose 2,6-bisphosphatase |
| Fd | ferredoxin | ferredoxin |
| Fhit | fragile histidine triad protein | fragile histidine triad protein |
| FMN | flavin mononucleotide | flavin mononucleotide |
| $FMNH_2$ | reduced (hydrogenated) FMN | $FMNH_2$ *or* reduced (*or* hydrogenated) FMN |
| Fp | flavoprotein | flavoprotein (Fp) |
| $G_0$ | quiescent state of cell cycle | $G_0$ phase |
| $G_1$ | growth *or* gap 1 phase of cell cycle | $G_1$ phase |
| $G_2$ | growth *or* gap 2 phase of cell cycle | $G_2$ phase |
| G protein | guanine triphosphate (GTP)–binding protein | G protein |
| Gα, Gβ, Gγ | G protein families | Gα, Gβ, Gγ protein or family |
| $Gα_{12}$, $Gα_{13}$ | members of Gα | $Gα_{12}$, $Gα_{13}$ protein |
| Gβγ, βγ | Gβ subunit *or* complex | Gβγ, βγ subunit or complex |

**Table 14.10-2.** Molecular Terms and Explanations (*continued*)

| Official term (alias[a]) | Explanation | Suggested usage at first mention |
|---|---|---|
| G1P, G6P | glucose 1-phosphate, glucose 6-phosphate | glucose 1-phosphate, glucose 6-phosphate |
| GalN | D-galactosamine | D-galactosamine |
| GalNAc | $N$-acetyl-D-galactosamine | $N$-acetyl-D-galactosamine |
| $G_i$ | inhibitory G protein | inhibitory G protein |
| Glc *or* D-Glc | D-glucose | glucose *or* D-glucose |
| $G_q$, $G_{q/11}$ | classes of G protein | $G_q$, $G_{q/11}$ protein |
| $G_s$ | stimulatory G protein | stimulatory G protein |
| GlcA | D-gluconic acid | gluconic acid *or* D-gluconic acid |
| GlcNAc (also NAG) | $N$-acetyl-D-glucosamine | $N$-acetyl-D-glucosamine GlcNAc |
| GlcUA | D-glucuronic acid | D-glucuronic acid |
| Grb2 | growth factor receptor–bound protein 2 | the protein Grb2 |
| $H_2F$ (also DHF) | dihydrofolate *or* 7,8-dihydrofolate | dihydrofolate ($H_2F$ *or* DHF) *or* 7,8-dihydrofolate ($H_2F$ *or* DHF) |
| $H_4F$ (also THF) | tetrahydrofolate *or* 5,6,7,8-tetrahydrofolate | tetrahydrofolate *or* 5,6,7,8-tetrahydrofolate |
| Hb | hemoglobin | hemoglobin |
| $HbA_{1a}$, $HbA_{1b}$, $HbA_{1c}$ | glycated (*not* glycosylated; Lyn Reynolds, editorial office director, *Diabetes*, email communication, May 21, 2013) hemoglobin fractions | preferred: glycated hemoglobin $A_{1c}$ ($HbA_{1c}$), etc (also: glycohemoglobin $A_{1c}$) |
| HbCO | carbon monoxyhemoglobin, carboxyhemoglobin | carbon monoxyhemoglobin |
| $HbO_2$ | oxyhemoglobin | oxyhemoglobin |
| HER2/neu | from human epidermal growth factor receptor 2; preferred term is now ERBB2; see 14.6.3, Oncogenes and Tumor Suppressor Genes | ERBB2 (formerly HER2 *or* HER2/neu) |
| HMG-CoA | β-hydroxy-β-methylglutaryl-CoA | β-hydroxy-β-methylglutaryl-CoA (*but* statins, not HMG-CoA inhibitors) |
| IKKβ | IκB kinase β (I: inhibitor) | IκB kinase β |
| CDKN2A (INK4) | inhibitors of CDK4 (see CDKI above and p16$^{Ink4}$, etc, below) | inhibitors of CDK4 |
| IGF-1, IGF-2 | insulinlike growth factor, type 1 and type 2 | insulinlike growth factor 1, insulinlike growth factor 2 |
| IGF-1R, IGF-22 | IGF-1 receptor, IGF-2 receptor | IGF-1 receptor, IGF-2 receptor |

(*continued*)

**Table 14.10-2.** Molecular Terms and Explanations (*continued*)

| Official term (alias[a]) | Explanation | Suggested usage at first mention |
|---|---|---|
| IP$_3$ | inositol 1,4,5-triphosphate | inositol 1,4,5-triphosphate |
| α-KG | α-ketoglutarate | α-ketoglutarate |
| lac | lactose | lactose |
| M | mitosis (phase of cell cycle) | M phase |
| Man | D-mannose | D-mannose |
| Mb | myoglobin (do not confuse with Mb, megabase, or MB, megabyte) | myoglobin |
| MbO$_2$ | oxymyoglobin | oxymyoglobin |
| M-CDK | M-cyclin–CDK complex | M-phase CDK |
| Mcm proteins | minichromosome maintenance proteins | Mcm proteins |
| M-cyclin | M-kinase–cyclin complex | M-cyclin |
| M-kinase | mitosis-phase kinase | M-kinase |
| Mur | muramic acid | muramic acid |
| Mur2Ac (also NAM) | N-acetylmuramic acid | N-acetylmuramic acid |
| NAD | nicotinamide adenine dinucleotide | nicotinamide adenine dinucleotide (NAD) *or* the nicotinamide coenzyme NAD |
| NAD$^+$ | oxidized NAD | NAD$^+$ |
| NADH | reduced (hydrogenated) NAD | reduced (*or* hydrogenated) NAD *or* NADH |
| NADH hydrogenase | NADH hydrogenase | NADH hydrogenase |
| NADP | NAD phosphate | NAD phosphate *or* NADP |
| NADPH | reduced (hydrogenated) NADP | reduced (*or* hydrogenated) NADP *or* NADPH |
| NAG | (*see* GlcNAc above) | |
| Neu5Ac | N-acetylneuraminic acid (sialic acid) | N-acetylneuraminic acid |
| NFκB | nuclear factor–κB | nuclear factor–κB (NF-κB *or* NF-B) |
| NMDA | N-methyl-D-aspartate | N-methyl-D-aspartate |
| NMN | nicotinamide mononucleotide | nicotinamide mononucleotide |
| NMN$^+$ | oxidized NMN | NMN$^+$ |
| NMNH | reduced (hydrogenated) NMN | reduced *or* hydrogenated NMN |
| NMP | nucleoside monophosphate | nucleoside monophosphate |
| NOx | nitrogen oxides, such as nitrate, nitrite, and nitrosothiols; nitric oxide (NO) metabolites | nitrogen oxides |

**Table 14.10-2.** Molecular Terms and Explanations (*continued*)

| Official term (alias[a]) | Explanation | Suggested usage at first mention |
|---|---|---|
| NPY | neuropeptide Y | neuropeptide Y |
| NT-proBNP | N-terminal fragment of the prohormone brain natriuretic peptide (see 14.6.1.5, Amino Acids) | N-terminal fragment of the prohormone brain natriuretic peptide |
| p16$^{Ink4}$, p15$^{Ink4B}$, p18$^{Ink4C}$, p19$^{Ink4D}$ | INK4s | the INK4 p16$^{Ink4}$, etc |
| CDKN1A (p21) | 21-kDa protein | the protein CDKN1A |
| p21$^{WAFI/CIP1}$, p27$^{KIP1}$, p57$^{KIP2}$ | other CDKI; WAFI: wild-type p53-activated protein 1; CIP1: CDK-interacting protein 1; KIP: kinase inhibitor protein | the CDKI p21$^{WAFI/CIP1}$, etc |
| TP53 (p53) | 53-kDa protein | the protein TP53 |
| CDKN1C (p57) | 57-kDa protein | the protein CDKN1C |
| PE, PPE | protein or gene family named for amino acid sequence motif (PE: Pro-Glu, PPE: Pro-Pro-Glu; see 14.6.1, Nucleic Acids and Amino Acids) | PE and PPE protein families, PE/PPE gene families, etc |
| P-gp | P-glycoprotein | P-glycoprotein |
| P$_i$ | inorganic phosphate | inorganic phosphate |
| PI | phosphatidyl inositol | phosphatidyl inositol |
| PIP$_2$ | phosphatidylinositol 4,5-bisphosphate | phosphatidylinositol 4,5-bisphosphate |
| Pol | polymerase (eg, DNA, RNA) | polymerase |
| PP$_i$ | inorganic pyrophosphate | inorganic pyrophosphate |
| pRb | retinoblastoma protein | retinoblastoma protein |
| PYY$_{3-36}$ | NPY receptor agonist (P: peptide; Y: NPY; Y: Y2 receptor; 3-36: 34 amino acid residue numbers) | peptide YY$_{3-36}$, the gut hormone PYY$_{3-36}$ |
| RANKL | receptor-activated nuclear factor–κB ligand | receptor-activated nuclear factor–κB ligand |
| RecA protein, RecA | recombinase A | recombinase A |
| RNAi | RNA interference | RNA interference |
| R point | restriction point (of cell cycle) | R point |
| RNase | ribonuclease | ribonuclease |
| rTpo | recombinant thrombopoietin | recombinant thrombopoietin |
| S | DNA synthesis phase of cell cycle | S phase *or* DNA synthesis phase |
| S-cyclin | S-kinase–cyclin complex | S-cyclin |

(*continued*)

**Table 14.10-2.** Molecular Terms and Explanations (*continued*)

| Official term (alias[a]) | Explanation | Suggested usage at first mention |
|---|---|---|
| sFlt-1 | soluble fms-like tyrosine kinase 1 (fms: McDonough feline sarcoma [oncogene]) | soluble fms-like tyrosine kinase 1 |
| S-kinase | synthesis-phase kinase | S-kinase |
| αSp22 | 22-kDa glycosylated form of α-synuclein | 22-kDa glycosylated α-synuclein |
| αSyn | α-synuclein | α-synuclein |
| TAF | TBP-associated factor | TATA-binding protein (TBP)–associated factor |
| TAF$_{II}$ | a class of TAFs | a class of factors associated with TBP |
| TATA box | a DNA sequence rich in adenine (A) and thymidine (T) | TATA box |
| TBP | TATA-binding protein | TATA-binding protein |
| TF$_{II}$D | complex of TBP and several TAF$_{II}$s | TBP-TAF$_{II}$ complex |
| UCP-1, UCP-2, UCP-3 | uncoupling proteins | uncoupling protein 1, and so on |
| UDP-Gal | uridine diphosphate galactose | UDP-galactose |
| UDP-Glc | UDP-glucose | UDP-glucose |
| uE$_3$ | unconjugated estriol | unconjugated E$_3$ |
| Wnt | named for *Drosophila melanogaster* wingless mutant integration site | the developmental protein Wnt, the Wnt signaling pathway, etc |

[a]Although these gene symbol aliases or nicknames, a result of their discovery before the completion of the Genome Project, may still be used by some, use of the approved gene symbol, not the alias, is strongly preferred. This usage will minimize confusion and make it possible to provide links to genomic databases for online versions of the article and to facilitate data retrieval in a number of databases. If an author insists on using an alias, provide the alias parenthetically after the approved gene symbol at first mention in text and abstract. This will link the two and provide a learning experience for those not yet familiar with the approved gene symbol.

The enzyme classes are as follows:

EC1     oxidoreductases

EC2     transferases

EC3     hydrolases

EC4     lyases

EC5     isomerases

EC6     ligases

Examples are shown in **Table 14.10-3**.

**Table 14.10-3.** Examples of Enzyme Class (EC) Names

| EC No. | Recommended name | Systematic name |
| --- | --- | --- |
| EC 1.11.1.7 | peroxidase | phenolic donor:hydrogen-peroxide oxidoreductase |
| EC 2.3.3.10 (formerly EC 4.1.3.5) | hydroxymethylglutaryl-CoA synthase | acetyl-CoA:acetoacetyl-CoA C-acetyltransferase |
| EC 2.7.1.1 | hexokinase | ATP:D-hexose 6-phosphotransferase |
| EC 3.1.1.7 | acetylcholinesterase | acetylcholine acetylhydrolase |
| EC 3.5.2.6 | β-lactamase | β-lactam hydrolase |
| EC 5.4.2.2 | phosphoglucomutase | α-D-glucose 1,6-phosphomutase |
| EC 6.5.1.1 | DNA ligase (ATP) | poly(deoxyribonucleotide):poly (deoxyribonucleotide) ligase (AMP-forming) |

**Principal Author:** Cheryl Iverson, MA

## ACKNOWLEDGMENT

Thanks to Boris C. Pasche, MD, PhD, Wake Forest Baptist Medical Center, Winston-Salem, North Carolina, and Mary L. (Nora) Disis, MD, *JAMA Oncology*, and Tumor Vaccine Medical Oncology, University of Washington, Seattle.

## REFERENCES

1. Biochemical Nomenclature Committees: International Union of Pure and Applied Chemistry and International Union of Biochemistry and Molecular Biology: IUPAC-IUBMB Joint Commission on Biochemical Nomenclature (JCBN) website. Updated July 23, 2019. Accessed August 1, 2019. https://www.qmul.ac.uk/sbcs/iubmb/

2. Nomenclature Committee of the International Union of Biochemistry and Molecular Biology (NC-IUBMB). Enzyme Nomenclature database. Updated July 23, 2019. Accessed August 1, 2019. https://www.qmul.ac.uk/sbcs/iubmb/enzyme/

3. National Center for Biotechnology Information website. Accessed August 1, 2019. https://www.ncbi.nlm.nih.gov

4. Medical Subject Headings (MeSH): National Library of Medicine. Accessed August 1, 2019. https://www.ncbi.nlm.nih.gov/mesh

5. Rigden DJ, Fernández-Suárez XM, Galperin MY. The 2016 database issue of *Nucleic Acids Research* and an updated molecular biology database collection. *Nucleic Acids Res.* 2016;44(D1):D1-D6. doi:10.1093/nar/gkv1356

6. HUGO Gene Nomenclature Committee (HGNC) website. Accessed August 1, 2019. https://www.genenames.org/

7. ADAMTS13 gene. Published April 20, 2015. Accessed May 8, 2018. https://ghr.nlm.nih.gov/gene/ADAMTS13

8. McDonald AG, Boyce S, Tipton KF. ExporEnz: the primary source of the IUBMB enzyme list. *Nucl Acids Res.* 2009;37:D593-D597. doi:10.1093/nar/gkn582. https://www.gmul.ac.uk./sbcs/iubmb/enzyme/

## 14.11 Neurology.

### 14.11.1 Nerves.
Most nerves have names (eg, ulnar nerve or nervus ulnaris). English names are preferred to Latin. For terminology, consult a medical dictionary, anatomy text, or *Terminologia Anatomica*.[1]

#### 14.11.1.1 Cranial Nerves.
The cranial nerves are listed in **Table 14.11-1**.
Use roman numerals or English names when designating cranial nerves:

> Cranial nerves III, IV, and VI are responsible for ocular movement.

> The oculomotor, trochlear, and abducens nerves are responsible for ocular movement.

Use ordinals when the numeric adjectival form is used:

> The third, fourth, and sixth cranial nerves are responsible for ocular movement.

#### 14.11.1.2 Vertebrae, Spinal Nerves, Spinal Levels, Dermatomes, and Somites.
These entities share a common nomenclature, deriving from spinal anatomic regions: cervical (neck), thoracic (trunk), lumbar (lower back), sacral (pelvis), and coccygeal (coccyx or tailbone).

Spinal nerves C1 through C7 are named for the vertebrae above which they emerge, while T1 through S5 are named for the vertebrae below which they emerge. Spinal nerve C8 emerges below vertebra C7; there is no C8 vertebra.

Vertebrae and spinal nerves are listed in **Table 14.11-2**. The alphanumeric terms need not be expanded and, when clear in context, *vertebra* and *nerve* need not be repeated:

**Table 14.11-1.** Cranial Nerves

| Nerve | English name | Latin name |
| --- | --- | --- |
| I | olfactory | olfactorius |
| II | optic | opticus |
| III | oculomotor | oculomotorius |
| IV | trochlear | trochlearis |
| V | trigeminal | trigeminus |
| VI | abducens | abducens |
| VII | facial | facialis |
| VIII | vestibulocochlear | vestibulocochlearis (acoustic) |
| IX | glossopharyngeal | glossopharyngeus |
| X | vagus | vagus |
| XI | accessory | accessorius |
| XII | hypoglossal | hypoglossus |

**Table 14.11-2.** Vertebrae and Spinal Nerves

| Region | Vertebrae | Spinal nerves |
|---|---|---|
| cervical | C1 through C7 | C1 through C8 |
| thoracic | T1 through T12 | T1 through T12 |
| lumbar | L1 through L5 | L1 through L5 |
| sacrum | S1 through S5 | S1 through S5 |
| coccyx | 4 fused, not individually designated | coccygeal nerve |

The first cervical vertebra is also known as the atlas, C2 as the axis, and C7 as the vertebra prominens.

Portions of a vertebra may be referred to as follows, ie, without the term *vertebra*:

C5 spinous process

L3 lamina

T12 transverse process

Hyphens are used for intervertebral spaces (including neural foramina) and intervertebral disks (**Table 14.11-3**).

Note: L4-5 diskectomy is correct usage. *Terminologia Anatomica* uses *disc*, not *disk*. See 11.0, Correct and Preferred Usage.

The sacrum, because its vertebrae are fused, does not contain intervertebral spaces. Its 4 paired foramina are commonly referred to as the first sacral foramen (or S1 foramen), second sacral foramen (or S2 foramen), etc.

Ranges of vertebrae are expressed as in the following examples; use letters for both the first and last vertebra in the indicated range:

C3 through C7    third through seventh cervical vertebrae (not C3 through 7)

T6 through S1    sixth thoracic through first sacral vertebrae

Ranges of vertebrae when used as modifiers have one or more hyphens, eg,

C1-C3 arthrodesis

C2-T1 spinous processes

**Table 14.11-3.** Intervertebral spaces and Disks

| Space | Disk |
|---|---|
| C2-3 (space between C2 and C3) | C2-3 disk |
| T2-3 (space between T2 and T3) | T2-3 disk |
| L2-3 (space between L2 and L3) | L2-3 disk |
| C7-T1 (space between C7 and T1) | C7-T1 disk |
| L5-S1 (space between L5 and S1) | L5-S1 disk |

C4-T3 fusion

L1-L2-L3 motion segments

L1-L4 bone mass density

L2-S1 canal stenosis

L3-L4-L5 fusion

L4-L5 laminectomy

erosion of T9-T12 vertebrae

The same abbreviations are used for spinal segments or levels, spinal dermatomes, and somites (mesodermal structures on either side of the developing spinal cord). Text should indicate which is being referred to, eg, vertebra, spinal nerve (or root, radiculopathy, or distribution), spinal level, dermatome, or somite. Within a clear context, as noted above, the words *vertebra, nerve,* etc, need not be repeated.

Serious injury of the cervical cord at the level of the C2-C5 vertebrae causes respiratory paralysis due to injury of spinal nerves C3 through C5.

The first patient had herpes zoster in the T9 dermatomal distribution, the second patient in the C5 distribution.

L1-S2 radiculopathy

L3-L4-L5 periradicular infiltration

**14.11.2** **Electroencephalographic Terms.** Guidelines for electroencephalography (EEG) are available through the American Clinical Neurophysiology Society (formerly the American Electroencephalographic Society)[2] and the International Federation of Clinical Neurophysiology[3] (formerly the International Federation of Societies for Electroencephalography and Clinical Neurophysiology).[4] Other helpful resources include *Adams and Victor's Principles of Neurology,*[5] the American Electroencephalographic Society guidelines in electroencephalography, evoked potentials, and polysomnography,[6] *Current Practice of Clinical Electroencephalography,*[7] and *Niedermeyer's Electroencephalography: Basic Principles, Clinical Applications, and Related Fields.*[8]

The International 10-20 System specifies placement of electrodes used in electroencephalography. The 10-20 system, which originated in the 1950s,[9,10] is so named because electrodes are spaced 10% or 20% apart along the head (**Figure 14.11-1**).

The terms used in the 10-20 system are widely used and recognized. They are systematically derived, as follows:

▪ Letters refer to anatomical areas (primarily of the skull, which do not necessarily coincide with the brain areas from which the electrodes register electrical activity).

▪ Odd numbers are for electrodes placed on the left side, even numbers are for electrodes placed on the right side, and the letter z ("zero") is for midline electrodes.

**Table 14.11-4** lists the electrode designations and locations.

**Figure 14.11-1.** Electroencephalographic Lead Positions

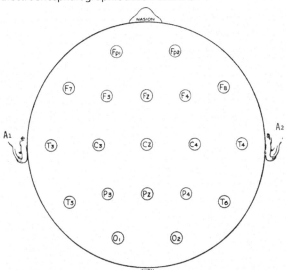

Reproduced from Hughes[11] by permission of Elsevier. Copyright Elsevier 1994.

Additional electrodes and other placement systems may be used, for instance, the "modified combinatorial nomenclature," also known as the 10-10 electrode system, which adds electrodes at intermediate 10% positions.[4,12-16] The same electrode may have a different name in the 10-20 and the 10% systems (eg, T3 and T4 in the 10-20 system are referred to as T7 and T8 in the 10% system).[7] The added electrodes result in additional numeric designations for existing regional electrodes (eg, C5, F10) and in new letters or letter-number combinations, as indicated in **Table 14.11-5**.

Neonatal electrodes may be placed differently (eg, the 12.5% to 25% system of the Children's Hospital of British Columbia) and may (or may not) have different designations,[7] as in the examples below:

**Table 14.11-4.** Electrode Designations and Locations

| Electrode designation | Location |
| --- | --- |
| A1, A2 | earlobe |
| Cz, C3, C4 | central |
| F7, F8 | lateral frontal (anterior temporal) |
| Fp1, Fp2 | frontopolar or prefrontal |
| Fz, F3, F4 | superior frontal |
| O1, O2 | occipital |
| Pz, P3, P4 | parietal |
| T3, T4 | midtemporal |
| T5, T6 | posterior temporal |

**Table 14.11-5.** Added Electrode Designations and Locations

| Added electrode designation | Location |
| --- | --- |
| AFz, AF3, AF4, AF7, AF8 | anterior frontal |
| C1, C2, C5, C6 | centrotemporal |
| CPz, CP1, CP2, CP3, CP4, CP5, CP6 | centroparietal |
| FCz, FC1, FC2, FC3, FC4, FC5, FC6, FC7, FC8, FC9, FC10 | frontocentral |
| Fpz | midprefrontal |
| FT7, FT8, FT9, FT10 | frontotemporal |
| Iz | inion |
| Nz | nasion |
| Oz | midoccipital |
| P1, P2, P5, P6 | parietal |
| P7, P8, P9, P10 | posterior temporal |
| POz, PO3, PO4, PO7, PO8 | parieto-occipital or temporal-occipital |
| Sp1, Sp2 | sphenoidal |
| T1, T2 | true anterior temporal |
| T7, T8, T9, T10 | midtemporal |
| TP7, TP8, TP9, TP10 | temporal-posterior temporal |

| | |
| --- | --- |
| LaF | left anterior frontal |
| LaT | left anterior temporal |
| LFC | left frontocentral |
| LO | left occipital |
| LP | left parietal |
| LST | left superior temporal |
| RaF | right anterior frontal |
| RaT | right anterior temporal |
| RFC | right frontocentral |
| RO | right occipital |
| RP | right parietal |
| RST | right superior temporal |

In figures showing EEGs, electrode symbols usually will be paired. Usually, the symbols will be beside and to the left of each channel of the tracing but may be above and below each channel with connecting lines. Authors should include with tracings a time marker and an indicator of voltage, as in the top tracing (**Figure 14.11-2**).

**Figure 14.11-2.** Sample Electroencephalographic Tracings

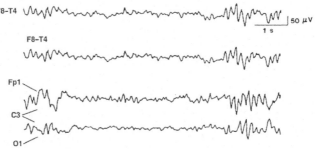

Descriptions of EEG potentials include many qualitative terms for waveforms and frequencies. The following are a few of numerous descriptive terms (note that Greek letters are spelled out):

alpha rhythm, beta activity, polymorphic delta activity, sleep spindles, spike-wave complexes, paroxysms, spikes, sharp waves, delta brush, frontal sharp transient, mu rhythm, lambda waves

A comprehensive glossary of EEG terms has been provided by the IFCN.[16]

Frequency is given per second (/s). For cycles (c) per second, hertz (Hz) is preferred to c/s (see 17.1, SI Units):

10-Hz alpha activity

a theta frequency of 5 to 7.5 Hz

15-Hz spindles

60-Hz artifact

background rhythm of 8 to 10 Hz

**14.11.3** **Evoked Potentials or Responses.** Several types of evoked potentials or responses (stimulated electrical signals)[5(pp13-39),6,17-20] may be recorded: brainstem auditory evoked potentials (BAEPs or BAERs), somatosensory evoked potentials (SSEPs, including various types such as the following, which are not mutually exclusive: short-latency, upper extremity, lower extremity, median nerve, posterior tibial nerve), and visual evoked potentials or responses (VEPs or VERs, including pattern shift [PSVEP] and flash [FVEP]). As in EEG, evoked potential testing uses recording electrodes and produces tracings.

Electrode terminology resembles that of EEGs (see above), with additional or modified electrodes such as the following,[6] which may be used without expansion:

BAEP electrodes

| | |
|---|---|
| Ac | contralateral earlobe |
| Ai | ipsilateral earlobe |
| EAM | external auditory meatus |
| EAMc | contralateral EAM |
| EAMi | ipsilateral EAM |

| M1, M2 | mastoid processes |
| Mc | contralateral M |
| Mi | ipsilateral M |

SSEP electrodes

| AC | anterior cervical |
| C1', C2', C3', C4' | near EEG C1, C2, C3, C4 |
| C2S, C5S | C2, C5 spinous processes |
| Cc | contralateral C3' or C4' |
| Ci | ipsilateral C3' or C4' |
| CP | midway between C3 or C4 and P3 or P4 |
| CPc | contralateral CP |
| CPi | ipsilateral CP |
| Cz' | near 10-20 Cz |
| EP | Erb point |
| EP1, EP2 | left and right EP |
| EPi | ipsilateral EP |
| Fpz' | near EEG Fpz |
| IC | iliac crest |
| L2S, L3S | L2, L3 spinous processes |
| LN | lateral neck |
| LNi | ipsilateral LN |
| PFd, PFp | popliteal fossa (distal, proximal) |
| REF | reference |
| T6S, T10S, T12S | T6, T10, T12 spinous processes |

VEP electrodes

| I | inion |
| LO | left occipital |
| LT | left posterior temporal |
| MF | midfrontal |
| MO | midoccipital |
| MP | midparietal |
| RO | right occipital |
| RT | right posterior temporal |
| V | vertex |

Waveforms recorded in evoked potential testing are identified with P for positive or N for negative plus a number indicating milliseconds between stimulus and response in neurologically normal adults:

VEP:    N75, N100, N155, P75, P100, P135

SSEP:   N9, N11, N13, N15, N18, N20, N34, N35, P9, P11, P13, P15, P27, P37

SSEPs were recorded from the brachial plexus (Erb point), cervical spine at C2 (N13), and the contralateral parietal area (N19) with a frontal (Fz) reference.

SSEPs showed normal Erb point and cervical potentials and significant delay of scalp components (N20 latency >>3 SDs, N13-N20 central conduction time >3 SDs, bilaterally).

Persistent delay of the P100 wave of the pattern-reversal VEP after an episode of optic neuritis is considered to be compatible with residual demyelination within the optic nerve.

An additional SSEP wave is the LP (lumbar potential).

Other waves, eg, in BAEP, are designated with roman numerals:

I through VII      vertex-positive waves

I′ through VI′     vertex-negative waves

BAEPs of the proband showed normal wave I, increased latency of waves II and III (>3 SDs), and absent IV and V components despite normal hearing acuity.

I-III interpeak interval

V/I amplitude ratio

14.11.4 **Polysomnography and Sleep Stages.** Polysomnography is the monitoring of various physiologic parameters simultaneously during sleep,[6,21] including the following:

- EEG: standard electrodes are used (see 14.11.2, Electroencephalographic Terms)

- Electro-oculogram (EOG): tracings are obtained from the left eye and right eye

- Electromyogram (EMG): submental (chin) EMG, leg muscle EMG, eg, left anterior tibialis, right anterior tibialis

- Respiratory function, eg, oxygen saturation ($Sao_2$), expired $CO_2$, and tidal volume ($V_T$) (see 14.16, Pulmonary and Respiratory Terminology)

- Electrocardiogram (ECG): see 14.3.1, Electrocardiographic Terms

Sleep stages are as follows[7,22]:

rapid-eye-movement sleep (REM sleep)

non–rapid-eye-movement (non-REM) sleep (NREM sleep)

sleep stage 1 (N1 sleep)

sleep stage 2 (N2 sleep)

sleep stage 3 (N3 sleep)

sleep stage 4 (N4 sleep)

**14.11.5** **Molecular Neuroscience.** The following terms are provided for reference (a major source is Nestler et al[23]) (see 14.10, Molecular Medicine). Terms should be expanded at first mention unless noted otherwise in the Expansion or Explanation column.

| Term | Expansion or explanation |
|---|---|
| $\alpha$-adrenergic receptor, $\alpha$ receptor (subtypes: $\alpha_{1A}$, $\alpha_{1B}$, $\alpha_{1D}$, $\alpha_{2A}$, $\alpha_{2B}$, $\alpha_{2C}$) | does not require expansion |
| $\alpha$-synuclein | does not require expansion |
| $A_1$, $A_2$ | neuropeptide adenosine receptors (also known as purine receptors $P_1$, $P_2$; see 14.6.1, Nucleic Acids and Amino Acids); does not require expansion |
| ACh | acetylcholine |
| AChE | acetylcholinesterase |
| AMPA | $\alpha$-amino-3-hydroxy-5-methyl-4-isoxazole propionic acid |
| $\beta$-adrenergic receptor, $\beta$ receptor (subtypes: $\beta_1$, $\beta_2$, $\beta_3$) | does not require expansion |
| BDNF | brain-derived neurotrophic factor |
| CCR3, CCR5, CXCR4 | chemokine receptors (see 14.8.1, Chemokines) |
| Ch1 through Ch8 | cholinergic nuclei |
| CNTF | ciliary neurotrophic factor |
| COMT | catechol-*O*-methyltransferase |
| cytokines | (see 14.8.4, Nomenclature, Immunology, Cytokines) |
| $\delta$-receptor | opioid $\delta$ receptor |
| $D_1$ through $D_5$ | dopamine receptors |
| DAT | dopamine transporters |

| EAAT1, EAAT2, EAAT3, EAAT4, EAAT5 | excitatory amino acid reuptake transporters |
|---|---|
| EGF | epidermal growth factor |
| GABA | γ-aminobutyric acid |
| $GABA_A$, $GABA_B$ | GABA receptor classes |
| GABAergic | GABA-mediated |
| GABA-T | GABA transaminase |
| GAT-1, GAT-2, GAT-3, GAT-4 | GABA family transporters |
| GDNF | glial cell line–derived neurotrophic factor |
| GFR | GDNF-neurturin receptor |
| GIRKs | G protein–coupled $K_{ir}3$ channels |
| $H_1$, $H_2$, $H_3$ | histamine receptors |
| 5-HT | 5-hydroxytryptamine, serotonin (preferred expansion) |
| $5\text{-HT}_{1A}$, $5\text{-HT}_{1B}$, $5\text{-HT}_{2A}$, $5\text{-HT}_{5B}$, $5\text{-HT}_7$ | 5-HT receptors |
| 5-HTT | serotonin transporter |
| 5HTTLPR | a polymorphism of the serotonin transporter gene (LPR: length polymorphism region) (see 14.6.2, Human Gene Nomenclature) |
| interleukins | (see 14.8.4, Cytokines) |
| $IP_3$ | inositol triphosphate |
| κ-receptor | opioid κ receptor |
| K(ATP) channel | potassium channel |
| K(Ca) | $Ca^{2+}$-gated $K^+$ channel |
| Kir1, Kir2, Kir3, Kir4, Kir5 | inwardly rectifying $K^+$ channels; does not require expansion |
| L channels, L-type channels | large-current or long-open-time $Ca^{2+}$ channels; does not require expansion |
| μ-receptor | opioid μ receptor |
| $M_1$ through $M_5$ | muscarinic receptors; does not require expansion |

| | |
|---|---|
| MAO | monoamine oxidase |
| $MAO_A$, $MAO_B$ | major forms of MAO |
| N channels | neuronal $Ca^{2+}$ channels; does not require expansion |
| nAChRs | nicotinic acetylcholine receptors |
| NET | norepinephrine GABA family transporter |
| neuromedin B | does not require expansion |
| neuromedin K | does not require expansion |
| neuropeptide Y | does not require expansion |
| NGF | nerve growth factor |
| $NK_1$, $NK_2$, $NK_3$ | neuromedin K tachykinin receptors |
| NMDA | $N$-methyl-D-aspartate |
| nNOS | neuronal nitric oxide synthetase |
| NSF | $N$-ethylmaleamide sensitive factor |
| NT-3, NT-4 | neurotrophin 3 and neurotrophin 4 |
| $NTS_1$, $NTS_2$ | neurotensin receptors |
| P channels | Purkinje $Ca^{2+}$ channels; does not require expansion |
| $P_1$, $P_2$ | neuropeptide purine receptors (also known as adenosine receptors $A_1$, $A_2$; see 14.6.1, Nucleic Acids and Amino Acids); does not require expansion |
| R-PTK | receptor-associated protein tyrosine kinase |
| σ-receptor | opioid σ receptor |
| SERT | serotonin GABA family transporter |
| SNAP-25 | synaptosomal-associated protein of 25 kDa |
| SNAP | soluble NSF attachment protein (note different expansion of SNAP than for SNAP-25) |
| SNARE proteins | SNAP receptors |
| SNAREpins | hairpin forms of SNARE proteins |
| substance P | does not require expansion |

| | |
|---|---|
| T channels | transient $Ca^{2+}$ channels; does not require expansion |
| t-SNARES | t: target membranes |
| VAChT | vesicular transporters of ACh |
| VAMP | vesicle-associated membrane protein, synaptobrevin |
| VGAT | vesicular transporter for GABA |
| VGLuT1 | vesicular transporter for glutamate |
| VMAT1 | vesicular transporter for monoamines |
| v-SNARE | v: vesicle |
| $Y_1$, $Y_2$, $Y_4$, $Y_5$, $Y_6$ | neuropeptide Y receptors |

Gene symbols for many of the above terms are found in the list of genes in 14.6.2, Human Gene Nomenclature. For reference, gene symbols are given in **Table 14.11-6** for terms in the preceding list whose abbreviations do not closely resemble the gene symbol.

**Table 14.11-6.** Gene Symbols in Genes Whose Abbreviations Do Not Closely Resemble the Gene Symbol

| Term | Gene symbol |
|---|---|
| $A_1$ | *ADORA1* |
| AMPA | *GRIA1* |
| δ receptor | *OPRD1* |
| D1 | *DRD1* |
| H1 | *HRH1* |
| $5\text{-HT}_{1A}$ | *HTR1A* |
| κ receptor | *OPRK1* |
| μ receptor | *OPRM1* |
| M1 | *CHRM1* |
| nAChR | *CHRNA1* |
| neuromedin K | *TAC3* |
| NMDA | *GRIN1* |
| σ receptor | *OPRS1* |
| substance P | *TAC1* |
| transporters (various) | *SLC* genes (various, eg, *SLC6A1*) |
| Y1 | *NPY1R* |

**Principal Author:** Cheryl Iverson, MA

ACKNOWLEDGMENT

Thanks to Roger N. Rosenberg, MD, formerly with *JAMA Neurology*, and Department of Neurology, University of Texas Southwestern, Dallas; Jeffrey L. Saver, MD, *JAMA*, and Geffen School of Medicine at UCLA, Los Angeles, California; and Christopher C. Muth, MD, *JAMA*. Thanks also to David Song, JAMA Network, for obtaining permissions.

REFERENCES

1. Federative Committee on Anatomical Terminology. *Terminologia Anatomica*. Georg Thieme Verlag; 1998.

2. American Clinical Neurophysiology Society. Accessed August 1, 2019. https://www.acns.org

3. International Federation of Clinical Neurophysiology (IFCN). Accessed August 1, 2019. https://www.ifcn.info/

4. Nuwer MR, Comi G, Emerson R, et al. IFCN standards for digital recording of clinical EEG. In: Deuschl G, Eisen A, eds. *Recommendations for the Practice of Clinical Neurophysiology: Guidelines of the International Federation of Neurophysiology*. *Electroencephalogr Clin Neurophysiol*. 1998;106(3):259-261.

5. Ropper AH, Samuels MA, Klein JP. Imaging, electrophysiologic, and laboratory techniques for neurologic diagnosis. In: *Adams and Victor's Principles of Neurology*. 10th ed. McGraw-Hill; 2014:13-39.

6. Gilmore RL, ed. American Electroencephalographic Society guidelines in electroencephalography, evoked potentials, and polysomnography. *J Clin Neurophysiol*. 1994;11(1):1-158.

7. Recording techniques. In: Ebersole JS, ed; Sinha SR, Husain AM, Nordli DR, assoc eds. *Current Practice of Clinical Electroencephalography*. 4th ed. Lippincott Williams & Wilkins; 2014:78-89.

8. Schomer DL, Lopes da Silva F, eds. *Niedermeyer's Electroencephalography: Basic Principles, Clinical Applications, and Related Fields*. 6th ed. Lippincott Williams & Wilkins; 2012.

9. Jasper HH. Report of the Committee on Methods of Clinical Examination in Electroencephalography: 1957. *Electroencephalogr Clin Neurophysiol*. 1958;10(2):370-375.

10. Rowan AJ, Tolunsky E. *Primer of EEG: With a Mini-Atlas*. Butterworth-Heinemann; 2003.

11. Hughes JR. *EEG in Clinical Practice*. 2nd ed. Butterworth-Heinemann 1994:2.

12. Sharbrough F, Chatrian G-E, Lesser RP, Lüders H, Nuwer M, Picton TW; Electrode Position Nomenclature Committee. American Electroencephalographic Society guidelines for standard electrode position nomenclature. *J Clin Neurophysiol*. 1991;8(2):200-202.

13. Chatrian G-E, Lettich E, Nelson PL. Modified nomenclature for the "10%" electrode system. *J Clin Neurophysiol*. 1988;5(2):183-186.

14. Nuwer MR. Recording electrode site nomenclature. *J Clin Neurophysiol*. 1987;4(2):121-133.

15. Acharya JN, Hani A, Cheek J, Thirumala P, Tsuchida TN. American Clinical Neurophysiology Society Guideline 2: Guidelines for Standard Electrode Nomenclature. *J Clin Neurophysiol*. 2016;33(4):308-311.

16. Noachtar S, Binnie C, Ebersole J, Mauguière F, Sakamoto A, Westmoreland B. A glossary of terms most commonly used by clinical electroencephalographers and proposal for the report form for the EEG findings. In: Deutschl G, Eisen A, eds. *Recommendations for the Practice of Clinical Neurophysiology: Guidelines of the International Federation of Neurophysiology. Electroencephalogr Clin Neurophysiol Suppl.* 1999;suppl 52:21-41.

17. American Association of Electrodiagnostic Medicine. Guidelines in electrodiagnostic medicine, 6: guidelines in somatosensory evoked potentials. *Muscle Nerve.* 1999;22(suppl 8):S111-S118.

18. Celesia GG, Bodis-Wollner I, Chatrian GE, Harding GFA, Sokol S, Spekreijse H. Recommended standards for electroretinograms and visual evoked potentials: report of an IFCN committee. *Electroencephalogr Clin Neurophysiol.* 1993;87(6):421-436.

19. Nuwer MR, Aminoff M, Goodin D, et al. IFCN recommended standards for brain-stem auditory evoked potentials: report of an IFCN committee. *Electroencephalogr Clin Neurophysiol.* 1994;91(1):12-17.

20. Deutschl G, Eisen A, eds. *Recommendations for the Practice of Clinical Neurophysiology: Guidelines of the International Federation of Neurophysiology. Electroencephalogr Clin Neurophysiol.* 1999;S52:1-304.

21. Radtke RA. Sleep disorders: laboratory evaluation. In: Ebersole JS, ed; Sinha SR, Husain AM, Nordli DR, assoc eds. *Current Practice of Clinical Electroencephalography.* 4th ed. Lippincott Williams & Wilkins; 2014:599-630.

22. American Academy of Sleep Medicine. *The International Classification of Sleep Disorders, Revised: Diagnostic and Coding Manual.* American Academy of Sleep Medicine; 2001.

23. Nestler EJ, Hyman SE, Holtzman DM, Malenka RC. *Molecular Neuropharmacology: A Foundation for Clinical Neuroscience.* 3rd ed. McGraw-Hill; 2015.

**14.12** **Obstetric Terms.** Two colloquial shorthand expressions quantify an individual's pregnancy history: GPA and TPAL. The GPA and TPAL expressions are familiar and widely used clinically. However, they are also recognized as imprecise and lacking in standardization.[1-3]

**14.12.1** **GPA.** The letters G, P, and A (or Ab) accompanied by numbers indicate number of pregnancies; number of pregnancies reaching viable gestational age, including live births and stillbirths; and number of spontaneous or induced abortions, respectively. Definitions of viability vary, however, and in articles "the outcome of any pregnancy that did not end normally"[4(pp194-195)] should be specified. In the expansions in **Table 14.12-1**, the clinical meaning accompanies its respective GPA shorthand.

For example, G3, P2, A1 indicates 3 pregnancies, 2 pregnancies reaching viable gestational age (including live births and stillbirths), and 1 abortion. In published articles, however, it is preferable to write out the expressions as follows:

gravida 3, para 2, aborta 1

Although some sources feature roman numerals with these expressions, use arabic numerals.

**Table 14.12-1.** Explanation of Abbreviations G, P, and A

| Letter | Expansion of letter | Clinical meaning |
|---|---|---|
| G | gravida | pregnancies |
| P | para | pregnancies reaching viable gestational age, including live births and stillbirths |
| A or Ab | aborta | abortions |

Quantifying prefixes combine with the terms *gravida* and *para* (see list below). Noun forms are *gravidity* and *parity* (with prefixes *nulligravidity, multiparity,* etc). Adjective forms are *gravid* and *parous* (with prefixes *multigravida, multiparous, primiparous,* etc).

| | |
|---|---|
| nulligravida | gravida 0 |
| primigravida | gravida 1 |
| secundigravida | gravida 2 |
| multigravida | gravida > 1 |
| nullipara | para 0 |
| primipara | para 1 |
| multipara | para > 1 |
| grand multipara | para ≥ 5 |

Even these Latin-derived terms are somewhat imprecise.[1,3] Therefore, in addition to use of expansions, further specifications (eg, single or multiple births, ectopic pregnancy) are required in scientific articles.

**14.12.2** **TPAL.** The letters in this expression indicate obstetric history as follows:

T    term births

P    premature births

A    abortions

L    living children

Often, 4 numbers separated by hyphens are recorded, as in the following:

TPAL: 3-1-1-4 *or* 3-1-1-4

This expression indicates 3 term births, 1 premature birth, 1 abortion, and 4 living children. However, the text of a manuscript should define the numerical expressions and not give the numbers alone.[4(p195)]

**14.12.3** **Apgar Score.** This score[4(pp594-595)-7] is an assessment of a newborn's physical well-being based on the 5 factors of heart rate, breathing, muscle tone, reflex irritability, and color, each of which is rated 0, 1, or 2; the 5 ratings are then summed. The Apgar score is often reported as 2 numbers, from 0 to 10, separated by a virgule, reflecting assessment at 1 minute and 5 minutes after birth. In general medical journals, however, it is best to specify the intervals, especially because the Apgar score may be assessed at other intervals (eg, 10, 15, or 20 minutes).

| | |
|---|---|
| *Ambiguous:* | Apgar score of 9/10 |
| *Preferred:* | Apgar score of 9/10 at 1 and 5 minutes, respectively *or* Apgar scores of 9 at 1 minute and 10 at 5 minutes |

The score is named after the late anesthesiologist, Virginia Apgar, MD; thus "Apgar" is *not* printed in all capital letters as though for an acronym (although versions of such an acronym, a backronym, have been created as a mnemonic device: appearance, pulse, grimace, activity, respiration[8]).

**14.12.4** **Birth Weight.** Birth weight is defined as the weight of a neonate immediately after delivery. It should be expressed to the nearest gram.[4(p3),5(p499)]

Low birth weight: weight less than 2500 g

Very low birth weight: weight less than 1500 g

Extremely low birth weight: weight less than 1000 g

**14.12.5** **Term Pregnancy.** The American College of Obstetrics and Gynecologists and the Society for Maternal-Fetal Medicine[9] discourage use of the general label *term pregnancy* and instead recommend more specific descriptions:

Early term: between 37 weeks 0 days and 38 weeks 6 days' gestation

Full term: between 39 weeks 0 days and 40 weeks 6 days' gestation

Late term: between 41 weeks 0 days and 41 weeks 6 days' gestation

Postterm: 42 weeks 0 days' gestation and beyond

**Principal Author:** Cheryl Iverson, MA

## ACKNOWLEDGMENT

Thanks to Frances E. Likis, DrPH, NP, CNM, *Journal of Midwifery & Women's Health*, Nashville, Tennessee, for reviewing and providing comments.

## REFERENCES

1. Summarizing the obstetric history. *JAMA*. 1991;266(23):3344. doi:10.1001/jama.1991.03470230104043
2. Pun TC, Ng JC. "Madame is a 30-year-old housewife, gravida X, para Y . . . ." *Obstet Gynecol*. 1989;73(2):276-277.
3. Woolley RJ. Parity clarity: proposal for a new obstetric shorthand. *J Fam Pract*. 1993;36(3):265-266.

4. Cunningham FG, Leveno KJ, Bloom SL, Hauth JC, Rouse DJ, Spong CY. *Williams Obstetrics*. 23rd ed. McGraw-Hill; 2010.
5. American Academy of Pediatrics, American College of Obstetricians and Gynecologists. *Guidelines for Perinatal Care*. 7th ed. American Academy of Pediatrics and American College of Obstetricians and Gynecologists; 2012.
6. Apgar V. A proposal for a new method of evaluation of the newborn infant. *Curr Res Anesth Analg*. 1953;32(4):260-267.
7. Apgar V, Holaday DA, James LS, Weisbrot IM, Berrien C. Evaluation of the newborn infant: second report. *JAMA*. 1958;168(15):1985-1988.
8. Butterfield J, Covery MJ. Practical epigram of the Apgar score. *JAMA*. 1962;181(4):353.
9. ACOG Committee Opinion No. 579: definition of term pregnancy. *Obstet Gynecol*. 2013;122(5):1139-1140. doi:10.1097/01.AOG.0000437385.88715.4a

**14.13** **Ophthalmology Terms.** Some terms described in this section are specific to ophthalmology, and others have special usage requirements in ophthalmology (see 11.0, Correct and Preferred Usage).

**adnexa oculi.** Although often used as a synonym for eyelids, the term *adnexa oculi* (which is plural) properly includes the eyelids, lacrimal apparatus, and other appendages of the eye and should be used with its inclusive meaning.

**diopter.** The diopter is a measure of the power of an optical lens and is the reciprocal of the focal length in meters. Diopter is abbreviated D when used with a number.

> diopter sphere
>
> diopter cylinder
>
> conversion from diopters to millimeters
>
> correction of 10.5 D

The prism diopter is a measure of the power of a prism and represents a 1-cm deflection of an image at a distance of 1 m. Its symbol, $\Delta$, may be used with numbers after first mention.

> The left eye showed an improvement, with only 25–prism diopter hypotropia.
>
> distance exotropia = 35 prism diopters ($\Delta$); near exotropia = 5$\Delta$

**disc, cup-disc ratio.** For the optic disc, spell as *disc* (not *disk*). The cup-disc ratio refers to the ratio of the diameter of the optic cup (a central area devoid of nerve fibers within the optic disc) to diameter of the optic disc.

> cup-disc ratio of 0.6

It can be useful to specify whether the ratio is vertical, horizontal, or other.

> The mean (SD) horizontal cup-disc ratio by contour estimated from stereophotography was 0.36 (0.18).

**disc diameters, disc areas.** Disc diameters (DDs) may be used to indicate location or dimension of findings on the ocular fundus with relative distances expressed as diameters of the optic disc.

> 2 DDs inferior to the fovea

> Lesions varied from 0.5 to 4.5 disc diameters (DDs; median, 2.0 DDs) for the first group, 0.75 to 7.5 DDs (median, 2.5 DDs) for the second group, and 1.0 to 9.0 DDs (median, 4.0 DDs) for the last group.

Disc areas (DAs) are also used to indicate relative sizes of findings on the ocular fundus, as well as in considerations of the size of the disc.

> A scar in the center of the retina, presumably from toxoplasmosis, occupied approximately 6 disc areas of the central macula.

> Substantial ischemia was defined as greater than 10 disc areas of retinal capillary nonperfusion.

> Disc areas (DAs) were measured using objective techniques. The mean DA for the patients in group 1 was 2.57 mm$^2$.

**electroretinogram, pattern electroretinogram.** Waves of the electroretinogram (ERG) are as follows:

> $a_1$ $\quad$ $a_2$ $\quad\quad$ b

An ERG may be described as normal, subnormal, or negative. Do not substitute one of these terms for another. (For visual evoked potentials, see 14.11.3, Evoked Potentials or Responses.)
Waves of the pattern electroretinogram (PERG)[1] are as follows:

> $a_{pt}$ $\quad$ $b_{pt}$ $\quad$ $c_{pt}$

Two main components of the PERG are the P50 wave, a positive-deflection waveform, and the N95 wave, a negative-deflection waveform. The terms P50 and N95 may be used without expansion.

**fovea, macula.** The center of the macula is the fovea. The terms *fovea* and *macula* should be used specifically and not interchangeably. Similarly, areas defined on imaging of the macula (such as on optical coherence tomography) should refer to the *center* point as the center of the image and *central* subfield as the central area of the image.

**Goldmann perimetry.** This is a method of assessing the visual field. The test stimuli are described by means of a 3-part term: spot size is designated with roman numerals I through V, and luminance is designated with arabic numerals 1 through 4 and letters a through e. For example:

> I-4-e isopter area

> I-2-e test object

> V-4-e light

**greatest linear dimension.** This is the greatest dimension between 2 points on the boundary of a lesion.

> Lesion size was less than or equal to 9 disc areas, and greatest linear dimension was less than or equal to 5400 μm.

**injection.** When used to indicate excess blood, engorgement, or dilation of a vessel, *injection* should be changed to *hyperemia* or *vasodilation* (eg, *conjunctival hyperemia* or *conjunctival vasodilation* [not *conjunctival injection*]).

**intraocular pressure.** Measurements of intraocular pressure (IOP) should include the method used (eg, Goldmann applanation tonometry) and, if determined, the corneal thickness measurement.

> Substantial postoperative astigmatism led to marked overestimation of the intraocular pressure (56 mm Hg) as measured with Goldmann aplanation tonometry with the mires in the standard horizontal position.

**intravitreous, intravitreal.** *Intravitreous* is an adjective and should precede nouns, such as an injection (eg, intravitreous injection). *Intravitreal* is an adverb and should precede verbs, unless part of a name in which *intravitreal* was used as an adjective (eg, dexamethasone intravitreal implant).

**lasers.** Lasers used in ophthalmology include the following:

> argon laser
>
> erbium:YAG laser
>
> eximer laser
>
> holmium:YAG laser
>
> krypton laser
>
> Nd:YAG laser
>
> photodynamic therapy laser
>
> Q-switched Nd:YAG laser
>
> transpupillary thermal therapy

The term Nd:YAG (neodymium:yttrium-aluminum-garnet) may be used without expansion.

**lids.** *Lids* should be changed to *eyelids*.

**masked.** *Masked* rather than *blinded* should be used in the ophthalmologic literature when referring to randomization or assessment of research participants or outcomes, if there could be confusion.

**OD, OS, OU.** These abbreviations may be used without expansion only with numbers (eg, 20/25 OU) or descriptive assessments of acuity (eg, counting fingers OS; see *Visual acuity, vision*) (Table 14.13-1).

Note that OU means each eye, not both eyes, although it is often used incorrectly to imply a vision measurement (eg, visual acuity or visual field) with both eyes at the same time (see *Visual acuity, vision*).

**Table 14.13-1.** Explanation of Acuity Abbreviations

| Abbreviation | Derivation | Meaning |
| --- | --- | --- |
| OD | Oculus dexter | Right eye |
| OS | Oculus sinister | Left eye |
| OU | Oculus uterque | Each eye |

**ophthalmoscopy.** *Ophthalmoscopy* refers to visualization of the eye with an ophthalmoscope; the term *funduscopy* is not considered a word because it would imply visualization with a "funduscope," which is not an instrument.

**orbit.** *Orbit* refers to the bony cavity that contains the eyeball and its adnexa (muscles, vessels, nerves). It should be clear to readers whether authors are referring to the orbit, the specific bones that compose it, the structures that fill the orbit, or a combination of these.

**visual acuity, vision.** Distinguish between *vision,* a general term, and *visual acuity,* measurable clearness of vision. If a measurement is given (eg, 20/20 [see below]), use *visual acuity.* Change "unaided vision" to "acuity without correction" (see 11.0, Correct and Preferred Usage). Authors should report the visual acuity in the manuscript using the same nomenclature that was used in the study. Typically, visual acuities are collected as logMAR (base 10 logarithm of the minimum angle of resolution) values, letter scores, decimal fractions, or Snellen fractions (using meters or feet). However, evidence[2] suggests that many readers, at least in the US, best understand visual acuity measurements when given as Snellen equivalents. For example, authors of manuscripts submitted to *JAMA Ophthalmology* are requested to provide the approximate Snellen equivalent in feet (20/20, 20/40, etc) in parentheses next to each visual acuity that is not in this Snellen format throughout the manuscript, including figures and tables.[3] The methods used to provide the appropriate Snellen equivalent visual acuities should be given in the Methods section of the manuscript and should be based on published data, for example, as provided by Ferris and colleagues[4] and the Diabetic Retinopathy Clinical Research Network.[5] Always list the visual acuity scores from best to worst when listing more than one (eg, 20/63 to 20/100) or letter scores of 60 (20/63) to 59 (29.100).

**distance acuity.** The Snellen eye chart is a well-known method of assessing distance visual acuity, resulting in the Snellen fraction, an expression such as 20/15, 20/20, or 20/60. The first number represents the testing distance from chart to patient; the second number represents the smallest row of letters that the patient can read. For example, acuity of 20/40 indicates that at 20 ft the smallest line read is readable by a normal eye at 40 ft. Do not add Snellen equivalents for differences in letter scores.

The units for distance acuity are feet (eg, 20 ft) or meters (eg, 6 m). By convention, acuity is expressed without these units specified (eg, 20/20). The JAMA Network journals follow the author's preference in expressing distance acuity equivalents as metric (eg, 6/6) or English (20/20) and do not convert English fractions to metric or vice versa. Only one type, English or metric, should be used throughout a manuscript.

Visual acuity is assessed separately for each eye. Other means are also used to assess visual acuity, such as counting fingers (CF), hand motions (HM), and light perception (LP), which may be expanded as LP with projection, LP without projection, or no LP (NLP). Express visual acuity, including numerical measures and other means, by using OD or RE (right eye) and OS or LE (left eye) (see *OD, OS, OU*).

The visual acuity was 20/40 OD and counting fingers OS.

Not: The visual acuity was 20/40 OD and counting fingers in the left eye.

Another method of assessing visual acuity makes use of the Bailey-Lovie or Early Treatment Diabetic Retinopathy Study (ETDRS) or electronic ETDRS (e-ETDRS) acuity charts and designates acuity using logMAR. A logMAR of 0.0 is equivalent to 20/20 Snellen (**Table 14.13-2**). LogMAR visual acuities always should be expressed in logMAR. Note that logMAR does not require expansion.

**letter scores vs letters.** Because Bailey-Lovie or ETDRS or e-ETDRS charts follow a protocol of recording letters read and then computing a letter score, visual acuities from these charts should provide visual acuities as letter scores, not letters (Table 14.13-3). For example,

**Table 14.13-2.** Table of Equivalent Visual Acuity Measurements[a]

| Snellen visual acuities | | | Decimal fraction | logMAR |
|---|---|---|---|---|
| 4 m | 6 m | 20 ft | | |
| 4/40 | 6/60 | 20/200 | 0.10 | +1.0 |
| 4/32 | 6/48 | 20/160 | 0.125 | +0.9 |
| 4/25 | 6/38 | 20/125 | 0.16 | +0.8 |
| 4/20 | 6/30 | 20/100 | 0.20 | +0.7 |
| 4/16 | 6/24 | 20/80 | 0.25 | +0.6 |
| 4/12.6 | 6/20 | 20/63 | 0.32 | +0.5 |
| 4/10 | 6/15 | 20/50 | 0.40 | +0.4 |
| 4/8 | 6/12 | 20/40 | 0.50 | +0.3 |
| 4/6.3 | 6/10 | 20/32 | 0.63 | +0.2 |
| 4/5 | 6/7.5 | 20/25 | 0.80 | +0.1 |
| 4/4 | 6/6 | 20/20 | 1.00 | 0.0 |
| 4/3.2 | 6/5 | 20/16 | 1.25 | −0.1 |
| 4/2.5 | 6/3.75 | 20/12.5 | 1.60 | −0.2 |
| 4/2 | 6/3 | 20/10 | 2.00 | −0.3 |

[a]Adapted with permission from Ferris et al.[4] Copyright 1982 Elsevier.

**Table 14.13-3.** Visual Acuity Score Conversion[a]

| Letter score | logMAR | Snellen equivalent |
|---|---|---|
| 0-3 | 1.70 to 1.64 | <20/800 |
| 4-8 | 1.62 to 1.54 | 20/800 |
| 9-13 | 1.53 to 1.44 | 20/640 |
| 14-18 | 1.42 to 1.34 | 20/500 |
| 19-23 | 1.32 to 1.24 | 20/400 |
| 24-28 | 1.22 to 1.14 | 20/320 |
| 29-33 | 1.12 to 1.04 | 20/250 |
| 34-38 | 1.02 to 0.94 | 20/200 |
| 39-43 | 0.92 to 0.84 | 20/160 |
| 44-48 | 0.82 to 0.74 | 20/125 |
| 49-53 | 0.72 to 0.64 | 20/100 |
| 54-58 | 0.62 to 0.54 | 20/80 |
| 59-63 | 0.52 to 0.44 | 20/63 |
| 64-68 | 0.42 to 0.34 | 20/50 |
| 69-73 | 0.32 to 0.24 | 20/40 |
| 74-78 | 0.22 to 0.14 | 20/32 |
| 79-83 | 0.12 to 0.04 | 20/25 |
| 84-88 | 0.02 to −0.06 | 20/20 |
| 89-93 | −0.08 to −0.16 | 20/16 |
| 94-97 | −0.18 to −0.24 | 20/12 |

[a]Adapted with permission from the Diabetic Retinopathy Clinical Research Network website.[5]

The best-corrected visual acuity letter score was 55 (approximate Snellen equivalent 20/80).

(Not: The best-corrected visual acuity was 55 letters.)

However, improvement or loss can be in letters. For example,

The mean change in visual acuity from baseline to 2 years among eyes assigned to laser treatment was 7 letters.

**near visual acuity.** Near visual acuity (reading vision) may be reported by means of Snellen equivalents or the Jaeger system (J values, ranging from J1 to J11). J2 is equivalent to Snellen 20/20.[6]

**visual field.** The extent of the visual field is described by means of degrees from a central point from 0° through 90°:

85° temporally

65° nasally

56° up and nasally

**vitreous.** *Vitreous* may be used as a noun or an adjective. Typically, avoid *vitreal* and *intravitreal* in all contexts (change *intravitreal* to *intravitreous*).

**Principal Author:** Cheryl Iverson, MA

### ACKNOWLEDGMENT

Thanks to Neil M. Bressler, MD, editor *JAMA Ophthalmology*, and Retina Division, Johns Hopkins Medicine, Baltimore, Maryland, for reviewing and providing comments. Thanks also to David Song, JAMA Network, for obtaining permissions.

### REFERENCES

1. Bach M, Brigell M, Hawlina M, et al. ISCEV standard for clinical pattern electroretinography (PERG): 2012 update. *Doc Ophthalmol*. 2013;126(1):1-7. doi:10.1007/s10633-012-9353-y
2. Lopes MS, Zayit-Soudry S, Moshiri A, Bressler SB, Bressler NM. Understanding and reporting visual acuity measurements in publications of clinical research. *Arch Ophthalmol*. 2011;129(9):1228-1229. doi:10.1001/archophthalmol.2011.248
3. Bressler N, Beck RW, Kass MA. *JAMA Ophthalmology* publication policies and procedures: fresh start for a new year. *JAMA Ophthalmol*. 2014;132(1):11-12. doi:10.1001/jamaophthalmol.2013.7874
4. Ferris FL III, Kassoff A, Bresnick GH, Bailey I. New visual acuity charts for clinical research. *Am J Ophthalmol*. 1982;94(1):91-96. doi:10.1016/0002-9394(82)90197-0
5. Information for investigators: visual acuity score conversion chart. Accessed August, 1, 2019. http://publicfiles/jaeb.org/drcrnet/Misc/VAScoreConversionChart.pdf
6. Visual acuity conversion chart. Accessed August 1, 2019. https://www.healio.com/~/media/Files/Journals/General/PDFs/JRSVACHART.pdf

## 14.14 ▪ Organisms and Pathogens.

### 14.14.1 ▪ Biological Nomenclature.

**14.14.1.1** **Scientific and Vernacular Names.** *Scientific names* are short terms used in place of lengthy descriptions of species of animals, plants, and organisms. A *scientific name* is typically derived from Latin and corresponds to a set of formally defined attributes. The meanings of scientific names are internationally understood.[1]

In contrast, *vernacular names* are typically based on the local language, using everyday, "common" words. Examples of vernacular names seen in medical publications include fungi, prokaryotes, meningococcus, and St John's wort. Vernacular names cannot be assumed to correspond to formally defined sets of attributes and vary by region and language. **Table 14.14.-1** gives examples of scientific and vernacular names.

In scientific writing, scientific names should be used when the labeled entity verifiably corresponds to the set of attributes associated with the scientific name, at least at first mention. Subsequently, vernacular names (including collective genus

**Table 14.14-1.** Examples of Scientific and Vernacular Names

| Scientific name | Vernacular name |
| --- | --- |
| *Ixodes scapularis* | deer tick |
| *Suscrofa domesticus* | domestic pig |
| *Rosimarinus officinalis* | rosemary |

terms, described later in this section) may be used. Parenthetical mention of the vernacular name when the scientific name is used, and vice versa, is helpful. Table 14.14-2 gives examples of first and subsequent mentions of scientific and vernacular names.

**14.14.1.2** **Biological Nomenclature.** Biological nomenclature is the scientific naming of organisms and is the source of scientific names. Taxonomy comprises the principles and practices of classifying organisms[1] to reflect their relatedness. Nomenclature "is the assignment of names to the taxonomic groups according to international rules."[2(p27)]

Biological nomenclature—the nomenclature of living things—derives from the paradigm of the 18th-century taxonomist Linnaeus, who used 2-word labels to replace the long descriptive Latin phrases appended to the genus name.[3,4] Since Linnaeus' time, international bodies have continued to formalize biological nomenclature, resulting in the current principal codes (**Table 14.14-3**). The codes contain principles, rules, and recommendations for name derivations, priority, validity, and spelling. For a name to have international standing, the codes stipulate valid publication according to specific requirements.

An effort has been made to unify biological nomenclature for all organisms with a single code, the BioCode, under the auspices of the International Committee for Bionomenclature (a joint committee of the International Union of Microbiological Societies and the International Union of Biological Sciences).[4,10-12] Another proposed unifying code is the PhyloCode, which is meant to reflect phylogeny and to be used concurrently with the extant codes, at least initially.[13,14]

**Table 14.14-2.** Examples of Scientific and Vernacular Name Usage

| First mention | Subsequent mention |
| --- | --- |
| St John's wort (*Hypericum perforatum*) | St John's wort |
| *Hypericum perforatum* (St John's wort) | *H perforatum,* or St John's wort, depending on context; eg, "participants given tablets prepared from a pure extract of *H perforatum*" |
| Indian tobacco (*Lobelia inflata*) | Indian tobacco |
| *Lobelia inflata* (Indian tobacco) | *L inflata,* commonly known as Indian tobacco, is a source of lobeline |

**Table 14.14-3.** Biological Nomenclature Principal Codes

| Code | Content |
|---|---|
| International Code of Zoological Nomenclature[5,6] | animals, including protozoa and parasites |
| International Code of Nomenclature for Algae, Fungi, and Plants[7] | fungi and noncultivated plants, including algae |
| International Code of Nomenclature of Bacteria[8] | bacteria |
| International Code of Nomenclature for Cultivated Plants[9] | cultivated plants |
| International Code of Virus Classification and Nomenclature | viruses (see 14.14.3, Virus Nomenclature) |

"The essence of the Linnaean revolution was the recognition that the function of the specific 'name' was merely to label a concept rather than to describe an entity."[4(p5)] Scientific names change when taxonomy changes but not when new knowledge indicates that the original name is no longer an apt descriptor. (For instance, it was learned several decades after its discovery that the bacterium *Haemophilus influenzae* did not cause influenza,[15] but the name was not changed.[8]) The stability of names is crucial, and name changes may cause harm.[4(p75)] "The *International Code of Nomenclature for Algae, Fungi, and Plants* aims at the provision of a stable method of naming taxonomic groups, avoiding and rejecting the use of names that may cause error or ambiguity or throw science into confusion."[7(preamble)] (See also "perilous name" in the bacteriologic code.[8])

**14.14.1.3** **Resources.** A useful source of names of organisms available on the web, particularly plant and animal names, is the Index to Organism Names.[16] Other resources are available at the National Center for Biotechnology Information Entrez Taxonomy home page.[17]

**14.14.1.4** **Style for Scientific Names.** This section presents style that applies to scientific names. The nomenclature codes differ in some style recommendations, but most publications, when possible, will apply style consistently for all scientific names (eg, will use abbreviations in the same way for animals, plants, and bacteria). Therefore, the recommended style to be applied to animals, plants, and bacteria is presented together in this section (see 14.14.2, Bacteria: Additional Terminology, and 14.14.3, Virus Nomenclature).

Organisms are classified in taxonomic groups, also called *taxa* (singular: taxon), within different ranks (**Table 14.14-4**):

**Table 14.14-4.** Examples of Ranks and Taxa

| Rank | Taxon |
|---|---|
| Genus | *Homo* |
| Species | *Homo sapiens* |

Major ranks, from most inclusive to most specific, are domain, kingdom, phylum or division, class, order, family, genus, and species.

Stylistic hallmarks of biological nomenclature differentiate scientific names from vernacular names.[1,3] These hallmarks are latinization, italics, and a 2-word term for species: the binomial, also called binary or binominal (eg, *Homo sapiens*). Within a code, the names of ranks above species usually must be unique; the same species designator, however, can be used with multiple genera, for example, *Klebsiella pneumoniae* and *Streptococcus pneumoniae*. Across codes, names may be the same at any rank, for example, the bacterial genus *Bacillus* and the stick and leaf insect genus *Bacillus*.

According to the international codes, initial capitals are used for all taxa, except for the second portion of the binomial. That portion is called the *specific name* in the zoological code and the *specific epithet* in the botanical and bacteriologic codes. Italics are always used for the genus and species components of the binomial. Diacritical marks (accents) and ligatures (eg, æ) are not used. Hyphens occasionally may be used in the specific epithet (eg, the butterfly *Polygonia c-album*, which has a *c*-shaped wing mark).[1]

All codes capitalize scientific names of taxa but differ on italicizing higher taxa. The bacterial code recommends italicizing all scientific names but recognizes that journals may wish to style all organism names similarly. Taxa above genus should not be italicized.

> Mucormycosis refers to an infection caused by fungi in the order Mucorales, which contains the genera *Mucor, Absidia*, and *Rhizopus*. These fungi are ubiquitous in the environment and are opportunistic pathogens that often cause fatal infections.

The following examples of the taxonomic classification according to the 3 codes illustrate style (see 10.3.6, Organisms). The suffixes are typical and specified in each code (eg, family: -idae [animals], -aceae [plants and bacteria]), although exceptions are found (**Table 14.14-5**).

**Table 14.14-5.** Examples of Taxonomic Classification

| Animal | | Fungi | | Bacteria | |
|---|---|---|---|---|---|
| **Rank** | **Taxon** | **Rank** | **Taxon** | **Rank** | **Taxon** |
| kingdom | Animalia | kingdom | Fungi (Mycota) | kingdom | Procaryotae |
| phylum | Chordata | phylum | Ascomycota | division | Firmicutes |
| class | Mammalia | class | Ascomycetes | class | Firmibacteria |
| order | Primates | order | Onygenales | order | (not applicable; ending: -*ales*) |
| family | Hominidae | family | Onygenaceae | family | Bacillaceae |
| genus | *Homo* | genus | *Ajellomyces* | genus | *Staphylococcus* |
| species | *Homo sapiens* | species | *Ajellomyces capsulatus* | species | *Staphylococcus aureus* |

**Table 14.14-6.** Examples of Subranks and Superranks

| Animal | | Fungi | |
|---|---|---|---|
| **Rank** | **Taxon** | **Rank** | **Taxon** |
| subphylum | Vertebrata | | |
| | | subclass | Peronosporomycetidae |
| suborder | Anthropoidae | | |
| superfamily | Hominoidae | | |

Another scheme for bacterial taxonomic rank uses domain and phylum rather than kingdom and division.[3] Subranks and superranks follow the same style, as shown in the examples in **Table 14.14-6** (see 14.14.1.6, Subgenus, and 14.14.1.8, Subspecific Ranks, Ternary Names).

14.14.1.5 **Abbreviation of Genus and Other Abbreviations.** As described in 13.11, Clinical, Technical, and Other Common Terms, treat each manuscript portion (title, abstract, text, etc) separately. After first mention of the binomial species name, abbreviate the genus portion of the name without a period. Do not abbreviate the specific name (eg, use *Clostridioides difficile* not *C diff*). Although the JAMA Network journals typically avoid beginning a sentence with an abbreviation, exceptions include a genus name that has already been expanded.

> *Staphylococcus aureus* is a common cause of hospital-acquired infection. Resistant *S aureus* infection is also a source of community-acquired infection. *S aureus* can be treated with a range of antibiotics.

When the genus name is repeated but used with a new specific name, do not abbreviate the genus name until subsequent mention.

> *Staphylococcus aureus* and *Staphylococcus epidermidis* may be components of normal flora or pathogens in clinically significant infections, although *S aureus* is the more serious pathogen of the two.

Do not abbreviate the specific name, and do not abbreviate the genus name when used alone.

> Avoid: *S au* is the more serious pathogen . . .

> Avoid: The more serious pathogen in the genus *S* . . .

When organisms with genus names that begin with the same letter are mentioned in the same article, genus is abbreviated after first mention, for instance:

> community-associated infections caused by *Staphylococcus aureus* and *Streptococcus pneumoniae* and bacteremia with *S aureus* and *S pneumoniae*

Style variations in such instances are permissible (eg, if the editor thinks there is any possibility of confusing genera), and author requests to expand the genus names should be honored.

Do not use multiletter abbreviations for genus name, for example:

*S aureus* and *S pneumoniae* (not *Sta aureus* or *Str pneumoniae*)

Do not use 2-letter abbreviations for the binomial; for example, do not use SA for *Staphylococcus aureus* or SE for *S epidermidis*. However, longer expressions that include the scientific name may be abbreviated:

CoNS    coagulase-negative *Staphylococcus* species

EHEC    enterohemorrhagic *Escherichia coli*

Hib    *Haemophilus influenzae* type b [vaccine or disease]

MRSA    methicillin-resistant *Staphylococcus aureus*

Abbreviations such as sp nov (*species nova,* new species), gen nov (*genus novum,* new genus), and subsp (subspecies) are used in published proposals of new genus and species designations, for example:

*Corynebacterium nigricans* sp nov

*Roseomonas mucosa* sp nov and *Roseomonas gilardii* subsp *rosea* subsp nov[18]

*Wigglesworthia glossinidia* sp nov[19]

*Wigglesworthia* gen nov[19]

New proposals for higher taxa are indicated as in the following examples[20-23]:

Cycliophora, new phylum

Eucycliophora, new class

Symbiida, new order

Symbiidae, new family

*Symbion* gen nov

*Symbion pandora* sp nov

*Pfiesteria piscicida* gen et sp nov (Pfiesteriaceae fam nov)

Parachlamydiaceae fam nov and Simkaniaceae fam nov

The "nov" abbreviations should be mentioned prominently in the article (eg, in the title) but need not be included with every mention of the organism name.

Synonyms are expressed as follows:

*Fugomyces cyanescens* (syn *Sporothrix cyanescens, Cerinosterus cyanescens*)

*Mesocestoides vogae* (syn *M corti*)

**14.14.1.6** **Subgenus.** Subgenus is capitalized, italicized, and placed in parentheses, sometimes with the abbreviation "subgen," for example:

*Mus (Mus) musculus*

*Moraxella* (subgen *Branhamella) catarrhalis*

**14.14.1.7** **Nomenclature, Organisms and Pathogens, Biological Nomenclature, Parentheses.** Parentheses can be used to indicate name changes (and a qualifier may be included, such as "formerly") or to clarify a name that may not be as familiar:

> *Bartonella* (formerly *Rochalimaea*) *henselae*
>
> *Helicobacter* (formerly *Campylobacter*) *pylori*
>
> *Cutibacterium acnes (Propionibacterium acnes)*
>
> *Issatchenkia orientalis* (anamorph *Candida krusei*)

Indicate a change in species name with the entire binomial in parentheses as follows:

> *Bacteroides ureolyticus* (formerly *Bacteroides corrodens*)
>
> *Pneumocystis jirovecii* (formerly *Pneumocystis carinii*) pneumonia

Authorship of the scientific name may be indicated by personal names, which are not italicized, following the species name. Sometimes parentheses are used. Within and among codes, conventions for such references vary. Editors should not restyle such terms but rather should verify with authors that the proper form has been used. "L." alone is the common abbreviation for "Linneaus" (eg, *Culex pipiens* L.), but "Linnaeus" should be written in full in publications whose readers are unlikely to know of this convention.

> *Aedes aegypti* (Linnaeus)
>
> *Culex pipiens* Linnaeus
>
> *Escherichia coli* (Migula) Castellani and Chalmers
>
> *Serratia marcescens* Bizio

The parentheses indicate that the organism, after initial description, was transferred into another genus by others, in the case of *E coli* by Castellani and Chalmers. Year of published discovery may be included.

> *Escherichia coli* (Migula 1895) Castellani and Chalmers 1919
>
> *Serratia marcescens* Bizio 1823

**14.14.1.8** **Subspecific Ranks, Ternary Names.** Subspecific ranks receive ternary or trinomial names. Subspecific designations are handled differently for animals, plants, and bacteria, as in the examples in **Table 14.14-7**. (The term *var* as a synonym for subspecies was removed from the bacterial nomenclature code in 1990.)

Plant names may use *var*, as above, *subsp*, *f* (form), and other subspecific epithets, which are not interchangeable, in ternary names, for example:

> *Satureja parnassica* subsp *parnassica*

Not all 3-word combinations are ternary names:

> *Ixodes scapularis* larvae
>
> *Legionella pneumophila* pneumonia
>
> *Schistosoma mansoni* miracidium
>
> *Trypanosoma brucei* procyclin

**Table 14.14-7.** Examples of Subspecific Designations for Animals, Plants, and Bacteria

| Type of organism | Subspecific rank (designator) | Example |
| --- | --- | --- |
| Animal | | |
|   Higher animal | subspecies (no designator) | *Mus musculus domesticus* |
|   Protozoon | | *Trypanosoma brucei gambiense* |
|   Fungus | variety (var) | *Cryptococcus neoformans* var *grubii* |
| Bacteria | | |
|   Bacterium | subspecies (subsp) | *Campylobacter fetus* subsp *fetus Mycobacterium avium* subsp *paratuberculosis* |

**14.14.1.9** **Infrasubspecific Subdivisions.** Subdivisions below the subspecies level (infrasubspecific subdivisions) include the serovar (serologically differentiated) and the biovar (biochemically or physiologically differentiated). The suffix *-type* is most often used in the clinical literature (eg, biotype, serotype). However, to avoid confusion with nomenclatural type ("the element of the taxon with which the name is permanently associated"[8(p17)]), the suffix -var is often preferred in microbiological literature.

Infrasubspecific subdivisions are designated with various numbers, letters, or terms; follow author usage:

> *Brucella suis* biovar 4
>
> *Cryptococcus neoformans* serovar A
>
> *Fusarium oxysporum* f sp *radices-lycopersici* [f sp: *forma specialis*]
>
> *Haemophilus influenzae* biotype I
>
> *Haemophilus influenzae* biotype VII
>
> *Pseudomonas fluorescens* biovar I
>
> *Staphylococcus aureus* subsp *aureus* biotype A
>
> *Staphylococcus simulans* biovar *staphylolyticus*
>
> *Ureaplasma urealyticum* parvo biovar
>
> *Ureaplasma urealyticum* T960 biovar
>
> *Yersinia enterocolitica* serovar O:8

**14.14.1.10** **Anglicized and Vernacular (Trivial, Common) Terms.** In medical publications, uncapitalized anglicized forms are often used for taxa in ranks above genus (see 9.5, Microorganisms) (**Table** 14.14-8).[24]

**14.14.1.11** **Collective Genus Terms.** Many organisms possess traditional generic plural designations, which are verifiable in the dictionary. Some also have special

**Table 14.14-8.** Anglicized and Formal Terms of Taxa

| Anglicized term | Formal term |
| --- | --- |
| vertebrates | Vertebrata |
| primates | Primates |
| hominids | Hominidae |
| fungi | Fungi |
| moniliaceous molds | Moniciliaceae |
| prokaryotes | Prokaryotae |
| mycobacteria | Mycobacteriaceae |
| chlamydiae | Chlamydiales |

adjectival forms. It is also acceptable to add the word *organisms* or *species* to the italicized genus name. See the examples in **Table 14.14-9**.

> a novel *Yersinia* species
>
> *Loxosceles* species (brown recluse) spider venom
>
> group A streptococcal infection
>
> viridans streptococcal endocarditis

**Table 14.14-9.** Examples of Plural and Adjectival Forms of Genus Names

| Genus | Plural noun form | Adjectival form |
| --- | --- | --- |
| *Chlamydia* | chlamydiae | chlamydial |
| *Cryptococcus* | *Cryptococcus* species | cryptococcal |
| *Escherichia* | *Escherichia* organisms | |
| *Legionella* | legionellae | |
| *Macaca* | macaques | |
| *Mycobacterium* | mycobacteria | mycobacterial |
| *Pseudomonas* | pseudomonads | pseudomona |
| *Salmonella* | salmonellae | |
| *Staphylococcus* | staphylococci | staphylococcal |
| *Streptococcus* | streptococci | streptococcal |
| *Treponema* | treponemes | treponemal |
| *Trypanosoma* | trypanosomes | trypanosomal |

Genus names often qualify other terms:

*Candida* endocarditis

*Lactobacillus* serogroups

*Legionella* pneumonia

**14.14.1.12** **Unspecified Species.** The name of a genus used alone implies the genus as a whole:

*Toxocara* infections are frequently acquired from household pets.

The term *species* is used in cases in which the genus is certain but the species cannot be determined. For instance, if an author knew that a skin test reaction indicated the presence of *Toxocara* organisms but was unsure whether the reaction resulted from *Toxocara canis* infection or *Toxocara cati* infection, the author might write:

The source of the patient's infection was *Toxocara* species.

In the latter example, *Toxocara* organisms would also be acceptable, but *Toxocara* alone would be incorrect.[25]

**14.14.1.13** **Name Changes.** Three relatively new names have faced different degrees of acceptance: *Chlamydophila* (see 14.14.2.3, *Chlamydia* and *Chlamydophila*), *Clostridioides difficile*, and *Pneumocystis jiroveci*.[26-29]

In 2016, CDC began using *Clostridioides difficile* instead of *Clostridium difficile*.[30]

The fungal genus *Pneumocystis* includes 2 authentic species. The name of the species infective of rats is *P carinii*. The human pathogen was transitionally named *P carinii* f sp *hominis* and is now known as *P jiroveci*.[26,27] The familiar abbreviation PCP may be retained for *Pneumocystis* pneumonia in human and nonhuman hosts.[26]

**14.14.1.14** **Usage.** In text dealing with infectious conditions, it is important to distinguish between the infectious agent and the condition. Infectious agents, infections, and diseases are not equivalent.

| | |
|---|---|
| *Incorrect:* | *Legionella pneumophila* may be serious or subclinical. |
| *Better:* | *Legionella pneumophila* infection may be serious or subclinical. |
| *Preferred:* | Infection with *Legionella pneumophila* may be serious or subclinical. |
| *Incorrect:* | *Legionella pneumophila* may be severe. |
| *Preferred:* | *Legionella pneumophila* pneumonia may be severe. |

**14.14.2** **Bacteria: Additional Terminology.**

**14.14.2.1** **General.** For general guidelines on biological nomenclature that apply to bacteria, see 14.14.1, Biological Nomenclature. Rules for bacterial nomenclature are found in the *International Code of Nomenclature of Bacteria*.[8] Sources of bacterial names available on the web are the List of Prokaryotic Names With Standing in Nomenclature[31] and the German Prokaryotic Nomenclature Up-to-Date search page.[32] General references consulted in preparation of this section are Jorgensen et al[33] and Carroll et al.[34]

**14.14.2.2** **Bacterial Genes.** Bacterial gene nomenclature is covered in 14.6.5, Nonhuman Genetic Terms.

**14.14.2.3** ***Chlamydia* and *Chlamydophila*.** A proposed change in taxonomy resulted in a number of changes, including name changes of 2 medically important organisms.[23,35] *Chlamydia pneumoniae* became *Chlamydophila pneumoniae* and *Chlamydia psitacci* became *Chlamydophila psitacci*. *Chlamydia trachomatis* remains so named. The proposal was questioned.[34(p359),36] The new terminology was originally adopted by the Centers for Disease Control and Prevention (CDC) and some major compendia of bacterial names.[32,37] However, this change was dropped, and the CDC today uses *Chlamydia* (Carolyn M. Black, PhD, director, Division of Scientific Resources, CDC, email, September 14, 2017). Writing in the 2015 *Manual of Clinical Microbiology,* Gaydos and Essis note, "Although the new taxonomy was validly published, the scientific chlamydia community has consistently rejected the use of the term *Chlamydophila*, and its use has been abandoned."[35(p1106)]

The TWAR biovar of *Chlamydophila pneumoniae* was named "after the laboratory designation of the first 2 isolates—TW-183 and AR-39."[38(p161)-40]

**14.14.2.4** ***Escherichia coli*.** The O:K:H serotype profile of *Escherichia coli* is based on the somatic O antigen, capsular K antigen, and flagellar H antigen. The O is a capital letter O, not a zero. The abbreviations O, K, and H within the terms need not be expanded. Expansion of other components is not necessary but can be helpful (NM, nonmotile; NT, not typeable; Orough, O antigen, rough). Note the following examples:

> *Escherichia coli* NM
>
> *E coli* O157:H7
>
> *E coli* O6:K13:H1
>
> O157:NM
>
> ONT:NM
>
> Orough:H9
>
> non-O157
>
> O111:NM Prominent serogroups include O26, O103, O111, and O128.

*E coli* strains associated with diarrhea are abbreviated as follows (expand at first mention in accordance with 13.11, Clinical, Technical, and Other Common Terms):

> EAEC          enteroaggregative *E coli*
>
> EIEC          enteroinvasive *E coli*

| EPEC | enteropathogenic *E coli* |
| ETEC | enterotoxigenic *E coli* |
| STEC | Shiga toxin–producing *E coli* (also called enterohemorrhagic *E coli* [EHEC]) |
| VTEC | verotoxigenic *E coli* |

Serotype and strain are often mentioned together in various combinations:

O157:H7 STEC

strains of STEC serotypes other than O157:H7

STEC O103

Note the following terms representing Shiga toxins:

stx1 (Shiga-like toxin 1)

stx2 (Shiga-like toxin 2)

**14.14.2.5** **Gram-Positive, Gram-Negative.** Bacteria are often grouped according to reaction to the Gram stain. Note capitalization style in the following (see 10.3, Proper Nouns):

gram-negative bacilli

gram-positive cocci

Gram stain

**14.14.2.6** ***Haemophilus.*** *Haemophilus influenzae* strains are defined by capsular antigens, designated types a through f, for instance:

*Haemophilus influenzae* type b (Hib)

The name of the vaccine should be expanded at first mention:

*Haemophilus influenzae* type b (Hib) vaccine . . . Hib vaccine

*H influenzae* type b (Hib) vaccination

*Haemophilus aegyptius* is closely related to *H influenzae* biotype III; *aegypticus* is a misspelling.

**14.14.2.7** **Laboratory Media.** Microorganism names applied to laboratory media use lowercase and roman letters:

bacteroides bile esculin agar

brucella agar

Capitalization indicates a product name:

Haemophilus ID Quad agar

**14.14.2.8** ***Lactobacillus* GG.** *Lactobacillus* GG refers to a strain of *Lactobacillus rhamnosus* named for the authors who isolated it.[41]

**14.14.2.9** **L Forms.** L phase variants, or L forms, are forms of various bacteria with deficient or defective cell walls. Examples of usage are as follows:

> *Helicobacter pylori* L-form infection
>
> L-form *Bacillus subtilis*
>
> L-form bioluminescence
>
> the L form of *Mycobacterium tuberculosis*

**14.14.2.10** **Macrolide Resistance.** Macrolide-resistant phenotypes are expressed as follows:

> M phenotype (M: macrolide)
>
> MLSB (L: lincosamides; SB: streptogramins B)
>
> cMLSB (c: constitutive, includes resistance to clindamycin)
>
> iMLSB (i: inducible by macrolides but not by clindamycin)

**14.14.2.11** ***Mycobacterium avium-intracellulare.*** This term indicates that in a particular context the 2 species *M avium* and *M intracellulare* are indistinguishable.

**14.14.2.12** ***Neisseria meningitidis.*** Clinically important serogroups of this organism include the following:

> serogroups A, B, C, X, Y, and W-135

The vernacular name of this organism is meningococcus.

**14.14.2.13** ***Salmonella.*** Nomenclature of salmonellae is complex and evolving.[31,42-44] The use of many models presented in the literature and the historical practice of considering different serotypes of *Salmonella* to be different species made the nomenclature used to describe *Salmonella* problematic for many years. However, the publication of Judicial Opinion 80 in the *International Journal of Systematic and Evolutionary Microbiology* in 2005 helped clarify nomenclature issues regarding the genus *Salmonella*.[43]

The main stylistic change is that the traditional binomial species designation is no longer applied to serotypes:

> *Salmonella* Typhi, *not Salmonella typhi*

Editors should query authors if the latter term and its like are used (except, for instance, in discussions of nomenclature) but otherwise should follow author preference and apply style as in the following examples. Note that nearly all *Salmonella* infections in warm-blooded animals are *Salmonella enterica* subspecies I.[33]

> Species:     *Salmonella enterica, S bongori* (formerly subspecies V)
>
> Subspecies, *S enterica:*
>
> *S enterica* subsp *enterica*          subspecies I
>
> *S enterica* subsp *salamae*          subspecies II

| | |
|---|---|
| *S enterica* subsp *arizonae* | subspecies IIIa |
| *S enterica* subsp *diarizonae* | subspecies IIIb |
| *S enterica* subsp *houtenae* | subspecies IV |
| *S enterica* subsp *indica* | subspecies VI |

Serotypes (serovars) are set roman, with the first letter capitalized[45]:

Use *Salmonella* serovar Typhimurium at first mention.

Thereafter, it may be given without the species name: *S* Typhimurium.

After first mention, ser may be omitted:

*Salmonella* Enteritidis

*Salmonella* Typhi

*Salmonella* Typhimurium

When the genus name is repeated, it may be abbreviated:

*S* Typhi

Serovars of *Salmonella* are defined by the O (somatic), Vi (capsular), and H (flagellar) antigens. Clinical diagnostic laboratories submit *Salmonella* isolates to state and territorial public health laboratories, where they are confirmed and serotyped according to the Kaufmann-White scheme,[46] using the following typical format (Ferric C. Fang, MD, Department of Laboratory Medicine and Microbiology, University of Washington School of Medicine, email, November 3, 2015):

Subspecies [space] O antigens[colon]phase 1 H antigen [colon] phase 2 H antigens

For example: I 4,5,12:i:1,2′ for *S enterica* serotype Typhimurium

Mucoid variants, which express a capsule that prevents immunologic detection of the O antigen, contain "Mucoid" instead of O in the antigenic formula: Mucoid:i:1,2. Rough variants are isolates that do not express the O antigen; rather "Rough" is used instead of the O antigen in the antigenic formula: Rough:i:1,2.[45(p23)] In contrast to *Escherichia coli* strains, when *Salmonella* serotype is expressed with those antigens, the letters O, H, and Vi are not included in the serotype designation. Colons separate the O, Vi, and H designations, which take a variety of forms (letter, numeric, etc):

*Salmonella enterica* subsp *salamae* ser 50:z:e,n,x

*Salmonella* serotype II 50:z:e,n,x

*Salmonella enterica* serotype IV 48:g,z51:–

*Salmonella* serotype IIIa 41:z4,z23:–

*Salmonella* subsp *arizonae* serovar 50:z4,z24:–

*Salmonella* Typhimurium 1,4,5,12:1:1,2

Alternatively, geographic or other designations are used:

*Salmonella* ser Brookfield

*Salmonella* Typhimurium MR-DT104

*Salmonella* Typhimurium DT204b

O antigen groups (O groups) are A, B, $C_1$, $C_2$, D, E, F, etc:

*Salmonella* group E

a group D *Salmonella* outbreak

O antigens have historically been designated by letter, but there are now more than 60 O antigen groups, so letters have been supplanted by numbers (at least by taxonomists; clinicians are still more used to seeing the letters). Numbers refer to subgroups; for example, serogroup D includes D1, D2, and D3. *Salmonella* Typhi is group D or group D1 if the subgroup is designated (Ferric C. Fang, MD, Department of Laboratory Medicine and Microbiology, University of Washington, email, November 3, 2015).

**14.14.2.14 Strain and Group Designations.** Strains and groups are designated in various ways, sometimes alone, sometimes following the binomial species name. These additional designations are not italicized. Strains are sometimes designated by the abbreviation of a culture collection repository and number. Such abbreviations need not be expanded when used in strain names only but should be otherwise.[25]

ATCC 27853 strain of *Pseudomonas aeruginosa*

CDC EO-2 [EO: eugonic oxidizer]

CDC group WO-2 [WO: weak oxidizer]

*Escherichia coli* ATCC 25922

*Staphylococcus aureus* NCTC 83

the control strain, NCTC 8325

*Geobacillus stearothermophilus* (DSMZ 22; equivalent to ATCC 12980)

cultures obtained from the American Type Culture Collection, Manassas, Virginia

**14.14.2.15 Streptococci.** Clinically important groups of streptococci are designated in various ways. Capital letters refer to Lancefield serologic groups, for example:

α-hemolytic streptococci

group A β-hemolytic streptococci

group A *Streptococcus pyogenes*

group B β-hemolytic streptococci (*Streptococcus agalactiae*)

group C streptococci

viridans streptococci

Proteins of *Streptococcus pyogenes* include the following:

> M protein
>
> class I M protein
>
> class II M protein
>
> P substance
>
> R protein
>
> T substance

The cell wall C polysaccharide of *Streptococcus pneumoniae* is the basis of the term "C-reactive protein" (an acute-phase inflammatory protein that reacts with the C polysaccharide).

Do not confuse the M protein with the M phenotype of various streptococci and other bacteria (see 14.14.2.10, Macrolide Resistance) or C polysaccharide with group C streptococci.

The vernacular name of *Streptococcus pneumoniae* is pneumococcus.

**14.14.2.16** **Vibrio.** *Vibrio cholerae* serogroups are expressed as in these 2 examples:

> *Vibrio cholerae* O1
>
> *V cholerae* O139

**Principal Author:** Cheryl Iverson, MA

## ACKNOWLEDGMENT

Thanks to Preeti Malani, MD, MSJ, *JAMA*, and Department of Internal Medicine, University of Michigan, Ann Arbor, and Ferric C. Fang, MD (*Salmonella*), University of Washington, Seattle, for reviewing and providing comments.

## REFERENCES

1. Jeffrey C. *Biological Nomenclature: For the Systematics Association*. 3rd ed. Cambridge University Press; 1992.
2. Brenner DJ, Staley JT, Krieg NR. Classification of procaryotic organisms and the concept of bacterial speciation. In: Boone DR, Castenholz RW, eds. *Bergey's Manual of Systematic Bacteriology*. 2nd ed. *Volume 1: The* Archaea *and the Deeply Branching and Phototrophic Bacteria*. Springer-Verlag; 2001:27-31.
3. Sneath PHA. Bacterial nomenclature. In: Boone DR, Castenholz RW, eds. *Bergey's Manual of Systematic Bacteriology*. 2nd ed. *Volume 1: The* Archaea *and the Deeply Branching and Phototrophic Bacteria*. Springer-Verlag; 2001:83-88.
4. Melville RV. *Towards Stability in the Names of Animals: A History of the International Commission on Zoological Nomenclature 1895-1995*. International Trust for Zoological Nomenclature; 1995.
5. International Commission on Zoological Nomenclature. *International Code of Zoological Nomenclature*. 5th ed. Accessed July 20, 2019. https://www.iczn.org/the-code/the-international-code-of-zoological-nomenclature/the-code-online/

6. International Commission on Zoological Nomenclature. ICZN Wiki. Accessed July 20, 2019. iczn.ansp.org/wiki/

7. McNeill J, Barrie FR, Buck WR, et al, eds; International Association for Plant Taxonomy. *International Code of Nomenclature for Algae, Fungi, and Plants (Melbourne Code)*. Koeltz Scientific Books; 2012. Updated September 12, 2012. Accessed May 24, 2018. https://www.iapt-taxon.org/nomen/main.php

8. Lapage SP, Sneath PHA, Lessel EF, Skerman VBD, Seeliger HPR, Clark WA. *International Code of Nomenclature of Bacteria and Statutes of the International Committee on Systematic Bacteriology and Statutes of the Bacteriology and Applied Microbiology Section of the International Union of Microbiological Societies*. International Union of Microbiological Societies, American Society for Microbiology; 1992.

9. Trehane P, Brickell CD, Baum BR, et al, eds. *International Code of Nomenclature for Cultivated Plants*. Quarterjack Publishing; 1995.

10. Greuter WS, Garrity G, Hawksworth DL, et al; International Committee for Bionomenclature (ICB). Draft BioCode (2011). Accessed July 20, 2019. www.bionomenclature.net/biocode2011.html

11. Ride WDL. Introduction. In: International Commission on Zoological Nomenclature. *International Code of Zoological Nomenclature*. 4th ed. International Trust for Zoological Nomenclature; 1999:xix-xxix.

12. International Union of Biological Sciences (IUBS) website. Accessed May 24, 2018. http://www.iubs.org

13. Robinson P, Kommedahl T. PhyloCode: a new system of nomenclature. *Science Editor*. 2002;25(2):52.

14. The PhyloCode. Modified May 14, 2019. Accessed July 20, 2019. https://www.ohio.edu/phylocode

15. Kolata G. *Flu: The Story of the Great Influenza Pandemic of 1918 and the Search for the Virus That Caused It*. Touchstone; 1999.

16. BIOSIS. Index to organism names (ION). Accessed August 1, 2019. https://organismnames.com/query.htm

17. NCBI Entrez Taxonomy home page. Accessed May 24, 2018. https://www.ncbi.nlm.nih.gov/taxonomy

18. Han XY, Pham AS, Tarrand JJ, Rolston KV, Helsel LO, Levett PN. Bacteriologic characterization of 36 strains of *Roseomonas* species and proposal of *Roseomonas mucosa* sp nov and *Roseomonas gilardii* subsp *rosea* subsp nov. *Am J Clin Pathol*. 2003;120(2):256-264.

19. Aksoy S. *Wigglesworthia* gen. nov. and *Wigglesworthia glossinidia* sp. nov., taxa consisting of the mycetocyte-associated, primary endosymbionts of tsetse flies. *Int J Syst Bacteriol*. 1995;45(4):848-851.

20. Funch P, Kristensen RM. Cycliophora is a new phylum with affinities to Entoprocta and Ectoprocta. *Nature*. 1995;378(6558):711-714.

21. Morris SC. A new phylum from the lobster's lips. *Nature*. 1995;378(6558):661-662.

22. Steidinger KA, Burkholder JM, Glasgow HB, et al. *Pfiesteria piscicida* gen. et sp. nov. (Pfiesteriaceae fam. nov.), a new toxic dinoflagellate with a complex life cycle and behavior. *J Phycol*. 1996;32(1):157-164.

23. Everett KD, Bush RM, Andersen AA. Emended description of the order Chlamydiales, proposal of Parachlamydiaceae fam. nov. and Simkaniaceae fam. nov., each containing one monotypic genus, revised taxonomy of the family

Chlamydiaceae, including a new genus and five new species, and standards for the identification of organisms. *Int J Syst Bacteriol.* April 1999;49:415-440.

24. Piqueras M, Guerrero R. Bacteriologic nomenclature. In: Smart P, Maisonneuve H, Polderman A, eds. *Science Editors' Handbook.* 2nd ed. European Association of Science Editors; 2013:59-65.

25. *ASM Style Manual for Journals and Books.* American Society for Microbiology: 1991.

26. Stringer JR, Beard CB, Miller RF, Wakefield AE. A new name (*Pneumocystis jiroveci*) for *Pneumocystis* from humans. *Emerg Infect Dis.* 2002;8(9):891-896.

27. Cushion MT. *Pneumocystis.* In: Jorgensen JH, Pfaller MA, Carroll KC, et al, eds. *Manual of Clinical Microbiology.* 11th ed. ASM Press; 2015:2015-2029.

28. Hughes WT. *Pneumocystis carinii* vs. *Pneumocystis jiroveci:* another misnomer (response to Stringer et al). *Emerg Infect Dis.* 2003;9(2):276-277.

29. Stringer JR, Beard CB, Miller RF, Cushion MT. A new name (*Pneumocystis jiroveci*) for *Pneumocystis* from humans (response to Hughes). *Emerg Infect Dis.* 2003;9(2):277-279.

30. Lawson PA, Citron DM, Tyrrell KL, Finegold SM. Reclassification of *Clostridium difficile* as *Clostridioides difficile. Anareobe.* August 2016;40:95-99. doi:10.1016/j.anaerobe.2016.06.008

31. Euzéby JP. List of prokaryotic names with standing in nomenclature. Updated June 18, 2015. Accessed May 24, 2018. http://www.bacterio.net

32. Deutsche Sammlung von Mikroorganismen und Zellkulturen GmbH (German Collection of Microorganisms and Cell Cultures GmbH). Prokaryotic Nomenclature Up-to-Date. Accessed May 24, 2018. http://www.dsmz.de/microorganisms/pnu/bacterial_nomenclature_mm.php

33. Jorgensen JH, Pfaller MA, Carroll KC, et al, eds. *Manual of Clinical Microbiology.* 11th ed. ASM Press; 2015.

34. Carroll KC, Brooks GF, Butel JS, Morse SA, Mietzner TA. *Jawetz, Melnick, & Adelberg's Medical Microbiology.* 26th ed. Lange Medical Books/McGraw-Hill; 2013.

35. Gaydos C, Essig A. *Chlamydiaceae.* In: Jorgensen JH, Pfaller MA, Carroll KC, et al, eds. *Manual of Clinical Microbiology.* 11th ed. ASM Press; 2015:1106-1121.

36. Schachter J, Stephens RS, Timms P, et al. Radical changes to chlamydial taxonomy are not necessary just yet. *Int J Syst Evol Microbiol.* 2001;51(pt 1):249.

37. Boone DR, Castenholz RW, eds. *Bergey's Manual of Systematic Bacteriology.* 2nd ed. *Volume 1: The* Archaea *and the Deeply Branching and Phototropoic Bacteria.* Springer-Verlag; 2001.

38. Grayston JT, Kuo C-C, Wang S-P, Altman J. A new *Chlamydia psittaci* strain, TWAR, isolated in acute respiratory tract infections. *N Engl J Med.* 1986;315(3):161-168.

39. Grayston JT, Kuo C-C, Campbell LA, Wang SP. *Chlamydia pneumoniae* sp. nov. for *Chlamydia* sp: strain TWAR. *Int J Syst Bacteriol.* 1989;39(1):88-90.

40. Saikku P, Wang SP, Kleemola M, Brander E, Rusanan E, Grayston JT. An epidemic of mild pneumonia due to an unusual strain of *Chlamydia psittaci. J Infect Dis.* 1985;151(5):832-839.

41. Gorbach SL, Chang TW, Goldin B: Successful treatment of relapsing *Clostridium difficile* colitis with *Lactobacillus* GG. *Lancet.* 1987;2(8574):1519.

42. Forsythe SJ, Abbott SL, Pitout J. *Klebsiella, Enterobacter, Citrobacter, Cronobacter, Serratia, Plesiomonas,* and Other Enterobacterioceae. In: Jorgensen JH, Pfaller MA, Carroll KC, et al, eds. *Manual of Clinical Microbiology.* 11th ed. ASM Press; 2015:714-737.

43. Strockbine NA, Bopp CA, Fields PI, Kaper BJ, Nataro JP. *Escherichia, Shigella,* and *Salmonella.* In: Jorgensen JH, Pfaller MA, Carroll CK, et al, eds. *Manual of Clinical Microbiology.* 11th ed. ASM Press; 2015:685-713.
44. Brenner FW, Villar RG, Angulo FJ, Tauxe R, Swaminathan B. Guest commentary: *Salmonella* nomenclature. *J Clin Microbiol.* 2000;38(7):2465-2467.
45. Grimont PAD, Weill F-X. Salmonella *Serovars.* 9th ed. WHO Collaborating Centre for Reference and Research on *Salmonella*; 2007.
46. Centers for Disease Control and Prevention. *National* Salmonella *Surveillance Overview.* US Dept of Health and Human Services; 2011.

**14.14.3** **Virus Nomenclature.** Most medical articles describe concrete viral entities and, therefore, use the common (vernacular, informal) names of viruses (eg, cytomegalovirus, Hantaan virus, orthopoxviruses). To indicate taxonomic groups, formal virus names are used (eg, *Human herpesvirus 5, Hantaan virus,* the genus *Orthopoxvirus*).

**14.14.3.1** **Style Rules.** A virus term that ends in *-virales, -viridae,* or *-virinae* should be capitalized (eg, change paramyxovirinae to Paramyxovirinae). Terms that end in *-virus* may or may not be formal terms (and may be genera, species, or subspecific entities); editors should follow author usage. Authors should distinguish formal and common terms and style them accordingly. It is useful to give the formal, taxonomic identity of a virus at first mention in an article; afterward the informal name is typically used (unless the article is discussing taxonomy per se). Formal names are used for species and above, so subspecific viral entities (eg, strains, serotypes, isolates) are not capitalized or italicized. Abbreviations may be used for common names.

Reference sources for viral terms include the latest nomenclature reports[1] and online databases.[2] See **Table 14.14-10**, which is based on these sources, for formal names, common names, and abbreviations of human (and related) viruses.

Background and further style specifics follow.

**14.14.3.2** **The Viral Code.** International virus taxonomy dates from 1966 and the first published report from 1971. Viral taxonomy and nomenclature are put forth by the International Committee on Taxonomy of Viruses (ICTV) in the International Code of Virus Classification and Nomenclature of ICTV.[1-3] (The ICTV is a committee of the Virology Division, International Union of Microbiology Societies.) The code is the work of more than 500 virologists worldwide, including 76 international study groups.[4] The ninth report was issued in 2012.[1]

Official virus names for species and higher taxa are available in book form,[1,3] with updates published in *Archives of Virology.* Online, official names and updates are available at ICTVdb.[2] The ICTVdb site also provides information about isolates (eg, serotypes, strains) with links to genome sequence databases. (It is hoped that this linkage will bring needed consistency between official viral nomenclature and viral entries in gene sequence databases.[4]) As with bacterial, animal, and plant nomenclature, viral nomenclature aims for stability and clarity (see 14.14.1, Biological Nomenclature). Names of viral taxa have standing when approved by the members of the full ICTV (https://talk.ictvonline.org).[5] Proposals for new names or changes should be submitted to the ICTV website.[2] The viral code applies to the ranks of order, family, subfamily, genus, and species (but not lower ranks). A virus may not

**Table 14.14-10.** Viruses of Humans

| Common and infraspecific names[a] | Formal species names | Basic abbreviation[b] | Genus | Family |
|---|---|---|---|---|
| adeno-associated virus | Adeno-associated virus-1, Adeno-associated virus-2, Adeno-associated virus-3, etc | AAV | Dependovirus | Parvoviridae (subfamily: Parvovirinae) |
| Alfuy virus | Murray Valley encephalitis virus | ALFV | Flavivirus | Flaviviridae |
| astrovirus | Human astrovirus | HAstV | Mamastrovirus | Astroviridae |
| Babanki virus | Sindbis virus | | Alphavirus | Togaviridae |
| BK virus | BK polyomavirus | BKPyV | Polyomavirus | Polyomaviridae |
| Bunyamwera virus | Bunyamwera virus | BUNV | Orthobunyavirus | Bunyaviridae |
| California encephalitis virus | California encephalitis virus | CEV | Orthobunyavirus | Bunyaviridae |
| Colorado tick fever virus | Colorado tick fever virus | CTFV | Coltivirus | Reoviridae |
| coronavirus (see human coronavirus) | | | | |
| COVID-19 virus (see SARS coronavirus 2) | | | | |
| coxsackieviruses (eg, coxsackievirus A10, coxsackievirus B6, coxsackievirus A24) | Human enterovirus A, Human enterovirus B, Human enterovirus C | CV | Enterovirus | Picornaviridae |
| Crimean-Congo hemorrhagic fever virus | Crimean-Congo hemorrhagic fever virus | CCHFV | Nairovirus | Bunyaviridae |
| cytomegalovirus | Human herpesvirus 5 | HHV-5 | Cytomegalovirus | Herpesviridae (subfamily: Betaherpesvirinae) |
| dengue virus | Dengue virus | DENV | Flavivirus | Flaviviridae |
| Desert Shield virus | Norwalk virus | Hu/NLV/DSV395 | Norovirus | Caliciviridae |
| Eastern equine encephalitis virus | Eastern equine encephalitis virus | EEEV | Alphavirus | Togaviridae |
| Ebola viruses (eg, Taï Forest ebolavirus–Côte d'Ivoire ebolavirus, Reston ebolavirus Pennsylvania, Sudan ebolavirus-Boniface, Zaire ebolavirus-Mayinga) | Côte d'Ivoire ebolavirus, Reston ebolavirus, Sudan ebolavirus, Zaire ebolavirus | TAFV-Côt RESTV-Penn SUDV-Bon, EBOV-May | Ebolavirus | Filoviridae |

(continued)

**Table 14.14-10.** Viruses of Humans (*continued*)

| Common and infraspecific names[a] | Formal species names | Basic abbreviation[b] | Genus | Family |
|---|---|---|---|---|
| echoviruses (eg, echovirus 1, echovirus 2) | *Human enterovirus B* | E | *Enterovirus* | Picornaviridae |
| enterovirus 68 enterovirus 70 | *Human enterovirus D* | EV | *Enterovirus* | Picornaviridae |
| Epstein-Barr virus | *Human herpesvirus 4* | HHV-4 | *Lymphocryptovirus* | Herpesviridae (subfamily: Gammaherpesvirinae) |
| Eyach virus | *Eyach virus* | EYAV | *Coltivirus* | Reoviridae |
| GB virus A GB virus C | *GB virus A, GB virus C* | GBV-A, GBV-C | unassigned | Flaviviridae |
| GB virus B | *GB virus B* | GBV-B | *Hepacivirus* (tentative) | Flaviviridae |
| Hantaan virus | *Hantaan virus* | HTNV | *Hantavirus* | Bunyaviridae |
| Hendra virus | *Hendravirus* | HeV | *Henipavirus* | Paramyxoviridae (subfamily: Paramyxovirinae) |
| hepatitis A virus | *Human hepatitis A virus* | HAV | *Hepatovirus* | Picornaviridae |
| hepatitis B virus hepatitis B virus-A hepatitis B virus-B, etc | *Hepatitis B virus* | HBV, HBV-A, HBV-B, etc | *Orthohepadnavirus* | Hepadnaviridae |
| hepatitis C virus HCV genotype 1a, etc | *Hepatitis C virus* | HCV, HCV-1, etc | *Hepacivirus* | Flaviviridae |
| hepatitis D virus | *Hepatitis delta virus* | HDV | *Deltavirus* | unassigned |
| hepatitis E virus | *Hepatitis E virus* | HEV | *Hepevirus* | Hepeviridae |
| hepatitis G virus | *GB virus C* | HGV | unassigned | Flaviviridae |
| herpes simplex virus type 1, herpes simplex virus type 2 | *Human herpesvirus 1, Human herpesvirus 2* | HHV-1, HHV-2 | *Simplexvirus* | Herpesviridae (subfamily: Alphaherpesvirinae) |
| herpesvirus simiae (also simian herpes B virus) | *Cercopithecine herpesvirus 2* | CeHV-2 | *Simplexvirus* *Simplexvirus* | Adenoviridae |
| human adenoviruses (eg, human adenovirus 2) | *Human adenovirus A* through *F* (eg, *Human adenovirus C*) | HAdV HAdV-2 | *Mastadenovirus* | |
| human coronavirus 229E, human coronavirus NL63 | *Human coronavirus 229E, Human coronavirus NL63* | HCoV 229E, HCoV NL63 | *Alphacoronavirus* | Coronaviridae |

**Table 14.14-10.** Viruses of Humans (*continued*)

| Common and infraspecific names[a] | Formal species names | Basic abbreviation[b] | Genus | Family |
|---|---|---|---|---|
| human herpesvirus 6, herpesvirus 7 | *Human herpesvirus 6, Human herpesvirus 7* | HHV-6, HHV-7 | *Roseolovirus* | Herpesviridae (subfamily: Betaherpesvirinae) |
| HIV 1 | *Human immunodeficiency virus 1, Human immunodeficiency virus 2* | HIV-1, HIV-2 | *Lentivirus* | Retroviridae (subfamily: Orthoretrovirinae) |
| human papillomavirus | *Human papillomavirus 5, etc* | HPV-5, etc | *Betapapillomavirus* | Papillomaviridae |
| human papillomavirus | *Human papillomavirus 4, etc* | HPV-4, etc | *Gammapapillomavirus* | Papillomaviridae |
| human papillomavirus | *Human papillomavirus 1, Human papillomavirus 63* | HPV-1, HPV-63 | *Mupapillomavirus* | Papillomaviridae |
| human papillomavirus | *Human papillomavirus 32, etc* | HPV-32 | *Alphapapillomavirus* | Papillomaviridae |
| human papillomavirus | *Human papillomavirus 41* | HPV-41 | *Nupapillomavirus* | Papillomaviridae |
| human T-lymphotropic virus 1 | *Primate T-lymphotropic virus 1* | HTLV-1 | *Deltaretrovirus* | Retroviridae (subfamily: Orthoretrovirinae) |
| human T-lymphotropic virus 2 | *Primate T-lymphotropic virus 2* | HTLV-2 | | |
| influenza A virus influenza A/PR/8/34 (H1N1) | *Influenza A virus* | FLUAV-A/ PR/8/34 | *Influenzavirus A* | Orthomyxoviridae |
| influenza B virus influenza B/Lee/40 | *Influenza B virus* | FLUBV-B/ Lee/40 | *Influenzavirus B* | Orthomyxoviridae |
| influenza C virus influenza C/Ann Arbor/1/50 | *Influenza C virus* | FLUCV-C/ Ann Arbor/1/50 | *Influenzavirus C* | Orthomyxoviridae |
| Japanese encephalitis virus | *Japanese encephalitis virus* | JEV | *Flavivirus* | Flaviridae |
| JC polyoma virus | *JC polyomavirus* | JCPyV | *Polyomavirus* | Polyomaviridae |
| Kaposi sarcoma–associated herpesvirus | *Human herpesvirus 8* | HHV-8 | *Rhadinovirus* | Herpesviridae (subfamily: Gammaherpesvirinae) |
| Kunjin virus | *West Nile virus* | KUNV | *Flavivirus* | Flaviviridae |

(*continued*)

**Table 14.14-10.** Viruses of Humans (*continued*)

| Common and infraspecific names[a] | Formal species names | Basic abbreviation[b] | Genus | Family |
|---|---|---|---|---|
| Kyasanur Forest disease virus | *Kyasanur Forest disease virus* | KFDV | *Flavivirus* | Flaviviridae |
| La Crosse virus | *California encephalitis virus* | LACV | *Orthobunyavirus* | Bunyaviridae |
| Lassa virus | *Lassa virus* | LASV | *Arenavirus* | Arenaviridae |
| Lebombo virus | *Lebombo virus* | LEBV | *Orbivirus* | Reoviridae |
| lymphocytic choriomeningitis virus | *Lymphocytic choriomeningitis virus* | LCMV | *Arenavirus* | Arenaviridae |
| Marburg virus | *Lake Victoria marburgvirus* | MARV | *Marburgvirus* | Filoviridae |
| measles virus | *Measles virus* | MeV | *Morbillivirus* | Paramyxoviridae (subfamily: Paramyxovirinae) |
| metapneumovirus | *Human metapneumovirus* | HMPV | *Metapneumovirus* | Paramyxoviridae (subfamily: Pneumovirinae) |
| Middle East respiratory syndrome | Middle East respiratory syndrome Coronavirus | MERS-CoV | *Betacoronavirus* | Coronaviridae |
| molluscum contagiosum virus | *Molluscum contagiosum virus* | MOCV | *Molluscipoxvirus* | Poxviridae (subfamily: Chordopoxvirinae) |
| monkeypox virus monkeypox virus Zaire-96-I-16 | *Monkeypox virus* | MPXV | *Orthopoxvirus* | Poxviridae (subfamily: Chordopoxvirinae) |
| mumps virus | *Mumps virus* | MuV | *Rubulavirus* | Paramyxoviridae (subfamily: Paramyxovirinae) |
| Murray Valley encephalitis virus | *Murray Valley encephalitis virus* | MVEV | *Flavivirus* | Flaviviridae |
| Nipah virus | *Nipah virus* | NiV | *Henipavirus* | Paramyxoviridae (subfamily: Paramyxovirinae) |
| Norwalk virus | *Norwalk virus* | NV | *Norovirus* | Calciviridae |
| O'nyong-nyong virus | *O'nyong-nyong virus* | ONNV | *Alphavirus* | Togaviridae |
| Omsk hemorrhagic fever virus | *Omsk hemorrhagic fever virus* | OHFV | *Flavivirus* | Flaviviridae |
| orf virus | *Orf virus* | ORFV | *Parapoxvirus* | Poxviridae (subfamily: Chordopoxvirinae) |
| Orungo virus | *Orungo virus* | ORUV | *Orbivirus* | Reoviridae |

**Table 14.14-10.** Viruses of Humans (*continued*)

| Common and infraspecific names[a] | Formal species names | Basic abbreviation[b] | Genus | Family |
|---|---|---|---|---|
| papillomavirus: see human papillomavirus | | | | |
| parainfluenza virus 1, parainfluenza virus 3 | *Human parainfluenzavirus 1, Human parainfluenzavirus 3* | HPIV-1, HPIV-3 | *Respirovirus* | Paramyxoviridae (subfamiliy: Paramyxovirinae) |
| parainfluenzavirus 2, parainfluenzavirus 4 | *Human parainfluenzavirus 2, Human parainfluenzavirus 4* | HPIV-2, HPIV-4 | *Rubulavirus* | Paramyxoviridae (subfamily: Paramyxovirinae) |
| parvovirus B19-A6 parvovirus B19-Au | *Human parvovirus B19* | B19V-A6 B19V-Au | *Erythrovirus* | Parvoviridae (subfamily: Parvovirinae) |
| poliovirus 1 poliovirus 2 poliovirus 3 | *Poliovirus* | PV | *Enterovirus* | Picornaviridae |
| rabies virus | *Rabies virus* | RABV | *Lyssavirus* | Rhabdoviridae |
| respiratory syncytial virus human respiratory syncytial virus A2 | *Human respiratory syncytial virus* | HRSV HRSV-A2 | *Pneumovirus* | Paramyxoviridae (subfamily: Pneumovirinae) |
| rhinoviruses (eg, rhinovirus A, human rhinovirus 37, rhinovirus B, human rhinovirus C) | *Human rhinovirus A, Human rhinovirus B, Human rhinovirus C* | HRV | *Enterovirus* | Picornaviridae |
| Rift Valley fever virus | *Rift Valley fever virus* | RVFV | *Phlebovirus* | Bunyaviridae |
| Ross River virus | *Ross River virus* | RRV | *Alphavirus* | Togaviridae |
| rotavirus | *Rotavirus B, Rotavirus C* | RV-B, HRV-C | *Rotavirus* | Reoviridae |
| rubella virus | *Rubella virus* | RUBV | *Rubivirus* | Togaviridae |
| Sagiyama virus | *Ross River virus* | RRV | *Alphavirus* | Togaviridae |
| Sapporo virus | *Sapporo virus* | SV | *Sapovirus* (formerly "Sapporo-like viruses") | Calciviridae |
| SARS virus or SARS-related coronavirus simian | *Severe acute respiratory syndrome coronavirus* | SARS-CoV | *Betacoronavirus* | Coronaviridae |
| SARS coronavirus 2 or COVID-19 virus (coronavirus disease 2019) | *Severe acute respiratory syndrome coronavirus 2* | SARS-CoV-2 | *Betacoronavirus* | Coronaviridae |

(*continued*)

**Table 14.14-10.** Viruses of Humans (*continued*)

| Common and infraspecific names[a] | Formal species names | Basic abbreviation[b] | Genus | Family |
|---|---|---|---|---|
| Simian hepatitis A virus | *Hepatitis A virus 1* | HAV-1 | *Hepatovirus* | Picornaviridae |
| simian herpes B virus (also herpesvirus simiae) | *Cercopithecine herpesvirus 2* | CeHV-2 | *Simplexvirus* | Herpesviridae (subfamily: Alphaherpesvirinae) |
| simian T-lymphotropic virus 1 | *Primate T-lymphotropic virus 1* | STLV-1 | *Deltaretrovirus* | Retroviridae (subfamily: Orthoretrovirinae) |
| Sin Nombre virus | *Sin Nombre virus* | SNV | *Hantavirus* | Bunyaviridae |
| Sindbis virus | *Sindbis virus* | SINV | *Alphavirus* | Togaviridae |
| St Louis encephalitis virus | *St Louis encephalitis virus* | SLEV | *Flavivirus* | Flaviridae |
| tanapox virus | *Tanapox virus* | TANV | *Yatapoxvirus* | Poxviridae (subfamily: Chordopoxvirinae) |
| tick-borne encephalitis virus | *Tick-borne encephalitis virus* | TBEV | *Flavivirus* | Flaviviridae |
| vaccinia virus, vaccinia virus Ankara, vaccinia virus Copenhagen | *Vaccinia virus* | VACV, VACV-ANK, VACV-COP | *Orthopoxvirus* | Poxviridae (subfamily: Chordopoxvirinae) |
| varicella-zoster virus | *Human herpesvirus 3* | HHV-3 | *Varicellovirus* | Herpesviridae (subfamily: Alphaherpesvirinae) |
| variola virus | *Variola virus* | VARV | *Orthopoxvirus* | Poxviridae (subfamily: Chordopoxvirinae) |
| Venezuelan equine encephalitis virus | *Venezuelan equine encephalitis virus* | VEEV | *Alphavirus* | Togaviridae |
| vesicular stomatitis Alagoas virus Indiana 3 | *Vesicular stomatitis Alagoas virus, Vesicular stomatitis Indiana virus 98COE, Vesicular stomatitis New Jersey virus* | VSAV-Ind3, VSIV-98COE, VSNJV | *Vesiculovirus* | Rhabdoviridae |
| West Nile virus | *West Nile virus* | WNV | *Flavivirus* | Flaviviridae |
| Western equine encephalitis virus | *Western equine encephalitis virus* | WEEV | *Alphavirus* | Togaviridae |
| yellow fever virus | *Yellow fever virus* | YFV | *Flavivirus* | Flaviviridae |

[a]Entries in this column are not complete listings of all members of the corresponding species. Entries may include species names, strains, serogroups, etc.
[b]Use abbreviations in accordance with recommendations in 13.0, Abbreviations.

yet be classified at each rank (eg, a viral species may belong to a family but not a genus), and a viral genus may not be assigned to a family. The rank of species was added to the code in 1991[6] and is reflected in the more than 2200 virus and viroid species distributed among 349 genera, 19 subfamilies, 87 families, and 6 orders.[6] International specialty groups are responsible for viral nomenclature below the rank of species (eg, types, strains). The code does not govern artificially created and laboratory hybrid viruses.

**14.14.3.3** **Formal vs Vernacular Virus Names.** Formal virus names are used for taxonomic groups (order, family, subfamily, genus, and species) in the abstract state.[1,7-9] Use of the formal name indicates that the group has official standing according to the ICTV code. Vernacular (common, informal) virus species names are used for actual entities (eg, laboratory material or outbreak specimens): "concrete viral objects that cause diseases. . . ."[9(p2247)]

**14.14.3.4** **Style of Virus Names.** For examples of the typographic conventions described in this section, see **Table 14.14-11**.[1,6,10,11] Typical endings for order, family, subfamily, genus, and species are listed in Table 14.14-11.

**14.14.3.5** **Latin and English forms.** Formal names of viral genus and above are latinized. English, the scientific lingua franca during the era of viral discovery, is used for formal virus species names no matter what the language of publication.

**14.14.3.6** **Initial capitals.** Formal virus names at each rank have initial capital letters. Other capitals are used when a proper noun is part of the name:

St Louis encephalitis virus

West Nile virus

Vernacular names do not use initial capitals unless a proper noun is part of the name:

La Crosse virus

**14.14.3.7** **Italics.** Although the viral nomenclature code recommends italicizing all scientific virus names (ie, species through order), codes for other organisms differ on

**Table 14.14-11.** Examples of Typical Endings for Order, Family, Subfamily, Genus, and Species

|  | Viruses | | Bacteria ending |
|  | Example | Ending | |
| --- | --- | --- | --- |
| Order | Mononegavirales | -virales | -ales |
| Family | Picornaviridae | -viridae | -aceae |
| Subfamily | Torovirinae | -virinae | -oideae |
| Genus | *Tenuivirus* | *-virus* | (varies) |
| Species | *Human parainfluenzavirus 1* | *-virus* | (varies) |

using italics for names of higher taxa. For example, for reasons of internal consistency, the JAMA Network journals do not italicize names of viral taxa above genus. The JAMA Network journals italicize formal viral genus and species names. The ICTVdb[2] recommends italic for species, with initial cap. It is consistent with style in other areas of biological nomenclature. Vernacular names are never italicized.

**14.14.3.8** **How to Style a Virus Term.** If a term ends in *-virales*, *-viridae*, or *–virinae*, the term would have an initial capital letter. For example, parvoviridae would be changed to Parvoviridae. Context will often determine whether a term ending in *-virus* is a formal or vernacular name and can be revised as necessary, querying the author. For instance, the term poliovirus might be left as is or might be changed to the formal species term *Poliovirus*. Terms for strains, types, serogroups, isolates, etc are never italicized or capitalized (see the section on those entities below). In figure legends in which actual viral entities are depicted (eg, electron micrographs), italics and capital letters would not be used for the actual entity depicted.[12] Legends to schematic depictions of viruses, however, probably refer to classes of virus, and formal style should be used.

**14.14.3.9** **Formal and Vernacular Names in Articles.** Formal names are used for abstract entities, vernacular names for physical entities:

> *West Nile virus* is a member of the genus *Flavivirus*. The presence of West Nile virus was confirmed in mosquitoes and dead crows.

> Polymerase chain reaction assays were used to detect RNA of West Nile virus (family Flaviviridae, genus *Flavivirus,* species *West Nile virus*).

It is useful, for purposes of identification, to include the formal name initially in an article that discusses actual viral entities (with the vernacular name used thereafter)[1,7,8,10]:

> *Hepatitis C virus* . . . hepatitis C virus

> *Human herpesvirus 4* . . . Epstein-Barr virus

> *Human herpesvirus 3* . . . varicella-zoster virus

> *Human immunodeficiency virus 1* . . . HIV-1

In such articles, the virus and its higher taxonomic classification may be usefully included early on:

> Most disease seen in the United States is caused by the Sin Nombre virus (family Bunyaviridae, genus *Hantavirus,* species Sin Nombre virus).

The formal name remains in English, the vernacular name in the language of publication[9,10]:

> *Measles virus* . . . virus de la rougeole . . .

> *Hepatitis B virus* . . . el virus de la hepatitis B

**14.14.3.10** **Abbreviations.** Formal viral species names should not be abbreviated. Common names of viral species names may be abbreviated. Recommended abbreviations are given in the international code (see Table 14.14-10).[1] Note that related gene symbols and virus abbreviations may differ (see 14.6.2, Human Gene Nomenclature):

| | |
|---|---|
| Gene symbol: | *HVBS4* |
| Gene description with virus abbreviation: | hepatitis B virus (HBV) integration site 4 |

The viral code recommends that rank always be specified with formal names and that it precede the virus name:

the family Paramyxoviridae

the genus *Respirovirus* (formerly the genus *Paramyxovirus*)

the species *Human parainfluenzavirus 1*

Virus names used as adjectives are not italicized[12]:

HIV infection

murine leukemia virus polymerase

vaccinia immune globulin

West Nile virus surveillance

Ebola virus

Official style calls for temporary names (recognized taxa whose names are not yet formally approved) to be presented in roman type within quotation marks:

*Sapovirus* (formerly "Sapporo-like virus")

"T4-like viruses"

Formal style is unambiguous. Vernacular style can be ambiguous because the ending -*virus* occurs in common names at all taxonomic ranks and in other informal designations (eg, arboviruses, which includes several families). It is therefore helpful for authors to specify rank with vernacular terms as well:

the family of retroviruses

Hantaan virus, a species of the genus *Hantavirus*

the paramyxovirus family

the paramyxovirus subfamily

**14.14.3.11** **Plant Virus Alternative.** Many plant virologists favor a different style for formal species names, which uses a binomial term that includes species and genus.[3,8,13] (Despite the designation "binomial," it may contain more than 2 words.) Plant virus names in this style consist of an English species name followed by the genus name:

| | |
|---|---|
| plant alternative: | Tobacco mosaic *tobamovirus* |
| ICTV style: | *Tobacco mosaic virus* (genus *Tobamovirus*) |

**14.14.3.12** **Binomial Proposal.** Formal virus species names do not currently follow the binomial style typical of other organisms (see 14.14.1, Biological Nomenclature), which includes the genus name and a specific epithet. Confusion exists between terms for abstract virus species and actual virus entities, which often are distinguished only typographically. Some virologists have indicated a preference for a binomial style for official virus species names.[7,9] Such a style would resemble the plant style described above, giving species and then genus. (For instance, *Measles virus* would become *Measles morbillivirus*. The vernacular term *measles virus* would remain in use for actual measles virus entities.) These differing ideas about scientific (vs common) names of viruses have long been a source of disagreement among virologists. After discussion of the proposal, the ICTV Executive Committee "overwhelmingly ascribe to the view that the disadvantages of renaming virus species on a large scale to conform to the NLBS [Non-Latinized Binomial System] or any other nomenclatural system greatly outweighs the potential advantages."[14]

**14.14.3.13** **Derivations.** For derivations of virus names, consult the reports of the ICTV.[2]

Some virus names are combinations of words; such names are known as *sigla*. Examples include *echovirus* (*e*nteric *c*ytopathic *h*uman *o*rphan *virus*) and picornavirus (*pico-, RNA virus*). Variant capitalization (eg, ECHOvirus, picoRNAvirus) is not used.

**14.14.3.14** **Strains, Types, and Isolates.** In clinical and laboratory articles that deal with actual entities, most terms will refer to strains, serotypes, serogroups, or viral isolates (ie, ranks below species). Such terms are not capitalized (unless they include proper nouns) or italicized. Such terms often contain numbers, letters, or names:

> coxsackievirus A1, coxsackievirus A24
>
> Desert Shield virus (a strain of *Norwalk virus*)
>
> enterovirus D68
>
> human adenovirus 2 (a strain of *Human adenovirus C*)
>
> human astrovirus 3, Berlin isolate
>
> human coronavirus 229E
>
> Hantaan virus 76-118 (a serotype of *Hantaan virus*)
>
> hepatitis C virus (HCV) genotype 1
>
> HCV subtype (or genotype) 3a
>
> hepatitis D virus genotype 1
>
> human poliovirus 1, poliovirus 1, or poliovirus type 1
>
> human poliovirus 2, poliovirus 2, or poliovirus type 2
>
> human poliovirus 3, poliovirus 3, or poliovirus type 3
>
> human respiratory syncytial virus A2
>
> La Crosse virus (a serotype of *California encephalitis virus*)
>
> Norwalk virus (a strain of *Norwalk virus*)

rotavirus B strain IDIR

tick-borne encephalitis virus European subtype

Formal species names may also include numbers or letters (eg, *Human herpesvirus 1*, *hepatitis B virus*; see Table 14.14-10).[15]

**14.14.3.15** **Hepatitis Terms.** Antigens of hepatitis B virus and antibodies to hepatitis B virus are expressed as given in **Table 14.14-12**.

Do not confuse hepatitis e antigen with hepatitis E virus or anti-HBe with anti–hepatitis E virus (anti-HEV).

**14.14.3.16** **Influenza Types and Strains.** Strains of influenza A virus are identified by antigenic subtypes, defined by the surface proteins hemagglutinin (H) and neuraminidase (N):

influenza A(H3N2)

There are 18 different hemagglutinin subtypes (H1-H18) and 11 different neuraminidase subtypes (N1-N11).[15]

The H,N suffix is used only for influenza A, but the 3 species of influenza virus may also contain suffixes with terms for the host of origin (if nonhuman), geographic origin (or a proper name in older strains), laboratory strain number, and year of isolation, separated by virgules (forward slashes) and, in the case of influenza A, followed by the H and N designations in parentheses:

influenza A/New York/55/2004 (H3N2)

influenza A/chicken/Hong Kong/317.5/01 (H5N1)

influenza B/Jiangsu/10/2003

influenza C/California/78

avian influenza A(H7N9)

avian influenza A/Anhui/01/2005 (H5N1)

novel influenza A (H1N1)

A virus that normally circulates in swine is called a *variant virus* when it is found in humans and is designated with "v": influenza A H3N2v.[16]

Influenza B viruses are not divided into subtypes but may be broken down into lineages and strains. Currently, circulating influenza B viruses belong to B/Yamagata and B/Victoria.

**Table 14.14-12.** Antigens and Antibodies of Hepatitis B Virus

| Antigen | Abbreviation | Antibody |
|---|---|---|
| hepatitis B surface antigen | HBsAg | anti-HBs |
| hepatitis B core antigen | HBcAg | anti-HBc |
| hepatitis B e antigen | HBeAg | anti-HBe |
| hepatitis B X antigen | HBxAg | anti-HBx |

**14.14.3.17** **Phages.** Phages are viruses that infect bacteria. The term *phage* is shortened from "bacteriophage." Although the current ICTV nomenclature code prohibits Greek letters in new virus names, older names with Greek letters have not been changed. Spelled-out Greek letters are also found, and letters may be uppercase or lowercase; follow author style. Vernacular terms often include the word *phage*:

> phage T4 *or* T4 phage

Phage groups or genera are sometimes referred to with general terms, such as the following: T-even phages, actinophages, coliphages, and T7 phage group.

Examples of formal phage names are given in **Table 14.14-13**.

All the above phage viruses have identically named strains, and many more strains belong to species of similar names. Follow author usage.

Enterobacteria phages Qβ and M11 are strains of *Enterobacteria phage Qβ*.

(For phage cloning vectors, see 14.6.1.4.4, Cloning Vectors.)

**14.14.3.18** **Genes.** For genes related to human viruses, see 14.6.2, Human Gene Nomenclature. For retrovirus gene terms, see 14.6.3, Oncogenes and Tumor Suppressor Genes, and 14.6.5, Nonhuman Genetic Terms.

**14.14.4** **Prions.** Disease names and abbreviations of spongiform encephalopathies are given in **Table 14.14-14**.[1,17-19]

(Do not confuse "kudu" and "kuru.")

The infectious agents of transmissible spongiform encephalopathies (TSEs) are known as *TSE agents* or *prions*. The term *prion* (from "proteinaceous infectious particle") reflects the agents' proposed association or identity with spongiform encephalopathy–related pathologic proteins. Follow author preference for the terms *TSE agent* and *prion*.

**Table 14.14-13.** Examples of Formal Phage Names

| Species | Abbreviation | Genus |
|---|---|---|
| *Acholeplasma phage L51* | L51 | *Plectrovirus* |
| *Enterobacteria phage λ* | λ | "λ-like viruses" |
| *Enterobacteria phage PRD1* | PRD1 | *Tectivirus* |
| *Enterobacteria phage Qβ* | Qβ | *Allolevivirus* |
| *Enterobacteria phage T1* | T1 | "T1-like viruses" |
| *Enterobacteria phage T4* | T4 | "T4-like viruses" |
| *Enterobateria phage Mu* | Mu | "Mu-like viruses" |
| *Halobacterium phage φH* | φH | "φH-like viruses" |
| *Lactococcus phage c2* | c2 | "c2-like viruses" |
| *Pseudomonas phage φ6* | φ6 | *Cystovirus* |

**Table 14.14-14.** Disease Names and Abbreviations of Spongiform Encephalopathies

| Disease | Abbreviation |
| --- | --- |
| bovine spongiform encephalopathy ("mad cow disease") | BSE |
| Creutzfeldt-Jakob disease | CJD |
| familial (genetic) CJD | fCJD |
| iatrogenic CJD | iCJD |
| sporadic CJD | sCJD |
| variant CJD (formerly new variant CJD [nvCJD]) | vCJD |
| chronic wasting disease of mule deer and elk | CWD |
| exotic ungulate encephalopathy (nyala, greater kudu, oryx) | EUE |
| fatal familial insomnia | FFI |
| feline spongiform encephalopathy | FSE |
| Gerstmann-Sträussler-Scheinker syndrome | GSS |
| kuru | |
| scrapie | |
| transmissible mink encephalopathy | TME |
| transmissible spongiform encephalopathy | TSE |

Proteins related to spongiform encephalopathies in humans are designated as follows:

| | |
| --- | --- |
| PrP | prion protein |
| PrP27-30 | PrP of 27-30 kDa |
| $PrP^C$ | cellular PrP |
| $PrP^{Sc}$ | scrapie-type PrP |
| PrP-res | protease-resistant PrP |
| PrP-sen | protease-sensitive PrP |
| rPrP | recombinant PrP |
| $BovPrP^{Sc}$ | (bovine) |
| $FePrP^{Sc}$ | (feline) |
| $HuPrP^{CJD}$ | (human) |
| $HuPrP^{Sc}$ | (human) |
| $MDePrP^{Sc}$ | (mule deer and elk) |
| $MkPrP^{Sc}$ | (mink) |
| MoPrP | (mouse) |

| NyaPrP$^{Sc}$ | (nyala and greater kudu) |
| OvPrP$^{Sc}$ | (ovine [scrapie]) |
| Tg(HuPrP) | (transgenic) |
| Tg(MoPrP-P101L) | |

The last term refers to a transgenic mouse line with a proline to leucine variation at residue 101 (see 14.6.1, Nucleic Acids and Amino Acids).

For prion-related genes, see 14.6.2, Human Gene Nomenclature.

**Principal Author:** Cheryl Iverson, MA

## REFERENCES

1. King AMQ, ed in chief; Adams MJ, Carstens EB, Lefkowitz EJ, eds. *Virus Taxonomy: Ninth Report of the International Committee on Taxonomy of Viruses.* Elsevier Academic Press; 2012.

2. Büchen-Osmond C. The Universal Virus Database (International Committee on Taxonomy of Viruses Database [ICTVdb]). *Computing Sci Eng.* 2003;5(3):16-25. doi:10.1109/MCISE.2003.1196303

3. Van Regenmortel MHV, Fauquet CM, Bishop DHL, et al, eds. *Virus Taxonomy: Classification and Nomenclature of Viruses: Seventh Report of the International Committee on Taxonomy of Viruses.* Academic Press; 2000.

4. Fauquet CM, Fargette D. International Committee on Taxonomy of Viruses and the 3,142 unassigned species. *Virol J.* 2005;2:64. doi:10.1186/1743-422X-2-64

5. Mayo MA, Fauquet CM, Maniloff J. Taxonomic proposals on the web: new ICTV consultative procedures. *Arch Virol.* 2003;148(3):609-611.

6. Kuhn JH. Virus nomenclature. In: Smart P, Maisonneuve H, Polderman A, eds. *Science Editors' Handbook.* 2nd ed. European Association of Science Editors; 2013:63-65.

7. Van Regenmortel MHV, Mahy BWJ. Emerging issues in virus taxonomy. *Emerg Infect Dis.* 2004;10(1):8-13.

8. Van Regenmortel MHV. Viruses are real, virus species are man-made, taxonomic constructions. *Arch Virol.* 2003;148(12):2481-2488.

9. Van Regenmortel MHV, Fauquet CM. Only italicised species names of viruses have a taxonomic meaning. *Arch Virol.* 2002;147(11):2247-2250.

10. Van Regenmortel MHV. On the relative merits of italics, Latin and binomial nomenclature in virus taxonomy. *Arch Virol.* 2000;145(2):433-441.

11. Van Regenmortel MHV, Mayo MA, Fauquet CM, Maniloff J. Virus nomenclature: consensus versus chaos. *Arch Virol.* 2000;145(10):2227-2232.

12. Van Regenmortel MHV. How to write the names of virus species. *Arch Virol.* 1999;144(5):1041-1042.

13. Van Regenmortel MHV. Perspectives on binomial names of virus species. *Arch Virol.* 2001;146(8):1637-1640.

14. Ball A [ICTV president]. Virus nomenclature: three steps forward, a half step back. Accessed May 24, 2018. https://talk.ictvonline.org/ictv1/f/general_ictv_discussions-20/399/virus-nomenclature-three-steps-forward-a-half-step-back

15. Centers for Disease Control and Prevention. Types of influenza viruses. Updated September 27, 2017. Accessed May 24, 2018. https://www.cdc.gov/flu/about/viruses/types/htm

16. Appiah GD, Blanton L, D'Mello T, et al. Influenza activity: United States, 2014-15 season and composition of the 2015-16 influenza vaccine. *MMWR Morb Mortal Wkly*

*Rep.* Updated June 5, 2015. Accessed May 24, 2018. https://www.cdc/gov/mmwr/preview/mmwrhtml/mm6421a5.htm

17. Glatzel M, Aguzzi A. Transmissible spongiform encephalopathies. In: Jorgensen JH, Pfaller MA, Carroll KC, et al, eds. *Manual of Clinical Microbiology.* 11th ed. ASM Press; 2015:1859-1866.

18. Prusiner SB. Novel proteinaceous infectious particles cause scrapie. *Science.* 1982;216(4542):136-144.

19. Prusiner SB. Prion diseases and the BSE crisis. *Science.* 1997;278(5336):245-251.

## 14.15     **Psychiatric Terminology.**

**14.15.1**    *Diagnostic and Statistical Manual of Mental Disorders (DSM).* The American Psychiatric Association has published 6 editions of a manual for the classification of mental disorders. Each edition has been titled *Diagnostic and Statistical Manual of Mental Disorders* and has used the abbreviation *DSM*:

     *DSM-I* (1952)

     *DSM-II* (1968)

     *DSM-III* (1980)

     *DSM-III-R* (1987)

     *DSM-IV* (1994)

     *DSM-5* (2013)

Note that with *DSM-5* the edition number changed from a roman numeral to an arabic numeral (*DSM-IV* to *DSM-5*). This change was made to facilitate incremental updates until a new edition is required. Incremental updates will be identified with decimals, for example, *DSM-5.1, DSM-5.2*.[1]

Using *DSM-5* as an example, these books should be cited as follows:

     American Psychiatric Association. *Diagnostic and Statistical Manual of Mental Disorders.* 5th ed. American Psychiatric Association; 2013.

A text revision of *DSM-IV* was published in 2000 as *Diagnostic and Statistical Manual of Mental Disorders, Fourth Edition, Text Revision*, abbreviated *DSM-IV-TR*. This book is a revision of the text describing the diagnostic and associated features, prevalence, course, and differential diagnosis of the disorders included in the *DSM-IV* diagnostic categories. However, the diagnostic classification and criteria in *DSM-IV-TR* are unchanged from those in the 1994 *DSM-IV* diagnostic manual. If *DSM-IV-TR* is cited for diagnostic criteria, it gives the misleading impression that the criteria used differ from those of *DSM-IV* and date from 2000 rather than 1994. Thus, a citation for the *DSM-IV* diagnostic criteria should be to *DSM-IV* (1994). There are no *DSM-IV-TR* diagnostic criteria per se. If a reference citation pertains to the updated descriptive material in *DSM-IV-TR*, that should be cited. If a citation pertains to both the *DSM-IV* criteria and the updated descriptive material in *DSM-IV-TR*, it would be best to clarify that in the text.

Beginning with *DSM-III*, the diagnostic system involved an assessment on several axes as follows:

| | |
|---|---|
| Axis I | Clinical Disorders |
| | Other Conditions That May Be a Focus of Clinical Attention |
| Axis II | Personality Disorders |
| | Mental Retardation |
| Axis III | General Medical Conditions |
| Axis IV | Psychosocial and Environmental Problems |
| Axis V | Global Assessment of Functioning |

However, "*DSM-5* has moved to a nonaxial documentation of diagnosis (formerly Axes I, II, and III), with separate notations for important psychosocial and contextual factors (formerly Axis IV) and disability (formerly Axis V)."[2(p16)] As Kupfer et al[3] note, "This is largely due to its [the multiaxial system's] incompatibility with diagnostic systems in the rest of medicine, as well as the result of a decision to place personality disorders and intellectual disability at the same level as other mental disorders."[3(p1691)]

The new recommendations in *DSM-5* have also attempted to ensure "greater harmony between this North American classification system and the *International Classification of Diseases (ICD)* system."[3(p1691),4]

*DSM-5* recommends that rather than the Global Assessment of Functioning scale, which had been recommended by *DSM-IV* for eligibility for short- and long-term disability compensation, the World Health Organization Disability Assessment Schedule[5] be used as "the best current measure of disability for routine clinical use."[6]

For proper expressions of editions of *DSM,* see 13.11, Clinical, Technical, and Other Common Terms.

**14.15.2** **Other Psychiatric Terminology.** For appropriate use of terms and terms to avoid, such as *addict, manic, schizophrenic,* and *hysterical,* see 11.1, Correct and Preferred Usage of Common Words and Phrases.

For molecular terms related to psychiatry and neuroscience, see 14.11.5, Molecular Neuroscience.

**Principal Author:** Cheryl Iverson, MA

### ACKNOWLEDGMENT

Thanks to the following for reviewing and providing comments: Donald C. Goff, MD, *JAMA*, and Department of Psychiatry, NYU Langone Medical Center, New York, New York; Stephan Heckers, MD, MSc, formerly with *JAMA Psychiatry*, and Department of Psychiatry and Behavioral Sciences, Vanderbilt University, Nashville, Tennessee; and Richard M. Glass, MD, formerly with *JAMA*.

### REFERENCES

1. *DSM-5* development: frequently asked questions. Accessed July 21, 2019. https://www.psychiatry.org/psychiatrists/practice/dsm/feedback-and-questions/ frequently-asked-questions

2. American Psychiatric Association. *Diagnostic and Statistical Manual of Mental Disorders*. 5th ed. American Psychiatric Association; 2013. Accessed April 23, 2018. https://www.psychiatry.org/practice/dsm/dsm5

3. Kupfer DJ, Kuhl EA, Regier DA. *DSM-5—the future arrived. JAMA*. 2013;309(16):1691-1692. doi:10.1001/jama.2013.2298

4. Using *DSM-5* in the transition to *ICD-10*. Accessed April 23, 2018. https://www.psychiatry.org/psychiatrists/practice/dsm/icd-10

5. WHO Disability Assessment Schedule (WHODAS 2.0). Last updated October 24, 2017. Accessed April 23, 2018. https://www.who.int/classifications/icf/whodasii/en

6. Kupfer DJ, Regier DA. *DSM-5* development. Accessed March 21, 2019. http://www.dsm5.org

**14.16** ■ **Pulmonary and Respiratory Terminology.** Standardization of symbols in respiratory physiology dates from at least 1950.[1]

Despite the familiarity of abbreviations in pulmonary and respiratory medicine, authors and editors are encouraged to expand all terms at first mention, except as noted.

Both symbols and abbreviations are used. Symbols consist of separate elements in various combinations whose letters may differ from the initial letters of the expansion, eg, Q (perfusion). Abbreviations are usually initialisms.

**14.16.1** ■ **Symbols.** Symbols and their subgrouping into main symbols and modifiers are consistent with approved nomenclature formulated circa 1980 by the Commission of Respiratory Physiology (International Union of Physiological Sciences) and the Publications Committee of the American Physiological Society.[2,3] The following groupings of pulmonary and respiratory symbols are adapted from Fishman,[2] Primiano and Chatburn,[4] West,[5,6] and Longo et al.[7]

Main symbols are typically capital letters set on the line and are the first elements of an expression. The same letter may stand for one entity in respiratory mechanics and another in gas exchange (eg, P stands for *pressure* in respiratory mechanics and *partial pressure* in gas exchange). The following are examples (note dots above some letters to indicate flow):

| | |
|---|---|
| C | compliance, concentration of gas in blood |
| D | diffusing capacity |
| F | fractional concentration in a dry gas |
| P | pressure or partial pressure |
| Q | volume of blood |
| $\dot{Q}$ | perfusion (volume of blood per unit time) |
| R | respiratory exchange ratio |
| S | saturation of hemoglobin with oxygen |
| sG | specific conductance |
| T | temperature |
| V | volume of gas |
| $\dot{V}$ | volume of gas per unit time |

Modifiers are set as small capitals (not subscript):

| | |
|---|---|
| A | alveolar |
| B | barometric |
| D | dead space |
| E | expired, expiratory |
| ET | end-tidal |
| I | inspired, inspiratory |
| L | lung |
| T | tidal |

Lowercase-letter modifiers (which are not subscript) follow small-capital modifiers, if both appear; note bar in last term:

| | |
|---|---|
| a | arterial |
| aw | airway |
| b | blood |
| c | capillary |
| c′ | end-capillary |
| i | ideal |
| max | maximum |
| p | pulse oximetry |
| v | venous |
| v̄ | mixed venous |

Gas abbreviations are usually the last element of the symbol, given as small capitals:

| | |
|---|---|
| CO | carbon monoxide |
| $CO_2$ | carbon dioxide |
| $N_2$ | nitrogen |
| $O_2$ | oxygen |

Note: At other times, when gas abbreviations are used on their own, large capitals are used (eg, carbon monoxide [CO]).

The main symbols and modifiers are combined in various ways to derive terms; common examples are listed in **Table 14.6-1**.

**Table 14.16-1.** Examples of Gas Symbols

| Term | Expansion | Typical units of measure[2,5-7] |
|---|---|---|
| $P_{CO_2}$[a] | partial pressure of carbon dioxide | mm Hg *or* kPa |
| $Pa_{CO_2}$[a] | partial pressure of carbon dioxide, arterial | mm Hg *or* kPa |
| $P_{O_2}$[a] | partial pressure of oxygen | mm Hg *or* kPa |
| $Pa_{O_2}$[a] | partial pressure of oxygen, arterial | mm Hg *or* kPa |
| $PA_{O_2}$ | partial pressure of oxygen, alveolar | mm Hg *or* kPa |
| $P\bar{v}_{O_2}$ | partial pressure of oxygen, mixed venous | mm Hg *or* kPa |
| $P_B$ | barometric pressure | mm Hg *or* kPa |
| $PA_{O_2} - Pa_{O_2}$ | alveolar-arterial difference (or gradient) in partial pressure of oxygen (preferred to AaD$_{O_2}$) | mm Hg *or* kPa |
| $Ca_{O_2}$ | oxygen concentration (or content), arterial | mL/dL *or* mmol/L |
| $Cc'_{O_2}$ | oxygen concentration (or content), pulmonary end-capillary | mL/dL |
| $C_L$ | lung compliance | L/cm $H_2O$ *or* L/mm Hg *or* L/kPa |
| $D_{LCO}$ | diffusing capacity of lung for carbon monoxide | mL·min$^{-1}$·mm Hg$^{-1}$ |
| $F_{E_{N_2}}$ | fractional concentration of nitrogen in expired gas | fraction |
| $F_{I_{O_2}}$ | fraction of inspired oxygen | fraction |
| $P_E max$ | maximum expiratory pressure | cm $H_2O$ *or* mm Hg |
| $P_I max$ | maximum inspiratory pressure | cm $H_2O$ *or* mm Hg |
| Raw | airway resistance | cm $H_2O$·L$^{-1}$·s$^{-1}$ *or* kPa·L$^{-1}$·s$^{-1}$ |
| $Sa_{O_2}$ | arterial oxygen saturation | % |
| sGaw | specific airway conductance | L·s$^{-1}$·cm $H_2O^{-1}$ *or* L·s$^{-1}$·kPa$^{-1}$ |
| $Sp_{O_2}$ | oxygen saturation as measured by pulse oximetry | % |
| $V_{DS}$ | volume of dead space | mL *or* L |
| $V_E$ | expired volume per unit time | L/min |
| $V_{O_2}$ | oxygen consumption | mL/min *or* L/min *or* mmol/min |
| $V_{O_2} max$ | maximum oxygen consumption | mL/min *or* L/min *or* mmol/min |
| V/Q̇ | ventilation perfusion ratio (also V/Q) | ratio |
| $V_T$ | tidal volume | mL *or* L |

[a]This term may be given without expansion at first mention (see also 14.11, Clinical, Technical, and Other Common Terms, and 18.0, Units of Measure).

Note: Sometimes quantities are given per unit body weight, eg, $V_T$ in liters per kilogram.

**14.16.2**     **Abbreviations.** Table 14.6-2 lists some common abbreviations from pulmonary function testing; they should always be expanded at first mention.

**Table 14.16-2.** Common Pulmonary Function Test Abbreviations

| Term | Expansion | Typical unit of measure |
| --- | --- | --- |
| CC | closing capacity | L |
| CV | closing volume | L |
| ERV | expiratory reserve volume | L |
| FEF | forced expiratory flow | L/min |
| $FEF_{25\%-75\%}$ | FEF, midexpiratory phase | L/min *or* L/s |
| $FEF_{200-1200}$ | FEF between 200 and 1200 mL of forced vital capacity | L/min *or* L/s |
| FEV | forced expiratory volume | L |
| $FEV_1$[a] | FEV in first second of expiration | L |
| $FEV_1$ (percent predicted)[a] | FEV in first second of expiration, taking into account age, height, sex, and race | % |
| $FEV_1/FVC$[a] | percent of FVC exhaled in first second | expressed as a ratio or a percent |
| FIVC | forced inspiratory vital capacity | L |
| FRC | functional residual capacity | L |
| FVC | forced vital capacity | L |
| IRV | inspiratory reserve volume | L |
| IVC | inspiratory vital capacity | L |
| MVV | maximum voluntary ventilation | L/min |
| PEF, PEFR | peak expiratory flow rate | L/min |
| RV | residual volume | L |
| TLC | total lung capacity | L |
| VC | vital capacity | L |

[a]Note that all 3 of these should be reported.

**14.16.3**   **Mechanical Ventilation.** The following should be expanded at first mention:

| | |
| --- | --- |
| APRV | airway pressure release ventilation |
| BiPAP | bilevel positive airway pressure (cm $H_2O$) |
| CPAP | continuous positive airway pressure (cm $H_2O$) |
| ECMO | extracorporeal membrane oxygenation |
| ET tube | endotracheal tube |
| HFV | high-frequency ventilation |
| NIPPV | noninvasive positive pressure ventilation |

| NIV | noninvasive ventilation |
|---|---|
| PAV | proportional assist ventilation |
| PEEP | positive end-expiratory pressure (cm $H_2O$) |
| VPAP | variable positive airway pressure (cm $H_2O$) |

**Principal Author:** Cheryl Iverson, MA

## ACKNOWLEDGMENT

Thanks to George T. O'Connor, MD, MS, *JAMA*, and Boston University School of Medicine, Boston, Massachusetts, for reviewing and providing comments.

## REFERENCES

1. Standardization of definitions and symbols in respiratory physiology. *Fed Proc.* 1950;9(3):602-605.
2. Fishman AP, ed. *Handbook of Physiology: A Critical, Comprehensive Presentation of Physiological Knowledge and Concepts.* Vol 2, section 3, pt 1. American Physiological Society; 1986:endpapers.
3. Macklem PT. Symbols and abbreviations. In: Fishman AP, ed. *Handbook of Physiology: A Critical Comprehensive Presentation of Physiological Knowledge and Concepts.* Vol 2, section 3, pt 1. American Physiological Society; 1986:ix.
4. Primiano FP Jr, Chatburn RL. Zen and the art of nomenclature maintenance: a revised approach to respiratory symbols and terminology. *Respir Care.* 2006;51(12):1450-1457.
5. West JB. *Pulmonary Pathophysiology: The Essentials.* 8th ed. Lippincott Williams & Wilkins; 2013.
6. West JB. *Respiratory Physiology: The Essentials.* 9th ed. Lippincott Williams & Wilkins; 2012.
7. Longo D, Fauci A, Kasper D, Hauser S, Jameson J, Loscalzo J, eds. *Harrison's Principles of Internal Medicine.* 18th ed. McGraw-Hill; 2011:3605, 3607.

**14.17** **Radiology.** Radiology, the medical specialty that uses imaging to diagnose and sometimes treat disease, is distinct from radiography, an imaging technique based on x-rays passing through tissue and emerging to "hit" film on the other side. Radiology comprises all types of medical imaging, including radiography. To help standardize nomenclature and abbreviations used in radiology, a short list of terms and their definitions and helpful resources is provided in this section.

**14.17.1** **Radiology Terms.** The following terms are commonly used in radiology.

*b* **value:** The "*b* value" (also occasionally referred to as the "*b* factor") is associated with diffusion-weighted magnetic resonance imaging (diffusion-weighted MRI or DWI). It measures "strength (intensity and timing) of the diffusion gradient,"[1,2] and the units are seconds per square millimeter.

maximum *b* value of 1221 $s/mm^2$

Four gradient strengths were applied, resulting in *b* values of 0 and 1000 $s/mm^2$ applied sequentially in the X, Y, and Z gradient directions.

**boost:** An additional dose of radiation delivered to a particular subset of the original treatment field, usually the tumor bed.[2]

**density:** *Density* should be used only in the photometric sense to refer to inherent characteristics of film or film blackening.[2] For describing the appearance on radiographic images, in most cases *density* should be changed to *opacity*, which is an area of whiteness. For computed tomography (CT) and magnetic resonance imaging (MRI), see *hyperattenuating* and *hyperintense*, respectively.

**Doppler:** See 14.3.6, Echocardiography.

**echo train:** A sequence of 2 or more echoes generated by the application of radiofrequency pulses or gradients. *Echo train* is not a unit of measure[2] but is expressed as in these examples:

> echo train length 5
>
> echo train length 18
>
> echo train length 16
>
> echo train length 20
>
> a long echo-train–length 3-dimensional fast-spin echo sequence

**excitations/signals:** Change "number of excitations" to "number of signals acquired" (applies to MRI). A signal is the component of an electrical current that contains information, as opposed to noise.[3]

**field of view:** The rectangular region superimposed over the area of the body from which MRI data are acquired.[4]

**field strength:** *Field* refers to the magnetic field generated by the MRI magnet (eg, high-field-strength imaging).[2]

**hyperattenuating, hypoattenuating:** CT images are described in terms of the relative attenuation of what is being measured. A *hyperattenuating* (or high-attenuation) lesion is more dense than surrounding tissue and appears as an area of whiteness on the CT image, whereas a *hypoattenuating* (low-attenuation) lesion appears as an area of blackness.

**hyperintense, hypointense:** In MRI, the image contrast is measured in terms of signal intensity, where *hyperintense* indicates areas of whiteness and *hypointense* indicates areas of blackness.[2]

**k-space:** This term refers to mathematical space with frequency and phase, rather than spatial data, as coordinates.[1]

> Our pulse sequences collected data spirally in k-space.
>
> k-space filtering
>
> k-space sampling

**lucency, lucent, radiolucent:** These terms refer to an area of blackness on a radiograph.[2]

**opacity:** An area of whiteness on a radiograph.[2]

**radiofrequency ablation:** A treatment technique that uses high-frequency alternating electrical current to destroy tissue cells by heating them.[5]

**T1, T1ρ, T2, T2\*:** These are types of relaxation time in MRI.[1,4] They need not be expanded.

| | |
|---|---|
| T1 | spin-lattice or longitudinal relaxation time |
| T1ρ | spin-lattice relaxation time in the rotating frame |
| T2 | spin-spin or transverse relaxation time |
| T2* | time constant for loss of phase coherence among spins |

**TE:** The time between the middle of 90° pulse and the middle of spin-echo production. Expand echo time (TE) as in this example:

Echo times (TEs) were 20 and 80 milliseconds.

**TR:** The time between the beginning of a pulse sequence and the beginning of the succeeding (essentially identical) pulse sequence. Expand repetition time (TR) as in this example:

Cardiac-gated repetition time (TR) was greater than 2400 milliseconds.

**14.17.2** ▪ **Resources.** Available radiologic glossaries include the following:

▪ Thoracic radiology: glossary of terms for thoracic radiology[6]

▪ Breast imaging: American College of Radiology *BI-RADS Atlas*[7]

▪ Magnetic resonance: *ACR Glossary of MRI Terms,*[4] glossary of magnetic resonance terms[1]

▪ Ultrasonography: *Recommended Ultrasound Terminology*[3]

▪ General, for laypersons and nonspecialists: RadiologyInfo glossary of terms[5]

In addition to the terms explained in this section, see 11.1, Correct and Preferred Usage of Common Words and Phrases, for terms such as *radiography, radiology, radiograph,* and *film;* 13.14, Radioactive Isotopes, and 17.0, for units such as H (Hounsfield) and keV (kiloelectron volt).

**Principal Author:** Cheryl Iverson, MA

## ACKNOWLEDGMENT

Thanks to Jennifer Eberhart, *Radiology*, Oak Brook, Illinois, and Philip Sefton, MS, ELS, *JAMA*, for reviewing and providing comments.

## REFERENCES

1. Rinck PA. Glossary. In: *Magnetic Resonance in Medicine: The Basic Textbook of the European Magnetic Resonance Forum.* 11th ed. 2017. Accessed July 22, 2019. https://www.magnetic-resonance.org/ch/22-01.html

2. Lang D. Usage and nomenclature. In: *Radiological Society of North America (RSNA) In-House Style Manual.* RSNA; 2005.

3. *Recommended Ultrasound Terminology.* 3rd ed. American Institute of Ultrasound in Medicine; 2008.

4. Hendrick RE, Bradley WG Jr, Harms SE, et al. ACR Revised Glossary 2005 (*ACR Glossary of MRI Terms*). American College of Radiology. Accessed August 5, 2019. https://www.acr.org/-/media/ACR/files/radiology-safety/MR-safety/MRGlossary.pdf

5. Glossary of terms. RadiologyInfo. Accessed April 25, 2018. https://www.radiologyinfo.org/en/glossary/browse-glossary.cfm?all=1

6. Hansell DM, Bankier AA, MacMahon H, McLoud TC, Müller NL, Remy J. Fleischner Society: glossary of terms for thoracic imaging. *Radiology*. 2008;246(3):697-722. doi:10.1148/radiol.2462070712

7. D'Orsi CJ, Sickles EA, Mendelson EB, et al. *BI-RADS Atlas*. 5th ed. American College of Radiology; 2013. Accessed April 25, 2018. https://www.acr.org/Quality-Safety/Resources/BIRADS

**14.18** **Terminology in Transition: Nephrology.** The global organization dedicated to developing and implementing evidence-based clinical practice guidelines in kidney disease, KDIGO (Kidney Disease: Improving Global Outcomes), is spearheading an international effort to revise the nomenclature used to describe kidney function and disease.

The effort will focus on making terminology more patient-centered and precise, with the goal of greater uniformity in medical practice, research, scientific publication, and public health.

Some of the terminology to be harmonized includes the following:

**Kidney vs renal**: Select the more patient-friendly term (ie, *kidney*). Also, using these in parallel leads to different abbreviations for the same condition (eg, RRT [renal replacement therapy] and KRT [kidney replacement therapy]).

**Kidney failure vs end-stage renal disease**: *Kidney failure* is the preferred term except when referring to eligibility for medical care under US legislation or other regulations. Patients with kidney failure should be further described by the presence or absence of therapy by dialysis, transplant, or conservative care and by symptom severity.

**Decreased glomerular filtration rate (GFR)**: Use this instead of *decreased kidney function*. Kidneys execute a variety of functions, not just glomerular filtration, so precision in terminology is preferred.

**Chronic kidney disease (CKD)**: This is not the same as decreased GFR. CKD is defined as decreased GFR or markers of kidney damage, such as elevated albuminuria or abnormalities of the urine sediment or kidney imaging. People with normal GFR may have CKD.

**Acute kidney disease (AKD)**: This is not the same as acute kidney injury (AKI). AKD conditions are present for less than 3 months, whereas AKI conditions have onset within a week.

The final recommendations and a complete glossary of related terms will be available in the near future and used to inform an update to this chapter in the manual online.

See also 13.0, Abbreviations.

# 15.0 Eponyms

**15.0** **Eponyms.** *Eponyms* are names or phrases derived from or including the name of a person or place. These terms are used in a descriptive or adjectival sense in medical and scientific writing to describe diseases, syndromes, signs, tests, methods, and procedures.

Eponyms often indicate the name of the describer or presumptive discoverer of the disease (Alzheimer disease) or sign (Murphy sign), the name of a person or kindred found to have the disease described (Christmas disease), or, when based on the name of a place (technically called *toponyms*), the geographic location in which the disease was found to occur (Lyme disease, Ebola virus). Historically, eponyms named after the describer or discoverer took the possessive form ('s) and those named for other persons or for places took the nonpossessive form. As the use of the possessive form for all eponyms has become progressively less common (see 15.2, Nonpossessive Form), this formal distinction has faded.

Correct use of eponyms should be considered with a view toward clarity and consistency, the awareness that meanings can change over time and across cultures, and a desire to minimize misunderstanding in the global medical community.

**15.1** **Eponymous vs Noneponymous Terms.** Use of eponyms in the biomedical literature should be considered with regard to their usefulness in transmitting medical information. Medical writing is replete with eponyms; however, descriptive terms are often more useful for a reader. For instance, the pancreatic duct is sometimes referred to as the duct of Wirsung, after its discoverer, but that term gives no useful information about the function or location of the duct. In any case, many eponyms can be replaced with a noneponymous term that consists of a descriptive word or phrase that designates the same disease, condition, or procedure. For example:

> osteitis deformans (instead of Paget disease of bone)
>
> hemolytic uremic syndrome (instead of Gasser syndrome)
>
> amyotrophic lateral sclerosis (instead of Lou Gehrig disease)

The use of the noneponymous term may provide information about location or function and facilitate international communication. It also helps avoid confusing distinctly different disease entities with similar eponymous names (eg, Paget disease of bone, Paget disease of the nipple).

In some cases, readers may be more familiar with the eponymous term. Placing the descriptive term(s) in parentheses after first mention of the eponymous term may be helpful in this instance. For example:

Stein-Leventhal syndrome (polycystic ovary syndrome)

Stevens-Johnson syndrome (bullous erythema multiforme)

Crohn disease (regional enteritis)

Eponyms, but not the nouns or articles that accompany them, should be capitalized.

Babinski sign

Osler nodes

the Fisher exact test

Adjectival forms of proper names are not capitalized.

parkinsonian gait (from Parkinson disease)

addisonian crisis (from Addison disease)

**15.2**    **Nonpossessive Form.** There is some continuing debate about the use of the possessive form for eponyms, but a transition toward the nonpossessive form has taken place. A major step toward preference for the nonpossessive form occurred when the National Down Syndrome Society advocated the use of *Down syndrome*, rather than *Down's syndrome*, explaining that the syndrome does not actually belong to anyone.[1] Previous editions of this manual,[2] the Council of Science Editors style manual,[3] and the 28th edition of *Stedman's Medical Dictionary*[4] recommend and use the nonpossessive form for eponymous terms. However, the 32nd edition of *Dorland's Illustrated Medical Dictionary* takes an intermediate position, stating, "The tendency in recent years has been to drop the *'s* from medical eponyms and to use the nonpossessive form of the personal name. . . .This decision should by no means, however, be taken as a proscription of the possessive eponym, and whether or not to use the possessive is very much a matter of individual preferences."[5] The use of the possessive form for eponyms is becoming progressively less common, and the entries for eponymic terms in dictionaries reflect this ongoing shift in usage.

One reason for preferring the nonpossessive form is that although eponyms are possessive nouns using proper names, they are structurally adjectival and should not convey a true possessive sense. For example, the name *Addison*, as used in describing "Addison's disease," is used as a noun modifier, with the sense of the modifier being clearly nonpossessive. Some possessive eponyms have evolved into the form of derived adjectives, as exemplified in the term *addisonian crisis*. Even when eponyms are used in an attributive sense, they have commonly lost possessive endings over time (eg, Nobel Prize). Thus, the transition of eponyms to the nonpossessive form is consistent with a linguistic perspective and with trends in English usage.

Use of the nonpossessive form of eponyms has become standard in medical genetics, and such usage, recommended by McKusick in *Mendelian Inheritance in Man: A Catalog of Human Genes and Genetic Disorders*,[6] is appropriate in other areas of medicine. McKusick's reasons for avoiding the possessive form of eponyms included the comment that "the eponym is merely a 'handle'; often the person whose name is used was not the first to describe the condition . . . or did not describe the full syndrome as it has subsequently become known." Hence, even the initial description may not belong to the named individual, providing an additional reason to avoid the possessive form.

Use of the nonpossessive form can avoid awkwardness that otherwise would occur in instances such as the following:

When the word following begins with a sibilant *c, s,* or *z* (*syndrome, sign, zone*)

When an eponym ends in *ce, s,* or *z*

When a hyphenated name is involved

> Brown-Séquard syndrome

When 2 or more names are involved:

> Charcot-Marie-Tooth disease

> Dejerine-Sottas dystrophy

> Tay-Sachs disease

When an article (*a, an, the*) precedes the term:

> an Opie paradox

> a Schatzki ring

Alternative stylings for eponymous terms may include the preposition *of*:

> angle of Virchow

> circle of Willis

The possessive form may be used when it is part of an established nonmedical eponymous name:

> Russell's viper

> St John's wort (*Hypericum perforatum*)

The possessive form is retained if it is part of the name of an organization or title or was used in the original quotation or citation:

> Alzheimer's Association

> *Dorland's Illustrated Medical Dictionary*

The possessive form is also retained for noneponymous terms that describe disorders characteristic of certain occupations or activities:

> woolsorter's disease

> gamekeeper's thumb

With the exceptions noted herein, the nonpossessive form should be used for eponymous terms.

**Principal Author:** Brenda Gregoline, ELS

## ACKNOWLEDGMENT

I thank Karen Boyd and Diane L. Cannon, formerly of JAMA Network; Barbara Gastel, MD, MPH, Texas A&M University, College Station; and Peter J. Olson, ELS, Sheridan Journal Services, Waterbury, Vermont, for their review of this chapter.

## REFERENCES

1. The National Down Syndrome Society. Preferred language guide. Accessed December 4, 2018. https://www.ndss.org/wp-content/uploads/2018/02/NDSS-Preferred-Language-Guide-2015.pdf

2. Iverson C, Christiansen S, Flanagin A, et al. *AMA Manual of Style: A Guide for Authors and Editors*. 10th ed. Oxford University Press; 2007.

3. Style Manual Committee, Council of Science Editors. *Scientific Style and Format: The CSE Manual for Authors, Editors, and Publishers*. 8th ed. University of Chicago Press/Council of Science Editors; 2014.

4. *Stedman's Medical Dictionary*. 28th ed. Lippincott Williams & Wilkins; 2005.

5. *Dorland's Illustrated Medical Dictionary*. 32nd ed. Saunders; 2012:xx-xxi.

6. McKusick VA. *Mendelian Inheritance in Man: A Catalog of Human Genes and Genetic Disorders*. 12th ed. Johns Hopkins University Press; 1998:xl, xlii.

# 16.0 Greek Letters

16.1 Greek Letter vs Word

16.2 Capitalization After a Greek Letter

16.3 Greek Alphabet

16.4 Page Composition and Electronic Formats

**16.0** **Greek Letters.** Greek letters are frequently used in statistical formulas and notations, mathematical composition, certain chemical names for drugs, and clinical and technical terms (see 13.12, Units of Measure; 14.0, Nomenclature; 19.0, Study Design and Statistics; and 20.0, Mathematical Composition).

> β-adrenergic
>
> κ light chain
>
> κ/λ light-chain ratio
>
> IFN-γ
>
> $\beta_2$-microglobulin
>
> $\chi^2$ test

**16.1** **Greek Letter vs Word.** Use of Greek letters rather than spelled-out words is preferred, unless common usage dictates otherwise (eg, *tau protein*). Consult *Dorland's* and *Stedman's* medical dictionaries for general terms. However, these sources may differ in the representation of terms (eg, *α-fetoprotein* in *Stedman's* and *alpha fetoprotein* in *Dorland's*).

For chemical terms, the use of Greek letters is almost always preferred.

> α-kanosamine
>
> metallo-β-lactamase
>
> ω-3 fatty acids

For electroencephalographic terms, use the word (see 14.11.2, Electroencephalographic Terms).

> The electroencephalographic activity showed 2 spectral peaks: one in the theta range and the other at higher frequencies (25-50 Hz).

For drug names that contain Greek letters, consult the sources listed in 14.4, Drugs, for preferred usage. In some cases, when the Greek letter is part of the word (as in *betamethasone*), the Greek letter is spelled out and set closed up. For some drug names, the approved nonproprietary name uses the word and not the letter, with an intervening space (as in *beta carotene*). (However, the chemical name for beta carotene is *β-carotene.*) Other drug names use the Greek letter (as in *β-lactam antibiotics*).

<table><tr><td>16.2</td></tr></table> **Capitalization After a Greek Letter.** In titles, subtitles (except in references), headings, and at the beginning of sentences, the first non-Greek letter after a lowercase Greek letter should be capitalized.

> β-Blockers help control heart rate and are also used in the treatment of abnormal heart rhythms.

Do not capitalize the Greek letter, unless the word normally includes a Greek capital letter. In that case, the first non-Greek letter after the capital Greek letter should be lowercase.

> B-Hemolytic streptococci are bacteria that can destroy red blood cells and cause a variety of diseases.

> Δ-9-tetrahydrocannabinol administered intravenously to marijuana smokers disappeared from the blood plasma with a half-life of 28 hours compared with 57 hours for nonusers of marijuana.

For hyphenation in words that contain Greek letters, consult 8.3.1.8, Hyphen, Special Combinations.

<table><tr><td>16.3</td></tr></table> **Greek Alphabet.** Capital and lowercase Greek letters are listed in **Table 16.3-1.**

**Table 16.3-1.** Capital and Lowercase Greek Letters

| Name of letter | Greek lowercase | Greek capital |
|---|---|---|
| Alpha | α | A |
| Beta | β | B |
| Gamma | γ | Γ |
| Delta | δ | Δ |
| Epsilon | ε | E |
| Zeta | ζ | Z |
| Eta | η | H |
| Theta | θ | Θ |
| Iota | ι | I |
| Kappa | κ | K |
| Lambda | λ | Λ |
| Mu | μ | M |
| Nu | ν | N |
| Xi | ξ | Ξ |
| Omicron | o | O |

**Table 16.3-1.** Capital and Lowercase Greek Letters (*continued*)

| Name of letter | Greek lowercase | Greek capital |
|---|---|---|
| Pi | π | Π |
| Rho | ρ | P |
| Sigma | σ | Σ |
| Tau | τ | T |
| Upsilon | υ | Y |
| Phi | φ | Φ |
| Chi | χ | X |
| Psi | ψ | Ψ |
| Omega | ω | Ω |

**16.4** ▬▬▬ **Page Composition and Electronic Formats.** If Greek letters need to be marked or modified on page proofs, this can be done by indicating the letters "Gk" in the margin, followed by a description of the character (eg, "Gk lowercase sigma").

Greek letters can pose problems for some web browsers. The best solution for publishers is to make sure they output Greek letters in a universal, platform-independent, nonproprietary standard for character encoding, such as Unicode. Most word processing and typesetting programs can generate Greek letters that are already Unicode encoded. Greek letters in running text should not be saved as graphics; these files are much larger than text and take longer to download.

**Principal Author:** Brenda Gregoline, ELS

## ACKNOWLEDGMENT

I thank Karen Boyd and Lila Haile, formerly of JAMA Network; Frances E. Liskis, DrPh, NP, CNM, *Journal of Midwifery & Women's Health*, Nashville, Tennessee; and Peter J. Olson, ELS, Sheridan Journal Services, Waterbury, Vermont, for comments on the chapter.

# Units of Measure

**17.0 Units of Measure.**

> *The English system of measurements appears to be the*
> *fever dream of a crazy person.*
> Samuel Arbesman[1]

The presentation of quantitative scientific information is an integral component of biomedical publication. Accurate communication of scientific knowledge and presentation of numerical data require a scientifically informative system for reporting units of measure.

**17.1 SI Units.** The International System of Units (le Système International d'Unités or SI) represents a modified version of the metric system that has been established by international agreement and currently is the official measurement system of most nations of the world.[2,3] The SI promotes uniformity of quantities and units, minimizes the number of units and multiples used in other measurement systems, and can express virtually any measurement in science, medicine, industry, and commerce.

In 1977, the World Health Organization recommended the adoption of the SI by the international scientific community. Since then, many biomedical publications throughout the world have adopted SI units as their preferred and primary method for reporting scientific measurements. Although SI units have long been the dominant measurement system used in science,[3] in the United States most physicians and other health care professionals use conventional units for many common clinical measurements (eg, blood pressure), and many clinical laboratories report most laboratory values by means of conventional units. Accordingly, some biomedical publications, including JAMA Network journals, have adopted an approach for reporting units of measure that includes a combination of conventional units and SI units (see 17.5, Conventional Units and SI Units in JAMA Network Journals). Authors, scientists, clinicians, editors, and others involved in preparing and processing manuscripts for biomedical publication should be familiar with appropriate use of units of measure and should ensure that the presentation and reporting of scientific information are clear and accurate, including any necessary conversion from conventional units to SI units or vice versa.

**17.1.1** **Base Units.** The SI is based on 7 fundamental units (base units) that refer to 7 basic quantities of measurement (**Table 17.1-1**). These units form the structure from which other measurement quantities are composed.

Although not included among the 7 base units, the liter is widely used in the SI as a fundamental measure of capacity or volume. The liter is the recommended unit for measurement of volume for liquids and gases, whereas the cubic meter is the SI unit of volume for solids. Although the kelvin is the SI unit for thermodynamic temperature, Celsius is used with the SI for temperature measurement in biomedical settings.

**17.1.2** **Derived Units.** Other SI measurement quantities are referred to as *derived units* and are expressed as products or quotients of the 7 base units. Certain derived SI units have special names and symbols and may be used in algebraic relationships to express other derived units (**Table 17.1-2**).

**17.1.3** **Prefixes** Prefixes are combined with base units and derived units to form multiples of SI units. The factors designated by prefixes are powers of 10, and most prefixes involve exponents that are simple multiples of 3, thereby facilitating conversion procedures using successive multiplications by $10^3$ or $10^{-3}$ (**Table 17.1-3**).

**Table 17.1-1.** The International System of Units (SI) Base Units and Symbols

| Quantity | Base unit name | SI unit symbol |
| --- | --- | --- |
| Length | meter | m |
| Mass | kilogram | kg |
| Time | second | s |
| Electric current | ampere | A |
| Thermodynamic temperature | kelvin | K |
| Luminous intensity | candela | Cd |
| Amount of substance | mole | mol |

**Table 17.1-2.** The International System of Units (SI) Derived Units and Symbols

| Quantity | Name | SI symbol | Derivation from base unit |
|---|---|---|---|
| Area | square meter | $m^2$ | $m^2$ |
| Volume | cubic meter | $m^3$ | $m^3$ |
| Speed, velocity | meter per second | m/s | m/s |
| Density, mass density | kilogram per cubic meter | $kg/m^3$ | $kg/m^3$ |
| Specific volume | cubic meter per kilogram | $m^3/kg$ | $m^3/kg$ |
| Concentration | mole per cubic meter | $mol/m^3$ | $mol/m^3$ |
| Frequency | hertz | Hz | $s^{-1}$ |
| Force | newton | N | $kg \cdot m \cdot s^{-2}$ |
| Pressure, stress | pascal | Pa | $kg \cdot m^{-1} \cdot s^{-2}$ ($N/m^2$) |
| Work, energy | joule | J | $kg \cdot m^2 \cdot s^{-2}$ ($N \cdot m$) |
| Luminous flux | lumen | lm | $m^2 \cdot m^{-2} \cdot cd = cd$ |
| Power, radiant flux | watt | W | $m^2 \cdot kg \cdot s^{-3}$ (J/s) |
| Electric potential | volt | V | $m^2 \cdot kg \cdot s^{-3} \cdot A^{-1}$ |
| Electric charge | coulomb | C | $A \cdot s$ |
| Electric resistance | ohm | $\Omega$ | $m^2 \cdot kg \cdot s^{-3} \cdot A^{-2}$ (V/A) |
| Capacitance | farad | F | $m^{-2} \cdot kg^{-1} \cdot s^4 \cdot A^2$ (C/V) |
| Magnetic flux | weber | Wb | $m^2 \cdot kg \cdot s^{-2} \cdot A^{-1}$ (V·s) |
| Magnetic flux density | tesla | T | $kg \cdot s^{-2} \cdot A^{-1}$ ($Wb/m^2$) |
| Inductance | henry | H | $m^2 \cdot kg \cdot s^{-2} \cdot A^{-2}$ |

**Table 17.1-3.** The International System of Units Prefixes

| Factor | Prefix | Symbol |
|---|---|---|
| $10^{24}$ | yotta | Y |
| $10^{21}$ | zetta | Z |
| $10^{18}$ | exa | E |
| $10^{15}$ | peta | P |
| $10^{12}$ | tera | T |
| $10^9$ | giga | G |
| $10^6$ | mega | M |
| $10^3$ | kilo | k |
| $10^2$ | hecto | h |

*(continued)*

**Table 17.1-3.** The International System
of Units Prefixes (*continued*)

| Factor | Prefix | Symbol |
|--------|--------|--------|
| $10^1$ | deka (deca) | da |
| $10^{-1}$ | deci | d |
| $10^{-2}$ | centi | c |
| $10^{-3}$ | milli | m |
| $10^{-6}$ | micro | μ |
| $10^{-9}$ | nano | n |
| $10^{-12}$ | pico | p |
| $10^{-15}$ | femto | f |
| $10^{-18}$ | atto | a |
| $10^{-21}$ | zepto | z |
| $10^{-24}$ | yocto | y |

Compound prefixes formed by the combination of 2 or more SI prefixes generally are not used. It is preferable to use an expression with a single prefix.

> *Avoid:*   mμm (millimicrometer)
>
> *Better:*   nm (nanometer)

The kilogram is the only SI base unit with a prefix as part of its name and symbol (kg). However, because compound prefixes are not recommended, prefixes relating to mass are combined with gram (g) rather than kilogram (kg).

> *Avoid:*   μkg (microkilogram)
>
> *Better:*   mg (milligram)

Note: For the abbreviation μ (micro), some use the abbreviation "mcg" instead, specifically when communicating medical information, owing to the possibility that the prefix μ (micro) might be misread as the prefix m (milli), resulting in a thousand-fold overdose. JAMA Network journals use the abbreviation μ.

**17.2**   **Expressing Unit Names and Symbols.** The SI includes conventions for expressing unit names and abbreviations (often referred to as symbols) and for displaying them in text.

**17.2.1**   **Capitalization.** The SI unit names are written lowercase (eg, kilogram) when spelled out, except for Celsius (as in "degrees Celsius"), which is capitalized. Abbreviations or symbols for SI units also are written lowercase, with the following exceptions:

▪ Abbreviations derived from a proper name should be capitalized (eg, N for newton, K for kelvin, A for ampere), although nonabbreviated SI unit names derived from a proper name are not capitalized (eg, newtons, amperes).

- An uppercase letter L is used as the abbreviation for *liter* to avoid confusion with the lowercase letter l and the number 1.

- Certain SI prefixes are capitalized to distinguish them from similar lowercase abbreviations:

  - M denotes the prefix *mega* ($10^6$), whereas m denotes the prefix *milli* ($10^{-3}$)
  - P denotes the prefix *peta* ($10^{15}$), whereas p denotes the prefix *pico* ($10^{-12}$)

**17.2.2 Products and Quotients of Unit Symbols.** The product of 2 or more SI units should be indicated by a space between them or by a raised multiplication dot. The multiplication dot must be positioned properly to distinguish it from a decimal point, which is set on the baseline (see 20.5, Expressing Multiplication and Division). When the unit of measure is the product of 2 or more units, either abbreviations (symbols) or nonabbreviated units should be used. Abbreviated and nonabbreviated forms should not be combined in products.

*Avoid:*   newton·m or N·meter

*Better:*   newton meter is expressed as newton meter or N m or N·m

When numerals are used to denote a quantity of measurement, it is preferable to use the abbreviated form of the SI unit.

*Avoid:*   50 newton meter

*Better:*   50 N·m

The quotient of SI unit symbols may be expressed by the forward slash or virgule (/) or by the use of negative exponents. If the derived unit is formed by 2 abbreviated units of measure (eg, μg/L), the quotient also may be expressed by means of the forward slash or negative exponents.

*Avoid:*   μg per L

*Better:*   μg/L or μg L$^{-1}$ or μg·L$^{-1}$

When the unit names are spelled out in a quotient or in text, the word *per* should be used.

*Avoid:*   The power output was measured in joules/second [or J/s].

*Better:*   The power output was measured in joules per second.

Expressions with 2 or more units of measure may require use of the forward slash, dot products, negative exponents, or parentheses (see 20.5, Expressing Multiplication and Division).

mL·kg$^{-1}$·min$^{-1}$ or mL/kg/min

m$^2$·kg·s$^{-2}$·A$^{-2}$ or (m$^2$·kg)/(s$^2$·A$^2$)

**17.3 Format, Style, and Punctuation.** The format, style, and punctuation guidelines generally apply for SI reporting but also are used for reporting most values in conventional units.

**17.3.1** **Exponents.** The SI reporting style uses exponents rather than certain abbreviations, such as *cu* and *sq*.

> *Preferred:* m²
> *Avoid:* sq m
>
> *Preferred:* m³
> *Avoid:* cu m

**17.3.2** **Plurals.** The same symbol is used for single and multiple quantities. Unit symbols are not expressed in the plural form.

> *Preferred:* 1 L 70 L
> *Avoid:* 1 Ls 70 Ls
>
> *Preferred:* 1 g 1500 g
> *Avoid:* 1 gs 1500 gs

**17.3.3** **Subject-Verb Agreement.** Units of measure are treated as collective singular (not plural) nouns and require a singular verb.

> To control the patient's fever, 500 mg of the medication was [not *were*] administered at the time of admission and 1000 mg was required 4 hours later.

**17.3.4** **Spelling Out Units of Measure.** A unit of measure that follows a number at the beginning of a sentence, title, or subtitle should not be abbreviated, even though the same unit of measure is abbreviated if it appears elsewhere in the same sentence (see 18.2.1, Beginning a Sentence, Title, Subtitle, or Heading, and 18.1.2, Common Fractions). Units of measure not immediately following a numeric value also should be spelled out.

> Fifty milligrams of medication was the baseline dose, which was titrated to 100 mg.
>
> Tumor sizes were measured in centimeters.
>
> Hundreds of milligrams of orlistat can be absorbed under certain conditions.

**17.3.5** **Abbreviations.** Most units of measure are abbreviated when used with numerals or in a virgule construction. Certain units of measure should be spelled out at first mention, with the abbreviated form in parentheses. Thereafter, the abbreviated form should be used in text (see 14.12, Units of Measure).

**17.3.6** **Punctuation.** Symbols or abbreviations of units of measure are not followed by a period, unless the symbol occurs at the end of a sentence.

> The patient's weight was 80 kg [not 80 kg.] and had increased by 10%.

**17.3.7** **Hyphens.** A hyphen is used to join 2 spelled-out units of measure.

> pascal-second
>
> person-years
>
> pack-years

Note: Capitalization for the above examples follows the style for temporary hyphenated compounds (see 10.2.2, Hyphenated Compounds) and appears as "Person-Years" in a title.

A hyphen is used to join a unit of measure and the number associated with it when the combination is used as an adjective (see 8.3.1.1, Temporary Compounds).

> an 8-L container
>
> a 10-mm strip

**17.3.8** **Spacing.** With the exception of the percent sign, the degree sign (for angles not temperatures), and normal and molar solutions (see 17.5.7, Solutions and Concentration), a full space should appear between the arabic numeral that indicates the quantity and the unit of measure.

> 140 nmol/L (not 140nmol/L)
>
> 135-150 nmol/L
>
> 3M sodium chloride
>
> 120 mm Hg
>
> 40% adherence rate
>
> 40%-50%
>
> 45° angle
>
> temperature of 37.5 °C (not 37.5°C)
>
> (temperature range, 38-39 °C)

Note: Ranges may use a hyphen when given in figures and tables and when given in parentheses in text.

When symbols are presented immediately adjacent to the value (eg, %), they repeat.

> 5%, 6%, and 7% (not 5, 6, and 7%)

**17.4** **Use of Numerals With Units.**

**17.4.1** **Expressing Quantities.** Arabic numerals are used for quantities with units of measure (see 18.1, Use of Numerals). By SI convention, it is preferable to use only numbers between 0.1 and 1000 and to use the appropriate prefix for expressing quantities. For example, 0.003 mL is expressed as 3 μL; 15 000 g is expressed as 15 kg.

Some clinical measurements are expressed in quantities and units that may have numbers outside this preferred range. For such values, the use of scientific notation is acceptable.

> 20 000 000 A may be expressed as 20 million amperes or as $2 \times 10^7$ A

Reported SI values should follow recommendations for preserving the proper number of significant digits (see 19.4.2, Rounding). The use of these increments is intended to eliminate reporting results beyond the appropriate level of precision.

**17.4.2** **Decimal Format.** The decimal format is recommended for numbers used with units of measure. Fractions should not be used with SI units.

> *Avoid:*   2½ kg
>
> *Better:*   2.5 kg

Mixed fractions occasionally are used in text to indicate less precise measurements and most commonly involve units of measure that represent time.

> After more than 7½ years of investigation, the effort to develop a new vaccine was abandoned.

The decimal format also could be used:

> After more than 7.5 years of investigation, the effort to develop a new vaccine was abandoned.

Numerical values less than 1 require placement of 0 before the decimal marker.

> *Avoid:*   .123
>
> *Better:*   0.123

However, certain statistical values, such as $\alpha$ levels and $P$ values, should be reported without the use of 0 before the decimal marker (see 18.7.1, Decimals, and 19.5, Glossary of Statistical Terms).

> The sample size was based on detecting a 10% difference in the primary outcome measure, using a 2-sided $\alpha$ level of .05.

> Statistical significance was defined as $P<.001$.

**17.4.3** **Number Spacing.** By SI convention, the decimal point is the only punctuation mark permitted in numerals, and it is used to separate the integer and decimal parts of the number. The SI does not use commas in numbers in particular because the comma is used in some countries as the decimal sign. Integers (whole numbers) with more than 4 digits are separated into groups of 3 (using a thin space, a space character that is usually 1⁄5 or 1⁄6 the width of an em dash; to insert a thin space using Unicode in Microsoft Word, type the code 2009 where the thin space should appear, set the cursor after "9," and press Alt + X on the keyboard) with respect to the decimal point. Four-digit integers are closed up (without a space). Decimal digits also are grouped in sets of 3 digits beginning at the decimal sign, with the same closed-up spacing for 4-digit groups (see 18.1.1, Numbers of 4 or More Digits to Either Side of the Decimal Point).

| Preferred | Avoid |
|---|---|
| 1234 | 1,234 |
| 123 456 | 123,456 |
| 12 345.678 901 | 12,345.678901 |
| 1234.567 89 | 1,234.56789 |
| 1 234 567.8901 | 1,234,567.8901 |

However, certain types of numerals that have more than 4 digits are expressed without spacing, such as street addresses, postal codes, page numbers, and numerals combined with letters, including trial registration identifiers.

Chicago, IL 60610

This study was supported by grant MCH-110624.

**Trial Registration**: ClinicalTrials.gov identifier: NCT00381954

**17.4.4 Multiplication of Numbers.** Multiplication of numbers should be indicated by the multiplication sign ($\times$) and may be used to express area (eg, a 15 $\times$ 35-cm$^2$ burn), volume (eg, a 5.2 $\times$ 3.7 $\times$ 6.9-m$^3$ cube), matrixes (eg, a 2 $\times$ 2 table), magnification ($\times$30 000), or scientific notation (eg, 3.6 $\times$ 10$^9$/L).

The multiplication sign in equations is set off by thin spaces on either side (see 20.9, Spacing With Mathematical Symbols). In situations such as expression of magnification (eg, original magnification $\times$30 000), it is set closed up to the number because this is not an equation.

**17.4.5 Indexes.** An index generally refers to a quantity derived from a ratio of 2 (or more) measurable quantities and often is used to compare individuals with each other or with normal values. Except for products or quotients that represent specific derived SI units of measure (see 17.2.2, Products and Quotients of Unit Symbols), the ratio of SI units used to create indexes does not represent an SI convention.

At first mention in the text, the formula used to calculate the index should be described; thereafter, the numerical value for the index may be given without units attached to it. For figures or tables, the formula should be included in legends or in footnotes, respectively. However, the formula used to calculate an index need not be included in the abstract of an article.

body mass index, calculated as weight in kilograms divided by height in meters squared (BMI of 30)

cardiac index, calculated as cardiac output in liters per minute divided by body surface area in square meters

**17.5 Conventional Units and SI Units in JAMA Network Journals.** In the United States, most physicians and other health care professionals use conventional units for most commonly encountered clinical measurements (eg, blood pressure), and most clinical laboratories report many laboratory values by means of conventional units. To serve these readers, but also to serve the needs of readers more familiar with JAMA Network journals have adopted an approach for reporting units of measure that includes a combination of SI units and conventional units.

**17.5.1** **Length, Area, Volume, Mass.** Measurements of length, area, volume, and mass are reported by means of metric units rather than English units (**Table 17.5-1**).

In less formal, nonscientific texts, such as essays, use of nonmetric units, such as miles or inches, and the use of idioms, such as "An ounce of prevention is worth a pound of cure" or "give an inch," are acceptable. In addition, if the nonmetric

**Table 17.5-1.** Conversions to Metric Measures

| Symbol | Known quantity | Multiply by | To find | Metric symbol |
|--------|----------------|-------------|---------|---------------|
| **Length** | | | | |
| in | inches | 2.54 | centimeters | cm |
| ft | feet | 30 | centimeters | cm |
| ft | feet | 0.3 | meters | m |
| yd | yards | 0.9 | meters | m |
| | miles | 1.6 | kilometers | km |
| **Area** | | | | |
| sq in | square inches | 6.5 | square centimeters | $cm^2$ |
| sq ft | square feet | 0.09 | square meters | $m^2$ |
| sq yd | square yards | 0.8 | square meters | $m^2$ |
| | square miles | 2.6 | square kilometers | $km^2$ |
| **Mass** | | | | |
| oz | ounces | 28 | grams | g |
| lb | pounds | 0.45 | kilograms | kg |
| **Volume** | | | | |
| tsp | teaspoons | 5 | milliliters | mL |
| tbsp | tablespoons | 15 | milliliters | mL |
| fl oz | fluid ounces | 30 | milliliters | mL |
| c | cups | 0.24 | liters | L |
| pt | US pints | 0.47 | liters | L |
| qt | US quarts | 0.95 | liters | L |
| gal | US gallons | 3.8 | liters | L |
| cu ft | cubic feet | 0.03 | cubic meters | $m^3$ |
| cu yd | cubic yards | 0.76 | cubic meters | $m^3$ |

unit was used as part of a survey or questionnaire, the original measure should be retained.

> The patients were asked, "Do you have difficulty walking 15 feet?"

Similarly, if data were measured in SI units and are displayed as such in an organized way (eg, cholesterol given in 5-mmol increments along a figure axis), the original measure may be retained, with a conversion given for the conventional unit.

**17.5.2** **Temperature.** The Celsius scale (°C) is used for temperature measurement rather than the base SI unit for temperature, the kelvin (K), which has little application in medicine. Although the kelvin and Celsius scales have the same interval value for temperature differences, they differ in their absolute values. For example, a temperature of 273.15 K is equal to 0 °C. Temperature values generally are reported in degrees Celsius, and values given in degrees Fahrenheit (°F) are converted to degrees Celsius (°C).

$$(°F - 32)(0.556) = °C$$

**17.5.3** **Time.** The SI unit for time is the second, although minute, hour, and day also are used. Other units of time, such as week, month, and year, are not part of the SI but also are used. The abbreviations for minute, hour, and day are min, h, and d, respectively, and the abbreviations for week, month, and year are wk, mo, and y, respectively. These abbreviations are used in tables, figures, and virgule constructions and are never capitalized (see 13.12, Units of Measure, and 8.4, Forward Slash [Virgule, Solidus]).

> The patient reported smoking 20 cigarettes/d.
>
> She had mild apnea, with 1 episode/h.
>
> Respirations were 60/min; pulse rate was 98/min.

**17.5.4** **Visual Acuity.** Visual acuity should be reported on the basis of how the measurement was determined. For example, using the Snellen fraction with English units, 20/20 or 20/100 indicates that the person being evaluated can see at 20 ft what a person with normal visual acuity can see at 20 ft or at 100 ft, respectively. The equivalent metric measurements for visual acuity are 6/6 and 6/30, respectively (see 14.13, Nomenclature, Ophthalmology Terms).

**17.5.5** **Pressure.** Blood pressure and intraocular pressure are reported in millimeters of mercury (mm Hg); cerebrospinal fluid pressure is reported as centimeters of water (cm $H_2O$). The pascal (newton per square meter [$N/m^2$]) is the recommended SI unit for pressure but generally is not used for reporting these common physiologic pressure measurements. Partial pressure of gases (eg, of oxygen and carbon dioxide) may be reported as millimeters of mercury (mm Hg) or as kilopascals (kPa) (see 14.16, Pulmonary and Respiratory Terminology).

**17.5.6** **pH.** Although SI nomenclature could be used to express values of hydrogen ion concentration (nmol/L), the pH scale (1-14) is used.

**17.5.7** **Solutions and Concentration.** A *molar* solution contains 1 mol (1 g molecular weight) of solute in 1 L of solution. The SI style for reporting molar solutions is mol/L; for solutions with millimolar concentrations, mmol/L is used; and for solutions with micromolar concentrations, μmol/L is used. The concentration is given as 4-mmol/L potassium chloride not 4 mmol/L *of* potassium chloride.

> The gel was incubated at 40 °C after applying 10 mL of a solution of 4-mmol/L potassium chloride and 5 mL of a solution of 1-mol/L sodium chloride.

Molar concentrations of solutions and reagents also may be expressed by using M to designate molar and SI prefixes to denote concentration (eg, mM for millimolar; μM for micromolar). Note that the molar concentration unit is set closed up to the number.

> The gel was incubated at 40 °C after applying 10 mL of a solution of 4mM potassium chloride and 5 mL of a solution of 1M sodium chloride.

A *normal* solution contains a concentration of 1 gram-equivalent of solute per liter.

To show the concentration of a solution in relation to normality (N), the abbreviation N is used, with no space between the numerical value and the N (eg, 3N). Half normal is indicated as 0.5N or N/2.

**17.5.8** **Energy.** The calorie is the unit of measure often used in chemistry and biochemistry for reporting heat energy. A value of 1 calorie is the amount of energy (heat) required to raise the temperature of 1 g of pure water by 1 °C. The joule is the preferred SI unit for energy, and calories and kilocalories may be converted to joules (J) and kilojoules (kJ) by using the following formulas:

> 1 calorie = 4.186 J
>
> 1 kilocalorie = 4.186 kJ

JAMA Network journals prefer to report heat energy in calories or kilocalories.

Formerly a distinction was made between the small calorie (with a lowercase c) and the large calorie, designated as Calorie (with a capital C and abbreviated Cal)[2] and equivalent to 1000 calories or 1 kilocalorie (kcal). In metabolic studies, the Calorie is the amount of heat energy required to raise or lower 1 kg of pure liquid water by 1 °C.[4] The Calorie also is used in nutrition to express the energy content of food.[5] By convention, the use of the capitalized C in dietary Calories indicates kilocalories (ie, 1 Cal is equivalent to 1 kcal or 1000 cal). For example, if the label on a food package indicates that a serving contains 300 Cal, that serving would yield 300 kcal (not 300 cal) of heat energy when subjected to complete combustion. JAMA Network journals prefer Calories or kilocalories for expressing the energy content of food.

Energy expenditure also is reported as Calories (or kilocalories) to reflect the amount of energy required for the work done. The values for Calorie expenditure are based on the metabolic cost, expressed as metabolic equivalents (METs). One MET represents the metabolic rate for an adult at rest (ie, set at 3.5 mL of oxygen consumed per kilogram of body mass per minute) or approximately 1 kcal/kg/h.[5] Activities with MET values near 1 are sedentary activities (eg, sitting quietly), whereas activities with higher MET values involve higher levels of energy expenditure (eg, brisk walking has a MET value of 3, or 3 times the resting metabolic rate).

**17.5.9** **Drug Doses.** Drug doses are expressed in conventional metric mass units (eg, milligrams or milligrams per kilogram) rather than in molar SI units. Moreover, certain drugs (such as insulin or heparin) may be prepared as mixtures and have no specific molecular weight, thereby precluding their expression in mass units. Although other drug dose units, such as drops (for ophthalmologic preparations), grains (for aspirin), and various apothecary system measurements (eg, teaspoonfuls, ounces, and drams), may be encountered clinically, these units generally are not used.

Another such example is cc for mL; cc is sometimes used in clinical settings, but to avoid confusion mL should be used in scientific publications. In addition, the units for drug doses are often different from the units used to measure drug concentrations, such as in therapeutic drug levels.

**17.5.10** **Laboratory Values.** In JAMA Network journals, laboratory values for clinical chemistry analyses, hematologic tests, immunologic assays, metabolic and endocrine tests, therapeutic drug monitoring, toxicology determinations, and urinalysis are reported by means of conventional laboratory units. **Table 17.5-2** provides examples of conventional units and SI units and is intended to facilitate conversion from conventional units to SI units (and vice versa). A conversion calculator is freely available online at www.amamanualofstyle.com.

Laboratory reference values and units vary considerably among individual laboratories and are highly dependent on the analytic methods used. For reports of diagnostic tests or interpretations, the reference range followed by the local laboratory should be included. Several resources[6-10] contain detailed information about these topics and tables with laboratory reference values and SI conversion factors.

For laboratory values reported in JAMA Network journals, factors for converting conventional units to SI units should be provided in the article. In text, the conversion factor should be given once, at first mention of the laboratory value, in parentheses following the conventional unit.

> The blood glucose concentration of 126 mg/dL (to convert to mmol/L, multiply by 0.0555) was used as a criterion for diagnosing diabetes.

For articles in which several laboratory values are reported in text, the conversion factors may be listed in a paragraph at the end of the Methods section but not in the abstract of the article. For figures or tables, the conversion factors should be included in legends or in footnotes, respectively, (see 4.1.3.10, Footnotes). For articles in which there is no Methods section, conversion factors can be given at first mention of the value, and reference ranges for the local laboratory can be included as well.

> When the results were returned, serum ammonia levels were markedly elevated at 643 µg/dL (to convert to µmol/L, multiply by 0.714). A subsequent hepatic panel was notable for mildly elevated levels of alanine aminotransferase (89 U/L; to convert to µkat/L, multiply by 0.0167) and γ-glutamyltransferase (81 U/L; to convert to µkat/L, multiply by 0.0167).

**Table 17.5-2.** Selected Laboratory Tests, With Conversion Factors[a]

| Analyte | Specimen | Conventional unit | Conversion factor (multiply by) | SI unit |
|---|---|---|---|---|
| Acetaminophen/paracetamol | Serum, plasma | μg/mL | 6.614 | μmol/L |
| Acetoacetate | Serum, plasma | mg/dL | 97.95 | μmol/L |
| Acetone | Serum, plasma | mg/dL | 0.172 | mmol/L |
| Acid phosphatase | Serum | U/L | 16.667 | nkat/L |
| Activated partial thromboplastin time (APTT) | Whole blood | s | 1.0 | s |
| Adenosine deaminase | Serum | U/L | 16.667 | nkat/L |
| Adrenocorticotropic hormone (ACTH) | Plasma | pg/mL | 0.22 | pmol/L |
| Alanine | Plasma | mg/dL | 112.2 | μmol/L |
| Alanine aminotransferase (ALT) | Serum | U/L | 0.0167 | μkat/L |
| Albumin | Serum | g/dL | 10 | g/L |
| Alcohol dehydrogenase | Serum | U/L | 16.667 | nkat/L |
| Aldolase | Serum | U/L | 0.0167 | μkat/L |
| Aldosterone | Serum, plasma | ng/dL | 27.74 | pmol/L |
| Alkaline phosphatase | Serum | U/L | 0.0167 | μkat/L |
| Alprazolam | Serum, plasma | ng/mL | 3.24 | nmol/L |
| Amikacin | Serum, plasma | μg/mL | 1.708 | μmol/L |
| α-Aminobutyric acid | Plasma | mg/dL | 96.97 | μmol/L |
| δ-Aminolevulinic acid | Serum | μg/dL | 0.0763 | μmol/L |
| Amiodarone | Serum, plasma | μg/mL | 1.55 | μmol/L |
| Amitriptyline | Plasma | ng/mL | 3.605 | nmol/L |
| Ammonia (as nitrogen) | Serum, plasma | μg/dL | 0.714 | μmol/L |

| | | | | |
|---|---|---|---|---|
| Amobarbital | Serum | µg/mL | 4.42 | µmol/L |
| Amphetamine | Serum, plasma | ng/mL | 7.4 | nmol/L |
| Amylase | Serum | U/L | 0.0167 | µkat/L |
| Androstenedione | Serum | ng/dL | 0.0349 | nmol/L |
| Angiotensin I | Plasma | pg/mL | 0.772 | pmol/L |
| Angiotensin II | Plasma | pg/mL | 0.957 | pmol/L |
| Angiotensin-converting enzyme | Serum | U/L | 16.667 | nkat/L |
| Anion gap $Na^+ - (Cl^- + HCO_3^-)$ | Serum, plasma | mEq/L | 1.0 | mmol/L |
| Antidiuretic hormone (ADH) | Plasma | pg/mL | 0.923 | pmol/L |
| Antithrombin III | Plasma | mg/dL | 10 | mg/L |
| $\alpha_1$-Antitrypsin | Serum | mg/dL | 0.184 | µmol/L |
| Apolipoprotein A-I | Serum | mg/dL | 0.01 | g/L |
| Apolipoprotein B | Serum, plasma | mg/dL | 0.01 | g/L |
| Arginine | Serum | mg/dL | 57.4 | µmol/L |
| Arsenic | Whole blood | µg/L | 0.0133 | µmol/L |
| Ascorbic acid (see vitamin C) | | | | |
| Asparagine | Plasma | mg/dL | 75.689 | µmol/L |
| Aspartate aminotransferase (AST) | Serum | U/L | 0.0167 | µkat/L |
| Aspartic acid | Plasma | mg/dL | 75.13 | µmol/L |
| Atrial natriuretic hormone | Plasma | pg/mL | 1 | ng/L |
| Bands (see white blood cell count) | | | | |
| Base excess | Whole blood | mEq/L | 1.0 | mmol/L |

(continued)

**Table 17.5-2.** Selected Laboratory Tests, With Conversion Factors (*continued*)

| Analyte | Specimen | Conventional unit | Conversion factor (multiply by) | SI unit |
|---|---|---|---|---|
| Basophils (see white blood cell count) | | | | |
| Bicarbonate | Serum | mEq/L | 1.0 | mmol/L |
| Bile acids (total) | Serum | µg/mL | 2.448 | µmol/L |
| Bilirubin, direct (conjugated) | Serum | mg/dL | 17.104 | µmol/L |
| Bilirubin, total | Serum | mg/dL | 17.104 | µmol/L |
| Biotin | Serum | pg/mL | 0.00409 | nmol/L |
| Bismuth | Whole blood | µg/L | 4.785 | nmol/L |
| Blood gases | | | | |
| Carbon dioxide, $PCO_2$ | Arterial blood | mm Hg | 0.133 | kPa |
| pH | Arterial blood | | 1.0 | |
| Oxygen, $PO_2$ | Arterial blood | mm Hg | 0.133 | kPa |
| Brain-type natriuretic peptide (BNP) | Plasma | pg/mL | 1.0 | ng/L |
| Bromide (toxic) | Serum | µg/mL | 0.0125 | mmol/L |
| C1 esterase inhibitor | Serum | mg/dL | 10 | mg/L |
| C3 complement | Serum | mg/dL | 0.01 | g/L |
| C4 complement | Serum | mg/dL | 0.01 | g/L |
| Cadmium | Whole blood | µg/L | 8.896 | nmol/L |
| Caffeine (therapeutic) | Serum, plasma | µg/mL | 5.15 | µmol/L |
| Calcitonin | Plasma | pg/mL | 0.292 | pmol/L |
| Calcium, ionized | Serum | mg/dL | 0.25 | mmol/L |

| Analyte | Specimen | Conventional unit | Factor | SI unit |
|---|---|---|---|---|
| Calcium, total | Serum | mg/dL | 0.25 | mmol/L |
| Cancer antigen (CA) 125 | Serum | U/mL | 1.0 | kU/L |
| Carbamazepine | Serum, plasma | μg/mL | 4.233 | μmol/L |
| Carbon dioxide (total) | Serum, plasma | mEq/L | 1.0 | mmol/L |
| Carboxyhemoglobin, toxic | Whole blood | % | 0.01 | Proportion of 1.0 |
| Carcinoembryonic antigen (CEA) | Serum | ng/mL | 1.0 | μg/L |
| β-Carotene | Serum | μg/dL | 0.01863 | μmol/L |
| Carotenoids | Serum | μg/dL | 0.01863 | μmol/L |
| Ceruloplasmin | Serum | mg/dL | 10 | mg/L |
| Chloramphenicol | Serum | μg/mL | 3.095 | μmol/L |
| Chlordiazepoxide | Serum, plasma | μg/mL | 3.336 | μmol/L |
| Chloride | Serum, plasma | mEq/L | 1.0 | mmol/L |
| Chlorpromazine | Plasma | ng/mL | 3.136 | nmol/L |
| Chlorpropamide | Plasma | mg/L | 3.61 | μmol/L |
| Cholecalciferol (see vitamin D) | | | | |
| Cholesterol | | | | |
| Total | Serum, plasma | mg/dL | 0.0259 | mmol/L |
| High-density lipoprotein (HDL) | Serum, plasma | mg/dL | 0.0259 | mmol/L |
| Low-density lipoprotein (LDL) | Serum, plasma | mg/dL | 0.0259 | mmol/L |
| Cholinesterase | Serum | U/mL | 1.0 | kU/L |
| Chorionic gonadotropin (β-hCG) (nonpregnant) | Serum | mIU/mL | 1.0 | IU/L |
| Chromium | Whole blood | μg/L | 19.232 | nmol/L |
| Citrate | Serum | mg/dL | 52.05 | μmol/L |

*(continued)*

**Table 17.5-2.** Selected Laboratory Tests, With Conversion Factors (*continued*)

| Analyte | Specimen | Conventional unit | Conversion factor (multiply by) | SI unit |
|---|---|---|---|---|
| Citrulline | Plasma | mg/dL | 57.081 | µmol/L |
| Clonazepam (therapeutic) | Serum | ng/mL | 3.167 | nmol/L |
| Clonidine | Serum, plasma | ng/mL | 4.35 | nmol/L |
| Clozapine | Serum | ng/mL | 0.003 | µmol/L |
| Coagulation factor I (Fibrinogen) | Plasma | g/dL | 29.41 | µmol/L |
| | Plasma | mg/dL | 0.01 | g/L |
| Coagulation factor II (prothrombin) | Plasma | % | 0.01 | Proportion of 1.0 |
| Coagulation factor V | Plasma | % | 0.01 | Proportion of 1.0 |
| Coagulation factor VII | Plasma | % | 0.01 | Proportion of 1.0 |
| Coagulation factor VIII | Plasma | % | 0.01 | Proportion of 1.0 |
| Coagulation factor IX | Plasma | % | 0.01 | Proportion of 1.0 |
| Coagulation factor X | Plasma | % | 0.01 | Proportion of 1.0 |
| Coagulation factor XI | Plasma | % | 0.01 | Proportion of 1.0 |
| Coagulation factor XII | Plasma | % | 0.01 | Proportion of 1.0 |
| Cobalt | Serum | µg/L | 16.968 | nmol/L |
| Cocaine (toxic) | Serum | ng/mL | 3.297 | nmol/L |
| Codeine | Serum | ng/mL | 3.34 | nmol/L |
| Coenzyme Q10 (ubiquinone) | Plasma | µg/mL | 1.0 | mg/L |
| Copper | Serum | µg/dL | 0.157 | µmol/L |
| Coproporphyrin | Urine | µg/24 h | 1.527 | µmol/d |
| Corticotropin | Plasma | pg/mL | 0.22 | pmol/L |

| | | | | |
|---|---|---|---|---|
| Cortisol | Serum, plasma | µg/dL | 27.588 | nmol/L |
| Cotinine | Plasma | µg/L | 5.675 | nmol/L |
| C-peptide | Serum | ng/mL | 0.331 | nmol/L |
| C-reactive protein | Serum | mg/dL | 10 | mg/L |
| Creatine | Serum | mg/dL | 76.25 | µmol/L |
| Creatine kinase (CK) | Serum | U/L | 0.0167 | µkat/L |
| Creatine kinase–MB fraction | Serum | ng/mL | 1.0 | µg/L |
| Creatinine | Serum, plasma | mg/dL | 88.4 | µmol/L |
| Creatinine clearance | Serum, plasma | mL/min/1.73 m$^2$ | 0.0167 | mL/s/m$^2$ |
| Cyanide (toxic) | Whole blood | µg/mL | 38.4 | µmol/L |
| Cyclic adenosine monophosphate (cAMP) | Plasma | ng/mL | 3.04 | µmol/L |
| Cyclosporine | Serum | ng/mL | 0.832 | nmol/L |
| Cystine | Plasma | mg/dL | 41.615 | µmol/L |
| D-dimer | Plasma | µg/mL | 5.476 | nmol/L |
| Dehydroepiandrosterone (DHEA) | Serum | ng/mL | 3.47 | nmol/L |
| Dehydroepiandrosterone sulfate (DHEA-S) | Serum | µg/dL | 0.027 | µmol/L |
| Deoxycorticosterone | Serum | ng/dL | 0.0303 | nmol/L |
| Desipramine | Serum, plasma | ng/mL | 3.754 | nmol/L |
| Diazepam | Serum, plasma | ng/mL | 0.0035 | µmol/L |
| Digoxin | Plasma | ng/mL | 1.281 | nmol/L |
| Diltiazem | Serum | mg/L | 2.412 | µmol/L |
| Disopyramide | Serum, plasma | µg/mL | 2.946 | µmol/L |
| Dopamine | Plasma | pg/mL | 6.528 | pmol/L |
| Doxepin | Serum, plasma | ng/mL | 3.579 | nmol/L |

(continued)

941

**Table 17.5-2.** Selected Laboratory Tests, With Conversion Factors (*continued*)

| Analyte | Specimen | Conventional unit | Conversion factor (multiply by) | SI unit |
|---|---|---|---|---|
| Electrophoresis (protein) | | | | |
| Proportion of total protein | | | | |
| Albumin | Serum | % | 0.01 | Proportion of 1.0 |
| $\alpha_1$-Globulin | Serum | % | 0.01 | Proportion of 1.0 |
| $\alpha_2$-Globulin | Serum | % | 0.01 | Proportion of 1.0 |
| $\beta$-Globulin | Serum | % | 0.01 | Proportion of 1.0 |
| $\gamma$-Globulin | Serum | % | 0.01 | Proportion of 1.0 |
| Concentration | | | | |
| Albumin | Serum | g/dL | 10.0 | g/L |
| $\alpha_1$-Globulin | Serum | g/dL | 10.0 | g/L |
| $\alpha_2$-Globulin | Serum | g/dL | 10.0 | g/L |
| $\beta$-Globulin | Serum | g/dL | 10.0 | g/L |
| $\gamma$-Globulin | Serum | g/dL | 10.0 | g/L |
| Eosinophils (see white blood cell count) | | | | |
| Ephedrine (toxic) | Serum | µg/mL | 6.052 | µmol/L |
| Epinephrine | Plasma | pg/mL | 5.459 | pmol/L |
| Erythrocyte count (see red blood cell count) | | | | |
| Erythrocyte sedimentation rate | Whole blood | mm/h | 1.0 | mm/h |
| Erythropoietin | Serum | mIU/mL | 1.0 | IU/L |
| Estradiol ($E_2$) | Serum | pg/mL | 3.671 | pmol/L |

| Analyte | Specimen | Conventional Unit | Conversion Factor | SI Unit |
|---|---|---|---|---|
| Estriol (E₃) | Serum | ng/mL | 3.467 | nmol/L |
| Estrogens (total) | Serum | pg/mL | 1.0 | ng/L |
| Estrone (E₁) | Serum, plasma | pg/mL | 3.698 | pmol/L |
| Ethanol (ethyl alcohol) | Serum, whole blood | mg/dL | 0.2171 | mmol/L |
| Ethchlorvynol (toxic) | Serum, plasma | µg/mL | 6.915 | µmol/L |
| Ethosuximide | Serum | mg/L | 7.084 | µmol/L |
| Ethylene glycol (toxic) | Serum, plasma | mg/dL | 0.1611 | mmol/L |
| Fatty acids (nonesterified) | Serum, plasma | mg/dL | 0.0355 | mmol/L |
| Fecal fat (as stearic acid) | Stool | g/d | 1.0 | g/24 h |
| Fentanyl | Serum | µg/mL | 2.972 | µmol/L |
| Ferritin | Serum | ng/mL | 1.0 | µg/L |
| α-Fetoprotein (AFP) | Serum | ng/mL | 1.0 | µg/L |
| Fibrin degradation products | Plasma | µg/mL | 1.0 | mg/L |
| Fibrinogen | Plasma | mg/dL | 0.01 | g/L |
| Flecainide | Serum, plasma | µg/mL | 2.413 | µmol/L |
| Fluoride | Whole blood | mg/dL | 0.5263 | mmol/L |
| Fluoxetine | Serum | ng/mL | 0.00323 | µmol/L |
| Flurazepam (toxic) | Serum, plasma | µg/mL | 2.578 | µmol/L |
| Folate (folic acid) | Serum | ng/mL | 2.266 | nmol/L |
| Follicle-stimulating hormone (FSH) | Serum, plasma | mIU/mL | 1.0 | IU/L |
| Fructosamine | Serum | mg/L | 5.581 | mmol/L |
| Fructose | Serum | mg/dL | 55.506 | µmol/L |
| Galactose | Serum, plasma | mg/dL | 0.0555 | mmol/L |
| Gastrin | Serum | pg/mL | 0.481 | pmol/L |

*(continued)*

**Table 17.5-2.** Selected Laboratory Tests, With Conversion Factors (*continued*)

| Analyte | Specimen | Conventional unit | Conversion factor (multiply by) | SI unit |
|---|---|---|---|---|
| Gentamicin | Serum | μg/mL | 2.090 | μmol/L |
| Glucagon | Plasma | pg/mL | 1.0 | ng/L |
| Glucose | Serum | mg/dL | 0.0555 | mmol/L |
| Glucose-6-phosphate dehydrogenase | Whole blood | U/g of hemoglobin | 0.0167 | nkat/g hemoglobin |
| Glutamic acid | Plasma | mg/dL | 67.967 | μmol/L |
| Glutamine | Plasma | mg/dL | 68.423 | μmol/L |
| γ-Glutamyltransferase (GGT) | Serum | U/L | 0.0167 | μkat/L |
| Glutethimide | Serum | μg/mL | 4.603 | μmol/L |
| Glycerol (free) | Serum | mg/dL | 0.1086 | mmol/L |
| Glycine | Plasma | mg/dL | 133.2 | μmol/L |
| Gold | Serum | μg/dL | 50.770 | nmol/L |
| Growth hormone (GH) | Serum | ng/mL | 1.0 | μg/L |
| Haloperidol | Serum, plasma | ng/mL | 2.66 | nmol/L |
| Haptoglobin | Serum | mg/dL | 10 | mg/L |
| Hematocrit | Whole blood | % | 0.01 | Proportion of 1.0 |
| Hemoglobin | Whole blood | g/dL | 10.0 | g/L |
| Mean corpuscular hemoglobin (MCH) | Whole blood | pg/cell | 1.0 | pg/cell |
| Mean corpuscular hemoglobin concentration (MCHC) | Whole blood | g/dL | 10 | g/L |
| Mean corpuscular volume (MCV) | Whole blood | μm³ | 1.0 | fL |
| Hemoglobin A₁c (glycated hemoglobin) | Whole blood | % of total hemoglobin (can be dual-reported as mmol/mol)[b] | 0.01 | Proportion of total hemoglobin |

| Analyte | Specimen | Conventional unit | Conversion factor | Proportion of 1.0 |
|---|---|---|---|---|
| Hemoglobin A$_2$ | Whole blood | % | 0.01 | Proportion of 1.0 |
| Histamine | Plasma | µg/L | 8.997 | nmol/L |
| Histidine | Plasma | mg/dL | 64.45 | µmol/L |
| Homocysteine | Plasma | mg/L | 7.397 | µmol/L |
| Homovanillic acid | Urine | mg/24 h | 5.489 | µmol/d |
| Hydrocodone | Serum | µg/mL | 3.34 | µmol/L |
| Hydromorphone | Serum | µg/mL | 3504 | nmol/L |
| β-Hydroxybutyric acid | Plasma | mg/dL | 96.06 | µmol/L |
| 5-Hydroxyindoleacetic acid (5-HIAA) | Urine | mg/24 h | 5.23 | µmol/d |
| Hydroxyproline | Plasma | mg/dL | 76.266 | µmol/L |
| Ibuprofen | Serum | µg/mL | 4.848 | µmol/L |
| Imipramine | Plasma | ng/mL | 3.566 | nmol/L |
| Immunoglobulin A (IgA) | Serum | mg/dL | 0.01 | g/L |
| Immunoglobulin D (IgD) | Serum | mg/dL | 10 | mg/L |
| Immunoglobulin E (IgE) | Serum | mg/dL | 10 | mg/L |
| Immunoglobulin G (IgG) | Serum | mg/dL | 0.01 | g/L |
| Immunoglobulin M (IgM) | Serum | mg/dL | 0.01 | g/L |
| Insulin | Serum | µIU/mL | 6.945 | pmol/L |
| Insulinlike growth factor | Serum | ng/mL | 0.131 | nmol/L |
| Iodine | Serum | µg/L | 7.880 | nmol/L |
| Iron | Serum | µg/dL | 0.179 | µmol/L |
| Iron-binding capacity | Serum | µg/dL | 0.179 | µmol/L |
| Isoleucine | Plasma | mg/dL | 76.236 | µmol/L |
| Isoniazid | Plasma | µg/mL | 7.291 | µmol/L |

*(continued)*

945

**Table 17.5-2.** Selected Laboratory Tests, With Conversion Factors (*continued*)

| Analyte | Specimen | Conventional unit | Conversion factor (multiply by) | SI unit |
|---|---|---|---|---|
| Isopropanol (toxic) | Serum, plasma | mg/L | 0.0166 | mmol/L |
| Kanamycin | Serum, plasma | µg/mL | 2.064 | µmol/L |
| Ketamine | Serum | µg/mL | 4.206 | µmol/L |
| 17-Ketosteroids | Urine | mg/24 h | 3.33 | µmol/d |
| Lactate | Plasma | mg/dL | 0.111 | mmol/L |
| Lactate dehydrogenase (LDH) | Serum | U/L | 0.0167 | µkat/L |
| LDH isoenzymes | | | | |
| LD$_1$ | Serum | % | 0.01 | Proportion of 1.0 |
| LD$_2$ | Serum | % | 0.01 | Proportion of 1.0 |
| LD$_3$ | Serum | % | 0.01 | Proportion of 1.0 |
| LD$_4$ | Serum | % | 0.01 | Proportion of 1.0 |
| LD$_5$ | Serum | % | 0.01 | Proportion of 1.0 |
| Lead | Serum | µg/dL | 0.0483 | µmol/L |
| Leucine | Plasma | mg/dL | 76.237 | µmol/L |
| Leukocytes (see white blood cell count) | | | | |
| Lidocaine | Serum, plasma | µg/mL | 4.267 | µmol/L |
| Lipase | Serum | U/L | 0.0167 | µkat/L |
| Lipoprotein(a) [Lp(a)]$^c$ | Serum | mg/dL | 0.1 | mg/L |
| Lithium | Serum | mEq/L | 1.0 | mmol/L |
| Lorazepam | Serum | ng/mL | 3.114 | nmol/L |
| Luteinizing hormone (LH) | Serum, plasma | mIU/mL | 1.0 | IU/L |
| Lycopene | Serum | mg/L | 1.863 | µmol/L |

**Lymphocytes (see white blood cell count)**

| | | | | |
|---|---|---|---|---|
| Lysergic acid diethylamide (LSD) | Serum | µg/mL | 3092 | nmol/L |
| Lysine | Plasma | mg/dL | 68.404 | µmol/L |
| Lysozyme | Serum, plasma | mg/dL | 10 | mg/L |
| Magnesium | Serum | mg/dL | 0.4114 | mmol/L |
| Manganese | Whole blood | µg/L | 18.202 | nmol/L |
| Maprotiline | Plasma | ng/mL | 1.0 | µg/L |
| Melatonin | Serum | ng/L | 4.305 | pmol/L |
| Meperidine | Serum, plasma | ng/mL | 4.043 | nmol/L |
| Mercury | Serum | µg/L | 4.985 | nmol/L |
| Metanephrine (total) | Urine | mg/24 h | 5.07 | µmol/d |
| Metformin | Serum | µg/mL | 7.742 | µmol/L |
| Methadone | Serum, plasma | ng/mL | 0.00323 | µmol/L |
| Methamphetamine | Serum | µg/mL | 6.7 | µmol/L |
| Methanol | Plasma | mg/dL | 0.312 | mmol/L |
| Methaqualone | Serum, plasma | µg/mL | 3.995 | µmol/L |
| Methemoglobin | Whole blood | g/dL | 155 | µmol/L |
| Methemoglobin | Whole blood | % of total hemoglobin | 0.01 | Proportion of total hemoglobin |
| Methicillin | Serum | mg/L | 2.636 | µmol/L |
| Methionine | Plasma | mg/dL | 67.02 | µmol/L |
| Methotrexate | Serum, plasma | mg/L | 2200 | nmol/L |
| Methyldopa | Plasma | µg/mL | 4.735 | µmol/L |
| Metoprolol | Serum, plasma | ng/mL | 3.74 | nmol/L |
| β$_2$-Microglobulin | Serum | mg/L | 1.0 | mg/L |

(continued)

**Table 17.5-2.** Selected Laboratory Tests, With Conversion Factors (*continued*)

| Analyte | Specimen | Conventional unit | Conversion factor (multiply by) | SI unit |
|---|---|---|---|---|
| Morphine | Serum, plasma | ng/mL | 3.504 | nmol/L |
| Myoglobin | Serum | µg/L | 0.05814 | nmol/L |
| Naproxen | Serum | µg/mL | 4.343 | µmol/L |
| Niacin (nicotinic acid) | Urine | mg/24 h | 8.123 | µmol/d |
| Nickel | Whole blood | µg/L | 17.033 | nmol/L |
| Nicotine | Plasma | mg/L | 6.164 | µmol/L |
| Nitrogen (nonprotein) | Serum | mg/dL | 0.714 | mmol/L |
| Nitroprusside (as thiocyanate) | | µg/mL | 17.2 | µmol/L |
| Norepinephrine | Plasma | pg/mL | 5.911 | pmol/L |
| Nortriptyline | Serum, plasma | ng/mL | 3.797 | nmol/L |
| Ornithine | Plasma | mg/dL | 75.666 | µmol/L |
| Osmolality | Serum | mOsm/kg | 1.0 | mmol/kg |
| Osteocalcin | Serum | ng/mL | 1.0 | µg/L |
| Oxalate | Serum | mg/mL | 11.107 | µmol/L |
| Oxazepam | Serum, plasma | µg/mL | 3.487 | µmol/L |
| Oxycodone | Serum | ng/mL | 3.171 | nmol/L |
| Oxygen, partial pressure (Po$_2$) | Arterial blood | mm Hg | 0.133 | kPa |
| Paraquat | Whole blood | µg/mL | 5.369 | µmol/L |
| Parathyroid hormone | Serum | pg/mL | 1 | ng/L |
| Pentobarbital | Serum, plasma | µg/mL | 4.419 | µmol/L |
| Pepsinogen | Serum | ng/mL | 1.0 | µg/L |

| | | | | |
|---|---|---|---|---|
| pH (see blood gases) | | | | |
| Phencyclidine (toxic) | Serum, plasma | ng/mL | 4.109 | nmol/L |
| Phenobarbital | Serum, plasma | µg/mL | 4.31 | µmol/L |
| Phenylalanine | Plasma | mg/dL | 60.544 | µmol/L |
| Phenylpropanolamine | Serum | µg/mL | 6613 | nmol/L |
| Phenytoin | Serum, plasma | mg/L | 3.968 | µmol/L |
| Phosphorus (inorganic) | Serum | mg/dL | 0.323 | mmol/L |
| Placental lactogen | Serum | µg/mL | 46.296 | nmol/L |
| Plasminogen (antigenic) | Plasma | mg/dL | 0.113 | µmol/L |
| Plasminogen activator inhibitor | Plasma | ng/mL | 22.19 | pmol/L |
| Platelet count (thrombocytes) | Whole blood | ×10³/µL | 1.0 | ×10⁹/L |
| Potassium | Serum | mEq/L | 1.0 | mmol/L |
| Prealbumin | Serum | mg/dL | 10 | mg/L |
| Pregnanediol | Urine | mg/24 h | 3.12 | µmol/d |
| Pregnanetriol | Urine | mg/24 h | 2.972 | µmol/d |
| Primidone | Serum, plasma | µg/mL | 4.582 | µmol/L |
| Procainamide | Serum, plasma | µg/mL | 4.25 | µmol/L |
| Progesterone | Serum | ng/mL | 3.18 | nmol/L |
| Prolactin | Serum | ng/mL | 1 | µg/L |
| Proline | Plasma | mg/dL | 86.858 | µmol/L |
| Propoxyphene | Plasma | µg/mL | 2.946 | µmol/L |
| Propranolol | Serum | ng/mL | 3.856 | nmol/L |
| Prostate-specific antigen | Serum | ng/mL | 1.0 | µg/L |

*(continued)*

949

**Table 17.5-2.** Selected Laboratory Tests, With Conversion Factors (*continued*)

| Analyte | Specimen | Conventional unit | Conversion factor (multiply by) | SI unit |
|---|---|---|---|---|
| Protein (total) | Serum | g/dL | 10.0 | g/L |
| Prothrombin time (PT) | Plasma | s | 1.0 | s |
| Protoporphyrin | Red blood cells | μg/dL | 0.0178 | μmol/L |
| Protriptyline | Serum, plasma | μg/dL | 3.787 | nmol/L |
| Pyridoxine (see vitamin B$_6$) | | | | |
| Pyruvate | Plasma | mg/dL | 113.56 | μmol/L |
| Quinidine | Serum | μg/mL | 3.082 | μmol/L |
| Red blood cell count | Whole blood | ×10$^6$/μL | 1.0 | ×10$^{12}$/L |
| Renin | Plasma | pg/mL | 0.0237 | pmol/L |
| Reticulocyte count | Whole blood | ×10$^3$/μL | 1.0 | ×10$^9$/L |
| Reticulocyte count | Whole blood | % of red blood cells | 0.01 | Proportion of red blood cells |
| Retinol (see vitamin A) | | | | |
| Riboflavin (see vitamin B$_2$) | | | | |
| Rifampin | Serum | mg/L | 1.215 | μmol/L |
| Salicylates | Serum, plasma | μg/mL | 7.24 | μmol/L |
| Selenium | Serum, plasma | μg/L | 0.0127 | μmol/L |
| Serine | Plasma | mg/dL | 95.156 | μmol/L |
| Serotonin (5-hydroxytryptamine) | Whole blood | ng/mL | 0.00568 | μmol/L |
| Sex hormone–binding globulin | Serum | μg/mL | 8.896 | nmol/L |
| Sodium | Serum | mEq/L | 1.0 | mmol/L |

| | | | | | |
|---|---|---|---|---|---|
| Somatomedin C (insulinlike growth factor) | Serum | ng/mL | 0.131 | nmol/L | |
| Somatostatin | Plasma | pg/mL | 0.611 | pmol/L | |
| Streptomycin | Serum | mg/L | 1.719 | µmol/L | |
| Strychnine | Whole blood | mg/L | 2.99 | µmol/L | |
| Substance P | Plasma | pg/mL | 0.742 | pmol/L | |
| Sulfate | Serum | mg/L | 10.41 | µmol/L | |
| Sulfmethemoglobin | Whole blood | % of total hemoglobin | 0.01 | Proportion of total hemoglobin | |
| Taurine | Plasma | mg/dL | 79.91 | µmol/L | |
| Testosterone | Serum | ng/dL | 0.0347 | nmol/L | |
| Tetrahydrocannabinol | Serum | µg/mL | 3.180 | µmol/L | |
| Theophylline | Serum, plasma | µg/mL | 5.55 | µmol/L | |
| Thiamine (see vitamin B$_1$) | | | | | |
| Thiopental | Serum, plasma | µg/mL | 4.144 | µmol/L | |
| Thioridazine | Serum, plasma | µg/mL | 2.699 | µmol/L | |
| Threonine | Plasma | mg/dL | 84 | µmol/L | |
| Thrombin time | Plasma | s | 1.0 | s | |
| Thrombocytes (see platelet count) | | | | | |
| Thyroglobulin | Serum | ng/mL | 1.0 | µg/L | |
| Thyrotropin | Serum | mIU/L | 1.0 | mIU/L | |
| Thyroxine, free (FT$_4$) | Serum | ng/dL | 12.87 | pmol/L | |
| Thyroxine, total (T$_4$) | Serum | µg/dL | 12.87 | nmol/L | |
| Thyroxine-binding globulin | Serum | µg/mL | 17.094 | nmol/L | |
| Tissue plasminogen activator | Plasma | IU/mL | 1000 | IU/L | |

(continued)

**Table 17.5-2.** Selected Laboratory Tests, With Conversion Factors (*continued*)

| Analyte | Specimen | Conventional unit | Conversion factor (multiply by) | SI unit |
|---|---|---|---|---|
| Tobramycin | Serum, plasma | µg/mL | 2.139 | µmol/L |
| Tocainide | Serum | µg/mL | 5.201 | µmol/L |
| α-Tocopherol (see vitamin E) | | | | |
| Tolbutamide | Serum | µg/mL | 3.70 | µmol/L |
| Transferrin | Serum | mg/dL | 0.123 | µmol/L |
| Triglycerides | Serum | mg/dL | 0.0113 | mmol/L |
| Triiodothyronine, free (FT$_3$) | Serum | pg/dL | 0.0154 | pmol/L |
| Triiodothyronine, total (T$_3$) | Serum | ng/dL | 0.0154 | nmol/L |
| Troponin I | Serum | ng/mL | 1.0 | µg/L |
| Troponin T | Serum | ng/mL | 1.0 | µg/L |
| Tryptophan | Plasma | mg/dL | 48.967 | µmol/L |
| Tyrosine | Plasma | mg/dL | 55.19 | µmol/L |
| Urea nitrogen | Serum | mg/dL | 0.357 | mmol/L |
| Uric acid | Serum | mg/dL | 0.0595 | mmol/L |
| Urobilinogen | Urine | mg/24 h | 1.7 | µmol/d |
| Valine | Plasma | mg/dL | 85.361 | µmol/L |
| Valproic acid | Serum, plasma | µg/mL | 6.934 | µmol/L |
| Vancomycin | Serum, plasma | µg/mL | 0.690 | µmol/L |
| Vanillylmandelic acid (VMA) | Urine | mg/24 h | 5.046 | µmol/d |
| Vasoactive intestinal polypeptide | Plasma | pg/mL | 0.296 | pmol/L |
| Vasopressin | Plasma | pg/mL | 0.923 | pmol/L |

| | Specimen | Conventional Unit | Conversion Factor | SI Unit |
|---|---|---|---|---|
| Verapamil | Serum, plasma | ng/mL | 2.20 | nmol/L |
| Vitamin A (retinol) | Serum | µg/dL | 0.0349 | µmol/L |
| Vitamin $B_1$ (thiamine) | Serum | µg/dL | 29.6 | nmol/L |
| Vitamin $B_2$ (riboflavin) | Serum | µg/dL | 26.6 | nmol/L |
| Vitamin $B_3$ | Whole blood | µg/mL | 4.56 | µmol/L |
| Vitamin $B_6$ (pyridoxine) | Plasma | ng/mL | 4.046 | nmol/L |
| Vitamin $B_{12}$ | Serum | pg/mL | 0.7378 | pmol/L |
| Vitamin C (ascorbic acid) | Serum | mg/dL | 56.78 | µmol/L |
| Vitamin D (1,25-dihydroxyvitamin D) | Serum | pg/mL | 2.4 | pmol/L |
| Vitamin D (25-hydroxyvitamin D) | Plasma | ng/mL | 2.496 | nmol/L |
| Vitamin E (α-tocopherol) | Serum | µg/mL | 2.322 | µmol/L |
| Vitamin K | Serum | ng/mL | 2.22 | nmol/L |
| Warfarin | Serum, plasma | µg/mL | 3.247 | µmol/L |
| White blood cell count | Whole blood | /µL | 0.001 | $\times 10^9$/L |
| Differential count | | | | |
| Neutrophils–segmented | Whole blood | /µL | 0.001 | $\times 10^9$/L |
| Neutrophils–bands | Whole blood | /µL | 0.001 | $\times 10^9$/L |
| Lymphocytes | Whole blood | /µL | 0.001 | $\times 10^9$/L |
| Monocytes | Whole blood | /µL | 0.001 | $\times 10^9$/L |
| Eosinophils | Whole blood | /µL | 0.001 | $\times 10^9$/L |
| Basophils | Whole blood | /µL | 0.001 | $\times 10^9$/L |
| Differential count (number fraction) | | | | |
| Neutrophils–segmented | Whole blood | % | 0.01 | Proportion of 1.0 |
| Neutrophils–bands | Whole blood | % | 0.01 | Proportion of 1.0 |
| Lymphocytes | Whole blood | % | 0.01 | Proportion of 1.0 |

*(continued)*

**Table 17.5-2.** Selected Laboratory Tests, With Conversion Factors (*continued*)

| Analyte | Specimen | Conventional unit | Conversion factor (multiply by) | SI unit |
|---|---|---|---|---|
| Monocytes | Whole blood | % | 0.01 | Proportion of 1.0 |
| Eosinophils | Whole blood | % | 0.01 | Proportion of 1.0 |
| Basophils | Whole blood | % | 0.01 | Proportion of 1.0 |
| Zidovudine | Serum, plasma | μg/mL | 3.7 | μmol/L |
| Zinc | Serum | μg/dL | 0.153 | μmol/L |

[a]The laboratory values are provided for illustration only and are not intended to be comprehensive or definitive. Each laboratory determines its own values. The information in this table is adapted from and based on the following sources: Kratz et al,[6] Young and Huth,[7] McPherson and Pincus,[8] Goldman and Schaeffer,[9] Longo et al,[10] Lipoprotein a Foundation,[11] and Laposata.[12]

[b]Most laboratories do not convert to molar units; conversion of Lp(a) is difficult unless the size (large or small) of an individual's Lp(a) molecules is known.

[c]For dual reporting hemoglobin A1$_c$ (HbA$_{1c}$) as both a percentage of total hemoglobin and mmol HbA$_{1c}$/mol Hb, see the NGSP website IFCC Standardization of HbA$_{1c}$.[13]

**Table 17.5-3.** Primary End Points

| Primary end point | CGM, mean (95% CI) | Conventional therapy, mean (95% CI) | Least square means or mean for difference: CGM–conventional treatment (95% CI) | P value |
|---|---|---|---|---|
| HbA$_{1c}$, %[a] | 7.92 (7.79 to 8.05) | 8.35 (8.19 to 8.51) | −0.43 (−0.57 to −0.29) | <.001 |
| HbA$_{1c}$, mmol/mol | 63 (61.6 to 64.5) | 68 (66.0 to 69.4) | −4.7 (−6.27 to −3.13) | |

Abbreviations: CGM, continuous glucose monitoring; HbA$_{1c}$, hemoglobin A$_{1c}$.

SI conversion factor: To convert percentage of total hemoglobin to proportion of total hemoglobin, multiply by 0.01.

[a]Values are reported as last observation carried forward with HbA$_{1c}$ measurement standardized by NGSP (http://www.ngsp.org/ifccngsp.asp).

Hematologic values should be reported by means of conventional units.

The complete blood cell count showed a hemoglobin level of 13.4 g/dL, hematocrit of 41%, platelet count of 180 000/μL, and white blood cell count of 6500/μL.

Standardization is emerging for reporting hemoglobin A$_{1c}$,[13] and we recommend dual reporting, as shown in **Table 17.5-3**.

For enzymatic activity, the international unit (IU) is used; 1 IU equals the amount of enzyme generating 1 μmol of product per minute.

The peak follicle-stimulating hormone level was 48 mIU/mL.

**17.5.11** **Radiation.** Measurements of ionizing radiation and radioactivity should be reported by means of SI units. The SI units for radiation are established by international agreement.[2] The unit for activity of a radionuclide is the becquerel; the absorbed dose of radiation (absorbed per unit weight of tissue) is the gray (Gy); and the dose equivalent used to indicate the detrimental effects of an absorbed radiation dose on biological tissue is the sievert (Sv).

A 1 Gy dose is equivalent to 1 joule (J) of radiation energy absorbed per kilogram of organ or tissue weight. The rad is the older, non-SI unit and is still in use as a unit of absorbed dose (100 rad = 1 Gy). However, equal doses of all types of ionizing radiation are not equally harmful. Alpha particles produce greater harm than beta particles, γ rays, and x-rays for a given absorbed dose. To account for this difference, radiation dose is expressed as equivalent dose in sieverts (Sv).[14]

SI units for radiation and factors to convert values from SI units to conventional units are given in **Table 17.5-4**.

Although SI units are preferred, authors of some articles, such as those reporting studies that involve nuclear medicine or radiation oncology, may prefer to report results in both SI units and non-SI units. As with units for laboratory results, conversion factors to convert radiation from SI units to conventional units should be provided in the text, footnotes to tables or figures, and/or the Methods section of the article.

**Table 17.5-4.** Measurement Units for Radiation, With Conversion Factors

| Quantity | SI unit (symbol) | Conversion factors | Non-SI unit |
|---|---|---|---|
| Radioactivity | becquerel (Bq) | 1 Bq = 2.7 × 10$^{-11}$ Ci (approx)<br>1 Ci = 3.7 × 10$^{10}$ Bq<br>1 Bq = 27 picocurie (pCi) | curie (Ci) |
| Absorbed dose | gray (Gy) | 1 Gy = 100 rad<br>1 rad = 0.01 Gy[a] | rad |
| "Dose" equivalent | sievert (Sv) | 1 Sv = 100 rem<br>1 rem = 0.01 Sv | rem |

[a]Although 1 rad = 1 cGy, the prefix *centi-* is generally not preferred in SI. Therefore, despite the appeal of one-to-one conversion, rad should be converted to gray not centigray.

**17.5.12** **Currency.** Amounts of money are expressed as a decimal number or whole number preceded by the symbol for the unit of measure for the currency.

> The cost-effectiveness analysis suggested a $7000 difference between the 2 treatment strategies.

Table 17.5-5 lists some international currencies and their symbols. Online currency converter programs are also available.[15,16]

**Table 17.5-5.** Selected International Currencies and Symbols

| Country | Currency | Symbol or abbreviation |
|---|---|---|
| Argentina | Argentine peso | $ |
| Australia | Australian dollar | A$ |
| Austria | euro | € |
| Bahamas | Bahamian dollar | B$ |
| Belgium | euro | € |
| Bermuda | Bermuda dollar | Bd$ |
| Bolivia | boliviano | $ |
| Brazil | Brazilian real | R$ |
| Canada | Canadian dollar | CAD$ |
| Chile | Chilean peso | Ch$ |
| China | yuan renminbi | ¥ |
| Colombia | Colombian peso | Col$ |
| Cuba | Cuban peso | $ |
| Czech Republic | Czech koruna | Kč |

**Table 17.5-5.** Selected International Currencies and Symbols (*continued*)

| Country | Currency | Symbol or abbreviation |
|---|---|---|
| Denmark | Danish krone | kr |
| Dominican Republic | Dominican peso | RD$ |
| Egypt | Egyptian pound | £ |
| Ethiopia | Ethiopian birr | ብር |
| European Union | euro | € |
| Finland | euro | € |
| France | euro | € |
| Germany | euro | € |
| Ghana | Ghana cedi | GH¢ |
| Greece | euro | € |
| Hong Kong | Hong Kong dollar | HK$ |
| Hungary | forint | ft |
| India | rupee | ₹ |
| Iran | rial | IRR |
| Iraq | new Iraqi dinar | IQD |
| Ireland | euro | € |
| Israel | Israeli new sheqel | ₪ |
| Italy | euro | € |
| Japan | yen | ¥ |
| Jordan | Jordanian dinars | JD |
| Lebanon | Lebanese pound | LBP |
| Luxembourg | euro | € |
| Malawi | kwacha | MK |
| Mexico | Mexican peso | Mex$ |
| The Netherlands | euro | € |
| New Zealand | New Zealand dollar | NZ$ |
| Nigeria | naira | ₦ |
| Norway | Norwegian krone | kr |
| Pakistan | rupee | Rs |
| Peru | nuevos soles | S/ |
| Poland | zloty | Zl |
| Portugal | euro | € |

(*continued*)

**Table 17.5-5.** Selected International Currencies and Symbols (*continued*)

| Country | Currency | Symbol or abbreviation |
|---------|----------|------------------------|
| Russia | ruble | R |
| Saudi Arabia | Saudi riyal | SR |
| Singapore | Singapore dollar | SGD |
| South Africa | rand | R |
| South Korea | won | ₩ |
| Spain | euro | € |
| Sweden | Swedish krona | Sk |
| Switzerland | Swiss franc | CHF |
| Taiwan | Taiwanese new dollar | NT$ |
| Thailand | baht | ฿ |
| Turkey | Turkish new lira | T£ |
| Uganda | shilling | USh |
| Ukraine | hryvnia | ₴ |
| United Kingdom | pound sterling | £ |
| United States of America | US dollar | $ |
| Vietnam | dong | đ |
| Zambia | kwacha | ZK |
| Zimbabwe | dollar | $ |

For amounts reported in non-US currency, the current exchange rate should be used to calculate the amount in US dollars, and that amount should be shown in parentheses.

> The baseline amount for the cost-benefit analysis was estimated from the procedure cost of CAD $3000 (US $2800).

> The projected cost of the new research laboratory was €25 million (US $47.7 million).

The following example shows how the currency appears as a unit of measure in a table stub.

> Household income, CAD$

**Principal Authors:** Lauren Fischer and Paul Frank

ACKNOWLEDGMENT

James C. Boyd, MD, University of Virginia Health System, Charlottesville, provided careful review of the SI conversion factors table. Hope J. Lafferty, AM, ELS, Hope

J. Lafferty Communications, Marfa, Texas; Trevor Lane, MA, DPhil, Edanz Group, Fukuoka, Japan; Rochelle Lodder, formerly of JAMA Network; and Peter J. Olson, ELS, Sheridan Services, Waterbury, Vermont, provided input on an earlier version of the chapter.

## REFERENCES

1. Arbesman S. Liters and followers. *Wall Street Journal.* August 2, 2014:C6.
2. Bureau International des Poids et Mesures. The International System of Units (SI). 9th ed. Updated 2019. Accessed August 18, 2019. https://www.bipm.org/en/publications/si-brochure/
3. Thompson A, Taylor BN. *Guide for the Use of the International System of Units (SI).* National Institute of Standards and Technology, US Dept of Commerce; 2008. Accessed September 23, 2015. https://physics.nist.gov/cuu/pdf/sp811.pdf
4. *Dorland's Illustrated Medical Dictionary.* 32nd ed. Elsevier Saunders; 2012.
5. Kriska AM, Caspersen CJ. Introduction to a collection of physical activity questionnaires. *Med Sci Sports Exerc.* 1997;29(6):S5-S9.
6. Kratz A, Ferraro M, Sluss PM, Lewandrowski KB. Normal reference laboratory values. *N Engl J Med.* 2004;351(15):1548-1563. doi:10.1056/NEJMcpc049016
7. Young DS, Huth EJ. *SI Units for Clinical Measurement.* American College of Physicians; 1998.
8. McPherson R, Pincus M, eds. *Henry's Clinical Diagnosis and Management by Laboratory Methods.* 22nd ed. Elsevier Saunders; 2012.
9. Goldman L, Schaeffer AI. *Goldman-Cecil Medicine.* 25th ed. Elsevier Saunders; 2015.
10. Longo D, Fauci A, Kasper D, Hauser S, Jameson J, Loscalzo J, eds. *Harrison's Principles of Internal Medicine.* 18th ed. McGraw-Hill Professional; 2011.
11. Lipoprotein a Foundation. Understand inherited lipoprotein(a). May 2017. Accessed August 1, 2019. https://www.lipoproteinafoundation.org/page/UnderstandLpa
12. Laposta M, ed. *Laboratory Medicine: The Diagnosis of Disease in the Clinical Laboratory.* 2nd ed. McGraw-Hill Education; 2014.
13. NGSP website. IFCC Standardization of HbA$_{1c}$. 2010. Accessed June 30, 2017. http://www.ngsp.org/ifccngsp.asp
14. Canadian Centre for Occupational Health and Safety. What is ionizing radiation? Accessed September 23, 2015. https://www.ccohs.ca/oshanswers/phys_agents/ionizing.html
15. ISO 4217 Currency codes. International Organization for Standardization; 2017. Accessed July 5, 2019. https://www.iso.org/iso-4217-currency-codes.html
16. Oanda.com Currency Converter. Accessed September 23, 2015. https://www.oanda.com/currency/converter

# Numbers and Percentages

**18.0** **Numbers and Percentages.** Any policy on the use of numbers in text must take into account the reader's impression that numbers written as numerals (symbols) appear to emphasize quantity more strongly than numbers spelled out as words. Because numerals convey quantity more efficiently than spelled-out numbers, they are generally preferable in technical writing. In literary writing, by contrast, spelled-out numbers may be more compatible with style. Despite these general principles, usage may appear inconsistent when a publication chooses to use numerals in some instances and words in others. The guidelines outlined in this section attempt to reduce these inconsistencies and avoid use of numerals that may be jarring to the reader. In situations that are not governed by these guidelines, common sense and editorial judgment should prevail.

**18.1** **Use of Numerals.** In scientific writing, numerals are used to express numbers in most circumstances (eg, 5 not five). Exceptions are the following:

- Numbers that begin a sentence, title, subtitle, or heading (see 18.2.1, Beginning a Sentence, Title, Subtitle, or Heading)

- Common fractions (see 18.1.2, Common Fractions)

- Accepted usage, such as idiomatic expressions and numbers used as pronouns (see 18.2.2, *One* Used as a Pronoun)

- Other uses of *one* in running text (text that is not part of an equation or otherwise separated from the main body of the text)

▣ Ordinals *first* through *ninth* (see 18.2.4, Ordinals)

▣ Numbers spelled out in quotes or article titles (see 18.2, Spelling Out Numbers)

Five Voices, One Story
Preventing Infections in the Intensive Care Unit: One Size Does Not Fit All

Note the following examples of numerals in text:

The relative risk of exposed individuals was nearly 3 times that of the controls.

In the second phase of the study, 3 of the investigators administered the 5 tests to the 7 remaining participants. The test scores showed a 2- to 2.4-fold improvement over those of the first phase.

In 2 of the 17 patients in whom both ears were tested, we were unable to obtain responses from either ear. While testing patient 3, we experienced technical problems that consisted of unmanageable electrical artifacts.

Groups 1 and 2 were similar in terms of demographic and clinical characteristics (Table 1). Table 2 lists the 4 tests that were performed.

A 3-member committee from the US Food and Drug Administration visited the researchers.

**18.1.1** **Numbers of 4 or More Digits to Either Side of the Decimal Point.** Commas are not used in large numbers. In 4-digit numbers, the digits are set closed up. For numbers of 10 000 or greater, a thin space is used to separate every 3 digits starting from the right-most integer (or, in numbers with decimals, from the left of the decimal point). For numbers with 5 or more digits to the right of the decimal point, a thin space is used between every 3 digits starting from the right of the decimal point (see 17.4, Use of Numerals With Units).

The exact weight of the salt was 8.453 98 g, but its reported value was rounded to 8.4540 g.

Our analytical sample included all 2455 community-dwelling individuals 65 years or older, representing 32 294 810 elderly persons in the United States.

**18.1.2** **Common Fractions.** Common fractions are written with a numerator and denominator in which both are integers (eg, 1/3, 1/2, 7/8). Where spelled out, simple common (where the numerator and denominator are nonzero integers, eg, 9/10) and nonsimple (when the numerator or denominator contain fractions) fractions are expressed with hyphenated words, whether the fraction is used as an adjective or a noun. Mixed fractions are typically expressed in numerals (see 18.1.3, Mixed Fractions).

Of those attending, nearly three-fourths were members of the association.

There is a half-second delay before the intensive care unit alarm triggers after an arrhythmia is detected.

The institutional review board committee requires a two-thirds majority to establish a consensus when voting on ethical matters.

The orthopedic surgeon asked for a seven-eighths-inch-diameter rod.

In some cases, fractions can be expressed with an indefinite article preceding the unit. Such constructions do not use the hyphen.

The test concluded after half an hour.

*A quarter* may be used in place of *one-fourth*.

A quarter of the consensus panel dissented.

Note: In scientific reports, precision is preferred (eg, 24% instead of "a quarter").

**18.1.3**    **Mixed Fractions.** Mixed fractions are the combination of a whole number and a fraction into a single, mixed number. They may be used for less precise measurements instead of decimals. These expressions usually involve time. Common fractions are typically spelled out (see 18.1.2, Common Fractions).

The surgery lasted 3¼ hours.

The patient was hospitalized for 5½ days.

Of the patients returning for a second visit, half received the intervention.

White women comprise approximately half of those who use the program for breast cancer screening, one-fourth are Hispanic women, and approximately 16% are Black women.

**18.1.4**    **Measures of Time.** Measures of time usually are expressed as arabic numerals (see 13.3, Days of the Week, Months, Eras). When dates are provided, numerals should be used for day and year; the month should be spelled out unless listed in a table. Conventional form for time and dates (11:30 PM on February 25, 1961) is preferred to European or military form (2330 on 25 February 1961). However, use of military time may clarify the time course in figures that depict a 24-hour experiment, times of drug dosing, and the like. For time, if the hour of the day is given, AM or PM is used and set in small capital letters (see 21.0, Editing, Proofreading, Tagging, and Display). When referring to time on the hour, the minutes may be omitted (eg, 3 PM). With 12 o'clock, simply use noon or midnight, whichever is intended.

At 5:45 AM, October 15, 2004, the researchers completed the final experiment.

The patient was admitted to the ward service just after midnight on January 1, 2016.

When referring to a position as it would appear on a clock face, express the position by means of numerals followed by *o'clock* (See 8.2.3.3, Colon, Numbers).

The needle was inserted at the 9-o'clock position.

The procedure was scheduled to begin at 9 AM.

**18.1.5** **Measures of Temperature.** Use the degree symbol with Celsius and Fahrenheit measures of temperature but not for Kelvin.[1] A space should appear between the number and the degree symbol (see 17.3.8, Spacing). Changes in temperature are expressed as higher and lower and not warmer or colder (see 18.4, Use of Digit Spans and Hyphens).

> The plates were cultured at 17 °C, which was 3 °C lower than usual.

> The patient was febrile (temperature, 38.8 °C).

> The thermodynamic temperature equivalent to 25 °C is 298.15 K.

**18.1.6** **Measures of Currency.** For sums of money, use the appropriate symbol to indicate the type of currency (eg, $, €, £, ¥; see 17.5.12, Currency).[1]

> His charge for the medication was $55.60 plus $0.95 for shipping.

> The equivalent sum in euros was €30.

**18.2** **Spelling Out Numbers.** Use words to express numbers that occur at the beginning of a sentence, title, subtitle, or heading; for common fractions; for accepted usage and numbers used as pronouns; for ordinals *first* through *ninth*; and when part of a published quote or title in which the number is spelled out. When spelling out numerals, hyphenate *twenty-one* through *ninety-nine* when these numbers occur alone or as part of a larger number. When numbers greater than 100 are spelled out, do not use commas or *and* (eg, one hundred thirty-two).

**18.2.1** **Beginning a Sentence, Title, Subtitle, or Heading.** Use words for any number that begins a sentence, title, subtitle, or heading. However, it may be better to reword the sentence so that it does not begin with a number.

> *Acceptable:*   Three hundred twenty-eight men and 126 women were included in the study.
>
> *Better:*   The study population comprised 328 men and 126 women.

> *Acceptable:*   **Participants:** Seventy-two thousand three hundred thirty-seven postmenopausal women aged 34 to 77 years.
>
> *Better:*   **Participants:** A total of 72 337 postmenopausal women aged 34 to 77 years.

> Three patients were identified; 2 had hypertension and 1 had diabetes.

Numerals may be used in sentences that begin with a specific year, but avoid beginning sentences with years if possible.

> *Acceptable:*   2008 marked the 80th anniversary of the discovery of penicillin.
>
> *Better:*   The year 2008 marked the 80th anniversary of the discovery of penicillin.

> *Acceptable:* 2012 was the medical school's centennial year.
>
> *Better:* The medical school's centennial year was 2012.

When a unit of measure follows a number that begins a sentence, it too must be written out, even if the same unit is abbreviated elsewhere in the same sentence. Because this construction can be cumbersome, rewording the sentence may be preferable (see 17.3, Format, Style, and Punctuation).

> *Acceptable:* Two milligrams of haloperidol was administered at 9 PM followed by 1 mg at 3:30 AM.
>
> *Better:* At 9 PM, 2 mg of haloperidol was administered followed at 3:30 AM by 1 mg.

**18.2.2** *One* **Used as a Pronoun.** The word *one* should be spelled out when used as a pronoun or noun.

> The investigators compared a new laboratory method with the standard one.

> These differences may be concealed if one looks only at the total group.

> William James uses the idea of the one and the many as the great challenge of the philosophical mind.

**18.2.3** **Accepted Usage.** Spell out numbers for generally accepted usage, such as idiomatic expressions. *One* frequently appears in running text without referring to a quantity per se and may appear awkward if expressed as a numeral. When *one* may be replaced by *a* or *a single* without changing the meaning, the word *one* rather than the numeral is usually appropriate. Other numbers, most often *zero, two,* and large rounded numbers, also may be written as words in circumstances in which use of the numeral would place an unintended emphasis on a precise quantity or would be confusing.

> Any one of the 12 individuals might have been holding the winning ticket. [In this example, *one* may be superfluous. Depending on the intent, the following may be an equivalent sentence: Any of the 12 individuals might have been holding the winning ticket.]

> The study was delayed by one problem after another.

> Models were developed to allow for the inclusion of one-time variables.

> The study participants frequently moved from one location to another.

> On the one hand, the blood glucose concentrations were substantially improved; on the other hand, the patient felt worse.

> Medical futility has become one of the dominant topics in medical ethics in recent years.

> In one recent case, the malpractice award was $1 million.

We ought to bring together in one place all that we have learned on a given subject.

The outcome was a zero-sum gain.

Please include an example or two of the following scales.

I would like to ask the patient a question or two about her perception of her illness.

She hoped to be a neurosurgeon one day.

He quoted the *Ten Commandments of Good Medical Practice*, a guidebook for resident physicians (see 10.0, Capitalization).

Many of the mass-vaccination campaigns have been large, with tens of thousands of persons immunized, and expensive, costing as much as a half-million dollars.

During one of the laboratory runs, it was observed that samples from cases 1, 3, and 9 had faint electrophoretic bands attributable to suboptimal DNA quality.

*But:* During 1 of the 17 laboratory runs, it was observed. . . . (See 18.3.2, Consecutive Numerical Expressions.)

**18.2.4**    **Ordinals.** Ordinal numbers generally express order or rank rather than a precise quantity. Because they usually address nontechnical aspects of the objects they modify, ordinals are often found in literary writing. The numerical expression of commonly used ordinals (1st, 2nd, 3rd, 4th, etc) may appear jarring and interrupt the flow of the text. For this reason, the ordinals *first* through *ninth* are spelled out.

The third patient was not available for reevaluation.

It finally has become second nature for the interns to establish an airway as the first part of any resuscitation effort.

The numeric form of ordinals greater than *ninth* is well established in literary texts (10th, 11th, and so on) except at the beginning of a sentence, title, subtitle, or heading. Use the following suffixes: *-st, -nd, -rd, -th*. The JAMA Network journals do not set these suffixes as superscripts.

Eleventh-hour negotiations resulted in the repeal of the Medicare Sustainable Growth Rate rule.

The pandemic will continue well into the 21st century.

He celebrated his 80th birthday while still in the hospital.

*But:* Some forms are spelled out by convention (eg, Twenty-fifth Amendment).

If a sentence contains 2 or more ordinals, at least 1 of which is greater than *ninth*, all should be expressed in numeric form.

Children in the 5th and 10th grades were included in the survey.

The first and third patients treated experienced complete remissions.

**18.3**    **Combining Numerals and Words.** Use a combination of numerals and words to express rounded large numbers and consecutive numerical expressions.

**18.3.1**    **Rounded Large Numbers.** Rounded large numbers, such as those starting with *million*, should be expressed with numerals and words.

> The disease affects 5 million to 6 million people. (Note that the word *million* is repeated to avoid ambiguity.)

The word *million* signifies the quantity $10^6$, whereas *billion* signifies the quantity $10^9$. Although *billion* has traditionally signified $10^{12}$ (1 million million) in Britain, many British medical journals[2] have used *billion* to indicate the quantity $10^9$. A number may be expressed in *million* rather than *billion* if the latter term could create ambiguity. In that case, the decimal should be moved 3 places to the right. *Trillion* should be used to denote the quantity $10^{12}$.

> The projected budget is £2.5 billion.
>
> *Or:* The projected budget is £2500 million.
>
> The budget deficit is expected to expand to $1 trillion by 2020.

**18.3.2**    **Consecutive Numerical Expressions.** When 2 numbers appear consecutively in a sentence, either reword the sentence or spell out 1 of the numbers for clarity.

> Study participants were provided twenty 5-mL syringes.

| | |
|---|---|
| *Avoid:* | In the cohort of 1500, 690 were men. |
| *Better:* | In the cohort of 1500 individuals, 690 were men. |
| *Or:* | In the cohort, 690 of the 1500 individuals were men. |

> When I first started out as an author, one had to send an envelope with 3 copies of a manuscript and one 3.5-in diskette to submit a manuscript for publication.

However, numerals may be listed consecutively if they refer to items in an array. As always, clarity and common sense should guide usage.

| | |
|---|---|
| *Acceptable:* | The life expectancy of groups 1, 2, and 3 was 69, 83, and 75 years, respectively. |
| *Better:* | The life expectancy was 69 years in group 1, 83 years in group 2, and 75 years in group 3. |

Abbreviations or symbols may follow numbers. In this case, if there is potential for misunderstanding, it is preferable to reword the sentence.

| | |
|---|---|
| *Acceptable:* | There are 2 $D_2$ dopamine receptor isoforms. |
| *Better:* | The $D_2$ dopamine receptor has 2 isoforms. |
| *Acceptable:* | The investigators were able to identify 3 γ-aminobutyric acid–mediated sites. |
| *Better:* | The investigators were able to identify 3 sites mediated by γ-aminobutyric acid. |

Superscripts that indicate references may be mistaken for exponents if they immediately follow a numeral.

Increased morbidity has been associated with a body mass index less than 18[2] and greater than 27.[3] [This can be reworded: Smith and Jones[2] found that a body mass index of less than 18 was associated with increased morbidity. They also found that patients with a BMI greater than 27 had increased morbidity.[3]]

**18.4** **Use of Digit Spans and Hyphens.** Digits should not be omitted when indicating a span of years or page numbers in the text. Hyphens may be used in text when a year span is used as the identifying characteristic of a study (eg, the 2010-2012 National Health and Nutrition Examination Survey) but only when the actual dates of the study have been defined previously in the text; if the dates are not defined in the text, the hyphen is ambiguous and may or may not mean that the dates indicated are inclusive. In certain circumstances, such as fiscal year or academic year, the actual span may be understood and no definition is required; in these cases, the hyphen is acceptable at first mention and throughout the text.

The students participated in the study during the 2010-2011 academic year.

Substantial profits were anticipated for fiscal years 2013-2015.

Helen B. Taussig, MD (1898-1986)

Use of *to* also may introduce ambiguity. *To* should be used rather than *through* only when the final digit is not included in the span and *through* instead of *to* when the final digit is included in the span. However, in some circumstances, such as life span, historical periods, fiscal or academic year, page numbers in text, or age ranges, the meaning is clear without making a distinction between *to* and *through*, and *to* may be used.

The participants ranged in age from 23 to 56 years.

The second enrollment period spanned January 30, 2012, to September 1, 2014. (In this example, the enrollment period ended on August 31.)

*Or:* The second enrollment period spanned January 30, 2012, through September 1, 2014. (In this example, the enrollment period ended on September 1, 2014.)

We looked at the following 3 periods: 1985 through 1989, 1990 through 2000, and 2001 through 2014.

Time spans may be referred to by means of hyphens between years once the meaning has been made clear at the first mention.

The mortality rate ratio of 2.01 (95% CI, 1.80-2.24) indicates that the mortality rate during 1990-2000 was approximately twice that during 2001-2014.

A hyphen may be used within parentheses or in tables to indicate spans, including CIs, without further definition, provided the meaning is clear. However, if one of the values in the span includes a minus sign (most commonly found in CIs), the word *to* should be used to avoid ambiguity (see 8.3, Hyphens and Dashes, and 19.4, Significant Digits and Rounding Numbers).

> The mean number of years of life gained was 1.7 (95% CI, 1.3-2.1).

> The mean number of years of disease-free life gained was 0.4 (95% CI, −0.1 to 0.9).

> After the drug was injected, the seizures continued for a brief period (20-30 seconds), then ceased.

> The fourth edition contains a discussion of recommended preventive measures (pp 1243-1296).

> The median age of the individuals in the sample was 56 years (range, 31-92 years).

If the unit of measure for the quantity is set closed up with the number, the unit should be repeated for each number.

> The differences between groups were relatively small (5%-8%).

> *But:* The pressure gradient varied widely (10-60 mm Hg) throughout the day.

If the unit of measure changes within the parentheses, the word *to* is used.

> Because of the wide range of measurements (2 mg to $3.7 \times 10^4$ kg), we displayed our results on a logarithmic scale.

**18.5** **Enumerations.** Indicate a short series of enumerated items by numerals run in and enclosed within parentheses in the text (see 8.5, Parentheses and Brackets).

> The testing format focused on 6 aspects: (1) alertness and concentration, (2) language, (3) naming, (4) calculations, (5) construction, and (6) memory.

For long or complex enumerations, indented numbers followed by a period, without parentheses, may be used.

> In response to other issues:
>
> 1. The study was conducted under 2 protocols that prespecified that the data would be pooled for the analyses.
> 2. A particular regression procedure (model selection stepdown) was applied individually for clinical outcomes.
> 3. The relative risk of all serious adverse events was similar to the relative risk at 6 months.

If enumerated items contain further enumerations of their own, it is best to provide this information in a box or table.

Bullets without enumeration may be used for emphasis and clarity when the specific order of the items is not important. If the items are complete sentences, begin each item with a capital letter and end it with a period.

The current labeling provides instructions as follows:

- Use should be limited to physicians experienced in emergency treatment of anaphylaxis.

- Initial dosage should be based on results of skin testing.

- The patient should be observed for at least 20 minutes after injection.

- Immunotherapy should be withheld when a β-blocker is used.

If the bulleted items are not complete sentences, no end punctuation is needed and the use of a capital or lowercase letter on the first word of each item is a matter of judgment, often determined by length (capital letters on initial letter of longer items, lowercase on initial letters of shorter items), with consistency within a single list.

Anorexia nervosa includes the following:

- Low body weight with refusal to maintain a healthy weight

- Fear of being overweight despite having an extremely low body weight

- Disturbed body image or denial of the degree of underweight

- In girls and women, absence of menstruation

Signs and symptoms of cardiogenic shock may include

- hypotension

- cold, clammy skin

- low urine output

- confusion

**18.6** ▪ **Abbreviating *Number*.**

| Variable | Drug | Placebo |
|---|---|---|
| No. of participants | 49 | 48 |

The word *number* may be abbreviated *No.* in the body of tables and line art or in the text when used as a specific designator. Do not use the number sign (#) in place of the abbreviation; this could be confused with the hashtag (#) used in social media. The word *number* should always be spelled out when it is used as a proper noun (eg, Social Security number).

A No. 10 catheter was placed in the femoral artery.

She was No. 1 in her graduating class.

When referring to numbers of individuals in a study—in tables and figures as well as within parentheses—the abbreviation $N$ is used when referring to the entire sample; $n$ refers to a subsample (see 19.5, Glossary of Statistical Terms).

Patients were enrolled at each study site (N = 2758) and randomly assigned to receive intervention (n = 1378) or placebo (n = 1380).

## 18.7     Forms of Numbers.

**18.7.1**     **Decimals.** The decimal form should be used when a fraction is given with an abbreviated unit of measure (eg, 0.5 g, 2.7 mm) to reflect the precision of the measurement (eg, 38.0 kg should not be rounded to 38 kg if the scale was accurate to tenths of a kilogram) (see 17.4.2, Decimal Format).

> The patient was receiving gentamicin sulfate, 3.5 mg/kg, every 8 hours. Her serum gentamicin level reached a peak of 5.8 µg/mL and a trough of 0.7 µg/mL after the third dose.

Place a zero before the decimal point in numbers less than 1, except when expressing the 3 values related to probability: $P$, $\alpha$, and $\beta$. These values cannot equal 1, except when rounding (see 19.5, Glossary of Statistical Terms). Because they appear frequently, eliminating the zero can save substantial space in tables and text. (Although other statistical values also may never equal 1, their use is less frequent, and to simplify usage, the zero before the decimal point is included.)

> $P = .16$
>
> $1-\beta = .80$
>
> Our predetermined $\alpha$ level was .05.
>
> *But:* $\kappa = 0.87$

Note, however, that $\alpha$ and $\beta$ may sometimes be used to indicate other statistics, and in some of these cases, their values may be 1 or greater.

> Cronbach $\alpha = 0.78$
>
> standardized $\beta$ coefficient = 2.34

By convention, a zero is not used in front of the decimal point of the measure of the bore of a firearm.

> .45-caliber semiautomatic handgun

Odds ratios, likelihood ratios, and relative risks are reported to the hundredth place unless the point estimate is very small.

> In unadjusted Cox proportional hazards regression, bariatric surgery was associated with reduced mortality (hazard ratio, 0.64; 95% CI, 0.51-0.80).

**18.7.2**     **Percentages.** The term *percent* derives from the Latin *per centum*, meaning by the hundred or in, to, or for every hundred. The term *percent* and the symbol % should be used with specific numbers. *Percentage* is a more general term for any number or amount that can be stated as a percent. *Percentile* is defined as the value on a scale of 100 that indicates the percentage of the distribution that is equal to or below it.

Ten percent of the work remained to be done.

Heart disease was present in a small percentage of the participants. (*But:* Five percent of the participants had heart disease.)

Her body mass index placed her in the 95th percentile of the study group.

Unless otherwise indicated, data in a table are expressed as number (percentage). If it is a table footnote, space is often saved by showing the data as "No. (%)."

Use arabic numerals and the symbol % for specific percentages. The symbol is set closed up to the numeral and is repeated with each number in a series or range of percentages. Include the symbol % with a percentage of zero.

A 5% incidence (95% CI, 1%-9%) was reported.

The prevalence in the populations studied varied from 0% to 20%.

At the beginning of a sentence, spell out both the number and the word *percent*, even if the percentage is part of a series or range. Often it is preferable to reword the sentence so that a comparison between percentages is more readily apparent.

| | |
|---|---|
| *Acceptable:* | Twenty percent to 30% of patients reported respiratory symptoms. |
| *Better:* | The percentage of patients who reported respiratory symptoms ranged from 20% to 30%. |
| *Or:* | Between 20% and 30% of the patients reported respiratory symptoms. |

When referring to a percentage derived from a study sample, include with the percentage the numbers from which the percentage is derived. This is particularly important when the sample size is less than 100 (see 19.4, Significant Digits and Rounding Numbers). To give primacy to the original data, it is preferable to place the percentage in parentheses.

Of the 26 adverse events, 19 (73%) occurred in infants.

Any discrepancy in the sum of percentages in a tabulation (eg, because of rounding numbers, missing values, or multiple procedures) should be explained.

The terms *percent change, percent increase*, and *percent decrease* are often used in place of *percentage of change*. Although these less formal terms are acceptable, their usage must be precise. They generally are computed as the difference between an index value and either an earlier or later value divided by the index value. Although a percent increase may exceed 100%, a percent decrease generally cannot. A percent decrease can also be expressed as a negative percent increase.

These terms must be differentiated from *percentage point change, increase,* or *decrease*, which are obtained by subtracting one percentage value from another. For example, a change in rate from 20% to 30% can be referred to either as an increase of 10 percentage points, as in "the intervention group improved 10 percentage points," or as a 50% increase (percent change), as in "the intervention group showed a 50% improvement" ([30% − 20%]/20%). The 2 terms are *not* interchangeable. Because the percent change does not indicate the actual beginning or ending values or the magnitude of the change, the actual values should be provided whenever possible.

**18.7.3** **Reporting Proportions and Percentages.** Whenever possible, proportions and percentages should be accompanied by the actual numerator ($n$) and denominator ($d$) from which they were derived. In text, the numerator and denominator should be expressed as "*n* of *d*" not by the virgule construction "*n/d*," which could imply that the numbers were computed in an arithmetic operation.

> Death occurred in 6 of 200 patients.

> *Not:* Death occurred in 6/200 patients.

For clarity, when a numerator and denominator are accompanied by a resulting proportion or percentage, the proportion or percentage should not intervene between the numerator and denominator.

> Death occurred in 6 of 200 patients (3%).

> Death occurred in 3% (6 of 200) of patients.

> Of the 200 patients, death occurred in 6 (3%).

> Of the 200 patients, 6 (3%) died.

> *Not:* Death occurred in 6 (3%) of 200 patients.

The denominator may be omitted if it is clear from the context.

> Death occurred in 10 patients (10%).

In expressing a series of proportions or percentages drawn from the same sample, the denominator need be provided only once.

> Of the 200 patients, 6 (3%) died, 18 (9%) experienced an adverse event, and 22 (11%) were lost to follow-up.

**18.7.4** **Reporting Rates and Ratios.** Use the virgule construction for rates when placed in parentheses (eg, 1/2) but never in running text. A colon is used for ratios (eg, 1:2). Rates should use the decimal format when the denominator is understood to be 100; otherwise, the denominator should be specified.

> Of all individuals exposed, children were affected at a rate of 0.05.

> The infant mortality rate was 3 per 10 000 live births.

> *Not:* The infant mortality rate was 3/10 000 live births.

**18.7.5** **Roman Numerals.** Use roman numerals with proper names (eg, Henry Ford III). Note that no comma is used before the numeral. However, arabic numerals should be used as designators in all other cases (eg, round 2, Table 4, year 5; see 10.4, Designators) unless roman numerals are part of formally established nomenclature (see 14.0, Nomenclature).

> Step I diet                  Schedule II drug
>
> level I trauma center        Axis I diagnosis
>
> NYHA class II
>
> But: type 2 diabetes, phase 3 study

Use roman numerals for cancer stages and arabic numerals for cancer grades (see 14.2, Cancer). In pedigree charts, use roman numerals to indicate generations and arabic numerals to indicate families or individual family members (see 4.2.2.4, Pedigrees). Roman numerals are also used for clotting factor and cranial nerve names. Roman numerals also may be used in outline format (see 4.1, Tables).

In bibliographic material (eg, references or book reviews), do not use roman numerals to indicate volume number, even though roman numerals may have been used in the original. However, if roman numerals were used in the original title or in an outline, refer to the title or outline as it was published, with roman numerals. Retain lowercase roman numerals that refer to pages in a foreword, preface, or introduction. Roman numerals may also be used to number supplements to journals so that roman numerals appear adjacent to page numbers in references to the work. In this case, the roman numerals should be retained.

For the use of roman numerals in biblical and classical references, follow the most recent edition of the *Chicago Manual of Style* (see 3.0, References).

The following list indicates the roman equivalents for arabic numerals. In general, roman numerals to the right of the greatest numeral are added to that numeral, and numerals to the left are subtracted. A horizontal bar over a roman numeral multiplies its value by 1000.

| | | | |
|---|---|---|---|
| 1 | I | 20 | XX |
| 2 | II | 30 | XXX |
| 3 | III | 40 | XL |
| 4 | IV | 50 | L |
| 5 | V | 60 | LX |
| 6 | VI | 70 | LXX |
| 7 | VII | 80 | LXXX |
| 8 | VIII | 90 | XC |
| 9 | IX | 100 | C |
| 10 | X | 200 | CC |
| 11 | XI | 300 | CCC |
| 12 | XII | 400 | CD |
| 13 | XIII | 500 | D |
| 14 | XIV | 600 | DC |
| 15 | XV | 700 | DCC |
| 16 | XVI | 800 | DCCC |
| 17 | XVII | 900 | CM |
| 18 | XVIII | 1000 | M |
| 19 | XIX | 5000 | $\overline{V}$ |

**Principal Author:** Edward H. Livingston, MD

## ACKNOWLEDGMENT

I thank Stephen J. Lurie, MD, PhD, and Margaret A Winker, MD, who wrote this chapter in the 10th edition of the *AMA Manual of Style,* on which this chapter is based. I also thank the following for their comments: Diane Cannon, formerly of the JAMA Network; Lila Haile, BA, *JAMA,* now with the Medical Council of Canada; Trevor Lane, MA, DPhil, Edanz Group, Fukuoka, Japan; and Ana Marušić, MD, PhD, *Journal of Global Health* and University of Split School of Medicine, Croatia.

## REFERENCES

1. Taylor BN, Thompson A. The International System of Units (SI). NIST special publication 330. 2008. Accessed December 6, 2018. https://www.nist.gov/sites/default/files/documents/2016/12/07/sp330.pdf
2. Billion bites the dust. *Nature.* 1992;358(6381):2. doi:10.1038/358002b0

## ADDITIONAL READINGS AND GENERAL REFERENCES

American Psychological Association. *Publication Manual of the American Psychological Association.* 6th ed. American Psychological Association; 2010.

*The Chicago Manual of Style.* 17th ed. University of Chicago Press; 2017.

Style Manual Committee, Council of Science Editors. *Scientific Style and Format: The CSE Manual for Authors, Editors, and Publishers.* 8th ed. University of Chicago Press/Council of Science Editors; 2014.

# 19.0 Study Design and Statistics

**19.0 Study Design and Statistics.**

*The essence of life is statistical improbability on a grand scale.*
Richard Dawkins[1]

*There are three kinds of lies: lies, damn lies, and statistics.*
Attributed to Disraeli by Mark Twain[1]

In medical and health research, the quality of the statistical analysis and the presentation of results are critical to a study's validity and influence. Decisions about statistical analysis are best made when studies are designed and should not occur after the data are collected. A fundamentally flawed study cannot be salvaged by statistical analysis. Regardless of the statistician's role, authors are responsible for the appropriate design, analysis, and presentation of the study's results.

Authors, journal editors, and manuscript editors of research manuscripts should have a general understanding of study designs, statistical terms and concepts, and the use of statistical tests and presentation. Statistical analyses should be completely summarized using brief but consistent language that will improve the reader's understanding of the analysis.

**19.1 The Manuscript: Presenting Study Design, Rationale, and Statistical Analysis.** Each portion of the manuscript should facilitate the reader's understanding of why and how the study was done and (1) clearly state a hypothesis or study question, (2) show that the methods adequately answer the research question and that the data were appropriately analyzed, (3) convince the reader that the results are valid and credible, and (4) place the implications of the research in context and show that the study limitations do not preclude interpretation of the results.

A *different font* is used in this chapter to denote words defined in the glossary (see 19.5, Glossary of Statistical Terms).

**19.1.1** **Abstract.** Many readers will read only the abstract of a research article, so it should include as precise a summary of the content as possible. In addition, because readers may decide to review the entire article based on information in the abstract, it should be well written and carefully constructed.

By imposing order on how material is presented, a structured abstract helps writers and readers systematically evaluate information. A structured abstract is one that contains specific subsections and headings.

- The structured abstract should enable the reader to quickly and easily identify the study type, hypothesis or question, and methods.[2]

- The study question or the hypothesis (objective) should be clearly stated (eg, "To determine whether enalapril reduces left ventricular mass . . . "); the study design, *population,* and setting from which the sample was drawn should be described; and the main outcome measures should be explained. The design or study type should be indicated (eg, randomized clinical trial, cohort study, meta-analysis).

- Study design and interventions should be specified.

- The results should include a brief description of the study participants or data included, and data should be presented in absolute numbers and some explanation of *effect size,* if appropriate, with *point estimates, confidence intervals,* and measures of statistical significance presented.

- The conclusions should follow from the results without overinterpreting the findings. A relevance statement should place the research findings in the context of the overall problem the research addresses and describe how the research findings might influence change or be used.

Abstracts are too brief for detailed explanation of statistical analyses, but a basic description may be appropriate (eg, "The screening test was validated by means of a *bootstrap method* and performance tested with a receiver operating characteristic curve.") (see 2.5, Abstract).

For clinical trials that have been registered in an appropriate public trial registry, the name of the registry and trial identification number should be provided at the end of the abstract (see 19.2, Randomized Clinical Trials).

The following is an example structured abstract for an observational study[3]:

> **Importance** The Third International Consensus Definitions Task Force defined sepsis as "life-threatening organ dysfunction due to a dysregulated host response to infection." The performance of clinical criteria for this sepsis definition is unknown.

**Objective** To determine the validity of clinical criteria to identify patients with suspected infection who are at risk for sepsis.

**Design, Setting, and Population** In a cohort study of 1.3 million electronic health record encounters from January 1, 2010, to December 31, 2012, at 12 hospitals in southwestern Pennsylvania, those with suspected infection in whom to compare criteria were identified. Confirmatory analyses were performed in 4 data sets of 706 399 out-of-hospital and hospital encounters at 165 US and non-US hospitals ranging from January 1, 2008, until December 31, 2013.

**Exposures** Sequential [Sepsis-related] Organ Failure Assessment (SOFA) score, systemic inflammatory response syndrome (SIRS) criteria, Logistic Organ Dysfunction System (LODS) score, and a new model derived using multivariable logistic regression in a split sample, the quick Sequential [Sepsis-related] Organ Failure Assessment (qSOFA) score (range, 0-3 points, with 1 point each for systolic hypotension [blood pressure ≤100 mm Hg], tachypnea [heart rate ≥22/min], or altered mentation).

**Main Outcomes and Measures** For construct validity, pairwise agreement was assessed. For predictive validity, the discrimination for outcomes (primary: in-hospital mortality; secondary: in-hospital mortality or intensive care unit [ICU] length of stay ≥3 days) more common in sepsis than uncomplicated infection was determined. Results were expressed as the fold change in outcome over deciles of baseline risk of death and area under the receiver operating characteristic curve (AUROC).

**Results** In the primary cohort, 148 907 encounters had suspected infection (n=74 453 derivation; n=74 454 validation) (mean [SD] age, 61 [19] years, 85 563 women [57%]) of whom 6347 (4%) died. Among ICU encounters in the validation cohort (n=7932 with suspected infection, of whom 1289 [16%] died), the predictive validity for in-hospital mortality was lower for SIRS (AUROC=0.64; 95% CI, 0.62-0.66) and qSOFA (AUROC=0.66; 95% CI, 0.64-0.68) vs SOFA (AUROC=0.74; 95% CI, 0.73-0.76; $P<.001$ for both) or LODS (AUROC=0.75; 95% CI, 0.73-0.76; $P<.001$ for both). Among non-ICU encounters in the validation cohort (n=66 522 with suspected infection, of whom 1886 [3%] died), qSOFA had predictive validity (AUROC=0.81; 95% CI, 0.80-0.82) that was greater than SOFA (AUROC=0.79; 95% CI, 0.78-0.80; $P<.001$) and SIRS (AUROC=0.76; 95% CI, 0.75-0.77; $P<.001$). Relative to qSOFA scores lower than 2, encounters with qSOFA scores of 2 or higher had a 3- to 14-fold increase in hospital mortality across baseline risk deciles. Findings were similar in external data sets and for the secondary outcome.

**Conclusions and Relevance** Among ICU encounters with suspected infection, the predictive validity for in-hospital mortality of SOFA was not significantly different than the more complex LODS but was statistically greater than SIRS and qSOFA, supporting its use in clinical criteria for sepsis. Among encounters with suspected infection outside the ICU, the predictive validity for in-hospital mortality of qSOFA was statistically greater than SOFA and SIRS, supporting its use as a prompt to consider possible sepsis.

From *JAMA*. 2016;315(8):762-774. doi:10.1001/jama.2016.0288

**19.1.2** **Introduction.** In the Introduction, briefly review the literature that documents the nature and importance of the research and rationale for the study. An extended full literature review belongs in the Discussion section. The study hypothesis or research question should be clearly stated in the last sentence(s) of the Introduction before the Methods section, preferably including the word *hypothesis* (or *question*). Introductions should be concise, generally 150 to 350 words, and should avoid reciting information about a topic that is generally known by readers (eg, "The incidences of obesity and diabetes are increasing in parallel throughout the world.").

Results or conclusions do not belong in the Introduction section of a manuscript.

**19.1.3** **Methods.** The Methods section should include enough information to enable a knowledgeable reader to replicate the study and, given the original data, verify the reported results. Analyses should follow the Enhancing the Quality and Transparency of Health Research (EQUATOR) Network reporting guidelines[4] and be consistent with the study protocol and statistical analysis plan or described as post hoc. Components should include as many of the following as are applicable to the study design:

- Study design (see 19.2, Randomized Clinical Trials; 19.3, Observational Studies; and 19.4, Significant Digits and Rounding Numbers).

- Year(s) (and exact dates, if appropriate) when the study was conducted or data were collected and when the data were analyzed.

- Disease or condition to be studied—how was it defined? State the specific case definition if there was one. If measurements were used to define cases, state what these were and what values were used to establish a diagnosis (eg, "Patients were diagnosed as having a myocardial infarction if their serum troponin level was more than 0.4 ng/mL.").

- Setting in which participants were studied (eg, community based, referral population, primary care clinic), as well as geographic location and, if applicable, name of institution(s).

- Type of research participants or other data studied. Who or what was eligible for inclusion in the study and who was excluded. Specify the *inclusion criteria* or *exclusion criteria*. If all participants were not included in each analysis, the reason for exclusions should be stated. If the methods or the results have been previously reported, provide citations for all reports or ensure that different reports of the same study can be easily identified (eg, by using a unique study name).

- For all studies (except meta-analyses), information about review and approval or waiver by institutional review board or ethics committee should be detailed when appropriate (see 5.8.1, Ethical Review of Studies and Informed Consent).

For studies that involve human participants, the method used to obtain informed consent should be reported, as well as whether consent was written or oral. Describe whether compensation or other incentives were provided to study participants.

- Intervention(s) or Exposure(s), including their duration. In general, sufficient detail should be provided to enable other investigators to replicate the interventions (including where to obtain the full study protocol) and to facilitate comparison with other studies. Treatments administered to or exposures experienced by control or comparison groups should also be described in detail.

- Ideally, there should be only 1 primary outcome *variable*, although on occasion there may be more than 1. All primary outcome variables should be specified. The primary outcome variable is the variable used to determine the study *sample* size. All other outcomes (such as prespecified secondary outcomes) and how they were measured should be described. The *reliability* of measures and whether investigators determining outcomes were *blinded* to which group received the intervention or underwent the exposure should also be provided. Because the terms *double-blinding* or *triple-blinding* have no specific definitions, authors should specifically identify each blinded group and how blinding was achieved (eg, when drugs are administered intravenously and the drugs have different colors, that the intravenous tubing was covered with foil).

- The Methods section should also describe what all the other variables were and how they were measured; for example, demographic variables and disease risk factors should be specified. These variables are often used to assess or adjust for *confounding* of the relationship or association between the *dependent variable* and *independent variables*. The unit of analysis should be explicitly stated.

- Preliminary analyses: if the study is a preliminary analysis of an ongoing study, the reason for publishing data before the end of the study should be clearly stated, along with information regarding whether and when the study is to be completed. Authors should indicate whether such analyses were preplanned at the time the study began.[5]

- Data to be analyzed in the study should be sufficiently described. For clinical trials, a data sharing statement is required. Data sharing statements can be provided for other study types as well (see 5.6.1.3, Data Sharing, Deposit, and Access Requirements of Journals).

- Sources of data not collected directly by the authors should be reported in the Methods section. For example, national census data may be used to calculate incidence rates. Database repositories or websites can be used to store or display data or information that could not be included in the manuscript, and they should be made publicly available, if possible. Information essential to the conduct of the study or its interpretation should be included in the manuscript. Authors should consider providing this information in an online supplement to the manuscript or depositing the relevant data in a publicly accessible repository (see 2.10.17, Additional Contributions).

▪ The end of the Methods section should include a Statistical Analysis subsection that describes all statistical methods, including procedures used for each analysis, all statistical tests used, and the statistical software, programs, modules, and versions of all these used to perform the statistical analysis. Define statistical terms, abbreviations, and symbols, if included. Tests used to calculate point estimates and CIs or other measures of variance should be described. The $\alpha$ level used to determine statistical significance should be specified, as should whether the tests were 1- or 2-sided. If analysis code is included, it should be placed in the online supplementary content.

The *power* of the study (which should have been calculated before the study was conducted to determine sample size) should be reported, as should assumptions made to calculate the study power. Data used to calculate power (eg, expected mean values for measurements and the SD) should be provided, along with a reference to prior publications relied on to make these assumptions. Authors should explicitly state why the minimal clinically important difference used for the study power calculation is assumed to be clinically relevant.

How and why data were transformed should be reported. Note that skewed data alone do not necessarily require transformation; transformation is usually required when the residual error is skewed. If *multiple comparisons* were performed, authors should specify how significance tests were adjusted to account for them. The exact steps used for developing models in *multivariable analysis* and pertinent references for statistical tests should also be specified. Detailed reporting of model fit statistics should be provided. In general, how well variation in the outcomes variable is explained by the model should be reported. Examples include reporting $R^2$ or pseudo-$R^2$ values ($R$ is italicized; see 21.9.4 Italics). Authors should list the assumptions underlying the use of all statistical tests and note how these assumptions were met. Test statistics should include *degrees of freedom* whenever applicable. It is always preferable for results to be presented in terms of *point estimates* and *confidence intervals*, which convey more information than do *P values* alone. Do not rely on hypothesis testing alone. If *P* values are to be reported for simple descriptive comparisons, the comparative data should always be reported along with the *P* values.

Procedures used for managing outliers, managing loss to or unavailability for follow-up, and modeling missing data should be specified. How outlying values were identified and treated should also be disclosed.

**19.1.4** **Results.** The Results section should begin with a brief description of the study participants or data assessed, with demographic information (eg, participants, mean [SD] age, and number [percentage] of female or male participants).

In the reporting of results, when possible, quantify findings and present them with appropriate indicators of measurement error or uncertainty, such as CIs. Authors should avoid relying solely on statistical hypothesis testing, such as the use of *P* values, which fails to convey important quantitative information. For most studies, *P* values should follow the reporting of comparisons of absolute numbers or rates and measures of uncertainty (eg, 0.8%, 95% CI, −0.2% to 1.8%; $P=.13$). *P* values should never be presented alone without the data that are being compared. If *P* values are reported, follow standard conventions for decimal places: for *P* values less than .001, report as $P < .001$; for *P* values between

.001 and .01, report the value to the nearest thousandth; for *P* values greater than or equal to .01, report the value to the nearest hundredth; and for *P* values greater than .99, report as *P* > .99. For studies with exponentially small *P* values (eg, genetic association studies), *P* values may be reported with exponents (eg, $P = 1 \times 10^{-5}$).

Authors should provide the numbers of observations in observational studies and the numbers randomized in randomized clinical trials. For randomized trials, provide the numbers randomly assigned. Losses to or unavailability for observation or follow-up should be reported. For multivariable models, all variables included in final models should be reported, as should model diagnostics and overall fit of the model when available.

Authors should avoid nontechnical uses of technical terms in statistics, such as *correlation, normal, predictor, random, sample, significant,* and *trend.* Inappropriate hedge terms, such as *marginal significance* or *trend toward significance,* for results that are not statistically significant should not be used. For observational studies, methods and results should be described in terms of association or correlation and should avoid cause-and-effect wording. Randomized trials may use terms such as *effect* and *causal relationship.* Also avoid uninformative modifiers of the strength of a finding, such as "strong association." If the association is statistically significant, use "significant association."

To give readers a sense of how the study population represents the overall population, the Results section should include the number of individuals (or other data units) initially screened for study inclusion, the number who were eligible for study entry, and the number who were excluded, had dropped out, or were lost to or unavailable for follow-up at each point in the study. For example, the JAMA Network journals require a figure that shows the flow of participants through clinical trials (see 19.2, Randomized Clinical Trials) or the studies included in a meta-analysis. The completeness of follow-up should be explicitly stated, as should the results of any missing data and outlier analysis. In general, multiple imputation is the preferred method for modeling missing data. Authors should provide a table of descriptive statistics about the sample and, if appropriate, the individual subgroups. Primary outcome measures should be discussed after the study population is described, followed by secondary outcome measures. Prespecified secondary outcomes should be reported after the primary outcome variable(s). If any prespecified outcomes are not being reported, explain why and if they have been or will be reported elsewhere.

*Post hoc analyses* may be presented, but they should be identified as such. Results of post hoc analyses may be unreliable, and thus such analyses should be used for generating rather than testing hypotheses (see *type I error*).

If 1 statistical test has been used throughout the manuscript, the test should be clearly stated in the Methods section. If more than 1 statistical test is used, the various statistical tests performed should be discussed in the Methods section and the specific test used reported along with the corresponding results. Tests of relative results (eg, *relative risk, odds ratio*) may overstate the real magnitude of differences between groups, particularly when absolute magnitudes are small. Thus, when presenting relative results, authors should also report an absolute difference along with a measure of the *central tendency* of the groups (eg, mean or median) and appropriate CIs.

Results should not be displayed only in a figure. Figures optimally display patterns and trends, but tables give exact values. Numerical results from a study's primary outcome variable and important secondary variables should be reported in a table, with the most important findings described in the text of the Results section.

**19.1.5** **Discussion.** Authors should address whether the hypothesis was supported or refuted by the study results or how the study question was answered. The study result should be placed in the context of published literature. The limitations of the study should be discussed, especially possible sources of *bias* and how these problems might affect conclusions and generalizability. Evidence to support or refute the problems introduced by the limitations should be provided. Sometimes, study limitations are presented in a separate subsection of the Discussion section. The implications for clinical practice, if any, and specific directions for future research may be offered (avoid generic uninformative recommendations, such as "future research is needed"; provide *specific* research recommendations). The conclusions should not go beyond the data and should be based on the study results and limited to the specific *population* represented by the study *sample*. The relevance for the findings as they pertain to clinical practice or the state of the science should be discussed.

One general approach to writing a Discussion section includes 7 parts:

1. Briefly summarize the study and the main results in a paragraph or two. Be sure to answer the research question posed in the introduction.

2. Interpret the results and suggest an explanation for them.

3. Describe how the results compare with what else is known about the problem; review the literature and put the results in context.

4. Suggest how the results might be generalized.

5. Discuss the implication of the results.

6. Under a separate subheading (Strengths and Limitations), describe the strengths and limitations of the study, their possible effects on the results, and, if possible, the steps taken to minimize their effects.

7. Under a separate subheading (Conclusions), report the conclusions.

**19.2** **Clinical Trials.** The International Committee of Medical Journal Editors (ICMJE) defines a clinical trial as "any research project that prospectively assigns human participants to intervention, with or without concurrent comparison or control groups, to study the relationship between a health-related intervention and a health outcome."[6] All clinical trials must be registered at an appropriate online public registry. Interventions include but are not limited to drugs, surgical procedures, devices, behavioral treatments, educational programs, dietary interventions, quality improvement interventions, process-of-care changes, and the like.

*Randomized clinical trials* (RCTs) generally yield the strongest inferences about the effects of medical treatments.[7,8] RCTs assess the efficacy of the treatment intervention in controlled, standardized, and highly monitored settings and usually among highly selected samples of patients. Thus, their results might not reflect the effects of the treatment in real-world settings or in other groups of individuals who were not enrolled in the trial. Treatment decisions will by necessity be made from a combination of information from RCTs and observational studies (see 19.3, Observational Studies).

As with any research, it is important to provide a detailed summary of an RCT's methods to facilitate a reader's understanding of the study's quality, replication of the study intervention, comparison of the study with other, similar studies, and the population to which the study relates. At a minimum, reports of RCTs should follow the CONSORT reporting guideline. The EQUATOR Network's CONSORT statement[9,10] has a checklist (**Table 19.2-1**) to facilitate complete reporting of RCT methods and results. The ICMJE recommends that authors complete the CONSORT checklist. Although completing the checklist does not guarantee that a study is high quality, it ensures that information critical to interpretation of the study and its limitations is accessible to readers, editors, and reviewers. The registration number should be reported in the manuscript's Abstract and/or Methods section. Journal editors may ask authors to provide a more detailed description of the study protocol. Many journals require that the original trial protocol and statistical analysis plan accompany the manuscript when it is submitted for publication. The ICMJE recommends that protocols be published with reports of clinical trials. For example, the JAMA Network journals and many journals publish trial protocols and statistical analysis plans in an online supplement to a published article.[11]

Reporting in the manuscript should be consistent with a prespecified outcome and prespecified analytic plan in the protocol and statistical analysis plan.

Flow diagrams provide an easy way for readers to understand how study participants flowed through the study, including when and why they dropped out or were lost to or unavailable for follow-up and how many participants were evaluated for the study end points. These diagrams are also useful for summarizing the sample selection process for both clinical studies and systematic reviews. Authors should include a flow diagram (typically as the first figure) in their manuscript, and, if the manuscript is accepted for publication, the CONSORT flow diagram (**Figure 19.2-1**) should be included in the published article (see 4.2.2, Diagrams). CONSORT is frequently updated to account for changes in how RCTs are performed.[10,12] Current information is available from the EQUATOR Network website.[4]

The report of an RCT should include a comparison of the participants' characteristics in the trial's different groups, usually as a table. Performing *significance* testing on the baseline differences between groups is controversial. Even with perfect random assignment, a mean of 1 in every 20 comparisons will appear to be "significant" at the .05 level by chance alone; such random findings illustrate the dangers of *post hoc analyses* (or ad hoc analyses). For this reason, reporting of statistical tests comparing the baseline characteristics of participants in RCTs is not recommended. Nevertheless, in randomized trials, baseline comparisons should be examined for statistical or clinical imbalances that may need to be addressed in the analysis.

In small studies, large differences may not be statistically significant because of small sample sizes and limited statistical *power*. Nonetheless, it may be helpful for authors to report statistical comparisons between groups. Such information should not be interpreted as a *null hypothesis* test of baseline differences between groups but rather as an estimate of the magnitude of any baseline differences that may cause difficulty in interpreting the intervention's true effect. These results should be

**Table 19.2-1.** CONSORT Checklist of Items to Include When Reporting a Randomized Trial[a]

| Section/topic | Item No. | Checklist item | Reported on page No. |
|---|---|---|---|
| **Title and abstract** | | | |
| | 1a | Identification as a randomized trial in the title | |
| | 1b | Structured summary of trial design, methods, results, and conclusions (for specific guidance see CONSORT for abstracts) | |
| **Introduction** | | | |
| Background and objectives | 2a | Scientific background and explanation of rationale | |
| | 2b | Specific objectives or hypotheses | |
| **Methods** | | | |
| Trial design | 3a | Description of trial design (such as parallel, factorial) including allocation ratio | |
| | 3b | Important changes to methods after trial commencement (such as eligibility criteria), with reasons | |
| Participants | 4a | Eligibility criteria for participants | |
| | 4b | Settings and locations where the data were collected | |
| Interventions | 5 | The interventions for each group with sufficient details to allow replication, including how and when they were actually administered | |
| Outcomes | 6a | Completely defined prespecified primary and secondary outcome measures, including how and when they were assessed | |
| | 6b | Any changes to trial outcomes after the trial commenced, with reasons | |
| Sample size | 7a | How sample size was determined | |
| | 7b | When applicable, explanation of any interim analyses and stopping guidelines | |
| Randomization | | | |
| Sequence generation | 8a | Method used to generate the random allocation sequence | |
| | 8b | Type of randomization; details of any restriction (such as blocking and block size) | |
| Allocation concealment mechanism | 9 | Mechanism used to implement the random allocation sequence (such as sequentially numbered containers), describing any steps taken to conceal the sequence until interventions were assigned | |
| Implementation | 10 | Who generated the random allocation sequence, who enrolled participants, and who assigned participants to interventions | |
| Blinding | 11a | If done, who was blinded after assignment to interventions (for example, participants, care providers, those assessing outcomes) and how | |
| | 11b | If relevant, description of the similarity of interventions | |

**Table 19.2-1.** CONSORT Checklist of Items to Include When Reporting a Randomized Trial (*continued*)

| Section/topic | Item No. | Checklist item | Reported on page No. |
|---|---|---|---|
| Statistical methods | 12a | Statistical methods used to compare groups for primary and secondary outcomes | |
| | 12b | Methods for additional analyses, such as subgroup analyses and adjusted analyses | |
| **Results** | | | |
| Participant flow (a diagram is strongly recommended) | 13a | For each group, the numbers of participants who were randomly assigned, received intended treatment, and were analyzed for the primary outcome | |
| | 13b | For each group, losses and exclusions after randomization, together with reasons | |
| Recruitment | 14a | Dates defining the periods of recruitment and follow-up | |
| | 14b | Why the trial ended or was stopped | |
| Baseline data | 15 | A table showing baseline demographic and clinical characteristics for each group | |
| Numbers analyzed | 16 | For each group, number of participants (denominator) included in each analysis and whether the analysis was by original assigned groups | |
| Outcomes and estimation | 17a | For each primary and secondary outcome, results for each group, and the estimated effect size and its precision (such as 95% confidence interval) | |
| | 17b | For binary outcomes, presentation of both absolute and relative effect sizes is recommended | |
| Ancillary analyses | 18 | Results of any other analyses performed, including subgroup analyses and adjusted analyses, distinguishing prespecified from exploratory | |
| Harms | 19 | All important harms or unintended effects in each group (for specific guidance see CONSORT for harms) | |
| **Discussion** | | | |
| Limitations | 20 | Trial limitations, addressing sources of potential bias, imprecision, and, if relevant, multiplicity of analyses | |
| Generalizability | 21 | Generalizability (external validity, applicability) of the trial findings | |
| Interpretation | 22 | Interpretation consistent with results, balancing benefits and harms, and considering other relevant evidence | |
| **Other information** | | | |
| Registration | 23 | Registration number and name of trial registry | |
| Protocol | 24 | Where the full trial protocol can be accessed, if available | |
| Funding | 25 | Sources of funding and other support (such as supply of drugs), role of funders | |

aFrom the JAMA Network Instructions for Authors.[11] Check the EQUATOR website for updates (http://www.equator-network.org/reporting-guidelines/consort/).

**Figure 19.2-1.** CONSORT Flow Diagram Showing the Progress of Patients Throughout the Trial

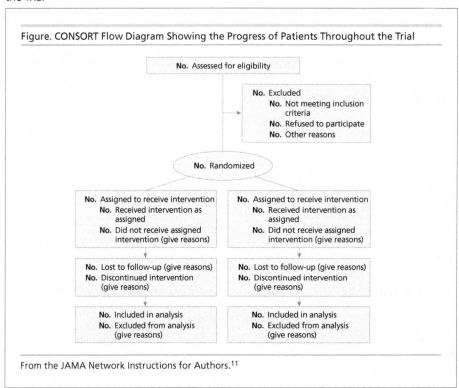

Figure. CONSORT Flow Diagram Showing the Progress of Patients Throughout the Trial

**No.** Assessed for eligibility

**No.** Excluded
 **No.** Not meeting inclusion criteria
 **No.** Refused to participate
 **No.** Other reasons

**No.** Randomized

**No.** Assigned to receive intervention
**No.** Received intervention as assigned
**No.** Did not receive assigned intervention (give reasons)

**No.** Assigned to receive intervention
**No.** Received intervention as assigned
**No.** Did not receive assigned intervention (give reasons)

**No.** Lost to follow-up (give reasons)
**No.** Discontinued intervention (give reasons)

**No.** Lost to follow-up (give reasons)
**No.** Discontinued intervention (give reasons)

**No.** Included in analysis
**No.** Excluded from analysis (give reasons)

**No.** Included in analysis
**No.** Excluded from analysis (give reasons)

From the JAMA Network Instructions for Authors.[11]

reported in a table or in running text. Information about baseline differences can help readers decide if the authors should have accounted for baseline differences in their statistical analysis of the prespecified outcomes.

*Intention-to-treat (ITT) analysis* is the preferred way to report randomized trial results.[13] Final results are based on analysis of data from all the participants who were originally randomly assigned, whether or not they completed the trial. Participants may have varying degrees of missing data, requiring some method for *imputation* to estimate the effect of missing results. Because patients in the standard treatment group of an ITT analysis may not adhere to the treatment regimen and have worse than expected outcomes, ITT analyses may overstate the equivalence of experimental conditions for noninferiority and equivalence trials.[13] *Noninferiority* and *equivalence trial* designs should report the outcomes for participants who completed the trial (known as per-protocol, as-treated analysis, or completers' analysis) (see 19.2.3, Equivalence Trials and Noninferiority Trials). A *per-protocol analysis* reports a study's results by the treatment received and not by the group into which the participants were randomly assigned. In general, per-protocol analyses are not advisable because the balance between groups achieved by random assignment may be lost (see 19.5, Glossary of Statistical Terms).

There is ongoing debate about when performance of an RCT may be unethical.[14,15] There is general agreement, however, that RCTs are unethical if the intervention is already known to be better than the control treatment received by the population under investigation, if there is an accepted standard of care that will not be provided to patients, or if participants could be unduly harmed by any condition in the experiment.

The decision to perform an interim analysis should be made before the study begins.[16] (Data and safety monitoring boards, however, may monitor adverse events continually throughout the study.) Investigators also usually define prospective *stopping rules* for such analyses; if the stopping rule is met, collection of additional data is not likely to change the interpretation of the study. If the criteria for the stopping rules have not been met, the results of interim analyses should not be reported unless the treatment has important adverse effects and reporting is necessary for patient safety. When a manuscript provides the results of an interim analysis, it should be clearly stated why the interim results are being reported. The a priori plans for an interim analysis and process for doing the interim analysis as described in the original study protocol should be reported in the manuscript. If the interim analysis deviates from the study protocol, the reasons for the change should be justified. If a manuscript reports the final results of a study for which an interim analysis was previously published, the reason for publishing both reports should be stated and the interim analysis referenced.

The *number needed to treat (NNT)* and *number needed to harm (NNH)* should be provided to make study results more accessible to clinicians and patients[7,8] (see 19.5, Glossary of Statistical Terms, for definitions of these terms). The NNT adds an easily understood perspective on the usefulness of a treatment by providing a number of patients who must receive treatment for 1 to benefit from it. Similarly, the NNH is the number of patients who will be exposed to a treatment or risk factor for 1 to be harmed by it.

*Publication bias* is the tendency of authors to submit and journals to preferentially publish studies with statistically significant results (see 19.3.6, Meta-analyses). To address the problem of publication bias, the ICMJE has required since July 1, 2005, that a clinical trial be registered in a public trials registry as a condition of publication.[6,17]

**19.2.1** **Parallel-Design, Double-blind Trials.** In parallel-design, double-blind trials, participants are assigned to only 1 treatment group of the study. These trials are generally designed to assess whether 1 or more treatments are more effective than the others. Participants and those administering the intervention should all be unaware of which intervention individual participants are receiving (double-blinding). Ideally, those rating the outcomes should also be blinded to treatment assignment (triple-blinding). Blinded parallel-design trials are often the optimal design to compare 2 or more types of drugs or other therapy because known and unknown potentially confounding factors should be randomly distributed between intervention and control groups. Reports of these types of trials should follow the CONSORT reporting guideline (http://www.equator-network.org/reporting-guidelines/consort/).[10] The CONSORT participant flow diagram should clearly indicate how many participants were assigned to each treatment group, how many were lost or unavailable at various stages of the trial, and the reasons that individuals did not complete the trial.[10] Methods of random assignment, allocation concealment, and assessment of the success of blinding should be reported. If there is no significant difference between groups, authors cannot claim that the treatments are equivalent; such a conclusion would require an equivalence or noninferiority trial design (see 19.2.3, Equivalence Trials and Noninferiority Trials). If the trial was not specifically designed as an equivalence trial, the absence of a difference between groups should be viewed as an inability to detect a difference, not as an indication that a difference does not exist.

**19.2.2 Crossover Trials.** In a *crossover* trial, participants receive more than 1 of the treatments under investigation, usually in a randomly determined sequence and with a prespecified amount of time (a *washout period*) between sequential treatments. The participants and the investigators are generally **blinded** to the treatment assignment (double-blinded). This experimental design is often used for evaluating drug treatments. Each participant serves as his or her own control, thereby eliminating variability when comparing treatment effects and reducing the sample size needed to detect a statistically *significant* effect. Most considerations of parallel-design randomized trials apply. Reports of these types of trials should follow the CONSORT reporting guideline (http://www.equator-network.org/reporting-guidelines/consort-within-person-randomised-trials/).[18] Rather than indicating which participants were assigned to which condition, the CONSORT participant flow diagram should indicate how many were assigned to each sequence of conditions (see Figure 4.2-22 in 4.2.2.1, Flowchart). Flow diagrams in the CONSORT recommendations are intended to be a flexible reporting device. The concept of flow diagrams (or visual summaries) are more important than using the exact diagram in the CONSORT statement.[19] Other information important to this study design includes possible carryover effects (ie, effect of intervention persists after completion of the intervention) and length of *washout period* (intervention effects should have ended completely before crossover to the other treatment). If the actual period of crossover differs from the original study protocol, how and why decisions were made to cross over to the alternate treatment and when the crossover occurred should be stated. The treatment sequence should be randomized to ensure that investigators remain blinded and that no systematic differences arise because of treatment order. Otherwise, unblinding is likely, treatment order may confound the analysis, and carryover effects will be more difficult to assess. If carryover effects are significant, or if a washout period with no treatment is undesirable or unethical, a parallel-group design (possibly with a larger sample size) may be necessary.

**19.2.3 Equivalence Trials and Noninferiority Trials.** It is sometimes desirable to compare a treatment or intervention that is already known to be effective with a treatment or intervention that is less expensive or has other advantages (eg, easier administration such as oral dosing).[20] In these cases, it would be unethical to expose participants to an inactive *placebo*. Thus, trial designs assess whether the treatment or intervention under study (the "new intervention") is the same as (for equivalence trials) and no worse than an existing alternative or "active control" (for noninferiority trials).[8,13,21-23] Reports of *equivalence trials* and *noninferiority trials* should follow the CONSORT reporting guideline (http://www.equator-network.org/reporting-guidelines/consort-non-inferiority/).[22]

In equivalence and noninferiority trials, authors must prespecify a margin of noninferiority (usually represent by the difference symbol Δ [delta]) within which the new intervention can be assumed to be no worse than the active control. There are a number of methods for arriving at the value Δ. Because different methods of estimating Δ may be more defensible in some situations than others, authors should provide clear explanations of their method and rationale for arriving at their value for Δ. Noninferiority trials test the 1-sided hypothesis that the effect of the new intervention is no more than Δ units less than the active control. Equivalence trials, which are less common than noninferiority trials, test the 2-sided hypothesis that the effect of the new treatment lies within the range of Δ to −Δ. For these trials, P values for noninferiority or P values for equivalence, respectively, should be calculated.

Although use of **ITT analysis** is optimal in trials that test whether one treatment is superior to another, use of such analysis can bias the results of equivalence and noninferiority trials. Analyzing a noninferiority trial by ITT could make an inferior treatment appear to be noninferior if poor patient adherence resulted in both treatments being similarly ineffective. Thus, when analyzing a noninferiority trial, both ITT and **per-protocol** analyses should be conducted. The results are most meaningful when both approaches demonstrate noninferiority.[21]

Interpretation of the results depends on the **confidence interval** for the difference between the new intervention and the active placebo, and whether this CI crosses Δ, −Δ, and 0. See the following examples and **Table 19.2-2**.[22,24]
Example for of how to report the results of an equivalence study:

> The event rate in the new treatment group was 37%, and the event rate in the standard treatment group was 42%, constituting a difference of 5% (95% CI, 2%-9%), which was within the equivalence margin of ±10%, meeting criteria for equivalence.

Example for how to report the results of a noninferiority study:

> The event rate in the new treatment group was 37%, and the event rate in the standard treatment group was 42%, constituting a difference of −5% (1-sided 97.5% CI, −infinity to 9%; P < .001 for noninferiority), which was within the noninferiority margin of 10%, meeting criteria for noninfinity.

**19.2.4** | **Cluster Trials.** *Cluster randomization* is undertaken when performance of the intervention risks contamination of the control group. Imagine a multifaceted intervention that involves sedation protocols and measures of arousal levels and readiness for weaning from a mechanical ventilator in a trial of extubation.[25] In this scenario, intensive care unit (ICU) personnel performing these functions may be influenced by the effectiveness of the interventions and consciously or unconsciously use them on patients assigned to the control group. In cases such as this, it is best to perform the intervention in one ICU and apply the control intervention in a separate ICU. Instead of randomizing individual patients to intervention or control groups, ICUs are randomized. Each ICU is considered a cluster of patients.

Cluster randomized trials cannot be truly blinded, so their use risks introduction of bias into the study.[26] They also violate one of the most important assumptions for most statistical tests: that the individuals in the study are independent of one another. For these reasons, studies using cluster techniques should specify why a cluster

**Table 19.2-2.** Checklist of Items for Reporting Noninferiority or Equivalence Trials (Additions or Modifications to the CONSORT Checklist Are Indicated in Footnotes)[a]

| Paper section and topic | Item No. | Noninferiority or equivalence trials |
|---|---|---|
| Title and abstract | 1[b] | How participants were allocated to interventions (eg, "random allocation," "randomized," or "randomly assigned"), specifying that the trial is a noninferiority or equivalence trial. |
| Introduction Background | 2[b] | Scientific background and explanation of rationale, including the rationale for using a noninferiority or equivalence design. |
| Methods Participants | 3[b] | Eligibility criteria for participants (details whether participants in the noninferiority or equivalence trial are similar to those in any trial[s] that established efficacy of the reference treatment) and the settings and locations where the data were collected. |
| Interventions | 4[b] | Precise details of the intervention intended for each group, detailing whether the reference treatment in the noninferiority or equivalence trial are identical (or very similar) to that in any trial(s) that established efficacy, and how and when they were actually administered. |
| Objectives | 5[b] | Specific objective and hypotheses, including the hypothesis concerning noninferiority or equivalence. |
| Outcomes | 6[b] | Clearly defined primary and secondary outcome measures, detailing whether the outcomes in the noninferiority or equivalence trial are identical (or very similar) to those in any trial(s) that established efficacy of the reference treatment and, when applicable, any methods used to enhance the quality of measurements (eg, multiple observations, training of assessors). |
| Sample size | 7[b] | How sample size was determined, detailing whether it was calculated using a noninferiority or equivalence criterion and specifying the margin of equivalence with the rationale for its choice. When applicable, explanation of any interim analysis and stopping rules (and whether related to a noninferiority or equivalence hypothesis). |
| Randomization Sequence generation | 8 | Method used to generate the random allocation sequence, including details of any restriction (eg, blocking, stratification). |
| Allocation concealment | 9 | Method used to implement the random allocation sequence (eg, numbered containers or central telephone), clarifying whether the sequence was concealed until interventions were assigned. |
| Implementation | 10 | Who generated the allocation sequence, who enrolled participants, and who assigned participants to their groups. |
| Blinding (masking) | 11 | Whether participants, those administering the interventions, and those assessing the outcomes were blinded to group assignment. When relevant, how the success of blinding was evaluated. |
| Statistical methods | 12[b] | Statistical methods used to compare groups for primary outcome(s), specifying whether a 1- or 2-sided confidence interval approach was used. Methods for additional analyses, such as subgroup analyses and adjusted analyses. |
| Results Participant flow | 13 | Flow of participants through each stage (a diagram is strongly recommended). Specifically, for each group report the numbers of participants randomly assigned, receiving intended treatment, completing the trial protocol, and analyzed for the primary outcome. Describe protocol deviations from trial as planned, together with reasons. |

**Table 19.2-2.** Checklist of Items for Reporting Noninferiority or Equivalence Trials (Additions or Modifications to the CONSORT Checklist Are Indicated in Footnotes) (*continued*)

| Paper section and topic | Item No. | Noninferiority or equivalence trials |
|---|---|---|
| Recruitment | 14 | Dates defining the periods of recruitment and follow-up. |
| Baseline data | 15 | Baseline demographic and clinical characteristics of each group. |
| Numbers analyzed | 16[a] | Number of participants (denominator) in each group included in each analysis and whether "intention-to-treat" and/or alternative analyses were conducted. State the results in absolute numbers when feasible (eg, 10 of 20, not 50%). |
| Outcomes and estimation | 17[a] | For each primary and secondary outcome, a summary of results for each group and the estimated effect size and its precision (eg, 95% CI). For the outcome(s) for which noninferiority or equivalence is hypothesized, a figure showing confidence intervals and margins of equivalence may be useful. |
| Ancillary analyses | 18 | Address multiplicity by reporting any other analyses performed, including subgroup analyses and adjusted analyses, indicating those prespecified and those exploratory. |
| Adverse events | 19 | All important adverse events or side effects in each intervention group. |
| Comment Interpretation | 20[a] | Interpretation of the results, taking into account the noninferiority or equivalence hypothesis and any other trial hypotheses, sources of potential bias or imprecision, and the dangers associated with multiplicity of analyses and outcomes. |
| Generalizability | 21 | Generalizability (external validity) of the trial findings. |
| Overall evidence | 22 | General interpretation of the results in the context of current evidence. |

[a]From the EQUATOR website.[22]
[b]Expansion of corresponding item on CONSORT checklist.[10,24] Authors should refer to specific CONSORT guidelines for reporting the design and results of equivalence and noninferiority trials.[4]

approach was used. They also should use analytic techniques that account for clustering, such as general estimating equations, mixed linear models, and hierarchical models. Studies that report the results of cluster randomized trials should explicitly state how clustering was accounted for in the statistical analysis.[26,27] The EQUATOR Network has guidance for the reporting of cluster trials, and reports of these types of trials should follow the CONSORT reporting guideline and its extension for cluster trials (http://www.equator-network.org/reporting-guidelines/consort-cluster/).[27]

Stepped-wedge cluster trials are a special class of cluster trials.[28] They are used when resources are limited and it is not feasible to apply an intervention at an individual patient level. Examples include a quality improvement intervention or implementation of a hospital-wide protocol, such as implementation of a new cleaning method. In a stepped-wedge design, all the clusters will eventually receive the intervention, and the randomization is based on the order in which clusters are entered into the study. Reports of these types of trials should follow the CONSORT reporting guideline and its extension for cluster trials (http://www.equator-network.org/reporting-guidelines/consort-cluster/) and adopt specific reporting elements for stepped-wedge designs.[27,29]

**19.2.5** **Nonrandomized Trials.** A *nonrandomized trial* prospectively assigns groups or populations to study the efficacy or effectiveness of an intervention but the assignment to the intervention occurs through self-selection or administrator selection rather than through randomization. Control groups can be historical, concurrent, or both. This design is sometimes called a quasi-experimental design. Reports of these trials should follow the Transparent Reporting of Evaluations With Nonrandomized Designs (TREND) reporting guideline (https://www.cdc.gov/trendstatement/).[30]

**19.3** **Observational Studies.** In an *observational study*, the researcher identifies a condition or outcome of interest and then measures factors that may be related to that outcome (**Table 19.3-1**). Although observational studies cannot lead to causal inferences, they may nonetheless generate hypotheses that may be tested (eg, if event A generally precedes event B, then it is possible that A may be responsible for causing B). Such studies may be either *retrospective* (the investigator tries to reconstruct what happened in the past) or *prospective* (the investigator identifies a group of individuals and then observes them for a specified period). Prospective studies generally yield more reliable conclusions than retrospective studies. Cause and effect cannot be established by observational studies; consequently, study findings from observational studies should not be presented using causal language. The term *association* should be used instead of causal terms, such as *effect* or *relationship*, when reporting and discussing variables in observational studies (see 2.1, Manuscript Preparation for Submission and Publication, Titles and Subtitles).

> Example: Change the title "*Effects* of Indulgent Descriptions on Vegetable Consumption" to "*Association* Between Indulgent Descriptions and Vegetable Consumption" because the study was an observational study and not a randomized trial.

Because individuals in observational studies are not randomly assigned to conditions, there are often large baseline differences between groups in such studies. For instance, individuals with better exercise habits often differ in several important ways (eg, educational level, income, diet, smoking) from those who do not exercise regularly. Because exercise and all these other factors influence health outcomes, exercise is *confounded* with these variables, and it is difficult to know whether exercise is responsible for any differences in health outcomes. Researchers may use several different statistical techniques to minimize the effects of confounding, including *matching*, *stratification*, *multivariable analysis*, *instrumental analysis*, and *propensity analysis*.

Even with the most extensive attempts to minimize confounding, it is always possible that results of observational studies may be attributable to variables that the authors did not measure. Because *residual confounding* is unavoidable in observational studies, findings from observational research are not as reliable as those from RCTs. Sometimes the results of observational studies may differ significantly from those of RCTs.[31] On the other hand, because observational studies are more often based on the outcomes of a large range of people in realistic situations, they may add useful insights to disease processes because they occur beyond the limited conditions of RCTs. Furthermore, observational studies may be the only

**Table 19.3-1.** Summary Description of Common Observational Study Designs

| Design | Brief description | Starting point | Assessment | Strengths | Weaknesses | Reporting guideline |
|---|---|---|---|---|---|---|
| Case-control | A case-control study, which is always retrospective, compares those who have had an outcome or event (cases) with those who have not (controls) | Outcome event status | Cohort | Overcomes temporal delays and the need for large sample sizes to accumulate rare events | Susceptible to recall bias | STROBE[32] |
| Case series | Case series describe characteristics of a group of patients or participants with a particular disease, disorder, signs, or symptoms or a group of patients or participants who have undergone a particular procedure or experienced a specific exposure or event | Consecutive series of patients or participants with similar characteristics receiving the same intervention or experiencing the same exposure | Characterizes a disease entity, treatment response, or exposure risk | Characterizes a disease or its treatment | Subject to selection bias if patients are not enrolled consecutively; no control group | Case series reporting guideline[33] |
| Cohort | A prospective cohort study follows a group, or cohort, of individuals who are initially free of the outcome of interest; a retrospective cohort study is a weaker design and investigators should be blinded to study outcomes when formulating the hypothesis and determining the dependent and independent variables | Exposure status | Outcome event status | Feasible when randomization of exposure not possible; generalizability | Susceptible to bias | STROBE[32] |
| Comparative effectiveness | Research attempting to understand how effective various interventions are when applied to patients in real-world settings | Groups of patients receiving different treatments | Treatment outcomes | Facilitates comparison of outcomes for different treatments of the same disease | Potential for selection bias | ISPOR[34] |

(continued)

**Table 19.3-1.** Summary Description of Common Observational Study Designs (*continued*)

| Design | Brief description | Starting point | Assessment | Strengths | Weaknesses | Reporting guideline |
|---|---|---|---|---|---|---|
| Cost-effectiveness analysis, cost-benefit analysis | Cost-effectiveness analysis determines all costs associated with an intervention relative to the benefits of that intervention; cost-benefit analysis determines the costs incurred to derive an effect of an intervention | Groups of patients receiving treatments | All costs associated with achieving the treatment outcomes | Facilitates awareness of the cost of treatments to achieve desired outcomes. This adds important context to clinical outcomes enabling clinicians to know if the costs associated with achieving those outcomes are worth it | Cost-effectiveness is an inherently subjective determination; how much should be expended to achieve a certain therapeutic goal is a matter of opinion; rarely do cost-effectiveness studies completely capture all costs associated with delivering an intervention | ISPOR RCT-CEA[35] |
| Cross-sectional | Examination of an entire population of participants at a single point in time or during a specific interval, in which exposure and outcome are ascertained simultaneously; study of groups or patients within the cross-section facilitates understanding of a risk factor's relationship with a disease | An entire population at one point in time | Presence of disease, disorder, or risk | Facilitates determination of the prevalence of disease, disorders, or risks; large samples of patients can be studied; can be used to examine the association between an exposure and disease when subpopulations are examined | Does not allow for observations at different times; length time bias: diseases with a long course will be overrepresented in the population at any given time | STROBE[32] |

| Design | Brief description | Starting point | Assessment | Strengths | Weaknesses | Reporting guideline |
|---|---|---|---|---|---|---|
| Diagnostic/ prognostic studies | Research describing the ability of diagnostic studies to confirm the presence of a disease; prognostic studies are those that examine the ability of some model to predict the presence or course of the disease | The point in the course of the disease where a test is obtained to establish a diagnosis; for prognostic studies, it is that point along the course of the disease where a prediction is made regarding some future outcome | Test the ability of a test to establish a diagnosis made by a reference standard; usually the sensitivity or specificity is used to determine how well the test performs; for prognostic models, various approaches are used such as the C index (area under the curve) or Akaike or Bayes Information Criteria; prognostic models should be validated in populations in which they will be used and should be different from the populations from which the models were derived | Diagnostic studies can be easily validated if high-quality references standards are available; prognostic studies are useful for counseling patients about risks of various outcomes given certain circumstances that, hopefully if modified, can result in better clinical outcomes | Many diagnostic studies have suboptimal sensitivity and specificity resulting in uncertain or inaccurate diagnoses; prognostic studies rarely account for all the factors that contribute to an outcome resulting in them being less than ideal for predicting outcomes in many circumstances | STARD,[36] TRIPOD[37] |
| Ecologic | Examine groups or populations of patients but not individual patients. Useful in understanding disease prevalence or incidence | Groups of people exposed to some factor | Outcome event status in the group | Facilitates analysis of large numbers of people. May uncover relationships between exposure factors and diseases. | Ecologic fallacy; group-level exposure and outcome may not relate well to individuals within that group; highly susceptible to bias | RECORD[38] |

*(continued)*

**Table 19.3-1.** Summary Description of Common Observational Study Designs (*continued*)

| Design | Brief description | Starting point | Assessment | Strengths | Weaknesses | Reporting guideline |
|---|---|---|---|---|---|---|
| Meta-analysis | Aggregation of results from similar studies to increase the power to make conclusions about the effectiveness of interventions | Published studies; the studies being compared should all begin at the same time point in a patient's course of disease or relative to when an intervention occurs | Summary point estimate for an effect of an intervention derived from several studies of that intervention; CIs should be included | Increases the ability to establish the efficacy of an effect when individual studies are too small to show that effect on their own | Methodology frequently abused; studies can only be aggregated if they have similar research designs and outcomes; conclusions may be misleading if the studies are heterogeneous | PRISMA,[39] MOOSE[40] |
| Qualitative research | Research about social interactions and personal experiences; intended to better understand people's perspectives about a topic | The time when someone experiences an event that the investigators want to better understand and how someone reacted to the event | Typically derived from interviews or surveys of individuals who were exposed to some intervention; these data cannot generally be assessed by statistical methodologies; they are summarized and reported as a subjective assessment of events. | Provides important information about how people perceive events/interventions, which may be as or more important than the physiological effects of the intervention | There may be incomplete reporting of key information; reporting of events might be biased by a person's perception of events | SRQR,[41] COREQ[42] |

| Design | Brief description | Starting point | Assessment | Strengths | Weaknesses | Reporting guideline |
|---|---|---|---|---|---|---|
| Quality improvement | Research on how systems works with the intent to improve their efficiency or safety | The time when an event occurs that the investigators want to study to improve processes that led to the event | Investigation of events occurring from some process is collected; this includes information about a particular scenario that is collected (medical record information, incident reports, interviews with participants, etc) and analyzed | When data are obtained from actual events, it may be high quality, actionable information facilitating interventions that can improve processes; the highest-quality information tends to be local and not multi-institutional | Findings may only relate to an individual institution or process and not generalizable to others; data obtained from administrative or other sources may not reliably represent the events being studied | SQUIRE[43] |
| Survey | A sample of a larger population is queried about a topic an investigator wants to understand about the larger population | The time when the survey is conducted or queries may be made about events that occurred in the past | Basic summary statistics of the answers acquired from the survey; population estimates with CIs representing the likelihood of the survey data being representative of the larger population are calculated | Obtain information from a large number of people, enhancing the generalizability of the findings; low cost to implement | Findings may be influenced by how questions are asked; difficult to get an adequate response rate to retain statistical validity; responders may be biased, resulting in their willingness to participate | AAPOR,[44] EQUATOR[45] |

way to investigate certain problems (eg, automobile crashes, exposure to toxic chemicals) for which it would be unethical to perform RCTs.

The EQUATOR Network's STROBE guidelines should be used to report most observational studies (http://www.equator-network.org/reporting-guidelines/strobe/)[32] (see 19.3.1, Cohort Studies).

**19.3.1** **Cohort Studies.** In a *cohort study*, a defined group of people (the cohort) is followed up over time to examine associations between different interventions and subsequent interventions. Cohort studies may be concurrent (prospective) or nonconcurrent (retrospective). A prospective cohort study follows up a group, or *cohort*, of individuals who are initially free of the outcome of interest. Individuals in a cohort generally share some underlying characteristic, such as age, sex, or exposure to a *risk factor*. Some studies may comprise several different cohorts. The study is usually conducted for a predetermined period, long enough for some members of the cohort to develop the outcome of interest. Individuals who developed the outcome are compared with those who did not. The report of the study should include a description of the cohort and the length of follow-up, what *independent variables* were measured and how, and what outcomes were measured and how. The number of individuals lost to or unavailable for follow-up and whether they differed from those with complete follow-up should also be included. All adverse events should be reported.

Any previous published reports of closely related studies from the same cohort should be cited in the text or should be clear from the study name (eg, the Framingham Study). All previous reports on the same or similar outcomes should be cited.

Retrospective cohort studies may be appropriate if investigators are blinded to study outcomes when formulating the *hypothesis* and determining the *dependent* and *independent variables*, but many of the strengths of prospective cohort studies are lost with retrospective studies, such as identifying the population to study and defining the variables and outcomes before the events occur.

Reports of cohort studies should follow the STROBE reporting guidelines (http://www.equator-network.org/reporting-guidelines/strobe/).[32]

**19.3.2** **Case-Control Studies.** *Case-control studies*, which are always retrospective, compare those who have had an outcome or event (*cases*) with those who have not (*controls*). Cases and controls are then evaluated for exposure to various *risk factors* and thus should not be selected on the basis of their exposure to the risk factors under investigation. Cases and controls generally are matched according to specific characteristics (eg, age, sex, duration of disease) to reduce *confounding* by these variables. However, if the matched variables are inextricably linked with the exposure of interest (not necessarily with the disease or outcome of interest), matching may confound the analysis (eg, matching on the consumption of cream substitutes instead of coffee drinking itself)[46] (see also *overmatching*). The *independent variable* is exposure to an item of interest (eg, a drug or disease). Information about the source of both cases and controls must be included, and *inclusion* and *exclusion criteria* must be listed for each. Cases and controls should be drawn from the same or similar *populations* to avoid *selection bias*. Pairs (1:1 match) or groups (eg, 1:2 or 1:3 match) of cases and controls may be matched on 1 or more variables. The analysis generally is unpaired, however, because of the difficulty in matching every important characteristic. Nonetheless, paired analysis reduces the necessary sample size to detect a difference and may be justified if individuals are well matched. *Recall bias* is common in all retrospective studies and is especially a concern when participants perceive that a factor related to the independent variable may be associated with the outcome. If recall bias may have occurred, the authors should discuss how they addressed this possibility.

In a *nested case-control study*, the cases and controls are drawn from some larger population or *cohort* that may have been convened for some other purpose. In these instances, authors should clearly indicate how the original sample was defined, the size of the original sample, and how the cases and controls were selected from it.

**19.3.3**    **Cross-sectional Studies.** *Cross-sectional studies* observe individuals at a single point or during a specific interval, in which exposure and outcome are ascertained simultaneously. Such studies may be helpful for suggesting associations among variables but cannot address whether one condition may precede or follow another. Thus, cross-sectional studies cannot establish *causation*, but they may nonetheless be helpful for suggesting hypotheses to guide more rigorous studies.

**Box 19.3-1.** Distinguishing Case Series From Cohort Studies

> It is common to confuse cohort and case series studies. For example, a study of 20 consecutive patients with a certain disease can be treated in 2 different ways. A study that divides the 20 patients into 2 groups according to the treatment received and compares the outcomes of these groups (eg, provides aggregated absolute risks per group or a risk ratio) would be probably classified as a cohort study. In contrast, a publication that describes the interventions received and outcomes for each patient/case separately would probably be classified as a case series.
>
> Summary of the distinction between cohort and case series studies proposed by Dekkers et al.[47]
>
> ---
>
> Cohort study: Patients are sampled on the basis of exposure. The occurrence of outcomes is assessed during a specified follow-up period.
>
> ---
>
> Case series: Patients with a particular disease or disease-related outcome are sampled. Case series exist in 2 types:
>
> ---
>
> 1. Sampling is based on a specific outcome and presence of a specific exposure.
>
> ---
>
> 2. Selection is based only on a specific outcome, and data are collected on previous exposures. Cases are reported regardless of whether they have specific exposures. This type of case series can be seen as the case group from a case-control study.
>
> ---
>
> Reports of case-control studies should follow the STROBE reporting guidelines (http://www.equator-network.org/reporting-guidelines/strobe/).[32]

**19.3.4** **Case Series.** In a *case series* study, observations are made on a series of individuals, before and after they have received the same intervention, exposure, or diagnosis but have no control group. Case series describe characteristics of a group of patients or participants with a particular disease, disorder, signs, or symptoms or a group of patients or participants who have undergone a particular procedure or experienced a specific exposure or event. A case series may also examine larger units, such as groups of hospitals or municipalities. Case series can be useful to formulate a case definition of a disease or describe the experience of an individual or institution in treating a disease or performing a type of procedure. Case series should comprise consecutive patients or observations seen by the individual or institution to minimize *selection bias*. Case series are not used to test a hypothesis because there is no comparison group. (Occasionally, comparisons are made with historical controls or published studies, but these comparisons are informal and should not include a formal statistical analysis.) A report of a case series should include the rationale for publishing the population described and inclusion and exclusion criteria. Case series are subject to several types of *biases*. Authors should be conservative regarding the conclusion drawn from case series analysis.

Box 19.3-1 describes how case series and cohort studies differ. A guideline for the appropriate reporting of uncontrolled case series is available and should be followed.[33]

**19.3.5** **Comparative Effectiveness Studies.** A *comparative effectiveness* study compares different interventions or strategies to prevent, diagnose, treat, and monitor health conditions to determine which work best for which patients and under what circumstances and which are associated with the greatest benefits and harms. Comparative effectiveness studies evaluate how effective existing therapies are in achieving various clinical outcomes. The outcomes may be tested by conducting RCTs or by observational analysis of existing data. Thus, from a study design perspective, they differ little from conventional studies of clinical efficacy.[48] The intent of comparative effectiveness studies is to inform patients, clinicians, and policy makers of the relative value of individual therapies when applied to certain groups of patients.[49]

Follow the International Society for Pharmacoeconomics and Outcomes Research (ISPOR) reporting guidelines for reports of comparative-effectiveness analyses.[34]

**19.3.6** **Meta-analyses.** A *meta-analysis* is a systematic, statistical pooling of the results of 2 or more similar studies to address a question of interest or hypothesis. According to Moher and Olkin,[50]

> [Meta-analyses] provide a systematic and explicit method for synthesizing evidence, a quantitative overall estimate (and CIs) derived from the individual studies, and early evidence as to the effectiveness of treatments, thus reducing the need for continued study. They also can address questions in specific subgroups that individual studies may not have examined.

A meta-analysis quantitatively summarizes the evidence regarding a treatment, procedure, or association. It is a more statistically powerful test of the null hypothesis than is provided by the separate studies themselves because the sample size is substantially larger than those in the individual studies.[51] However, as detailed herein, there are controversies associated with meta-analyses.[52-57] Meta-analyses of RCTs should follow the Preferred Reporting Items for Systematic Reviews and Meta-Analyses (PRISMA) reporting guidelines, and meta-analyses of observational studies should follow the Meta-analysis of Observational Studies in Epidemiology (MOOSE) reporting guidelines; both guidelines include recommendations for including flow diagrams and checklists.[39,40]

To ensure that a meta-analysis accurately reflects all the available evidence, the methods of identifying possible studies for inclusion should be explicitly stated (eg, literature search, reference search, contacting authors regarding other or unpublished work). Authors should state the dates covered by their search and the search terms used (see 21.9.4 Italics). A search strategy that includes several approaches to identify articles is preferable to a single database search.[58] Authors should make all attempts to include results of non–English-language articles. Collaborating with a medical librarian can greatly facilitate this process.[59]

Meta-analyses are considered observational such that causation cannot be implied from the results of a meta-analysis, including meta-analyses of RCTs; only associations among various risk factors, interventions, and outcomes can be determined. There are conflicting views on whether individual RCTs provide better evidence of the effect of treatments relative to a well-conducted meta-analysis. The statistical power of a meta-analysis is increased by aggregating results, but heterogeneity among studies can result in misleading conclusions, as can varying, subjective interpretations of study bias.[60,61] One particularly powerful method of aggregating data is to obtain original trial data on original patients from various studies and aggregate them into a single analysis: an individual patient meta-analysis. This requires use of reporting techniques that account for this type of study design: the PRISMA-IPD (individual patient data).[62,63]

*Publication bias*, or the tendency of authors and journals to publish articles with positive results, is a potential limitation of any systematic review of the literature.[64] Unpublished studies may be included in meta-analyses if they meet predefined inclusion criteria. One approach to addressing whether publication bias might affect the results is to define the number of negative studies that would be needed to change the results of a meta-analysis from positive to negative. Authors may also provide *funnel plots*, which can also reveal publication bias (see 4.2.1.12, Funnel Plot).

Other controversial issues include which study designs are acceptable for inclusion, whether and how studies should be rated for quality,[65] and whether and how to combine results from studies with disparate study characteristics. When data from the same study are reported in several publications, the various publications should be assessed to determine how to include the information in the meta-analysis. Options include linking information from several reports or assessing the individual reports to determine which should be included or not included in the meta-analysis.[66] Although few would disagree that meta-analysis of RCTs is most appropriate when possible, many topics include too few RCTs to permit meta-analysis or cannot be studied in a trial.

Gerbarg and Horwitz[67] have suggested that criteria for combining studies should be similar to those for multicenter trials and should include similar prognostic factors, which would justify combining them. Whether studies can be appropriately combined can be determined statistically by analyzing the degree of *heterogeneity* (ie, the variability in outcomes across studies). Assessment of heterogeneity includes examining the *effect size*, the sample size in each group, and whether the effect sizes from different studies are homogeneous. A commonly used test for the degree of heterogeneity is the *Cochran Q* statistic.[7] This is calculated by summing the squares of the difference between the mean effect size for all the studies and the square of the effect size of the individual studies. These differences are multiplied by the inverse of the variance of the individual studies to minimize the influence of small studies that will have a large variance. Conceptually, it is easier to understand the amount of heterogeneity by calculating the $I^2$ *statistic*, and the $I^2$ statistic is preferred because it focuses on the magnitude of variability rather than the statistical significance of the variability.[68] $I^2$ is calculated as follows: $I^2 = 100 \times (Q - df)/Q$. The *degrees of freedom*, *df* (see 21.9.4, Editing, Proofreading, Tagging, and Display, Specific Uses of Fonts and Styles, Italics), equal the number of included studies minus 1. Negative values of $I^2$ are considered equal to 0. $I^2$ ranges from 0 (no heterogeneity) to 1 (complete heterogeneity).

If statistically significant heterogeneity is found, then combining the studies into a single analysis may not be valid.[69] Another concern is the influence a small number of large trials may have on the results; large trials in a small pool of studies can dominate the analysis, and the meta-analysis may reflect little more than the individual large trial. In such cases, it may be appropriate to perform *sensitivity analyses* comparing results with and without inclusion of the large trial(s).

Meta-analyses are often analyzed by means of both *fixed-effects* and *random-effects models* to determine how different assumptions affect the results. An example of how results of a meta-analysis may be depicted graphically is shown in Figure 4.2-17 in 4.2.1.11, Forest Plots). The more conservative random-effects model is generally preferred.

A *network meta-analysis* provides a mechanism for assessment of the relative efficacy of an intervention compared with another, neither of which was directly tested against each other in clinical trials.[70] For example, a study might have compared drug A with placebo and a different study compared drug B with placebo. A network meta-analysis facilitates comparison of the relative efficacy of drug A with drug B.

A meta-analysis is useful only as long as it reflects current literature. Thus, a concern of meta-analysts and clinicians is that the meta-analysis should be updated as new studies are published. One international effort, the Cochrane Collaboration, publishes and frequently updates a large number of systematic reviews and meta-analyses on a variety of topics,[71] as does the US Preventive Services Task Force.[72]

**19.3.7** **Economic Analyses.** Although a treatment or screening technique may be proven effective in an RCT, it still may not be clinically useful. Some interventions are prohibitively expensive, may benefit only a small fraction of a population, or may lead to significant downstream costs that preclude short-term savings or benefits.

*Cost-effectiveness analyses* and *cost-benefit analyses* comprise a set of mathematical techniques to model these complex consequences of medical interventions.[73,74] A cost-effectiveness analysis "compares the net monetary costs of a health care intervention with some measure of clinical outcome or effectiveness such as mortality rates or life-years saved."[75] A cost-benefit analysis is similar but converts clinical measures of outcomes into monetary units, allowing both costs and benefits to be expressed on a single scale. This use of a common metric thus enables comparisons between different treatment or screening strategies.

The results of a cost-effectiveness analysis are usually expressed in terms of a cost-effectiveness ratio, for example, the cost per year of life gained. The use of *quality-adjusted life-years (QALYs)* or *disability-adjusted life-years (DALYs)* permits direct comparison of different types of interventions using the same measure for outcomes. The use of such composite measures allows researchers to weigh the relative benefits of length and quality of life.

The complexity of these analyses and the many decisions required when selecting data and choosing assumptions may be of particular concern when the analysis is performed by an investigator or company with financial interest in the treatment being evaluated.[76] Such analyses may have biases that are difficult to detect even with the most rigorous peer review process.[77]

One approach frequently used by cost-effectiveness analysts is to define a base case that represents the choices to be considered, perform an analysis for the base case, and then perform *sensitivity analyses* to determine how varying the data used and assumptions made for the base case affects the results. Sometimes authors test their conclusions by performing *bootstrap method* or *jackknife test* analyses. This involves taking a large number of repeated random samples from the data and then observing whether this procedure generally replicates the previous analytic conclusions. Several journals have published guidelines and approaches to cost-effectiveness analyses, but consensus has yet to emerge on their reporting[78-81] or interpretation.[74] Nonetheless, authors should clearly indicate all sources of data for both treatment effects and costs. Graphical approaches may help readers better understand the basic conclusions of the analysis.[73] The JAMA Network journals require authors of cost-effectiveness analyses and decision analyses to submit a copy of the decision tree comprising their model. Although this need not be included in the body of the published article, such information is necessary for reviewers and editors to assess the details of the model and its analysis.

Standards for reporting economic evaluations are available from the EQUATOR Network and are known as Consolidated Health Economic Evaluation Reporting Standards (CHEERS).[82]

**19.3.8** **Studies of Diagnostic and Prognostic Tests.** Diagnostic and prognostic studies are designed to develop, validate, or update the diagnostic or prognostic accuracy of a test or model. Correct treatment depends on accurate diagnosis. Diagnoses may be made based on a patient's history, physical signs or physical examination findings, or procedures such as blood tests and radiologic imaging. Few diagnostic tests, however, can be relied on to yield accurate diagnoses 100% of the time. Thus, it is important to study the performance of diagnostic tests.[83]

Studies to determine the diagnostic accuracy of a test are a vital part in this evaluation process. The EQUATOR Network recommends that authors use the Standards for Reporting of Diagnostic Accuracy (STARD) guideline or the Transparent Reporting of a Multivariable Prediction Model for Individual Prognosis or Diagnosis (TRIPOD) guideline for studies of diagnostic and prognostic tests.[36,37] As an example, The Rational Clinical Examination series in *JAMA* provides detailed information about the usefulness of many clinical findings and diagnostic tests and has information about how to best assess the utility of diagnostic tests.[84]

Studies of diagnostic and prognostic tests generally yield estimates of *likelihood ratios*, *sensitivity*, *specificity*, *positive predictive values*, and *negative predictive values*. Authors should report *confidence intervals* associated with these statistics. It is also common for these studies to report *receiver operating characteristic curves*, such as *area under the curve*.

Table 19.3-2 shows how aggregated diagnostic studies can be displayed.[85]

Receiver operating characteristic curves show the association between a test's cutoff point for being positive or negative and its sensitivity and specificity (**Figure 19.3-1**). The test's sensitivity (reflecting the true positive rate) is plotted against 1 − specificity (the false-positive rate). When results are pooled, these curves are generated by regression methods.

**19.3.9** **Survey Studies.** In a survey study, a representative sample of individuals is asked to describe their opinions, values, or behaviors.[87] For surveys of behavior (eg, diet, exercise, smoking), authors should provide evidence that the survey correlates with the actual, observed behaviors of a similar sample of individuals. That is, the survey should have been shown to have *validity*. If the survey instrument is different in any way from that given to the previous validation sample (eg, wording, order, omission of questions), then it may no longer be a valid measure of those behaviors.

For surveys, as for other studies, it is critical to provide detailed inclusion and exclusion criteria and describe how and when individuals no longer participated in the survey once they were initially identified. Flow diagrams can be a useful way of presenting this information. There is currently no standard reporting format for survey studies, however, and authors have usually reported no more than a single *response rate* for their survey. To address this situation, the American Association for Public Opinion Research (AAPOR) has published a set of expanded definitions.[44] The AAPOR document defines response rate as "the number of complete interviews with reporting units divided by the number of eligible reporting units in the sample." The document points out that this general definition allows for at least 6 different ways of actually computing this statistic, depending on how the numbers of "complete interviews" and the "number of eligible reporting units" are defined. There are also several ways to define cooperation rates (the proportion of all cases interviewed of all eligible units ever contacted), refusal rates (the proportion of all cases in which a housing unit or respondent refuses to do an interview), and contact rates (the proportion of all cases in which some responsible member of the housing unit was reached by the survey). Thus, authors should be clear about how they assigned individuals to categories and which categories they used to compute these statistics.

The AAPOR document defines specific reporting procedures for the 3 most common survey designs: random-digit-dial telephone surveys, in-person surveys, and mail surveys. The AAPOR recently reviewed online surveys and highlighted challenges posed by low response rates, systematic bias in responses (certain types of individuals may not have internet access), and respondents not paying careful attention to the questions.

**Table 19.3-2.** Accuracy of the White Blood Cell Count for the Diagnosis of Infectious Mononucleosis

| | No. of studies and reference No. | | Sensitivity (95% CI)[b] | Specificity (95% CI)[b] | Positive LR (95% CI)[b] | Negative LR (95% CI)[b] |
|---|---|---|---|---|---|---|
| | Only sensitivity[a] | Sensitivity and specificity | | | | |
| **Atypical lymphocytosis** | | | | | | |
| ≥40% | 0 | 1[22] | 0.25 (0.19-0.32) | 1.0 (0.98-1.0) | 50 (38-64) | 0.75 (0.68-0.81) |
| ≥20% | 0 | 1[22] | 0.56 (0.49-0.64) | 0.98 (0.94-0.99) | 26 (9.6-68) | 0.45 (0.38-0.53) |
| ≥10% | 0 | 3[23,24,26] | 0.66 (0.52-0.78) | 0.92 (0.71-0.98) | 11 (2.7-35)[c] | 0.37 (0.26-0.51)[d] |
| ≥50% Lymphocytes and ≥10% atypical lymphocytes | 0 | 3[22,23,26] | 0.43 (0.23-0.65) | 0.99 (0.92-1.0) | 54 (8.4-189)[e] | 0.58 (0.39-0.77)[f] |
| Lymphocytosis (≥4 × 10^9/L lymphocytes) by age group, y | 0 | 1[27] | 0.84 (0.71-0.93) | 0.94 (0.92-0.96) | 15 (11-21) | 0.17 (0.09-0.32) |
| ≥18 | 0 | 1[27] | 0.97 (0.82-0.99) | 0.96 (0.84-0.98) | 26 (17-42) | 0.04 (0.01-0.25) |
| <18 | 0 | 1[27] | 0.65 (0.43-0.84) | 0.88 (0.83-0.93) | 5.6 (3.4-9.2) | 0.39 (0.22-0.69) |
| **Ratio of lymphocytes to WBC count** | | | | | | |
| >0.50 | 0 | 4[23-26] | 0.55 (0.44-0.67) | 0.92 (0.81-0.97) | 8.5 (2.8-20)[g] | 0.49 (0.36-0.64)[g] |
| >0.45 | 0 | 1[25] | 0.65 (0.61-0.69) | 0.93 (0.90-0.95) | 9.3 (6.7-13) | 0.38 (0.33-0.43) |
| >0.40 | 0 | 1[25] | 0.74 (0.70-0.78) | 0.86 (0.83-0.89) | 5.3 (4.2-6.6) | 0.30 (0.26-0.35) |
| >0.35 | 0 | 1[25] | 0.84 (0.80-0.87) | 0.72 (0.68-0.76) | 3.0 (2.6-3.5) | 0.22 (0.18-0.27) |
| Monocytosis (>1 × 10^9/L monocytes) | 0 | 2[26,27] | 0.14-0.33 | 0.95-0.98 | 2.9-14 | 0.69-0.90 |
| Leukocytosis (>10 × 10^9/L WBC count) | 1[29] | 3[24,26,27] | 0.40 (0.28-0.53) | 0.87 (0.62-0.96) | 2.7 (1.2-5.7)[c] | 0.79 (0.73-0.85)[h] |

Abbreviations: LR, likelihood ratio; WBC, white blood cell.

[a]Some of the studies were case series and were not studies of diagnostic accuracy; therefore, the data could only be used to calculate sensitivity. Heterogeneity ($I^2$ statistic) is only reported for LRs when there are at least 3 studies providing data.

[b]If there are only data from a single study, the point estimate and a 95% CI are presented. If there are data from 2 studies, ranges are presented. For 3 studies, data from a univariate meta-analysis (calculated using data from Comprehensive Meta-Analysis) are presented. For 4 or more studies, data from a bivariate meta-analysis (using the metandi procedure in Stata version 13.1) are presented.

[c]$I^2$ = 88%.

[d]$I^2$ = 80%.

[e]$I^2$ = 71%.

[f]$I^2$ = 76%.

[g]$I^2$ = 100%.

[h]$I^2$ = 0%.

**Figure 19.3-1.** Receiver Operating Characteristic Curves

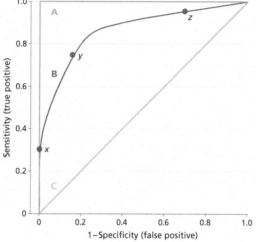

Figure. Receiver Operating Characteristic Curve and Area Under the Curve

Three hypothetical curves are shown. Curve A represents the discriminatory capacity of the ideal test. The test or model correctly identifies all patients experiencing an event without misclassifying any patients who do not experience an event (AUC = 1.0). Curve B shows a more typical curve of a potentially useful test. The model correctly classifies more patients with events than misclassifies patients without events (AUC = 0.8). Curve C shows a test that it is no better than chance. The model has similar chances of correctly classifying patients with vs patients without events (AUC = 0.5). Point x on curve B represents a model with a high threshold for a positive result (ie, requiring a high-risk score before predicting the patient will have an event) and no false-positive results; however, only 30% of those destined to have the event will be correctly identified. Point y represents an example of a model with increased sensitivity but at the cost of more false-positive results (sensitivity of 75%, 20% are false-positive results). Point z represents a model with a high sensitivity (95%) but with limited ability to identify patients who will not experience an event (70% are false-positive results). Reproduced from Alba et al.[86]

Survey studies may be longitudinal (the same respondents are surveyed at several time points) or cross-sectional. Causality may be cautiously inferred from longitudinal surveys but never from cross-sectional surveys. Case-control studies (see 19.3.2, Case-Control Studies) and cohort studies (see 19.3.1, Cohort Studies) may exclusively use survey methods to obtain their *dependent variables*, and thus in practice, the distinction between observational studies and survey studies may be nuanced.

As a general rule, survey response rates should exceed 60% to ensure an adequate sampling of the study population.[88]

**19.3.10** **Qualitative Research.** *Qualitative studies* are based on observations and interviews with individuals. Qualitative studies discover, interpret, and describe rather than test and evaluate. Mixed-methods studies are included in this category that combine quantitative and qualitative designs in a sequential or concurrent manner.

Qualitative studies should be reported using Standards for Reporting Qualitative Research (SRQR) reporting guidelines or Consolidated criteria for reporting qualitative research (COREQ) reporting guidelines.[41,42]

**19.3.11** **Quality Improvement Studies.** Quality improvement studies involve examination of health care systems and how specific changes in processes or procedures can improve the quality of health care delivery. These studies use methods that differ from other medically related studies, such as iterative changes using plan-do-study-act cycles in a single health care system, randomized trials (usually cluster randomized trials), and retrospective observational analyses of quality improvement interventions in various health care systems.

Standards for reporting quality improvement studies are available from the EQUATOR Network and are known as the Standards for Quality Improvement Reporting Excellence (SQUIRE).[43]

**19.3.12** **Ecologic Studies.** *Ecologic studies* examine groups or populations of patients but not the individuals themselves. They are useful for understanding disease prevalence or incidence and facilitating analysis of large numbers of people. These studies may uncover associations between exposure factors and diseases. Ecologic studies are limited by the *ecologic fallacy*. Group-level exposure and the outcome may not relate well to individuals within that group. These studies are highly susceptible to bias.

**19.3.13** **Mendelian Randomization Studies.** *Mendelian randomization* uses genetic variants to determine whether an observational association between a risk factor and an outcome is consistent with a potential causal effect.[90,91] Mendelian randomization relies on the natural, random assortment of genetic variants during meiosis, yielding a random distribution of genetic variants in a population. Individuals are naturally assigned at birth to inherit a genetic variant that affects a risk factor (eg, a gene variant that raises low-density lipoprotein cholesterol [LDL-C] levels) or not to inherit such a variant. Individuals who carry the variant and those who do not are then followed up for the development of an outcome of interest. Because these genetic variants may be unassociated with confounders, differences in the outcome between those who carry the variant and those who do not can be attributed to the difference in the risk factor. For example, a genetic variant associated with higher LDL-C levels that also is associated with a higher risk of coronary heart disease may provide supportive evidence to infer a potential causal effect of LDL-C on coronary heart disease.

Mendelian randomization rests on 3 assumptions: (1) the genetic variant is associated with the risk factor, (2) the genetic variant is not associated with confounders, and (3) the genetic variant influences the outcome only through the risk factor. The second and third assumptions are collectively known as independence from pleiotropy. *Pleiotropy* refers to a genetic variant that influences the outcome through pathways independent of the risk factor. The first assumption can be evaluated directly by examining the strength of association of the genetic variant with the risk factor. The second and third assumptions, however, cannot be empirically proven and require judgment by the investigators and the performance of various sensitivity analyses.

**19.3.14** **Mediation Analysis.** In studies that use *mediation analysis*, the relationship between intervention and outcome is partitioned into indirect and direct effects or associations. These relationships are often shown in a diagram[89] (see **Figure 19.3-2**). Mediation analysis can estimate indirect and direct relationships and the

**Figure 19.3-2.** Pathways of Relationships in a Mediation Analysis

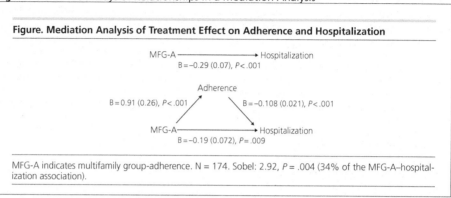

**Figure. Mediation Analysis of Treatment Effect on Adherence and Hospitalization**

MFG-A ⟶ Hospitalization
$B = -0.29\ (0.07),\ P < .001$

Adherence

$B = 0.91\ (0.26),\ P < .001$     $B = -0.108\ (0.021),\ P < .001$

MFG-A ⟶ Hospitalization
$B = -0.19\ (0.072),\ P = .009$

MFG-A indicates multifamily group-adherence. N = 174. Sobel: 2.92, $P = .004$ (34% of the MFG-A–hospitalization association).

proportion mediated, a statistical measure estimating how much of the total intervention works through a particular mediator.

The explicit objective of mediation analyses is to demonstrate potential causal relationships; however, this may not be possible and requires that specific assumptions be met. In a mediation analysis, the intervention-outcome, intervention-mediator, and mediator-outcome relationships must be unconfounded to permit valid causal inferences. In a randomized trial, participants are randomly assigned to intervention groups, so the intervention-outcome and intervention-mediator effects can be assumed to be unconfounded. However, trial participants are not usually randomly assigned to receive or not receive the mediator, so the mediator-outcome relationship may be confounded, even in randomized trials. To overcome this potential source of bias, investigators can control for known confounders of the mediator-outcome effect by using techniques such as regression adjustment. However, unmeasured confounding may still introduce bias even if known confounders have been adjusted for. Sensitivity analyses should be used to assess the potential bias caused by unmeasured confounding in mediation analyses. The risk of confounding in mediation analyses is greater in observational studies than in randomized trials, and in these cases, caution is required when interpreting findings and is best reported as interpreting estimates of indirect and direct associations.[89]

**19.4**     **Significant Digits and Rounding Numbers.** When numbers are expressed in scientific and biomedical articles, they should reflect the degree of accuracy of the original measurement. Numbers obtained from mathematical calculations should be rounded to reflect the original degree of precision.

**19.4.1**     **Significant Digits.** The use of a numeral in a numbers column (eg, the ones column, the tens column) implies that the method of measurement is accurate to that level of precision. For example, when a reporter attempts to estimate the size of a crowd, the estimate might be to the nearest tens of number of people but would not be expressed as an exact number, such as 86, unless each individual was counted. Similarly, when an author provides a number with numerals to the right of the decimal point, the numerals imply that the measurement used to obtain the number is accurate to the last place a numeral is shown. Therefore, numbers should be rounded to reflect the precision of the instrument or measurement; for example, for a scale accurate to 0.1 kg, a weight should be expressed as 75.2 kg, not 75.23 kg. Similarly, the instrument used to measure a concentration is accurate only to a given fraction of the concentration, for example, 15.6 mg/L, not 15.638 mg/L (see Table 17.5-2 in 17.5.10, Laboratory Values, for the appropriate number of significant digits). Numbers that result from calculations, such as means and SDs, should be expressed to no more than 1 significant digit beyond the accuracy of the instrument. Thus, the mean (SD) of weights of individuals weighed on a scale accurate to 0.1 kg should be expressed as 62.45 (4.13) kg. Adult age is reported rounded to 1-year increments (eg, 52 years), so the mean could be expressed as, for example, 47.7 years.

*Odds ratios*, *risk ratios*, *hazard ratios*, and 95% CIs should have significant digits extending to the one hundredths place (eg, 1.01, 5.26, 9.85, 0.15). Numbers extending beyond the one hundredth place should be rounded.

**19.4.2** **Rounding.** The digits to the right of the last significant digit are rounded up or down. If the digit to the right of the last significant digit is less than 5, the last significant digit is not changed. If the digit is greater than 5, the last significant digit is rounded up to the next higher digit. (For example, 47.746 years is rounded to 47.7 years and 47.763 years is rounded to 47.8 years.) If the digit immediately to the right of the last significant digit is 5, with either no digits or all zeros after the 5, the last significant digit is rounded up if it is odd and not changed if it is even. For example, 47.7500 would become 47.8; 47.65 would become 47.6. If the digit to the right of the last significant digit is 5 followed by any number other than 0, the last significant digit is rounded up (47.6501 would become 47.7).

*P* values and other statistical expressions raise particular issues about rounding. For more information about how and why to round *P* values and other statistical terms, see ***P value*** in 19.5, Glossary of Statistical Terms. Briefly, *P* values should be expressed to 2 digits to the right of the decimal point (regardless of whether the *P* value is significant), unless *P* < .01, in which case the *P* value should be expressed to 3 digits to the right of the decimal point. (One exception to this rule is when rounding *P* from 3 digits to 2 digits would result in *P* appearing nonsignificant, such as *P* = .046. In this case, expressing the *P* value to 3 places is preferred. The same holds true for rounding CIs that are significant before rounding but nonsignificant after rounding.) The smallest *P* value that should be expressed is *P* <.001 because additional zeros do not convey useful information.[92] *P* values are expressed without a 0 preceding the decimal point.

*P* values may be expressed to more than 3 decimal places in genome-wide association and other genetics studies (eg, *P* = $1 \times 10^{-5}$), studies that involve the Bonferroni correction (eg, A Bonferroni-corrected significance threshold of .0083 was used to account for . . . ), and other types of studies with adjustments for ***multiple comparisons***, and when the level of significance in a study is defined as a small number much less than *P* < .05.

*P* values should never be rounded up to 1.0 or down to 0; rather, the *P* value should be expressed as *P* > .99 or *P* < .001, respectively. Although such a procedure might be justified arithmetically, the results are misleading. *P* values may approach infinitely close to these upper and lower bounds but never close enough to establish that the associated observation was absolutely predestined (*P* = 1.0) or absolutely impossible (*P* = 0) to occur because the value represents a probability.

See also 19.1.4, Results.

**19.5**    **Glossary of Statistical Terms.** In the glossary that follows, terms defined elsewhere in the glossary are displayed in *boldface and italic font*. An arrow ($\rightarrow$) indicates points to consider in addition to the definition. For detailed discussion of these terms, the referenced texts and the additional reading at the end of the chapter are useful sources.

Eponymous names for statistical procedures often differ from one text to another (eg, the Newman-Keuls and Student-Newman-Keuls test). The names provided in this glossary follow the *Dictionary of Statistical Terms*,[93] published for the International Statistical Institute. Although some statistical texts use the possessive form for most eponyms, the possessive form for eponyms is not recommended in AMA style (see 15.0, Eponyms).

Most statistical tests are applicable only under specific circumstances, which are generally dictated by the scale properties of both the independent variable and dependent variable. **Table 19.5-1** presents a guide to selection of commonly used statistical techniques. This table is not meant to be exhaustive but rather to indicate the appropriate applications of commonly used statistical techniques.

**abscissa:** horizontal or *x-axis* of a graph. The *y-axis* is referred to as the *ordinate*.

**absolute difference:** the difference between an event rate before an intervention and the event rate after the intervention. For example, if the influenza rate in a population is 20% before a vaccination program is implemented and it decreases to 15% after the program is initiated, the absolute difference is 5%. Absolute differences are subtracted numbers, whereas *relative differences* are fractions. Absolute differences are useful because they provide the absolute magnitude of

**Table 19.5-1.** Selection of Commonly Used Statistical Techniques[a]

| | Scale of measurement | | |
|---|---|---|---|
| | Interval[b] | Ordinal | Nominal[c] |
| 2 Treatment groups | Unpaired *t* test | Mann-Whitney rank sum test | $\chi^2$ Analysis-of-contingency table; Fisher exact test if <5 in any cell |
| ≥3 Treatment groups | Analysis of variance | Kruskal-Wallis statistic | $\chi^2$ Analysis-of-contingency table; Fisher exact test if <5 in any cell |
| Before and after treatment in same individual | Paired *t* test | Wilcoxon signed rank test | McNemar test |
| Multiple treatments in same individual | Repeated-measures analysis of variance | Friedman statistic | Cochran *Q* |
| Association between 2 variables | Linear regression and Pearson product moment correlation | Spearman rank correlation | Contingency coefficients |

[a]Adapted with permission from *Primer of Biostatistics*.[94] ©McGraw-Hill.
[b]Assumes normally distributed data. If data are not normally distributed, then rank the observations and use the methods for data measured on an ordinal scale.
[c]For a nominal dependent variable that is time dependent (such as mortality over time), use life-table analysis for nominal independent variables and Cox proportional hazards regression for continuous and/or nominal independent variables.

an effect, whereas small absolute differences can appear to be very large when expressed as relative differences. The inverse of the absolute difference is the *number needed to treat*.

**absolute risk:** probability of an event occurring during a specified period. The absolute risk equals the *relative risk* times the average probability of the event during the same time, if the *risk factor* is absent.[95] See *absolute risk reduction*.

**absolute risk reduction (ARR):** proportion in the control group experiencing an event minus the proportion in the intervention group experiencing an event. The inverse of the absolute risk reduction is the *number needed to treat*. See *absolute risk*.

**accuracy:** ability of a test to produce results that are close to the true measure of the phenomenon.[95] Generally, assessing accuracy of a test requires that there be a *criterion standard* (or reference standard) with which to compare the test results. Accuracy encompasses a number of measures, including *reliability*, *validity*, and lack of *bias*. *Accuracy* should be distinguished from *precision*, which refers to the variability or how close together successive measurements of the same phenomenon are.[96]

**actuarial life-table method:** see *life table*, *Cutler-Ederer method*.

**adjustment:** statistical techniques used after the collection of data to adjust for the effect of known or potential *confounding variables*.[95] A typical example is adjusting a result for the independent effect of age of the participants (age is an *independent variable*). In this case, adjustment has the effect of holding age constant. Some outcomes may be age dependent, but statistical adjustment yields a result that would occur if the age effect were not present. Typically, this is performed by including the variable to be adjusted as an independent variable in a regression procedure.

**aggregate data:** data accumulated from disparate sources.

**agreement:** statistical test performed to determine the equivalence of the results obtained by 2 tests when one test is compared with another (one of which is usually but not always a *criterion standard* [or reference standard]). Agreement also occurs in studies where evaluators provide judgments of, say, medical images (radiographs, slides). A measure of agreement, such as the κ statistic or concordance, should also be provided in such situations.

→ Agreement should not be confused with *correlation*. Correlation is used to test the degree to which changes in a variable are related to changes in another variable, whereas agreement tests whether 2 variables are equivalent. For example, an investigator compares results obtained by 2 methods of measuring hematocrit. Method A gives a result that is always exactly twice that of method B. The correlation between A and B is perfect because A is always twice B, but the agreement is poor; method A is not equivalent to method B. One appropriate way to assess agreement has been described by Bland and Altman[97] (see *Bland-Altman plot*).

**Akaike information criterion (AIC):** Method for determining which of various models best fits an observed data set. Used for models fit by maximum likelihood. The likelihood function is penalized by the number of parameters fit to account for the fact that any model will fit better if it has more parameters.

→ *L* is the maximum value of the model's **likelihood function** and *k* is the number of parameters estimated. When fitting several models, the model that fits best has the lowest AIC. Used in conjunction with the Bayes information criteria (BIC). These criteria are among the preferred ways to establish which model fits the data best when fit by maximum likelihood methods.

**algorithm:** systematic process performed in an ordered, typically branching sequence of steps; each step depends on the outcome of the previous step.[98] An algorithm may be used clinically to guide treatment decisions for an individual patient on the basis of the patient's clinical outcome or result.

**α (alpha), α level:** the threshold for statistical significance. It is the size of the likelihood acceptable to the investigators that an association observed between 2 variables is due to chance (the probability of a *type I error*); usually $\alpha = .05$. If $\alpha = .05$, $P < .05$ will be considered significant. When presenting α levels, do not include zero before the decimal point (but see *Cronbach α*).

**analysis of covariance (ANCOVA):** statistical test used to examine data that include both *continuous* and *nominal independent variables* and a continuous *dependent variable*. It is basically a hybrid of *multiple regression* (used for continuous independent variables) and *analysis of variance* (used for nominal independent variables).[95] In general, when analyzing a change of some factor when compared with a baseline value, it is better to use ANCOVA than report the outcome as the subtracted value of the outcome-baseline value because regression to the mean occurs for baseline values that are too high or low. ANCOVA provides a better mechanism when baseline differences exist in the experimental subjects.[99]

**analysis of variance (ANOVA):** statistical method used to compare a *continuous dependent variable* and more than 1 *nominal independent variable*. When *multiple comparisons* between groups is necessary, ANOVA avoids problems inherent in using *t tests* for *multiple comparisons* of independent observations. The null hypothesis for ANOVA is that there are no differences in the means between any groups within a sample that is studied. This hypothesis is tested by calculating the variance between the means of the groups and dividing it by the variance of the total population. Because only 1 hypothesis is tested (ie, that there are no differences between any of the group's mean values), the problem of repeated testing is avoided. The greater the differences between the means of the groups, the larger the variance will be between the groups, resulting in a larger ratio. The *null hypothesis* in ANOVA is tested by means of the *F test*. In ANOVA, the null hypothesis only tests that there are no differences between any mean values of the groups tested. If a significant difference is found by *F* testing, contrasts or *multiple comparison* testing procedures are required to know which of the groups differ.

In 1-way ANOVA, there is a single *nominal independent variable* with 2 or more levels (eg, age categorized into strata of 20-39 years, 40-59 years, and ≥60 years). When there are only 2 mutually exclusive categories for the nominal independent variable (eg, male or female), the 1-way ANOVA is equivalent to the *t test*.

A 2-way ANOVA is used if there are 2 independent variables (eg, age strata and sex), a 3-way ANOVA if there are 3 independent variables, and so on. If more than 1 independent variable is analyzed, the process is called *factorial ANOVA*, which assesses the *main effects* of the independent variables as well as their *interactions*.

For example, if the effect of age category and sex on systolic blood pressure (SBP) is tested, the independent effect of age categories on SBP and those for sex can be tested as *main effects*. An *interaction* exists when the effect of combined groups is larger than the sum of the effect of both groups. In a factorial 3-way ANOVA with independent variables *A*, *B*, and *C*, there is one 3-way interaction term (*A* × *B* × *C*), 3 different 2-way interaction terms (*A* × *B*, *A* × *C*, and *B* × *C*), and 3 main effect terms (*A*, *B*, and *C*). A separate *F* test must be computed for each different main effect and interaction term.

If *repeated measures* are made on an individual (such as measuring blood pressure over time), a statistical method should be used that does not depend on complete independence of samples (because serial measurement from the same individual are not statistically independent from one another) and capitalizes on the fact that the measures are from the same individual. This is accomplished by use of repeated-measures *ANOVA*, which has the added benefit of facilitating control for confounding factors (such as age or socioeconomic status). Randomized-block ANOVA is used if treatments are assigned by means of *block randomization*.[95,100]

→ An ANOVA can establish only whether a significant difference exists among groups, not which groups are significantly different from each other. If hypotheses are generated before the experiment is performed about which groups might differ, ANOVA can be performed together with contrasts to establish if significant differences exist between individual groups. If hypotheses were not established before the experiment, the statistical significance of group differences can be determined by a pairwise analysis of variables by the *Newman-Keuls test* or *Tukey test* or one of several other tests. These *multiple comparison procedures* avoid the potential of a *type I error* that might occur if the *t* test were applied at this stage.

Multiple comparison tests explore what groups are significantly different from the others after an ANOVA has found a significant *F* test result. They either test for differences between all possible pairs of subgroups (*t*, Duncan, Student-Newman-Keuls, Tukey-Kramer, Bonferroni, etc) or between a control and all the remaining groups (*t*, Dunnett, Bonferroni, etc).

→ The *F* ratio of ANOVA is the ratio of the variance observed between the group means and the variance of the entire population and is a number between 0 and infinity. The *F* ratio is compared with tables of the *F distribution*, taking into account the $\alpha$ *level* and *degrees of freedom (df)* for the numerator and denominator, to determine the *P* value.

> *Example:* The difference was found to be significant by 1-way ANOVA ($F_{2,63} = 61.07$; $P < .001$).[100]

The *df*s are provided along with the *F* statistic. The first subscript (2) is the *df* for the numerator; the second subscript (63) is the *df* for the denominator. The *P* value can be obtained from an *F* statistic table that provides the *P* value that corresponds to a given *F* and *df*. In practice, however, the *P* value is generally calculated by a computerized *algorithm*. A statistically significant ANOVA test means only that there is a difference between some of the groups included in the analysis. It does not determine which groups are significantly different from each other; to find out, a *multiple comparisons procedure* must be performed.[100] Other models, such as *Latin square*, may also be used.

**ANCOVA:** see *analysis of covariance*.

**ANOVA:** see *analysis of variance*.

**Ansari-Bradley dispersion test:** rank test to determine whether 2 distributions known to be of identical shape (but not necessarily of *normal distribution*) have equal *parameters* of scale.[101]

**area under the curve (AUC):** technique used to measure the performance of a test plotted on a *receiver operating characteristic (ROC) curve* to assess the integrated response of a hormone's release, such as insulin during a glucose tolerance test, or to measure drug clearance in pharmacokinetic studies.[98] See also *receiver operating characteristic (ROC) curve*.

When measuring hormone release or drug clearance, the AUC assesses the total release of a hormone or exposure of an individual to the drug as measured by levels in blood or urine over time. The AUC is also used to calculate the drug's half-life.

→ The method used to determine the AUC should be specified (eg, the trapezoidal rule).

**artifact:** Something measured in a study that is not really present but results from the way the study was conducted.[95]

> *Example:* The hemoglobin level of 4.0 g/d was incorrect because the blood was drawn from just above the patient's intravenous catheter.

**assessment:** in the statistical sense, evaluating the outcome(s) of the *study* and *control groups*.

**assignment:** process of distributing individuals to study and control groups. See also *randomization*.

**association:** statistically significant relationship between 2 variables in which one does not necessarily cause the other. When 2 variables are measured simultaneously, association rather than *causation* generally is all that can be determined.

> *Example:* After confounding factors were controlled for by means of multivariate regression, a significant association remained between age and disease prevalence. However, these methods do not allow one to conclude that age causes differences in disease prevalence.

**as-treated analysis:** see *per-protocol analysis*

**attributable risk:** the difference in the rate of disease when a *risk factor* is present from what the disease rate is when the risk factor is absent. It is the amount of disease attributable to the risk factor.[95] Attributable risk assumes a causal relationship (ie, the factor to be eliminated is a cause of the disease and not merely associated with the disease). See *attributable risk percentage* and *attributable risk reduction*.

**attributable risk percentage:** the percentage of risk associated with a given *risk factor*.[95] For example, risk of stroke in an older person who smokes and has hypertension and no other risk factors can be divided among the risks attributable to smoking, hypertension, and age. Attributable risk percentage is often determined for a *population* and is the percentage of the disease related to the risk factor. See *population attributable risk percentage*.

**attributable risk reduction:** the number of events that can be prevented by eliminating a particular *risk factor* from the *population*. Attributable risk reduction is a function of 2 factors: the strength of the *association* between the risk factor and the disease (ie, how often the risk factor causes the disease) and the frequency of the risk factor in the *population* (ie, a common risk factor may have a lower attributable risk in an individual than a less common risk factor but could have a higher attributable risk reduction because of the risk factor's high prevalence in the *population*). Attributable risk reduction is a useful concept for public health decisions. See also *attributable risk*.

**average:** the arithmetic mean; one measure of the *central tendency* of a collection of measurements. The word *average* is often used synonymously with *mean* but can also imply the *median*, *mode*, or some other statistic. Thus, the word *average* should generally be avoided in favor of a more precise term.

**Bayes information criteria (BIC):** see *Akaike information criteria (AIC)*. Like the AIC, the BIC is a means for determining which of several models best fit data using maximum likelihood analysis. It penalizes the result more than the AIC does to lessen the influence of overfitting.

$$BIC = \ln(n) \times k - 2 \ln(L)$$

where $n$ indicates the number of data points; $k$, the number of parameters; and $L$, the maximum likelihood function for the model. The model with the lowest AIC or BIC should be selected as the best-fitting model.

**bayesian analysis:** a statistical method that uses prior knowledge combined with new data to obtain a new probability. The general approach assumes that something is known about what is being assessed before any tests are performed. For example, the prevalence of HIV in intravenous drug abusers enrolled in treatment programs is 8%.[102] When testing for HIV in such a patient, the *prior probability* of having a positive HIV test result is 8% because it is known that 8% of that population of patients has the disease. A positive or negative HIV test result will either increase or decrease the 8% likelihood of having HIV, resulting in a new probability called the *posterior probability*.

**β (beta), β error or type II error:** probability of showing no significant difference when a true difference exists; a false acceptance of the *null hypothesis*.[98] One minus β is the statistical *power* of a test to detect a true difference between groups; a value of .20 for β is equal to .80 or 80% power. The test has an 80% probability of detecting a difference between groups if one exists. A β of .10 or .20 is most frequently used in power calculations. Power is important when no difference is found between groups after an intervention. If the power is low, then there is the possibility that a true difference exists but that the tests performed could not detect the difference. When the power is high (usually resulting from a large sample size) and no difference between groups is found, there is greater confidence in concluding that no difference actually exists between the groups. The β error is synonymous with *type II error*.[100]

**bias (or systematic error):** a systematic situation or condition that causes a result to depart from the true value in a consistent direction. Bias refers to defects in study design (often *selection bias*) or measurement.[95] One method to reduce measurement bias is to ensure that the investigator measuring outcomes for a participant is unaware of the group to which the participant belongs (ie, *blinded assessment*). The following list summarizes the types of bias that exist.[7]

| Types of Bias[a] | |
|---|---|
| Berkson's bias | A type of selection bias where both cases and controls are derived from a subpopulation, resulting in both groups being different than the main population. For example, if both the cases and controls come from a group of hospitalized patients, they may not represent the population at large because of some factor that resulted in the members of the groups being hospitalized. See Cutter et al[103] for examples. |
| Channeling effect or channeling bias | The tendency of clinicians to prescribe treatment according to a patient's prognosis. As a result of this behavior in observational studies, treated patients are more or less likely to be high-risk patients than untreated patients, leading to a biased estimate of treatment effect. |
| Data completeness bias | Using a computer decision support system (CDSS) to log episodes in the intervention group and using a manual system in the non-CDSS control group can create variation in the completeness of data. |
| Detection bias (or surveillance bias) | The tendency to look more carefully for an outcome in one of the comparison groups. |
| Differential verification bias (or verification bias or workup bias) | When test results influence the choice of the reference standard (eg, test-positive patients undergo an invasive test to establish the diagnosis, whereas test-negative patients undergo long-term follow-up without application of the invasive test), the assessment of test properties may be biased. |
| Expectation bias | In data collection, an interviewer has information that influences his or her expectation of finding the exposure or outcome. In clinical practice, a clinician's assessment may be influenced by previous knowledge of the presence or absence of a disorder. |
| Incorporation bias | Occurs when investigators use a reference standard that incorporates a diagnostic test that is the subject of investigation. The result is a bias toward making the test appear more powerful in differentiating target-positive from target-negative patients than it actually is. |
| Interviewer bias | Greater probing by an interviewer of some participants than others, contingent on particular features of the participants. |

| | |
|---|---|
| Lead-time bias | Occurs when outcomes such as survival, as measured from the time of diagnosis, may be increased not because patients live longer but because screening lengthens the time that they know they have disease. |
| Length-time bias | Occurs when patients whose disease is discovered by screening may appear to do better or live longer than people whose disease presents clinically with symptoms because screening tends to detect disease that is destined to progress slowly and that therefore has a good prognosis. |
| Observer bias | Occurs when an observer's observations differ systematically according to participant characteristics (eg, making systematically different observations in treatment and control groups). |
| Partial verification bias | Occurs when only a selected sample of patients who underwent the index test is verified by the reference standard, and that sample is dependent on the results of the test. For example, patients with suspected coronary artery disease whose exercise test results are abnormal may be more likely to undergo coronary angiography (the reference standard) than those whose exercise test results are normal. |
| Publication bias | Occurs when the publication of research depends on the direction of the study results and whether they are statistically significant. |
| Recall bias | Occurs when patients who experience an adverse outcome have a different likelihood of recalling an exposure than patients who do not experience the adverse outcome, independent of the true extent of exposure. |
| Referral bias | Occurs when characteristics of patients differ between one setting (such as primary care) and another setting that includes only referred patients (such as secondary or tertiary care). |
| Reporting bias (or selective outcome reporting bias) | The inclination of authors to differentially report research results according to the magnitude, direction, or statistical significance of the results. |
| Social desirability bias | Occurs when participants answer according to social norms or socially desirable behavior rather than what is actually the case (eg, underreporting alcohol consumption). |

| Spectrum bias | Ideally, diagnostic test properties are assessed in a population in which the spectrum of disease in the target-positive patients includes all those in whom clinicians might be uncertain about the diagnosis, and the target-negative patients include all those with conditions easily confused with the target condition. Spectrum bias may occur when the accuracy of a diagnostic test is assessed in a population that differs from this ideal. Examples of spectrum bias would include a situation in which a substantial proportion of the target-positive population has advanced disease and target-negative participants are healthy or asymptomatic. Such situations typically occur in diagnostic case-control studies (for instance, comparing those with advanced disease vs healthy individuals). Such studies are liable to yield an overly sanguine estimate of the usefulness of the test. |
|---|---|
| Surveillance bias | see *detection bias* |
| Verification bias | see *differential verification bias* |
| Workup bias | see *differential verification bias* |

[a]From *Users' Guides to the Medical Literature.*[7]

**biased estimator:** an estimator is a function that results in a value that represents some property of a distribution. For example, an estimator for the mean value is some function that takes individual numbers, sums them, and divides by how many numbers there were, resulting in the mean value. A biased estimator is one that systematically results in an estimate for some value that is incorrect.

**bimodal distribution:** the normal distribution is characterized by the bell-shaped curve. A bimodal distribution has 2 peaks with a valley between them. There are 2 *modal values* (the most common number in a distribution of numbers). The *mean* (the number representing the central tendency of a group of numbers) and *median* (the number that has half the numbers larger than it and half smaller than it) may be equivalent, but neither is a good representation of the data. A *population* composed entirely of schoolchildren and their grandparents might have a mean age of 35 years, although there would be 1 bell-shaped curve representing the ages of the grandchildren and another representing the grandparents' ages.

**binary variable:** variable that has 2 mutually exclusive subgroups, such as male/female or pregnant/not pregnant; synonymous with *dichotomous variable.*[104]

**binomial distribution:** probability distribution that characterizes binomial data; used for modeling cumulative *incidence* and *prevalence* rates[98] (eg, the probability of a person having a stroke in a given *population* during a given period; the outcome must be stroke or no stroke). In a binomial sample with a probability ($p$) of the event and number (n) of participants, the predicted mean is $p \times n$ and the predicted variance is $p(p - 1)$.

**biological plausibility:** assumption that a causal relationship may be present because a known biological phenomenon exists that can explain the relationship. Statistically, this can be expressed as evidence that an *independent variable* may exert a biological effect on a *dependent variable* with which it is associated. For example, studies in animals were used to establish the biological plausibility of adverse effects of passive smoking.

**bivariable analysis:** used when the effect of a single *independent variable* on a single *dependent* variable is assessed.[95] Common examples include the *t test* for 1 *continuous variable* and 1 *binary variable* and the $\chi^2$ *test* for 2 binary variables. Bivariate analyses can be used for hypothesis testing in which only 1 independent variable is taken into account, to compare baseline characteristics of 2 groups or to develop a model for multivariable regression. See also *univariable* and *multivariate analysis*.

**bivariate analysis:** bivariate analysis implies that there is more than 1 dependent variable, a situation that may arise when ANOVA is performed. The suffix *–ate* in *bivariate* implies that something acts on the variables, which implies that *bivariate* refers to the dependent and not independent variables. See also *bivariable analysis, multivariate analysis*.

**Bland-Altman plot (also known as the Tukey mean difference plot):** a method to assess *agreement* (eg, between 2 tests) developed by Bland and Altman.[97] The difference between measures for the same subject is plotted on the y-axis against the mean of the 2 observations on the x-axis. This yields a scatterplot that graphically shows if one of the tests is unreliable compared with the other (example from Hoffmann et al[105]).

→ Sample wording: **Methods:** A Bland-Altman assessment for agreement was used to compare computed tomography measurement of coronary calcium with angiography. A range of agreement was defined as a mean bias of ± 2 SDs. **Results:** The Bland-Altman analysis indicates that the 95% limits of agreement between computed tomography coronary calcium measurement and angiography ranged from −19% to +43%. Note: When the Bland-Altman plot shows that the variables are NOT similar, one could say, "The 2 methods do not consistently provide similar measures because there is a level of disagreement that includes clinically important discrepancies of up to XX" [fill in the threshold value for the measure that exceeds what is considered clinically important].

**blinded (masked) assessment:** evaluation or categorization of an outcome in which the person assessing the outcome is unaware of the treatment assignment.

**blinded (masked) assignment:** assignment of individuals participating in a prospective study (usually random) to a study group and a *control group* without the investigator or the participants being aware of the group to which they are assigned. Studies may be single-blind, in which either the participant or the person administering the intervention does not know the treatment assignment, or double-blind, in which neither knows the treatment assignment. The term *triple-blind* is sometimes used to indicate that the persons who analyze or interpret the data are similarly unaware of treatment assignment. Authors should indicate who exactly was blinded.

The term *masked assignment* is preferred by some investigators and journals, particularly those in ophthalmology. Assessors may be blinded to things other than the treatment group, such as the purpose of the study or patient characteristics.

→ Blinded assessment is important to prevent *bias* on the part of the investigator performing the assessment, who may be influenced by the study question and consciously or unconsciously expect a certain test result.

**block randomization:** type of *randomization* in which the unit of randomization is not the individual but a larger group, sometimes stratified on particular variables, such as age or severity of illness, to ensure even distribution of the variable between randomized groups.

**Bonferroni adjustment:** one of several statistical adjustments to the *P value* that may be applied when *multiple comparisons* are made. The $\alpha$ *level* (usually .05) is divided by the number of comparisons to determine the $\alpha$ level that will be considered statistically significant. Thus, if 10 comparisons are made, an $\alpha$ of .05 would become $\alpha = .005$ for the study. Alternatively, the *P* value may be multiplied by the number of comparisons, while retaining the $\alpha$ of .05.[104] For example, a *P* value of .02 obtained for 1 of 10 comparisons would be multiplied by 10 to get the final result of $P = .20$, a nonsignificant result.

→ The Bonferroni test is a conservative adjustment for large numbers of comparisons (ie, less likely than other methods to give a significant result) but is simple and used frequently.

**bootstrap method (resampling method):** statistical method for validating a new *parameter* in the same group from which the parameter was derived. This method is typically used to estimate CIs. Values from a data set are randomly sampled, creating a new data set that is the same size as the original one. The mean of the new sample is calculated. This is repeated many times, and the 95% CIs of the new collection of data sets are calculated. These CIs are then used as the CIs of the original data set.[98]

→ Sometimes the bootstrap approach is used to validate a new statistical model. After a model is built, it is repeated many times using randomly sampled data from the original data from which the model was derived. The model may be considered reliable if it provides results with each bootstrap run similar to those obtained from the original model. In general, this is not an ideal approach for model validation because the data used to create the model may differ somewhat from data obtained from other cohorts. It is best to validate models on data other than those from which the model was constructed.

**Brown-Mood procedure:** test used with a *regression* model that does not assume a *normal distribution* or common variance of the errors.[93] It is an extension of the median test.

**C statistic: (also referred to as the C index or concordance statistic):** a measure of the area under a *receiver operating characteristic curve*.[106,107] The C statistic is commonly used in logistic regression procedures. The C statistic is the probability that, given 2 individuals (one who experiences the outcome of interest and the other who does not or who experiences it later), the model will yield a higher risk for the first patient than for the second. It is a measure of concordance (hence, the name C statistic) between model-based risk estimates and observed events. C statistics measure the ability of a model to rank patients from high to low risk but do not assess the ability of a model to assign accurate probabilities of an event occurring (that is measured by the model's calibration). C statistics generally range from 0.5 (random concordance) to 1 (perfect concordance).

The C statistic is calculated by evaluating each pair of data points against one another and determining whether the model's predicted probability is higher for an individual who had an event relative to one who did not experience the event. If the model always results in a higher risk of an event for individuals who experience the event, the C statistic will equal 1.0. If the model completely fails, it will equal 0.5 because there is a 50-50 chance that the model will predict a higher risk for individuals with event by chance alone.

Note: Do not hyphenate C statistic.

**case:** in a study, an individual with the outcome or disease of interest.

**case-control study:** *retrospective study* in which individuals with the disease (*cases*) are compared with those who do not have the disease (*controls*). Cases and controls are identified without knowledge of exposure to the risk factors under study. Cases and controls are matched on certain important variables, such as age, sex, and year in which the individual was treated or identified. A case-control study on individuals already enrolled in a cohort study is referred to as a nested case-control study.[98] This type of case-control study may be an especially strong study design if characteristics of the cohort have been carefully ascertained (see 19.3.2, Case-Control Studies).

→ Cases and controls should be selected from the same *population* to minimize confounding by factors other than those under study. Matching cases and controls on too many characteristics may obscure the association of interest, because if cases and controls are too similar, their exposures may be too similar to detect a difference (see *overmatching*). For example, if only males are studied, the effect of sex on an intervention cannot be determined. Similarly, if the participants are matched on age, the effect of age on outcome cannot be determined. Case-control studies also have risk for recall bias, where a patient's memory of events before the disease may differ from the memory of a control patient without the disease who may have paid less attention to factors that contribute to the disease being evaluated. Patients with a disease may have had more intense data collection than control patients. Patients and controls may have been selected from special populations (eg, people who happen to be admitted to certain hospitals) that may not represent all the relevant populations at risk for a disease.

**case-fatality rate:** probability of death among people who have a disease. The rate is calculated as the number of deaths during a specific period divided by the number of persons with the disease at the beginning of that period.[104]

**case series:** retrospective descriptive study in which clinical experience with a number of patients is described (see 19.3.4, Case Series).

**categorical data:** categorical data have nonnumerical values (they are named or nominal). For example, sex and race are categorical data. They are often represented by numbers when used for statistical analysis. For example, sex is male or female and may be represented in a database as 0 or 1. Categorical data that only have 2 categories are known as dichotomous[93] (eg, sex or race/ethnicity). The categories have no numerical importance. Categorical data are summarized by proportions, percentages, fractions, or simple counts. Categorical data are synonymous with *nominal data*. Analyzing categorical data is less optimal than leaving the data continuous because the high and low categories might be influenced by outliers. There are difficulties in interpreting the importance of results for values that are adjacent to the cutoff points that create the categories. For example, if a cutoff is created for cardiovascular risk categories at 5-year intervals, the resultant risk score may assign a very different risk for a 49-year-old patient than one who is 51 years old, yet their risk is probably very similar.

**cause, causation:** something that brings about an effect or result; to be distinguished from *association*, especially in observational studies. To establish something as a cause it must be known to precede the effect. The concept of causation includes the *contributory cause*, the *direct cause*, and the *indirect cause*. In general, causality should be assumed only from randomized clinical trials. Observational studies demonstrate associations and usually not causation. Wording in manuscripts should be consistent with these distinctions.

**censored data:** data in which the true value is replaced by some other value. Censoring has 2 different statistical connotations: (1) data in which extreme values are reassigned to some predefined, more moderate value and (2) data in which values have been assigned to individuals for whom the actual value is not known, such as in *survival analyses* for individuals who have not experienced the outcome (usually death) at the time the data collection was terminated.

The term *left-censored data* means that data were censored from the low end or left of the distribution. Typically, it means that the start time for some event is not known. For example, if studying the age at which women get breast cancer, a patient is enrolled who had breast cancer already and the age at onset is unknown, that observation would be left-censored. This also means that all that is known about the age at onset of the breast cancer is that it was less than the age of the woman when she was enrolled.

*Right-censored data* come from the high end or right of the distribution[98] (eg, in survival analyses). For right-censored data, the end time is not known, and all that is known is that it is greater than some value. If studying the age at death from breast cancer in a woman who was still alive at the end of the study, that observation would be right-censored because all that is known about how old she will be when she dies is that it will be older than she was at the end of the study.

**central limit theorem:** the means of random samples from any distribution will themselves have a normal distribution. Increasing the number of values increases the probability that the calculated mean value is the same as the real one for the population. Stated another way: the probability that any calculated mean value is the same as the actual total population mean value decreases as the sample size becomes smaller.[108] This is the basis for the importance of the normal distribution in statistical testing.[93]

**central tendency:** measures such as the mean, mode, and median that provide a single numerical value attempting to characterize a data set.[108] The mean characterizes a gaussian distribution of numbers as the average value. When data are not distributed in a gaussian distribution, the mean should not be used. In that case, it is best to use the median value, which is the value with half the numbers being greater than it and half being smaller than it. The mode is the most common number in a distribution of numbers.[98]

**$\chi^2$ test (chi-square test):** a test of significance of categorical data based on the $\chi^2$ statistic. The square of the expected values subtracted from the observed values is divided by the expected values. The sum of all these is called the $\chi^2$ statistic. The $\chi^2$ test assumes there is no association between the observed and expected numbers. When they are close to one another, the $\chi^2$ value is small, and when they are far apart, it is large.

→ The $\chi^2$ test can be used to assess the *goodness of fit* for a model by comparing the values of some parameter estimated by a model with those actually observed in the original data. The $\chi^2$ test can also compare an observed *variance* with hypothetical variance in normally distributed samples.[91] In the case of a continuous *independent variable* and a nominal *dependent variable*, the $\chi^2$ test for trend can be used to determine whether a linear relationship exists (eg, the relationship between systolic blood pressure and stroke).[95]

→ If there are multiple categories of data and there is a question of there being a trend in the data such that the categories increase or decrease in a consistent way, the $\chi^2$ test is modified to test for the presence of the trend. This is known as the Cochran-Armitage test for trend.

→ The *P value* for the $\chi^2$ test is determined from $\chi^2$ tables with the use of the specified $\alpha$ level and the *df* calculated from the number of cells in the $\chi^2$ table. The $\chi^2$ statistic should be reported to no more than 1 decimal place; if the *Yates correction* was used, that should be specified. See also *contingency table*.

> *Example:* The exercise intervention group was least likely to have experienced a fall in the previous month ($\chi^2_3 = 17.7$, $P = .02$). [See 21.9.4 Editing, Proofreading, Tagging, and Display, Specific Uses of Fonts and Styles, Italics.]

> *Example:* We compared the responses of attending physicians and advanced practice nurses with the use of the $\chi^2$ test of significance at the level of $P < .05$.

Note that the *df* for $\chi^2_3$ is specified using a subscript 3; it is derived from the number of cells in the $\chi^2$ table (for this example, 4 cells in a 2 × 2 table). The value 17.7 is the $\chi^2$ value. The *P* value is determined from the $\chi^2$ value and *df*.

Results of the $\chi^2$ test may be biased if there are too few observations (generally <5) per cell. In this case, the *Fisher exact test* is preferred.

**choropleth map:** map of a region or country that uses shading to display quantitative data[98] (see 4.2.3, Maps).

**chunk sample:** subset of a *population* selected for convenience without regard to whether the sample is random or representative of the population.[93] Synonymous with *convenience sample,* which is the more commonly used term.

**cluster randomization:** the assignment of groups (eg, schools, clinics) rather than individuals to intervention and control groups. This approach is often used when assignment by individuals is likely to result in contamination (eg, if adolescents within a school are assigned to receive or not receive a new sex education program, it is likely that they will share the information they learn with one another; instead, if the unit of assignment is schools, entire schools are assigned to receive or not receive the new sex education program). Cluster assignment is typically randomized, but it is possible (although not advisable) to assign clusters to the treatment or control by other methods.

**Cochran-Armitage test for trend:** when there are multiple categories of data and there is a question of the existence of a trend in the data such that the categories increase or decrease in a consistent way, the $\chi^2$ test is modified to test for the presence of the trend.

**Cochran Q test:** used when there is binary (yes/no) data and the question is if the percentage of successes (*yes* answers or *1*s) is not different between 2 or more groups. The groups must be matched (ie, have the same number of participants). The analysis results in a *Q* statistic, which, with the *df*, determines the *P value*; if significant, then the hypothesis that the proportion of successes between groups is the same is disproven, and one concludes that the variation between the 2 or more groups cannot be explained by chance alone.[93] Often used to determine whether different observers of the same phenomenon yield consistent observations. See also *interobserver bias* and *$I^2$ statistic*.

**coefficient of determination:** square of the *correlation coefficient*, used in linear or multiple *regression analysis*. This statistic indicates the proportion of the variation of the *dependent variable* that can be predicted from the *independent variable*.[95] If the analysis is *bivariate*, the correlation coefficient is indicated as *r* and the coefficient of determination is *$r^2$*. If the correlation coefficient is derived from *multivariate analysis*, the correlation coefficient is indicated as *R* and the coefficient of determination is *$R^2$*. See also *correlation coefficient*.

> *Example:* The sum of the $R^2$ values for age and body mass index was 0.23. Twenty-three percent of the variance could be explained by those 2 variables. The correlation coefficient between body mass index and systolic blood pressure was 0.8. There is a 64% chance that systolic blood pressure can be predicted from a body mass index value.

**coefficient of variation:** ratio of the *standard deviation (SD)* to the *mean*. The coefficient of variation is expressed as a percentage and is used to compare *dispersions* of different *samples*. It is typically used to determine how consistent a measure is when repeated many times. The smaller the coefficient of variation, the greater the *precision of the measurement*.[100] The coefficient of variation is also used when the SD is dependent on the mean (eg, the increase in height with age is accompanied by an increasing SD of height in the *population*). The coefficient of variation has no units of measure.

**cohort:** a group of individuals who share a common exposure, experience, or characteristic, or a group of individuals followed up or traced over time in a *cohort study*.[93]

**cohort effect:** change in rates that can be explained by the common experience or characteristic of a group or *cohort* of individuals. A cohort effect implies that a current pattern of variables may not be generalizable to a different cohort.[93]

> *Example:* The decline in socioeconomic status with age was a cohort effect explained by fewer years of education among the older individuals.

**cohort study:** study of a group of individuals, some of whom are exposed to a variable of interest (eg, a drug treatment or environmental exposure), in which participants are followed up over time to determine who develops the outcome of interest and whether the outcome is associated with the exposure. Cohort studies may be concurrent (prospective) or nonconcurrent (retrospective)[95] (see 19.3.1, Cohort Studies).

→ Whenever possible, a participant's outcome should be assessed by individuals who do not know whether the participant was exposed. See also *blinded assessment*.

**concordant pair:** pair in which both individuals have the same trait or outcome (as opposed to *discordant pair*). Used frequently in twin studies.[98]

**conditional probability:** *probability* that an event (*E*) will occur given the occurrence of *F*, called the conditional probability of *E* given *F*. The reciprocal is not necessarily true: the probability of *E* given *F* may not be equal to the probability of *F* given *E*.[104]

**confidence interval (CI):** range within which one can be confident (usually 95% confident, to correspond to an *α level* of .05) that the *population* value the study is intended to estimate lies.[95] The CI is an indication of the precision of an estimated population value.

→ Confidence intervals used to estimate a population value usually are symmetric or nearly symmetric around a value, but CIs used for *relative risks* and *odds ratios* may not be. Confidence intervals are preferable to *P values* because they convey information about *precision* as well as statistical significance of point estimates.

→ Confidence intervals are expressed with a hyphen separating the 2 values. To avoid confusion, the word *to* replaces hyphens if one of the values is a negative number. Units that are closed up with the numeral are repeated for each CI; those not closed up are repeated only with the last numeral (see 19.4, Significant Digits and Rounding Numbers, and 18.4, Use of Digit Spans and Hyphens).

> *Example:* The odds ratio was 3.1 (95% CI, 2.2-4.8). The prevalence of disease in the *population* was 1.2% (95% CI, 0.8%-1.6%).

**confidence limits (CLs):** upper and lower boundaries of the *confidence interval*, expressed with a comma separating the 2 values.[98]

> *Example:* The mean (95% confidence limits) was 30% (28%, 32%).

**confounding:** (1) a situation in which the apparent effect of an exposure on risk is caused by an *association* with factors other than those that are being studied and can influence the outcome; (2) a situation in which the effects of 2 or more causal factors as shown by a set of data cannot be separated to identify the unique effects of any of them; (3) a situation in which the measure of the effect of an exposure on risk is distorted because of the association of exposure with another factor(s) that influences the outcome under study[98] See also *confounding variable.*

**confounding variable:** variable that can cause or prevent the outcome of interest, is not an intermediate variable, and is associated with the factor under investigation. Unless it is possible to adjust for confounding variables, their effects cannot be distinguished from those of the factors being studied. *Bias* can occur when adjustment is made for any factor that is caused in part by the exposure and also is correlated with the outcome.[98] *Multivariate analysis* is used to control the effects of confounding variables that have been measured but cannot account for unmeasured confounding variables.

**contingency coefficient:** the coefficient $C$ (not to be confused with the *C statistic*), used to measure the strength of *association* between 2 characteristics in a *contingency table*.[104]

**contingency table:** table created when *categorical variables* are used to calculate expected frequencies in an analysis and to present data, especially for a $\chi^2$ *test* (2-dimensional data) or *log-linear models* (data with at least 3 dimensions). A typical 2 × 2 table might represent patients having a disease in the columns and those with a positive test result in the rows. Each of the 4 cells would have the number of patients who do or do not have the disease and do or do not have a positive test results. A 2 × 3 contingency table has 2 rows and 3 columns. The *df* are calculated as (number of rows − 1)(number of columns − 1). Thus, a 2 × 3 contingency table has 6 cells and 2 *df.*

**continuous data:** data that contain all possible real number values that may exist between 2 boundaries. Examples of measures using continuous data include blood pressure, height, and weight. This differs from categorical data, which have non-numerical values (they are named or nominal). Sex and race are examples of categorical data.[95] There are 2 kinds of continuous data: ratio data and interval data. Ratio-level data have a true zero, and thus numbers can meaningfully be divided by one another (eg, weight, systolic blood pressure, cholesterol level). For instance, 75 kg is half as heavy as 150 kg. Interval data may be measured with a similar precision but lack a true zero point. Thus, 32 °C is not half as warm as 64 °C, although temperature may be measured on a precise continuous scale. Continuous data include more information than *categorical, nominal,* or *dichotomous data.* Use of parametric statistics requires that continuous data have a normal distribution or that the data can be transformed to a *normal distribution* (eg, by computing logarithms of the data).

**contrast:** procedure used in *ANOVA* to determine if statistically significant differences exist between groups. Weights are assigned to each group that add up to zero. If there are 3 groups, the one to determine whether it is different than the others might be assigned a value of 1.0 and each of the 2 remaining groups assigned values of 0.5.

**contributory cause:** *independent variable* (cause) that is considered to contribute to the occurrence of the *dependent variable* (effect), typically in a randomized clinical trial. That a cause is contributory should not be assumed unless all of the following have been established: (1) a relationship exists between the putative cause and effect, (2) the cause precedes the effect in time, and (3) altering the cause alters the probability of occurrence of the effect.[95] Other factors that may contribute to establishing a contributory cause include the concept of *biological plausibility*, the existence of a *dose-response relationship*, and consistency of the relationship when evaluated in different settings.

**control:** in a *case-control study*, the designation for an individual without the disease or *outcome* of interest; in a *cohort study*, the individuals not exposed to the *independent variable* of interest; and in a *randomized clinical trial*, the group receiving a placebo, sham treatment, or standard treatment rather than the **intervention** under study.

**control group:** a group that does not receive the experimental intervention. In many studies, the control group receives either usual care or a placebo.

**controlled clinical trial:** study in which a group receiving an experimental treatment is compared with a *control* group receiving a placebo or an active treatment other than the experimental one (see 19.2.1, Parallel-Design Double-blind Trials).

**convenience sample:** sample of participants selected because they were available for the researchers to study, not because they are necessarily representative of a particular *population*.

→ Use of a convenience sample limits generalizability and can confound the analysis, depending on the source of the sample. For instance, if a sample of patients is selected from a group of patients who had undergone cardiac catheterization or echocardiography to compare cardiac auscultation, echocardiography, and cardiac catheterization, the patients are unlikely to resemble the population at large. This is because patients undergo the tests that served as the basis for which they were selected because they have already been found to have cardiac abnormalities. Consequently, the spectrum of cardiac auscultatory findings in the convenience sample will differ from that of the general population and, most likely, will show many more abnormalities than found in unselected patients.

**correlation:** a general term meaning that there is an association between 2 variables.[95] The strength of the association is described by the *correlation coefficient*. There are many reasons why 2 variables may be correlated, but it is important to remember that correlation alone does not prove *causation*. See also *agreement*.

→ The *Kendall τ rank correlation test* is used when testing 2 *ordinal* variables, the *Pearson product moment correlation* is used when testing 2 normally distributed **continuous variables**, and the *Spearman rank correlation* is used when testing 2 nonnormally distributed continuous variables.[100]

→ Correlation is often depicted graphically by means of a scatterplot of the data (see Figure 4.2-4 in 4.2.1.3, Statistical Graphs). The more circular a scatterplot, the smaller the correlation; the more linear a scatterplot, the greater the correlation.

**correlation coefficient:** measure of the association between 2 variables. The coefficient falls between −1 and 1; the sign indicates the direction of the relationship and the number indicates the magnitude of the relationship. A plus sign indicates that the 2 variables increase or decrease together; a minus sign indicates that increases in one are associated with decreases in the other. A value of −1 or 1 indicates that the sample values fall in a straight line, whereas a value of 0 indicates no relationship. The correlation coefficient should be followed by a measure of the significance of the correlation, and the statistical test used to measure correlation should be specified.

*Example:* Body mass index increased with age (Pearson $r = 0.61$; $P < .001$); years of education decreased with age (Pearson $r = −0.48$; $P = .01$).

→ When 2 variables are compared, the correlation coefficient is expressed by $r$; when more than 2 variables are compared by *multivariate analysis*, the correlation coefficient is expressed by $R$. The symbol $r^2$ or $R^2$ is termed the *coefficient of determination* and indicates the amount of variation in the *dependent variable* that can be explained by knowledge of the *independent variable*.

For example, if the correlation coefficient is 0.5, then the coefficient of determination is 0.25. This means that 25% of the variance of one variable can be explained by the other. Another way to express the relationship is that if one variable is known, there is a 25% chance of accurately predicting the value of the other variable.

**cost-benefit analysis:** economic analysis that compares the costs accruing to an individual for some treatment, process, or procedure and the ensuing medical consequences, with the benefits of reduced loss of earnings resulting from prevention of death or premature disability. The cost-benefit ratio is the ratio of marginal benefit (financial benefit of preventing 1 case) to marginal cost (cost of preventing 1 case)[98] (see 19.3.7, Study Design and Statistics, Observational Studies, Economic Analyses).

**cost-effectiveness analysis:** comparison of strategies to determine which provides the most clinical value for the cost.[100] A preferred intervention is the one that will cost the least for a given result or be the most effective for a given cost.[79] Outcomes are expressed by the cost-effectiveness ratio, such as cost per year of life saved (see 19.3.7, Economic Analyses).

**cost-utility analysis:** form of economic evaluation in which the outcomes of alternative procedures are expressed in terms of a single utility-based measurement, most often the *quality-adjusted life-year (QALY)*.[98]

**covariates:** a variable that may influence an outcome of interest but is not the main variable being studied. Controlling for a covariate may improve the understanding between the variable of interest and the outcome being studied. For example, if the relationship between the degree of hypertension and stroke occurrence is examined, other factors, such as age or cholesterol level, will influence stroke outcomes and are considered covariates. How hypertension influences stroke is better understood when age and cholesterol levels are controlled for by including them in statistical analyses.

**Cox-Mantel test:** a nonparametric method for comparing 2 survival curves. This method does not assume any one particular distribution of data,[104] similar to the *log-rank test.*[95]

**Cox proportional hazards regression model (Cox proportional hazards model):** model used to assess rate data (number of items per unit time) as opposed to proportions, which are analyzed by logistic regression. In addition to an outcome such as alive or dead, the time it takes to experience that outcome (time to event) is incorporated in Cox proportional hazards regression, adding power to the analysis above that available from logistic regression. The hazard is the probability that if a person survives to a certain time, that person will not survive to make it into the next observed interval.

Cox proportional hazards regression assesses the influence some exposure has on the time it takes for an outcome to occur. Individuals with and without the exposure are compared with the assumption that the exposure's influence will be proportional in both groups (ie, that changes beyond the baseline hazard will be multiples of one another). When the hazards are proportional, the groups with and without the exposure will be represented as parallel lines when the outcome is graphed as a function of time. An indicator that the proportional hazards assumption is not met is when *Kaplan-Meier* curves of the exposed and unexposed groups are not parallel and cross one another. One of the several procedures that test the proportionality of the data should be used when Cox proportional hazards regression is performed. Although Cox proportional hazards regression assumes that the hazards are proportional, corrections can be made to account for nonproportionality.

Accounting for proportionality is important because the mathematics for the analysis depend on a ratio that erases the baseline risk from the equation. As a consequence, results from Cox proportional hazards regression can only provide relative risks and not absolute risks because the absolute risk of an event relies on knowing the event's baseline risk. Because it is a regression procedure, covariates can be added (as they are in logistic regression) to assess the influence of the exposure variable while assuming that the added covariates are held constant and do not influence the outcome.[92,104]

**criterion standard (also known as reference standard):** test considered to be the diagnostic standard for a particular disease or condition, used as a basis of comparison for other (usually noninvasive) tests. An outdated term is *gold standard*, which refers to a time when the monetary system was based on the value of gold. This is no longer the case and the term is obsolete.[98] Ideally, the *sensitivity* and *specificity* of the criterion standard for the disease should be 100%. See also *diagnostic discrimination*.

**Cronbach $\alpha$:** used to determine the consistency between scores when they are used together to generate an aggregate score. For example, if there is a 10-question quality-of-life instrument with each of the 10 questions having answers ranging from 1 to 5 and the overall score representing the quality of life is the sum of all 10 scores, then the 10 questions should be consistent with one another. Statistically, each of them should be highly correlated with one another.[98] The Cronbach $\alpha$

ranges from 0 (little internal consistency between the questions) to 1 (the questions are highly consistent with each other).[104]

**cross-design synthesis:** method for evaluating outcomes of medical interventions, developed by the US General Accounting Office, which pools results from databases of randomized clinical trials and other study designs. It is a form of meta-analysis (see 19.3.6, Meta-analyses).[98]

**cross-level bias:** a mechanism underlying the ecologic fallacy. Ecologic fallacy occurs when individual effects that exist are not found when data are examined at a group level. One cause for this is cross-level bias. Examples include confounders being distributed differentially between groups or the baseline prevalence of the disorder differs between groups and the risk for disease depends on the group prevalence. Cross-level bias occurs when an intervention that is known to be effective on an individual level is administered at different rates in different facilities to patients with the disease the intervention is intended to treat. This occurs when clinicians apply differing criteria for administering a treatment based on their own practice patterns.

**crossover design:** method of comparing 2 or more treatments or interventions. Individuals initially are randomized to one treatment or the other; after completing the first treatment, they are crossed over to 1 or more other *randomization* groups and undergo other courses of treatment being tested in the experiment. Advantages are that a smaller sample size is needed to detect a difference between treatments because a paired analysis is used to compare the treatments in each individual, but the disadvantage is that an adequate washout period is needed after the initial course of treatment to avoid carryover effect from the first to the second treatment. Order of treatments should be randomized to avoid potential bias[104] (see 19.2.2, Crossover Trials).

**cross-sectional study:** study that identifies participants with and without the condition or disease under study and the characteristic or exposure of interest at the same point in time.[95]

→ Causality is difficult to establish in a cross-sectional study because the outcome of interest and associated factors are simultaneously assessed. Demonstrating causality requires an experimental and a control group, an intervention, and then an observation period that follows delivery of the intervention.

**crude death rate:** total deaths during a year divided by the midyear population. Deaths are usually expressed per 100 000 persons.[104]

**cumulative incidence:** number of people who experience onset of a disease or outcome of interest during a specified period; may also be expressed as a rate or ratio.[98]

**Cutler-Ederer method (also known as the actuarial life-table method):** form of *life-table* analysis that uses actuarial techniques. The method assumes that the times at which follow-up ended (because of death or the outcome of interest) are uniformly distributed during the period, as opposed to the *Kaplan-Meier method*, which assumes that termination of follow-up occurs at the end of the time block. Therefore, Cutler-Ederer estimates of risk tend to be slightly higher than Kaplan-Meier estimates.[109] Often an intervention and *control group* are depicted on 1 graph, and the curves are compared by means of a *log-rank test*.

**cut point:** in testing, the arbitrary level at which "normal" values are separated from "abnormal" values, often selected at the point 2 *SDs* from the mean. See also *receiver operating characteristic curve.*[98]

**DALY:** see *disability-adjusted life-years.*

**data:** collection of items of information.[98] (*Datum*, the singular form of this word, is rarely used.) See 7.5.2, False Singulars.

**data dredging (also known as a "fishing expedition"):** jargon meaning *post hoc analysis*, with no a priori *hypothesis*, of several variables collected in a study to identify variables that have a statistically significant association for purposes of publication. One form of this is called HARKing (hypothesizing after the results are known).

→ Although post hoc analyses occasionally can be useful to generate hypotheses, data dredging increases the likelihood of a *type I error* and should be avoided. If post hoc analyses are performed, they should be declared as such and the number of post hoc comparisons performed specified. They should always be considered exploratory analyses.

**decision analysis:** process of identifying all possible choices and outcomes for a particular set of decisions to be made regarding patient care. Decision analysis generally uses preexisting data to estimate the likelihood of occurrence of each outcome. The process is displayed as a decision tree, with each node depicting a branch point that represents a decision in treatment or intervention to be made (usually represented by a square at the branch point) or possible outcomes or chance events (usually represented by a circle at the branch point). The relative worth of each outcome may be expressed as a utility, such as the *quality-adjusted life-year.*[98]

**degrees of freedom (df):** see *df.*

**dependent variable:** outcome variable of interest in any study; the outcome that one intends to explain or estimate[95] (eg, death, myocardial infarction, or reduction in blood pressure). *Multivariable analysis* controls for *independent variables* or *covariates* that might modify the occurrence of a single dependent variable (eg, age, sex, and other medical diseases or risk factors). When there is more than 1 dependent variable, regressions should be referred to as multivariate.

**descriptive statistics:** method used to summarize or describe data with the use of the *mean, median, SD, SE,* or *range* or to convey in graphic form (eg, by using a *histogram*, shown in Figure 4.2-5 in 4.2.1.4, Statistical Graphs) for purposes of data presentation and analysis.[104]

**df (degrees of freedom)** (*df* is not expanded at first mention): the number of arithmetically independent comparisons that can be made among members of a sample. In a *contingency table*, *df* is calculated as (number of rows − 1)(number of columns − 1).

Another definition for *df* was put forth by Sir Ronald Fisher. It is the number of independent values needed to determine a system. For example, for the 4-number system defining the average, $(1 + 2 + 3 + 4)/4 = 2.5$, the *df* is the number of observations (4) minus the parameter that is the mean value (there is 1 mean) = 3 *df*. The reason being that the system can be recreated from 3 values. If 3 values are selected, any combination of 1, 2, 3, or 4, the fourth has to be the remaining number if the mean is to be 2.5.

For a *t* test or regression analysis, it is the number of observations minus the number of unknown parameters to be estimated. When regression results are reported as "adjusted," it means that the sample size used in calculations is the number of observations (n) minus the number of parameters estimated. These adjusted values are the ones that should be reported as the regression result.

→ The *df* should be reported as a subscript after the related statistic, such as the *t test*, *analysis of variance*, and $\chi^2$ *test* (eg, $\chi^2_3$ = 17.7, *P* = .02; in this example, the subscript 3 is the *df*).

**diagnostic discrimination:** statistical assessment of how the performance of a clinical diagnostic test compares with the *criterion standard* (or reference standard). To assess a test's ability to distinguish an individual with a particular condition from one without the condition, the researcher must (1) determine the variability of the test, (2) define a *population* free of the disease or condition and determine the normal range of values for that population for the test (usually the central 95% of values, but in tests that are quantitative rather than qualitative, a *receiver operating characteristic curve* may be created to determine the optimal cut point for defining normal and abnormal), and (3) determine the criterion standard for a disease (by definition, the criterion standard should have 100% sensitivity and specificity for the disease) with which to compare the test. Diagnostic discrimination is reported with the performance measures *sensitivity*, *specificity*, *positive predictive value*, and *negative predictive value*; *false-positive rate*; and the *likelihood ratio*.[95]

→ Because the values used to report diagnostic discrimination are ratios, they can be expressed either as the ratio, using the decimal form, or as the percentage, by multiplying the ratio by 100.

*Example:* The test had a sensitivity of 0.80 and a specificity of 0.95; the false-positive rate was 0.05.

*Or:* The test had a sensitivity of 80% and a specificity of 95%; the false-positive rate was 5%.

→ When the diagnostic discrimination of a test is defined, the individuals tested should represent the full spectrum of the disease and reflect the population on which the test will be used. For example, if a test is proposed as a screening tool, it should be assessed in the general population.

**dichotomous variable:** a variable with only 2 possible categories (eg, male/female, alive/dead); synonymous with *binary variable*.[104]

→ A variable may have a *continuous* distribution during data collection but is made dichotomous for purposes of analysis (eg, one group being younger than 65 years and the other being 65 years or older). This is done most often for nonnormally distributed data. Note that the use of a *cut point* generally converts a *continuous variable* to a dichotomous one (eg, normal vs abnormal). Data may be categorized by establishing several cut points and separating the data into quantiles.

If there is only 1 cut point, the resultant data are dichotomous. Analyses of continuous data are much more powerful than categorized data and are always preferred (see *categorical variables*).

**difference in differences:** determines whether there is a statistically significant effect of some change that was made at a discrete time on some outcome. For example, to determine whether the implementation of a policy requiring Center of Excellence status for Medicare coverage of bariatric surgery was effective, the progressively decreasing rate of complications was analyzed in facilities before and after the policy was implemented. The control group included facilities that were not Centers of Excellence, and the experimental group included facilities that became Centers of Excellence after the policy was implemented. If the slope of the outcomes from the 2 groups deviates after the policy is implemented, then that policy is considered to be associated with the outcomes. The change in slope is determined by the statistical significance of an interaction term in a regression equation.[110,111]

**direct cause:** *contributory cause* that is considered to be the most immediate cause of a disease. The direct cause is dependent on the current state of knowledge and may change as more immediate mechanisms are discovered.[95]

> *Example:* Although several other causes were suggested when the disease was first described, HIV is the direct cause of AIDS.

**disability-adjusted life-years (DALY):** quantitative indicator of burden of disease that reflects the years lost because of premature mortality and years lived with disability, adjusted for severity.[112]

**discordant pair:** pair in which the individuals have different *outcomes*. In twin studies, only the discordant pairs are informative about the *association* between exposure and disease.[98] The antonym is *concordant pair*.

**discrete variable:** variable that is counted as an integer; no fractions are possible.[104] Examples are counts of pregnancies or surgical procedures, or responses to a *Likert scale*.

**discriminant analysis:** analytic technique used to classify participants according to their characteristics (eg, the *independent variables*, signs, symptoms, and diagnostic test results) to the appropriate *outcome* or *dependent variable*,[104] also referred to as discriminatory analysis.[92] This analysis tests the ability of the independent variable model to correctly classify an individual in terms of outcome. For example, if studying 3 possible outcomes after discharge for congestive heart failure (no readmission, readmission within 30 days, death within 30 days) and information is available about the patients (eg, age, sex, socioeconomic status), discriminant analysis would be used to determine which variables can best predict which patients have 1 of the 3 outcomes. In this example, age may prove to be the best predictor for death and socioeconomic status the best predictor for readmission.

**dispersion:** degree of scatter shown by observations. For continuous data, dispersion is best represented by the SD. For nonnormally distributed data or categorical data, it is best shown by interquartile ranges (or some other quantile, such as terciles, or quintiles) or by some other form of *percentiles*.[93]

**distribution:** the frequency and pattern of all possible values for some variable.[95] Distributions may have a *normal distribution* (bell-shaped curve) or a *nonnormal distribution* (eg, *binomial* or *Poisson distribution*).

**dose-response relationship:** relationship in which changes in levels of exposure are associated with changes in the frequency of an *outcome* in a consistent direction. This supports the idea that the agent of exposure (most often a drug) is responsible for the effect seen.[93] May be tested statistically by using a $\chi^2$ test for trend.

**Duncan multiple range test:** modified form of the *Newman-Keuls test for multiple comparisons*. It is a test for determining which pairs of groups have statistically significant different mean values when there are more than 2 means to be compared. This test is not dependent on first having found that any difference exists between any means values by the *F test of ANOVA*.[104]

**Dunn test:** *multiple comparisons procedure* based on the *Bonferroni adjustment*.[104]

**Dunnett test:** *multiple comparisons procedure* intended for comparing each of a number of treatments with a single *control*.[104]

**Durbin-Watson test:** test to determine whether the *residuals* from *linear regression* or *multiple regression* are independent or, alternatively, are serially (auto) correlated.[104] If the Durbin-Watson value is less than 2, then the data are positively autocorrelated; greater than 2, the data are negatively autocorrelated. When the Durbin-Watson statistic equals 2, there is no autocorrelation. Because conventional regression procedures assume data independence, they should not be used in autocorrelated data. When autocorrelation is present, time series statistics (eg, autoregressive integrated moving average [ARIMA] models) should be used for the analysis. Data that are commonly autocorrelated include incidence rates for disease measured in successive periods.

**ecologic fallacy:** error that occurs when the existence of a group association is used to imply, incorrectly, the existence of a relationship at the individual level.[95] Alternatively, there may be a strong individual effect of an exposure that is not observed when assessed at a group level. For example, when 1930 US Census data were used to assess the relationship between being foreign born and literacy, higher rates within states of being foreign born were unexpectedly associated with higher literacy rates. When the analysis was performed on an individual and not a state level, the expected relationship between being foreign born and low literacy rates was found. This apparent paradox, or ecologic fallacy, occurred because low-literacy immigrants tended to immigrate to regions with high literacy rates.[113]

**ecologic study:** examination of groups or populations of patients but not the individuals themselves. Ecologic studies are useful for understanding disease prevalence or incidence and facilitate analysis of large numbers of people. These studies may uncover relationships between exposure factors and diseases. These studies are limited by the *ecologic fallacy*. Group-level exposure and the outcome may not relate well to individuals within that group. These studies are highly susceptible to bias.

**effectiveness:** extent to which an intervention is beneficial when implemented under the usual conditions of clinical care for a group of patients,[95] as distinguished from *efficacy* (the degree of beneficial effect seen in a clinical trial) and *efficiency* (the intervention effect achieved relative to the effort expended in time, money, and resources).

**effect of observation:** bias that results when the process of observation alters the outcome of the study.[95] See also *Hawthorne effect*.

**effect size:** observed or expected change in *outcome* as a result of an intervention. Whereas statistical significance provides only an indication that a difference between groups exists, it does not provide an indication of how important that effect is. Effect size provides a measure of the magnitude of the differences between groups and should always be considered in addition to the statistical significance. Effect size is calculated from the absolute difference between groups divided by a measure of the variation in the data, such as the SD. Effect size can assist in understanding the clinical significance of research findings.

→ Expected effect size is used during the process of estimating the sample size necessary to achieve a given *power*. Given a similar amount of variability among individuals, a large effect size will require a smaller sample size to detect a difference than will a smaller effect size.[114]

**efficacy:** degree to which an intervention produces a beneficial result under the ideal conditions of an investigation,[95] usually in a randomized clinical trial; it is usually greater than the intervention's *effectiveness*.

**efficiency:** effects achieved in relation to the effort expended in money, time, and resources. Statistically, the precision with which a study design will estimate a *parameter* of interest.[98]

**effort-to-yield measures:** amount of resources needed to produce a unit change in *outcome*, such as *number needed to treat*[100]; used in cost-effectiveness and cost-benefit analyses (see 19.3.7, Economic Analyses).

**equivalence trial:** trials that estimate treatment effects that exclude any patient-important superiority of interventions under evaluation. Equivalence trials require a priori definition of the smallest difference in outcomes between these interventions that patients would consider large enough to justify a preference for the superior intervention (given the intervention's harms and burdens). The CI for the estimated treatment effect at the end of the trial should exclude that difference for the authors to claim equivalence (ie, the confidence limits should be closer to zero than the minimal patient-important difference). This level of precision often requires investigators to enroll large numbers of patients with large numbers of events. Equivalence trials are helpful when investigators want to see whether a cheaper, safer, simpler (or increasingly often, better method to generate income for the sponsor) intervention is neither better nor worse (in terms of efficacy) than a current intervention. Claims of equivalence are frequent when results are not significant, but one must be alert to whether the CIs exclude differences between the interventions that are as large as or larger than those patients would consider important. If they do not, the trial is indeterminate rather than yielding equivalence.[11,22]

**error:** difference between a measured or estimated value and the true value. Three types are seen in scientific research: a false or mistaken result obtained in a study; measurement error, a random form of error; and systematic error that skews results in a particular direction.[98]

**estimate:** value or values calculated from sample observations that are used to approximate the corresponding value for the *population*.[95]

**event:** end point or outcome of a study; usually the *dependent variable*. The event should be defined before the study is conducted and assessed by an individual masked to the intervention or exposure category of the study participant.

**exclusion criteria:** characteristics of potential study participants or other data that will exclude them from the study sample (such as being younger than 65 years, history of cardiovascular disease, expected to move within 6 months of the beginning of the study). Like *inclusion criteria*, exclusion criteria should be defined before any individuals are enrolled.

**expectation:** the summation or integration of all possible values of a random variable; synonymous with the mean value.

**explanatory variable:** variable that helps explain the phenomenon represented by the dependent variable. It is synonymous with *independent variable* but preferred by some because "independent" in this context does not refer to statistical independence.[93]

**extrapolation:** conclusions drawn about the meaning of a study for a *target population* that includes types of individuals or data not represented in the study sample.[95] The value of a missing or unknown variable may be derived from other known variables by extrapolation. This is often performed by fitting a regression equation.

**face validity:** the extent to which a measurement instrument appears to measure what it is intended to measure.

**factor analysis:** procedure used to group related variables to reduce the number of variables needed to represent the data. This analysis reduces complex correlations between a large number of variables to a smaller number of independent theoretical factors. The researcher must then interpret the factors by looking at the pattern of "loadings" of the various variables on each factor.[100] Loadings describe the relationship between the variables and the factors. Weak factors have little effect on the variable and have small numerical values for the loading values. In theory, there can be as many factors as there are variables, and thus the authors should explain how they decided on the number of factors in their solution. The decision about the number of factors is a compromise between the need to simplify the data and the need to explain as much of the variability as possible. There is no single criterion on which to make this decision, and thus authors may consider a number of indexes of *goodness of fit*. There are a number of *algorithms* for rotation of the factors, which may make them more straightforward to interpret. Factor analysis is commonly used for developing scoring systems for rating scales and questionnaires.

**false negative:** negative test result in an individual who has the disease or condition as determined by the *criterion standard* (or reference standard).[95] See also *diagnostic discrimination*.

**false-negative rate:** proportion of test results found or expected to yield a false-negative result; equal to 1 minus sensitivity.[95] See also *diagnostic discrimination*.

**false positive:** positive test result in an individual who does not have the disease or condition as determined by the *criterion standard* (or reference standard).[95] See also *diagnostic discrimination*.

**false-positive rate:** proportion of tests found to or expected to yield a false-positive result; equal to 1 minus specificity.[95] See also *diagnostic discrimination*.

**F distribution:** ratio of the distribution of 2 normally distributed independent variables; synonymous with *variance ratio distribution*. It is used for *ANOVA*.[98]

**Fisher exact test (also known as the Fisher-Yates test and the Fisher-Irwin test[93]):** assesses the independence of 2 variables by means of a 2 × 2 *contingency table*; used when the frequency in at least 1 cell is small[104] (<5).

**fixed-effect model:** when used in the context of multilevel (eg, hierarchical) analysis, refers to a standard regression equation that characterizes one level of a system. For example, if modeling the effect of teaching on student performance, if a model is constructed only at the student level, it would be a fixed-effect model. If the model is constructed to include the student and school levels, then it would be a random-effects model. Random-effects models represent the synthesis of 2 or more regression equations into a single regression model and allow the slope or intercept terms to vary.

→ Fixed-effect models are also used to generate a summary estimate of the magnitude of effect in a meta-analysis that restricts inferences to the set of studies included in the meta-analysis and assumes that a single true value underlies all the primary study results. The assumption is that if all studies were infinitely large, they would yield identical estimates of effect; thus, observed estimates of effect differ from one another only because of random error. This model takes only within-study variation into account and not between-study variation.[115] The antonym is *random-effects model*.

Because the model involves a single level, it should be referred to as the singular fixed-effect. Multilevel models should be referred to by the plural, random effects.

**forest plot:** graphical representation of the results of a series of studies when their results are summarized into a single graph; usually used for showing the results of meta-analyses. Each horizontal line represents the point estimate and 95% CIs for a single study. The size of the symbol that represents the study results' point estimate is proportional to the weight that study was given in the meta-analysis. These weights are usually the inverse of the study variance (see Figure 4.2-16 in 4.2.1.11, Statistical Graphs). A vertical line is placed where the intervention being assessed has no effect. For hazard ratios, risk ratios, and odds ratios, this is a dotted line at 1.0. For standardized mean differences, this point would be a solid line at zero. A vertical dashed line may be placed at the point estimate for the overall summary finding from a meta-analysis.

**Friedman test:** a *nonparametric* test for a design with 2 factors that uses the ranks rather than the values of the observations.[93] Nonparametric analog to *analysis of variance*.

**F test (score):** alternative name for the *variance ratio* test (or *F* ratio),[98] which results in the *F* score. The *F* test is used to test the significance of *analysis of variance*.[104] When ANOVA is performed, if the *F* test is statistically significant, there is a difference in the variance between 2 or more groups, but the test does not specify which groups are different. To determine which groups are different, a *multiple comparison* test, such as the *Dennett*, *Tukey*, or other tests, is performed.

> *Example:* There were differences by academic status in perceptions of the quality of both primary care training ($F_{1,682} = 6.71$; $P = .01$) and specialty training ($F_{1,682} = 6.71$; $P = .01$). (The numbers set as subscripts for the *F* test are the *df* for the numerator and denominator, respectively.) In the medical literature, the subscripted values are often not included when reporting the results of *F* tests.

**funnel plot:** a graphic technique for assessing the possibility of publication bias in a systematic review. The effect measure is typically plotted on the horizontal axis and a measure of the random error associated with each study on the vertical axis. In the absence of publication bias, because of sampling variability, the graph should have the shape of a funnel. If there is bias against the publication of null results or results showing an adverse effect of the intervention, one quadrant of the funnel plot will be partially or completely missing (see Figure 4.2-17 in 4.2.1.12, Funnel Plot).

**gaussian distribution:** see *normal distribution*.

**genome-wide association study:** a study that evaluates the association of genetic variation with outcomes or traits of interest by using 100 000 to 1 000 000 or more markers across the genome.

**gold standard:** See *criterion standard*.

**goodness of fit:** agreement between an observed set of values and a second set derived from a statistical model.[93] It is considered good statistical practice to test the goodness of fit of any statistical model to assess how well it models the phenomena it is purported to represent. For regressions solved by a least-squares approach (used when the dependent variable is a continuous value, such as cost of care), the goodness of fit is represented by the coefficient of determination ($R^2$). $R^2$ is calculated by subtracting the residual sum of the squares (RSS) by the total sum of the squares (TSS) and dividing this quantity by the total sum of the squares. The closer this value is to 1, the better the model fit. The coefficient of determination should not be confused with the correlation coefficient ($r$), which measures the association between 2 variables. See *correlation coefficient*.

Models fit with maximum likelihood (ML) are more difficult to assess. A pseudo-$R^2$ can be calculated, but it is not equivalent to the $R^2$ calculated for ordinary linear regression models. How the addition of variables to the model improves its fit can be assessed by *likelihood ratios* (LRs), where the likelihood of the model with the added variable is divided by the likelihood for the model without the variable. This ratio has a $\chi^2$ distribution, and statistical significance of the improved model can be statistically tested by $\chi^2$ with 2 *df*. Because addition of variables to models generally improves the fit, when model fits are compared, they should be penalized by the number of variables they contain. This is done by the *Akaike information criteria* (AIC) or *Bayes information criteria* (BIC). When models with different numbers of variables are compared, the model with the lowest AIC or BIC is generally considered to have the optimal fit.

The *Hosmer-Lemeshow* test is often used to assess the maximum likelihood ratio model fit for frequency data. This test divides the observed and expected data into deciles. A $\chi^2$ test is performed with the null hypothesis that no difference exists between any of the 10 deciles. If the Hosmer-Lemeshow test has $P > .05$, then no difference between observed and expected data is concluded, suggesting a good model fit. The Hosmer-Lemeshow test is not optimal because there is a substantial loss of analytic power when the data are aggregated into deciles; the Hosmer-Lemeshow test may not accurately reflect the goodness of fit for models with large amounts of data.

**group association:** situation in which a characteristic and a disease both occur more frequently in one group of individuals than another. The association does not mean that all individuals with the characteristic necessarily have the disease.[95]

**group matching (also known as frequency matching[95]):** process of matching during assignment in a study to ensure that the groups have a nearly equal distribution of particular variables. The closeness of the match should be shown by providing the standardized difference (differences divided by pooled SDs).[116]

**Hartley test:** test for the equality of variances of a number of *populations* that are *normally distributed* based on the ratio between the largest and smallest sample variations.[93]

**Hawthorne effect:** effect produced in a study because of the participants' awareness that they are participating in a study. The term usually refers to an effect on the *control group* that changes the group in the direction of the outcome, resulting in a smaller effect size.[104] A related concept is *effect of observation*. The Hawthorne effect is different from the *placebo effect*, which relates to participants' expectations that an intervention will have specific effects. The Hawthorne effect is commonly seen in quality assurance investigations where measures of certain outcomes are collected and data collection processes are changed because those collecting the data are aware that these measures are now being evaluated.

**hazard rate, hazard function:** theoretical measure of the likelihood that if individuals enter a certain period they will experience an event before the end of the designated period.[98] A number of hazard rates for specific intervals can be combined to create a hazard function.

**hazard ratio:** the ratio of the hazard rate in one group to the hazard rate in another. It is calculated from the *Cox proportional hazards model*. The interpretation of the hazard ratio is similar to that of the *relative risk*. In Cox proportional hazards regression, the ratio is calculated to avoid needing to know the baseline hazard to model how various factors affect the hazard of an event. Because the calculation depends on the ratio, the hazards should change in time at the same rate (have the same slope). This is known as the proportional hazards assumption. When a Cox proportional hazards regression is performed, a test should be performed to ensure that the proportional hazard assumption is met. If the curves cross, the hazards are not proportional. If they are not proportional, the model must be adjusted to account for the lack of proportionality.[117,118]

**hierarchical model:** See *mixed-model analysis*.

**heterogeneity:** qualities of groups that are aggregated are not similar. The term is commonly used in meta-analysis to denote that the studies aggregated in a single analysis are not similar to one another. The degree of heterogeneity is measured with the *Q test* or the *$I^2$ test*. The antonym is *homogeneity*.

**heteroscedasticity:** systematic deviation of data rather than the data being randomly distributed. See *homoscedasticity*. Heteroscedasticity in data violates the assumptions for linear regression analysis.

**histogram:** graphical representation of data in which the frequency (quantity) within each class or category is represented by the area of a rectangle centered on the class interval. The heights of the rectangles are proportional to the observed frequencies (see Figure 4.2-5 in 4.2.1, Statistical Graphs).

**Hoeffding independence test:** *bivariable* test of *nonnormally distributed continuous data* to determine whether the elements of the 2 groups are independent of each other.[98]

**Hollander parallelism test:** determines whether 2 *regression lines* for 2 *independent variables* plotted against a *dependent variable* are parallel. The test does not require a *normal distribution*, but there must be an equal and even number of observations corresponding to each line. If the lines are parallel, then both independent variables predict the *dependent variable* equally well. The Hollander parallelism test is a special case of the *signed rank test*.[93]

**homogeneity:** the qualities of individuals aggregated into groups are similar to one another. In meta-analyses, homogeneity means that the individual studies that are combined in a single analysis are similar to one another. Homogeneity also refers to the equality of a quantity of interest (such as *variance*), specifically in a number of groups or *populations*.[93] See antonym *heterogeneity* for a discussion of measures of homogeneity in meta-analysis.

**homoscedasticity:** statistical determination that the variance of the different variables under study is equal.[98] Homoscedasticity can be assessed by plotting the error (difference between observed data and the regression line) against the independent variables and looking for systematic deviations. If the errors are randomly distributed, then the data are homoscedastic; if not, they are heteroscedastic, and the regression results are invalid. See also *heterogeneity*.

**Hosmer-Lemeshow goodness-of-fit test:** a series of statistical steps used to assess *goodness of fit* for logistic regression analyses. The observed and modeled observations are aggregated into equal-sized groups, and usually 10 groups are used. A $\chi^2$ test is performed, and if there is a significant difference found between the observed and modeled groups of data, the model is considered to not fit well. Thus, if $P < .05$, the model is considered to not fit well, and $P$ values above this level suggest a good fit to the model. The Hosmer-Lemeshow test has limited power to detect differences between observed and fitted data because only 10 groups are compared rather than the much larger number of values involved in the regression itself. The Hosmer-Lemeshow test does not perform well as a goodness-of-fit test for large data sets.[119]

**Hotelling *T* statistic:** generalization of the *t test* for use with *multivariate data*; results in a *T* statistic. Significance can be tested with the *variance ratio distribution*.[93]

**hypothesis:** an educated guess about some phenomenon; a supposition that leads to a prediction that can be tested and found to be supported or refuted.[98,120] The *null hypothesis* in statistical analysis states that no difference exists between groups. Statistically significant differences between groups are assessed by comparing them and finding if the chance that any observed differences between groups has a probability of being observed that is less than 5% ($P < .05$). Hypothesis testing includes (1) generating the study hypothesis and defining the null hypothesis, (2) determining the level below which results are considered statistically significant, or *α level* (usually $\alpha = .05$), and (3) identifying and applying the appropriate statistical test to accept or reject the null hypothesis.

**$I^2$ statistic:** the $I^2$ statistic is a test of heterogeneity. $I^2$ can be calculated from Cochran $Q$ according to the formula $I^2 = 100\% \times$ (Cochran $Q - df$). Any negative values of $I^2$ are considered equal to 0, so that the range of $I^2$ values is 0% to 100%, indicating no heterogeneity to high heterogeneity.

**imputation:** a group of techniques for replacing missing data with values that are likely to have been observed if they were present. Among the simplest methods of imputation is last observation carried forward, in which missing values are replaced by the last observed value. This provides a conservative estimate in cases in which the condition is expected to improve on its own but may be overly optimistic in conditions that are known to worsen over time. In general, last observation carried forward should not be performed. Missing values may also be imputed based on the patterns of other variables. In *multiple imputation*, missing data are modeled for a data set based on other data to provide the best guess for what the values for the missing data should have been. The process of guessing what the missing data should be is repeated many times, resulting in a large number of data sets. From the multiple data sets, parameters are estimated, as are the CIs for those parameters. Multiple imputation is the preferred method for modeling missing data. Complete case analysis is performed by excluding cases with missing data and only analyzing cases that have all the data of interest. This can result in biased results and/or can be associated with a substantial loss in analytic power and should not be done.[121,122]

**incidence:** number of new cases of disease among persons at risk that occur over time,[98] as contrasted with *prevalence*, which is the total number of persons with the disease at any given time. Incidence is usually expressed as a percentage of individuals affected during an interval (eg, year) or as a rate calculated as the number of individuals who develop the disease during a period divided by the number of person-years at risk.

> *Example:* The incidence rate for the disease was 1.2 cases per 100 000 per year.

**inclusion criteria:** characteristics a study participant must possess to be included in the study population (such as age of 65 years or older at the time of study enrollment and willing and able to provide informed consent). Like *exclusion criteria*, inclusion criteria should be defined before any participants are enrolled in a study, and such criteria should be mentioned in the Methods section of research articles.

**independence, assumption of:** assumption that the occurrence of one event is in no way linked to another event. Many statistical tests depend on the assumption that each *outcome* is independent.[98] This may not be a valid assumption if repeated tests are performed on the same individuals (eg, blood pressure is measured sequentially over time), if more than 1 outcome is measured for a given individual (eg, myocardial infarction and death or all hospital admissions), or if more than 1 intervention is made on the same individual (eg, blood pressure is measured during 3 different drug treatments). Tests for *repeated measures* may be used in those circumstances. If a *Durbin-Watson test* suggests that autocorrelation is present, then the data should be analyzed using autoregression techniques.

**independent variable:** variable postulated to influence the *dependent variable* within the defined area of relationships under study.[98] The term does not refer to statistical independence, so some use the term *explanatory variable* instead.[93]

> *Example:* Age, sex, systolic blood pressure, and cholesterol level were the independent variables entered into the multiple logistic regression that assessed how these characteristics influenced the dependent variable, mortality.

**indirect cause:** a factor $X$ can cause an effect on $Y$ directly, but if $X$ acts on some other factor $Z$ that in turn affects $Y$, $X$ acts on $Y$ as an indirect cause.[95]

> *Example:* Overcrowding in the cities facilitated transmission of the tubercle bacillus and precipitated the tuberculosis epidemic. (Overcrowding is an indirect cause; the tubercle bacillus is the direct cause.)

**inference:** conclusions arrived at on the basis of evidence and reasoning.[98]

> *Example:* Intake of a high-fat diet was significantly associated with cardiovascular mortality; therefore, we infer that eating a high-fat diet increases the risk of cardiovascular death.

**instrument error:** error introduced in a study when the testing instrument is not appropriate for the conditions of the study or is not accurate enough to measure the study *outcome*[95] (may be attributable to deficiencies in such factors as calibration, *accuracy*, and *precision*).

**instrumental variable analysis:** a method used in observational studies that minimizes the risk of confounding. An instrument is some factor that is correlated with the type of treatment received but not with the outcome. For example, a patient may live near a hospital that only performs one type of intervention but not another. If the patient only goes to the nearest hospital and receives one or the other treatment, then the distance the person lives from the facility or their zip/postal code might be used as an instrumental variable. In this instance, an analysis of outcomes stratified by zip/postal code will yield results that mimic those for randomized trials because patients will only receive one or another intervention based on where they live and not on their clinical condition.

**intention-to-treat (ITT) analysis, intent-to-treat (ITT) analysis:** analysis of outcomes for individuals based on the treatment group to which they were randomized rather than on which treatment they actually received and whether they completed the study.[13] When groups are assessed by the actual treatment received rather than the one they were intended to get, the analysis is referred to as a per-protocol analysis. The ITT analysis maintains an equal distribution of the study group's baseline characteristics and generally avoids bias associated with changes in treatment plans that occur after the study was initiated. ITT is the preferred main analysis approach for randomized trials. ITT can increase the risk for bias in noninferiority trials, and although ITT should be the primary analytic approach for noninferior trials, a *per-protocol analysis* should also be presented[123] (see 19.2, Randomized Clinical Trials).

→ Although other analyses, such as evaluable patient analysis or per-protocol analyses, are often performed to evaluate outcomes based on treatment actually received, the ITT analysis should be presented regardless of other analyses because the intervention itself may influence whether treatment was changed and whether participants dropped out. ITT may bias the results of equivalence and noninferiority trials; for those trials, additional analyses should be presented (see 19.2.3, Equivalence Trials and Noninferiority Trials).

**interaction:** when 2 variables affect one another in a nonlinear way. It is common for 2 variables to have an additive effect. When the 2 variables are working in concert with one another and have an effect that is greater than what each one adds to an effect by itself, an interaction is present. An example might be that as a person ages he or she becomes more susceptible to hypoglycemia and that when insulin is given hypoglycemia may occur. The effect of insulin on hypoglycemia in older people may be greater than in younger people and greater than expected from studying the hypoglycemic effects of insulin or age alone. See *interactive effect*, *interaction term*.

**interaction term:** variable used in *analysis of variance, analysis of covariance,* and regression analysis in which 2 independent variables interact with each other (eg, when assessing the effect of energy expenditure on cardiac output, the increase in cardiac output per unit increase in energy expenditure might differ between men and women; the interaction term would enable the analysis to take this difference into account). The term is created by multiplying the 2 interacting variables into a single variable. For example, if age is one variable and insulin dose is another, the interacting term will be age by insulin dose (the age variable multiplied by the insulin dose variable). If the interaction variable is statistically significant in a regression analysis, an interaction between variables is assumed to be present.[95]

**interactive effect:** effect of 2 or more *independent variables* on a *dependent variable* in which the effect of one independent variable is influenced by the presence of another.[93] The interactive effect may be additive (ie, equal to the sum of the 2 effects present separately), synergistic (ie, the 2 effects together have a greater effect than the sum of the effects present separately), or antagonistic (ie, the 2 effects together have a smaller effect than the sum of the effects present separately).

**interim analysis:** data analysis performed during a clinical trial to monitor treatment effects. Interim analysis should be prespecified in the study protocol before patient enrollment and the *stopping rules* if a particular treatment effect is reached. Each time an interim analysis is performed, the $\alpha$ level set for establishing statistical significance of the outcome should be adjusted just as one would do for a repeated-measures analysis. This is because each time the data are assessed and a statistical significance test is performed, each successive look at the data increases the likelihood of falsely concluding that a statistically significant result is present when it really is not (type I error). The process for adjusting the $\alpha$ level is called $\alpha$ expenditure.[15]

**interobserver bias:** likelihood that one observer is more likely to give a particular response than another observer because of factors unique to the observer or instrument. For example, one physician may be more likely than another to identify a particular set of signs and symptoms as indicative of religious preoccupation on the basis of his or her beliefs, or a physician may be less likely than another physician to diagnose alcoholism in a patient because of the physician's expectations.[104] The *Cochran Q test* is used to assess interobserver bias.[104]

**interobserver reliability:** test used to measure agreement among observers about a particular measure or *outcome*.

→ Although the proportion of times that 2 observers agree can be reported, this does not take into account the number of times they would have agreed by chance alone. For example, if 2 observers must decide whether a factor is present or absent, they should agree 50% of the time according to chance. The *κ statistic* assesses agreement while taking chance into account and is described by the equation [(observed agreement) − (agreement expected by chance)]/(1 − agreement expected by chance). The $\kappa$ value may range from 0 (poor agreement) to 1 (perfect agreement) and may be classified by various descriptive terms, such as slight (0-0.20), fair (0.21-0.40), moderate (0.41-0.60), substantial (0.61-0.80), or near perfect (0.81-0.99).[123]

→ In cases in which disagreement may have especially grave consequences, such as one pathologist rating a slide "without disease" and another rating a slide "invasive carcinoma," a weighted $\kappa$ may be used to grade disagreement according to the severity of the consequences.[123] See also *Pearson product moment correlation.*

**interobserver variation:** see *interobserver reliability*.

**interquartile range (IQR):** the distance between the 25th and 75th percentiles, which is used to describe the dispersion of values for categorical data. Like other quantiles (eg, tertiles, quintiles), expressing the range of data is preferred when the data are *nonnormally distributed*. Data that are not normally distributed should not have their distribution expressed as the *SD*. The interquartile range describes the inner 50% of values; the interquintile range (20th to 80th percentile) describes the inner 60% of values; the interdecile range (10th to 90th percentile) describes the inner 80% of values.[93]

**interrater reliability:** reproducibility among raters or observers; synonymous with *interobserver reliability*.

**interval estimate:** see *confidence interval*.[95]

**intraobserver reliability (or variation):** reliability (or, conversely, variation) in measurements by the same person at different times.[95] Similar to *interobserver reliability*, intraobserver reliability is the agreement between measurements by one individual beyond that expected by chance and can be measured by means of the *κ statistic* or the *Pearson product moment correlation*.

**intrarater reliability:** synonymous with *intraobserver reliability*.

**jackknife test:** technique for estimating the *variance* and *bias* of an estimator. An estimator is a process that results in a numerical value that characterizes a distribution. For example, there are processes that calculate the mean and variance of a sample, and the processes that do the calculation are called estimators. If the estimators are biased, they may result in incorrect estimates of the mean and variance. The jackknife method detects bias in estimators. The jackknife technique calculates a mean by calculating the mean of a sample leaving 1 value out, repeating this n − 1 times and calculating the mean of those estimates. If the estimate obtained by the jackknife method differs from the mean calculated by some other method, there is bias in the method used to calculate the mean. A similar process can be used to detect bias in variance estimates. *Bootstrapping* performs a similar function, but instead of leaving one value out of a subset of the sample, sampling of subsets is repeated many times, and a new mean or variance is calculated.[123]

**Kaplan-Meier method (also known as the product-limit method):** *nonparametric* method of estimating survival functions and compiling *life tables*.[118] Kaplan-Meier survival curves (see Figure 4.2-3 in 4.2.1.2, Survival Plots) show the fraction of patients surviving or experiencing an event in any given interval after some sort of intervention. Unlike the *Cutler-Ederer method*, the Kaplan-Meier method assumes that termination of follow-up occurs at the end of the time block. Therefore, Kaplan-Meier estimates of risk tend to be slightly lower than Cutler-Ederer estimates.[95] The horizontal lines on the plots represent the known survival time for the patients being studied. Patients who are *censored* (ie, those who do not experience the event of interest) are represented as tick marks on a Kaplan-Meier plot. Each vertical line represents an individual patient experiencing an event. Often an *intervention* and *control group* are depicted on one graph, and the groups are compared by a *log-rank test*. Because the method is nonparametric, there is no attempt to fit the data to a theoretical curve. Thus, Kaplan-Meier plots have a jagged appearance, with discrete drops at the end of each interval in which an event occurs.

**κ (kappa) statistic:** statistic used to measure nonrandom agreement between observers or measurements. It is calculated by subtracting the probability of 2 observers randomly agreeing with one another from the observed frequency that they agree with each other and dividing this quantity by (1 minus the probability that they agree with one another randomly). When κ = 1, there is perfect agreement; if κ = 0, there is no agreement.[98] See *interobserver* and *intraobserver reliability*.

**Kendall τ (tau) rank correlation:** method used to determine if an association exists between 2 ordinal (ie, categorical data that can be ordered from high to low) or ranked variables. Pairs of data between the 2 variables are compared, and if the values of one variable are consistently higher or lower than the other, a correlation between the 2 variables is assumed to exist. When τ = 1, the raters always agreed; if τ = −1, they never agreed; and if τ = 0, the different rankings between raters was completely random.[123,124]

**Kolmogorov-Smirnov test:** test used to determine if the distribution of a data set matches a particular probability distribution. This test is performed by subtracting the observed continuous probability distribution from a theoretical one. Typically, this test is used to determine if sample data fit the normal probability distribution. If $P \leq .05$, then the observed distribution is different than the theoretical distribution it is thought to conform with.[104] The Kolmogorov-Smirnov test may be used to assess *goodness of fit*.[98]

**Kruskal-Wallis test:** is the nonparametric equivalent of the 1-way *ANOVA* test and does not require normally distributed data assumptions of equal variance. Used to compare 3 or more groups, this test tests the null hypothesis that there are no differences in the distributions of any group. Like ANOVA, the Kruskal-Wallis test determines only that there are no differences between any group. If differences are found, then a multiple comparison test, such as a *Tukey* or multiple *Mann-Whitney test* using a *Bonferroni correction,* can be used to determine if differences exist between individual groups.[104] The Kruskal-Wallis test is a *nonparametric* analog of *ANOVA* and generalizes the 2-sample *Wilcoxon rank sum test* to the multiple-sample case.[93]

The Kruskal-Wallis test is performed by ranking all the data from highest to lowest and then separating into the various prespecified groups. The mean rank for each group is compared by $\chi^2$ analysis using n − 1 groups as the number of degrees of freedom.

→ Sample wording: **Methods:** A Kruskal-Wallis test was used to test for differences among the 7 different drug doses for their effect on antibody response because normality was questionable and sample sizes within each group were small. **Results:** The Kruskal-Wallis test for comparison of different drug doses indicates that there was a statistically significant difference in the distribution of antibody responses between the groups ($\chi^2_6 = 15.3$, $P = .02$).[124]

**kurtosis:** the way in which a unimodal curve deviates from a *normal distribution*; may be more peaked (leptokurtic) or more flat (platykurtic) than a normal distribution.[104] The measure of the normal distribution's kurtosis is 3. The other assessment of the shape of a distribution is its *skewness* (the deviation from being symmetric or how much of the distribution exists in its tails).

**Latin square:** form of complete treatment crossover design used for crossover drug trials that eliminates the effect of treatment order. Each patient receives each drug, but each drug is followed by another drug only once in the array. For example, in the following 4 × 4 array (**Table 19.5-2**), letters A through D correspond to each of 4 drugs, each row corresponds to a patient, and each column corresponds to the order in which the drugs are given.[16]

See 19.2.2, Crossover Trials.

**Table 19.5-2.** Latin Square

|  | First drug | Second drug | Third drug | Fourth drug |
|---|---|---|---|---|
| Patient 1 | C | D | A | B |
| Patient 2 | A | C | B | D |
| Patient 3 | D | B | C | A |
| Patient 4 | B | A | D | C |

**lead-time bias:** artifactual increase in survival time that results from earlier detection of a disease, usually cancer, during a time when the disease is asymptomatic. Lead-time bias produces longer survival from that of diagnosis but not longer survival from the time of onset of the disease.[95] Imagine that 2 patients develop small tumors at the same time, of which they will die irrespective of any treatment in 10 years. Then imagine that this particular tumor would become obvious at 7 years. One patient gets screened at 5 years, the tumor is detected, and treatment administered. This patient dies 5 years after screening. The other patient receives treatment at 7 years when the tumor is obvious and only lives for 3 years after treatment. It appears that screening resulted in 2 additional years of life, but this is an artifact because there was a 2-year lead in making a diagnosis. Making a diagnosis did not result in a longer life, but it made cancer screening appear effective. See also *length-time bias*.

→ Lead-time bias may give the appearance of a survival benefit from screening when in fact the increased survival is only artifactual. Lead-time bias is used more generally to indicate a systematic error that arises when follow-up of groups does not begin at comparable stages in the natural course of the condition.

**least significant difference test:** one of the multiple comparison tests assessing differences in individual groups when the null hypothesis for an *analysis of variance* is proven false, meaning that the group variances are not all equal. An extension of the *t test*.[95]

**least-squares method:** method of estimation, particularly in *regression analysis*, that minimizes the sum of the differences between the observed responses and the values predicted by a model.[104] The regression line is created so that the sum of the squares of the *residuals* is as small as possible.

**left-censored data:** see *censored data*.

**length-time bias:** bias that arises when a sampling scheme is based on patient visits because patients with more frequent clinic visits are more likely to be selected than those with less frequent visits. In a screening study of cancer, for example, screening patients with frequent visits is more likely to detect slow-growing tumors than would sampling patients who visit a physician only when symptoms arise.[104] Another scenario is if one patient has a rapidly growing form of a tumor, the time between when the cancer becomes symptomatic and the patient dies is short. The rapid course may make it less likely that the patient gets screened. Another patient might have a slower-growing form of the same tumor, get screened, and live a long time until he or she dies. Screening appears effective because the patient who had a tumor with a more benign course lived longer than the one who had a rapidly growing tumor and who was less likely to undergo screening because of the rapidity of the tumor's growth. See also *lead-time bias*.

**life table:** method of organizing data that allows examination of the experience of 1 or more groups of individuals over time with varying periods of follow-up. For each increment of the follow-up period, the number entering, the number leaving, and the number dying of disease or developing disease can be calculated. In contrast to Kaplan-Meier analysis, where changes in survival probability are calculated for each patient having events, in life-table analysis arbitrary intervals are selected and the survival probability for all the patients having events within that interval is calculated. An assumption of the life-table method is that a censored individual (eg, not completing follow-up, dying during the interval from a cause other than the event) is exposed for half the incremental follow-up period.[104] Thus, the number of patients at risk for the event at the beginning of the interval is adjusted by half the number censored during that interval. (The *Kaplan-Meier method* and the *Cutler-Ederer method* are also forms of life-table analysis but make different assumptions about the length of exposure.)

→ The clinical life table describes the outcomes of a cohort of individuals classified according to their exposure or treatment history. The cohort life table is used for a cohort of individuals born at approximately the same time and followed up until death. The current life table is a summary of mortality of the population during a brief (1- to 3-year) period, classified by age, often used to estimate life expectancy for the population at a given age.[98]

**likelihood ratio:** probability of getting a certain test result if the patient has the condition relative to the probability of getting the result if the patient does not have the condition. The greater the likelihood ratio, the more likely that a positive test result will occur in a patient who has the disease. A ratio of 2 means a person with the disease is twice as likely to have a positive test result as a person without the disease.[100] The likelihood ratio test is based on the ratio of 2 likelihood functions and is used to assess the model fit for regression models fit by maximum likelihood modeling, as is done in logistic regression.[93] For *dichotomous variables*, this is calculated as *sensitivity*/(1 − *specificity*). See also *diagnostic discrimination*.

**Likert scale:** scale often used to assess opinion or attitude, ranked by attaching a number to each response, such as 1, strongly agree; 2, agree; 3, undecided or neutral; 4, disagree; and 5, strongly disagree. The score is a sum of the numerical responses to each question.[93]

**Lilliefors test:** test of normality (using the *Kolmogorov-Smirnov test* statistic) in which *mean* and *variance* are estimated from the data.[93]

**linear regression:** statistical method used to compare *continuous dependent* and *independent variables*. When the data are depicted on a graph as a *regression line*, the independent variable is plotted on the *x-axis* and the dependent variable on the *y-axis*. The *residual* is the vertical distance from the data point to the regression line[100]; analysis of residuals is a commonly used procedure for *linear regression* (see Figure 4.2-4 in 4.2.1.3, Scatterplots). This method is frequently performed using *least-squares* regression.[92]

→ The description of a linear regression model should include the equation of the fitted line with the estimated value for the slope and its 95% CI if possible, the $r^2$, the fraction of variation in $y$ explained by each of the $x$ variables (correlation and partial correlation), and the variances of the fitted coefficients $a$ and $b$ (and their *SDs*).[92,125]

*Example:* The regression model identified a significant positive relationship between the dependent variable weight and height (slope = 0.25; 95% CI, 0.19-0.31; $y = 12.6 + 0.25x$; $t_{451} = 8.3$; $P < .001$; $r^2 = 0.67$).[100]

(In this example, the slope is positive, indicating that as one variable increases the other increases; the *t test* with 451 *df* is significant; the regression line is described by the equation and includes the slope 0.25 and the constant 12.6. The coefficient of determination $r^2$ demonstrates that 67% of the variance in weight is explained by height.)[100]

→ Four important assumptions are made when linear regression is conducted: the dependent variable is sampled randomly from the population; the spread or dispersion of the dependent variable is the same regardless of the value of the independent variable (this equality is referred to as homogeneity of variances or *homoscedasticity*); the relationship between the 2 variables is linear; and the independent variable is measured with complete precision.[95]

**LOESS (locally estimated scatterplot smoothing) or LOWESS (locally weighted scatterplot smoothing):** method for fitting a curve to data that does not depend on knowing what mathematical function (if any) describes the data (such as the data following a linear or exponential relationship).[126] Each data point is fitted by a regression equation finding the best estimate for the mean and variance for that point based on fitting a curve to the point and some window around the data. Larger windows result in smaller variances for these estimates but result in greater data smoothing. In contrast, smaller windows yield fitted data points that more closely follow the trends within the data but have large variances associated with the point estimates. LOESS is used to find patterns and trends within data.[126]

*Example:* Mortality rates for Medicare beneficiaries were measured between 1999 to 2013 (**Figure 19.5-1**). The symbols represent the observed mortality rates for each year. The solid lines represent estimates for these rates derived from LOESS method and the shaded areas show the 95% CI for those estimates as determined by LOESS.[127]

**Figure 19.5-1.** LOESS Method to Fit a Curve to the Data

Figure. Trends in Observed All-Cause Mortality Rates in the Medicare Population, 1999-2013

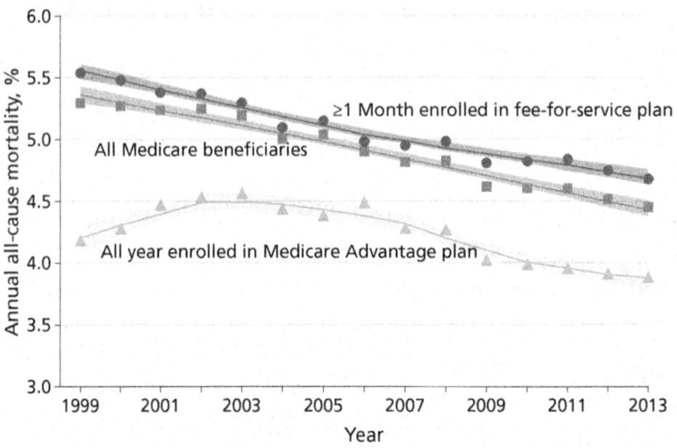

The symbols around each trend line represent the observed mortality rates for each year. All Medicare beneficiaries aged ≥65 years, Medicare beneficiaries aged ≥65 years who were enrolled in the fee-for-service plan for ≥1 month, and Medicare beneficiaries aged ≥65 years who were enrolled in a Medicare Advantage program for the full duration for the year are shown. The shaded areas around each line represent 95% CIs. Lines were smoothed using the LOESS method (local regression).[127]

**logistic regression:** type of regression model used to analyze the relationship between a *binary dependent variable* (eg, alive or dead, complication or no complication) and 1 or more *independent variables*. Often used to determine the independent effect on the dependent variable of one of the explanatory variables while simultaneously controlling for several other factors that are included as independent variables in the regression equation. Results are usually expressed by *odds ratios* and 95% *CIs*.[95] (The multiple logistic regression equation may also be provided, but because these involve exponents they are substantially more complicated than linear regression equations. Therefore, in journals, the equation is generally not published but can be made available on request from authors. Alternatively, it may be placed in supplementary tables.)

→ To be valid, a multiple regression model must have an adequate sample size for the number of variables examined. A rough rule of thumb is to have 10 to 20 events (eg, deaths, complications) for each explanatory variable examined.[128]

→ When using logistic regression, the Methods section of a manuscript should include wording such as the following: "To examine the effect of the type of analgesia used and chest tube size on complications of pleurodesis, multiple logistic regression was used." The results should be stated as follows: "The odds ratio for using a 12F chest tube and having complications of pleurodesis was 1.9 (95% CI, 0.7-5.1) relative to placing a 24F chest tube." It is always good practice to state what the absolute risks are: "In 55 patients with 12F chest tubes, there were 13 complications (24%), and in the 56 patients with 24F chest tubes, there were 8 complications (12%)."

**log-linear model:** models where the logarithm of the dependent variable is a linear combination of the independent variables. In general, the dependent variable is shown in terms of being equal to the exponent of the right side of the regression equation. These may be used for the analysis of *categorical data*.[93]

$$\rightarrow \ln(Y) = \alpha + \beta_1 X_1 + \beta_2 X_2 + \beta_3 X_{3 \ldots} + \epsilon$$

$Y = \exp(\alpha + \beta_1 X_1 + \beta_2 X_2 + \beta_3 X_{3 \ldots} + \epsilon)$ are examples of log-linear models.

**log-rank test:** method to compare differences between survival curves for different treatments; same as the *Mantel-Haenszel test*.[93] If $P < .05$, then it is concluded that there is a less than 5% chance that any observed discrepancies between 2 survival curves are due to chance alone.

**main effect:** estimate of the independent effect of an explanatory (*independent*) variable on a *dependent variable* in *analysis of variance* or *analysis of covariance*. In a factorial-designed experiment, several interventions can be tested simultaneously. For each intervention (eg, a drug dose), there can be a single level of the dose (comparing drug vs no drug) or several levels of the drug (different doses). With this design, several drugs can be tested in one large experiment to determine their influence on some outcome. The *main effect* is the effect of one of the factors (drugs) on the outcome inclusive of all the various doses and excluding the effect of the other factors (drugs). *Interactions* can be tested between factors (drugs) in the same experiment. The interaction is tested for by creation of a variable that multiplies the factors being compared. When an interaction exists (eg, the interaction variable is statistically significant), the factors have an effect that is greater than what would be expected by the addition of each when they act alone.[104]

**Mann-Whitney test:** *nonparametric* equivalent of the *t test*, used to compare *ordinal dependent variables* with *nominal independent variables* or *continuous independent variables* converted to an ordinal scale.[98] Similar to the *Wilcoxon rank sum test*.

**MANOVA:** multivariate *analysis of variance*. This involves examining the overall *significance* of all *dependent variables* considered simultaneously and thus has less risk of *type I error* than would a series of *univariable analysis of variance* procedures on several dependent variables. See also *ANOVA*.

**Mantel-Haenszel test:** another name for the *log-rank test*.

**Markov process:** process of modeling possible events or conditions over time that assumes that the probability that a given state or condition will be present depends only on the state or condition immediately preceding it and that no additional information about previous states or conditions would create a more accurate estimate.[104] These models account for patients moving from one state or condition to another. For example, if there is a 2% stroke rate per year in a population, Markov models facilitate modeling how many patients with stroke will be present after a number of years. They do this by assuming that starting with 100 patients there will be 2 with a stroke after the first year and 98 left who are at risk for stroke. After the second year there will be 4 patients with stroke in the population and 96 eligible to have a stroke in the next year. Markov models estimate how many patients will be in each state (stroke or no stroke) for any given number of years (or cycles) that the investigator wants to model.

**masked assessment:** synonymous with *blinded assessment*.

**masked assignment:** synonymous with *blinded assignment*.

**matching:** process of making study and *control groups* comparable with respect to factors other than the factors under study, generally as part of a *case-control study*. Matching can be done in several ways, including frequency matching (matching on frequency distributions of the matched variable[s]), category (matching in broad groups, such as young and old), individual (matching on individual rather than group characteristics), and pair matching (matching each study individual with a control individual).[98] Attempts to approximate matching in observational studies are performed by **propensity** methods, where the propensity to be in one group or another is calculated (usually by multivariable regression) and used to match patients into one group or another. After matching, the baseline characteristics of the 2 groups before and after the match should be shown.[129]

**McNemar test:** form of the $\chi^2$ *test* for *binary* responses in comparisons of matched pairs.[98] The ratio of *discordant* to *concordant pairs* is determined; the greater the number of discordant pairs with the better *outcome* being associated with the treatment intervention, the greater the effect of the intervention.[104]

**mean:** sum of values measured for a given variable divided by the number of values; a measure of *central tendency* appropriate for *normally distributed data*.[130] The *SD* should always be displayed along with mean values (*m*). The SD shows how much dispersion there is around the estimate of the data's central tendency. In general, if the SD is larger than the mean value, the data should be assumed to be not normally distributed. Means should not be used to represent the central tendency of data that are not normally distributed because the mean itself assumes that data are normally distributed. *Kurtosis* and *skewness* are measures of how much a data distribution deviates from a normal distribution. See also *average*.

→ If the data are not normally distributed, the *median* should be used as a measure of central tendency and should be displayed along with the 25% and 75% interquartile range to provide a sense for how much scatter there is in the data.

**measurement error:** estimate of the variability of a measurement. Variability of a given *parameter* (eg, weight) is the sum of the true variability of what is measured (eg, day-to-day weight fluctuations) plus the variability of the instrument or observer measurement or variability caused by measurement error (error variability, eg, the scale used for weighing).

**median:** midpoint of a distribution chosen so that half the values for a given variable appear above and half occur below.[95] For data that do not have a *normal distribution*, the median provides a better measure of *central tendency* than does the mean because it is less influenced by *outliers*.[119] Medians should be displayed along with measures of uncertainty, such as 25% and 75% interquartile ranges.

**median test:** *nonparametric* rank-order test for 2 groups.[93]

**mediation analysis:** a method used to assess a pathway in which 1 variable associated with a second variable in turn is associated with a third variable, in which the second variable mediates the association between the first 2 variables (Figure 19.3-2).

**mendelian randomization:** a means for mimicking the results of randomized trials by using genetic variations that exist between individuals that influence health outcomes that are not subject to the confounding or reverse-causation bias that can distort observational findings. An example might be genetic variation that results in high or low high-density lipoprotein cholesterol (HDL-C) levels and assessing the effect of that genetic variation on cardiovascular outcomes to test the potential effect of HDL-C on those outcomes.

**meta-analysis:** a method of aggregating statistical results and deriving a single estimate for an effect based on a number of similar studies. To perform a meta-analysis, the studies should be similar, with little heterogeneity. When there is a great deal of heterogeneity, data aggregation as a meta-analysis should not be performed, and the various studies should be assessed as a systematic review. Meta-analyses should be viewed like any research study and have a detailed Methods section. Heterogeneity among studies should be reported as $I^2$ and the point estimate for comparing the studies reported along with 95% CIs. Showing the effects of individual studies is facilitated by including a *forest plot* (see Figure 4.2-16 in 4.2.1.11, Forest Plots, and 19.3.6, Meta-analyses).

**missing data:** incomplete information on individuals resulting from any of a number of causes, including loss to follow-up, refusal to participate, and inability to complete the study. Although the simplest approach would be to remove such participants from the analysis, this introduces bias in the analysis and should not be done. Furthermore, certain health conditions may be systematically associated with the risk of having missing data, and thus removal of these individuals could *bias* the analysis. It is generally better to model the missing data with multiple *imputation*, which is then included in the analysis.[121,122]

**mixed-methods analysis (also known as multimethod research):** study design using a variety of methods, both qualitative and quantitative, to answer a research question.

**mixed-model analysis (also known as hierarchical analysis):** statistical model having both fixed and random effects. Regression analyses assume that individual data are independent of one another. When the data are not independent (ie, correlated), mixed models may be used. This occurs when data are clustered (eg, patients in one hospital may have effects related to the hospital that differ from those of patients treated in another hospital) or repeated measures are performed (one measure taken after another from the same person will be correlated). Fixed and random effects are characteristics of data. Data are random if they can be considered to be drawn randomly from some distribution and are expected to vary from one subject to another. For example, if the effect of an intervention on patients who are in various hospitals is being studied, the variable representing hospitals may be modeled as a random effect because the hospitals were randomly selected from the universe of all hospitals. However, the intervention is the same for all patients and all hospitals, so it is considered a fixed effect. Variables that do not change between individuals are considered fixed effects.[131]

**mode:** in a series of values of a given variable, the number that occurs most frequently; used most often when a distribution has 2 peaks (*bimodal distribution*).[130] This is also appropriate as a measure of *central tendency* for *categorical data*.

**Monte Carlo simulation:** a family of techniques for modeling complex systems for which it would otherwise be difficult to obtain sufficient data. In general, Monte Carlo simulations will randomly resample data from a larger data set to mimic the random selection that occurs in experiments. Instead of doing actual experiments, Monte Carlo simulations use a computer *algorithm* to generate a large number of observations that are randomly selected. The patterns of these numbers are then used to assess probabilities of events occurring and for any irregularities that might arise.

**mortality rate:** death rate described by the following equation: [(number of deaths during period) × (period of observation)]/(number of individuals observed). For values such as the crude mortality rate, the denominator is the number of individuals observed at the midpoint of observation. See also *crude death rate*.[104]

→ Mortality rate is often expressed in terms of a standard ratio, such as deaths per 100 000 persons per year.

**Moses rank-like dispersion test:** rank test of the equality of scale of 2 identically shaped populations, applicable when the population *medians* are not known.[93]

**multilevel model:** models in which the data are aggregated into groups. Students may be clustered into a classroom, which is clustered into a school, which is clustered into a school district. Because data organized like this will not meet the assumption of independence, regression analyses examining characteristics of these groups should be modeled using *mixed-models* analysis.

**multiple analyses problem:** problem that occurs when several statistical tests are performed on one group of data because of the potential to introduce a *type I error*. Multiple analyses are problematic when the analyses were not specified as primary *outcome* measures. Multiple analyses can be appropriately adjusted for by means of a *Bonferroni adjustment* or any of several *multiple comparison procedures*.

**multiple comparison procedures:** If many tests for statistical significance are performed on a data set, there is a risk of falsely concluding that a difference exists when it does not. For example, when the first test is performed and the null hypothesis is rejected (concluding that the groups are different) at the $P < .05$ level, there is a 5% chance that the observed difference between the groups was attributable to chance alone. If another test is performed on the same data using the same assumptions, the chance that the null hypothesis is rejected by chance alone this second time is not 5% but 5% + 5% = 10%, meaning that when 2 tests for significance are performed, the chance of rejecting the null hypothesis (ie, concluding falsely that a difference exists when it does not) is 10%. One way to correct for this problem is to divide the $P$ value used for significance by the number of statistical tests performed. This is called the *Bonferroni* correction and, for our example of 2 tests, 0.05/2 would yield an $\alpha$ value of .025 for a significance threshold.[132,133]

The same problem exists when performing statistical significance tests for multiple groups as is done for *ANOVA*. The first test establishes only that significant differences exist between groups but does not specify which groups. Finding out which groups are different from one another post hoc becomes a multiple comparison problem.

→ Some tests for multiple comparisons result in more conservative estimates (less likely to be significant) than others. More conservative tests include the *Tukey test* and the *Bonferroni adjustment*; the *Duncan multiple range test* is less conservative. Other tests include the *Scheffé test*, the *Newman-Keuls test*, and the Gabriel test,[93] as well as many others. There is ongoing debate among statisticians about when it is appropriate to use these tests.

**multiple regression:** general term for analysis procedures used to estimate values of the *dependent variable* for all measured *independent variables* that are found to be associated. The procedure used depends on whether the variables are *continuous* or *nominal*. When all variables are continuous variables, multiple *linear regression* is used and the mean of the dependent variable is expressed using the equation $Y = \alpha + \beta_1\chi_1 + \beta_2\chi_2 + \cdots + \beta_k\chi_k$, where $Y$ is the dependent variable and $k$ is the total number of independent variables. When independent variables may be either nominal or continuous and the dependent variable is continuous, *analysis of covariance* is used. (Analysis of covariance often requires an *interaction term* to account for differences in the relationship between the independent and dependent variables.) When all variables are nominal and the dependent variable is time dependent, *life-table* methods are used. When the independent variables are either continuous or nominal and the dependent variable is nominal and time dependent (such as incidence of death), the *Cox proportional hazards model* may be used. Nominal dependent variables that are not time dependent are analyzed by means of *logistic regression* or *discriminant analysis*.[92]

**multivariable analysis:** the name means many variables. Any statistical test that deals with 1 *dependent variable* and at least 2 *independent variables*. It may include *nominal* or *continuous* variables, but *ordinal* data must be converted to a nominal scale for analysis. The multivariate approach has 3 advantages over bivariate analysis: (1) it allows for investigation of the relationship between the dependent and independent variables while controlling for the effects of other independent variables; (2) it allows several comparisons to be made statistically without increasing the likelihood of a *type I error*; and (3) it can be used to compare how well several independent variables individually can estimate values of the dependent variable.[95] Examples include *analysis of variance, multiple (logistic or linear) regression, analysis of covariance, Kruskal-Wallis test, Friedman test, life table*, and *Cox proportional hazards model*.

**multivariate analysis:** similar to multivariable analysis except that there is more than 1 dependent variable. The term *multivariate* is frequently incorrectly used in the scientific literature when multivariable analysis is meant. Multivariate analysis is seen with repeated-measures experiments when an outcome variable is repeatedly measured in different periods. It is also seen in hierarchical and cluster statistical models when there are many individuals in a single cluster. The suffix *–ate* added to "variable" indicates that something is done to the variables, implying that the variables in question are on the left side of the equation.

**N:** total number of units (eg, patients, households) in the sample under study.

> *Example:* We assessed the admission diagnoses of all patients admitted from the emergency department during a 1-month period (N = 127).

**n:** number of units in a subgroup of the sample under study.

> *Example:* Of the patients admitted from the emergency department (N = 127), the most frequent admission diagnosis was unstable angina (n = 38).

**natural experiment (also known as "found" experiment):** investigation in which a change in a risk factor or exposure occurs in one group of individuals but not in another. The distribution of individuals into a particular group is non-random, and as opposed to controlled clinical trials, the change is not brought about by the investigator.[95] The natural experiment is often used to study effects that cannot be studied in a controlled trial, such as the incidence of medical illness immediately after an earthquake.

**naturalistic sample:** set of observations obtained from a sample of the population in such a way that the distribution of *independent variables* in the sample is representative of the distribution in the *population*.[95]

**necessary cause:** characteristic whose presence is required to bring about or cause the disease or *outcome* under study.[134] A necessary cause may not be a *sufficient cause*.

**negative predictive value:** the probability that an individual does not have the disease (as determined by the *criterion standard*) if a test result is negative.[95] This measure takes into account the *prevalence* of the condition or the disease. A more general term is *posttest probability*. See *positive predictive value, diagnostic discrimination*.

**nested case-control study:** *case-control study* in which cases and controls are drawn from a *cohort study*. The advantages of a nested case-control study over a case-control study are that the controls are selected from participants at risk at the time of occurrence of each case that arises in a cohort, thus avoiding the *confounding* effect of time in the analysis, and that cases and controls are by definition drawn from the same *population*[95] (see 19.3.1, Cohort Studies, and 19.3.2, Case-Control Studies).

**Newman-Keuls test:** a type of *multiple comparisons procedure*, used to compare more than 2 groups. It first compares the 2 groups that have the highest and lowest means, then sequentially compares the next most extreme groups, and stops when a comparison is not significant.[94]

**n-of-1 trial:** randomized trial that uses a single patient and an *outcome* measure agreed on by the patient and physician. The n-of-1 trial may be used by clinicians to assess which of 2 or more possible treatment options is better for the individual patient.[134]

**nocebo:** negative effects on treatment efficacy and tolerability induced or driven by psychological factors. For example, in a study of migraine treatment when patients were told that a study drug was a placebo, the patients perceived that it had less effect than in patients who believed the study drug was pharmacologically active.[135]

**nominal variable (also called categorical variable):** There is no arithmetic relationship among the categories, and thus there is no intrinsic ranking or order between them, variables that can be named (eg, sex, gene alleles, race, eye color). The nominal or discrete variable usually is assessed to determine its frequency within a *population*.[95] The variable can have either a *binomial* or *Poisson distribution*.

**nomogram:** a visual means of representing a mathematical equation. For example, in the nomogram in **Figure 19.5-2**, hospital readmission within 30 days after discharge is predicted. Points are assigned for each variable by drawing a line upward from the corresponding variable to the points line. The sum of the points plotted on the total points line corresponds with the prediction of 30-day readmission.

**Figure 19.5-2.** Nomogram Predicting Postsurgery Survival

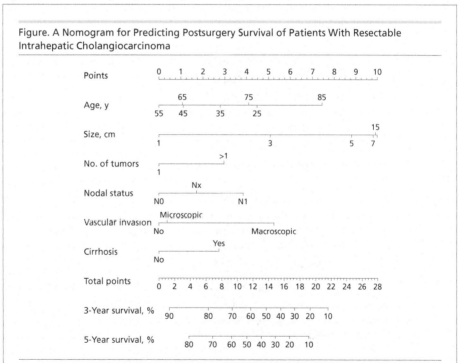

Figure. A Nomogram for Predicting Postsurgery Survival of Patients With Resectable Intrahepatic Cholangiocarcinoma

To calculate predicted survival, the patient's age is located on the row labeled "Age, y" and a straight line is drawn up to the row labeled "Points" to determine the corresponding points. This process is repeated for each of the remaining factors by drawing a straight line to the "Points" row to determine the points associated with each factor. After summing the total points, one locates the appropriate total point number and draws a straight line from this to the rows labeled "3-Year survival, %" and "5-Year survival, %" to determine the patient's predicted survival probability.

**nonconcurrent cohort study:** *cohort study* in which an individual's group assignment is determined by information that exists at the time a study begins. The extreme of a nonconcurrent cohort study is one in which the *outcome* is determined retrospectively from existing records.[95]

**noninferiority trial:** A study that examines the effect of a treatment believed to reduce adverse effects, toxic effects, or burdens of treatment relative to an existing standard treatment. The issue of such a treatment is the extent to which it maintains the primary benefits of the existing standard treatment. Unlike equivalence trials, which aim to establish that a novel treatment is neither better nor worse than standard treatment beyond a specified margin, a noninferiority trial endeavors to show that the novel treatment is "not much worse" than standard treatment. Noninferiority trials test whether the new treatment is not as good as the standard treatment by some noninferiority margin. The noninferiority margin is an estimate of how much worse the outcomes can be yet remain acceptable because they are offset by the benefits of the new treatment (eg, less cost, fewer adverse effects, simplified dosing regimens).[20-22] See also *equivalence trials*.

**nonnormal distribution:** data that do not have a *normal* (bell-shaped curve) *distribution*; examples include the *binomial*, *Poisson*, and exponential distributions.

→ Nonnormally distributed continuous data must be either transformed to a normal distribution to use parametric methods or, more commonly, analyzed by nonparametric methods.

**nonparametric statistics:** statistical procedures that do not assume that the data conform to any theoretical distribution. Nonparametric tests are most often used for *ordinal* or *nominal* data or for nonnormally distributed continuous data converted to an ordinal scale[95] (eg, weight classified by tertile). Although these tests are useful for data that are not normally distributed, they are less powerful than parametric statistics for determining whether significant differences exist between groups.

**nonrandomized trial:** prospectively assigns groups or populations to study the efficacy or effectiveness of an intervention but in which the assignment to the intervention occurs through self-selection or administrator selection rather than through randomization. Control groups can be historical, concurrent, or both. This design is sometimes called a quasi-experimental design. Reports of these trials should follow the Transparent Reporting of Evaluations with Nonrandomized Designs (TREND) reporting guideline (https://www.cdc.gov/trendstatement/).[30]

**normal distribution (also known as gaussian distribution):** *continuous data* distributed in a symmetrical, bell-shaped curve with the mean value corresponding to the highest point of the curve. This distribution of data is assumed in many statistical procedures.[95,108]

→ Descriptive statistics, such as *mean* and *SD*, can be used to accurately describe data only if the values are normally distributed or can be transformed into a normal distribution. When not normally distributed, the central tendency for data should be displayed as the median value and the distribution by the interquartile range.

**normal range:** range of values for a diagnostic test found among patients without a disease. *Cut points* for abnormal test results are arbitrary and are often defined as the central 95% of values, or the *mean* of values ±2 *SDs*.

**null hypothesis:** statement used in statistics asserting that no true difference exists between comparison groups.[95,120] In general, statistical tests do not prove that the null hypothesis is true; rather, the results of statistical testing can reject the null hypothesis at the stated $\alpha$ likelihood of a *type I error*.

→ In the Methods section, it is usually stated that the null hypothesis was rejected if $\alpha < .05$. Under these circumstances, the null hypothesis stating that no difference exists between groups is rejected if there is a less than 5% chance that any such observed difference was found because of chance alone.

→ There is an adage in statistics that the absence of evidence does not mean the evidence of absence. Not showing that the null hypothesis of there being no difference between groups is true is not the same as proving that there is no difference between groups, only that the study was unable to demonstrate that a difference exists.

**number needed to harm (NNH):** computed similarly to *number needed to treat*, but number of patients who, after being treated for a specific period, would be expected to experience 1 bad *outcome*. The NNH is calculated by inverting the absolute risk of harm. The absolute risk of harm is the proportion of patients harmed by an intervention subtracted from the proportion of patients experiencing harm who did not receive the intervention.

→ The NNH should be reported along with CIs and the absolute risk information used in its calculation. It should be expressed in a way that the reader can easily interpret the NNH concept; for example, "During follow-up, there were 1746 acute myocardial infarctions (21.7% fatal), 1052 strokes (7.3% fatal), 3307 hospitalizations for heart failure (2.6% fatal), and 2562 deaths from all causes among cohort members. For the composite of acute myocardial infarction, stroke, heart failure, or death, the attributable risk was 1.68 (95% CI, 1.27-2.08) excess events per 100 person-years of rosiglitazone compared with pioglitazone treatment. The corresponding number needed to harm for this composite end point was 60 (95% CI, 48-79) persons treated for 1 year to generate 1 excess event." The NNT of 60 was calculated by taking the inverse of the attributable (ie, absolute) risk of 0.0168.

**number needed to treat (NNT):** number of patients who must receive an intervention for a specific period for 1 patient to benefit from the intervention.[95] The NNT is the reciprocal of the *absolute risk reduction*, the difference between event rates in the intervention and placebo groups in a clinical trial. See also *number needed to harm*.

→ The NNT is preferably reported along with its CI and absolute risks and expressed in a way that is intuitively obvious to the reader; for example, "Meta-analysis using a random-effects model showed that corticosteroids alone were associated with a reduced risk of unsatisfactory recovery (relative risk [RR], 0.69 [95% CI, 0.55-0.87]; $P = .001$) (number needed to treat to benefit 1 person, 11 [95% CI, 8-25])."

→ The study patients from whom the NNT is calculated should be representative of the *population* to whom the numbers will be applied. The NNT does not take into account adverse effects of the intervention.

**observational study:** An observational study can be used to describe many designs that are not randomized trials (eg, cohort studies or case-control studies that have a goal of establishing causation, studies of prognosis, studies of diagnostic tests, and qualitative studies) (see 19.3, Observational Studies). For example, the term is commonly used in the context of cohort studies and case-control studies in which patient or caregiver preference, or happenstance, determines whether a person is exposed to an intervention or putative harmful agent or behavior (in contrast to the exposure's being under the control of the investigator, as in a randomized trial). Observational studies are also commonly performed using large administrative or clinical databases. Because the data are not usually collected for the purpose of the study and treatments are given based on a patient's clinical condition and not randomly allocated, observational studies are limited in what they can conclude because of selection bias or unmeasured confounding.[116,136] Causation cannot be concluded from observational studies, and it is best to refer to the relationships between risk factors and outcomes as associations and not use causative language.

**odds ratio (OR):** ratio of 2 odds. Odds ratio may have different definitions, depending on the study, and therefore should be defined. For example, it may be the odds of having the disease if a particular risk factor is present to the odds of not having the disease if the risk factor is not present, or the odds of having a risk factor present if the person has the disease to the odds of the risk factor being absent if the person does not have the disease.

→ The OR typically is used for a case-control or cohort study. For a study of incident cases with an infrequent disease (eg, <2% incidence), the OR approximates the *relative risk*.[96] When the incidence is relatively frequent, the OR may be arithmetically corrected to better approximate the *relative risk*.[137]

→ The OR is usually expressed by a point estimate and expressed with a measure of uncertainty, such as the 95% *confidence interval*. An OR for which the CI includes 1 indicates no statistically significant effect on risk; if the point estimate and CI are both less than 1, there is a statistically significant reduction in risk (eg, 0.75; 95% CI, 0.60-0.87); if the point estimate and CI are both greater than 1, there is a statistically significant increase in risk (eg, 1.25; 95% CI, 1.10-1.40).

**1-tailed test:** test of statistical significance in which deviations from the *null hypothesis* in only 1 direction are considered.[95,120] Most commonly used for the *t test*.

→ One-tailed tests are more likely to produce a statistically significant result than are *2-tailed tests*. The use of a 1-tailed test implies that the intervention can move only in 1 direction (ie, beneficial or harmful). Thus, the use of a 1-tailed test must be justified.

**ordinal data:** type of data with a limited number of categories with an inherent ordering of the category from lowest to highest but without fixed or equal spacing between increments.[95] Examples are Apgar scores, heart murmur rating, and cancer stage and grade. Ordinal data can be summarized by means of the *median* and *quantiles* or *range*.

→ Because increments between the numbers for ordinal data generally are not fixed (eg, the difference between a grade 1 and a grade 2 heart murmur is not quantitatively the same as the difference between a grade 3 and a grade 4 heart murmur), ordinal data should be analyzed by *nonparametric statistics*.

**ordinate:** vertical or *y-axis* of a graph. The *x-axis* is referred to as the *abscissa*.

**outcome:** *dependent variable* or end point of an investigation. In retrospective studies, such as case-control studies, the outcomes have already occurred before the study is begun; in prospective studies, such as cohort studies and controlled trials, the outcomes occur during the time of the study.[95] Primary outcomes are the main object of a study and are usually identified by the study hypothesis. Ideally, there should only be a single primary outcome. Study power is calculated based on the primary outcome. Secondary outcomes are outcomes other than the primary outcome that investigators wish to observe in the results of studies. Secondary outcomes are specified for analysis before the study is performed. Exploratory outcomes are those that an investigator elects to analyze after an experiment is performed but had not prespecified in the analytic plan.

**outliers (outlying values):** values at the extremes of a *distribution*. Because the *median* is far less sensitive to outliers than is the *mean*, it is preferable to use the median to describe the *central tendency* of data that have extreme outliers. Outliers can have a large influence on analytic techniques, such as regression analysis. They can also substantially influence study results that break down data into groups (quantiles) and compare high vs low quantiles. Whenever these analyses are performed, investigators should carefully assess the potential influence of outliers.

→ If outliers are excluded from an analysis, the rationale for their exclusion should be explained in the text. A number of tests are available to determine whether an outlier is so extreme that it should be excluded from the analysis.

**overfit:** a perfect fit between the data and outcome variables will occur if the number of variables in a regression equals the number of data points. In other words, the more variables present in a regression equation, the better the fit will be. Inclusion of an excessive number of variables will result in fits for statistical models that are good but misleading. In general, it is best to include only the fewest number of variables necessary to develop a statistical model. When comparing the results of regression analyses using different numbers of variables, this phenomenon should be corrected for by penalizing the comparator statistic by the number of variables present in the regression equation. This is done in the *Akaike* and *Bayes information criteria* processes.

**overmatching:** the phenomenon of obscuring by the matching process of a case-control study a true causal relationship between the *independent* and *dependent variables* because the variable used for matching is strongly related to the mechanism by which the independent variable exerts its effect.[95] For example, matching cases and controls for residence within a certain area could obscure an environmental cause of a disease. Overmatching may also be used to refer to matching on variables that have no effect on the dependent variable, and therefore are unnecessary, or the use of so many variables for matching that no suitable controls can be found.[98]

**oversampling:** in survey research, a technique that selectively increases the likelihood of including certain groups or units that would otherwise produce too few responses to provide reliable estimates. For example, Hispanic individuals comprise approximately 17% of the US population. When trying to understand something about the Hispanic population, if one created a statistical sample from the overall US population, the likelihood of finding significant factors relating to Hispanic individuals would be low because there are relatively few Hispanic individuals. In oversampling, a larger number of Hispanic individuals than White individuals would be sampled to increase the likelihood that factors important to whatever is being studied as they relate to Hispanic individuals can be identified.

**paired samples:** form of matching that can include self-pairing, where each participant serves as his or her own *control*, or artificial pairing, where 2 participants are matched on prognostic variables.[98] Twins may be studied as pairs to attempt to separate the effects of environment and genetics. Paired analyses provide greater power to detect a difference for a given sample size than do nonpaired analyses because interindividual differences are minimized or eliminated. Pairing may also be used to match participants in *case-control* or *cohort studies*. See Table 19.3-1.

**paired t test:** *t test* for paired data.

**parameter:** measurable characteristic of a *population*. One purpose of statistical analysis is to estimate population parameters from sample observations.[95] The statistic is the numerical characteristic of the sample; the parameter is the numerical characteristic of the population. *Parameter* is also used to refer to aspects of a model (eg, a regression model).

**parametric statistics:** tests used for continuous data that require the assumption that the data being tested are *normally distributed*, either as collected initially or after transformation to the ln or log of the value or other mathematical conversion.[95] The *t test* is a parametric statistic. See Table 19.5-1.

**Pearson product-moment correlation:** test of *correlation* between 2 groups of *normally distributed* data. See *diagnostic discrimination*. The Methods section should specify that this test was performed. For example, "A Pearson product-moment correlation coefficient was calculated between last survey year and change in prevalence of BMI lower than 16 to detect whether there was an association between these variables." The Results section should show the correlation value; for example, "For 13 countries where DHS program data also contained men, the Pearson product-moment correlation coefficient between rates of BMI lower than 16 among men and women was $r = 0.88$."

→ The square of the Pearson correlation coefficient gives the probability of observing one value given another. For the example above, where $r = 0.88$, given a value for the last survey year there is a 0.77% (calculated by squaring 0.88) probability of obtaining the corresponding value of the change in prevalence of BMI lower than 16.

**percentile:** see *quantile*.

**per-protocol analysis:** analysis of patients in a clinical trial analyzed by the treatment they received rather than which group they were initially randomized into (which would be intention to treat). This approach compromises the prognostic balance that randomization achieves and is therefore likely to provide a biased estimate of treatment effect. See also *intention to treat*.

**placebo:** a biologically inactive substance administered to some participants in a clinical trial. A placebo should ideally appear similar in every other way to the experimental treatment under investigation. Assignment, allocation, and assessment should be *blinded*. See also *nocebo*.

**placebo effect:** refers to specific expectations that participants may have of the intervention. These expectations can make the intervention appear more effective than it actually is. Comparison of a group receiving *placebo* vs those receiving the active intervention allows researchers to identify effects of the intervention itself because the placebo effect should affect both groups equally.

**point estimate:** single value calculated from sample observations that is used as the estimate of the *population* value, or *parameter*,[95] and should be accompanied by an interval estimate (eg, 95% *confidence interval*).

**Poisson distribution:** distribution that occurs when a *nominal* event (often disease or death) occurs rarely.[98] This distribution is used when there are count data, such as the number of events per unit measure. For example, when assessing the procedure volume–outcome relationship, the number of procedures per hospital studied would follow a Poisson distribution. The Poisson distribution is present when the mean equals the variance of a distribution. The Poisson distribution is used instead of a *binomial distribution* when sample size is calculated for a study of events that occur rarely.

**population:** any finite or infinite collection of individuals from which a sample is drawn for a study to obtain estimates to approximate the values that would be obtained if the entire population were sampled.[104] A population may be defined narrowly (eg, all individuals exposed to a specific traumatic event) or widely (eg, all individuals at risk for coronary artery disease).

**population attributable risk percentage:** percentage of risk within a *population* that is associated with exposure to the *risk factor*. Population *attributable risk* takes into account the frequency with which a particular event occurs and the frequency with which a given risk factor occurs in the population. Population attributable risk does not necessarily imply a cause-and-effect relationship. It is also called *attributable fraction*, *attributable proportion*, and *etiologic fraction*.[95] The population attributable risk percentage is the percent of the incidence of a disease in the population that would be eliminated if exposure were eliminated. The population attributable risk is calculated by subtracting the incidence of a disease in a population of patients not exposed to some risk factor ($I_u$) from the incidence of disease in the total population (both exposed and unexposed) ($I_p$):

$$PAR = I_u - I_p$$

When this is divided by $I_p$ and multiplied by 100, the result is the population attributable risk percentage.

**positive predictive value (PPV):** proportion of those participants or individuals with a positive test result who have the condition or disease as measured by the *criterion standard*. This measure takes into account the **prevalence** of the condition or the disease. Clinically, it is the probability that an individual has the disease if the test result is positive. Although sensitivity is often used to assess the efficacy of a diagnostic test in establishing a diagnosis, it is the proportion of test results that will be positive when someone has a disease. When patients are first seen, it is not known if they have the disease. In this context, the PPV provides a better assessment of how a test will perform for establishing a diagnosis. The disease prevalence influences the PPV. Rare diseases have a low PPV and common ones have higher PPVs. The preferred measure for a test's ability to establish a diagnosis is its *likelihood ratio (LR)*.[95] See Table 19.3-2 and *diagnostic discrimination*.

**posterior probability:** in *bayesian analysis*, the probability obtained after the *prior probability* is combined with the probability from the study of interest.[98] If one assumes a *uniform prior* (no useful information for estimating probability exists before the study), the posterior probability is the same as the probability from the study of interest alone.

→ The prior probability is the probability of some events occurring before new information is obtained. For example, the probability of being bitten by a mosquito in the Amazon might be 50%. However, if you learn that this region was sprayed with an insecticide and the mosquito population reduced, application of a mathematical operation reflecting the probability of getting bitten as a function of the mosquito population will change the probability to some other value. If the new value is 15% after spraying, this new value is called the posterior probability.

**post hoc analysis (also known as ad hoc analysis):** performed after completion of a study and not based on a hypothesis considered before the study. Such analyses should be performed without prior knowledge of the relationship between the *dependent* and *independent variables*. A potential hazard of post hoc analysis is the *type I error*. In general, post hoc analyses are not as definitive as prespecified analyses and should be considered as exploratory. It is important not to use causal language when describing the results of post hoc analyses and to refer to relationships between variables and outcomes as associations.

→ While post hoc analyses may be used to explore intriguing results and generate new hypotheses for future testing, they should not be used to test hypotheses because the comparison is not hypothesis driven. See also *data dredging*.

**posttest probability:** the probability that an individual has the disease if the test result is positive (*positive predictive value*) or that the individual does not have the disease if the test result is negative (*negative predictive value*).[95]

**power:** ability to detect a statistically significant difference with the use of a given sample size and *variance*; determined by frequency of the condition under study, magnitude of the effect, study design, and sample size.[95] Power should be calculated before a study is begun. If the sample is too small to have a reasonable chance (usually 80% or 90%) of rejecting the *null hypothesis* if a true difference exists, then a negative result may indicate a *type II error* rather than a true failure to reject the null hypothesis.[138]

→ Power calculations should be performed as part of the study design. A statement providing the power of the study should be included in the Methods section of all randomized clinical trials (Table 19.2-1) and is appropriate for many other types of studies. A power statement is especially important if the study results are negative, to demonstrate that a *type II error* was unlikely to have been the reason for the negative result. Performing a post hoc power analysis is controversial, especially if it is based on the study results. Nonetheless, if such calculations were performed, they should be described in the Discussion section and their post hoc nature clearly stated.

→ The study power determines the sample size. The more powerful a study, the more confidence one has that a difference between groups does not truly exist when that is the study result. In general, larger sample sizes are required when the expected differences between groups are small or there is a great deal of variation in the data. When reporting the results of a power analysis, it is important to show the rationale (including citations to published reports) for the anticipated differences between the groups and variation in the data. This is to avoid the appearance of predicting an artificially small variance or anticipating an unreasonably large difference between the groups to minimize the necessary sample size for a study. The observed difference between groups and group variances should be roughly the same as was predicted when the power calculation was made, before patients were enrolled in the study. If not, the sample size calculation might have been in error.

*Example:* The statistical power to demonstrate a superior success rate (1-sided hypothesis test) in the primary end point for the coil group vs the usual care group was 90% with a significance of $\alpha = .05$ and a total sample size of 100 patients.[139] This was based on achieving the end point of 37% of patients having improved function in the coil group and 5% in the usual care group, with 30% of patients unable to perform the 6-minute walk test or lost to follow-up at 6 months. The hypothesis of a 37% primary end-point achievement in the coil group was based on data provided by PneumRx in 2012. One-sided statistical tests were considered appropriate in view of the favorable results of previous smaller studies and confirmed by a recent meta-analysis. The sample size was calculated using Nquery software, version 7.0 (Statistical Solutions Ltd).

*Example:* A sample size of 136 participants was planned to have 90% power to detect a difference in change in hemoglobin $A_{1c}$ between treatment groups, assuming a population difference of 0.5%, SD of 26-week values of 1.0%, correlation between baseline and 26-week values of 0.56, type I error rate of 5% (2-sided), and no more than a 15% loss to follow-up.

**precision:** inverse of the *variance* in measurement (see *measurement error*)[98]; *precision* refers to the variability or how close together successive measurements of the same phenomenon are. Note that precision and *accuracy* are independent concepts; if a blood pressure cuff is poorly calibrated against a standard, it may produce measurements that are precise (successive measurements are very close to one another) but inaccurate (the measured blood pressure deviates from the true blood pressure).

**pretest probability:** same as *prevalence*.

**prevalence (also known as pretest probability):** proportion of persons with a particular disease at a given point in time. Prevalence can also be interpreted to mean the likelihood that a person selected at random from the population will have the disease.[95] See also *incidence*.

**principal components analysis (PCA):** procedure used to group related variables to help describe data. The variables are grouped so that the original set of correlated variables is transformed into a smaller set of uncorrelated variables called the principal components.[98] Variables are not grouped according to *dependent* and *independent variables*, unlike many forms of statistical analysis. Principal components analysis is similar to *factor analysis* and is used to detect patterns in a collection of data.

**prior probability:** in *bayesian analysis*, the probability of an event based on previous information before the study of interest is considered. The prior probability may be informative, based on previous studies or clinical information, or not, in which case the analysis uses a *uniform prior* (no information is known before the study of interest). A reference prior is one with minimal information, a clinical prior is based on expert opinion, and a skeptical prior is used when large treatment differences are not expected.[104] When bayesian analysis is used to determine the *posterior probability* of a disease after a patient has undergone a diagnostic test, the prior probability may be estimated as the prevalence of the disease in the *population* from which the patient is drawn (usually the clinic or hospital population).

**probability:** in clinical studies, the number of times an event occurs in a study group divided by the number of individuals being studied.[95]

**product-limit method:** see *Kaplan-Meier method*.

**propensity analysis:** in observational studies, a way of minimizing *bias*. The propensity for an individual to be in one group or another is calculated from variables available to the investigator by regression analysis.[116] Individuals are then matched based on the propensity score. To determine how closely the groups are matched, it is best to display their baseline characteristics as both unmatched and matched.[129] The closeness of the match is also assessed by showing the standardized difference between the means or proportions of the various groups. Rather than match, balance can be achieved by calculating the propensity score and then using it as an independent variable in a regression analysis to adjust for the differences between groups.

→ Although propensity analysis helps balance groups in observational studies, it is limited by the variables available to describe the phenomena being studied. Unmeasured confounding can never be overcome, so even propensity-matched groups will not be as well balanced as those from randomized trials. Consequently, propensity-matched groups can only show associations and not causality. Some investigators have criticized propensity methods as not being inherently better than multivariable methods to achieve statistical adjustment.

**proportionate mortality ratio:** number of individuals who die of a particular disease during a span of time, divided by the number of individuals who die of all diseases during the same period.[95] This ratio may also be expressed as a rate, that is, a ratio per unit of time (eg, cardiovascular deaths per total deaths per year).

**prospective study:** study in which participants with and without an exposure are identified and then followed up over time; the *outcomes* of interest have not occurred at the time the study commences.[104] Antonym is *retrospective study*.

**pseudorandomization:** assigning of individuals to groups in a nonrandom manner, for example, selecting every other individual for an intervention or assigning participants by a government identification number or birth date.

**publication bias:** tendency of articles reporting positive and/or "new" results to be submitted and published and studies with negative or confirmatory results not to be submitted or published; especially important in meta-analysis but also in other systematic reviews. Substantial publication bias has been demonstrated from the "file-drawer" problem.[140] See also *funnel plot*.

**purposive sample:** set of observations obtained from a *population* in such a way that the sample distribution of independent variable values is determined by the researcher and is not necessarily representative of distribution of the values in the population.[95]

**_P_ value:** probability of obtaining the observed data (or data that are more extreme) if the *null hypothesis* were exactly true.[104] Also expressed as the probability that the observed result was obtained by chance alone. For example, if it is said that the difference between groups was statistically significant with $P = .046$ then the probability that the difference observed was from chance alone is 4.6%.

→ Although *hypothesis* testing often results in the $P$ value, $P$ values themselves can only provide information about whether the null hypothesis is rejected. *Confidence intervals* are much more informative because they provide a plausible range of values for an unknown *parameter*, as well as some indication of the *power* of the study as indicated by the width of the CI.[92] (For example, an odds ratio of 0.5 with a 95% CI of 0.05 to 4.5 indicates to the reader the [im]precision of the estimate, whereas $P = .63$ does not provide such information.) CIs are preferred whenever possible. Including both the CI and the $P$ value provides more information than either alone.[92] This is especially true if the CI is used to provide an interval estimate and the $P$ value to provide the results of hypothesis testing.

→ When any $P$ value is expressed, it should be clear to the reader what parameters and groups were compared, what statistical test was performed, and the *degrees of freedom (df)* (when appropriate) and whether the test was *1-tailed* or *2-tailed* (if these distinctions are relevant for the statistical test).

→ For expressing $P$ values in manuscripts and articles, display $P$ as a capital, italicized letter. The actual value for $P$ should be expressed to 2 digits for $P = .01$, whether or not $P$ is *significant*. (When rounding a $P$ value would make the $P$ value nonsignificant, such as $P = .049$ rounded to .05, the $P$ value can be left as 3 digits.) If $P < .01$, it should be expressed to 3 digits. The actual $P$ value should be expressed ($P = .04$), rather than expressing a statement of inequality ($P < .05$), unless $P < .001$. In general, expressing $P$ to more than 3 significant digits does not add useful information to $P < .001$ because precise $P$ values with extreme results are sensitive to biases or departures from the statistical model.[92]

Exceptions to the 2-digit rule exist in several situations. In genetic studies (particularly genome-wide association studies [GWASs] and in studies in which there are adjustments for multiple comparisons, such as **Bonferroni adjustment**, and the definition of level of significance is substantially less than $P < .05$), it may be important to express $P$ values to more significant digits. For example, if the threshold of significance is $P < .0004$, then by definition the $P$ value must be expressed to at least 4 digits to indicate whether a result is statistically significant. GWASs express $P$ values to very small numbers, using scientific notation. If a manuscript you are editing defines statistical significance as a $P$ value substantially less than .05, possibly even using scientific notation to express $P$ values to very small numbers, it is best to retain the values as the author presents them.

> *Example:* A single-nucleotide variant on chromosome 19 was significantly associated with posttraumatic stress disorder in the European American samples of the New Soldier Study (genetic sequence: rs11085374; odds ratio [OR], 0.77; 95% CI, 0.70-0.85; $P = 4.59 \times 10^{-8}$).[141]

> *Example:* A Bonferroni adjustment was made to account for having 6 outcomes such that the $P$ value for statistical significance is .0083 (.05/6) and 99.17% CIs are presented around the effect estimates to reflect the adjusted $\alpha$ level (ie, $1 - .0083 = .9917$).[142]

$P$ values should not be listed simply as "not significant" or "NS" because for **meta-analysis** the actual values are important and not providing exact $P$ values is a form of incomplete reporting.[92] Because the $P$ value represents the result of a statistical test and not the strength of the association or the clinical importance of the result, $P$ values should be referred to simply as statistically significant or not significant; phrases such as "highly significant" and "very highly significant" should be avoided.

$P$ values should never be reported alone. Because the $P$ value refers only to the probability that something is statistically significant or not, it is necessary to assess the $P$ value in the context of other statistical information, such as absolute or relative risks and CIs. Findings that are statistically significant can be clinically unimportant; however, this cannot be determined from $P$ values alone.

Best practice is to not use a zero to the left of the decimal point because statistically it is not possible to prove or disprove the null hypothesis completely when only a sample of the population is tested ($P$ cannot equal 0 or 1, except by rounding). If $P < .00001$, $P$ should be expressed as $P < .001$ as discussed. If $P > .999$, $P$ should be expressed as $P > .99$.

**Q statistic:** See *Cochran Q test*.

**qualitative data:** data that fit into discrete categories according to their attributes, such as *nominal* or *ordinal data*, as opposed to *quantitative data*.[98]

**qualitative study:** form of study based on observation and interview with individuals that uses inductive reasoning and a theoretical sampling model, with emphasis on *validity* rather than *reliability* of results. Qualitative research is used traditionally in sociology, psychology, and group theory but also occasionally in clinical medicine to explore beliefs and motivations of patients and physicians.[143]

**quality-adjusted life-year (QALY):** a method used to adjust the survival someone might experience by the quality of life he/she has during that survival period. The number of years survived is multiplied by a *utility,* which is some measure of the quality of life that ranges from 0 to 1.0. For example, if someone is expected to live 5 years but has a disability that is expected to reduce his/her quality of life by 0.5, he/she would have 2.5 quality-adjusted life-years (QALYs).[98]

**quantile:** method used for grouping and describing dispersion of data. Commonly used quantiles are the tertile (3 equal divisions of data into lower, middle, and upper ranges), quartile (4 equal divisions of data), quintile (5 divisions), and decile (10 divisions). Quantiles are also referred to as *percentiles*.[93] In general, analyses should use continuous data when they are available and not with the data grouped into quantiles. Analyzing quantile data reduces statistical power, and outliers tend to heavily influence the uppermost and lowest quantiles.

→ Data may be expressed as median (quantile range); for example, length of stay was 7.5 days (interquartile range, 4.3-9.7 days). See also *interquartile* range.

**quantitative data:** data in numerical quantities, such as *continuous data* or counts[98] (as opposed to *qualitative data*). *Nominal* and *ordinal data* may be treated either qualitatively or quantitatively.

**quasi-experiment:** experimental design in which variables are specified and participants assigned to groups, but interventions cannot be controlled by the experimenter. One type of quasi-experiment is the *natural experiment*.[98]

*r:* correlation coefficient for *bivariable analysis*.

*R:* correlation coefficient for *multivariable analysis*.

*$r^2$:* coefficient of determination for *bivariable analysis*. See also *correlation coefficient*.

*$R^2$:* coefficient of determination for *multivariable analysis*. See also *correlation coefficient*.

**random-effects model:** used to allow the slope or intercept to vary in a multilevel (hierarchical) model. The model refers to more than 1 layer of analysis. An example might be examining effects on students grouped into schools modeled with a series of regression equations.

Random effects models can also provide a summary estimate of the magnitude of effect in a meta-analysis. These models assume that the included studies are a random sample of a population of studies addressing the question posed in the meta-analysis. Each study estimates a different underlying true effect, and the distribution of these effects is assumed to be normal around a mean value. Because a random-effects model takes into account both within-study and between-study variability, the CI around the point estimate is, when there is appreciable variability in results across studies, wider than it could be if a fixed-effects model were used.[51,144]

When there is heterogeneity in a meta-analysis, random-effects models can be used to help determine the sources of heterogeneity.

Because random effects refer to many layers of a model, the term should be used in the plural. Conversely, because fixed-effect models refer to a single layer of a model, the term is singular. Antonym to random-effects model is *fixed-effects model*. See *fixed-effect model* for more detail. See also *meta-analysis*.

**randomization:** method of assignment in which all individuals have the same chances of being assigned to the conditions in a study. Individuals may be randomly assigned at a 2:1 or 3:1 frequency, in addition to the usual 1:1 frequency. Participants may or may not be representative of a larger *population*.[92] Simple methods of randomization include coin flip or use of a random numbers table. See also *block randomization*.

**randomized clinical trial:** A trial in which the participants are randomly assigned to one group or another before the intervention is given, in contrast to an observational trial in which participants are separated into groups based on what intervention they may or may not have gotten after they received treatment. Also distinguished from a case-control trial in which groups are assigned based on whether a patient had some outcome (see 19.2.1, Parallel-Design, Double-blind Trials).

**random sample:** method of obtaining a sample that ensures that every individual in the population has a known (but not necessarily equal, for example, in weighted sampling techniques) chance of being selected for the sample.[95]

**range:** the highest and lowest values of a variable measured in a sample.

> *Example:* The mean age of the participants was 45.6 years (range, 20-64 years).

**rank sum test:** see *Mann-Whitney test* or *Wilcoxon rank sum test*.

**rate:** measure of the occurrence of a disease or outcome per unit of time, usually expressed as a decimal if the denominator is 100 (eg, the surgical mortality rate was 0.02) (see 18.7.3, Reporting Proportions and Percentages).

**ratio:** fraction in which the numerator is not necessarily a subset of the denominator, unlike a proportion[95] (eg, the assignment ratio was 1:2:1 for each drug dose [twice as many individuals were assigned to the second group as to the first and third groups]).

**realization:** in statistics, a realization is the actual observed value of a random variable. By convention, the random variable is designated by capital letters and the realization by lowercase letters. A random variable, $X$, can have many values, but after some process (draw a number at random) it takes on a definite value, $x$, its realization.

**recall bias:** systematic error resulting from individuals in one group being more likely than individuals in the other group to remember past events.[98]

→ Recall bias is especially common in *case-control studies* that assess risk factors for serious illness in which individuals are asked about past exposures or behaviors, such as environmental exposure in an individual who has cancer.[95]

**receiver operating characteristic curve (ROC curve):** graphic means of assessing the extent to which a test can be used to discriminate between persons with and without disease[98] and to select an appropriate cut point for defining normal vs abnormal results. The ROC curve is created by plotting *sensitivity* vs (1 − *specificity*). The area under the curve provides some measure of how well the test performs; the larger the area, the better the test. The *C statistic* is a measure of the area under the ROC curve.

Diagnostic tests can be assessed by a graph of the ROC (Figure 19.3-1). The value for what is called a positive test result can be varied to optimize the tradeoff between false-positive and false-negative results. The closer the curve comes to the upper-left corner of the graph, the better the overall test performance.[86]

→ The appropriate cut point is a function of the test. A screening test would require high *sensitivity*, whereas a diagnostic or confirmatory test would require high specificity. See Table 19.5-3 and *diagnostic discrimination*.

**Table 19.5-3.** Diagnostic Discrimination

| Test result | Disease by criterion standard | Disease-free by criterion standard |
|---|---|---|
| Positive | a (true positives) | b (false positives) |
| Negative | c (false negatives) | d (true negatives) |
| | *a + c* = total number of persons with disease | *b + d* = total number of persons without disease |
| | Sensitivity = *a/(a+c)* | Specificity = *d(b+d)* |
| | Positive predictive value = *a(a+b)* | Negative predictive value = *d(c+d)* |

**reference group:** group of presumably disease-free individuals from which a sample of individuals is drawn and tested to establish a range of normal values for a test.[95]

**regression analysis:** statistical techniques used to describe a *dependent variable* as a function of 1 or more *independent variables*; often used to control for confounding variables.[95] See also *linear regression* and *logistic regression*.

**regression line:** diagrammatic presentation of a *linear regression* equation, with the independent variable plotted on the x-axis and the *dependent variable* plotted on the *y-axis*. As many as 3 variables may be depicted on the same graph.[98]

**regression to the mean:** the principle that extreme values are unlikely to recur. If a test that produced an extreme value is repeated, it is likely that the second result will be closer to the mean. Thus, after repeated observations results tend to "regress to the *mean*." A common example is blood pressure measurement; on repeated measurements, individuals who are initially hypertensive often will have a blood pressure reading closer to the *population* mean than the initial measurement was.[95]

**relative risk (RR):** probability of developing an *outcome* within a specified period if a risk factor is present divided by the probability of developing the outcome in that same period if the risk factor is absent. The relative risk is applicable to randomized clinical trials and *cohort studies*[95]; for *case-control studies*, the *odds ratio* can be used to approximate the relative risk if the outcome is infrequent.

→ The relative risk should be accompanied by *confidence intervals*.

*Example:* The individuals with untreated mild hypertension had a relative risk of 2.4 (95% CI, 1.9-3.0) for stroke or transient ischemic attack. [In this example, individuals with untreated mild hypertension were 2.4 times as likely as were individuals in the comparison group to have a stroke or transient ischemic attack.]

**relative risk reduction (RRR):** proportion of the control group experiencing a given outcome minus the proportion of the treatment group experiencing the outcome divided by the proportion of the control group experiencing the outcome.

**reliability:** ability of a test to replicate a result given the same measurement conditions, as distinguished from *validity*, which is the ability of a test to measure what it is intended to measure.[98]

**repeated measures:** analysis designed to take into account the lack of independence of events when measures are repeated in each participant over time (eg, blood pressure, weight, or test scores). This type of analysis emphasizes the change measured for a participant over time rather than the differences between participants over time. A traditional analytic technique rarely in use now for repeated measures is *ANOVA* with repeated measures. Repeated measures are correlated and therefore violate the regression analysis requirement that data be independent. This correlation can be accounted for by using multilevel models when performing regression. The repeated measures are considered clustered within the individual from whom the measure was obtained. With multilevel modeling, the first level is the repeated measure and the second level is the individual who had repeated measures.

**repeated-measures ANOVA:** see *analysis of variance (ANOVA)*.

**reporting bias:** a *bias* in assessment that can occur when individuals in one group are more likely than individuals in another group to report past events. Reporting bias is especially likely to occur when different groups have different reasons to report or not report information.[95] For example, when examining behaviors, adolescent girls may be less likely than adolescent boys to report being sexually active. See also *recall bias*.

**reproducibility:** ability of a test to produce consistent results when repeated under the same conditions and interpreted without knowledge of the prior results obtained with the same test[95]; synonymous with *reliability*.

**residual:** measure of the discrepancy between observed and predicted values. The residual *SD* is a measure of the *goodness of fit* of the *regression line* to the data and gives the uncertainty of estimating a point $y$ from a point $x$.[93]

**residual confounding:** in observational studies, the possibility that differences in *outcome* may be caused by unmeasured or unmeasurable factors.[136]

**response rate:** number of complete interviews with reporting units divided by the number of eligible units in the sample[88] (see 19.3.9, Survey Studies). See also *participation rate*.

**retrospective study:** study performed after the *outcomes* of interest have already occurred[98]; most commonly a *case-control study* but also may be a retrospective *cohort study* or *case series* or *observational study*. Antonym is *prospective study*.

**right-censored data:** see *censored data*.

**risk:** probability that an event will occur during a specified period. Risk is equal to the number of individuals who develop the disease during the period divided by the number of disease-free persons at the beginning of the period.[95]

**risk factor:** characteristic or factor that is associated with an increased probability of developing a condition or disease. Also called a risk marker, a risk factor does not necessarily imply a causal relationship. A modifiable risk factor is one that can be modified through an intervention[98] (eg, stopping smoking or treating an elevated cholesterol level, as opposed to a genetically linked characteristic for which there is no effective treatment).

**risk ratio:** the ratio of 2 risks. See also *relative risk*.

**robustness:** term used to indicate that a statistical procedure's assumptions (most commonly, normal distribution of data) can be violated without a substantial effect on its conclusions.[98]

**root-mean-square:** see *standard deviation*.

**rule of 3:** method used to estimate the number of observations required to have a 95% chance of observing at least 1 episode of a serious adverse effect. For example, to observe at least 1 case of penicillin anaphylaxis that occurs in approximately 1 in 10 000 cases treated, 30 000 treated cases must be observed. If an adverse event occurs 1 in 15 000 times, 45 000 cases need to be treated and observed.[95]

**run-in period:** a period at the start of a trial when no treatment is administered (although a *placebo* may be administered). This can help to ensure that patients are stable and will adhere to treatment. This period may also be used to allow patients to discontinue any previous treatments and so is sometimes also called a *washout period*.

**sample:** subset of a larger *population*, selected for investigation to draw conclusions or make estimates about the larger population.[140]

**sampling error:** error introduced by chance differences between the estimate obtained from the *sample* and the true value in the *population* from which the sample was drawn. Sampling error is inherent in the use of sampling methods and is measured by the *standard error*.[95]

**Scheffé test:** see *multiple comparisons procedures*.

**SD:** see *standard deviation*.

**SE:** see *standard error*.

**SEE:** see *standard error of the estimate*.

**selection bias:** bias in assignment that occurs when the way the study and *control groups* are chosen causes them to differ from each other by at least 1 factor that affects the *outcome* of the study.[95]

→ A common type of selection bias occurs when individuals from the study group are drawn from one population (eg, patients seen in an emergency department or admitted to a hospital) and the control participants are drawn from another (eg, clinic patients). Regardless of the disease under study, the clinic patients will be healthier overall than the patients seen in the emergency department or hospital and will not be comparable controls. A similar example is the "healthy worker effect": people who hold jobs are likely to have fewer health problems than those who do not, and thus comparisons between these groups may be biased.

**SEM:** see *standard error of the mean*.

**sensitivity:** proportion of individuals with the disease or condition as measured by the *criterion standard* (or reference standard) who have a positive test result (individuals with true-positive results divided by all those with the disease).[95] See Table 19.5-3 and *diagnostic discrimination*.

→ Although sensitivity is the most commonly cited measure of a test's efficacy in establishing a diagnosis, it is not the best to use to determine the clinical efficacy of a test. This is because it measures how often a test result is positive when a patient has a disease. When patients are seen in clinic, it is not known what they have, and tests are obtained to make a diagnosis. What must be known is how often a patient for whom the diagnosis is not known has a positive result and has the disease in question (ie, the positive predictive value of the test). Better yet, use *likelihood ratios* to determine the efficacy of a test in establishing diagnoses.

→ One way to remember how to best use test sensitivity and specificity is SNOUT/SPIN: SNOUT means when the result of a highly *S*ensitive test is *N*egative the disease is essentially ruled *OUT* (because highly sensitive tests have few false-negative results). SPIN means that the result of a highly *S*pecific test when *P*ositive rules a disease *IN* (because highly specific tests have few false-positive results).

**sensitivity analysis:** method to determine the *robustness* of an assessment by examining the extent to which results are changed by differences in methods, values of variables, or assumptions[95]; applied in *decision analysis* to test the robustness of the conclusion to changes in the assumptions. It is performed by inserting a range of values into the variables of a statistical model and assessing how they influence the model's output. Because regression models are only valid with the range of data used to build them, the data inserted for a sensitivity analysis should only be within the same ranges.

**signed rank test:** See *Wilcoxon signed rank test*.

**significance:** statistically, the testing of the *null hypothesis* of no difference between groups. A significant result rejects the null hypothesis. Statistical significance is highly dependent on sample size and provides no information about the clinical significance of the result. Large samples will almost always have statistically significant differences. Consequently, it is better to assess the effect size of the difference rather than its statistical significance when determining clinical significance.[114,138] Clinical significance also involves a judgment as to whether the *risk factor* or intervention studied would affect a patient's *outcome* enough to make a difference for the patient. The level of clinical significance considered important is sometimes defined prospectively (often by consensus of a group of physicians) as the minimal clinically important difference, but the cutoff is arbitrary. Avoid the use of phrases such as "marginal significance" or "trend toward significance" or speculative words such as "highly significant."

**sign test:** a *nonparametric* test of significance that depends on the signs (positive or negative) of variables and not on their magnitude; used when combining the results of several studies, as in *meta-analysis*.[98] See also *Cox-Stuart trend test*.

**skewness:** the degree to which the data are asymmetric on either side of the *central tendency*. Data for a variable with a longer tail on the right of the *distribution* curve are referred to as positively skewed; data with a longer left tail are negatively skewed.[104]

**snowball sampling:** a sampling method used in qualitative research in which survey respondents are asked to recommend other respondents who might be eligible to participate in the survey. This may be used when the researcher is not entirely familiar with demographic or cultural patterns in the population under investigation.

**Spearman rank correlation (ρ):** statistical test used to determine the covariance between 2 *nominal* or *ordinal variables*.[104] The nonparametric equivalent to the *Pearson product moment correlation*, it can also be used to calculate the *coefficient of determination*.

**specificity:** proportion of those without the disease or condition as measured by the *criterion standard* who have negative results by the test being studied[95] (individuals with true-negative results divided by all those without the disease). See Table 19.5-3 and *diagnostic discrimination*.

**standard deviation (SD):** commonly used descriptive measure of the spread or *dispersion* of data. It is calculated by obtaining the positive square root of the *variance*.[95] One SD incorporates 68% of the data, and 2 SDs represents the middle 95% of values obtained. It may be represented by the Greek letter sigma ($\sigma$) when referring to a population or *s* when referring to a sample. In contrast to the variance, the units of the SD are the same as are those of the original data, easing the interpretation of the SD as it relates to the original data.[108]

→ Describing data by means of SD implies that the data are *normally distributed*; if they are not, then the median value and *interquartile range* or a similar measure involving *quantiles* is more appropriate to describe the data. One indication that data are not normally distributed is when the SD is larger than the mean (eg, mean [SD] length of stay = 9 [15] days or mean [SD] age at evaluation = 4 [5.3] days). When this occurs, the mean and SD should not be used to represent the central tendency of the data; quantiles should be used. Note that the format mean (SD) should be used.

**standard error (SE):** positive square root of the *variance* of the sampling distribution of the statistic.[93] The SE provides an estimate of the precision with which a parameter (such as the mean value) can be estimated. There are several types of SE; the type intended should be clear. See also *standard error of the mean (SEM)*.[108,120]

In text and tables that provide descriptive statistics, *SD* rather than *SE* is usually appropriate; by contrast, *parameter* estimates (eg, regression coefficients) should be accompanied by SEs. In figures where error bars are used, the 95% *confidence interval* is preferred (see Figure 4.2-8 in 4.2.1.5, Bar Graphs).

**standard error of the difference:** measure of the dispersion of the differences between samples of 2 *populations*, usually the differences between the *means* of 2 *samples*; used in the *t test*.

**standard error of the estimate (SEE):** *SD* of the observed values about the *regression line*.[93]

**standard error of the mean (SEM):** an inferential statistic, which describes the certainty with which the mean computed from a random *sample* estimates the true mean of the *population* from which the sample was drawn.[94] If multiple samples of a population were taken, then 95% of the samples would have means that fall within 2 SEMs of the mean of all the sample means. Larger sample sizes will be accompanied by smaller SEMs because larger samples provide a more precise estimate of the population mean than do smaller samples.[108,120]

→ The SEM is not interchangeable with *SD*. The SD generally describes the observed dispersion of data around the mean of a sample. By contrast, the SEM provides an estimate of the precision with which the true population mean can be inferred from the sample mean. The mean itself can thus be understood as either a descriptive or an inferential statistic; it is this intended interpretation that governs whether it should be accompanied by the SD or SEM. In the former case the mean simply describes the *average* value in the sample and should be accompanied by the SD, whereas in the latter it provides an estimate of the population mean and should be accompanied by the SEM. The interpretation of the mean is often clear from the text, but authors may need to be queried to discern their intent in presenting this statistic.

→ When many samples are obtained from a population, the mean of each sample will differ somewhat from the true population mean. The spread (or SD) of this set of mean values is characterized by the SE. Larger samples sizes will result in a smaller SE. The SEM is calculated by dividing the sample SD by the square root of the number of data points in the sample. The units of the SE are the same as those for the original data.

**standard error of the proportion:** *SD* of the *population* of all possible values of the proportion computed from *samples* of a given size.[94]

**standardization (of a rate):** adjustment of a rate to account for factors such as age or sex.[95]

**standardized mortality ratio:** ratio in which the numerator contains the observed number of deaths and the denominator contains the number of deaths that would be expected in a comparison *population*. This ratio implies that confounding factors have been controlled for by means of indirect *standardization*. It is distinguished from *proportionate mortality ratio*, which is the mortality rate for a specific disease.[95]

**standard normal distribution:** a *normal distribution* in which the raw scores have been recomputed to have a mean of 0 and an *SD* of 1.[104] Such recomputed values are referred to as *z scores* or *standard scores*. The *mean, median,* and *mode* are all equal to zero. The variance equals 1 (eg, unit variance, $\sigma^2 = 1$).

**standard score:** see *z score*.[93]

**statistic:** value calculated from *sample* data that is used to estimate a value or *parameter* in the larger *population* from which the *sample* was obtained,[95] as distinguished from *data*, which refers to the actual values obtained via direct observation (eg, measurement, medical record review, patient interview).

**stepped-wedge design:** The sequential rollout of a quality improvement (QI) intervention to study units (clinician, organizations) during a number of periods so that by the end of the study all participants have received the intervention, usually in a *cluster randomized trial*. The order in which participants receive the intervention may be randomized (similar rigor to cluster randomized designs). Data are collected and outcomes measured at each point at which a new group of participants ("step") receives the QI intervention. Observed differences in outcomes between the control section of the wedge with those in the intervention section are attributed to the intervention.

**stochastic:** type of measure that implies the presence of a random variable.[93]

**stopping rule:** rule, based on a test *statistic* or other function, specified as part of the design of the trial and established before patient enrollment, that specifies a limit for the observed treatment difference for the primary *outcome* measure, which, if exceeded, will lead to the termination of the trial or one of the study groups.[145-147] The stopping rules are designed to ensure that a study does not continue to enroll patients after a significant treatment difference has been demonstrated that would still exist regardless of the treatment results of subsequently enrolled patients.

**stratification:** division into groups. Stratification may be used to compare groups separated according to similar *confounding* characteristics. Stratified sampling may be used to increase the number of individuals sampled in rare categories of *independent variables* or to obtain an adequate sample size to examine differences among individuals with certain characteristics of interest.[46]

**Student-Newman-Keuls test:** see *Newman-Keuls test*.

**[Student] t test:** see *t test*. W. S. Gossett, who originated the test, wrote under the name Student because his employment as a statistician with the Guinness brewing company precluded individual publication.[98] Simply using the term *t* test is preferred.[120]

**study group:** in a *controlled clinical trial*, the group of individuals who undergo an intervention; in a *cohort study*, the group of individuals with the exposure or characteristic of interest; and in a *case-control study*, the group of cases.[95]

**sufficient cause:** characteristic that will bring about or cause the disease.[95]

**superiority trial:** trial designed to show that a treatment is better than another treatment or placebo. Superiority trials can be thought of as nonequivalence trials.

Superiority trials investigate whether a new therapy is better or worse than an established therapy or placebo. Because the new therapy may be better or worse than what it is being compared with, statistical tests should be 2-tailed. These trials tend to require large numbers of patients to have adequate power to be assured that no difference exists when the statistical test shows no significant difference between groups.[20-22,148] See also *equivalence trial*.

**supportive criteria:** substantiation of the existence of a contributory cause. Potential supportive criteria include the strength and consistency of the relationship, the presence of a *dose-response relationship*, and *biological plausibility*.[95]

**surrogate end points:** in a clinical trial, *outcomes* that are not of direct clinical importance but that are believed to be related to those that are. Such variables are often physiologic measurements (eg, blood pressure) or biochemical (eg, cholesterol level). Such end points can usually be collected more quickly and economically than clinical end points, such as myocardial infarction or death, but their clinical relevance may be less certain.

**survival analysis:** statistical procedures for estimating the survival function and for making inferences about how it is affected by treatment and prognostic factors.[98] See also *life table*.

**target population:** group of individuals to whom one wishes to apply or extrapolate the results of an investigation, not necessarily the *population* studied.[95] If the target population is different from the population studied, whether the study results can be extrapolated to the target population should be discussed.

**τ (tau):** see *Kendall τ rank correlation*.

**Total sum of the square (TSS):** sum of the squared difference between an observed value and the overall mean value for a data set. It is used in regression analysis to calculate how well the regression line fits the data and in *ANOVA* for calculating the variance (which is the TSS divided by the degrees of freedom, which, in turn, is the number of data points minus 1).

**trend, test for:** see *$\chi^2$ test*.

**trial:** controlled experiment with an uncertain *outcome*[93]; used most commonly to refer to a randomized study.

**triangulation:** in qualitative research, the simultaneous use of several different techniques to study the same phenomenon, thus revealing and avoiding *biases* that may occur if only a single method were used.

**true negative:** negative test result in an individual who does not have the disease or condition as determined by the *criterion standard*.[95] See also Table 19.5-3.

**true-negative rate:** number of individuals who have a negative test result and do not have the disease by the *criterion standard* divided by the total number of individuals who do not have the disease as determined by the criterion standard; usually expressed as a decimal (eg, the true-negative rate was 0.85). Synonymous with a test's specificity. See also Table 19.5-3.

**true positive:** positive test result in an individual who has the disease or condition as determined by the *criterion standard*.[95] See also Table 19.5-3.

**true-positive rate:** number of individuals who have a positive test result and have the disease as determined by the *criterion standard* divided by the total number of individuals who have the disease as measured by the criterion standard; usually expressed as a decimal (eg, the true-positive rate was 0.92). Synonymous with a test's *sensitivity*. See also Table 19.5-3.

**t test:** statistical test used to determine whether the means of 2 groups that have continuous data with equal variances are statistically different from one another. Use of the *t* test assumes that the variables have a *normal distribution*; if not, *nonparametric statistics* must be used.[95,120]

→ Usually the *t* test is *unpaired*, unless the data have been measured in the same individual over time. A paired *t* test is appropriate to assess the change of the *parameter* in the individual from baseline to final measurement; in this case, the dependent variable is the change from one measurement to the next. These changes are usually compared against 0, on the *null hypothesis* that there is no change from time 1 to time 2.

→ Presentation of the *t* statistic should include the *degrees of freedom (df)*, whether the *t* test was paired or unpaired, and whether a *1-tailed* or *2-tailed test* was used. Because a 1-tailed test assumes that the study effect can have only 1 possible direction (ie, only beneficial or only harmful), justification for use of the 1-tailed test must be provided. (The 1-tailed test at $\alpha = .05$ is similar to testing at $\alpha = .10$ for a 2-tailed test and therefore is more likely to give a significant result.)

*Example:* The difference was significant by a 2-tailed test for paired samples ($t_{15} = 2.78$, $P = .05$).

→ The *t* test can also be used to compare different *coefficients of variation*.

**Tukey test:** a type of *multiple comparisons procedure* used to determine which groups are different from one another in an *ANOVA* procedure.

**2-tailed test:** test of statistical *significance* in which deviations from the *null hypothesis* in either direction are considered.[95] For most *outcomes*, the 2-tailed test is appropriate unless there is a plausible reason why only 1 direction of effect is considered and a *1-tailed test* is appropriate. Commonly used for the *t test* but can also be used in other statistical tests. Synonymous with 2-sided test.

**type I error:** a result in which the *sample* data lead to a rejection of the *null hypothesis* despite the fact that the null hypothesis is actually true in the *population*. The $\alpha$ level is the size of a type I error that will be permitted, usually .05. Essentially the same as saying that a difference between groups is found when it does not really exist.

→ A frequent cause of a type I error is performing *multiple comparisons*, which increases the likelihood that a significant result will be found by chance. To avoid a type I error, one of several *multiple comparisons* procedures can be used.

**type II error:** the situation where the *sample* data lead to a failure to reject the null hypothesis despite the fact that the null hypothesis is actually false in the *population*. Essentially the same as concluding that there is no difference between groups when one really exists.

→ A frequent cause of a type II error is insufficient sample size. Therefore, a *power* calculation should be performed when a study is planned to determine the sample size needed to avoid a type II error.

**uncensored data:** *continuous data* reported as collected, without adjustment, as opposed to *censored data*.

**uniform prior:** assumption that no useful information regarding the *outcome* of interest is available before the study and thus that all individuals have an equal prior *probability* of the outcome. See also *bayesian analysis*.

**unity:** a *relative risk* of 1 is a relative risk of unity, and a *regression line* with a slope of 1 is said to have a slope of unity. Synonymous with the number 1.

**univariable analysis:** statistical tests that involve only 1 *dependent variable* and no independent variables. Uses measures of *central tendency* (*mean* or *median*) and location or *dispersion*. The term may also apply to an analysis in which there are no *independent variables*. In this case, the purposes of the analysis are to describe the sample, determine how the sample compares with the *population*, and determine whether chance has resulted in a skewed distribution of 1 or more of the variables in the study. If the characteristics of the sample do not reflect those of the population from which the sample was drawn, the results may not be generalizable to that population.[95] It is common to use the incorrect term *univariate*. The suffix *-ate* means to act on. Because no variable is acted on in a univariable analysis, *univariable* is a more appropriate term than *univariate* when there is only a single variable involved. See also *multivariable* and *multivariate analysis*.

**unpaired analysis:** method that compares 2 treatment groups when the 2 treatments are not given to the same individual. Most *case-control studies* also use unpaired analysis.

**unpaired t test:** see *t test*.

***U* test:** see *Wilcoxon rank sum test*.

**utility:** in decision theory and clinical decision analysis, a scale used to judge the preference of achieving a particular *outcome* (used in studies to quantify the value of an outcome vs the discomfort of the intervention to a patient) or the discomfort experienced by the patient with a disease.[98] Commonly used methods are the time trade-off and the standard gamble. The result is expressed as a single number along a continuum from death (0) to full health or absence of disease (1.0). This quality number can then be multiplied by the number of years a patient is in the health state produced by a particular treatment to obtain the *quality-adjusted life-year* (see 19.3.7, Economic Analyses).

**validity (of a measurement):** degree to which a measurement is appropriate for the question being addressed or measures what it is intended to measure. For example, a test may be highly consistent and reproducible over time, but unless it is compared with a *criterion standard* or other validation method, the test cannot be considered valid. *Construct validity* refers to the extent to which the measurement corresponds to theoretical concepts. Because there are no criterion standards for constructs, construct validity is generally established by comparing the results of one method of measurement with those of other methods. *Content validity* is the extent to which the measurement samples the entire domain under study (eg, a measurement to assess delirium must evaluate cognition). *Criterion validity* is the extent to which the measurement is correlated with some quantifiable external criterion (eg, a test that predicts reaction time). Validity can be concurrent (assessed simultaneously) or predictive (eg, ability of a standardized test to predict school performance).[98] See also *diagnostic discrimination*.

→ Validity of a test is sometimes mistakenly used as a synonym of *reliability*; the two are distinct statistical concepts and should not be used interchangeably. Validity is related to the idea of *accuracy* or how close the measured value is to the real value, whereas reliability is related to the idea of *precision* or how close to one another successive measures are.

**validity (of a study):** *internal validity* means that the observed differences between the control and comparison groups may, apart from sampling error, be attributed to the effect under study; *external validity* or *generalizability* means that a study can produce unbiased inferences regarding the target *population*, beyond the participants in the study.[98]

**Van der Waerden test:** *nonparametric* test that is sensitive to differences in *location* for 2 samples from otherwise identical *populations*.[93]

**variable:** characteristic measured as part of a study. Variables may be *dependent* (usually the *outcome* of interest) or *independent* (characteristics of individuals that may affect the dependent variable).

**variance:** variation measured in a set of data for one *variable*, defined as the sum of the squared deviations (the difference between each data point and the mean of the variable) divided by the *degrees of freedom* (number of observations in the sample minus 1).[104] The *SD* is the square root of the variance. The units for the variance are the square of the units of the data from which the variance was calculated.

**variance components analysis:** process of isolating the sources of variability in the *outcome* variable for the purpose of analysis.

**variance ratio distribution:** synonymous with *F distribution* and is used for *ANOVA*.[98]

**visual analog scale:** scale used to quantify subjective factors, such as pain, satisfaction, or values that individuals attach to possible outcomes. Participants are asked to indicate where their current feelings fall by marking a straight line with 1 extreme, such as "worst pain ever experienced," at one end of the scale and the other extreme, such as "no pain," at the other end. The feeling (eg, degree of pain) is quantified by measuring the distance from the mark on the scale to the end of the scale.[98]

**washout period:** see 19.2.2, Crossover Trials.

**Wilcoxon rank sum test:** a *nonparametric* test that ranks and sums observations from combined samples and compares the result with the sum of ranks from

1 sample.[93] _U_ is the statistic that results from the test. Synonymous with *Mann-Whitney test*.

**Wilcoxon signed rank test:** *nonparametric* test in which 2 treatments that have been evaluated by means of matched samples are compared. Each observation is ranked according to size and given the sign of the treatment difference (ie, positive if the treatment effect was positive and vice versa) and the ranks are summed.[93]

**Wilks Λ (lambda):** a test used in *multivariate analysis of variance (MANOVA)* that tests the effect size for all the dependent variables considered simultaneously. It thus adjusts significance levels for *multiple comparisons*.

**x-axis:** horizontal axis of a graph. By convention, the *independent variable* is plotted on the x-axis. Synonymous with *abscissa*.

**Yates correction:** continuity correction used to bring a distribution based on discontinuous frequencies closer to the continuous $\chi^2$ distribution from which $\chi^2$ tables are derived.[98]

**y-axis:** vertical axis of a graph. By convention, the *dependent variable* is plotted on the y-axis. Synonymous with *ordinate*.

**_z_ score:** score used to analyze *continuous variables* that represents the deviation of a value from the mean value, expressed as the number of *SDs* from the mean. The _z_ score is frequently used to compare children's height and weight measurements, as well as behavioral scores.[98] Synonymous with *standard score*.

**19.6** **Statistical Symbols and Abbreviations.** The following may be used without expansion except where noted. For a term expanded at first mention, the abbreviation may be placed in parentheses after the expanded term and the abbreviation used thereafter (see 13.11, Clinical, Technical, and Other Common Terms). Most terms other than mathematical symbols can also be found in 19.5, Glossary of Statistical Terms.

| Symbol or abbreviation | Description |
| --- | --- |
| $\lvert x \rvert$ | absolute value |
| $\Sigma$ | sum |
| $>$ | greater than |
| $\geq$ | greater than or equal to |
| $<$ | less than |
| $\leq$ | less than or equal to |
| $\wedge$ | hat, used above a parameter to denote an estimate |
| ANOVA | analysis of variance (expand at first mention) |
| ANCOVA | analysis of covariance (expand at first mention) |

| Symbol or abbreviation | Description |
| --- | --- |
| AR | autoregression |
| $\alpha$ | alpha, probability of type I error |
| $1 - \alpha$ | confidence coefficient |
| $\beta$ | beta, probability of type II error or population regression coefficient |
| $1 - \beta$ | power of a statistical test |
| $b$ | sample regression coefficient |
| CI | confidence interval |
| C statistic | concordance statistic (same as C index) |
| $\chi_3^2$ (chi-square) | $\chi^2$ test or statistic, with 3 $df$ shown as an example |
| CV | coefficient of variation $(s/\bar{x}) \times 100$ (expand at first mention) |
| $d$ | Cohen $d$ |
| D | difference |
| $df$ | degrees of freedom ($v$ is the international symbol[149] and also may be used if familiar to readers) |
| $D^2$ | Mahalanobis distance, distance between the means of 2 groups |
| $\Delta$ | delta, change, difference |
| $\delta$ | delta, true sampling error |
| $\epsilon$ | epsilon, true experimental error |
| $e$ | exponential |
| $E(x)$ | expected value of the variable $x$ |
| f | frequency or a function of, usually followed by an expression in parentheses, eg, $f(x)$ |
| $F$ | $F$ test, ratio of 2 variances. This test can be represented by $F_{v1, v2(1-\alpha)}$, where $df = v1$, $v2$ for numerator and denominator, respectively, and $(1 - \alpha)$ = confidence coefficient |
| $G^2(df)$ | likelihood ratio $\chi^2$ |
| HR | hazard ratio (expand at first mention) |
| $H_0$ | null hypothesis |

| Symbol or abbreviation | Description |
| --- | --- |
| $H_1$ | alternate hypothesis; specify whether 1- or 2-sided |
| $I^2$ | test for heterogeneity |
| $\kappa$ | kappa statistic |
| $\lambda_i$ | lambda, hazard function for interval $i$; eigenvalue; or estimate of parameter for log-linear models |
| $\Lambda$ | Wilks lambda |
| ln | natural logarithm |
| log | logarithm to base 10 ($\log_{10}$) |
| MANOVA | multivariate analysis of variance (expand at first mention) |
| $\mu$ | population mean |
| n | size of a subsample |
| N | total sample size |
| $n!$ | ($n$) factorial |
| OR | odds ratio (expand at first mention) |
| $P$ | statistical probability |
| $r$ | bivariable coefficient of determination |
| $R$ | multivariable correlation coefficient |
| $r^2$ | bivariable coefficient of determination |
| $R^2$ | multivariable coefficient of determination |
| RR | relative risk (expand at first mention) |
| $\rho$ | rho, population correlation coefficient |
| $s^2$ | sample variance |
| $\sigma^2$ | sigma squared, population variance |
| $\sigma$ | sigma, population SD |
| SD | standard deviation of a sample, can also mean standardized difference |
| SE | standard error |
| SEM | standard error of the mean |
| $t$ | $t$ test; specify $\alpha$ level, $df$, 1-tailed vs 2-tailed |
| $\tau$ | Kendall tau |

| Symbol or abbreviation | Description |
| --- | --- |
| $T^2$ | Hotelling $T^2$ statistic |
| $U$ | Mann-Whitney $U$ (Wilcoxon) statistic |
| $\bar{x}$ | arithmetic mean |
| $z$ | z score |

**Principal Author:** Edward H. Livingston, MD

## ACKNOWLEDGMENT

Thanks to the following for reviewing and providing comments to improve the manuscript: Miriam Cintron, *JAMA*; Trevor Lane, MA, DPhil, Edanz Group, Fukuoka, Japan; Tom Lang, MA, Tom Lang Communications, Kirkland, Washington; and Ana Marušić, MD, PhD, *Journal of Global Health* and University of Split School of Medicine, Croatia.

## REFERENCES

1. Knowles E. *The Oxford Dictionary of Quotations*. 5th ed. Oxford University Press; 1999.
2. Haynes RB, Mulrow CD, Huth EJ, Altman DG, Gardner MJ. More informative abstracts revisited. *Ann Intern Med*. 1990;113(1):69-76. doi:10.7326/0003-4819-113-1-69
3. Seymour CW, Liu VX, Iwashyna TJ, et al. Assessment of clinical criteria for sepsis: for the Third International Consensus Definitions for Sepsis and Septic Shock (Sepsis-3). *JAMA*. 2016;315(8):762-774. doi:10.1001/jama.2016.0288
4. The EQUATOR Network. Accessed January 26, 2019. http://www.equator-network.org/
5. CONSORT: Pilot and Feasibility Trials. Accessed August 11, 2018. http://www.consort-statement.org/extensions/overview/pilotandfeasibility
6. International Committee of Medical Journal Editors. Recommendations for the conduct, reporting, editing, and publication of scholarly work in medical journals. Updated December 2018. Accessed January 9, 2019. http://www.icmje.org/
7. Guyatt G, Rennie D, Meade MO, Cook DJ. *Users' Guides to the Medical Literature: A Manual for Evidence-Based Clinical Practice*. 3rd ed. McGraw-Hill Education; 2015.
8. JAMAevidence. Accessed January 26, 2019. https://jamaevidence.mhmedical.com/
9. Calvert M, Blazeby J, Altman DG, et al. Reporting of patient-reported outcomes in randomized trials: the CONSORT PRO extension. *JAMA*. 2013;309(8):814-822. doi:10.1001/jama.2013.879
10. CONSORT 2010 statement: updated guidelines for reporting parallel group randomised trials. Updated January 24, 2019. Accessed January 25, 2019. http://www.equator-network.org/reporting-guidelines/consort/
11. JAMA Network Instructions for Authors. Accessed August 6, 2019. https://jamanetwork.com/journals/jama/pages/for-authors
12. Campbell MJ. Extending CONSORT to include cluster trials. *BMJ*. 2004;328(7441):654-655. doi:10.1136/bmj.328.7441.654

13. Detry MA, Lewis RJ. The intention-to-treat principle: how to assess the true effect of choosing a medical treatment. *JAMA*. 2014;312(1):85-86. doi:10.1001/jama.2014.7523

14. Weijer C, Shapiro SH, Cranley Glass K. For and against: clinical equipoise and not the uncertainty principle is the moral underpinning of the randomised controlled trial. *BMJ*. 2000;321(7263):756-758. doi:10.1136/bmj.321.7263.756

15. Hellman D. Evidence, belief, and action: the failure of equipoise to resolve the ethical tension in the randomized clinical trial. *J Law Med Ethics*. 2002;30(3):375-380.

16. Meinert CL. *Clinical Trials Dictionary: Terminology and Usage Recommendations.* 2nd ed. John Wiley & Sons Inc; 2012.

17. DeAngelis CD, Drazen JM, Frizelle FA, et al. Clinical trial registration: a statement from the International Committee of Medical Journal Editors. *JAMA*. 2004;292(11):1363-1364. doi:10.1001/jama.292.11.1363

18. CONSORT 2010 statement: extension checklist for reporting within person randomised trials. Updated January 24, 2019. Accessed January 26, 2019. http://www.equator-network.org/reporting-guidelines/consort-within-person-randomised-trials/

19. Young P, Bailey M, Beasley R, et al. Effect of a buffered crystalloid solution vs saline on acute kidney injury among patients in the intensive care unit: the split randomized clinical trial. *JAMA*. 2015;314(16):1701-1710. doi:10.1001/jama.2015.12334

20. Kaji AH, Lewis RJ. Noninferiority trials: is a new treatment almost as effective as another? *JAMA*. 2015;313(23):2371-2372. doi:10.1001/jama.2015.6645

21. Mulla SM, Scott IA, Jackevicius CA, You JJ, Guyatt GH. How to use a noninferiority trial: Users' Guides to the Medical Literature. *JAMA*. 2012;308(24):2605-2611. doi:10.1001/2012.jama.11235

22. Reporting of noninferiority and equivalence randomized trials: extension of the CONSORT 2010 statement. Updated January 24, 2019. Accessed January 26, 2019. http://www.equator-network.org/reporting-guidelines/consort-non-inferiority/

23. Piaggio G, Elbourne DR, Pocock SJ, Evans SJ, Altman DG, Group C. Reporting of noninferiority and equivalence randomized trials: extension of the CONSORT 2010 statement. *JAMA*. 2012;308(24):2594-2604. doi:10.1001/jama.2012.87802

24. Moher D, Schulz KF, Altman D, Group C. The CONSORT statement: revised recommendations for improving the quality of reports of parallel-group randomized trials. *JAMA*. 2001;285(15):1987-1991. doi:10.1001/jama.298.7.776

25. Curley MQ, Wypij D, Watson R, et al. Protocolized sedation vs usual care in pediatric patients mechanically ventilated for acute respiratory failure: a randomized clinical trial. *JAMA*. 2015;313(4):379-389. doi:10.1001/jama.2014.18399

26. Meurer WJ, Lewis RJ. Cluster randomized trials: evaluating treatments applied to groups. *JAMA*. 2015;313(20):2068-2069. doi:10.1001/jama.2015.5199

27. CONSORT 2010 statement: extension to cluster randomised trials. Updated January 24, 2019. Accessed January 26, 2019. http://www.equator-network.org/reporting-guidelines/consort-cluster/

28. Ellenberg SS. The stepped-wedge clinical trial: evaluation by rolling deployment. *JAMA*. 2018;319(6):607-608. doi:10.1001/jama.2017.21993

29. Hemming K, Haines TP, Chilton PJ, Girling AJ, Lilford RJ. The stepped wedge cluster randomised trial: rationale, design, analysis, and reporting. *BMJ*. 2015;350:h391. doi:10.1136/bmj.h391

30. Transparent Reporting of Evaluations with Nonrandomized Designs (TREND). CDC website. Updated September 26, 2018. Accessed January 25, 2019. https://www.cdc.gov/trendstatement/

31. Rossouw JE, Anderson GL, Prentice RL, et al. Risks and benefits of estrogen plus progestin in healthy postmenopausal women: principal results from the Women's Health Initiative randomized controlled trial. *JAMA*. 2002;288(3):321-333. doi:10.1001/jama.288.3.321

32. The Strengthening the Reporting of Observational Studies in Epidemiology (STROBE) Statement: guidelines for reporting observational studies. Updated November 15, 2018. Accessed January 26, 2019. http://www.equator-network.org/reporting-guidelines/strobe/

33. Kempen JH. Appropriate use and reporting of uncontrolled case series in the medical literature. *Am J Ophthalmol*. 2011;151(1):7-10. doi:10.1016/j.ajo.2010.08.047

34. Good research practices for comparative effectiveness research: defining, reporting and interpreting nonrandomized studies of treatment effects using secondary data sources. Updated October 23, 2013. Accessed March 27, 2018. http://www.equator-network.org/reporting-guidelines/good-research-practices-for-comparative-effectiveness-research-defining-reporting-and-interpreting-nonrandomized-studies-of-treatment-effects-using-secondary-data-sources-the-ispor-good-research-pr/

35. Good research practices for cost-effectiveness analysis alongside clinical trials: the ISPOR RCT-CEA Task Force report. Accessed March 29, 2018. http://www.equator-network.org/reporting-guidelines/good-research-practices-for-cost-effectiveness-analysis-alongside-clinical-trials-the-ispor-rct-cea-task-force-report/

36. STARD 2015: An Updated List of Essential Items for Reporting Diagnostic Accuracy Studies. Updated November 1, 2018. Accessed January 26, 2019. http://www.equator-network.org/reporting-guidelines/stard/

37. Transparent reporting of a multivariable prediction model for individual prognosis or diagnosis (TRIPOD): the TRIPOD statement. Accessed March 16, 2018. http://www.equator-network.org/reporting-guidelines/tripod-statement/

38. The Reporting of studies Conducted using Observational Routinely-collected health Data (RECORD) Statement. Accessed March 29, 2018. http://www.equator-network.org/reporting-guidelines/record/

39. Preferred Reporting Items for Systematic Reviews and Meta-Analyses: The PRISMA Statement. Updated September 6, 2018. Accessed January 26, 2019. http://www.equator-network.org/reporting-guidelines/prisma/

40. Meta-analysis of Observational Studies in Epidemiology: a proposal for reporting. Accessed January 27, 2019. http://www.equator-network.org/reporting-guidelines/meta-analysis-of-observational-studies-in-epidemiology-a-proposal-for-reporting-meta-analysis-of-observational-studies-in-epidemiology-moose-group/

41. Standards for Reporting Qualitative Research: a synthesis of recommendations. Accessed March 16, 2018. http://www.equator-network.org/reporting-guidelines/srqr/

42. Consolidated Criteria for Reporting Qualitative Research (COREQ): a 32-item checklist for interviews and focus groups. Accessed March 16, 2018. http://www.equator-network.org/reporting-guidelines/coreq/

43. SQUIRE 2.0 (Standards for Quality Improvement Reporting Excellence): revised publication guidelines from a detailed consensus process. Updated February 1, 2017. Accessed January 26, 2019. http://www.equator-network.org/reporting-guidelines/squire/

44. American Association for Public Opinion Research (AAPOR). *Standard Definitions*. Accessed August 6, 2019. https://aapor.org/Publications-Media/AAPOR-Journals/Standard-Definitions.aspx

45. Good practice in the conduct and reporting of survey research. Accessed January 27, 2019. http://www.equator-network.org/reporting-guidelines/good-practice-in-the-conduct-and-reporting-of-survey-research/

46. Rothman KJ, Greenland S, Lash TL. *Modern Epidemiology*. 3rd ed. Wolters Kluwer Health/Lippincott Williams & Wilkins; 2008.

47. Dekkers OM, Egger M, Altman DG, Vandenbroucke JP. Distinguishing case series from cohort studies. *Ann Intern Med*. 2012;156(1):37-40. doi:10.7326/0003-4819-156-1-201201030-00006

48. Concato J. Is it time for medicine-based evidence? *JAMA*. 2012;307(15):1641-1643. doi:10.1001/jama.2012.482

49. Golub RM, Fontanarosa PB. Comparative effectiveness research: relative successes. *JAMA*. 2012;307(15):1643-1645. doi:10.1001/jama.2012.490

50. Moher D, Olkin I. Meta-analysis of randomized controlled trials: a concern for standards. *JAMA*. 1995;274(24):1962-1964. doi:10.1001/jama.1995.03530240072044

51. Murad M, Montori VM, Ioannidis JA, et al. How to read a systematic review and meta-analysis and apply the results to patient care: Users' Guides to the Medical Literature. *JAMA*. 2014;312(2):171-179. doi:10.1001/jama.2014.5559

52. Bailar JC III. The practice of meta-analysis. *J Clin Epidemiol*. 1995;48(1):149-157. doi:10.1016/0895-4356(94)00149-K

53. Shapiro S. Meta-analysis/shmeta-analysis. *Am J Epidemiol*. 1994;140(9):771-778.

54. Petitti DB. Of babies and bathwater. *Am J Epidemiol*. 1994;140(9):779-782.

55. Greenland S. Can meta-analysis be salvaged? *Am J Epidemiol*. 1994;140(9):783-787.

56. Chalmers TC, Lau J. Meta-analytic stimulus for changes in clinical trials. *Stat Methods Med Res*. 1993;2(2):161-172. doi:10.1177/096228029300200204

57. Jadad AR, McQuay HJ. Meta-analyses to evaluate analgesic interventions: a systematic qualitative review of their methodology. *J Clin Epidemiol*. 1996;49(2):235-243. doi:10.1016/0895-4356(95)00062-3

58. Sampson M, Barrowman NJ, Moher D, et al. Should meta-analysts search Embase in addition to Medline? *J Clin Epidemiol*. 2003;56(10):943-955. doi:10.1016/S0895-4356(03)00110-0

59. Rethlefsen ML, Murad M, Livingston EH. Engaging medical librarians to improve the quality of review articles. *JAMA*. 2014;312(10):999-1000. doi:10.1001/jama.2014.9263

60. Berlin JA, Golub RM. Meta-analysis as evidence: building a better pyramid. *JAMA*. 2014;312(6):603-606. doi:10.1001/jama.2014.8167

61. Shaw P. Quantifying the benefits and risks of methylphenidate as treatment for childhood attention-deficit/hyperactivity disorder. *JAMA*. 2016;315(18):1953-1955. doi:10.1001/jama.2016.3427

62. Stewart LA, Clarke M, Rovers M, et al. Preferred Reporting Items for a Systematic Review and Meta-analysis of individual participant data: the PRISMA-IPD statement. *JAMA*. 2015;313(16):1657-1665. doi:10.1001/jama.2015.3656

63. Golub RM, Fontanarosa PB. Researchers, readers, and reporting guidelines: writing between the lines. *JAMA*. 2015;313(16):1625-1626. doi:10.1001/jama.2015.3837

64. Easterbrook PJ, Berlin JA, Gopalan R, Matthews DR. Publication bias in clinical research. *Lancet*. 1991;337(8746):867-872. doi:10.1371/annotation/a65c0f61-eb99-42f0-828b-5a8662bce4f7

65. Dickersin K, Scherer R, Lefebvre C. Identifying relevant studies for systematic reviews. *BMJ*. 1994;309(6964):1286-1291. doi:10.1136/bmj.309.6964.1286

66. Higgins JPT, Green S. *Cochrane Handbook for Systematic Reviews of Interventions.* Version 5.1.0. Updated March 2011. Cochrane Collaboration; 2011. https://www.handbook.cochrane.org

67. Gerbarg ZB, Horwitz RI. Resolving conflicting clinical trials: guidelines for meta-analysis. *J Clin Epidemiol.* 1988;41(5):503-509. doi:10.1016/0895-4356(88)90053-4

68. Murad MH, Montori VM, Ioannidis JPA, et al. Understanding and applying the results of a systematic review and meta-analysis. In: Guyatt G, Rennie D, Meade MO, Cook DJ, eds. *Users' Guides to the Medical Literature: A Manual for Evidence-Based Clinical Practice.* 3rd ed. McGraw-Hill Education; 2015.

69. Thompson SG. Why sources of heterogeneity in meta-analysis should be investigated. *BMJ.* 1994;309(6965):1351-1355. doi:10.1136/bmj.309.6965.1351

70. Mills EJ, Ioannidis JPA, Thorlund K, Schünemann HJ, Puhan MA, Guyatt G. Network meta-analysis. In: Guyatt G, Rennie D, Meade MO, Cook DJ, eds. *Users' Guides to the Medical Literature: A Manual for Evidence-Based Clinical Practice.* 3rd ed. McGraw-Hill Education; 2015.

71. Bero L, Rennie D. The Cochrane Collaboration. Preparing, maintaining, and disseminating systematic reviews of the effects of health care. *JAMA.* 1995;274(24):1935-1938. doi:10.1001/jama.1995.03530240045039

72. Bauchner H, Fontanarosa PB, Golub RM. *JAMA* welcomes the US Preventive Services Task Force. *JAMA.* 2016;315(4):351-352. doi:10.1001/jama.2015.18448

73. Mark DH. Visualizing cost-effectiveness analysis. *JAMA.* 2002;287(18):2428-2429. doi:10.1001/jama.287.18.2428

74. Saha S, Hoerger TJ, Pignone MP, et al. The art and science of incorporating cost effectiveness into evidence-based recommendations for clinical preventive services. *Am J Prev Med.* 2001;20(3):36-43. doi:10.1016/S0749-3797(01)00260-4

75. Udvarhelyi I, Colditz GA, Rai A, Epstein AM. Cost-effectiveness and cost-benefit analyses in the medical literature: are the methods being used correctly? *Ann Intern Med.* 1992;116(3):238-244. doi:10.7326/0003-4819-116-3-238

76. Kassirer JP, Angell M. The journal's policy on cost-effectiveness analyses. *N Engl J Med.* 1994;331(10):669-670. doi:10.1056/NEJM199409083311009

77. Hill SR, Mitchell AS, Henry DA. Problems with the interpretation of pharmacoeconomic analyses: a review of submissions to the Australian Pharmaceutical Benefits Scheme. *JAMA.* 2000;283(16):2116-2121. doi:10.1001/jama.283.16.2116

78. Russell LB, Gold MR, Siegel JE, Daniels N, Weinstein MC. The role of cost-effectiveness analysis in health and medicine. *JAMA.* 1996;276(14):1172-1177. doi:10.1001/jama.1996.03540140060028

79. Siegel JE, Weinstein MC, Russell LB, Gold MR. Recommendations for reporting cost-effectiveness analyses. *JAMA.* 1996;276(16):1339-1341. doi:10.1001/jama.1996.03540160061034

80. Drummond M, Jefferson T. Guidelines for authors and peer reviewers of economic submissions to the *BMJ. BMJ.* 1996;313(7052):275-283. doi:10.1136/bmj.313.7052.275

81. Drummond MF, Richardson WS, O'Brien BJ, Levine M, Heyland D. Users' Guides to the Medical Literature, XIII: how to use an article on economic analysis of clinical practice, A: are the results of the study valid? *JAMA.* 1997;277(19):1552-1557. doi:10.1001/jama.1997.03540430064035

82. Consolidated Health Economic Evaluation Reporting Standards (CHEERS) statement. Updated February 1, 2017. Accessed January 26, 2019. http://www.equator-network.org/reporting-guidelines/cheers/

83. Bossuyt PM, Reitsma JB, Bruns DE, et al. Towards complete and accurate reporting of studies of diagnostic accuracy: the STARD initiative. *BMJ*. 2003;326(7379):41-44. doi:10.1136/bmj.326.7379.41

84. Simel DL, Rennie D. A primer on the precision and accuracy of the clinical examination. In: *The Rational Clinical Examination: Evidence-Based Clinical Diagnosis*. McGraw-Hill Education; 2016.

85. Ebell MH, Call M, Shinholser J, Gardner J. Does this patient have infectious mononucleosis? the Rational Clinical Examination systematic review. *JAMA*. 2016;315(14):1502-1509. doi:10.1001/jama.2016.2111

86. Alba A, Agoritsas T, Walsh M, et al. Discrimination and calibration of clinical prediction models: Users' Guides to the Medical Literature. *JAMA*. 2017;318(14):1377-1384. doi:10.1001/jama.2017.12126

87. Johnson TP, Wislar JS. Response rates and nonresponse errors in surveys. *JAMA*. 2012;307(17):1805-1806. doi:10.1001/jama.2012.3532

88. Livingston EH, Wislar JS. Minimum response rates for survey research. *Arch Surg*. 2012;147(2):110-110. doi:10.1001/archsurg.2011.2169

89. Lee H, Herbert RD, McAuley JH. Mediation analysis. *JAMA*. 2019;321(7):697-698. doi:10.1001/jama.2018.21973

90. Emdin CA, Khera AV, Kathiresan S. Mendelian randomization. *JAMA*. 2017;318(19):1925-1926. doi:10.1001/jama.2017.17219

91. Davey Smith G, Paternoster L, Relton C. When will mendelian randomization become relevant for clinical practice and public health? *JAMA*. 2017;317(6):589-591. doi:10.1001/jama.2016.21189

92. Bailar JC, Mosteller F. *Medical Uses of Statistics*. 2nd ed. NEJM Books; 1992.

93. Marriott FHC, Kendall MG, International Statistical Institute. *A Dictionary of Statistical Terms*. 5th ed. Longman Publishing Group; 1990.

94. Glantz SA. *Primer of Biostatistics*. McGraw-Hill; 1981.

95. Riegelman RK, Riegelman RK. *Studying a Study & Testing a Test: Reading Evidence-Based Health Research*. 6th ed. Wolters Kluwer/Lippincott Williams & Wilkins Health; 2013.

96. Eisenhart C. Realistic evaluation of the precision and accuracy of instrument calibration systems. *J Res Natl Bur Stand*. 1963;67C:161-187.

97. Bland JM, Altman D. Statistical methods for assessing agreement between two methods of clinical measurement. *Lancet*. 1986;327(8476):307-310. doi:10.1016/S0140-6736(86)90837-8

98. Last JM, Abramson JH, International Epidemiological Association. *A Dictionary of Epidemiology*. 3rd ed. Oxford University Press; 1995.

99. Vickers AJ, Altman DG. Statistics notes: analysing controlled trials with baseline and follow up measurements. *BMJ*. 2001;323(7321):1123-1124. doi:10.1136/bmj.323.7321.1123

100. Lang TA, Secic M. *How to Report Statistics in Medicine: Annotated Guidelines for Authors, Editors, and Reviewers*. 2nd ed. American College of Physicians; 2006.

101. Ansari AR, Bradley RA. Rank-sum tests for dispersions. *Ann Math Statist*. 1960;31(4):1174-1189. https://projecteuclid.org/euclid.aoms/1177705688

102. Watters JK, Bluthenthal RN, Kral AH. HIV seroprevalence in injection drug users. *JAMA*. 1995;273(15):1178-1178. doi:10.1001/jama.1995.03520390036028

103. Cutter GR, Mutti DO, Zadnik K. Optometric care and undetected eye disease: a case of Berkson's bias? *Arch Intern Med*. 1995;155(4):427-429. doi:10.1001/archinte.1995.00430040102015

104. Everitt B. *The Cambridge Dictionary of Statistics in the Medical Sciences*. Cambridge University Press; 1995.

105. Hoffmann MK, Shi H, Schmitz BL, et al. Noninvasive coronary angiography with multislice computed tomography. *JAMA*. 2005;293(20):2471-2478. doi:10.1001/jama.293.20.2471

106. Pencina MJ, D'Agostino RB Sr. Evaluating discrimination of risk prediction models: the C statistic. *JAMA*. 2015;314(10):1063-1064. doi:10.1001/jama.2015.11082

107. Meurer WJ, Tolles J. Logistic regression diagnostics: understanding how well a model predicts outcomes. *JAMA*. 2017;317(10):1068-1069. doi:10.1001/jama.2016.20441

108. Livingston EH. The mean and standard deviation: what does it all mean? *J Surg Res*. 2004;119(2):117-123. doi:10.1016/j.jss.2004.02.008

109. Riegelman RK, Hirsch RP. *Studying a Study and Testing a Test: How to Read the Medical Literature*. 2nd ed. Little Brown; 1989.

110. Dimick JB, Nicholas LH, Ryan AM, Thumma JR, Birkmeyer JD. Bariatric surgery complications before vs after implementation of a national policy restricting coverage to centers of excellence. *JAMA*. 2013;309(8):792-799. doi:10.1001/jama.2013.755

111. Dimick JB, Ryan AM. Methods for evaluating changes in health care policy: the difference-in-differences approach. *JAMA*. 2014;312(22):2401-2402. doi:10.1001/jama.2014.16153

112. The disability-adjusted life year (DALY) definition, measurement and potential use. Accessed November 30, 2018. https://documents.worldbank.org/curated/en/482351468764408897/The-disability-adjusted-life-year-DALY-definition-measurement-and-potential-use

113. Robinson WS. Ecological correlations and the behavior of individuals. *Int J Epidemiol*. 2009;38(2):337-341. doi:10.1093/ije/dyn357

114. Livingston EH, Elliot A, Hynan L, Cao J. Effect size estimation: a necessary component of statistical analysis. *Arch Surg*. 2009;144(8):706-712. doi:10.1001/archsurg.2009.150

115. Ingelfinger JA. *Biostatistics in Clinical Medicine*. 3rd ed. McGraw-Hill; 1994.

116. Haukoos JS, Lewis RJ. The propensity score. *JAMA*. 2015;314(15):1637-1638. doi:10.1001/jama.2015.13480

117. Tolles J, Lewis RJ. Time-to-event analysis. *JAMA*. 2016;315(10):1046-1047. doi:10.1001/jama.2016.1825

118. Allison PD. *Survival Analysis Using SAS: A Practical Guide*. 2nd ed. SAS Institute; 2010.

119. Hosmer DW, Lemeshow S, Sturdivant RX. *Applied Logistic Regression*. 3rd ed. Wiley; 2013.

120. Livingston EH. Who was student and why do we care so much about his *t*-test? *J Surg Res*. 2004;118(1):58-65. doi:10.1016/j.jss.2004.02.003

121. Li P, Stuart EA, Allison DB. Multiple imputation: a flexible tool for handling missing data. *JAMA*. 2015;314(18):1966-1967. doi:10.1001/jama.2015.15281

122. Newgard CD, Lewis RJ. Missing data: how to best account for what is not known. *JAMA*. 2015;314(9):940-941. doi:10.1001/jama.2015.10516

123. Everitt B, Everitt B. *Statistical Methods in Medical Investigations*. 2nd ed. Halsted Press; 1994.

124. Elliott AC, Woodward WA. *Statistical Analysis Quick Reference Guidebook: With SPSS Examples.* Sage Publications; 2007.

125. Cohen J, Cohen P, West SG, Aiken LS. *Applied Multiple Regression/Correlation Analysis for the Behavioral Sciences.* 3rd ed. Lawrence Erlbaum Associates; 2003.

126. Cleveland WS, Devlin SJ. Locally weighted regression: an approach to regression analysis by local fitting. *J Am Stat Assoc.* 1988;83(403):596-610.

127. Krumholz HM, Nuti SV, Downing NS, Normand ST, Wang Y. Mortality, hospitalizations, and expenditures for the Medicare population aged 65 years or older, 1999-2013. *JAMA.* 2015;314(4):355-365. doi:10.1001/jama.2015.8035

128. Harrell FE. *Regression Modeling Strategies: With Applications to Linear Models, Logistic Regression, and Survival Analysis.* Springer; 2001.

129. Stukel TA, Fisher ES, Wennberg DE, Alter DA, Gottlieb DJ, Vermeulen MJ. Analysis of observational studies in the presence of treatment selection bias: effects of invasive cardiac management on AMI survival using propensity score and instrumental variable methods. *JAMA.* 2007;297(3):278-285. doi:10.1001/jama.297.3.278

130. Colton T. *Statistics in Medicine.* Little Brown; 1974.

131. Detry MA, Ma Y. Analyzing repeated measurements using mixed models. *JAMA.* 2016;315(4):407-408. doi:10.1001/jama.2015.19394

132. Cao J, Zhang S. Multiple comparison procedures. *JAMA.* 2014;312(5):543-544. doi:10.1001/jama.2014.9440.

133. Elashoff JD. Down with multiple t-tests. *Gastroenterology.* 1981;80(3):615-620.

134. Guyatt G, Sackett D, Taylor DW, Chong J, Roberts R, Pugsley S. Determining optimal therapy--randomized trials in individual patients. *N Engl J Med.* 1986;314(14):889-892. doi:10.1056/NEJM198604033141406

135. Bingel U; for the Placebo Competence Team. Avoiding nocebo effects to optimize treatment outcome. *JAMA.* 2014;312(7):693-694. doi:10.1001/jama.2014.8342

136. Agoritsas T, Merglen A, Shah ND, O'Donnell M, Guyatt GH. Adjusted analyses in studies addressing therapy and harm: Users' Guides to the Medical Literature. *JAMA.* 2017;317(7):748-759. doi:10.1001/jama.2016.20029

137. Zhang J, Yu KF. What's the relative risk? a method of correcting the odds ratio in cohort studies of common outcomes. *JAMA.* 1998;280(19):1690-1691. doi:10.1001/jama.280.19.1690

138. Livingston EH, Cassidy L. Statistical power and estimation of the number of required subjects for a study based on the *t*-test: a surgeon's primer. *J Surg Res.* 2005;126(2):149-159. doi:10.1016/j.jss.2004.12.013

139. Deslée G, Mal H, Dutau H, et al. Lung volume reduction coil treatment vs usual care in patients with severe emphysema: the REVOLENS randomized clinical trial. *JAMA.* 2016;315(2):175-184. doi:10.1001/jama.2015.17821

140. Scherer RW, Dickersin K, Langenberg P. Full publication of results initially presented in abstracts: a meta-analysis. *JAMA.* 1994;272(2):158-162. doi:10.1001/jama.1994.03520020084025

141. Stein MB, Chen C-Y, Ursano RJ, et al. Genome-wide association studies of post-traumatic stress disorder in 2 cohorts of US Army soldiers. *JAMA Psychiatry.* 2016;73(7):695-704. doi:10.1001/jamapsychiatry.2016.0350

142. Kypri K, Vater T, Bowe SJ, et al. Web-based alcohol screening and brief intervention for university students: a randomized trial. *JAMA.* 2014;311(12):1218-1224. doi:10.1001/jama.2014.2138

143. Pope C, Mays N. Reaching the parts other methods cannot reach: an introduction to qualitative methods in health and health services research. *BMJ.* 1995;311(6996):42-45. doi:10.1136/bmj.311.6996.42

144. Murad MH, Montori VM, Ioannidis JPA, Prasad K, Cook DJ, Guyatt G. Fixed-effects and random-effects models. In: Guyatt G, Rennie D, Meade MO, Cook DJ, eds. *Users' Guides to the Medical Literature*. 3rd ed. McGraw-Hill; 2015.

145. Schomer DL, Lewis RJ. Stopping seizures early and the surgical epilepsy trial that stopped even earlier. *JAMA*. 2012;307(9):966-968. doi:10.1001/jama.2012.251

146. Bassler D, Briel M, Montori VM, et al. Stopping randomized trials early for benefit and estimation of treatment effects: systematic review and meta-regression analysis. *JAMA*. 2010;303(12):1180-1187. doi:10.1001/jama.2010.310

147. Viele K, McGlothlin A, Broglio K. Interpretation of clinical trials that stopped early. *JAMA*. 2016;315(15):1646-1647. doi:10.1001/jama.2016.2628

148. Kaji AH, Lewis RJ. Are we looking for superiority, equivalence, or noninferiority? asking the right question and answering it correctly. *Ann Emerg Med*. 2010;55(5):408-411. doi:10.1016/j.annemergmed.2010.01.024

149. Halperin M, Hartley HO, Hoel PG; COPSS Committee on Symbols and Notation. Recommended standards for statistical symbols and notation. *Am Stat*. 1965;19(3):12-14. doi:10.2307/2681417

## ADDITIONAL READING AND GENERAL REFERENCES

Elliott AC, Woodward WA. *Statistical Analysis Quick Reference Guidebook: With SPSS Examples*. Sage Publications; 2007.

Guyatt G, Rennie D, Meade M, Cook D, American Medical Association. *Users' Guides to the Medical Literature: A Manual for Evidence-Based Clinical Practice*. 3rd ed. McGraw-Hill Education Medical; 2015.

Livingston EH, Lewis RJ. *JAMA Guide to Statistics and Methods*. McGraw-Hill Education; 2020.

JAMAevidence. Accessed November 9, 2019. https://jamaevidence.mhmedical.com

Motulsky H. *Intuitive Biostatistics: A Nonmathematical Guide to Statistical Thinking*. 3rd ed. Oxford University Press; 2014.

Riegelman RK, Riegelman RK. *Studying a Study & Testing a Test: Reading Evidence-Based Health Research*. 6th ed. Wolters Kluwer/Lippincott Williams & Wilkins Heath; 2013.

Rothman KJ, Greenland S, Lash TL. *Modern Epidemiology*. 3rd ed. Wolters Kluwer Health/Lippincott Williams & Wilkins; 2008.

# 20.0 Mathematical Composition

**20.0** **Mathematical Composition.** Mathematical formulas and other expressions that involve special symbols, character positions, and relationships may present difficulties in clarity in print and online publications. Avoid ambiguity through proper use of parentheses and brackets and adhere to typographic conventions and capitalization rules in equations (see 8.5, Parentheses and Brackets, and 21.0, Editing, Proofreading, Tagging, and Display). Some software applications, such as MathType,[1] and document markup languages, such as LaTeX,[2] provide support for typesetting, formatting, and displaying complex mathematical notation and equations.

**20.1** **Displayed vs Run-in.** Simple formulas may remain within the text of the manuscript if they can be set on the line (ie, run in; see 20.2, Stacked vs Unstacked Fractions or Formulas):

> The pulmonary vascular resistance index (PVRI) was calculated as follows: PVRI = (MPAP − PCWP)/CI, where MPAP indicates mean pulmonary artery pressure; PCWP, pulmonary capillary wedge pressure; and CI, cardiac index.

Long or complicated formulas should be set off and centered on a separate line.

> For any given sample, $s$, we then defined the smoking index score, $\mathrm{SI}(s)$, as

$$\mathrm{SI}(s) = \frac{1}{n} \sum_{c}^{n} w_c \frac{\beta_{cs} - \mu_c}{\sigma_c},$$

> where $w_c$ is +1 (−1) if the smoking-associated CpG, $c$, is hypermethylated (hypomethylated) in smokers and where $\beta_{cs}$ is the β-methylation value of the CpG $c$ in sample $s$.

Whether run in to the text or set below it and centered, an equation is an element of the sentence that contains it. Punctuation and grammatical rules thus apply, just as they do for all other sentence elements. For example, if the equation is the last element in a sentence, it must be followed by a period. If there are 3 equations in a list, they must be separated by commas, and the final equation must be preceded by "and."

If there are numerous equations in a manuscript or if equations are related to each other or are referred to after initial presentation, they should be numbered consecutively. Numbered equations should each be set on a separate line, centered, with parenthetical numbers set flush left or flush right. More complex equations can be numbered sequentially and displayed in a separate box. See examples in **Box 20.1-1**.

**Box 20.1-1.** Examples of Complex Equations

Equation 1. Full model

$$\left(\sum_{j=1}^{J}\sum_{k=1}^{2}\sum_{t=1}^{T_{j,k}}\left\{\sum_{l=1}^{2}p\left(S_{j,k,l,m=1}\cap\text{tx}\right)\right.\right.$$
$$\left.+\left[1-\sum_{l=1}^{2}p(S_{j,k,l,m=1}\cap\text{tx})\right]\sum_{l=1}^{2}p(S_{j,k,l,m=2}\cap\text{tx})\right\}\right)$$
$$+\sum_{u=1}^{U}p(I_{u}\cap\text{tx})$$

Equation 2. Probabilities of sexual transmission

$$p(S_{j,k,l,m}\cap\text{tx})$$
$$= p(S_{j,k,l,m})\times p(D_{j,k,l})$$
$$\times\left(1-\left\{1-\left[p(\text{tx})\times\text{RR}_{S_{j,m}}\right][1-(l-1)c]\right\}^{A,j,k,m}\right)$$

Equation 3. Probability of IDU transmission

$$p(I_{u}\cap\text{tx}) = p(D_{u})\times(1-\{1-[p(\text{tx})\times\text{RR}_{I}]\}^{F})$$

Equation 4. Per-act transmission risk, vaginal sex

$$p(\text{tx}) = 0.0000173\times 2.89^{\log_{10}(VL)}$$

$A_{j,k,m}$ indicates annual per-partner number of episodes for sex act or role; $c$, proportion of transmissions averted by condom use (condom effectiveness); $D_{j,k,l}$, sex partner serodiscordance; $D_{u}$, drug partner serodiscordance; $F$, annual per-partner episodes of IDU distributive sharing; $I_{u}$, injection drug use (IDU); $j$, partner sex (1 if male, 2 if female); $J$, maximum number of partner sex types (1 if partner is female, 2 if male); $k$, partner main or casual type; $l$, protected or unprotected sex partner (1 if unprotected, 2 if protected); $m$, insertive or receptive sex role; $RR_{I}$, per-act relative risk of needle sharing compared with vaginal sex; $RR_{S_{j,m}}$, per-act relative risk of act and role compared with vaginal sex; $S_{j,k,l,m}$, vaginal or anal act or role with partner; $T_{j,k}$, total partners of sex $j$ and type $k$; tx, transmission; and $U$, total IDU-sharing partners.

(1) $$x = r\ \cos\theta,$$

(2) $$y = r\ \sin\theta,$$

(3) $$z = (x + y).$$

Standard abbreviations should be used in expressing units of measure (see 13.12, Units of Measure). For short, simple equations, it may be preferable to express an equation as words in the running text rather than to set it off as an actual formula:

> Attributable risk is calculated by subtracting the incidence among the nonexposed from the incidence among the exposed.

Note: Do not present a formula or equation as a unit of measure (eg, do not use kg/m² as a unit of measure for body mass index, which is calculated as weight in kilograms divided by height in meters squared, because it is the actual equation that is used to determine body mass index). Therefore, the sentence "His BMI was 30.0 kg/m²" is incorrect; instead, the sentence should read, "His BMI was 30.0."

**20.2** **Stacked vs Unstacked Fractions or Formulas.** Both stacking of fractions (ie, separating numerator and denominator by a horizontal line) and unstacking of fractions (ie, using a slash in place of the horizontal line) are acceptable as long as clarity is not lost (see 8.4.4, Forward Slash [Virgule, Solidus], In Equations).

$$y = (x_1 + x_2)/(x_1 - x_2) \quad \text{or} \quad y = \frac{x_1 + x_2}{x_1 - x_2}$$

Whenever a fraction is unstacked, parentheses, brackets, and braces (collectively called "fences" in mathematical notation) should be used as appropriate to avoid ambiguity. For instance, the expression

$$a + \frac{b + c}{d} + e,$$

if written as $a + b + c/d + e$, is ambiguous and could have several interpretations, such as

$$\frac{a + b + c}{d + e}$$

or

$$a + b + \frac{c}{d} + e.$$

The expression's meaning is unambiguous if presented as follows:

$$a + \left[(b + c)/d\right] + e.$$

Parentheses should be used to set off simple expressions. If additional fences are needed for clarity, parenthetical expressions should be set off in brackets, and bracketed expressions should be set off with braces. Note that parentheses are thus always the innermost fences (see 8.5.2.3, Brackets, In Formulas). All fences should be present in matched pairs.

$$E = 1.96 \{ [P(1-P)] / m \}^{1/2}$$

## 20.3   Exponents.

### 20.3.1   Fractional Exponents vs Radicals.

Use of radicals (eg, any expression that contains a radical symbol: $\sqrt{\phantom{x}}$) may sometimes be avoided by substituting a fractional exponent:

$$(a^2 - b^2)^{1/2} \text{ instead of } \sqrt{a^2 - b^2}.$$

As with unstacking fractions, if clarity is sacrificed by making the equation fit within the text, it is preferable to set it off. For example, $E = 1.96\{[P(1-P)]/m\}^{1/2}$ may fit within the text, but the equation set off and centered as below might be more easily understood:

$$E = 1.96 \sqrt{\frac{P(1-P)}{m}}.$$

### 20.3.2   Negative Exponents.

A negative exponent denotes the reciprocal of the expression, as illustrated in these examples:

$$x^{-n} = 1/x^n, \ A^{-1} = 1/A, \ B^{-2} = 1/B^2;$$

$$\frac{A}{(x+y)^2} \text{ may also be written as } A(x+y)^{-2} \text{ or } A/(x+y)^2.$$

### 20.3.3   Logarithmic Expressions.

The term *log* is an abbreviation of *logarithm*. A system of logarithms may be based on any number, although logarithmic systems based on the numbers 10, 2, and the irrational number *e* are most common. The base should be subscripted and follow the word *log*. In the following examples, note that logarithms are always computed from exponents of the number that forms their basis.

$$\log_{10} 1000 = 3 \text{ because } 10^3 = 1000$$

$$\log_2 8 = 3 \text{ because } 2^3 = 8$$

Logarithms based on *e* are called *natural logarithms* and are often represented as *ln*.

$$\ln 2.71 = 1$$

The terms "$e^x$" and "exp *x*" are identical in meaning and are interchangeable. The latter is preferable for constructions that involve additional subscripts or superscripts. For instance, exp $(x^3 - 1)$ is identical to $e^{x^3-1}$, but the former is preferred because it is easier to read and typeset.

**20.4** **Long Formulas.** Long formulas may be given in 2 or more lines by breaking them at operation signs outside brackets or parentheses and keeping the indention the same whenever possible (some formulas may be too long to permit indention). If lines begin with an operation sign, they should be lined up with the first character to the right of the operation sign in the line above.

$$Y = \left[(a_1 + b_1)/(a_2 - b_2)\right]$$
$$+ \left[(\sigma_1 + \sigma_2)/(\sigma_2 - \sigma_1)\right]$$
$$+ \left[(s_1 + s_2)/(t_1 + t_2)\right]$$

However, if a formula loses comprehensibility by being unstacked and broken up and/or if it fits the width of the column, it is preferable to leave it stacked.

$$\text{Percent Excess Weight Loss} = (\text{Baseline Weight} - \text{Ideal Weight})$$
$$- \frac{(\text{Follow-up} - \text{Ideal Weight})}{\text{Baseline Weight} - \text{Ideal Weight}} \times 100$$

**20.5** **Expressing Multiplication and Division.** The product of 2 or more terms, including units of measure, is conventionally indicated by a raised multiplication dot (·) (eg, 7 kg · m²) or by 2 or more characters closed up (eg, $y = mx + b$). However, in scientific notation the times sign (×) is used (eg, $3 \times 10^{-10}$ cm) (see 17.4.4, Units of Measure, Use of Numerals With Units, Multiplication of Numbers). An asterisk should not be used to represent multiplication despite its use in this role in computer programs. However, there may be occasions on which the asterisk may be used to provide the reader with the exact equation used in the analysis (eg, regression models).

A forward slash, a horizontal line, a negative exponent, or the word *per* may be used to express rates, which are generally obtained by dividing one unit by another. For example, velocity (meters per second) may be expressed as follows:

$$\text{m/s} \quad \text{or} \quad \frac{\text{m}}{\text{s}} \quad \text{or} \quad \text{m} \cdot \text{s}^{-1}.$$

Complex rates involve division of a rate by another unit. Complex rates that are used frequently are conventionally indicated by 2 forward slashes in the same expression.

The dose was 25 mg/kg/d.

Plasma renin activity was 1.3 ng/mL/h.

Acceleration at the surface of the earth is 9.8 m/s/s (or 9.8 m/s²).

Negative exponents may also be used to express such a rate when appropriate: 2 mL · kg⁻¹ · min⁻¹ (see 17.2.2, Products and Quotients of Unit Symbols). Common sense and clarity should guide this decision.

**20.6** ███████ **Commonly Used Symbols.** Use mathematical symbols in running text only if they are presented with a numerical value within parentheses. These symbols can be used in figures, tables, and boxes with no explanatory footnotes. Some commonly used symbols are as follows:

| Symbol | Description |
|---|---|
| $>$ | greater than |
| $\geq$ | greater than or equal to |
| $<$ | less than |
| $\leq$ | less than or equal to |
| $\pm$ | plus or minus (This symbol should not be used to indicate variability around a central tendency, eg, "The control group had a mean [SD] value of 12 [7]," not "The control group had a mean of $12 \pm 7$.") |
| $\int_a^b$ | integral from value of $a$ to value of $b$ |
| $\sum_{a=1}^{30}$ | summation from $a = 1$ to $a = 30$ |
| $\prod_{a=1}^{30}$ | product of $a = 1$ to $a = 30$ |
| $\Delta$ | delta (change, difference between values) |
| $f$ | function |
| $\neq$ | not equal to |
| $\approx$ | approximately equal to |
| $\sim$ | similar to (reserve for use in geometry and calculus, when it can be used in equations to mean "is distributed as"; use words in other cases where "approximately" is meant) |
| $\cong$ | congruent to |
| $\equiv$ | defined as |
| $\therefore$ | therefore |
| $\infty$ | infinity |
| $!$ | factorial, eg, $n! = n(n - 1)(n - 2) \ldots 1$ |

The following symbols are usually reserved for specific values:

| | |
|---|---|
| $\pi$ | pi (approximately 3.1416; do not confuse with uppercase $\Pi$) |
| $e$ | base of the system of natural logarithms (approximately 2.7183; see 20.3.3, Logarithmic Expressions; in statistical equations, however, "e" represents the error term in a regression equation) |
| $i$ | the square root of $-1$ |

For a list of additional symbols that are used in statistics, see 19.6, Statistical Symbols and Abbreviations.

The following are examples of these commonly used mathematical expressions:

$>10^5$ CFUs/mL

$24.5 \pm 0.5$

$L \approx 2 \times 10^{10}$ m

$f(x) = x + \Delta x$

$y = dx/dt$

$P < .001$

$P < 10 \times 3^{-10}$ (for very small $P$ values, do not use "e" to represent the exponent; see 19.4.2, Rounding)

$$\sum_{i=1}^{n} a_i x_i$$

$$\int_{10}^{13} 2x \, dx$$

$$F \sim \frac{m_1 m_2}{r^2}$$

$r! \, (n - r)!$

$(e^x + e^{-x})/2$

$Y = \beta_1 + \beta_2 + e$

$kg \cdot m \cdot s^{-2}$

$x_{r_1}$

$x_{r^2}$

$x_{2^1}^x$

$x + \dfrac{x^2}{2} + \dfrac{x^3}{3} + \dfrac{x^4}{4} + \cdots + \dfrac{x^n}{n}$  (in this case the operation sign is indicated on both sides of the ellipses)

Any symbols rendered in HTML should be compatible across most commonly used browser platforms.

**20.7** ▌ **Typography and Capitalization.** In general, variables, unknown quantities, and constants (eg, $x$, $y$, $z$, $A$, $B$, $C$) are set in italics, whereas units of measure (eg, kg, mL, s, m), symbols (including Greek characters [see 16.0, Greek Letters]), and numbers are set roman. In addition, subscripts or superscripts used as modifiers are set roman:

$C_{in}$ = clearance of inulin.

Note: Do not display forms of statistical analysis as subscript, such as $P_{interaction} < .001$. Better: $P < .001$ for interaction (see 19.0, Study Design and Statistics).

Arrays (A) and vectors (V) should be set boldface. Mathematical functions, such as sin, cos, ln, and log, are set roman.

$$\mathbf{V} = oai + bj + ck$$

$$\mathbf{A} = \begin{bmatrix} a_{11} & a_{12} & a_{13} \\ a_{21} & a_{22} & a_{23} \\ a_{31} & a_{32} & a_{33} \end{bmatrix}$$

For equations that are set off from the text, the words and letters should be set roman and the equation should be capitalized by the same rules that apply to titles (see 10.2, Titles and Headings).

$$U = \frac{\text{Efficacy}}{\text{Toxicity} - \text{Risk}} \times \frac{\text{Money Saved by Its Use}}{\text{Cost of Contrast Medium}}$$

$$\text{Age-Specific Attributable Risk} = \left( RR_i - 1 \right) / RR_i$$

**20.8 Punctuation.** Punctuation after a set-off equation is helpful and often clarifies the meaning. Display equations are often preceded by punctuation.

In the linear quadratic equation model, the survival probability for cells receiving a $j$ increment of radiation, $D_j$, is as follows:

$$S = \exp(-\alpha D_j - \beta D_j),$$

where $\alpha$ and $\beta$ are the variables of the linear quadratic equation model.

Do not use periods after a set-off equation if the equation is preceded by a period.

**20.9 Spacing With Mathematical Symbols.** Thin spaces (a space character that is usually 1/5 or 1/6 the width of an em dash; the Unicode value for the 1/6 em space is 2009) should be used before and after the following mathematical symbols when they are used as verbs, conjunctions, or operators: $\pm$, $=$, $<$, $>$, $\leq$, $\geq$, $+$, $-$, $\div$, $\times$, $\cdot$, $\approx$, $\sim$, $\cap$, $\int$, $\prod$, $\Sigma$, and $|$. Examples follow.

$a \pm b, a = b, a + b, a - b, a \div b, a \times b, a \cdot b, a > b, a < b$

$P < .001$

$2 + 3 = 5$

When symbols are used as adjectives, they are set close to the number.

A temperature of $-2$ °C

$2 + -3 = -1$

The choice of $<.05$ as the value for statistical significance is essentially arbitrary.

All large polyps ($\geq 20$ mm) were resected.

The following are more examples of symbols set close to numbers, superscripts and subscripts, and parentheses, brackets, and braces.

$2a$      $(a+b)$
$a_2$      $[a+b]$
$x^2$      $<75$ years
$(a-b)$

**Principal Authors:** Lauren Fischer and Paul Frank

## ACKNOWLEDGMENT

Thanks to Karen Boyd, formerly with JAMA Network, Rochelle Lodder, formerly with JAMA Network, and Paul Ruich, JAMA Network, for careful review of this chapter.

Additional Information: Coauthor Paul Frank died in 2015.

## REFERENCES

1. Design Science. MathType. Accessed November 30, 2018. http://www.dessci.com/en/products/mathtype/
2. The LaTeX Project. LaTeX–a document preparation system. 2015. Accessed July 23, 2019. https://latex-project.org/

## ADDITIONAL READINGS

Style Manual Committee, Council of Science Editors. *Scientific Style and Format: The CSE Manual for Authors, Editors, and Publishers.* 8th ed. University of Chicago Press/Council of Science Editors; 2014.

Swanson E, O'Sean A, Schleyer A. *Mathematics Into Type.* Updated ed. American Mathematical Society; 1999. Accessed July 23, 2019. https://www.ams.org/publications/authors/mit-2.pdf

# 21.0 Editing, Proofreading, Tagging, and Display

**21.1** **Electronic Editing.** Publishers and editors need to be cognizant of the various modes of delivery of their content (digital and/or print) and how the content will be used; they should then customize their processes accordingly.[1] Many have discovered the benefits of having both print and digital products derived from a single source, which minimizes the possibility of discordant versions and allows for publication to different outputs quickly and accurately.

In addition to editing the content of a document, manuscript and technical editors often need to add structure (eg, markup or styles) and linking (internal and external links) to facilitate typesetting and publication and to ensure that the content can be archived and reused.

There are many different markup languages and approaches; one of the most common approaches used by scientific and technical publications is discussed briefly here.

Note: Many of the terms used in this chapter are defined in Publishing Terms, chapter 22.

**21.1.1** **Editing With XML.** XML (extensible markup language) is both machine and human readable, creating a structure and avenue for data exchange, transformation, and reuse. It provides rules for naming and defining parts of a document and their relationship with each other.[1] XML uses tags in start-end pairs (such as <title>Title of the Article</title> and <body> </body>) to define the elements in that piece of content. In XML, all the content is enclosed with tags that identify what the data are (eg, the article's title is tagged <title>Title of Article</title>). The tagged content can be validated using a schema or DTD (document-type definition). The DTD defines the overall structure of content and helps ensure consistency across documents. For example, the JAMA Network journals use a DTD based on the National Library of Medicine (NLM) DTD, which is endorsed by the National Information Standards Organization.[2]

XML resulted from the need for publishers to simultaneously output print and electronic content.[1] XML is used to define the structure of a document, rather than simply its appearance.[3] Because journals tend to use the same or similar content structures and styles from issue to issue or article to article, XML is ideal for providing both consistent structure via tagging and the flexibility to output in various modes (eg, print, website, app). XML is freely available[4] and does not require specific software.

Editing in XML can be performed using an XML editor, software with added functionality to facilitate the editing of XML, or a plain text editor. XML editors have added facilities, such as tag completion and menus for tasks, that are common in XML editing based on data supplied via the DTD.

The JAMA Network journals accept author-submitted documents (typically created in Microsoft Word) and export valid XML from those files with tagging that conforms to the NLM/JATS (Journal Article Tag Suite) DTD. At that point, the content can be used to create proofs for print, PDFs for digital publication, and HTML (hypertext markup language) for the journal website and apps and to deposit with databases such as PubMed and CrossRef. For more on JATS tagging, see https://jats.nlm.nih.gov/publishing/tag-library/1.2.

**21.2** **Electronic Editing Workflow.** Many software programs have text editing functionality that allows users to view edits and track changes. It is common for insertions to be underlined and deletions to be struck through. Each program offers tools to show or hide the editing marks, notes about formatting, and embedded comments. Some newer software programs permit collaborative writing and editing. How users (eg, authors and editors) respond to the editing depends on not only the software program but also the technologies and workflow involved. For example, manuscript editors at the JAMA Network send edited manuscripts to authors showing text insertions and deletions as well as embedded comments and questions as a PDF file. Authors can respond by using editing or commenting tools directly on the PDF; by printing it out, marking up the copy, scanning it, and returning via email; or by outlining corrections and query answers in an email. Authors are also provided with proofs that are generated programmatically to look like a composed proof for initial review before final composition and publication.

The JAMA Network journals, as well as other publications, have created efficiencies by using a single-source workflow. In this process, content remains in the original document format (eg, Word) and is stored with the XML file and related content (eg, supplemental files, multimedia). Because XML is the basis of this workflow and content, any changes required (before, during, or even after publication in the form of a correction) must be made in the source document and new XML generated. If an individual output is corrected but the source file is not, any current and future versions of that content will not reflect the change. For example, if a correction is made to the digital (HTML) version only, and the source file is not updated, the PDF will not contain the updated content.

**21.3** **Editing and Proofreading Marks.** Corrections often need to be marked on manuscripts and typeset copy. The following marks are common in publishing and used by manuscript editors, production editors, proofreaders, and others involved in correcting copy.

*Insertion and Deletion*

| | |
|---|---|
| Caret (insert) | ∧ |
| Close up space | ⌒ |
| Correct typographical error | corre**k**t ⎯⎯⎯ c |
| Delete | ℯ |
| Delete and close up | ℯ |
| Delete underline | Word⎯⎯⎯ ℯ |
| Spell out | (sp) |
| Stet text (let stand as set) | (stet) |

*Positioning*

| | |
|---|---|
| Align | ‖ or = |
| Break line | ⌐ |
| Center | ] [ |
| Flush left | [ or (fl) |
| Hanging indent | ⌐1⌐ ] |
| Justify | → |
| Move left | [ |
| Move right | ] |
| Lower | ⌐⌐ |
| Raise | ⌐⌐ |
| Transpose | ∿ (tr) |

*Punctuation*

| | | |
|---|---|---|
| Period | ⊙ | |
| Comma | ⌃, | |
| Colon | ⌃: | |
| Semicolon | ⌃; | |
| Apostrophe | ⌄' | |
| Single quotation marks | ⌄' | ⌄' |
| Double quotation marks | ⌄" | ⌄" |
| Prime sign | ⌄' | (prime) |
| Hyphen | = | |
| Equals sign | = | (equals) |
| Minus sign | — | (minus) |
| Plus sign | + | |
| Plus/minus sign | ± | |
| Em dash | $\frac{1}{M}$ | |
| En dash | $\frac{1}{N}$ | |
| Parentheses | ⤙ / ⤚ | |
| Brackets | ⊦ / ⊧ | |
| Braces | { / } | |
| Slash | / | |
| Backslash | \ | |
| Bullet | • | (bullet) |

*Queries*

Query to author                      (Au?)

Set when known                 (swk)

*Spacing*

Insert space                        (#)

Insert thin space                (thin #)

Equalize space                  (eq #)

Indent 1 em space            [1]

Begin a new paragraph        ¶

Run in text (no paragraph)

*Style of Type*

Wrong font                      (wf)

Lowercase                     (lc)    or    Word

Lowercase with initial capitals    (c + lc)      an example

Capitalize                    (CAP)      word

Set roman or regular type (lightface;
     not bold or italic)               (rom)   or   (lf)

Set in *italic* type               (ital)       word

Set in **boldface** type          (bf)       word

Set in ***boldface italic*** type     (bf ital)      word

Small caps                    (sc)      word

Small caps with initial full capitals    (c + sc)     an example

Subscript letter or number        $\hat{2}$

Superscript letter or number      $\check{2}$

**21.4** **Proofreading Sample.** The following example shows how a proof was marked for corrections and how the corrected text appears in the revised proof.

Most US soldiers currently deployed in war zones are in Afghanistan or Iraq where malaria transmission is seasonal and varies geographically. While Plasmodium vivax historically accounts for 80% to 90% of indigenous cases in Afghanistan and 95% of cases in Iraq, with *P* falciparum causing the majority of the remaining cases 13,14 these numbers are likely to be inaccurate due to unreliable reporting in the last five years from these war torn areas

Most US soldiers currently deployed in war zones are in Afghanistan or Iraq where malaria transmission is seasonal and varies geographically. While *Plasmodium vivax* historically accounts for 80% to 90% of indigenous cases in Afghanistan and 95% of cases in Iraq, with *Plasmodium falciparum* causing the majority of the remaining cases,[13,14] these numbers are likely to be inaccurate due to unreliable reporting in the last 5 years from these war-torn areas.

**21.5** **Basic Elements of Design.**

> *The rules of typography are centuries old, and although the technologies have changed, the goal has always remained the same: a beautiful setting in the service of a pleasant and fruitful reading experience.*
> James Felici[5]

Typography is broadly defined as the composed arrangement and appearance of text and other elements on a surface that involves elements of design. The editor and graphic designer often cooperate in the process of creating the typography and design for a book, monograph, or journal (print or digital), with the goal of achieving a balance of form and readability.

According to typographer Edmund Arnold, good design and typography for English-language publications should follow the linear flow of the Latin alphabet and support the act of reading.[6] According to Arnold, when an individual reads in the English language (or others based on the Latin alphabet), the eyes first fall naturally to the top left corner and then move across and down the page, first from left to right and then in a right-to-left sweep to the next line, until reaching the bottom right corner. Any design or typographic element that forces the reader to work against this natural flow (reading gravity) interrupts the reading rhythm and should be avoided. Wheildon[6] conducted a controlled study in which half of the participants read an article with a design that followed

Arnold's "reading gravity" principles and half read the same article but with a design that did not follow these principles. Rates of comprehension for those reading the article designed to comply with the principles of reading gravity were better (67% good, 19% fair, and 14% poor) than for those reading the same article when the principles of reading gravity were disregarded (32% good, 30% fair, and 38% poor).

Typography for reading on a computer or other digital medium should follow the basic principles of reading as described above. There are a number of shared design considerations (eg, consistency and size of typeface; use of boldface for emphasis, subheadings, or calling out citations to tables or figures in text; concerns about overly long or wide tables or figures). However, digital typography has additional attributes and concerns and must reflect standards that address a different set of reading, browsing, and searching habits. For example, a web page must work across different computer platforms, browsers, and screen sizes, and the publisher cannot control how the typographic elements (such as typeface, font, size, and color) appear on different users' screens. The web is designed for interactivity and scrolling, so links and navigational buttons need to be clearly indicated.

This chapter focuses primarily on typography for the printed page and for Latin character sets. Resources for design and typography for the web are listed in the Additional Resources and General References at the end of the chapter. Whether print or digital, typography should follow standards, consistent hierarchy and display of elements, style rules, and style sheets.

Good design arranges text and objects in a manner that invites and leads the reader through the composed page or material and enhances legibility and comprehension.[6,7] The basic elements of design that affect typography in print and digitally include the following:

- **Contrast:** This refers to the contrast between dark and light type and large and small units of information (such as title and byline, sideheads and subheads, and text). In addition, the evenness of darkness or blackness of letters and characters affects legibility; this evenness depends on the specific typeface used as well as spacing between letters, words, and lines (see 21.3, Spacing).[7]

- **Rhythm:** The rhythm of the design refers to repetition of similar units in both opposition and juxtaposition (eg, spacing and proportion of type to the page or screen and size of screen, eg, desktop or mobile) and other design elements and repetition of graphic contrasts or similarities.

- **Size:** The size of type and other elements affects legibility and the overall appearance of a composed page. The size relationships within the design refer to the optical images of the type and graphic elements and the relevant and proportional manners in which they appear on the page.

- **Color:** In this context, color has 2 meanings: (1) the darkness or density of the type (letters and characters) and the typeset page and (2) the use of contrasting nonblack colors, which attracts attention and creates associations.

- **Movement and Focal Points:** The elements of a page or screen should guide the reader's eye along the lines of composition unconsciously, from large to small,

**Figure 21.6-1.** Layout of Pages 1 to 2 of a *JAMA* Article

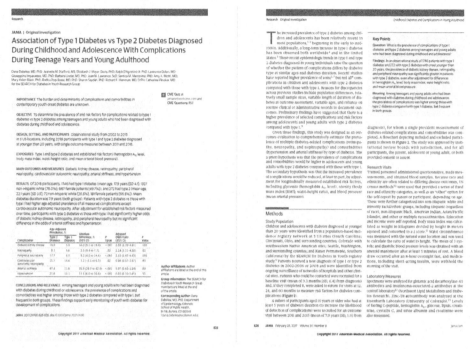

from top to bottom, from left to right, and from dark to light, and should follow the gravity of reading.

In scholarly publishing, a number of typographic and design elements, such as prescribed text format, titles and headings, bylines, abstracts, tables, figures, lists, equations, block quotations, reference citations and lists, navigational elements, and internal and external links, must be considered and incorporated. Consistent use of typographic style within a specific work (eg, journal, book) enhances readability and is recommended for scholarly publications. This consistency often requires programmed style sheets based on standards for a specific publication.

The examples of journal pages shown in **Figure 21.6-1** include some of these typographic elements of design as they are used in the print and PDF versions of the JAMA Network journals.

**21.6** **Typefaces, Fonts, and Sizes.** A typeface is a design for a set of characters (eg, Times Roman, Arial). A font of type is the complete assortment of characters, qualities (eg, size, pitch, and spacing), and styles (eg, bold, italics) of a particular typeface. Note: The term *font* is often used incorrectly as a synonym for *typeface*.

A family of type:

Times New Roman

*Times New Roman Italic*

**Times New Roman Bold**

***Times New Roman Italic Bold***

There are 2 common forms of typeface: serif and sans serif. Serif typefaces (eg, Times Roman) have a short, light line (serif) projecting from a letter's main strokes. Sans serif typefaces (eg, Arial) are unadorned letters without the short line projections. Serif type is generally believed to be more readable than sans serif type for large amounts of printed text because serifs on the letters guide the eyes along a line of copy and the modulated thick and thin strokes of serif types help distinguish individual letters and words to be read. Thus, for print publications, serif type is generally used for body text because of its readability; sans serif type is used for contrasting and complementary elements and to attract attention (eg, titles, headings).[1,3,4] For electronic display, sans serif typefaces often display better and are more legible than serif typefaces.[1]

The font for a publication typically includes 7 styles:

| | |
|---|---|
| roman capitals (uppercase letters) | ABCD |
| roman lowercase letters | abcd |
| boldface capitals | **ABCD** |
| boldface lowercase letters | **abcd** |
| italic capitals | *ABCD* |
| italic lowercase letters | *abcd* |
| small capitals | ABCD |

Each of these styles may also include different weights or heaviness of stroke (eg, light, regular, heavy, black, extra bold, condensed). Each font also includes numerals, punctuation marks, symbols and diacritical marks (eg, accents, tildes, umlauts), and ligatures and diphthongs (≥2 letters joined together; ligatures [eg, *œ* and *fi*] may be vowels and consonants, whereas diphthongs [eg, *æ*] are vowels only). Not all serif and sans serif typefaces share similar characteristics, and not all typefaces include all font characteristics. For more discussion on typeface characteristics, see Bringhurst's *The Elements of Typographic Style*.[7]

Increasingly, web fonts are being created that are designed for electronic display, particularly on low-resolution devices, such as smartphones and tablets.[5] Two examples of such typefaces are Georgia and Verdana. These feature better character fitting and larger x-height,[5] both qualities that offer better onscreen readability (but not necessarily for print).

The size of type is conventionally referred to as its point size. The height of characters in a specific font is measured in points; each point is approximately 1/72 inch (0.35 mm), 12 points equals 1 pica, and 6 picas equals 1 inch (25.4 mm). Picas are used in the dimensions of a page, including spacing between columns and other elements. However, the overall dimensions of a page may be provided in inches by publishers and printers who still work with conventional (nonmetric) units.[3]

The height of a letter in a specific font is measured by its x-height (so named because it is derived from the height of a lowercase *x*). The x-height is the distance between the baseline of a line of type and the top of the main part of the lowercase letter, not including ascenders and descenders. An ascender is the part of a letter that rises above the x-height of the font as seen in the letters *b, d, f, h, k,* and *t*. A descender refers to the part of the letter that dips below the baseline (eg, *p, q, y,* and *Q*) (**Figure 21.6-2**). The width of a specific character is measured by pitch, which refers to how many characters can fit in an inch.

**Figure 21.6-2.** The x-Height, Ascenders, and Descenders of Letters

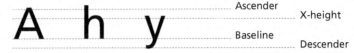

Typefaces are commonly available and used in 6-point to 72-point sizes. In print, type sizes below 14 points are generally used for body text, and sizes of 14 points and above are generally used for display types (eg, titles and headlines). Optimal text type sizes vary, depending on the medium and the content.[8] The JAMA Network journals, for example, use Guardian Egyptian 8 point for regular body text and Guardian Sans 15 point, medium weight, for article titles.

Online, the lower resolution of display would make smaller point sizes difficult to read. Thus, 14-point type is often used onscreen, which causes the reader to scroll more but makes the copy more legible.[5]

Points are also used to measure the space between lines of type (leading). The pica is used to measure the length of a line and the depth of the type area.

The horizontal spacing of type is measured in *ems*, which is a measure for each size of type whose value varies with size, specifically the size of a lowercase *m*. For example, in 9-point type, the em is 9 points; for 12-point type, the em is 12 points.[7] Multiple conventions suggest an optimal number of characters per line for speed and comprehension of reading of journal articles and books and to avoid excessive hyphenation or a page spotted with erratic and distracting white spaces between words (eg, ladders, rivers).[5,7] The optimal number varies according the typeface, type size, column format (eg, 3-, 2-, or 1-column format), and publication (journal vs book). One convention suggests that readability is best when 45 to 75 characters (including punctuation and spaces) fit on 1 line of the column.[7,8] Higher numbers of characters are best suited to single-column designs. For multiple-column formats, such as those used in scholarly journals, conventions suggest that 40 to 50 characters per line is ideal or that the column width should accommodate 1½ alphabets (approximately 39 characters) of the typeface per line. In each case, a column width that is too narrow results in excessive hyphenation at line endings, whereas one that is too wide results in a line too long for the eye to easily complete.

**21.7** ▮ **Spacing.** Readability of type depends on the spacing between letters, words, and lines; none of these is independent of the others.

**21.7.1** ▮ **Letterspacing.** *Letterspacing* refers to the space between letters and other characters. Ideally, the spaces between letters should be balanced. There are no absolute values for optimal letterspacing, but type size and column width are interdependent in design and may affect reading comprehension. *Kerning* (adjusting the space between characters) is often used to modify spacing between pairs of characters to bring letters closer together or farther apart in an attempt to fit words into a defined space (ie, in text that uses justified columns rather than ragged right line ends). Kerning is typically done in units of 1, 2, or 3. The more kerning units used, the closer the letters become. Kerning should be used cautiously to avoid the merging of letters and reducing legibility.[5,7]

Examples of changes in the appearance of a line of type that occur by changing the letterspacing are as follows:

No letterspacing:     *JAMA* is published weekly.

2-Point letterspacing: *JAMA* is published weekly.

4-Point letterspacing: *JAMA* is published weekly.

**21.7.2** **Word Spacing.** Typefaces have predetermined spacing between words that is dictated by the point size and width of a typestyle, the darkness or density of the typeface, and the openness or tightness of the letterspacing. For text set ragged right (unjustified), word spacing may be fixed and unchanging. However, for text that is set flush left and flush right (justified), the spacing may need to be more flexible. For justified text, an average word space of a fourth of an em is ideal, with a minimum and maximum range of a fifth of an em to half an em.[4]

**21.7.3** **Line Spacing.** *Line spacing* refers to the vertical distance between the base of 1 line of text and the base of the next line of text. Line spacing is traditionally known as *leading* for the strips of lead once used between lines of printer type. The space between lines of type is measured in points. Generally, leading is 20% to 45% larger than the copy size.[5] For example, 10-point copy would be set on 12 points of leading or line spacing (10/12), as is shown for the body copy in Figure 21.6-1. Optimal line spacing requires consideration of the type size, layout density, and line length. Generally, longer lines call for increased line spacing for optimal readability. See below for different examples of changes in line spacing that change the appearance of the text. More open line spacing also calls for wider margins; tighter line spacing can be done within narrower margins.

*No extra line spacing:*
The type size and style are identical
in each line; only the space between
the lines changes.

*2-Point line spacing:*
The type size and style are identical
in each line; only the space between
the lines changes.

*4-Point line spacing:*
The type size and style are identical

in each line; only the space between

the lines changes.

The conventions for letterspacing and word spacing vary, depending on the amount of spacing between lines, column width and depth, and whether the text is justified (set as a squared-off block) or unjustified (set with a ragged right margin). For example, a smaller type size may be used on a wider column if the line spacing is adequate for readability. The nature of the composed material will suggest whether variations in typography may be effectively used.

**21.8** **Layout.** *Layout* is the arrangement of all the elements of design and typography on the page or screen for optimal readability, taking into account the context and aesthetic requirements of the content. To create emphasis, complementary typefaces and various fonts within a typeface may be used. However, only a few compatible typefaces should be used at once. Multiple typefaces on a single page can compete for attention, are distracting, and impede readability.[6,8] Two typefaces (a serif for body text and a sans serif for titles and subheads) with appropriate use of styles, such as bold and italics, will most often suffice for a print scholarly publication. The type size and weight create emphasis or continuity, as needed. Headings and subheadings create the outline within the text to frame the article.

In page layout for a scholarly journal, all the elements of design and typography are governed by style and composition rules, often directed by the tagging of the XML. See Figure 21.6-1 for examples. HTML and cascading style sheets are often used to direct the structure and layout. Good web design will be optimized for mobile use. For more details on overall design elements, see resources at the end of this chapter and chapter 22.0, Publishing Terms.

**21.9** **Specific Uses of Fonts and Styles.**

**21.9.1** **Lowercase.** Lowercase (minuscule) letters are smaller than capital (or uppercase) letters and are differently configured (eg, a, A). The term *lowercase* originates from the earlier use of manually set wooden or metal characters that were kept by compositors in 2 cases; the lower case contained the smaller letters and the upper case contained the larger capital letters.[9] Sentences are typically set with the initial letter of the first word of a sentence as a capital letter and all other letters lowercase.

In titles, the initial letter of each major word is set as a capital letter and all other letters are lowercase. Some publications use sentence-style lowercase for titles, with only the initial letter of the first word being a capital. For example, the JAMA Network journals use a mix of initial uppercase and lowercase letters for titles (see 10.2, Titles and Headings).

> Use of Clinical Prediction Rules for Guiding Use of Computed Tomography in Adults With Head Trauma
>
> Potential Mechanisms for Cancer Resistance in Elephants and Comparative Cellular Response to DNA Damage in Humans
>
> Pharmacologic Management of Irritable Bowel Syndrome

The format recommended herein for bibliographic references follows sentence-style lowercase for journal article titles and mixed capitals and lowercase for book titles:

1. Chetty R, Stepner M, Abraham S, et al. The association between income and life expectancy in the United States, 2001-2014. *JAMA*. 2016;315(16):1750-1766. doi:10.1001/jama.2016.4226

2. National Academies of Sciences, Engineering, and Medicine. *Pain Management and the Opioid Epidemic: Balancing Societal and*

*Individual Benefits and Risks of Prescription Opioid Use.* National Academies Press; 2017.

(See 3.9.1, English-Language Titles.)

The case of words (lowercase and uppercase) for titles, headings, and labels in tables and figures is addressed in 4.1.3, Table Components, and in 4.2.6, Components of Figures.

**21.9.2**    **Capital (Uppercase).** Capital (majuscule) letters are larger than lowercase letters and are used as initial letters in the first word of sentences and for proper names. They are also often used as the initial letter of major words in titles, headings, and subheadings. (*Caput* is Latin for head.[6]) Use of all capital letters in large blocks of text should be avoided because legibility is decreased; other means of emphasis should be used if needed, such as bold type. For this reason, the JAMA Network journals use all-capital letters sparingly (eg, for sideheads in print/PDF abstracts).

A *drop cap* (a form of *initial cap*) is an oversized capital letter of the first word that begins a paragraph and drops through several lines of text. It may be used to draw the reader's attention to the beginning of an article, chapter, or important section (see Figure 21.6-1 for an example). An initial cap may also be a raised cap when the capital letter is raised above the main line of text.

**21.9.3**    **Boldface.** A general scheme of headings and side headings may call for the use of boldface type for first- and second-level headings and for first-level side headings in the text, although heading styles and formats vary among publications (see 2.8, Parts of a Manuscript, Headings, Subheadings, and Side Headings). For example, the JAMA Network journals use the following headings:

### Methods (level 1 head, flush left, bold cap and lowercase, larger size)

**Statistical Analysis** (level 2 head, bold cap and lowercase, set in journal color)

**Clustering Data** (level 3 head, bold caps and lowercase)

Boldface may also be used in text to call out references to figures or tables (usually only at first mention):

Demographic data for the participants in the study are given in **Table 1**.

**21.9.4**    **Italics.** *Italics* is a form of roman type style that slants to the right. Italics have multiple uses. However, setting large blocks of body text in italics should be avoided because legibility is reduced. Use italics as follows:

- For level 4 heads (second-level sideheads)

- When terms are described as terms and letters as letters (see 8.6.7, Coined Words, Slang, and 8.7.5, Using Apostrophes to Form Plurals):

  The page number is called the *folio*.

  In his handwriting, the *n*'s look like *u*'s.

- For titles of books and journals, proceedings, symposia, plays, paintings, long poems, video games, musical compositions, movies, space vehicles, planes, and ships (see 10.2, Titles and Headings):

  *JAMA Psychiatry*

  USS *Constitution*

  Verdi's *Requiem*

  *Spirit of St Louis* (plane)

  *Microbe Invader* (video game)

- For legal cases (see 3.16, US Legal References), eg, *Roe v Wade*

- For epigraphs set at the beginning of a work

- For search terms (see 2.6, Keywords):

  Search terms included both subject headings and keywords for *aortic diseases, intramural hematoma, aortic dissection, penetrating ulcer, aortic ulcer, aortic syndrome, optimal medical therapy, open repair, endovascular treatment, stent graft, therapy,* and *diagnosis.*

- For some non-English words and phrases (see 12.1.1, Use of Italics) that are not shown among English terms in the current edition of *Merriam-Webster's Collegiate Dictionary* or in accepted medical dictionaries (eg, *de Qi* sensation). Italics are not used if words or phrases are considered to have become part of the English language (eg, café au lait, in vivo, in vitro, en bloc).

- For lowercase letters used in alphabetic enumerations of items or topics (the parentheses are set roman): (*a*), (*b*), (*c*), etc.

- For genus and species names of some microorganisms, plants, and animals when used in the singular and the names of a variety or subspecies. Plurals, adjectival forms, and taxa above genus (eg, class, order, family) are not italicized (see 14.14, Organisms and Pathogens):

  Bacillaceae

  *Staphylococcus*

  *Staphylococcus aureus*

  staphylococci

  staphylococcal

  *Streptococcus* (*But:* organisms, streptococcal, streptococci)

- For portions of restriction enzyme terms (see 14.6.1, Nucleic Acids and Amino Acids):

  *Hpa*I

  *Bam*HI

- For gene symbols but not gene names (see 14.6.2, Human Gene Nomenclature; 14.6.3, Oncogenes and Tumor Suppressor Genes; and 14.6.5, Nonhuman Genetic Terms):

  *ERBB2*

  *CFTR*

- For chemical prefixes (*N*-, *cis*-, *trans*-, *p*-, etc) (see 14.4.4, Chemical Names, and 15.10, Molecular Medicine)

- For mathematical expressions, such as lines, variables, unknown quantities, and constants (see 20.0, Mathematical Composition). Numerals or abbreviations for trigonometric functions and differentials are not italicized:

  $\sin x = a/b$

- For some statistical terms (see 19.6, Statistical Symbols and Abbreviations):

  *P* value

  $R^2$

  *t* test

- For the abbreviation for acceleration due to gravity, *g*, to distinguish it from g for gram (see 13.11, Clinical, Technical, and Other Common Terms)

- For the term *sic* (see also Insertions in Quotations in 8.5.2, Brackets)

- In formal resolutions, for *Resolved*

- Sparingly, for emphasis

**21.9.5** **Small Caps.** In this typeface style, all the letters take the shape of a capital letter. However, in the place of lowercase letters, smaller capital letters are used. The small caps generally, but not always, align with the same x-height as the regular roman face, in the same typeface. Use small capital letters as follows:

- AM and PM in time (see 17.5.3, Time)

- BC, BCE, CE, and AD (see 13.3, Days of the Week, Months, Eras)

- Some prefixes in chemical formulas (L for levo-, D for dextro-) (see 14.4.4, Chemical Names, and 14.10, Molecular Medicine)

**21.9.6** **Color.** Although not technically a font type, color is another option to add emphasis, create hierarchy, and organize elements in a publication. Colored type on a white background does not have the same contrast as black type, so the white spaces around the letters can lose their clarity.[5] To compensate, the typeface should be larger or bolder. At typical body text sizes, color is not particularly effective. Letter forms do not cover much surface area, so colored text is difficult to notice unless it is highly contrasting.[8] Some journals use different colors of text or shading to indicate hyperlinks to other content. However, in scientific publications (whether print or digital), colored text should be used sparingly.

**Principal Author**: Stacy L. Christiansen, MA

## ACKNOWLEDGMENT

Thank you to the following for their review and guidance: Karen Adams-Taylor, JAMA Network; David Antos, JAMA Network; Erin Kato, JAMA Network; Trevor Lane, MA, DPhil, Edanz Group, Fukuoka, Japan; Chris Meyer, JAMA Network; and Monica Mungle, JAMA Network.

## REFERENCES

1. *Chicago Manual of Style*. 17th ed. University of Chicago Press; 2017.
2. NLM Journal Archiving and Interchange Tag Suite. Updated September 13, 2012. Accessed July 22, 2018. https://dtd.nlm.nih.gov/
3. Council of Science Editors. *Scientific Style and Format: The CSE Manual for Authors, Editors, and Publishers*. 8th ed. University of Chicago Press/Council of Science Editors; 2014.
4. Extensible markup language (XML). W3C (World Wide Web Consortium). Updated October 11, 2016. Accessed July 22, 2018. https://www.w3.org/XML/
5. Felici J. *The Complete Manual of Typography*. 2nd ed. Peachpit; 2012.
6. Wheildon C. *Type & Layout: Are You Communicating or Just Making Pretty Shapes?* Worsley Press; 2005.
7. Bringhurst R. *The Elements of Typographic Style, Version 4.0*. Hartley & Marks; 2013.
8. Butterick M. *Butterick's Practical Typography*. 2019. Accessed August 12, 2019. https://practicaltypography.com
9. Haley A. Lowercase letters. Fonts.com website. Accessed January 2, 2016. https://www.fonts.com/content/learning/fontology/level-1/type-anatomy/lowercase-letters

## ADDITIONAL RESOURCES AND GENERAL REFERENCES

Ambrose G, Harris P. *The Fundamentals of Typography*. 2nd ed. AVA Publishing; 2011.

Craig J, Scala IK. *Designing With Type: The Essential Guide to Typography*. 5th ed. Watson-Guptill Publishers; 2006.

Kasdorf WE, ed. *The Columbia Guide to Digital Publishing*. Columbia University Press; 2003.

Lynch PJ, Horton S. *Web Style Guide: Basic Design Principles for Creating Web Sites*. 3rd ed. Yale University; 2009.

National Center for Biotechnology Information, National Library of Medicine. Journal Publishing Tag Library, NISO JATS Version 1.2 (ANSI/NISO Z39.96-2019). May 2019. Accessed August 12, 2019. https://jats.nlm.nih.gov/publishing/tag-library/1.2/

**22.1**   **Glossary of Publishing Terms.** This glossary is intended to define terms commonly encountered during editing and publishing as well as some industry terms that also have a more common vernacular meaning. The glossary is not all-inclusive. New terms and new usage of existing terms will emerge with time and advances in technology.

**abstract:** A brief summary of a research article, thesis, review, or conference proceeding used to help the reader quickly ascertain the paper's purpose. Abstracts should stand alone and contain sufficient information for a reader to understand the main hypothesis, results, and conclusions of a paper without any further information. See also *extract* and *call-out*.

**acid-free paper:** Paper made by alkaline sizing, a treatment that improves the paper's resistance to liquid and vapor and improves the paper's permanence.

**acknowledgment:** The part of a book or article that thanks people, other than the authors, who had a role in the writing, research, collection, and review of data or other tasks related to the published work.

**advertorial:** Promotional or advertising content that has the appearance of editorial content (see 5.12.3, Advertorials).

**align:** To place text and/or graphics to line up horizontally or vertically with related elements.

**analytics:** Data monitored to assess the performance of an online publication or website, which includes usage (such as views, downloads, and visitors), citations, media coverage, social media activity, interactions such as subscriptions or account creation, and other metrics.

**ANSI:** American National Standards Institute.

**API:** Application program interface. A series of action-oriented functions that programmers use to pass data and objects between different applications and operating systems.

**application:** A computer program that enables the user to perform a specific task, such as a word processor, a web browser, or a graphic tool. Applications that are primarily used on mobile devices are typically called *apps*.

**archive:** To copy files for backup purposes or to store files or data in a repository.

**art repair, art rebuilding:** Replacing text, symbols, arrows, and lines on line art to produce illustrations that are consistent in format, type, and size.

**article processing charge (APC):** A fee charged to authors to make a work publicly available by open access. See also *open access*.

**ascender:** The part of lowercase letters, such as *d, f, h*, and *k*, that extends above the midportion or x-height of the letter.

**ASCII:** American Standard Code for Information Interchange. A code representing an alphanumeric group of characters that is recognized by most computers and computer programs.

**attribute:** XML term for a name-value pair associated with an XML element that modifies certain features of the element. For example, in JATS XML tagging, the tag name "@corresp" is used for the attribute named "Corresponding Author." See also *element*.

**author's editor:** An editor who substantially edits an author's manuscript and prepares it to meet the requirements for publication in a particular journal.

**back up:** Save copies of digital files in the cloud or on disk, tape, or other medium.

**backstrip:** A strip of paper affixed to the bound edges of paper that form a journal's spine.

**bad break:** A poor or potentially confusing arrangement of type at the end of a line or the bottom or top of a page or column. Examples include a paragraph that ends with 1 or 2 words at the top of a page or column (widow) or the first line of a paragraph that starts at the bottom of a page or column (orphan), a heading that falls on the last line of a page or column, an improperly hyphenated word or acronym, or the second part of a properly hyphenated word starting a page.

**bandwidth:** The capacity of a communication system in transferring data.

**banner:** A rectangular graphic at the top of a web page. Also, in advertising, a banner advertisement is typically a rectangular advertisement placed on a website above or below (or on a side of) the site's main content and may be linked to the advertiser's website. Vertical banner advertisements are sometimes called tower advertisements or skyscraper advertisements.

**baseline:** The imaginary line on which the letters in a line of type appear to rest.

**basis weight:** The weight of paper determined by the weight in pounds of a ream (500 sheets) of paper cut to a standard size for a specific grade. For example, 500 sheets, 25 × 38 in, of 80-lb coated paper will weigh 80 lb.

**baud rate:** In telecommunications and electronics, the signaling rate; a baud is the number of changes to the transmission media per second in a modulated signal.

**binary system:** A system of numbers using only the digits 1 and 0 for all values; it is the basis for digital computers.

**binding:** (1) The process by which printed units or pages are attached to form a book, journal, or pamphlet, including operations such as folding, collating, stitching, or gluing. Types of binding include loose-leaf binding, perfect binding, saddle-stitch binding, and selective binding. (2) The cover and spine of a book or journal.

**bit:** A binary digit, either 0 or 1; the smallest unit of digital information.

**bitmap (bmp):** Also called raster graphic image or digital image, a data file or structure that represents a generally rectangular grid of pixels, or points of color, on a computer monitor, paper, or other display device.

**bitmap fonts:** Low-resolution fonts designed for computer screens, whose characters are represented by bitmaps or by a pattern of dots.

**blanket:** Fabric coated with rubber or other material that is clamped around a printing cylinder to transfer ink from the press plate to the paper.

**bleed:** A printed image that runs off the edge of a printed page. A partial bleed extends above, below, or to the side of the established print area but does not continue off the page.

**blind folio:** A page number counted but not printed on the page.

**blind image:** An image that fails to print because of ink receptivity error.

**blind review:** A process in which reviewer names (single blind) or reviewer and author names (double blind) are kept anonymous during peer review.

**blog:** Short for weblog. A blog is a journal-style website that is frequently updated and intended for general public consumption. Blogs generally represent the personality of their authors.

**blueline(s):** The proof sheet(s) of a book or magazine printed in blue ink that shows exactly how the pages will look when they are printed.

**blueprint, blackprint:** A photoprint made from film that is used to check the position and relative arrangement of text and image elements.

**body type:** The type characteristics used for the main body text of a work.

**boilerplate:** A section of text that can be reused without changes, often program matically inserted into content.

**boldface (bf):** A typeface that is heavier and darker than the text face used.

**bps:** Bits per second. A measurement of the speed with which data travel from one place to another.

**broadside:** Printed text or illustrations positioned on the length rather than the width of the page, requiring the reader to turn the publication on its side to read it; usually used for tables and figures that are wider than the normal width of a publication. Also called landscape orientation.

**browser:** A program for searching and accessing information on the web.

**bug:** Something that causes an error in computer software or hardware.

**bullet:** A dot of a heavy weight (•) used to highlight individual elements in a list.

**byline:** A line of text at the beginning of an article listing the authors' names (see 2.2, Author Bylines and End-of-Text Signatures, and 5.1.1, Authorship: Definition, Criteria, Contributions, and Requirements).

**byte:** A unit of digital information that can code for a single alphanumeric symbol; 1 byte equals 8 to 64 bits.

**calibrate:** To adjust a device, such as a scanner or a monitor, image setter, or printing press, to more precisely reproduce color.

**caliper:** Thickness of paper or film measured in terms of thousandths of an inch (mils or points); also the tool used to measure the thickness of paper.

**call-out:** Reprinted text, usually bolder and larger than that of the original text, used to place emphasis, improve design, or fill white space. See also *extract* and *pullout quotes*.

**camera-ready:** Copy, including graphics and text, that is ready to be photographed for reproduction without further composition or alteration. Although photo offset printing has been largely replaced by digital-to-plate printing and desktop publishing, the term is still used to signify that a document is ready to be made into a printing plate.

**Cap:** As a proofreading or editing mark, short for capital letter.

**caption:** The text accompanying an illustration or photograph (see 4.0, Tables, Figures, and Multimedia).

**cascading peer review:** Process by which a manuscript is transferred from one journal to another within a group of journals or publisher.

**cascading style sheet (CSS):** Programmable guide for adding style (type, font, color, spacing) to web pages and documents.

**cell:** In tables or spreadsheets, a unit in an array formed by the intersection of a column and a row (see 4.0, Tables, Figures, and Multimedia).

**central processing unit (CPU):** The component in a computer that interprets instructions and processes data contained in software.

**CEPS:** Color electronic prepress systems. Electronic color equipment used to perform electronic retouching and pagination.

**character:** A letter, numeral, symbol, or punctuation mark.

**character count:** The number of characters and spaces in a document. A manual character count is done by counting the number of characters and spaces in an average line of the manuscript, multiplying that number by the number of lines on the manuscript page, and multiplying that number by the total number of manuscript pages. Word-processing programs can provide an exact character count and word count.

**circulation:** The total number of copies (if printed) of a publication sold and distributed. Opinions differ on metrics of online "circulation" and the field is evolving—number of page views, minutes spent reading, unique visitors, and "shares" and "mentions" (promotion and amplification of the article or website in other media) have all been used as ways to quantify readers.

**citation:** A specific reference to a source for substantiation in a scholarly paper.

**citation analysis:** An analysis of the number of times a published article is cited in the reference list of subsequently published articles.

**cloud:** Internet-based computing, in which shared resources and information are provided to computers and other devices on demand. Instead of buying dedicated hardware and having it depreciate, organizations can share computing and digital storage infrastructure and pay as they go. Storing information "in the cloud" refers to this model of off-site digital storage.

**CMYK:** Abbreviation for the 4 process printing colors: cyan, magenta, yellow, and black.

**collaborator:** Nonauthor contributor to a work, typically a member of a group-authored manuscript.

**collective work:** A publication, such as an anthology or encyclopedia or other collection, in which a number of contributions are assembled into a collective whole. There are 2 types of authorship in a collective work: (1) authorship of the collective work as a whole, which may include revisions, editing, compilation, and similar authorship that went into putting the work into final form, and (2) authorship of the individual contributions (see 5.6, Intellectual Property: Ownership, Access, Rights, and Management).

**colophon:** A summary of information about the publication or the publication's production methods or specifications; also the publisher's emblem or trademark.

**color breaks:** Separating elements of a piece of artwork that will print in more than 1 color. A second or third color proof may be attached to a black proof to show the color screen on artwork.

**color correct:** To change the color values in a set of film separations or, using a software application, to correct or compensate for errors in photography, scanning, separation, and output.

**color separation:** Separation of artwork into component films of cyan, magenta, yellow, and black (CMYK) in preparation for printing.

**compilation:** A section of a publication that is made up of a group of items, for example, letters or book reviews that are run together as opposed to each article starting on a new page.

**composite figure:** A figure that is composed of more than 1 type of element (eg, halftone, line art, 4-color).

**composition:** The arrangement of type, graphics, and typographic characteristics for printing or display in an electronic image of text (such as a PDF).

**compression:** A computer technique of eliminating redundant information, such as blank lines from a document or white space from an image, to reduce the file size for faster transmission or more compact storage of data.

**computer-assisted composition:** A process in which text in digital form is processed through a set of typesetting strictures that dictate the type size and font, hyphenation and justification, character and word spacing, and all typographical requirements needed to typeset the text. The data stream created from this process is used to drive an image setter for typesetting and printing a page of text.

**condensed type:** A narrow version of a typeface, designed to fit more text on each line (see 21.0, Editing, Proofreading, Tagging, and Display).

**content management system (CMS):** Software that enables management, storage, and tracking of content and workflows.

**context-sensitive editor:** A software program that uses document structure to determine which elements are appropriate to insert in a particular context within a document (such as an XML editor).

**continuous tone:** An image that has gradations of tone from dark to light, in contrast to an image formed of pure blacks and whites, such as a pen-and-ink drawing or a page of type (see also *halftone* and *duotone*).

**controlled circulation:** Copies of or access to a publication distributed to a select list of recipients, usually without charge.

**cookie:** Message given to a web browser by a server to identify users.

**copy:** Any matter, including a manuscript in handwritten, typescript, or digital format, artwork, photographs, tables, and figures, to be set or reproduced for printing.

**copy editor:** An editor who prepares a document or other copy for publication, making alterations and corrections to ensure accuracy, consistency, and uniformity. Also called a manuscript editor.

**copy fitting:** Estimating the space required to display a given amount of text in a specific type size, typeface, and format.

**copyright:** The law protecting rights to published and unpublished works (see 5.6.3, Copyright: Definition, History, and Current Law).

**corrupted:** Refers to data that have been damaged in some way.

**cover:** The front and back pages of a publication. The 4 pages making up the covers in a print publication are often designated covers 1, 2, 3, and 4. Covers 1 and 4 are outside pages, and covers 2 and 3 are inside pages.

**cover stock:** Paper used for the cover, usually heavier than the paper used for the body of the publication.

**Creative Commons (CC):** A public copyright license that enables the free distribution of an otherwise copyrighted work. There are different levels of copyright within the Creative Commons license. Some allow for editing and building on a work, some do not, and some make a distinction as to whether such reuse is for commercial or noncommercial purposes. For more on Creative Commons, see https://creativecommons.org.

**crop:** To trim a photograph, illustration, or other element to fit a desired design or format or to cut off unwanted portions.

**crop marks:** Lines placed on the sides, top, and bottom of a photograph or illustration that indicate the size or area of the image to be reproduced.

**CTP:** Computer-to-plate. A printing process that transmits a digital image directly from a computer file to a plate used on a press, eliminating the need for film or negatives.

**cursor:** An on-screen indicator, such as a blinking line, arrow, hollow square, or other image (usually mouse or keystroke driven), that marks a designated place on the screen and indicates current point of data entry or modification, menu selection, or program function.

**database:** A collection of stored data from which information can be extracted and organized in various forms and formats.

**debug:** To trace and correct errors in a computer program.

**demand printing, print on demand:** A part of the publishing industry that creates short-run, customized print publications quickly and on individual request.

**demographic versions:** Different versions of an issue of a publication that contains specific inserts or content targeted for specific readers; the inserts are usually advertisements but can also include targeted editorial content.

**derivative work:** Work based on one or more preexisting works, such as a translation, musical arrangement, dramatization, fictionalization, motion picture version, sound recording, art reproduction, or abridgment.

**descender:** The part of such letters as *p, q,* and *y* that extends below the main body of the letter or baseline (compare *ascender* and see *x-height*).

**desktop color separation:** A computer file format that separates an EPS (encapsulated PostScript) color file into the 4 color elements: cyan, magenta, yellow, and black (CMYB).

**desktop publishing:** A computer-based publishing system, including page layout software.

**digital asset management:** A centralized system for archiving, searching, and retrieving digital files and associated metadata.

**digitize:** To transform a printed character or image into bits or binary digits so that it can be entered into and manipulated in a computer.

**display type:** Type that differs from the body type of the text of a printed work. Display type is used in titles, headings, and subheadings and is usually larger than the body type.

**document:** Organized content in written, printed, or digital format.

**DOI:** Digital object identifier. A means of identifying a physical file or internet file or document. A DOI provides a means of persistently identifying a piece of intellectual property on a digital network and associating it with related current data in a structured extensible way.

**domain:** The name that identifies an internet site or server location (eg, jamanetwork.com). Domain names have 2 or more parts separated by dots, which move from specific to general. Domains are also used in the last part of an email address following the @ symbol. The middle-level domain identifies the server or device. The top-level domain identifies the machine name but is recognized often as the type of business (eg, .com, .net, .edu, .org, .mil, .gov) or letters that indicate a country (eg, .ca, .uk, .fr.).

**dot:** In a halftone, an individual printing element or spot (see also *dot gain* and *dots per inch*).

**dot gain:** A printing defect that causes dots to print larger than they should, resulting in darker tone and color than intended.

**dots per inch (DPI):** A measure of the resolution of a printed image.

**double spread:** Printed material (text, tables, illustrations) that extends across 2 pages (left- and right-hand pages); also called a spread or a 2-page spread.

**download:** The process of transferring digital files from a remote server to a local computer. Can be used as a metric to count the number of times content is accessed. See also *views* and *visitors*.

**DRM:** Digital rights management. A system used to protect the copyrights of data distributed or accessed via the internet or other digital media. A DRM system protects intellectual property by encrypting the data or marking the content with a digital watermark so that the content cannot be distributed.

**drop cap, dropped cap:** The initial letter of a word (usually beginning a paragraph) set in boldface, larger than the body text.

**drop folio:** A page number printed at the bottom of the page.

**DSL:** Digital subscriber line. Provides an extremely high-speed internet connection with the same wires as a regular telephone line.

**DTD:** Document type definition. Defines the structure of content (ie, journals or books) with a list of elements (ie, title, author, abstract, paragraphs). The DTD is the blueprint for XML documents.

**dummy:** A layout of a page or an entire journal, to represent the size and appearance after printing.

**duotone:** A 2-color halftone reproduction from a black-and-white photograph; usually reproduced in black and 1 other color.

**DVD:** Digital video disk. An optical disk storage media format that can be used for data storage, including movies with high video and sound quality.

**editor:** (1) Someone who directs a publication or heads an editorial staff and/or decides on the acceptability of a document for publication (eg, editor, editor in chief); manages a publication (eg, managing editor); or prepares a document for publication by altering, adapting, and refining it (eg, manuscript editor, copy editor, author's editor). (2) In computer terminology, a program used to create text files or make changes to an existing file. Text or full-screen editors allow users to move through a document with direction keys, keystrokes, and a mouse- or command-driven cursor. Line editors allow the user to view the document as a series of numbered lines.

**editorial:** (1) Of or relating to an editor or editing. (2) A written expression of opinion that may or may not reflect the official position of the publication. (3) Published material that is not promotional (eg, not an advertisement).

**e-ISSN:** Electronic ISSN, as distinguished from a print ISSN (p-ISSN). See also *ISSN*.

**element:** XML term for a component of a journal article. Can be as small as an abbreviation or as large as an abstract or table, or even the entire article. See also *attribute*.

**ellipsis:** A series of 3 periods ( . . . ) used to indicate an omission or that data are not available (see also 8.8, Ellipses).

**em:** A measurement used to specify to the typesetter the amount of space desired for indention, usually equal to the square body of the type size (eg, a 6-point em is 6 points wide).

**em dash:** A punctuation mark (—) used to indicate an interruption or break in thought in a sentence; also used after introductory clauses and before closing clauses or designations (see 8.3, Hyphens and Dashes).

**embargo:** Agreement between journals and news reporters not to report information contained in a manuscript that has been accepted but not yet published until a specified date and time in exchange for advance access to the information.

**embedding:** Inserting code or links to display multimedia (audio or video) in an article or online content.

**emulsification:** A condition in offset printing that results from a mixing of the water-based fountain solution and oil-based ink on the press.

**emulsion side:** The side of a photographic film to which a chemical coating is applied and on which the image is developed.

**en:** Half an em.

**en dash:** A punctuation mark (–) (longer than a hyphen and half the length of an em dash) used in hyphenated or compound modifiers (see 8.3, Hyphens and Dashes).

**enamel:** The surface of shiny, coated paper.

**end mark:** A symbol, such as a dash (—) or an open square (□), to indicate the end of an article; often used in news stories.

**e-print:** A digital version of a research document that is available for download online. See also *reprint*.

**EPS (encapsulated PostScript):** EPS is a file extension for a graphics file format used in vector-based images in Adobe Illustrator. Can contain text and images.

**e-publication:** Electronic publication; a work published in digital format that is accessed via the internet.

**expanded type:** Type in which the characters are wider than normal (see 21.0, Editing, Proofreading, Tagging, and Display).

**export:** To convert and transfer data from one application into another application.

**extract:** A portion of content, called out or quoted for emphasis or to introduce a reader to content. May include the first set portion of an article (eg, the first 50 words). See also *abstract*, *pullout quotes*, and *call-out*.

**face:** Typeface; style of type (see also *font*).

**fair use:** A legal doctrine that permits limited use of copyrighted works without obtaining permission from the rights holders. It usually refers to the use of a copyright work for a limited and transformative purpose, such as to comment on, criticize, or parody (see 5.6, Intellectual Property: Ownership, Access, Rights, and Management).

**F&G:** Folded and gathered signatures of a publication for final review before publication.

**FAQs:** Frequently asked questions. Often used by web page designers to help users access and search for information and resolve common problems.

**figure:** A visual presentation, such as an illustration, photograph, drawing, or graph (see 4.0, Tables, Figures, and Multimedia).

**filler:** (1) Editorial content used to fill white space created by articles or advertisements not filling an entire page. (2) Chemicals used to fill the spaces between fibers in paper to improve the paper's opacity.

**finish:** The surface of paper.

**firewall:** A security software program or device that blocks or restricts entry into a local area network from the internet.

**flush:** Lines of type aligned vertically along the left margin (flush left) or the right margin (flush right).

**flush and hang:** To set the first line flush left on the margin and indent the remaining lines.

**flyleaf:** Any blank page at the front or back of a book.

**folio:** A page number placed at the bottom or top of a printed page.

**font:** The complete assortment of qualities (eg, size, pitch, and spacing) and styles (eg, boldface, italic) of a particular typeface (see 21.0, Editing, Proofreading, Tagging, and Display).

**foot, footer, running foot:** Standardized text at the bottom of each page of a publication.

**footnote:** An ancillary piece of information printed at the bottom of a page or below a table.

**form, press form:** A group of assembled pages (usually 8, 12, 16, or 32 pages), printed at the same time, then folded into consecutively numbered pages.

**format:** The shape, size, style, margins, type, and design of a publication.

**fountain:** In offset (lithographic) printing, the part of the press that contains the dampening device and solution (usually water, buffered acid, gum, and alcohol); in nonoffset printing, the part of the press that contains the ink.

**FPO:** For position only. Refers to low-resolution graphics used in place of high-resolution graphics to show placement of artwork and photographs before printing.

**FTP:** File transfer protocol. A method for exchanging files between computers on the internet.

**function key:** A key on a computer keyboard that gives an instruction to the machine or computer, as opposed to the keys for letters, numbers, and punctuation marks; often labeled F (eg, F1, F2).

**galley proof:** A proof of typeset text copy run 1 column wide before being made into a page.

**gatefold:** A foldout page.

**ghost author:** An author who meets all criteria for authorship but is not named in the byline of a publication (see 5.1.2, Authorship Responsibility, Guest and Ghost Authors and Other Contributors).

**ghost writer:** A person who has written an article or major parts of it but who is not listed in the Acknowledgment section for this contribution.

**ghosting:** Shadows produced by uneven ink coverage (variations are caused by wide contrasts in the colors or tones being printed).

**GIF (.gif):** Graphics interchange format. A compressed graphic file normally used for images that do not require many colors (maximum, 256).

**glossy:** A photograph or line art printed on smooth, shiny paper.

**gold open access:** Work that is immediately available free of charge at the site of publication to any member of the public.

**gradation:** A transition of shades between black and white, between one color and another, or between one color and white.

**grain direction:** The direction of the fibers in a sheet of paper created when the paper is made.

**granularity:** The level of specificity with which parts of a digital document are identified by a context-sensitive editor.

**graphical user interface (GUI):** Pronounced [goo-ee]; a computer display format that allows the user to select commands, run programs, and view lists of files and other options by pointing a cursor to icons or menus (text lists) of items on the screen. Ubiquitous now; was invented as an alternative to command-line programming.

**graphics:** A catch-all term for illustrative material, such as photographs, drawings, and statistical graphs, intended for publication.

**grayscale:** A range of grays with gradations from white to black. A grayscale image contains various shades of gray.

**greeking:** (1) A simulation of a reduced-size page used by word-processing applications during the print preview function because it is usually not possible to shrink text size in proportion to the page size. The graphic symbols used to represent text resemble Greek letters; hence the term *greeking*. Also called lorem ipsum or lipsum. (2) Refers to nonsense text or gray bars inserted in a page to check the layout.

**green open access:** Work that is made publicly available free of charge in a repository, whether institutional or subject based, perhaps after an embargo period.

**gutter:** The 2 inner margins of facing pages of a publication, from printed area to binding.

**hairline:** The thinnest stroke of a character.

**hairline rule:** A thin rule, usually measuring half of a point.

**halftone:** A black-and-white continuous-tone artwork, such as a photograph, that has shades of gray (see 4.0, Tables, Figures, and Multimedia).

**halftone screen:** A grid used in the halftone process to break the image into dots. The fineness of the screen is denoted in terms of lines per inch (eg, 120, 133, 150).

**H&J:** Hyphenation and justification. The determination of line breaks and the division of words into lines of prescribed measurement.

**handwork:** Extra work the printer does by hand, such as stripping in type or making part of a page opaque.

**hard copy:** Printed copy, in contrast to copy stored in digital format.

**head, header, running head:** Standardized text at the top of each page of a publication.

**head margin:** Top margin of a page.

**homepage:** The first screen a user views when connecting to the main domain of a site on the web.

**HTML:** Hypertext markup language. Codes (tags) used to prepare a file that contains text and graphics for placement on the internet via the web.

**http:** Hypertext transfer protocol. Used at the beginning of a web address to connect with a website and transfer information and graphics across the web.

**https:** Hypertext transfer protocol, secure. This protocol is used for performing financial and other types of transactions that require secure transmission of information.

**hybrid open access:** A publication model in which some of the articles in a journal are open access. This status typically requires the payment of a publication fee (also called an article processing charge or APC) to the publisher.

**hyperlink:** (v) The nonlinear relating of information, images, and sounds that allows a computer user to jump quickly from one topic, item, or representation to another by clicking on a highlighted word or icon; (n) the highlighted word or icon.

**icon:** A small graphic image displayed on a computer screen that represents common computer commands (eg, a trash can that represents a command for deleting unwanted text, files, or applications).

**image setter:** A device that plots an array of dots or pixels onto photosensitive material (film) line by line, until an entire page is created (including text, graphics, and color). The film can be output as a negative or positive with resolutions from 300 to 3000 dots per inch.

**impact factor:** A measure of the frequency with which the average article in a journal has been cited in a particular year. It helps to evaluate a journal's relative importance when compared with others in the same field. The impact factor is calculated by dividing the number of current citations to all articles published in the 2 previous years by the total number of countable articles published in those 2 years. See also *citation* and *citation analysis*.

**import:** Using data produced by one application in another, for example, importing data from a spreadsheet and using it to produce a report in a word-processing document.

**imposition:** The process of arranging pages or press forms of a publication so that the pages will be in sequential order when printed, folded, and bound into a publication; a guide or list of the sequential order of pages.

**impression:** The transfer of an ink image by pressure from type, plate, or blanket to paper. The speed of a sheet-fed printing press is measured by the number of impressions printed per hour.

**imprint:** The name of the publishing house or entity that issues a book; the imprint is typically found at the bottom of the title page. It may or may not be the same as the name of the publishing company, and a publishing company may have various imprints.

**indent:** To set a line of type or paragraph in from the margin or margins (see 21.0, Editing, Proofreading, Tagging, and Display).

**initial:** A large letter, the first letter of a word used to begin a paragraph, chapter, or section. A "sunken" or "dropped" initial cuts 2 or 3 lines down into the text; a "stickup" initial aligns at the bottom with the first line of text and sticks up into the white space above.

**ink fountain:** Device on the press that supplies the ink to the inking rollers.

**insert:** Printed material (a piece of paper or multiple pages) that is positioned between the numbered pages of a publication during the binding process. The insert is usually printed on different paper than that used in the publication; it is often an advertisement.

**instant messaging:** Text-based messaging that allows the user to communicate with others in real time through the internet.

**international paper sizes:** The range of standard metric paper sizes as determined by the International Organization for Standardization (ISO).

**internet:** A global network connecting millions of computers for communications and data transfer purposes.

**intranet:** A private network with access restricted to specific users (eg, employees of a company or members of an organization).

**IP address:** Internet Protocol address. A unique identifier for each device that sends or receives data over the internet.

**ISBN:** International Standard Book Number. A 13-digit number that uniquely identifies books and booklike products published internationally (eg, the ISBN for this manual is 978-0-19-024655-6).

**ISO:** The International Standards Organization.

**ISSN:** International Standard Serial Number. An 8-digit number that identifies periodical publications as such, including electronic serials (eg, the ISSN for *JAMA* in print is 0098-7484, and for *JAMA* online, 1538-3598).

**italic:** A typestyle with characters slanting upward and to the right (italic) as opposed to roman type (see 21.0, Editing, Proofreading, Tagging, and Display).

**JATS:** Journal Article Tag Suite. A standard from NISO (the National Information Standards Organization) that defines a set of XML elements and attributes for tagging scientific literature.

**Java:** A general programming language.

**JPG or JPEG (.jpg):** Joint Photographic Experts Group. A JPEG is a compressed graphic file (usually with the file extension .jpg or .jpeg) normally used for images that require many colors (eg, photographs).

**JSON:** JavaScript Object Notation. An alternative to XML that has the advantages of being simpler, more readable by humans, better suited to data interchange, and object-oriented rather than document-oriented.

**justify:** To add or delete space between words or letters to make copy align at the left and right margins (see 21.0, Editing, Proofreading, Tagging, and Display).

**kerning:** Modification of spacing between characters, usually to bring letters closer together, to improve overall appearance.

**keyline:** Tissue or acetate overlay separating or defining elements and color for line art or halftone artwork.

**ladder:** Four or more hyphens that appear at the end of consecutive lines; a typographic pattern to be avoided.

**landscape:** A layout in which the dimensions for width are greater than those for height. Compare portrait, the usual orientation of a page.

**LaTeX:** A free document preparation system for typesetting, composition, or online display of scientific content.

**layout:** A drawing that shows a conception of the finished product; includes sizing and positioning of the elements.

**leaders:** A row of dots or dashes designed to guide the reader's eye across space or a page.

**leading:** Pronounced [led-ding]; the spacing between lines of type (also called line spacing); a carryover term from hot metal composition. For example, 9-point type on 11 points of line space allows 2 points of leading below the type (see 21.0, Editing, Proofreading, Tagging, and Display).

**legend:** Descriptive text that accompanies a figure, photograph, or illustration; also a list (key) that explains symbols on a map or chart (see 4.0, Tables, Figures, and Multimedia). See also *caption*.

**ligature:** Two or more letters, such as æ, set as connected (see 21.0, Editing, Proofreading, Tagging, and Display).

**line art:** Illustration composed of lines and/or lettering, for example, charts, graphs (see 4.0, Tables, Figures, and Multimedia).

**lines per inch (LPI):** A measure of printing resolution for halftone screens.

**listserve:** A digital mailing list program that manages email addresses of an online discussion group. The listserve program duplicates the messages sent by individual users and automatically sends them to every user in the group. *Listserv* is a registered trademark.

**live area:** The area of a page within the margins.

**logo:** One or more words or other combinations of letters or designs often used for easy recognition and promotion of company names, trademarks, and so on.

**long page:** In makeup, a page that runs longer than the live area or margins of the page.

**loose-leaf binding:** Binding that permits pages to be readily removed and inserted.

**lossy:** Image compression method that removes minor tonal and/or color variations, causing loss of information (detail) at high compression ratios.

**lowercase:** Letters that are not capitalized.

**macro:** A series of automatically executed computer commands activated by a few programmed keystrokes; useful for repetitive tasks.

**makeready:** The part of the printing process that immediately precedes the actual press run, in which colors, ink coverage, and register are adjusted to produce the desired quality; may also apply to the binding process.

**makeup:** The arrangement of type lines and illustrations into pages or press forms for review or printing (see also *imposition*; compare *live area*).

**manuscript:** A typed (or occasionally handwritten) composition before it is published.

**margin:** The section of white space that surrounds typed, composed, or printed copy.

**mark up:** The process of marking manuscript copy with directions for tagging, style, and composition.

**master proof:** The set of galley proofs or page proofs that carries all corrections and alterations.

**masthead:** A listing of editorial, production, and publishing staff; editorial boards; contact information; subscription and advertising information; and important disclaimers.

**matte finish:** The surface of dull-coated paper.

**measure:** The length of the line (width of the column) in which type is composed or set, usually measured in picas and points.

**megabyte (MB):** A unit of computer storage, equal to approximately 1 million bytes.

**memory:** The part of a computer in which digital information is permanently stored.

**MeSH:** Medical Subject Headings. The US National Library of Medicine's controlled-vocabulary thesaurus used for indexing articles in MEDLINE.

**metadata:** Data about data. For example, a content management system contains information (metadata) about publications (data). Metadata are used in markup languages, such as HTML and XML.

**MHz:** Abbreviation for megahertz, a unit that measures a computer system's cycle speed; 1 MHz equals 1 million cycles per second.

**mobile device:** A small, typically handheld computer, such as a smartphone or a tablet.

**modem:** Modulator-demodulator. An electronic telecommunication device that converts computer-generated data (digital signals) into analog signals that can be carried over telephone lines.

**moiré pattern:** An undesirable wavy pattern caused by incorrect screen angles, overprinting halftones, or superimposing 2 geometric patterns.

**MOV:** QuickTime video file format.

**MPEG:** Motion Picture Experts Group. As a file format, refers to video and audio compression and transmission.

**MSL:** Must start left. Indicates that an article must start on a left-hand page.

**MSR:** Must start right. Indicates that an article must start on a right-hand page.

**network:** Two or more computers connected to share resources.

**NISO:** National Information Standards Organization. A US nonprofit standards organization that develops, maintains, and publishes technical standards related to publishing, bibliographic, and library applications.

**nonlossy:** Image compression without loss of quality.

**nonproportional spacing:** Spacing that does not allow for the adjustment of space between characters to eliminate extra white space; all letters have the same space, which creates more space around narrow letters and decreases readability.

**offset, offset printing:** Commonly used term for offset lithographic printing; a printing method in which an image is transferred from an inked plate cylinder to a blanket made of rubber or other synthetic material and then onto a sheet of paper.

**opacity:** (1) A quality of paper that prevents type or images printed on one side from showing through on the other side. (2) The covering power of ink in printing.

**opaque:** To block out (on the film negative) those areas that are not to be printed.

**open access:** A publication model that permits immediate, free access without restrictions (such as a subscription or access fee) and permits use and reuse without restrictions (such as certain copyright and license restrictions). See also *gold open access, green open access*, and *hybrid open access*.

**optical character recognition (OCR):** An OCR input device is capable of scanning a typescript and replicating the typed characters, which creates a digital document that can be edited and searched (as opposed to a scanner, which simply transfers images from paper to a digital file).

**orphan:** One or 2 short words at the end of a paragraph that fall on a separate line at the bottom of a page or column or a single line of type that starts at the bottom of a page or column.

**outline halftone:** A portion taken from a halftone that is the shape or modified shape of a subject.

**overlay:** A hinged flap of paper or transparent plastic covering for a piece of artwork. It may protect the work and/or allow for instructions or corrections to be marked for the printer or camera operator.

**overprinting:** Printing over an area or page that has already been printed.

**overrun:** Production of more copies than the number ordered.

**paginate:** To number, mark, or arrange the pages of a document, manuscript, article, or book.

**Pantone Matching System:** A color identification system that matches specific shades of approximately 500 colors with numbers and formulas for the corresponding inks, developed by Pantone Inc.

**paragraph:** A unit of text set off by indention, horizontal space, bullets, or other typographical device.

**parse:** To analyze files by checking tags (codes) to ensure that they are used correctly.

**pasteup:** An assembly of the elements of type and artwork as a guide to the printer for makeup.

**PDF:** Portable document format. A proprietary file format that shows the elements of a printed document as an electronic image that can be viewed, navigated, annotated, or printed.

**peer review:** The process by which editors ask experts to read, assess, and comment on the suitability of a manuscript and other content for publication (see 6.0, Editorial Assessment and Processing, and 5.11.4, Editorial Responsibility for Peer Review).

**peer-reviewed journal:** A journal that contains editorial content that is peer reviewed.

**perfect binding:** Process in which signatures are collated, the gutter edge is cut and ground, adhesive is applied to the signatures, and the cover is applied.

**perforate:** To punch lines of small holes or slits in a sheet so that it can be torn off with ease.

**pica:** A unit of measure; 1 pica equals approximately ⅙ inch or 12 points.

**pica type:** Type that equals 10 characters to the inch.

**pitch:** In fixed-pitch fonts, pitch refers to the number of characters per inch. Common pitch values are 10 and 12. Proportional-pitch fonts have no pitch value because different characters have different widths, for example, the letter *M* is wider than the letter *I*.

**pixel:** A unit in a digital image; the smallest point of a bit-mapped screen that can be assigned independent color and intensity.

**plate:** (1) A sheet of metal, plastic, rubber, paperboard, or other material used as a printing surface; the means by which an image area is separated from a nonimage area. (2) A full-page, color book illustration, often printed on paper different from that used for the text.

**PMID:** PubMed identification number. The unique identifying number assigned to a record when it is entered into PubMed.

**PNG:** Portable network graphic file format.

**pockets:** Sections on a binder in which individual signatures are placed and then selected as required for each copy to be bound.

**point:** The printer's basic unit of measurement, often used to determine type size; 1 point equals approximately $\frac{1}{72}$ inch; 12 points equal 1 pica.

**PostScript:** A page description language and programming language used primarily in the electronic and desktop publishing areas.

**PowerPoint:** Microsoft software, used to make slide show presentations. File format extensions are the default .ppt (presentation), .pot (template), and .pps (PowerPoint Show).

**ppi:** Pixels per inch. Unit of measurement for digital images.

**preprint:** An article or part of a book printed and distributed or posted online before formal publication and/or review.

**preprint server:** A database or repository that hosts preprints.

**press plates:** The plates used to print multiple copies on the press.

**press run:** The total number of copies of journals, books, or other materials printed.

**print order:** The number of copies of printed material ordered.

**printout:** Paper output of a printer or other device that produces normal-reading copy from computer-stored data.

**proof:** A hard copy of the text and graphic material of a document used to check accuracy of text, composition, positioning, and/or typesetting.

**proofreader:** One who reads or reviews proofs for errors.

**proportional spacing:** Spacing that allows for the adjustment of character spacing based on character width and increases readability.

**protocol:** (1) A system for transmitting data between 2 devices that establishes the type of error checking to be used; data compression structures; how the sending device will indicate that it has finished sending a message; and how the receiving device will indicate that it has received a message. (2) A detailed plan for a scientific study.

**PSD:** Photoshop (Adobe) file format.

**publisher:** An entity or person who directs the production, dissemination, and sale of selected information.

**PubMed:** A searchable database of scientific and biomedical literature compiled by the US National Library of Medicine.

**PubMed Central:** A free digital repository that archives publicly accessible full-text scholarly articles that have been published within the biomedical and life sciences journal literature.

**pullout quotes, pull quote:** Sections of text, usually bolder and larger than the original text, used to emphasize content, improve design, or fill white space.

**ragged right:** Type set with the right-hand margin unjustified (or ragged).

**RAM:** Random access memory. Temporary computer memory used by a computer to hold data currently being processed or created that are lost when the computer is shut down.

**raster:** A digitized image that is mapped into a grid of pixels; therefore, the image is resolution dependent. The color of each pixel is defined by a specific number of bits.

**raster image processor (RIP):** A device that produces a digital bitmap to show an image's position on a page before printing.

**ream:** Five hundred sheets of paper.

**recto:** A right-hand page.

**redlining:** A software program that shows changes made in a document on screen and on a printed typescript for review by the editor and author. Also called revision marking, track changes, or strikethrough/replace.

**register:** To print an impression on a sheet in correct relationship to other impressions already printed on the same sheet, for example, to superimpose exactly the various color impressions. When all parts or inks match exactly, they are in register; when they are not exactly aligned, they are out of register.

**reprint:** A reproduction of an original printing in paper or digital format. See also *e-print*.

**reproduction proof:** A high-quality proof for use in photoengraving or offset lithography.

**resin-coated paper:** Paper used in composition to produce a type proof of the quality needed for photographic reproduction.

**resolution:** A measurement of the visual quality of an image according to discrimination between distinct elements; the fineness of detail that can be distinguished in an image.

**responsive design:** Flexible web page creation that permits readability and use of online content regardless of screen size or device.

**reverse-out, reverse text, reverse image:** Text or image that appears in white surrounded by a solid block of color or black.

**river:** A streak of white space that runs down through lines of type, breaking up the even appearance of the page; to be avoided.

**ROB:** Run-of-book. Advertising term meaning a regular page, as opposed to an advertisement insert. Can also refer to placement anywhere space is available in the publication.

**roman:** A typestyle with upright characters, as opposed to italic (see 21.0, Editing, Proofreading, Tagging, and Display).

**RSS:** Really Simple Syndication or Rich Site Summary. An XML format for syndicating web content.

**run in:** To merge a paragraph with the preceding paragraph.

**runaround:** Type composed or set to fit around an illustration, box, or other design element.

**running foot, footer:** A line of copy, usually giving publication name, subject, title, date, volume number, and/or authors' names, that appears at the bottom of consecutive pages.

**running head, header:** A line of copy, usually giving publication name, subject, title, date, volume number, and/or authors' names, that appears at the top of consecutive pages.

**runover:** Material that does not fit in the space allowed (see also *live area* and *long page*).

**saddle-stitch binding:** Process by which signatures, or pages, and covers are assembled by inserting staples into the centerfold.

**sans serif:** An unadorned typeface; a letter without a short line that projects from the top or bottom of the main stroke of the letter (see 21.0, Editing, Proofreading, Tagging, and Display). See also *serif*.

**scaling:** Determining the appropriate size of an image and the amount of reduction or enlargement needed for the image to fit in a specific area.

**scanner:** A device that uses an electronic reader to transform type, characters, and images from a printed page into a digital form.

**scholar's margin:** A margin/area to the right or left of the main text area wide enough to make notes. Useful for placing go-with slugs, thumbnails, bylines, and other article elements.

**score:** To indent or mark paper or cards slightly so they can be folded exactly at certain points.

**scribe:** Thin strips of nonprinting areas, such as those between figure parts.

**search engine:** A program that enables users to search for documents on the web.

**selective binding:** A method of binding in which specific contents of each copy produced are determined by instructions transmitted electronically from a computer. Signatures, or specific groups of pages, are selected to produce a copy for a specific recipient or recipient group.

**self-cover:** A cover for a publication that is made of the same paper used for the text and printed as part of a larger press form.

**serif:** An adorned typeface; a short, light line that projects from the top or bottom of a main stroke of a letter (see 21.0, Editing, Proofreading, Tagging, and Display). See also *sans serif*.

**server:** A computer software package or hardware that provides specific services to other computers.

**short page:** In makeup, a page that runs shorter than the established live area.

**show-through:** Inking that can be seen on the opposite side of the paper because of the heaviness of the ink or the thinness of the paper.

**sidebar:** Text or graphics placed in a box and printed on the right or left side of a page.

**signature:** (1) A printed sheet composed of several pages that have been folded so that the pages are in consecutive order according to pagination. (2) A line of text that appears at the bottom of an article that lists the names of the author(s).

**signature block:** A block of text that appears at the bottom of an email message, discussion group, and/or forum post that contains the writer's name and may also include the writer's title, company name, location, email address, and personal message; also sometimes used after letters, book reviews, and other small items of copy.

**sink:** Starting type below the top line of the live area, which leaves an area of white space.

**site license:** (1) A licensing agreement that permits access and use of digital information at a specific site. (2) A fee paid to a software company to allow multiple users at a site to access or copy a piece of software.

**sizing:** Adding material to a paper to make it more resistant to moisture.

**slug:** One or more lines of copy inserted to draw the attention of the reader, for example, direction to see a related article or editorial.

**small caps:** Capital letters that are smaller than the typical capital letters of a specific typeface, usually the size of the x-height of the font (see 21.0, Editing, Proofreading, Tagging, and Display).

**software:** Programs and procedures required to enable a computer to perform a specific task, as opposed to the physical components of the system.

**solid:** Style of type set with no space between lines.

**spacing:** Lateral spaces between words, sentences, or columns; also paragraph indentions (see also *leading*).

**spam:** Unsolicited junk email sent to numerous recipients.

**specifications (specs):** Instructions given to the printer that include numbers of copies (press run or print order); paper stock, coating, and size; and color, typography, and design.

**spider, web crawler:** Software that regularly checks the internet for web pages to feed a search engine.

**spine:** The backbone of a perfect-bound journal or book. The width of the spine depends on the number and thickness of pages in the publication.

**spiral binding:** A process of binding a publication with wires or plastic in a spiral form inserted through holes along the binding side.

**spot color:** One or more extra colors on a page.

**spread:** Two pages that face each other.

**STM:** Scientific, technical, and medical fields.

**stet:** Instruction that marked or crossed-out copy or type is to be retained as it originally appeared.

**stock:** Type of paper for printing.

**straight copy:** Material that can be set in type with no handwork or special programming (copy that contains no mathematical equations, tables, and so on).

**strapline:** The "subtitle" portion of a logo or slogan.

**strikethrough:** To mark a character or some text for deletion by superimposing a line through the main body of the character(s).

**strip:** To join film in a unit according to a press imposition before platemaking.

**stub:** The left-most column of the table, which usually contains the list of topics, variables, or instances to which the values in the table body apply.

**style:** A set of uniform rules to guide the application of grammar, spelling, typography, composition, and design.

**stylesheet:** A file or form that defines the layout of a document or web page, including parameters such as margins, fonts, and type sizes.

**subhead:** A subordinate heading (see 21.0, Editing, Proofreading, Tagging, and Display).

**subscript:** A number or symbol that prints partly below the baseline, for example, $A_2$ (also called inferior).

**subscription:** The price for a publication; usually set in annual terms.

**superscript:** A number or symbol that prints partly above the baseline, for example, $A^2$.

**supplement:** Material that is deemed not integral to understanding a scientific paper but provided online for deeper exploration. Supplementary material can include, for example, audio or video clips, large tables or figures, lengthy and detailed methods or protocols, or computer code. Supplementary material should be peer reviewed along with the main article but is often not typeset or copyedited in the same way as the main article.

**SWK:** "Set when known." Used to indicate information (such as page numbers) that will be inserted later in the production process.

**tag:** To insert a style or composition code in a computer file or document or the code inserted in a computer file or document.

**text:** The main body of type in a page, manuscript, article, or book. Also used for electronic files that contain only characters, no formatting or illustrations.

**text editor:** An application used to create, view, and edit text files.

**thin space:** A space character that is usually $^1/_5$ or $^1/_6$ of an em in width, inserted with Unicode 2009.

**thumbnail:** A miniature display of a page or graphic.

**TIFF (or TIF):** Tagged image file format. A file format that allows bitmapped images to be exchanged among different computer applications.

**tints:** Various even tone areas of a solid color, usually expressed in percentages.

**tip, tip-in:** A sheet or several sheets of paper glued or affixed to another before binding a periodical or book.

**toner:** Imaging material or ink used in photocopiers and computer printers.

**trademark:** A legally registered word, name, symbol, slogan, or any combination of these, used to identify and distinguish products and services and to indicate the source and marketer of those products and services (see 5.6.16, Intellectual Property: Ownership, Access, Rights, and Management, Trademark).

**transparency:** (1) A transparent object, such as a photographic slide, that is viewed by shining light through it; color-positive film (traditional/conventional). (2) Effect created by pixels turned "off" or by a mask.

**transpose (tr):** A proofreading and editing term meaning to reverse the positions of 2 elements (eg, characters, words, sentences, or paragraphs).

**trap, trapping:** The process of printing one ink on top of another to produce a third color or to avoid thin white spaces between colors.

**trim:** The edges that are cut off 3 sides—the top (head), bottom (foot), and right (face)—of a publication after binding.

**trim line, trim marks:** The line or marks indicated on copy to show where the page ends or needs to be cut.

**trim size:** The final size of the publication.

**turnaround time:** The period between any 2 events in publishing (eg, between manuscript submission and acceptance, between manuscript scanning and tele-communication to the printer).

**type gauge:** A type-measurement tool calibrated in picas and points.

**typescript:** A manuscript output by a computer printer or in typewritten form (see also *hard copy*).

**typesetter:** A person, firm, or machine that sets type.

**typestyle:** An additional style performed on characters set in type, such as bold, italics, shadow, or strikethrough (see 21.0, Editing, Proofreading, Tagging, and Display).

**typo:** A typographical error in a published work, such as a misspelling or missing letter.

**uc/lc:** Editing mark used to mean uppercase/lowercase (letters), for example, New York, New York, rather than NEW YORK, NEW YORK.

**underrun:** Production of fewer printed copies than was ordered.

**Unicode:** A set of characters and symbols with corresponding codes, able to be used by many software and typesetting programs.

**unjustified:** A ragged or uneven margin (see 21.0, Editing, Proofreading, Tagging, and Display).

**upload:** To transfer a digital file or data from a local computer to a remote computer.

**uppercase:** A capital letter.

**URL:** Uniform resource locator. An address for a document or information available via the internet or web (eg, http://www.jamanetwork.com/journals/jama).

**vector graphics:** The use of geometric primitives, such as points, lines, curves, and polygons, to represent images in computer graphics; resolution-independent graphic images that can be defined by mathematical equations and scaled with no loss of quality.

**verso:** A left-hand page.

**views:** A usage metric that counts the number of times an online page is viewed. See also *visitors* and *downloads*.

**virgule:** A forward slanted line (/) used to separate numbers, letters, or other characters (also called forward slash; see 8.4, Forward Slash [Virgule, Solidus]).

**visitors:** A usage metric that refers to the number of people who view a web page. See also *views* and *downloads*.

**watermark:** (1) An image or set of characters produced by thinning a specific area of paper that is visible when the paper is held up to light; often used to show a company logo. (2) Faint characters imposed over type or images on a page to prevent unauthorized copying or distribution.

**web:** (1) An offset lithographic printing press. (2) A continuous roll of paper used in printing.

**website:** A group of web pages and other content usually containing hyperlinks to each other, identified with a domain name, and made available on a web server.

**web press:** A lithographic press that prints on a continuous roll (web) of paper.

**well:** A part of a journal, usually the middle pages, in which advertising is not allowed; usually reserved for important scientific and clinical articles in biomedical journals. Regular features, such as news articles, essays, letters, and book reviews, are typically run outside the editorial well, where advertisement interspersion may be allowed.

**wf:** Abbreviation for wrong font; incorrect or inconsistent type size or typeface.

**white space:** The area of a page that is free of any text or graphics.

**widow:** A short line that ends a paragraph and is positioned at the top of a page or column; to be avoided.

**Wi-Fi:** A wireless local area network that uses radio waves to connect computers and other devices to the internet.

**word processor:** A general term for a computer program with which text that consists of words and figures can be input, edited, recorded, stored, and printed.

**wrong-reading:** Produced to read as a mirror image (from left to right) of the original copy; usually refers to film.

**WYSIWYG:** "What you see is what you get" (pronounced wizzy-wig). What is displayed on the computer screen is essentially how the final product will appear after printing.

**x-height:** A vertical measurement of a letter, usually equal to the height of a lowercase letter without ascenders or descenders (eg, *x*).

**XML:** Extensible Markup Language. Describes content by means of user-defined tags and a DTD to describe the content.

**XSL:** Extensible Stylesheet Language. A file that describes how to display an XML document of a given type.

**zip:** (n) A compressed file archive that appears as a single file. (v) To compress files by means of a data compression format that allows files to take up less space on a disk or hard drive.

**Principal Author:** Brenda Gregoline, ELS

ACKNOWLEDGMENT

Thanks to the following for their comments on this chapter: Helene M. Cole, MD, formerly of *JAMA*; Barbara Gastel, MD, MPH, Texas A&M University, College Station; Trevor Lane, MA, DPhil, Edanz Group, Fukuoka, Japan; and Peter J. Olson, ELS, Sheridan Journal Services, Waterbury, Vermont.

**23.0    Resources.** The resources listed in this chapter are provided for information only and do not imply an endorsement by the *AMA Manual of Style*.

## 23.1    General Dictionaries.

Acronym Finder. https://www.acronymfinder.com

*The American Heritage Dictionary of the English Language*. 5th ed. Houghton Mifflin Harcourt Trade; 2011. https://ahdictionary.com

Dictionary.com. https://www.dictionary.com

*Merriam-Webster's Collegiate Dictionary*. 11th ed. Merriam-Webster Inc; 2003. [continuously updated] https://merriam-webster.com

OneLook. https://www.onelook.com [searches many dictionaries with one search]

Oxford English Dictionary. https://oed.com

## 23.2    Medical and Scientific Dictionaries.

*Dorland's Illustrated Medical Dictionary*. 33rd ed. Elsevier; 2019.

*Stedman's Medical Dictionary*. 28th ed. Lippincott Williams & Wilkins; 2005. https://stedmansonline.com

## 23.3    General Style and Usage.

Brooks BS, Pinson JL, Wilson JG. *Working With Words: A Concise Handbook for Media Writers and Editors*. 7th ed. Bedford/St Martin's Press; 2009.

*The Chicago Manual of Style: The Essential Guide for Writers, Editors, and Publishers*. 17th ed. University of Chicago Press; 2017. https://www.chicagomanual ofstyle.org

Fowler HW, Burchfield RW, ed. *The New Fowler's Modern English Usage*. 3rd rev ed. Oxford University Press; 2004.

Garner BA, ed. *A Dictionary of Modern English Usage*. 2nd ed. Oxford University Press; 1998.

Garner BA. *Garner's Modern American Usage*. 3rd ed. Oxford University Press; 2009.

Stilman A. *Grammatically Correct: The Essential Guide to Spelling, Style, Usage, Grammar, and Punctuation*. Writer's Digest; 2010.

Walker JR, Taylor T. *The Columbia Guide to Online Style*. 2nd ed. Columbia University Press; 2006.

## 23.4 Medical/Scientific Style and Usage.

American Psychological Association. *Publication Manual of the American Psychological Association*. 7th ed. American Psychological Association; 2019. https://apastyle.apa.org

Coghill AM, Garson LR. *The ACS Style Guide: Effective Communication of Scientific Information*. 3rd ed. American Chemical Society; 2006.

Cohn V, Cope L. *News & Numbers: A Writer's Guide to Statistics*. 3rd ed. Wiley-Blackwell; 2011.

Davis NM. *Medical Abbreviations: 32,000 Conveniences at the Expense of Communication and Safety*. 15th ed. Neil M Davis Associates; 2011.

Lang TA, Secic M. *How to Report Statistics in Medicine: Annotated Guidelines for Authors, Editors, and Reviewers*. 2nd ed. American College of Physicians; 2006.

Smart P, Maisonneuve H, Polderman A, eds. *Science Editors' Handbook*. 2nd ed. European Association of Science Editors; 2013. https://www.ease.org.uk

Style Manual Committee, Council of Science Editors. *Scientific Style and Format: The CSE Manual for Authors, Editors, and Publishers*. 8th ed. University of Chicago Press/Council of Science Editors; 2014. https://scientificstyleandformat.org

## 23.5 Writing.

Casagrande J. *The Best Punctuation Book, Period: A Comprehensive Guide for Every Writer, Editor, Student, and Businessperson*. Crown Publishing Group; 2014.

Day RA, Sakaduski N. *Scientific English: A Guide for Scientists and Other Professionals*. 3rd ed. Greenwood Press; 2011.

Gastel B, Day RA. *How to Write and Publish a Scientific Paper*. 8th ed. Greenwood Press; 2016.

Lindsay D. *Scientific Writing = Thinking in Words*. CSIRO Publishing; 2011.

Lunsford AA. *EasyWriter*. 5th ed. Bedford/St Martin's Press; 2013.

Norris M. *Between You & Me: Confessions of a Comma Queen*. WW Norton & Co; 2015.

O'Conner PT. *Woe Is I: The Grammarphobe's Guide to Better English in Plain English*. 3rd ed. Riverhead Books; 2010.

Penrose AM, Katz SB. *Writing in the Sciences: Exploring Conventions of Scientific Discourse.* 3rd ed. Longman; 2010.

Pinker S. *The Sense of Style: The Thinking Person's Guide to Writing in the 21st Century.* Viking; 2014.

Schimel J. *Writing Science: How to Write Papers That Get Cited and Proposals That Get Funded.* Oxford University Press; 2011.

Truss L. *Eats, Shoots and Leaves: The Zero Tolerance Approach to Punctuation.* Gotham Books; 2006.

## `23.6` Ethical and Legal Issues.

*AP Stylebook Online.* Briefing on media law. https://www.apstylebook.com/

Beauchamp TL, Childress JF. *Principles of Biomedical Ethics.* 7th ed. Oxford University Press; 2013.

Committee on Publication Ethics. A code of conduct and best practice guidelines for journal editors. https://publicationethics.org/resources/code-conduct

Council of Science Editors. White Paper on Publication Ethics: CSE's White Paper on Promoting Integrity in Scientific Journal Publications. Updated 2018. https://www.councilscienceeditors.org/resource-library/editorial-policies/white-paper-on-publication-ethics/

Fischer MA, Perle EG, Williams JT. *Perle, Williams, & Fischer on Publishing Law.* 4th ed. Wolters Kluwer Law and Business; 2015.

Hart JD. *Internet Law: A Field Guide.* 6th ed. BNA Books; 2008.

International Committee of Medical Journal Editors. Recommendations for the Conduct, Reporting, Editing, and Publication of Scholarly Work in Medical Journals. http://www.icmje.org

US Copyright Office. https://copyright.gov

World Association of Medical Editors. Resources. www.wame.org/resources

World Medical Association. World Medical Association Declaration of Helsinki: Ethical Principles for Medical Research Involving Human Subjects. *JAMA.* 2013;310(20):2191-2194. doi:10.1001/jama.2013.281053

## `23.7` Peer Review.

Godlee F, Jefferson T, eds. *Peer Review in Health Sciences.* 2nd ed. BMJ Books; 2003.

Hames I. *Peer Review and Manuscript Management in Scientific Journals: Guidelines for Good Practice.* Wiley-Blackwell; 2007.

International Congress on Peer Review and Scientific Publication. https://peerreviewcongress.org

## 23.8 Illustrations/Displaying Data.

Frankel F. *Envisioning Science: The Design and Craft of the Science Image.* MIT Press; 2002.

Hodges ERS. *The Guild Handbook of Scientific Illustration.* 2nd ed. Wiley-Blackwell; 2003.

Nicol AAM, Pexman PM. *Displaying Your Findings: A Practical Guide for Creating Figures, Posters, and Presentations.* 6th ed. American Psychological Association; 2010.

Tufte ER. *The Cognitive Style of PowerPoint.* Graphics Press; 2003.

Tufte ER. *Envisioning Information.* Graphics Press; 1990.

Tufte ER. *The Visual Display of Quantitative Information.* Graphics Press; 1983.

Tufte ER. *Visual Explanations: Images and Quantities, Evidence and Narrative.* Graphics Press; 1997.

## 23.9 Websites.

Centers for Disease Control and Prevention. https://www.cdc.gov

Cochrane Library. https://www.cochranelibrary.com/

HUGO Gene Nomenclature Committee. https://www.genenames.org

Human Genome Variation Society. https://www.hgvs.org

National Academy of Medicine. https://www.nationalacademies.org

National Academy of Sciences. http://www.nasonline.org

US National Library of Medicine Databases. https://www.nlm.nih.gov [includes MEDLINE, National Center for Biotechnology Information (NCBI), NLM Gateway, and PubMed]

World Health Organization. https://www.who.int/en

## 23.10 Guidelines.

Committee on Publication Ethics (COPE). https://publicationethics.org

Declaration of Helsinki. https://www.wma.net/policies-post/wma-declaration-of-helsinki-ethical-principles-for-medical-research-involving-human-subjects/

EQUATOR Network. https://www.equator-network.org/

Good Publication Practice for Communicating Company-Sponsored Medical Research: GPP3. *Ann Intern Med.* 2015;163(6):461-464. doi:10.7326/M15-0288

International Committee of Medical Journal Editors (ICMJE) Uniform Requirements. http://www.icmje.org

World Association of Medical Editors (WAME) Policy Statements. www.wame.org/policies-and-resources

## 23.11 Professional Scientific Writing, Editing, and Communications Organizations and Groups.

American Copy Editors Society (ACES)
https://aceseditors.org

American Medical Writers Association (AMWA)
https://www.amwa.org

Association of Earth Science Editors (AESE)
http://www.aese.org

Association of Learned and Professional Society Publishers (ALPSP)
https://www.alpsp.org

Board of Editors in the Life Sciences (BELS)
https://www.bels.org

Committee on Publication Ethics (COPE)
https://www.publicationethics.org

Council of Science Editors (CSE)
https://www.councilscienceeditors.org

European Association of Science Editors (EASE)
https://ease.org.uk

European Medical Writers Association (EMWA)
https://www.emwa.org

International Committee of Medical Journal Editors (ICMJE)
http://www.icmje.org

International Society of Managing & Technical Editors
https://www.ismte.org

Society for Scholarly Publishing (SSP)
https://www.sspnet.org

Society for Technical Communication (STC)
https://www.stc.org

World Association of Medical Editors (WAME)
https://www.wame.org

**Principal Author:** Brenda Gregoline, ELS

# Index

National Science and Technology Council, 213
National Science Foundation, 213
*Native American,* usage, 547
natural experiment (found experiment),
    1058, 1071
naturalistic sample, statistical definition, 1058
natural killer cells, 829
natural logarithms, 1100
"natural" products, proprietary names, 683
*nauseous* vs *nauseated,* usage, 526
Navy, US, 561-562
NBD Code. *See* NASPE/BPEG
    Defibrillator Code
NBG Code (NASPE/BPEG Generic Code), 672
NBL Code (NASPE/BPEG Pacemaker-Lead
    Code), 673
NC-IUBMB (Nomenclature Committee of
    International Union of Biochemistry and
    Molecular Biology), 842
near visual acuity, 871
necessary cause, 1058
Nederlands Trial Register, 36
*needlestick,* usage, 537
*negative,* usage, 506
negative exponents, 1100, 1101
negative numbers, in tables, 129
negative predictive value
    for diagnostic discrimination, 1034
    diagnostic/prognostic studies, 1006
    posttest probability and, 1066
    statistical definition, 1058
negatives, double, 433
*Neisseria meningitidis,* 884
nematode, gene terminology, 782
*neonates,* usage, 540
nephrology nomenclature, 914
nerve terminology, 850-852
nested case-control study, 1001, 1058
network (computer), 1138
network maps, 148, 154, 155
network mcta-analysis, 1004
neurology
    electroencephalographic terms, 852-855
    evoked potentials or responses, 855-857
    gene terminology, 748-750
    molecular neuroscience, 858-861
    nerves, 850-852
    polysomnography and sleep stages, 857-858
*newborns,* usage, 540
*New Era Publications International, ApS v
    Henry Holt and Company, Inc,* 273
Newman-Keuls test
    analysis of variance and, 1015
    Duncan multiple range test and, 1036
    statistical definition, 1058
news agencies, external pressure on editors
    from, 337
news articles, format, 5

news embargo, 395, 398-400
news media, 318
    author interactions with, 399-401
    reference citation format for
        publications, 87-88
    science coverage, 392-393
newspapers, reference citation format, 87-88
news releases
    public information, 401-406
    reference citation format, 102-103
news reports
    acceptable duplicate reports, 204
    libel/defamation, 328-329
    meeting presentation, 202-203
    patients' rights, 319
news summaries, 202
*New York Times Co v Sullivan,* 324, 326
NIH. *See* US National Institutes
    of Health
NISO. *See* National Information Standards
    Organization
NLM. *See* US National Library of Medicine
NNH (number needed to harm), 989, 1061
*No.* (number abbreviation), 970
*no,* quotation marks and, 482
nocebo, statistical definition, 1059
node, in TNM staging system, 658
n-of-1 trial, statistical definition, 1058
nomenclature
    blood groups
        ISBT name and number, 652-654
        traditional nomenclature, 646-652
    cancer terminology
        *The Bethesda System for Reporting Cervical
            Cytology,* 661-663
        cancer stages, 657-661
        molecular cancer terminology, 663, 664
        multiple endocrine neoplasia, 663
        TNM staging system, 657-661
    cardiology terminology
        cellular and molecular cardiology,
            675-677
        coronary artery angiographic
            classifications, 668
        echocardiography terms, 670-671
        electrocardiographic terms, 665-668
        electrogram terms, 668
        heart disease classification and scoring,
            673-675
        heart sounds, 669
        implanted cardioverter-defibrillator codes,
            672, 673
        jugular venous pulse contours, 669-670
        murmurs, 669
        pacemaker codes, 672
        pacemaker-lead codes, 673
    defined, 642-644
    devices, 699-700

references (*cont.*)
  video, 93-95
  webinars, 90-91
  websites, 98
reference standard, statistical definition, 1031
referral bias, 1019
referral systems, for rejected manuscripts,
    359-360, 362
Reflections, 5
reflexive pronouns, 426
refusal rate, survey study, 1006
*regardless,* usage, 525
*regime* vs *regimen,* usage, 529
regional reporters, legal, 105-106
regions, chromosome, 761-762
register, publishing definition, 1141
registration
  copyright, 270-271
  trademark, 289-290
regression analysis
  Brown-Mood procedure, 1022
  coefficient of determination, 1026
  least-squares method, 1049
  statistical definition, 1073
  total sum of the square, 1080
regression coefficient, on scatterplots, 134
regression line(s)
  Hollander parallelism test, 1042
  linear regression, 1051
  residual standard deviation and, 1074
  slope of unity, 1082
  standard error of the
      estimate, 1078
  statistical definition, 1073
regression to the mean, statistical
    definition, 1073
Regulations for the Protection of Human
    Subjects (Common Rule), 309-313
regulatory genes, retroviral, 783-784
rejection of a manuscript
  appeal of decision, 356, 361, 417-418
  cascading systems for rejected manuscripts,
      299, 359-360, 362
  duplicate submission, 207
  editorial assessment and, 416
  editorial responsibilities, 361-362
  peer review and confidentiality, 300
  record retention, 253
  unethical studies, 207
*relationship,* usage, 511
relative difference, 1012
relative pronouns, 427-429
relative risk (RR)
  absolute risk and, 1013
  confidence intervals, 1027
  hazard ratio and, 1042
  manuscript, 983
  odds ratio and, 1062

statistical definition, 1073-1074
  of unity, 1082
relative risk reduction (RRR), 1074
relevance
  in manuscript preparation, 39
  in structured abstract, 33-35
reliability
  accuracy and, 1013
  manuscript, 981
  qualitative study, 1070
  reproducibility and, 1074
  statistical definition, 1074
  validity of measurement vs, 1083
religious clergy, abbreviations, 573
reminder advertisements, 381
*renal,* usage, 914
*(R)*-enantiomers, 687
Rennie, Drummond, 212, 224
repeated measures, 1044, 1074
repeated-measures ANOVA, 1015
repeating nucleotide sequences, 707
repeating single-nucleotide pairs, 707
*repeat* vs *repeated,* usage, 529
reporting (selective outcome reporting) bias,
    1019, 1074
reporting guidelines
  print and online, 14
  research reports, 2
  study types and, 6-11
repositories
  depositing articles in, 421
  papers in, 246-256
  reference citation format for papers in,
      75-76, 80
reprints, 389-390, 421, 1141
reproduced figures, 164
reproducibility, statistical definition, 1074
reproduction permission, 273, 275-276
reproduction proof, 1141
republication of text
  abstracts, 78
  libel/defamation, 328-329
  permission, 276
reputation, protection of, 323-324
resampling method. *See* bootstrap method
research, defined, 310
research and review articles, 183, 413
research letters, 2, 5, 365
research misconduct, 213-214
research participant(s)
  acknowledgments, 54
  Common Rule, 309-313
  data sharing, 50
  in manuscript, 980
  institutional review board, 310-311, 313-315
  rights of participants
      informed consent, 310-311
      journal policies and procedures, 312-315